PENGUIN HEALTH

THE NEW OUR BODIES, OURSELVES

Angela Phillips is a freelance journalist specializing in subjects to do with women and health. She works for national newspapers, women's magazines and occasionally television. She is also a member of the Maternity Alliance Management Committee, City and Hackney Community Health Council Women's Group, and the Childcare Now campaign, and was a founder member of the National Abortion Campaign. She is the mother of two children and lives in London. Her other publications include *Your Body Your Baby Your Life* and *Who Cares For Europe's Children?*

Jill Rakusen originally trained as a musician and has realized surprisingly late in life the connection between music and health. She has worked for many years on women's health issues – writing, teaching, counselling and running groups, and was a founder member of the Women's Health Information Centre. Her main interests now are the promotion of mental health, including facilitating the healing and growing process (both her own and others'), and she loves running her own brand of workshop designed to help people (re)discover their potential, through exploring their relationship to sound and to music. Her publications include *Menopause: a Guide for Women of All Ages*. She lives in Yorkshire and currently works in Health Promotion for North Manchester Health Authority.

Both writers have been actively involved in the Women's Liberation Movement for many years.

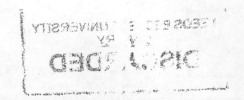

LONDON TELEPHONE CODES

The 01 London telephone code has been replaced by 071 for inner London and 081 for outer London. If you are unsure of the correct code for any of the London numbers in this book, please refer to the British Telecom literature.

THE BOSTON WOMEN'S HEALTH BOOK COLLECTIVE
BRITISH EDITION BY ANGELA PHILLIPS AND JILL RAKUSEN

THE NEW
OUR BODIES, OURSELVES

A HEALTH BOOK BY AND FOR WOMEN

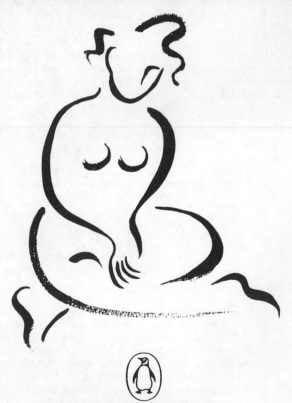

PENGUIN BOOKS

FREDERICK WARNE

Published by the Penguin Group
27 Wrights Lane, London W8 5TZ, England
Penguin Books USA Inc., 375 Hudson Street, New York, N.Y. 10014, USA
Penguin Books Australia Ltd, Ringwood, Victoria, Australia
Penguin Books Canada Ltd, 10 Alcorn Avenue, Toronto, Ontario, Canada M4V 3B2
Penguin Books (N.Z.) Ltd, 182–190 Wairau Road, Auckland 10, New Zealand

Penguin Books Ltd, Registered Offices: Harmondsworth, Middlesex, England

First published in the USA, under the title *Our Bodies, Ourselves,*
by Simon and Schuster 1973
British edition first published in hardback by Allen Lane The Penguin Press 1978
Published simultaneously in paperback by Penguin Books

Revised edition first published in the USA by Simon and Schuster 1984
First published in Australia, with an Australian and New Zealand directory,
by Penguin Books 1985
Second British edition, with Australian and New Zealand directories, first published
by Penguin Books 1989
3 5 7 9 10 8 6 4

Filmset in Linotron 202 Electra by
Wyvern Typesetting Ltd, Bristol

Printed and bound in Great Britain by
William Clowes Limited, Beccles and London
Text design by Sonia Alexis

CONTENTS

PART IV

CHILDBEARING

PART V

WOMEN GROWING OLDER

PART VI

SOME COMMON AND UNCOMMON MEDICAL AND HEALTH PROBLEMS

PART VII

WOMEN AND THE MEDICAL SYSTEM

INTRODUCTION

This book is enormous, and rather forbidding, even to us (and we know it inside out). So here are some suggestions for those who are wondering where to begin.

A good place to start is Chapter 1, *A Good Story* – not just because it *is* a good story but also because you'll get to know a bit about the original authors and how the book started from such small beginnings. Next, *Body Image* may help you make connections with what many women find most difficult about being a woman; this can be reassuring and enlightening. Part VII: *Women and the Medical System* will give you an overview of how our system works and doesn't work, and why, plus how to find your way around the NHS.* Chapter 7, *Alternative and Complementary Approaches to Health and Healing*, provides an overview of how you can help yourself – and be helped – within a holistic framework, plus a discussion of the advantages and limitations of 'alternative' medicine. These chapters will provide a basis from which you can best use the rest of the book.

The other chapters are mostly intended to be read if you want to find out more about specific issues/problems. However, we would like to single out Chapter 4, *Food*, as worthy of a look, if only to reassure anyone who feels oppressed by the countless exhortations which assault us from all sides – whether from advertisers, health freaks or health educators: here, we have tried to provide some context within which to understand the dilemmas we face, and some practical solutions which we hope go some way towards relieving the guilt so many of us feel when confronted with the issue of food.

Producing a new British edition of *Our Bodies, Ourselves* has been a mammoth task. We had been asked to do a 'simple' editing job on the American edition and to produce a British appendix. However, we knew from the experience of the last edition that this would be inadequate. An American health book is in so many ways inappropriate to British women. In the spirit of the original we consulted widely. Our view was confirmed over and over again by the many women we asked to comment on the different chapters.

As we progressed, we found ourselves changing more and more of the new American text, as well as our previous text. For a start we had to do a lot of updating. However, we were also concerned that without the willingness to make changes, our wide consultation would have been a hollow and token exercise. We use the pronoun 'we' through most of the book. That 'we' refers to the collective experience of all the women who have contributed to this book. Obviously we do not all agree with every statement, and it has not been possible to incorporate every suggestion and wish into the text; as editors, we have had the responsibility for trying to produce a considered, consistent and coherent whole.

The great extent to which this book diverges from the American edition does not necessarily represent our disagreement with the American authors so much as our differences. We may speak a common language but we live with different cultural assumptions, different health-care systems, a different political framework, different laws, and the history of our respective health movements is different too.

So we were faced with having to produce a completely new British edition within the budget which our publishers had set aside for a much smaller job. While it has often been demoralizing and frustrating, and even overwhelming at times, our sense of excitement about the value and importance of this book has, like last time, kept us going. We also felt that we owed it to the original authors and to our wide readership to ensure that a book which has become a feminist classic retained its value and reputation.

While we were delighted to see that the new US edition had taken up some of the ideas from our last British edition, for us it is time to move on. So, for example, we have greatly expanded 'alternative' approaches to health and healing, partly because we feel that the issues raised are

---

*While it may not be up to date by the time you read this (the present Thatcher Government's intentions are ominous to say the least), the chapter will provide a basis for understanding the issues that face women whatever our health-care system.

pivotal to our whole experience of health and illness, and partly because it is so hard to get access to relevant material which has a critical, and feminist, perspective.

The very nature of our health-care system has meant that, so far, alternative medicine is rarely available on the National Health Service. While we are committed to the NHS and profoundly critical of attempts to privatize it, we see this chapter as part of a debate about the content of health care and in no way as an endorsement of private medical practice. In line with this approach we have expanded the section on cancer (in Chapter 25) to include a considered discussion of alternative, complementary and self-help approaches.

Other significant changes from the US edition include, for example, making room for a substantial chapter on mental health (Chapter 8) rather than confining ourselves, as the American authors did, to a discussion of psychotherapy. The section on relationships gives more attention to issues in lesbian relationships because we feel that within a homophobic society lesbians need particular support and validation. We have also broadened Chapter 10, *Violence against Women*, for example to make links with racist harassment, prison violence and the peace movement. The chapter from the US edition on new reproductive technologies has been absorbed into the chapters on infertility and the health-care system in an attempt to provide a coherent analysis of both infertility and of issues involving technology in general; and we have also included illegal as well as prescription drugs in Chapter 5, *Alcohol, Nicotine and Other Mood-altering Drugs*. Inevitably we have had to cut back in some places to make room for these changes.

Because of the many constraints under which we have had to work, we have had to make some compromises and, inevitably, some decisions that we would prefer we didn't have to live with. We would like to have had the financial resources to include black women and women with disabilities as paid co-editors of the book. Instead, we have had to rely on a lot of voluntary help and that inevitably has meant that volunteers had less power over the content of the book than we (both white, middle class and, to date, able-bodied) have had. We have also had to leave unexplored the question of coping with heart disease – a major issue for women in the West: we felt it was crucial to present the issues concerning prevention adequately and hope that what is missing from the 'treatment' and 'self-help' aspects can be made up to some extent by the resources listed, by Chapter 7's discussion of healing and to some extent by the section on cancer in Chapter 25 which is relevant to women facing any kind of serious disease.

Given the speed of change in the field of health, some material will be out of date before this edition is even printed. We have listed where possible further reading and organizations to contact for up-to-date information.* Yet many things never change, particularly the importance of sustaining a critical feminist perspective, and of feeling positive about ourselves so that we are confident enough to challenge those who set themselves up as 'experts' and sit in judgement upon us.

We believe that our new edition is a testament to the original ideas of the book: women's health is political and women without medical training are capable of learning enough about health issues to challenge the 'experts'. It is also a testament to the commitment of feminists. Virtually all the people who have contributed their time have done so as a generous gift to other women. A gesture of faith in the feminist tradition of knowledge sharing. We have been able to draw on far more feminist expertise this time, many women having commented on each chapter – both before and after rewrites – and some women having prepared contributions too. A sure sign that feminist ideas are far-reaching.

We would like particularly to thank: Pip Beck, Carole Booth, Cathy Cobham, Claire Cribb, Mary Currie, Lyn Durwood, Kath Fraser, Chris Gowdridge, Kate Holden, Sue Hunt, Janet Law, Marianne Leverton, the Maternity Alliance, Sisterwrite Bookshop, Marilyn Warnick and the librarians at Swansea Medical Library who provided invaluable practical support at various times; Marge Berer, Angie Cotter, Sue Dimond, Jane Hawksley, Virginia Laurence, Jan McKinley, Sue O'Sullivan, Jean Robinson, Jane Sheppard and Carol Smith who gave general help with many specific areas; and Maggie Eisner who made her usual rigorous and forthright comments on many sections, and provided us with material in some instances too.

We are particularly grateful to Alex and Rachel Sturrock, who stoically allowed us to take over their play-space with vast amounts of paper, and to North Manchester Health Authority, who enabled Jill to finish her work on the book after she had joined their staff, to Marion Bruce-Quay and Joyce Leeson who facilitated this, and to Jill's colleagues who accepted this so stoically, particularly Caroline Bedale, Carnell Bell, Marcia Dooley, Judith Emanuel, Graham Heafford and Madge Strong; to David Player, then of the Health Education Council, who kindly made a financial contribution to our costs (with no strings attached); and to Linda Patterson, Arnold Rakusen and Philippa Rakusen who also provided much-needed financial support.

The following people helped in myriad and diverse ways, not always knowingly: Anne-Marie from Cardiff, Linda Chase Broda, Sam Collett, Angie Cotter, Joy Courtney, Sue Crawshaw, Rachel Dimond, George-Anne Lamont, Judy Ledward, Brenda Mallon, Sue Napolitano, Sue O'Sullivan, Gretchen Pyves, Jo Spence and Jill Sutcliffe. Thanks go to them, to Gyandharm, who was willing to give so much, not least because he believed in this book, and to the other seven 'celebrants' of 1986 – Cathy, Marie, Mo,

---

*The listing of items in Resources (to be found at the end of the relevant chapters) does not necessarily mean that we wholeheartedly endorse them. It will be clear why those mentioned in the text are listed. Others are listed because we believe they have something to offer.

Nigel, Ray, Rita and Sylvia – who in no small way enabled it to be finished.

Many people helped on specific chapters, and we would like to acknowledge their help in the following respects: Micheline Mason commented on *Body Image*, Fiona McCloskey helped with the *Anatomy* chapter; Marion Bowman, Melanie Miller, the London Women and Food Group, Maggie Sanderson, Aubrey Sheiham, Julie Shepherd, Kiran Shukla, Carol Smith and Peggy Wynn helped with *Food*; Sue Clements and Jan Fuller rewrote the chapter on *Drugs*, and Sue Barlow and Bobbie Jacobson also gave invaluable input. Liz Merrick rewrote *Women in Motion*, with help from Maggie Pether; Lynn Fitzgerald also provided some last-minute input.

In the preparation of *Alternative and Complementary Approaches to Health and Healing*, Jill would like to acknowledge her indebtedness to members of the Alternative Medicine Sub-group of the Politics of Health Group, of which she was a member throughout its short but valuable history, and to Angie Cotter and Sue Dimond, who helped her develop a coherent strategy for tackling the complex issues involved within a feminist framework. Angie also helped with refining the connections between this and the mental health chapter. The following also helped with specific sections: Jean Freer, Kate Holden, National Federation of Spiritual Healers, Dell Round, Karen Payne (healing), Alison Howarth (herbs), Rima Handley (homoeopathy), Stella King, Alison West, Jan Resnick (acupuncture), Mary Lynne Ellis (art), Rosie Fisher (music), Sue Thame (Alexander Technique), Maggie MacKenzie (massage), Amber Lloyd (relaxation) and Robin Munro (yoga). Linda Chase Broda wrote the section on T'ai Chi, and Richenda Power and *Self and Society* enabled us to use her material on naturopathy.

Annie Brackx, Angie Cotter, Helen Crisp, Sue Dimond, Karen Newbigging, Sue O'Sullivan, Kath Prior and Pam Trevithick were all very helpful and encouraging during the preparation of *Women and Mental Health*. Leighton Cole, Sos Dance, Kate Holden, Karen Payne, Betty Smith, Jan Resnick, Mary Lynne Ellis, Nicola Rowe, and several women who prefer to remain anonymous helped by commenting on or being interviewed for specific sections, and Robina Shah contributed the section on black women.

Sue Barlow, Barbara Harrison and other members of the Women and Work Hazards Group were very helpful in the preparation of *Occupational and Environmental Health*, as were Francis Carter, Claire Holman and the London Hazards Centre. Kath Fraser and Shirley Henderson of Scottish Women's Aid were especially helpful during the preparation of *Violence against Women*, while Sue Dimond, Jean Freer, the Greenham woman hitching on the M1 in 1986, Gill Lewis, Joan Miller, Sue O'Sullivan, Abida Parveen, Maggie Scott, Prue Stevenson, Penny Windsor and Women in Prison also helped in various ways. Sue O'Sullivan and Sue Dimond helped greatly with planning the integration of the section on *Relationships and Sexuality*. The following commented, contributed or agreed to be interviewed: Marion Bruce-Quay, Kooj Chu-han, Jude Connor, Eleanor Green, Lynne Harne, Ingrid McClements, Micheline Mason, North London Lesbian Mothers' Group, the Older Lesbian Network, Pratibha Parmar, Rights of Women Lesbian Custody Group, Lori Streich, Neomi Thomas and Ruth Wallsgrove. Marge Berer, Katherine Gieve, Jeanne Saint and Wendy Savage helped with various aspects of *Controlling Our Fertility*; we are particularly grateful to Marge, who redrafted Chapter 15, *Contraception*, and who in turn extends special thanks to Toni Belfield for sharing her knowledge and days of time; Valerie Beral, Peter Huntingford and Jean Robinson also commented on aspects of the text, and Fiona McCloskey drafted the section on natural birth control. We are grateful to them all.

The following helped with various aspects of the *Childbearing* section: Elizabeth Anionwu, Juliet Ashe, Marge Berer, Jane Coomber, Miki David, Melanie Davies, Renata Duelli-Klein, Lyn Durwood, Maggie Eisner, Jo Garcia, Shamin Habibullah, Maj Hulten, Peter Huntingford, Ailie Kerrane, Sheila Kitzinger, Caroline McKeith, Mona and Rory O'Moore, Maggie Pearson, Naomi Pfeffer, Melanie Pleaner, Kulbir Randhawa, Tricia from the Infertility Support Group, Judy Walder and Anne Woollett. Fiona Poland kindly stepped in to help with rewriting *Women Growing Older*, and the following helped with their comments: Sheila Adam, Marjorie Lee, the London Menopause Collective, Ingrid McClements, Kathy Meade, Linda Patterson and Ellen Smith.

Many people helped with the chapters on *Common* and *Uncommon Medical Problems*: the Endometriosis Association, the PID Support Group and Vicky Whelan kindly contributed material; Elizabeth Anionwu, Carnell Bell, Anona Blackwell, Marcia Dooley, Maggie Eisner, the Herpes Association, Joyce Leeson, J. K. Oates, Katie Simmons and Carol Smith helped in a variety of respects. Anne Carrick wrote a first draft of the cervix section but unfortunately had to leave the country before she could complete the text; Tina Posner and Connie Smith gave their time freely and patiently as various aspects of this section were worked on, and Chris Bennett helped finalize the sections on cervical cell abnormality and screening. Valerie Beral, Lesley Doyal, Katrina and Jeanie from Australia, Virginia Laurence, Linda Patterson, Jean Robinson and Lisa Saffron also helped by reading and commenting on aspects of the cervix section at some point during its development. Mel Bartley, Wendy Farrant and Jill Russell helped enormously in orientating the text on heart disease; Maggie Eisner, Joyce Leeson and Linnie Price also provided helpful comments. Many people provided helpful comments for the section on cancer: Sue Barlow, Penny Brohn, Ute Brookman, Anne Carrick, Angie Cotter, Lesley Doyal, Maggie Eisner, Bernard Greenwood, Virginia Laurence, Joyce Leeson, Pat Pilkington, Laura Potts, Sadhya Rippon and Jo Spence. Many others helped by agreeing to be interviewed; for the most part they have to remain anonymous. The Trans-Pennine Breast Cancer Group kindly agreed to our using some material on 'living with cancer' that was originally drafted for the breast cancer section. We are grateful particularly to the Bristol Cancer Help Centre, which graciously enabled Jill to spend time there, and to those staff and residents who gave of their time and of themselves with trust: they helped her deepen her understanding of the connections between illness and creativity which she hopes has been reflected in some way in at least some of the text, and in her work ever since. Having had the privilege to stay at Bristol is something she continues to treasure, and to build on personally and politically.

We are grateful to the Trans-Pennine Breast Cancer Group – Judith Emanuel, Laura Potts, Lesley Thompson and Mary Twomey – for the immense amount of work they put into the section on breast cancer, to Helena, Jo, Joan, Josephine, Laura, Rita and Sue, who, in talking about their experiences, helped them develop their understanding; to Mary Turner, who deciphered and typed the first draft; and to Valerie Beral, Virginia Laurence, Maureen Roberts and Jean Robinson for their time, energy and helpful comments. Mary Chamberlain, Lesley Doyal, Mary Ann Elston, Kath Fraser, Helen Rosenthal and Fidelma Winkler kindly contributed to the final section, *Women and the Medical System*; we are grateful also to Helen Allinson, Marge Berer, Anjona Buckman, Carolyn Faulder, Isis/Wicce, the London Black Women's Health Action Project and John Yudkin for their help on various aspects of it, and, finally, to Freda Davis for kindly allowing us to use her beautiful poem.

Those women who took responsibility for preparing material in this book are indicated at the beginning of each chapter and/or section. The following women were responsible for the original American chapters: Fran Ansley, Laurie Ansorge, Terrie Antico, Susan Bell, Trude Bennet, Pamela Berger, Sarah Berndt, Gene Bishop, Edith Bjornson Sunley, Kris Brown, Paula Brown Doress, Barbara A. Burg, Edith Butler-Hallstein, Lucy Candib, Dina Carbonell, Loly Carrillo, Diane Clapp, Adele Clark, Robin Cohen, Louise Corbett, Mary Crowe, Sasha Curran, Irene Davidson, Letitia Davis, DES Action, Cheri DesMarais, Vilunya Diskin, Joan Ditzion, Alice Downey, Julia Doyle Sukenik, Carol Driscoll, J. W. Duncan, Buffy Dunker, Barbara Eck Menning, Endometriosis Association, Mickey Friedman, Deanna Forist, Alice Friedman, Dana Gallagher, Lois Glass, Janet Golden, Ginger Goldman, Suzanne Gosselin, D. Hamer, Lois Harris, Nancy P. Hawley, Meg Hickey, Barbara Horgan, Ruth Hubbard, Jane Hyman Wegscheider, Roxanne Hynek, Jane Jewell, Janet Jones, Susan Keady, Dlana Klugman, Margaret Lazarus, Sherry Leibowitz, Patricia Logan, Nancy London, B. J. Louison, Carol McEldowney, Elizabeth McGee, Kathleen MacPherson, Sandra Malasky, Caroline Mamber, Jenny Mansbridge, Debbie Milligan, Marian Marbury, Betty Mitchell, Judy Norris, Judy Norsigian, Gwendolyn Parker, Barbara Perkins, Jane Pincus, Bebe Poor, Laura Punnett, Kathleen Quinlan, Margaret Quinn, Joan Rachlin, Esther Rome, Mariana Romo-Carmona, Annette Rosen, Lynn Rubinett, Marty Ruedi, Sheryl Ruzek, Hilary Salk, Marian Sandmaier, Wendy Sanford, Cathy Schwartz, Lynn Scott, Ann Shepardson, Lena Sorensen, Jill Stanzler, Mary Stern, Norma Swenson, Terry Thorsos, Nancy Todd, Ruth Weber, Peggy Nelson Wegman, Denise Wells, Nancy Wilbur, Dennie Wolf, Jill Wolhandler, Susan Woskie and Nancy Zimmet.

We hope it is now clear that this book is not simply a product of our own time and energy! It would not have been possible without the input of many, many people.

Every effort has been made to locate and contact the owners of all the illustrations that appear in this text but a few people had not come back to us when this edition went to press. Any outstanding contributors will be credited in the next edition.

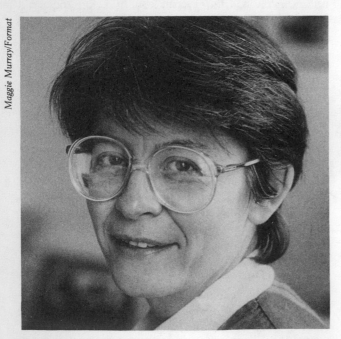

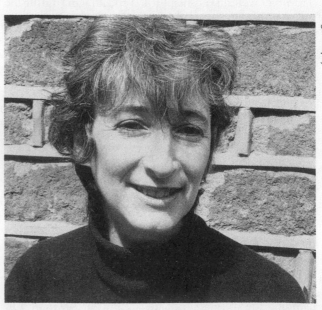

ANGELA PHILLIPS and JILL RAKUSEN, May 1988

A GOOD STORY – A MESSAGE FROM BOSTON, MASSACHUSETTS

The history of this book is lengthy and satisfying. It began in 1969 in a small discussion group called 'Women and Their Bodies' at a Women's Conference in Boston, USA. For many of us, talking to women in this way was a totally new experience and we decided to go on meeting as a group to continue the discussion.

We had all experienced frustration and anger towards specific doctors and the medical maze in general, and initially we wanted to do something about this. As we talked we began to realize how little we knew about our own bodies, so we decided to do further research, to prepare papers in groups and then to discuss our findings together. We learned both from professional sources (medical text-books, journals, doctors, nurses) and from our own experience.

For instance, many of us had 'learned' about the menstrual cycle in science or biology classes. But most of us did not remember much of what we had learned. This time when we read in a text that the onset of menstruation is a normal and universal occurrence in young girls, we started to talk about our first menstrual periods. We found that, for many of us, beginning to menstruate had not felt normal at all, but scary, embarrassing, mysterious. We realized that what we had been told about menstruation and what we had not been told – even the tone of voice it had been told in – had all had an effect on our feelings about being female.

The results of our findings were used to present courses for other women. We would meet in any available free space, in schools, nurseries, church halls, in our own homes. As we taught, we learned from other women, and as they learned, they went on to give courses to others. We saw it as a never-ending process always involving more and more women.

Some people have asked us why the book is only about women. As women we do not consider ourselves experts on men (as men through the centuries have considered them-selves experts on us). We feel that it would be best for men to do what we have done for themselves.

After teaching the first course we decided to duplicate our papers for other women to use. This led to the first inexpensive edition of the book, which was published by the New England Free Press. There was so much demand for the book that in time it seemed logical to publish commercially to reach even more women. Over time we have revised and updated the material several times, using the royalties from sales to support health education work.

Knowledge has freed us to an extent. It has freed us, for example, from playing the role of mother if it is not a role that fits us. It has given us room to discover the energy and talents that are in us. We want to help make this freedom available to every woman. This is why people in the women's movement have been so active in fighting legal restrictions, the imperfections of available contraceptives, poor sex education, and poorly administered health care that keep too many women from having this crucial control over their bodies.

For us, body education is core education. Our bodies are the physical bases from which we move out into the world; ignorance, uncertainty – even, at worst, shame – about our physical selves create in us an alienation from ourselves that keeps us from being the whole people that we should be.

HOW THE EXPERIENCE CHANGED US

Since most of us had patterned our lives around men, working together was a liberating experience. Like most women's groups we talked to each other about how it felt growing up female; this gave us a basis to discuss what we thought and felt about ourselves and how we wanted to change. At first it was rather scary admitting that we were not completely satisfied with our lives. Some of us were afraid that commitment to the women's movement and to the group would weaken our ties with men, children, jobs, lifestyles; that we might lose control of our lives. We came to realize that this fear was unrealistic. No one could take from us what we did not want to give up.

Probably the most valuable thing we learned was to speak

for ourselves and be ourselves. Many of us feared discussing personal details of our lives and relationships, we feared being ridiculed by others, but we soon learned that we had a lot in common. By facing up to our ambivalent feelings and being honest and open, we were able to build up more trusting relationships.

We discovered four cultural notions of femininity which we have in some sense shared: woman as inferior, passive, beautiful object, wife and mother. We realized how severely these notions had constricted us, how humanly limited we felt at being passive dependent creatures with no identities of our own. Gradually, with each other's support, we began to rediscover ourselves.

REDISCOVERING ANGER

As we were changing we found we were frequently feeling angry. This surprised us and embarrassed us. We had grown up feeling that we needed to love everyone and be loved by everyone. If we got angry with someone or they with us, we felt in some sense that we were failures.

We shared memories of our pasts. Nearly all of us had had a hard time expressing anger verbally or physically. We began to admit that we had felt angry during our lives but that we had been using the anger against ourselves in hating ourselves. There were many ways we had learned to cover up our anger. It had built up for so long inside us that we were afraid we would explode if we let it out. We realized that there are many aspects of our lives that make us angry. Until we know and feel our own oppression we are not motivated to try to create constructive alternative ways of being and living. Many have accused us of being shrill. Our mood is far more complex. Our critics hear only the anger, and anger separated from real issues is a distortion. The anger that is in us is a starting point for creative change and growth.

LEARNING TO VALUE OURSELVES

When we started talking to each other we realized how deeply ingrained was our sense of being less valuable than men. At school we had learned that though we were expected to do well our real vocation was to be wife and mother. Boys were being trained for the important work in society. We learned that what our culture labelled work was not for us, and what we did was not seen as important. The few of us who did *not* stay out of 'male' work suffered the consequences.

> *For me the evidence of my mental competence was unavoidable, and I never had any trouble defending or voicing my opinions with men, because I beat them in all the tests. Consequently none of them would come near me in my first seventeen years of life.*

It was as if to be considered women we had to keep our inferior place. If we challenged this we were treated badly

and came to think of ourselves in negative ways. Our learned sense of inferiority affected the way we thought about our bodies – our physical selves.

We had lived our lives as though we were inferior but we learned that this personal sense of inferiority was in fact shared and that it was merely a reflection of the way power is distributed in society. While men continue to hold on to this power, women will continue to be denigrated. When we looked at our own lives we realized that we were partly responsible for the problem. We did not sufficiently respect ourselves or our needs and we did not sufficiently respect each other. By accepting society's view of us we were perpetuating it.

We all went through a time when we rejected our old selves and took on new qualities exclusively. For a while we became distortions, angry all the time or fiercely independent. It was as though we had partly new selves, and we had to find out what they were like. But ultimately we realized that rejecting our 'feminine qualities' was simply another way of accepting our culture's sexist values.

We began to reassess what we had felt were our weaknesses and to see them as strengths. As women we had been brought up to be sensitive to the problems of others and to take care of their emotional and physical needs. In the past we had lived mainly for others; we now recognized the need to live also for ourselves. We looked again at our passivity and dependence and recognized the value of being able to sit back when we need to, and we realized that dependence is an integral part of any interdependent, intimate relationship. We learned to incorporate the traditional 'female' characteristics so that we could use them instead of *being* them. As we explore and change we discover things that we don't like about ourselves, but we realize that these things do not reflect our inferiority, they are part of being human.

Although we learned to value the essentially servicing work that we do, we wanted also to incorporate more product-oriented work into our lives. This book falls into that category. It has been exciting to collaborate on a

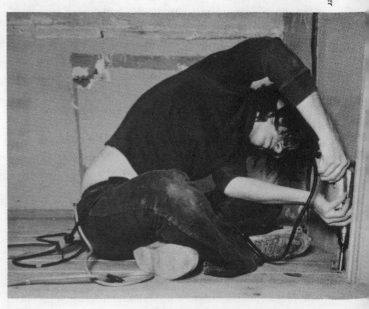

Jean Raisler

tangible product, but throughout the process we have in no way sacrificed the quality of our relationships with one another as men often do when they work together. We have genuinely collaborated and devised new ways of working together within the social context that we created. Along with this new, task-oriented activity has come a new sense of wanting to succeed, to get recognition for what we do. As women we had been taught to want to fail or at least not to excel.

Our new confidence has led us to rediscover physical activity, climbing, canoeing, karate and car maintenance, and to take care of ourselves. We no longer feel the need for constant support from our families, particularly men. We can choose to be alone and to seek support when we need it; we realize that we are no longer powerless, helpless children. Nevertheless we are for ever fighting a constant inner struggle to give up and become weak, dependent and helpless again.

FIFTEEN YEARS LATER

The first publication of *Our Bodies, Ourselves* helped spark many women to explore the health issues most important to them. Since then, women throughout the world have generated such a wealth of information and resources that this time around we turned to *them* for help in rewriting the book.

The New Our Bodies, Ourselves, reflects our Collective's long-time commitment to keeping the book up to date. We emphasize what we as women can do for ourselves and for one another, and we often discuss non-medical perspectives and remedies as well as medical ones. The thousands of women who contact us in person, in letters and by phone have opened up whole new subjects and issues for revisions: 'I looked in your book for a discussion of *in vitro* fertilization and couldn't find it.' 'You've got to include the experiences of differently-abled [disabled] women next time.' 'This is what happened to me when I got PID [pelvic inflammatory disease]; tell other women about it so they will be forewarned and know how to get the right kind of treatment.' 'Could you please say more about lesbians and medical care?' It was difficult to decide what to cut, especially when every chapter turned out to be twice as long as we had room for. To include and condense so much information has meant oversimplifying some subjects and short-changing others.

After noting that in previous editions our discussions of the life cycle always ended with menopause, older women vehemently told us that indeed there *is* life after menopause. Together with them we wrote an all-new chapter on growing older. The chapter on international issues grew out of our correspondence and conversations with women abroad and women who visit our office. While this continues to be a book written primarily by white women, it includes experiences and information gathered by black women.

Our Collective consists of the same core group who worked on the 1973 edition of *Our Bodies, Ourselves* (minus one). We have become a kind of family to one another. We have looked after each other's children, had family picnics and celebrations, played music together and met for meals, given workshops with each other throughout the USA and spent hours in long conversations. Four new babies were born in the past two years, making twenty-one children in all. We have seen one another through four divorces and three marriages, one case of hot flushes and some long, dramatic affairs with men and women. Three children have gone off to college and nine are in the midst of adolescence. We have comforted each other the best we could through four parents' deaths and the illnesses of several others. Most of us have other work in addition to working for the Collective. Now that revisions are over, we plan to do more public speaking. Most important, we will be raising funds to keep our health information centre going and vital. Now, more than ever before, we hold to our original goals:

- to fit as much information on women's health between the covers of this book as we can;
- to let women's different voices and experiences speak out in its pages;
- to reach as many women as possible with the tools which will enable them to take greater charge of their own health care and their lives, deal with the existing medical system and fight whenever possible for improvements and changes;
- to support those women and men working for change both within and outside the existing system of health and medical care;
- to work to create a more just society in which good health is a right, not a luxury, a society which does not perpetuate unequal relationships between the sexes;
- above all, we want to encourage women to get together – to meet, talk and listen to each other.

As we have come to feel separate, we have tried to change old relationships and/or enter new relationships in new ways. We now also feel positive about our needs to be dependent and to connect with others. We have come to value long-term commitments, which we find increasingly rare in such a changing society, just as we value our new separateness.

We are increasingly proud of our dependence upon one another in a culture which so prizes independence. Yet our efforts (along with so many others') to form a community of women are still evolving and, despite their strengths, are quite fragile. A competitive society like ours makes it difficult to work collectively, to be open, to trust one another. It is more difficult to be a feminist these days than it was in the optimistic climate of the early seventies. And when the many women with backgrounds and experiences different from our own speak up and tell the truth about their lives, they make it clear just how diverse this huge community is. Sometimes the great differences between us – race, class, ethnicity, sexual preference, values and strategies – turn us against one another. Keeping in mind our common ground as women must be one of our main tasks. Acknowledging the past and present hurts, the inner fears of difference and the external realities which separate us can enable us to learn to hear each and every woman's voice clearly, to nurture each and every woman's life.

> Remember the dignity
> of your womanhood.
> Do not appeal,
> do not beg,
> do not grovel.
> Take courage,
> join hands,
> stand beside us,
> Fight with us . . .
>
> CHRISTABEL PANKHURST
> (Suffragette, 1858–1928)

From
Norma	Nancy	Vilunya	Wendy
Pam	Paula	Esther	Joan
Judy	Ruth	Jane	

465 Mt Auburn Street
Watertown, MA 02172
USA

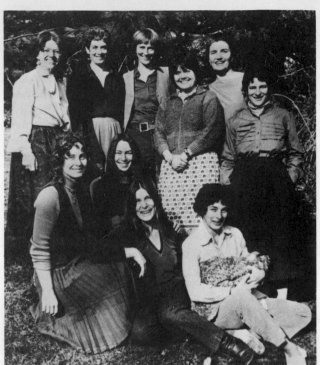

Elizabeth Cole

Boston Women's Health Book Collective

OUR FACES BELONG TO OUR BODIES

Our faces belong to our bodies.
Our faces belong to our lives.

Our faces are blunted.
Our bodies are stunted.
We cover our anger with smiles.

Our faces belong to our bodies.
Our faces belong to our lives.

Our anger is changing our faces, our bodies.
Our anger is changing our lives.

Women who scrub have strong faces
Women who type have strong faces
Women with children have strong faces
Women who love have strong faces

Women who laugh have strong faces
Women who fight have strong faces
Women who cry have strong faces
Women who die have strong faces.

Our love is changing our faces, our bodies.
Our love is changing our lives.

Our sisters are changing our faces, our bodies.
Our sisters are changing our lives.

Our anger is changing our faces, our bodies.
Our anger is changing our lives.

Our power is changing our faces, our bodies.
Our power is changing our lives.

Our struggle is changing our faces, our bodies.
Our struggle is changing our lives.

While the information contained in *Our Bodies, Ourselves* will hopefully empower you and give you useful tools and ideas, this book is not intended to replace professional health and medical care.

This book has cost a great deal to produce, the major part of which has been underwritten by the Boston Women's Health Book Collective, a non-profit-making organization devoted to education about women and health. The collective runs two women's health centres (one based at a women's prison), and distributes free materials extensively to women in the USA and abroad. Royalties from the sale of *Our Bodies, Ourselves* world-wide is not sufficient to support their work, and royalties from this book are unlikely to be sufficient even to cover the authors' costs. Readers wishing to see women benefit from the proceeds of this book are therefore invited to make a donation to **Women's Way UK**, which comprises the following small, national women's charities.

Creative and Supportive Trust. Helps women released from prison and psychiatric hospitals, and with drug and alcohol rehabilitation.

Maternity Alliance. Works for improvements in rights and services for mothers, fathers and babies.

Midwives' Information and Resource Unit (MIDIRS). Run by midwives to promote and advise on clinical and professional developments in maternity care.

National Childcare Campaign. Aims to improve day-care options for women.

New Ways to Work. Informs on flexible working arrangements and alternatives to full-time work.

Women's Health and Reproductive Rights Information Centre. A central resource on women's health issues and reproductive rights.

Women's Legal Defence Fund. Encourages and supports women bringing sex discrimination cases.

Women's Way operates a 'Give as You Earn' scheme and offers the opportunity to choose which organization to donate to. Send a stamped, self-addressed envelope to Women's Way UK, 26 Bedford Square, London WC1B 3HU for more information. Or, if you are salaried or waged, make a copy of the form below, fill it in and give it to your accounts department.

- -

Name ....

Address ....

Payroll Number ....

Employer's Address ....

....

.... Tel ....

As a contribution to the production of **Our Bodies, Ourselves**, I would like to join the 'Give as You Earn' scheme. Please deduct the following sum from my gross earnings before tax each pay day until further notice (*tick appropriate box*)

☐ £1   ☐ £4   ☐ £10   ☐ £15   ☐ £20   ☐ other (*please insert*) £   .   p
and pay it to: **Women's Way UK**, 26 Bedford Square, London, WC1B 3HU

Signature .... Date ....

- -

PART I

TAKING CARE OF OURSELVES

INTRODUCTION

Rewritten by
JILL RAKUSEN

The following chapters offer some of the basic information we as women need to take care of our health. Though medical care sometimes helps us when we are ill, it does not keep us healthy. To a great extent what makes us healthy or unhealthy is how we are able to live our daily lives – what we eat, how we exercise, how much rest we get, how much stress we live with, how much we use alcohol, cigarettes or drugs, how safe or hazardous our workplaces are, whether we experience the threat or reality of sexual violence. Some of these things are under our control as individuals. Many, however, are not; we can influence them only by working with others to bring changes, as we discuss in this book. Many of these daily health factors are dependent on how much money we have: in an unjust society some people can afford to take better care of their health than others. It is a major aim of the feminist movement to make the crucial tools for health and survival available to everyone.

While we do need medical help at times (even when drugs, surgery and crisis intervention are not necessarily the best approaches), there is a lot that we ourselves can do – for ourselves, each other – in staying healthy, healing ourselves, working for change. Yet while we can do a lot, as we discuss particularly in this section, we can also take 'self-help' too far: for becoming actively concerned about our health can lead us to an overly-individualistic approach that ignores social and economic reality – except in so far as it puts money in the hands of those who profit from it. As the US National Center for Health Education has pointed out, 'Health is certainly selling, but who is profiting?'

Individual responsibility for health, though clearly a factor that needs recognition, fits in with the current economic and political climate. Self-reliance and self-help can become dangerously close to the philosophy currently being employed by our government to dismantle the NHS. 'Healthism' – the over-emphasis on keeping healthy – is also another questionable extension of the self-help philosophy. Social critic Robert Crawford[1] suggests that people have become preoccupied with controlling the more manageable health factors like smoking or diet because they feel powerless to change major factors like financial uncertainty or potential nuclear disaster. When we are overly focused on healthiness or a 'healthy lifestyle' as goals to strive for (or as the measure of a 'healthy' society), we deflect attention from the more important goals of social justice and peace.

Crawford also points out that even though prevention is crucial, and dangerously glossed over by conventional medicine, it, too, can be over-emphasized. In expanding the concept of prevention ever further, we risk defining more and more aspects of life in terms of health and illness – that is, according to a medical model. We may end up seeing exercise, eating, meditation, fresh air, dance, for example – all pleasures in their own right – simply as measures of our potential health or non-health. In this way, ironically, we further medicalize our lives.

Keeping healthy can also become a moral issue. We are made to feel guilty for getting ill. People shake their heads disapprovingly over those who 'don't take care of themselves'. In many cases this amounts to blaming the victim; it shows a failure to recognize the social and economic influences on health habits and illness. With personal habits, too, a certain judgemental tone creeps in: 'She *should* have more control over her smoking' or 'She *should* get more exercise, stop eating so much sugar.' Even when these are matters of personal choice, a moralistic healthism is inappropriate. And it doesn't help us change, even when we may want to.

Healthism is a bandwagon that has been jumped on and given a huge push by the burgeoning 'health and fitness' industry. Even the word 'natural' has become abused for marketing purposes. *Looking* healthy has become a fashionable end in itself (with the right clothing, of course), and through the phenomenon of healthism, women are now on the receiving end of having to look desirably healthy as well as desirably attractive. As Rosalind Coward says in her book, *Female Desire*:

> While [the] ideology of health and fitness has clearly affected men and women of all ages, it has nevertheless been directed at women in a particular way,

enmeshing with other very definite attitudes towards the body and appearance . . . the new emphasis on overall health . . . is also a new kind of obsession, which has the effect of making the female body a particular site of concern for Western culture. This new obsession makes women the bearers of a whole series of preoccupations about sex and health.[2]

The ideology of health and fitness may well in itself be a source of stress for many women.

STRESS

Stress is a major health issue. Humans, like all animals, have innate stress-alarm systems originally designed to help us fight or run away when faced with danger. In earlier, simpler times this fight-or-flight response was appropriate. In today's world, however, the dangers are no longer so obvious or so simple. We experience multiple, prolonged, often ambiguous stresses (see below) for which immediate action is often impossible. We squelch the fight-or-flight response over and over again in the course of a single day. It

is an increasingly accepted theory that years of failing to discharge the body's stress response can damage the body's immune (disease-fighting) system and result in many different kinds of ill health. Possible long-term consequences of living with too much stress include ulcers, high blood pressure, higher risk of coronary heart disease, rheumatoid arthritis and cancer.

We can minimize the effects of stress in various ways, such as exercise, healthy food, massage, meditation, etcetera, which we discuss in this section. Regular time to ourselves, without interruption, is also important – but since as yet this is impossible for many women, we need to find ways of supporting each other's needs in this area and insisting that we have as much right to solitude as men do. It also helps to complain when we need to, to discharge pent-up feelings (methods for doing this can include bashing pillows or learning co-counselling, see p. 121), and to laugh – the value of laughter cannot be underestimated, as Norman Cousins so graphically shows in his book.[4] Having pets (whether cats, dogs or even fish) appears to reduce stress too. This is probably connected with the sense of unambivalent love and affection that they engender in us; people with pets also appear to live longer. As Professor Aaron

---

SOME CAUSES OF STRESS

- financial insecurity
- job loss
- death of somebody we love and/or need
- ending or beginning of a relationship
- job changes; a new job
- having a baby
- moving home
- being discriminated against because of race, class, age, looks, sexual preference or physical disability
- an illness for which we can find no appropriate care
- a diet low in fresh foods and high in sugar, white flour, caffeine, additives and salt
- environmental pollution
- the threat of nuclear war

STRESSES SPECIFIC TO WOMEN

- A majority of women now combine outside jobs with full responsibility for home and children. In addition, we may feel – from others, from ourselves – the pressure to be 'perfect' at each of these.
- Most jobs pay women little and don't allow us to use our abilities.*

- Many women are single parents; many are poor.
- Some of us are at home all day with small children.
- We face sexual harassment and abuse on the street, in workplaces, at home.

SYMPTOMS OF EXCESSIVE STRESS

- headaches
- neck, back and shoulder pains
- nervous twitches, 'tics'
- sleeplessness
- skin rashes
- greater susceptibility to colds, influenza or other illnesses
- worsening of existing conditions or illnesses
- depression, anxiety, irritability, nervousness, despair
- jaw pains and toothaches (from grinding teeth)
- cold sores
- stomach aches, diarrhoea, loss of or increase in appetite

*Illnesses caused by stress are more likely to strike manual and clerical workers, particularly women.[3]

A SELF-HELP CHECKLIST*
FOR THOSE WHO FEEL 'ONE DEGREE UNDER'
BUT HAVE NO PARTICULAR SYMPTOMS

By MAGGIE EISNER

AM I GETTING THE BALANCE RIGHT?

- Do I pay attention to what I eat, and do I make peaceful, pleasant mealtimes for myself? If not, is it possible to do this?
- Do I have satisfying work to do?
- Do I get some fresh air and physical exercise every day?
- Do I have a relationship with someone I can trust and confide in?
- Do I have any satisfying spare-time activities?

HAVE I GOT ANY LONG-TERM STRESSES?

These make people feel ill. Even if you can't do anything about them, it *is* useful to identify and be aware of them.

- Have I got enough money to live on?
- Have I got a decent place to live?
- Do I have any hurtful, stressful relationships?
- Am I being oppressed as a member of a minority group?
- Does my job expose me to risks (such as noise, chemicals, VDU screens)?
- Have I got a lot of people who are dependent on me or make demands on me (children, elderly relatives, neighbours)?

HAVE THERE BEEN ANY SIGNIFICANT CHANGES IN MY LIFE RECENTLY? SUCH AS:

- death or serious illness of a close friend or relative

- moving house
- redundancy
- changing job
- retirement
- starting a relationship
- ending a relationship
- having a child
- child leaving home

DO I HAVE ANY UNHEALTHY HABITS? SUCH AS:

- 'social' drugs (including smoking, alcohol, tea or coffee drinking)
- over-the-counter drugs
- prescribed drugs
- bad posture

SCREENING TESTS

If you have no symptoms, there are a few routine tests which are particularly useful:

- checking blood pressure
- testing urine for sugar
- cervical smear
- STD check (if you or your partner are sexually active with more than one person)
- weighing yourself

In addition, some women may wish to perform breast self-examinations (see p. 543) and, if you are generally tired, thyroid function tests and a blood count for anaemia are valuable.

*This self-help checklist may help you find reasons for the way you feel. It doesn't necessarily suggest solutions.

Katcher has found, people have more problems being affectionate than in having sex.* Stroking animals reduces blood pressure and heart rates, as does talking to them. They can make excellent therapists (this was written by someone who lives with one adorable dog and two very therapeutic goldfish!).

*He also observed that the concept of women using dogs as a substitute for maternal care is an invidious sexist stereotype – both women and men respond to dogs and other pets in similar ways.

In our attempts to minimize stress, we must also beware, paradoxically, of causing ourselves greater stress. Suddenly to deprive ourselves of coping mechanisms, such as smoking or binge eating can, in the words of Arabella Melville and Colin Johnson, be like 'taking the lid off a pressure cooker without cooling it first'.[5] So we must be careful not to take it too much to heart when we receive admonitions from health personnel who can so easily make us feel guilty or inadequate because of our 'bad habits'. Instead, we need to support each other, and seek support, particularly for dealing with the root causes of stress in our lives, so that our own bad habits may become less highly charged, and ultimately even redundant.

NOTES

1. Robert J. Crawford. 'Healthism and Medicalization of Everyday Life', *International Journal of Health Services*, vol. 10, no. 3, 1980.
2. Rosalind Coward. *Female Desire – Women's Sexuality Today*. London: Granada, 1984, p. 21.
3. Labour Research Department. *Stress at Work*, 1988 (available from LRD, 78 Blackfriars Road, London SE1 8HF). See also *Women's Health, Work and Stress*, a WHIC broadsheet available from WHRRIC (see p. 638).
4. Norman Cousins. *Anatomy of an Illness*. London: Corgi, 1981.
5. Arabella Melville and Colin Johnson. *The Long-Life Heart: How to Avoid Heart Disease and Live a Longer Life*. London: Century, 1985.

CHAPTER
2

BODY IMAGE

Prepared by
JILL RAKUSEN

Imagine yourself naked in front of a mirror. Turn around slowly. Do you like what you see? Stroke your body's contours. Do you like what you feel? Try saying something appreciative to each part of yourself. It may be difficult at first. Almost every woman judges some part of her body – sometimes all of it – as 'not right', tries to hide it from view, feels ashamed of it even with friends or lovers.

We often feel negative about our physical selves. Our hair is too straight or too curly, nose too small or too large, breasts too big or too small, stomach or thighs too fat, frame too bony. We don't like our body hair or odours. Our genitals – well, we just try to ignore them; after all, they really 'belong' to lovers or doctors, not to us. We often compare ourselves to others; we're never OK the way we are. We feel ugly, inadequate. If others say we are beautiful, we don't/can't believe it, or we worry about losing our beauty. We spend precious time and money trying to change our looks. We may also subject ourselves to health hazards: cosmetics and vaginal deodorants which contain dangerous chemicals, low-calorie diets which deprive us of needed nutrients, hair dyes with cancer-causing ingredients, clothes which severely hamper movement, shoes which damage our feet and even our backs, and questionable plastic surgery on our faces or breasts. Looks are too often a matter of survival: many employers require that we look a particular way in order to get or keep our jobs. It's hard not to judge ourselves – and each other – on the 'acceptability' of our bodies.

Talking with other women about body image helps us see that we can come to think differently about our bodies and come to accept ourselves more fully. It's a process which we can begin at any point in our lives and continue as long as we live.

It helps to examine the pressures on us to look a certain way. Growing up, we learn to think of our bodies mainly in terms of *how we look*. Early on we get the message: you've got to look good in order to be acceptable, to please men.

My husband gave me a full-length mirror for my

thirtieth birthday, to remind me I'd better keep an eye on my looks.

Every society throughout history has had standards of beauty, but at no time before has there been such an intense media blitz telling us what we *should* look like. Magazine covers, films, TV shows, advertisement hoardings surround us with images which fail to reflect the tremendous diversity among us. Never before have there been hundreds of profitable businesses set up to convince us we don't look good enough. Whole industries depend on selling us products through slick ads depicting 'beautiful' women, playing on our insecurities and fears of imperfection.

We naturally want to look and feel good, to wear colours and materials that are beautiful to us, to feel attractive and appreciated. The trouble is that the media define 'looking good' so narrowly that few of us ever feel we have made it. Picture for yourself the 'ideal' woman in our dominant culture today. She is almost without exception thin, shapely, white, able-bodied, smooth-skinned, young and glamorous. She may change from decade to decade (sometimes breasts are out, sometimes they are in), yet we always have to measure up to some image. * Media images do have less impact if friends and family like us as we are.

If we are passably close to the current media image of beauty we may not be aware of the intense pressures working on us. But if we are more obviously 'different' – fat, old, women of colour or physically disabled, for instance – we encounter the pressures more openly and every day. Women who don't 'fit' the image experience painfully the negative judgements, fears and hatreds which in subtle or unsubtle ways make it hard for nearly every woman in our society to love and accept herself as she is.

---

*Those of us who are feminists and/or lesbians may not worry so much about pleasing men. Yet we may replace one ideal with another, substituting muscular for shapely, for instance, or Amazon for cover-girl, so that there is still an image we feel we have to live up to. Those of us who are non-white or non-Anglo-Saxon often feel torn between the dominant culture's standards and those of our own community.

PHYSICAL DISABILITY AND THE PRESSURE TO BE PHYSICALLY 'PERFECT'

AUTHORS' NOTE: Several women from Boston Self-Help (a self-help organization for people with physical disabilities) were generous with their time in talking with us, suggesting books and articles and reading over what we'd written here. Many of us in the Collective had never known women with physical disabilities; our meetings with the Boston Self-Help group began to change both how we see disabled women and how we see ourselves. We have chosen to use the pronouns 'we' and 'us' in this section because both groups discovered at those meetings that many of the issues we face as women are similar, because the women in the group said that to use the third-person 'they' would be too distancing, and because it is important to them that able-bodied women be conscious that they are only 'temporarily' able-bodied. By remembering that this state could change at any time through accident or illness, we are more likely to see disabled women as sisters rather than turn away from them in indifference or fear.

Thousands of women in this country walk with a limp, move in a wheelchair or with crutches, have impaired sight, speech or hearing, have lost a limb to fire or accident or disease, need special assistance with simple bodily

Jean Gillespie

This woman is post-polio and has no use of her arms and hands. She takes care of her daughter using her teeth and toes and love.

functions or wear the scars of some damaging event. Many of these women are silent and invisible – many of us choose to hide in order to avoid the pain of being stared at and objectified, and the public, in fear, does not acknowledge and accept us.

With a body that doesn't 'measure up', we learn pretty quickly what our culture really wants from women.

Having a disability made me very aware at an early age of the messages I was receiving from the larger society about how I was supposed to look and how you're supposed to be. Also, as the doctors poked and studied me endlessly, I learned more quickly than some non-disabled women that I'm seen as an object.

My family's thing was that girls dated in order to find a prospective mate. Since I had cerebral palsy, they assumed I was never going to marry. So why should I date? And I've only just begun to wear a dress this year, because I was always encouraged to wear trousers. There was no reason for me to dress like a woman because I wasn't one. That wasn't part of my identity.

The more we vary from the norm, the less families, friends, doctors expect or allow us to be sexual. (See Sex and Physical Disabilities, p. 253.) If we can't have children, we are pitied for not being 'real' women. If we aren't 'pleasing' to look at, we are expected to compensate, and we come to expect it of ourselves: we learn to smile a lot and be sweet, or clown around, so people won't feel so uncomfortable around us. Or, believing in our own unworthiness, we fall into the background.

Other 'female' stereotypes surface quickly – we are weak, less intelligent, need protection. If we can't control our movements or bodily functions people think we are mentally incompetent. ('My family thinks of epilepsy as a mental illness.' 'People see my body and don't expect me to be intelligent.') Like many women, only more so, we are treated like children far into our adult lives. ('People will pinch me on the cheek and use words that you would use to a child.' 'The doctors still talk to my parents or to the person with me instead of directly to me, as though I'm a child, and I'm sick of it.') As women with physical disabilities, it is difficult but important to assert our adulthood, our power, our individuality and intelligence. This process is crucial for *all* women.

Severe job discrimination penalizes us for having 'unacceptable' bodies and creates a strong economic incentive for 'fitting in' and minimizing differences. This pressure to keep a low profile if we are disabled makes us feel isolated and less free to get the help we need and deserve both physically and emotionally. It also means we have a hard time becoming economically independent. As one woman said, 'We are not disabled; it is society which disables us by being so unsupportive.'

Sooner or later, if we're lucky, we realize how angry we

are at always having had to hide our true feelings and the realities of our lives.

> *After I got my braces removed at age twelve, I did everything I could to hide my skinny, scarred legs, including wearing knee socks or trousers in the hottest weather. Slowly my anger grew at the restrictions I was accepting. Partly with the help of other disabled women, I came to see my underlying feeling that if people saw my legs they'd not only reject me for being ugly, but they'd somehow see the years in the hospital or how dependent and scared I'd been. I began to re-evaluate these experiences as simply things that had happened, not who I am. I wear shorts when I want to now, and I like my legs the way they are.*

If coming to love and accept our bodies is a difficult process for every woman in this society, it is especially hard with a disability.

> *Finally I like my body, and because of my disability that statement has added significance. There is something 'WRONG' with my body, so how can I possibly feel good about it or enjoy life in it? Simple answers are:* I have no choice *and* I want to. *The more complex answer is that* there is nothing wrong with my body. *It falls within the wide range of human experience and is therefore both natural and normal. I've been in this body all my life. I was born with it and I'll die with it. It's part of who I am, and I'd be someone else without this body just the way it is.*

Dialogue between disabled and non-disabled women reveals that we have much in common. A woman with a brittle bone condition writes:

> *I can't quite pin-point when I began to listen to the experiences of able-bodied women and relate them to my own. It may have been when someone said that she couldn't go out of the house because her skin was so spotty, or when a beautiful black woman told me how all her life she had wanted to be white and blotchy like her friend at school, or it could have been when a friend of mine who had always been my envy for being followed around by drooling men said that she was so lonely because people only reacted to her stunning body and never to the person inside it. It may have been when my family began to talk about one of its female members who had put on weight and had, in their eyes, become not only unattractive but somehow outrageously undutiful in her role as an ornament. It may have been none of this that made the turning point for me, but instead it could have been the way some of the women put their arms around me and called me their beautiful sister that made me begin to see that we are not so different after all. We are all*

made to feel that our role is firstly to be beautiful in a highly stereotyped way, secondly to be interesting and amusing company to men and thirdly, good servants. My experience of finding that I was not necessarily any of those things is the experience of most women sooner or later. I have been lucky enough to discover that I am still a whole and worthwhile person and feel that all those dark years linked me profoundly to other women.[1]

BODY IMAGE AND WEIGHT*

In most cultures and historical periods women have been proud to be large – being fat was a sign of fertility, of prosperity, of the ability to survive. Yet fear of fat and bigness reigns in most sectors of our culture today. Media images of women insist that 'Thin is beautiful'. The medical world blames a whole range of problems on 'overweight'. Fat women encounter daily hostility and discrimination.

No wonder so many of us worry about our weight no matter what we weigh, spend precious hours counting calories, feel guilty when we 'splurge'.

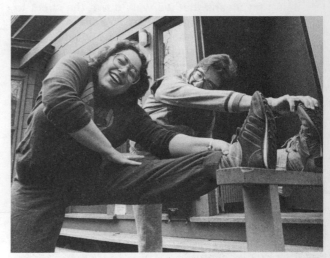

Bonnie Burt

> *I don't like myself heavy. I want to feel thin, streamlined and spare, and not like a toad. I have taken anti-fat thinking into myself so deeply that I hate myself when I am even ten pounds 'overweight', whatever* that *means.*

Fat activists suggest that making women afraid to be fat is a form of social control. Fear of fat keeps women preoccupied, robs us of our pride and energy, keeps us from *taking*

---

*For more on this topic, especially on health issues and low-calorie dieting, see Chapter 4.

up space. Activist Vivian Mayer sees 'Mass starvation of women' as our culture's equivalent of foot-binding, lip-stretching and other forms of female mutilation.[2]

Recent research indicates that the 'ideal' body weight for each woman is at least ten pounds higher than that stated by medical charts, and that no one at this point *knows* a given woman's 'ideal' weight.[3] Many health problems blamed on overweight turn out to have a more complex relationship to weight than doctors once assumed. Studies suggest that dieting is usually not successful in the long run, and that repeated low-calorie dieting is a major cause of ill health.

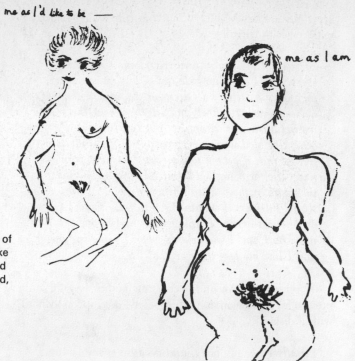

me as I'd like to be ——

me as I am

We did an excercise in the group once: drawing a picture of ourselves as we really are and our fantasy of how we'd like to be. Then we talked about our bodies as we had pictured them – the colours we had used, how the bits were related, what was missing . . .

BEING FAT IN AN ANTI-FAT SOCIETY*

Being fat means that we walk down the street to comments like 'fat bitch' or 'pig'. We are expected to laugh at fat jokes. People laugh at us when we try to be physically active or if we show an interest in sex. Friends and family try to get us to diet instead of helping us love ourselves. At public events the seats are too small and uncomfortable. We search for days to find clothes that fit and have a harder time than thin women finding a job or getting into college. Like many other minorities, we never see *our* image on TV or in films except as comic or pathetic characters. We often hear that our fatness is the cause of everything that goes wrong in our lives. We are judged as weak-willed or morally lax because we 'indulge' ourselves. We live for long stretches in a state of starvation (called 'being on a diet') because our appearance touches people's fear of their own appetites.

If we are fat, health practitioners often attribute our health problems to 'obesity', postpone treatment until we lose weight, accuse us of cheating if we don't, make us so ashamed of our size that we don't go for help and make all kinds of assumptions about our emotional and psychological state ('She must have emotional problems to be so fat'). In fact, much of our ill health as fat women results from the *stress* of living with fat-hatred – social ridicule and hostility, isolation, financial pressures resulting from job discrimination, lack of exercise due to harassment and, perhaps most important, the hazards of repeated dieting.

Fat women have begun to form support groups. Here are suggestions from some members of Fat Liberation:

No matter what anyone says to you (or what you fear they are saying about you), you have the *right* to go anywhere and do anything you like: to eat whatever you want in restaurants, to go dancing, to enjoy life. If someone or some place makes you feel uncomfortable (by rude remarks, aisles too narrow or chairs too small) it is up to *them* to change, not you.

You have the right to respond angrily to the nasty things people say to you or about you. Practise a few good withering glances or comebacks.

Take up all of the space your body occupies – no more hunching or slumping to try to look smaller. Stand up tall and relax. Practise being big. Or pretend you're a lion afraid of nothing and very, very strong. Move around your house remembering to breathe deeply, keeping your shoulders and back straight. Be loose and big in your movements. Work to create the feeling that you are entitled to go wherever you want and the world should make room for your wonderful presence. Whatever the size of your stomach (thighs, rear end), stop sucking in your stomach muscles. Insist on the right to be comfortable all the way out to your skin. Try to buy clothes that fit easily. Pleated pants or ones with elastic in the waist are less likely to bind your stomach in. Tight clothes don't make us look thinner – but they do make it harder to get out and move around.[4]

*Thanks especially to Judith Stein and Rea Rea Sears of Boston Area Fat Liberation.

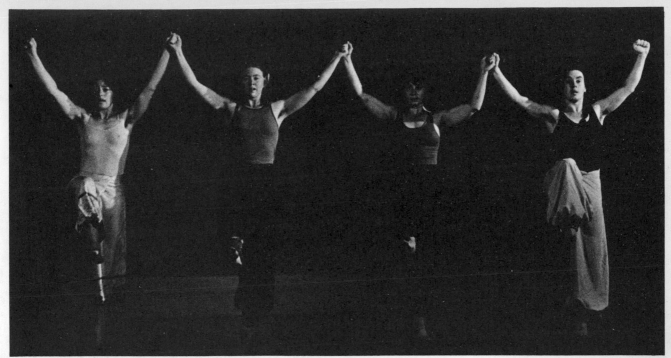

Members of Wallflower Order Dance Collective

These developments offer women a chance to become more relaxed about weight:

- by experimenting with what weight feels *comfortable* to us;
- by being more accepting of weight variations through the life cycle;
- by developing a clearer understanding of which health problems are truly associated with weight; we must learn to distinguish what facts exist among the many, often damaging fictions;
- by exercising and eating nutritious food to feel healthy, and letting our body weight set itself accordingly;
- if we do diet, by choosing a programme which emphasizes exercise and helps us change eating patterns but doesn't starve us.

WORKING TOGETHER FOR CHANGE

In moving towards a more positive self-image, we are stronger if we can talk with other women. We need each other's help to change the deeply entrenched attitudes which make us dislike our bodies. Here are some things groups of women can do together:

- Look at ads and criticize how they demean women and limit our ideas of beauty. Find ways to make your protest known to the companies advertised* and to let the media know you want to see more varied and realistic images of women.

- Learn more about how our bodies work, through self-help sessions† and/or discussion.
- Plan together how to challenge men who judge, choose and discard women on the basis of appearance.
- Form or join a working-women's organization; work on ways to pressurize employers into accepting a wider range of looks and dress.
- Work together on tackling the fears and stereotypes which make us all discriminate against people who are 'different'. (This is a long process. One step is being painfully honest about our own prejudices; another is learning not to blame ourselves for them; another is getting to know women who are different – in race, age, physical ability.)

If we can begin to eliminate the hatred and ridicule levied against women who don't fit the 'norm', we can lessen the stress of 'not fitting in' and, with it, a lot of stress-related illness. We also open the possibility of building a social-change movement of many different kinds of women. Working together to change the attitudes and conditions which restrict us, we feel proud and more able to take control of our lives.

A better self-image doesn't pay the rent or cook supper or prevent nuclear war. Feeling better about ourselves doesn't change the world by itself, but it can give us more energy to do what we want and can to work for change.

*See Chapter 10 for an example.

†See Chapter 27.

NOTES

1. Micheline in Jo Campling (ed.). *Images of Ourselves: Women with Disabilities Talking*. London: Routledge and Kegan Paul, 1981, pp. 26–7.
2. Aldebran Vivian Mayer. 'Uptight and Hungry: the Contradiction in Psychology of Fat', *The Radical Therapist: Journal of Radical Therapy*, London: Penguin Books, 1974, p. 6.
3. See, in particular, William Bennett and Joel Gurin. *The Dieter's Dilemma: Eating Less and Weighing More*. New York: Basic Books, 1982.
4. Cited in an unpublished manuscript by Judith Stein and others.

RESOURCES
PUBLICATIONS

Campling, Jo (ed.). *Images of Ourselves: Women with Disabilities Talking*. London: Routledge and Kegan Paul, 1981.

Chernin, Kim. *Womansize: the Tyranny of Slenderness*. London: Women's Press, 1983.

Corbette, K., A. Cupolo and V. Lewis. *No More Stares: Role Model Book for Disabled Teenage Girls*. Disability Rights Defense Fund (2023 San Pablo Avenue, Berkeley, CA 94702, USA), 1982.

Coward, Rosalind. *Female Desire – Women's Sexuality Today*. London: Granada, 1984.

Cross, Merry. 'Feminism and the Disability Movement – a Personal View' in Joy Holland (ed.). *Feminist Action 1*. London: Battle Axe Books, 1984.

Duffy, Yvonne. *All Things are Possible*. A.J. Garvin and Associates (PO Box 7525, Ann Arbor, MI 48107, USA), 1981.

Glasman, Claire. *True Confessions of a Raspberry*. Centrepiece pamphlet no. 4 (available from WinVisible, see Organizations).

Haug, Frigga (ed.). *Female Sexualization – A Collective Work of Memory*. London: Verso, 1987. An impressive book that explores far more than we are able ways of understanding our attitudes to our physical selves.

Mason, Micheline. *Women's Health and Disability*. Broadsheet (available from WHRRIC, see Organizations).

Orbach, Susie. *Fat is a Feminist Issue II* (rev. ed.). London: Hamlyn, 1984.

Robertson S. (ed.). *Disability, Rights Handbook*. London: Disability Alliance (see Organizations), 1986.

Schoenfielder, Lisa and Barb **Wieser** (eds.). *Shadow on a Tightrope: Writings by Women about Fat Oppression*. Aunt Lute Book Co. (PO Box 2723, Iowa City, IA 52244, USA).

In from the Cold. A liberation magazine for people with disabilities produced by the Liberation Network for People with Disabilities (see below).

ORGANIZATIONS

Campaign for Press and Broadcasting Freedom, 9 Poland Street, London W1. Tel: 01–437 2795. Concerned, among other things, with media portrayals of women and of people with disabilities.

Compulsive Eating Groups – contact Women's Therapy Centre (see below).

Disability Alliance, 25 Denmark Street, London WC2 8NJ. Tel: 01–240 0806. Educational and research association.

Fat Women's Group, c/o London Women's Centre, Wesley House, 4 Wild Court, London WC2B 5AU

Gemma (Lesbians with and without Disabilities), BM 5700, London WC1N 3XX. A national friendship information and support group. Quarterly newsletter (on tape). Inquiries – sae; tape or braille – welcome.

Liberation Network for People with Disabilities, Merry Cross, 1 Lewey House, Bow Common Lane, London E1.

PHAB – Physically Handicapped and Able-bodied, Tavistock House, North Tavistock Square, London WC1H 9AX. Tel: 01–388 1963.

Sisters Against Disablement, 162 Evelyn Court, Amhurst Road, London E8.

Union of Physically Impaired Against Segregation (UPIAS), c/o John Mason, Secretary, Flat 2, 98 Woodhill, Woolwich, London, SE18 5JL. Tel: 01–854 8431.

WinVisible (Women with Visible and Invisible Disabilities), c/o King's Cross Women's Centre, 71 Tonbridge Street, London WC1H 9DZ. Tel: 01–837 7509.

Women's Monitoring Network, c/o London Women's Centre, Wesley House, 4 Wild Court, London WC2B SAU. Concerned with oppressive role of media.

Women's Therapy Centre, 6 Manor Gardens, London N7. Tel: 01–263 6200.

Women's Health and Reproductive Rights Information Centre, 52–54 Featherstone Street, London EC1Y 8RT. Tel: 01–251 6580/6332.

THE ANATOMY AND PHYSIOLOGY OF SEXUALITY AND REPRODUCTION*

Prepared by
JILL RAKUSEN

FINDING OUT ABOUT OURSELVES

When we first began to prepare this material, many of us didn't know the names of parts of our anatomy. Some of us had learned bits and pieces of information, but it was not permissible to find out too much. The taboos were strongest in the areas of reproduction and sex, which is why our book concentrates on them.

> *The first month I was at college some of my friends were twittering about a girl down the hall. She was having a painful time trying to learn to put in a tampon. Finally someone helped her and found she was trying to put it in her anus.*

Knowing the facts about our anatomy and physiology has been very exciting for us. It's exhilarating to discover that the material is not as difficult as we once thought. Knowing the language of doctors makes them less mysterious and frightening. We now feel more confident when asking questions; we have information that enables us to become active participants in our own health care.

It's important to become as familiar with the appearance of our sexual organs, both inside and outside, as we are with other parts of our bodies. With just a mirror we can see how we look on the outside. See page 32 for how we can look inside at our vaginal walls and cervix (lower part of the uterus).

> *I'll never forget the first time I did self-examination. I looked in the mirror at my vagina – all brown on the outside and bright pink within. I was absolutely amazed. I realized I'd got no idea what colour I was inside.*

*Anatomy is the physical shape and placement of our organs; physiology is how our organs work.

It has taken a while for some of us to get over our inhibitions about seeing or touching our genitals.

> *When someone first said to me two years ago, 'You can feel the end of your own cervix with your finger,' I was interested but flustered. I had hardly ever put my finger in my vagina at all, and felt squeamish about touching myself there, in that place 'reserved' for lovers and doctors. It took me two months to get up my nerve to try it, and then one afternoon, pretty nervously, I squatted down in the bathroom and put my finger in deep, back into my vagina. There it was(!), feeling slippery and rounded, with an indentation at the centre through which, I realized, my menstrual flow came. It was both very exciting and beautifully ordinary at the same time. Last week I bought a plastic speculum so I can look at my cervix. Will it take as long this time?*

PELVIC ORGANS

The following description will mean much more if you look at yourself with a mirror while you read the text. It is written as if you were squatting and looking into a hand mirror. If you are uncomfortable in that position sit as far forward on the edge of a chair as you comfortably can. Make sure you have plenty of light and enough time and privacy to feel relaxed.

First you will see your *vulva*, or outer genitals.† This includes all of the sexual and reproductive organs you can see in your crotch. The most obvious feature on an adult woman is the *pubic hair*, the first wisps of which are one of

†See Betty Dodson's *Liberating Masturbation: A Meditation on Self Love* (New York: Bodysex Designs, 1974) for drawings of vulvas, showing how much variety there can be in the proportions of the different parts; Suzanne Gage's drawings in *A New View of a Woman's Body* by the Federation of Feminist Women's Health Centers; and Tee Corinne's *Labiaflowers* (both listed in Resources).

WOMAN WITH PELVIC ORGANS

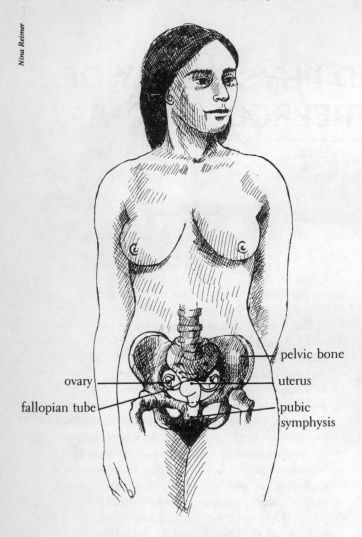

Nina Reimer

ovary
fallopian tube
pelvic bone
uterus
pubic symphysis

Starting from the front, right below the mons area the inner lips join to form a soft fold of skin, or *hood*, over and connecting to the *glans*, or tip of the *clitoris* (klit'-or-is). †
Gently pull the hood up to see the glans. This is the most sensitive spot in the entire genital area. It is made up of erectile tissue which swells during sexual arousal. Let the hood slide back over the glans. Extending from the hood up to the pubic symphysis, you can now feel a hardish, rubbery, movable cord right under the skin. It is sometimes sexually arousing if touched. This is the *shaft* of the clitoris. It is connected to the bone by a *suspensory ligament*. You cannot feel this ligament or the next few organs described, but they are all important in sexual arousal and orgasm. At the point where you can no longer feel the shaft of the clitoris it divides into two parts, spreading out wishbone fashion, but at a much wider angle, to form two *crura* (singular: *crus*), the two anchoring wing-tips of erectile tissue which attach to the pelvic bones. The crura are about three inches long. Starting from where the shaft and crura meet, and continuing along down the sides of the vestibule are two bundles of erectile tissue called the *bulbs of the vestibule*. These, along with the whole clitoris and an extensive system of connecting veins throughout the pelvis, become firm and filled with blood (pelvic congestion) during sexual arousal. Some pelvic congestion, giving a feeling of fullness or heaviness in the pelvic region can occur before your period comes. Both the crura of the clitoris and the bulbs of the vestibule are wrapped in muscle tissue. This muscle helps to create tension and fullness during arousal and contracts during orgasm, playing an important role in the involuntary spasms felt at the time. The whole clitoris and vestibular bulbs are the only organs in the body solely for sexual sensation and arousal.

Vestibular or *Bartholin's glands* are two small rounded bodies on either side of the vaginal opening and to the rear of the vestibular bulbs. They sometimes get infected and swell. You can feel them then. Once these glands were thought to provide lubrication during sex, though in fact they only produce a few drops of fluid.

You will notice that the inner lips attach to the underside of the clitoris. This is important for sexual stimulation. Right below this attachment is a small dot or slit. This is the *urinary opening*, the outer opening of a short (about an inch and a half), thin tube leading to your *bladder*. Below that is a larger opening, the *vaginal opening*. Because the urinary opening is so close to the vagina, it can become irritated from prolonged or vigorous sex and you may feel some discomfort while urinating. ** Around the vaginal opening you may be able to see the *hymen*. When you were born it was a thin membrane surrounding the vaginal opening, partially blocking it and very occasionally covering the opening completely. Hymens come in widely

the early signs of puberty. After menopause, the hair thins out. It grows from the soft fatty tissue called the *mons*. The mons area lies over the *pubic symphysis*. This is the joint of the pubic bones, which are part of the *pelvic bones*, or hip girdle. You can see that the hair continues between your legs and probably on around your *anus* (the opening of the *rectum*, or large intestine). The hair-covered area between your legs is also fatty, like the mons. This fatty area is called the *outer lips* (*labia majora*). * They surround some soft flaps of skin which are hairless. These are the *inner lips* (*labia minora*). They are sensitive to touch. With sexual stimulation they swell and change colour. The area between the inner lips and the anus is the *perineum*.

As you gently spread the inner lips apart, you can see that they protect a delicate area between them (the *vestibule*).

---

*The formal medical term is included in parentheses if it is different from the English term. We are not including slang terms in the text. They often represent a male view of a woman's body and have been used to put women down. We can make up new words of our own, or find old words with a gentler sound, like 'yoni', or use the common words, like 'pussy' or 'cunt', in a more positive and loving way.

†The glans of the clitoris is commonly referred to as 'the clitoris'. We will follow that convention, but please remember that the clitoris referred to here as 'the whole clitoris' is really a much more extensive organ, consisting of the glans, shaft and crura, all described in the text.[1]

**See Chapter 23, p. 507, on urinary problems.

Nina Reimer

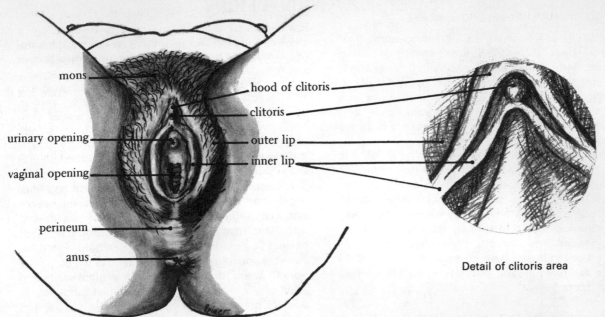

mons

hood of clitoris

clitoris

urinary opening

outer lip

inner lip

vaginal opening

perineum

anus

Detail of clitoris area

VULVA

varying sizes and shapes. The hymen can be stretched before intercourse by using a tampon, or simply by gentle finger pressure. Even when stretched by intercourse, little folds of hymen tissue remain.

Nina Reimer

SOME HYMEN VARIATIONS

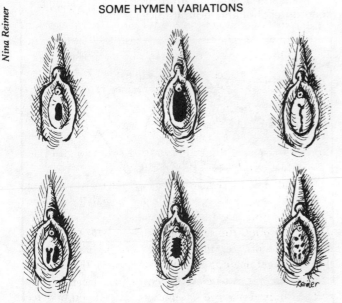

Now insert a finger or two into your *vagina*. Notice how the vaginal walls which were touching each other now spread around your fingers and hug them. Feel the soft folds of skin. These folds allow the vagina to mould itself around what is inside it, whether around fingers, a tampon, a penis, or a baby. The walls of the vagina may be almost dry to very wet. Dryer times usually occur before puberty, often during lactation and after menopause, as well as during that part of the cycle right after the flow. Wetter times are around ovulation, pregnancy and when sexually aroused. These continuous secretions provide lubrication,

help keep the vagina clean, and maintain the acidity of the vagina to prevent infections. Push gently all around against the walls of the vagina and notice where you feel particularly sensitive. For some women it is only the outer third; in others it is most or all of the vagina. Now put your finger halfway in and try to grip your finger with your vagina. It might help if you imagine you are stopping the flow of urine. You are contracting the *pelvic floor muscles*. These muscles hold the pelvic organs in place and provide support for your other organs all the way up to your diaphragm, which is stretched across the bottom of your rib cage. If these muscles are weak you may have trouble having an orgasm, controlling your urine flow (urinary incontinence) or have prolapse of your pelvic organs. See p. 347 for ways to strengthen these muscles.

There is only a thin wall of skin separating the vagina from the rectum, so you may be able to feel a bump on one side of your vagina if you have some stool in the rectum, a small haemorrhoid or perhaps a prolapsed organ pushing on your vagina.

Now slide your middle finger as far back into your vagina as you can. Notice that your finger goes in towards the small of your back at an angle, not straight up the middle of your body. With your finger you may be able to just feel the end of your vagina. This part of the vagina is called the *fornix*. (If you are having trouble reaching it, bring your knees and chest closer together so your finger can slide in further. However, some women still may not be able to do this.) A little before the end of the vagina you can feel your *cervix*. It feels like a nose with a small dimple in its centre. If you've had a baby the cervix may feel more like a chin. The cervix is the base of the *uterus*, or womb. The uterus changes position and shape during the menstrual cycle and during sexual excitement, as well as during puberty and menopause, so the place where you feel the cervix one day may be slightly different from where you feel it the next. Some days you can barely reach it. The dimple you felt is the *os*, or opening into the uterus. It is about the diameter of

SELF-EXAMINATION

Over the past few years an increasing number of women have discovered the benefits of doing vaginal and cervical self-examination. By examining yourself regularly you can learn more about what is 'normal' for you; what your discharges look like; the colour, size and shape of your cervix; and the changes in your mucus during different stages of your menstrual cycle.

Doing self-examination, we see parts of our bodies that we have learned to ignore or fear. By using a speculum ourselves we use a small part of medical technology to gain back some control over our bodies. Many women have taken self-examination a step further by talking about their experiences and sharing their knowledge with other women in self-help groups.

For self-examination you will need only a few basic items:

- a light source that can be directed, such as a strong torch;
- a speculum (plastic specula are inexpensive and easier to get than metal); you can get one with ease from the Women's Health and Reproductive Rights Information Centre (see p. 638), or with less ease from some medical suppliers;
- a lubricant such as K-Y Jelly or warm water;
- a mirror with a long handle;
- antiseptic soap or alcohol.

Find a comfortable setting and get into a relaxed position on the floor or couch, etc. Some women prefer sitting on the floor with a pillow at their back for support.

Familiarize yourself with the speculum and then lie back with your knees bent and your feet placed wide apart. You may want to lubricate the speculum (see above). Hold the speculum in a closed position with the handle pointing upward. Some women prefer to place the speculum into the vagina sideways and then turn it. Experiment until you discover the most comfortable variation for you.

Once you have fully inserted the speculum, grasp the handle and firmly pull its shorter section towards you. This opens the blades of the speculum inside your vagina. Now hold the speculum steady and push down on the outside section until you hear a click; this means that the speculum is locked into place.

For some women placing the speculum and finding the cervix may take some effort. Breathe deeply and manipulate the speculum gently while looking into the mirror. Focus the light source on the mirror to help you see better. (A friend can help with this.) With the speculum in the correct position you will be able to see both the folds in the vaginal walls and your cervix, which looks pink, bulbish and wet. (If you are pregnant your cervix will have a bluish tint and if you are menopausal or breastfeeding it may be quite pale.) Depending on where you are in your menstrual cycle, your secretions may be white and creamy or clear and stretchy. By learning what is 'normal' for you, you will more easily be able to identify any changes that may indicate ovulation, an infection or pregnancy.

Some women prefer to remove the speculum while it is still in its open position, and others close the blades first. Clean it afterwards with antiseptic soap or alcohol and store it for later use.

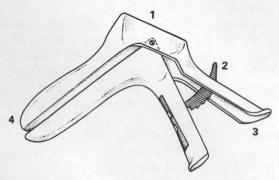

A closed speculum

1 spy-hole
2 Ratchet – which holds blades in place when the handles are pushed together to open them
3 Handles
4 Blades of the speculum (these are inserted into the vagina in the closed position).

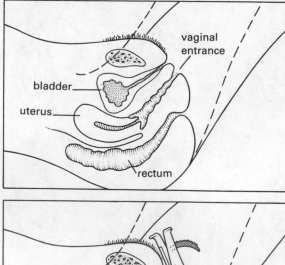

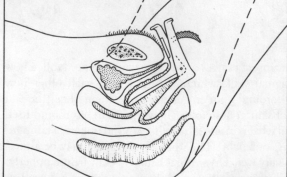

(Above) An open speculum in place in the vagina so that the cervix and sides of the vagina can be seen.

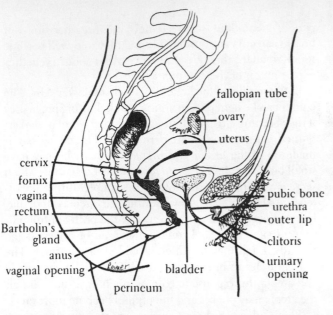

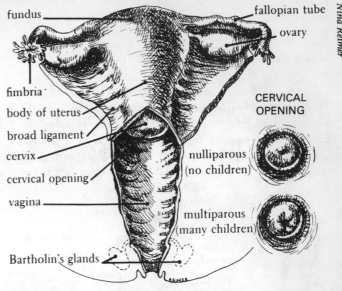

Nina Reimer

CERVICAL OPENING

nulliparous (no children)

multiparous (many children)

side view

a very thin straw. No tampon, finger, or penis can go through it, although it is capable of expanding to allow a baby through.

You will probably not be able to feel the rest of the organs. The non-pregnant uterus is about the size of a fist. Its thick walls have some of the most powerful muscles in the body. It is located between the bladder and the rectum (see diagram). The walls of the uterus touch each other unless pushed apart by a growing foetus or by an abnormal growth. The upper end of the uterus is called the *fundus*.

Extending outwards and back from the upper end of the uterus are the two *fallopian tubes* (or *oviducts*; literally, 'egg tubes'). They are approximately four inches long and look like ram's horns, facing backwards. The connecting opening from the inside of the uterus to the fallopian tube is as small as a fine needle. The other end of the tube is fringed (fimbriated) and funnel-shaped. The wide end of the funnel wraps part way around the *ovary* but does not actually attach to it.

The ovaries are about the size and shape of unshelled almonds, located on either side and somewhat behind the uterus. They are about four or five inches below your waist. They are held in place by connective tissue and are protected by a surrounding mass of fat. They have a twofold function: to produce germ cells (eggs) and to produce female sex hormones (*oestrogen*, *progesterone* and many other hormones, only some of whose function is understood). The small gap between the ovary and the end of the corresponding tube allows the egg to float freely after it is released from the ovary. The finger-like ends (*fimbria*) of the fallopian tube move to set up currents which wave the egg into the tube. In rare cases when the egg is not 'caught' by the tube, it can be fertilized outside the tube, resulting in an abdominal pregnancy. See ectopic (misplaced) pregnancy in Chapter 21, p. 439, for more on this.

Parallels in Female and Male Pelvic Organs

All female and male organs, including sexual and reproductive organs, are similar in origin, homologous (developed from the same embryonic tissue) and analogous (similar in function). Female and male foetuses appear identical during the first six weeks in the uterus. The following are examples of corresponding organs.

FEMALE	MALE
outer lips	scrotum
inner lips	bottom side of penis
glans of clitoris	glans of penis
shaft of clitoris	corpus cavernosum
ovaries	testes
bulb of vestibule	bulb of penis and corpus spongiosum
Bartholin's glands	Cowper's glands (bulbo-urethral glands)

MALE PELVIC ORGANS

Nina Reimer

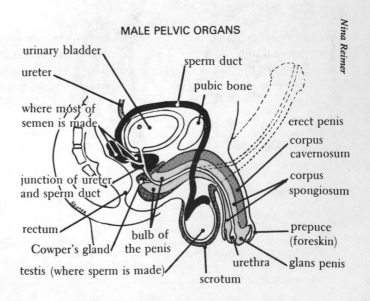

BREASTS

When we look at our breasts in the mirror we will most likely notice that they are not the same size and shape. * Often the right one is smaller than the left. If we observe our breast shape over time we will also notice that they usually become droopier over the years as our skin becomes less elastic. This happens even faster after menopause. For some of us there are pronounced changes during the menstrual cycle, with the most fullness right before our

periods. Also, during pregnancy and breastfeeding our breasts can enlarge considerably and they may well become much smaller as breastfeeding stops. After about a year they regain much of their former size.

In the middle of the breast is a circle of darker skin. The colour can be light pink to almost black. During pregnancy it may become larger and, in light-skinned women, darker. Sometimes the changes are permanent. This darker skin is made up of the *areola* and *nipple*. The areola may have small bumps on it. These are *sebaceous* or *oil glands* which secrete a lubricant that protects the nipple during breast-feeding. Hairs often grow around our areolas and may increase over time or with the use of the birth control pill. Our nipples may stick out, lie flat or be inverted (go inward). Each may be different and all are normal. The only muscles in our breasts are directly under the nipple and areola. In response to cold or touch or sexual arousal, the areola may pucker and the nipples become more erect.

The inside of the breast consists of *fat, connective tissue* and a *milk-producing (mammary) gland*. The gland is made up of *milk-producing areas* and *ducts* which during lactation carry the milk from these areas to the nipple. During the reproductive years, even when we are not nursing, these glands may periodically produce small amounts of fluid which flow from the nipples.

With the great increase of sex hormones during adolescence, the glandular tissue in the breasts starts to develop and increase in size to about the amount of a spoonful. All women have approximately the same amount of glandular tissue at the same points in their reproductive life cycles. Most of the breast consists of fat over and between sections of the gland and connective tissue. The amount of fat collected in the breasts is partly determined by heredity. This fat makes breast size vary and explains why breast size is not related to the sexual responsiveness of the breast area or to the amount of milk produced after giving birth. Because sex hormone levels change during the menstrual cycle, when starting and stopping birth control pills, during pregnancy, during lactation and after meno-pause, there can be variations in a particular woman's breast size and shape.

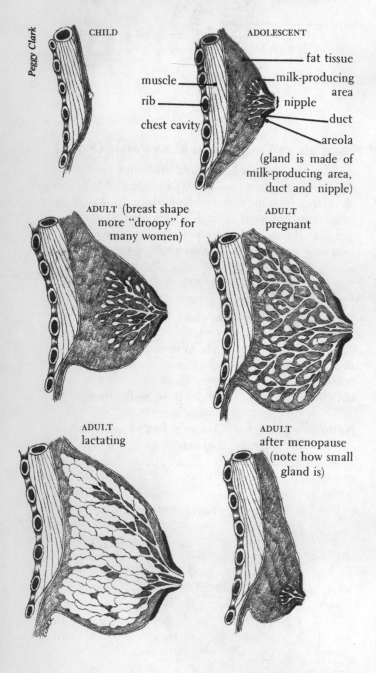

Peggy Clark

CHILD

ADOLESCENT

fat tissue

muscle

rib

milk-producing area

nipple

chest cavity

duct

areola

(gland is made of milk-producing area, duct and nipple)

ADULT (breast shape more "droopy" for many women)

ADULT pregnant

ADULT lactating

ADULT after menopause (note how small gland is)

STAGES IN THE REPRODUCTIVE CYCLE

In childhood our bodies are immature. During puberty we make the transition from childhood to maturity. In women, puberty is characterized by decreased bone growth; by growth of breasts, pubic and armpit (axillary) hair. Ovulation and menstruation (menarche) start near the end of puberty, generally when we are about twelve and a half, though any time from nine to eighteen years is normal. To menstruate, a girl must generally reach about 7½ stone (47½ kg), at which point about a quarter of her body weight is fat. In order to sustain menstrual cycles, a woman must maintain a slightly higher weight than when she first

*For stories of how women feel about their breasts and many pictures of breasts see Ayalah and Weinstock, *Breasts: Women Speak About Their Breasts and Their Lives.*

menstruated. Menstruation and ovulation continue until the average age of forty-eight or forty-nine, with a range of between forty and fifty-five as normal. When they stop, menopause has occurred. The transition between the reproductive and post-reproductive stages, called menopause or the climacteric, often takes place over as many as fifteen years.

This entire reproductive cycle is regulated by hormones, chemical messengers and initiators in the body. The levels of sex hormones are low during childhood, increase tremendously during the reproductive years and then become somewhat lower and in a different balance after menopause. The signs and symptoms of the transitional periods are thought to be caused by the changing levels of hormones.

During the reproductive years there are monthly fluctuations of hormones which determine the timing of ovulation and menstruation. This cycle prepares a woman's body for the possibility of pregnancy every month.

THE OVARIAN CYCLE: OVULATION

The ovaries at birth contain about 400,000 follicles, which are balls of cells with an immature egg in the centre. Only about 300 to 500 of these will develop into mature eggs.

Each month during our reproductive years, several (ten to twenty) follicles begin maturing under the influence of hormones (see Appendix). Usually only one develops fully and becomes a mature ovum ready for fertilization. The others degenerate before completing their development. One of the cell layers in the follicle secretes oestrogen. The follicle, with the maturing egg inside, moves towards the surface of the ovary. During ovulation the follicle and the ovarian surface disintegrate at a particular point, allowing the egg to float out. If women feel this, it usually is as a twinge or cramp in the lower abdomen or back, sometimes with vaginal discharge, perhaps bloody. This is *Mittelschmerz* ('middle pain'). A few women have headaches, gastric pains or sluggishness. The symptoms can be severe enough to be confused with appendicitis or ectopic pregnancy. Cervical mucus usually changes at this time, too (see box over page).

Just before ovulation the same cell layer in the follicle starts secreting progesterone as well as oestrogen. After ovulation the empty follicle is called a *corpus luteum* ('yellow body', referring to the yellow fat in it). If the woman becomes pregnant, the hormones produced by the corpus luteum help to maintain the pregnancy. If no pregnancy occurs, the follicle degenerates. After several months only a whitish scar remains near the surface of the ovary. It is then called the *corpus albicans* ('white body') and eventually disappears entirely.

After ovulation the released egg is trapped by the funnel-shaped end of one of the fallopian tubes (oviducts) and begins its several-day journey to the uterus, moved along by wavelike (peristaltic) contractions of the tube. Conception (see box) usually occurs within one day of ovulation. There is a growing number of women in whom the fertilized egg implants itself in the fallopian tube instead of in the uterus because the tube has been scarred or unusually twisted by infection. Tubal pregnancy requires surgery before the tube ruptures (see p. 439).

If the egg is not fertilized, it disintegrates or is sloughed off in the vaginal secretions, usually before menstruation. You won't notice it.

Although it is unusual, *a woman can get pregnant from having intercourse during her period* (see Natural Birth Control, p. 278).

ENDOMETRIAL CHANGES AND MENSTRUATION

Oestrogen, made by the maturing follicle in the ovary, causes the uterine lining (*endometrium*) to proliferate (grow, thicken and form glands) and increases the uterine blood supply (proliferating phase). Progesterone, made by the ruptured follicle after the egg is released, causes the glands in the endometrium to begin secreting embryo-nourishing substances (secretory phase). A fertilized egg can implant only in a secretory lining, not in a proliferative one. If all goes well, the egg, after its approximately six-and-a-half-day journey, should find a well-developed secretory lining.

If conception has not occurred, the ruptured follicle, or corpus luteum, will produce oestrogen and progesterone for only about twelve days, with the amount dwindling in the last few days. As the oestrogen and progesterone levels drop, the tiny arteries and veins in the uterus pinch themselves off. The lining is no longer nourished and is shed. This is menstruation, the menstrual period or flow. During menstruation, most of the lining is shed; the bottom third remains to form a new lining. Then a new follicle starts growing and secreting oestrogen, a new uterine lining grows and the cycle begins again.*

Any cycle that is more or less regular is normal. The length of the cycle usually ranges from twenty to thirty-six days, the average being twenty-eight days. (Menstruation is from the Latin *mensis*, for 'month'.) Some women have alternating long and short cycles. There are spontaneous small changes, and there can be major ones when a woman is under a great deal of stress. As you get older or after you have a baby, you may notice marked changes. A period can last two to eight days, with four to six days being the average. The flow stops and starts, though this may not always be evident. A usual discharge for a menstrual period is about four to six tablespoons, or two to three ounces.

The menstrual fluid contains cervical mucus, vaginal secretions, mucus and cells and degenerated endometrial particles as well as blood (sometimes clotted), but this mixed content is not obvious since the blood stains everything red or brown. This regular loss of blood, even though small, can cause anaemia. The fluid usually does not smell

*See illustration on p. 38. It is possible to menstruate without ovulating (anovulatory period) even after cycles have been established. In young women, anovulatory cycles average once a year, increasing to eight to ten a year as menopause approaches.

HOW PREGNANCY HAPPENS
Prepared together with
FIONA McCLOSKEY
BRISTOL WOMEN'S HEALTH GROUP

Pregnancy depends on the combined fertility of a man and a woman. During sexual intercourse (see Chapter 14) sperm are ejaculated through a man's penis into a woman's vagina, or through 'alternative insemination' they are inserted there (see p. 432). If uninterrupted, and if the woman's mucus facilitates this (see below), some of the sperm travel through the cervical opening, through her uterus and into the fallopian tubes. It is also possible for sperm deposited in or near the lips around the vagina during sex play to reach the vagina and follow the route to fertilize the egg. If sperm and egg meet in the outer third of the fallopian tube, a sperm may unite with the egg (fertilization). After fertilization, the new bundle of cells, or zygote, takes several days to move down the fallopian tube to the uterus, where it implants and grows, eventually becoming a baby if the pregnancy is not interrupted. The zygote does not always implant, however, and sometimes it may implant in the tube or elsewhere – resulting in an 'ectopic pregnancy', which is dangerous (see p. 439).

There are thus three essential elements to understanding how pregnancy happens – sperm, egg and the woman's fertile mucus. The importance of fertile mucus is often forgotten.

THE EGG

During our fertile years, we ovulate – release an egg – approximately once per month or 'cycle' (see 'ovulation').* After the egg leaves the ovary it is picked up by the fallopian tubes and travels down to the uterus. There are only approximately twenty-four hours after an egg's release in which it is capable of fertilization. However, because fertile mucus (see below) may keep sperm alive for up to a week, genital contact with live sperm during the preceding five to seven days could lead to pregnancy.

FERTILE MUCUS

Several days before an egg is released, the mucus glands in a woman's cervix become very active, secreting 'fertile' mucus into the vagina. This mucus helps protect sperm from acid secretions in the vagina, and can keep sperm alive for several days, guiding them towards the entrance of the uterus, and chemically preparing them for fertilization. Fertile mucus is an essential link between sperm and egg, and pregnancy cannot happen without it. Scant or absent fertile mucus is a common cause of fertility problems.

THE SPERM

Sperm are made in a man's testicles ('balls'), throughout a man's life – from puberty to old age. Through sexual stimulation, blood flows into erectile tissue inside the penis, causing the penis to become stiff, hard and erect. A few sperm can come out in the drops of liquid that may come from the penis soon after the erection occurs. Continued sexual stimulation, e.g. through intercourse, can cause the man to have an orgasm. As ejaculation begins, the sperm travel up the sperm ducts, over the bladder and through the prostate gland into the urethra and then are propelled out of the urethra by rhythmic contractions which are very pleasurable to the man. This is called orgasm. Up to 300 million sperm come out in one ejaculation. So many will die on the way to the egg that this great number is needed to ensure that reproduction can occur.

Sperm come out fast. They travel an inch in eight minutes, and can reach an egg in less than thirty minutes, possibly even in as little as ninety seconds. If the woman is not at the fertile time of her cycle, the sperm will die in the vagina within a matter of hours.

*If two ovulations occur in any one cycle, the second will happen within twenty-four hours of the first.

until it makes contact with the bacteria in the air and starts to decompose. Towards the end of the flow, some of the discharge may have an unpleasant odour.

Women in different cultures have handled their menstrual flow in many ways. Sometimes they don't use anything. Since earliest times, women have made tampons and pads from available materials, often washing and reusing special cloths or rags. Today, some women make them from gauze or cotton balls. Most women use commercial sanitary towels and tampons. Directions come with the products. (Toxic shock syndrome, TSS – see p. 566 – has been linked to the use of tampons, and occasionally to sponges and diaphragms.) Do not use tampons between your periods or ones that are more absorbent than you need during your period. Unfortunately, absorbency labelling is not uniform; one brand's 'regular' can be more absorbent than another's 'super'. It is too absorbent if it is hard to pull out or shreds when you remove it or if your vagina becomes

FERTILITY AWARENESS

Prepared by
FIONA McCLOSKEY
BRISTOL WOMEN'S HEALTH GROUP

Increasing numbers of us are realizing that it is possible to develop an understanding of our menstrual and fertility cycles. While this understanding – fertility awareness – has mostly been seen as relevant only as a means of birth control ('natural' birth control), it is useful in other respects as well:

- it can help us *become* pregnant when we want to;
- it can help people who are having problems conceiving (see Infertility, p. 422);
- it can generally help demystify our bodies;
- it can be a useful tool in the prevention and treatment of any gynaecological ill health we may experience;
- it can help us understand what's going on if our menstrual pattern changes, e.g. in the run-up to menopause, or if we are under stress;
- it can enable us to establish if we have become pregnant at an earlier date than the standard pregnancy test;
- by enabling us to pinpoint ovulation, if we become pregnant a very accurate estimate can be made of the delivery date (the standard method works well for women who have twenty-eight day cycles, but for those of us with longer or shorter cycles the standard calculations are often unnecessarily inaccurate).

In contrast to the medical view that women's biology is chaotic and difficult to understand, fertility awareness stresses the ordered and comprehensible patterns of women's fertility. It sees the menstrual cycle as a positive and important part of human experience, one that can be worked with rather than against.

DEVELOPING OUR FERTILITY AWARENESS

To be aware of our fertility, we first need to understand how we can become pregnant (see How Pregnancy Happens, box on p. 36). While fertility awareness is a very effective method of birth control (see Chapter 15), please do not try using it in this way unless you have been properly taught. The summary we give below is not enough on its own.

The best and most effective way to learn fertility awareness is by finding a teacher who is trained in observation of the mucus, cervix and temperature changes discussed below. Another approach is to form a women's group and invite a teacher along for some or all of the sessions. In this way you get to see more patterns of change in the cycle over a shorter space of time. Learning fertility awareness takes from three to six cycles on average. Although a number of books are available (the more useful ones are listed on p. 306), it is not possible to get sufficiently detailed information to interpret your own cycle from a book.

In all fertile menstrual cycles there are changes in the uterus, vaginal secretions and temperature. These are the main indications of fertility, whereas changes such as breast tenderness, spotting and 'ovulation' pain are so-called minor indications because they do not occur in all women in all menstrual cycles and cannot therefore be relied upon.

Uterus. The lower part of the uterus, the cervix, changes in position, texture and opening. Many women are familiar with their cervixes through using tampons or caps. One way of learning about your cervix is to feel it over several cycles so that you can become familiar with how it changes. As far as the uterus itself is concerned, it often softens and opens, moving generally upwards in the pelvic area as ovulation approaches. At ovulation or immediately after it, the uterus tends to become firmer, to close and to move downwards. Some women do not experience all of these changes, although it is rare not to experience any. It may take practice before you can detect them, but gradually a regular pattern of change will emerge.

Vaginal secretions. One of the earliest signs of approaching puberty for girls is an increase in vaginal secretions. This starts before the first menstruation but few girls in Western societies are told to expect anything other than blood, let alone given a positive explanation of what our secretions mean. Besides menstrual blood there are three main normal secretions which we may notice.

1. A silvery fluid that is lubricative and comes from the lower part of the vagina when we are sexually excited.

2. A white creamy secretion which keeps the vagina healthy and is slightly acidic. It may appear watery or milky at certain times or thicker and more clotted at other times of the cycle. When it flows out of the vagina on to underwear it sometimes turns more yellow in colour.

3. A clear stretchy secretion from the womb – the fertile mucus.

The amount, colour and consistency of the secretions changes as ovulation approaches. A common pattern of change is that for five or six days before ovulation there is an increase in amount, a feeling of wetness, and a clearer and stretchier consistency. The mucus from the cervix at this time is considered

continues over

to be fertile because it is capable of keeping sperm alive until ovulation.

After ovulation there is usually a fairly abrupt decline in the amount of secretions. There may again be a feeling of wetness for a few days before menstruation due to the fall in progesterone (see p. 40).

Temperature. The background temperature of our bodies at rest changes from a lower level prior to ovulation to a slightly higher one after ovulation. This small change can be measured with a fertility thermometer, which has an expanded scale of

measurement in contrast to an ordinary clinical thermometer. Fertility thermometers are available free on prescription or at Family Planning Clinics (DH FPN 175 is the reference for this free provision should you be questioned about it), or you can buy one over the counter in most large chemists.

The importance of the temperature change is that it can provide an easy objective confirmation that ovulation has taken place. This is especially useful and reassuring if a woman is trying to find out exactly when she is fertile.

Nina Reimer

ENDOMETRIUM AT FOUR STAGES OF MENSTRUAL CYCLE

day 5

day 14 (ovulation)

day 19

day 1 of new cycle
(day 1 is first day of menstrual period).

dry. Tampons can cause sores you probably are not able to notice on the vaginal walls when used under those circumstances. Some women ouxperience vaginal irritation, itching, soreness, unusual odour or bleeding while using tampons. If you do, stop using them or change brands or

absorbencies to see if that helps. There is no pre-market safety testing of tampons. Most research is done by the manufacturers, who keep it secret.

Recently, women have rediscovered natural sponges (not cellulose) which are reusable and economical. A sponge is soft and comfortable and when damp takes the shape of your vagina, eliminating the dryness and irritation so common with commercial tampons. Unfortunately, because sponges grow in the oceans where so many pollutants are dumped, we don't know what the sponge has been exposed to, how much pollutant it has absorbed or whether residual pollutants may cause us problems. Almost no testing has been done.*

Dampen the sponge before insertion. When you think the sponge is full, pull it out with your finger. Wash it well in cool water. Before reinserting, squeeze it to remove excess water. Some women tie a string on to the sponge, but as with tampons, the string may act as a wick for bacteria from outside the vagina. To make things simpler in public toilets, carry an extra sponge in a plastic bag. If the sponge develops an odour, rinse it in a mild solution of vinegar and water. The sponge does not have to be made sterile. (Tampons are not sterile.) However, if you have an infection, do not reuse your sponge. Discard the sponge when it begins to fall apart.

Some women are also using a diaphragm or cap as a cup to collect the menstrual fluid. Use a little lubricating jelly on the rim if it is hard to put in. You will learn from experience when it is full. Then remove, wash and reinsert it. If it is left in too long it will overflow.

Those of us who have limited sensation in the lower part of our bodies or are confined to wheelchairs often find all of these methods either irritating or difficult to use. There is no satisfactory solution to this yet.

> Sanitary product companies are always introducing 'new, improved' products. Avoid *deodorized* or *scented* tampons, sanitary towels and feminine deodorant sprays. Many women have allergic reactions to the chemicals in them.

ATTITUDES TO MENSTRUATION

Cultural, religious and personal attitudes to menstruation are a part of our menstrual experience and often reflect negative attitudes towards women. Consider for a moment the ways you have been influenced by attitudes and customs about menstruation. How did you first hear about it? How else have you found out about it: family, friends, advertising, lovers, books, films, teachers, nurses, doctors, taboos, slang, names, jokes? What particular experiences stand out in your mind? How did they make you feel? Are your current experiences different? How is menstruation a part of your life now?

Certain cultures have isolated women entirely, or put them only in the company of other women, during their periods, because people thought menstrual blood was

---

*Different researchers, using only a few sponge samples each, have obtained contradictory results. Caribbean or Florida sponges grow in *generally* less polluted waters than Mediterranean sponges.

> # LEARNING MORE ABOUT YOUR CYCLE
>
> A good way to start learning more about your own cycle and what is usual and normal for you is to keep a simple chart. Note the start of your flow on a calendar. Add whatever else you are interested in or make a separate chart or journal. Some things you might consider looking at more carefully are colour, texture, taste, clots, cervical changes, breast changes, fluctuations in your general physical, emotional or sexual state. You may find no pattern where you thought there was one, or you may find that some changes occur at particular times in your cycle.
>
> Charts are available from Wellwoman Information (see Organizations in Resources); the *Spare Rib Diary* also contains a chart (see p. 63).

'unclean' and gave menstruating women supernatural powers, sometimes good but more often destructive. Women themselves may have started these practices to give themselves a time for meditation or to give older women a chance to pass on special women's secrets to younger ones.

Current taboos include refraining from exercise, showers and sexual intercourse, or hiding the fact of menstruation entirely. Notice the wording in ads for menstrual products to see how this is reinforced in our country.

In the belief that the whole menstrual cycle makes women unstable or less capable, some people deny jobs to women and treat us as inferior. The idea that women lose a lot of time from work is largely unsupported. One study of nurses shows that they lost very little time because of menstrual problems.[2] Most women do not have any measurable difference in their thinking capacity throughout their cycles[3] or in their ability to perform tasks.[4] We still work where we are 'needed' – at home, in factories, in offices – with no concessions in schedules or routines to take account of individual differences in our cycles. Men, however, who are much more prone to seriously incapacitating and unpredictable diseases, such as heart problems, continue in highly responsible positions.

FEELINGS ABOUT MENSTRUATION

Many of us were scared or even embarrassed when we first started to menstruate. We grew up with little or no knowledge about where the blood and tissue were coming from and why it came and why it sometimes hurt. Some of us thought we were dying when we first saw our menstrual blood. Some of us were desperately afraid that a teacher or boy would notice when we had our period. On the other hand, some of us felt inadequate if we didn't menstruate.

I used to worry about having my period. It seemed that all my friends had started already, or were

*just having it. I felt left out. I began to think of it
as a symbol: when I got my period, I would
become a woman.*

Beginning and ending menstruation will always be different for each person – welcome to some, not to others.
We do know that as we feel better about our bodies and
learn more about ourselves, our experiences of our cycles
can change. During times when we feel especially good
about ourselves, we may experience our periods as self-affirming, creative and pleasurable.

*I really love getting my period. It's like the
changing seasons. I feel a bond with other women.
I feel fertile and womanly and empowered because
of my potential to make a life. I even like the little
aches I get because it's a reminder of having my
period.*

Some of us will pay less attention to menstruation and
others will explore it further through art, songs, writings
and new rituals. We want to be sure to tell both our
daughters and sons about the many changes of the life cycle
so that they can be comfortable and open about them in a
way that we were not. (For menstrual problems, see
p. 510.)

APPENDIX: HORMONES OF THE MENSTRUAL CYCLE

During the reproductive part of a woman's life, baseline
levels of all the sex hormones are being continuously
produced. In addition to those levels, there are fluctuations
which establish the menstrual cycle. The main organs
involved in the cycle are the *hypothalamus* (a part of the
brain) and the *pituitary* and the *ovaries* (both glands). The
hypothalamus signals the pituitary, which then signals the
ovaries, which in turn signal the hypothalamus. The
signalling is done by hormones secreted by the different
organs and carried from one part of the body to another
through the blood.

The hypothalamus is sensitive to the fluctuating levels of
hormones produced by the ovaries. When the level of
oestrogens, primarily oestradiol beta 17, drop below a
certain level, the hypothalamus releases GnRH, gonadotropin-releasing hormone. This stimulates the pituitary to
release FSH, follicle-stimulating hormone. This triggers
the growth of ten to twenty of the ovarian follicles. Only
one of these will mature fully; the others will start to
degenerate sometime before ovulation. The ones that
degenerate are called 'atretic'.

As the follicles grow they secrete oestrogens in increasing
amounts. The oestrogens affect the lining of the uterus,
signalling it to grow, or proliferate (proliferatory phase).

When the egg approaches maturity inside the follicle that
will develop fully, the follicle secretes a burst of progesterone in addition to the oestrogens. The oestrogens
probably trigger the hypothalamus to secrete GnRH. This
releasing factor signals the pituitary to secrete simultaneously large amounts of FSH and LH, luteinizing
hormone. The FSH-LH peak probably signals the follicle
to release the egg (ovulation). Under the influence of LH,
the follicle changes its function. Now called a corpus
luteum, the follicle secretes decreasing amounts of oestrogens and increasing amounts of progesterone. The progesterone influences the oestrogen-primed uterine lining to
secrete fluids nourishing to the egg if it is fertilized
(secretory or luteal phase). Immediately after the peak that
triggers ovulation, FSH returns to a baseline level. LH
declines as the progesterone increases. If the egg is
fertilized, the corpus luteum continues to secrete oestrogens and progesterone to maintain the pregnancy.
However, the corpus luteum is stimulated to do this by
HCG, human chorionic gonadotropin, a hormone which
is secreted by the developing placenta. HCG so far appears
to be chemically identical to LH, so it's not surprising it has
the same function.

If the egg is not fertilized, the corpus luteum degenerates
until it becomes non-functioning; it is then called a corpus

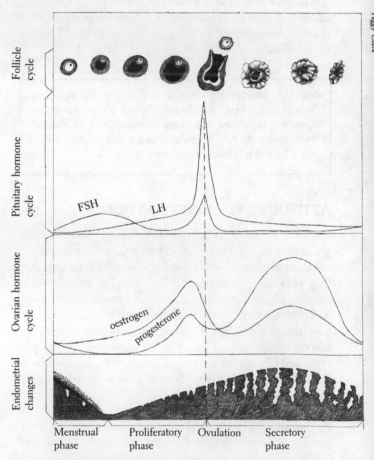

THE MENSTRUAL CYCLE – relationship between follicle
development, hormone cycles and endometrial (uterine
lining) build-up and disintegration. The cervical mucus gets
progressively wetter from the menstrual phase to ovulation,
then becomes drier during the secretory phase.

albicans. As the degeneration occurs, the levels of hormones from the corpus luteum decline. The declining levels fail to maintain the uterine lining, which leads to

menstruation. When the level of oestrogens reaches a low enough point, the hypothalamus releases GnRH and the cycle starts again.

NOTES

1. For a discussion of attitudes towards the clitoris see Ruth and Edward Brecher's excellent summary of the Masters and Johnson findings, *An Analysis of Human Sexual Response*. New York: Signet, 1966; see also Mary Jane Sherfey. *The Nature and Evolution of Female Sexuality*. New York: Vintage Books, 1972.
2. Jean Garling and Susan Jo Roberts. 'An Investigation of Cyclic Distress among Staff Nurses', in Alice Dan et al. *The Menstrual Cycle: Vol. 1*. New York: Springer, 1980, pp. 305–11.
3. Sharon Golub. 'Premenstrual Changes in Mood, Personality and Cognitive Function', in Dan et al., op. cit., pp. 237–46.
4. Effie A. Graham. 'Cognition as Related to Menstrual Cycle Phase and Estrogen Level', in Dan et al., op. cit., pp. 190–208.

RESOURCES
PUBLICATIONS

Ayalah, Daphna, and Isaac **Weinstock**. *Breasts: Women Speak About Their Breasts and Their Lives*. New York: Summit Books, 1979. Photos of breasts and women's feelings about their own.
Bell, Ruth, et al. *Changing Bodies, Changing Lives: A Book for Teens on Sex and Relationships*. New York: Random House, 1980. Excellent.
Blume, Judy. *Are You There, God? It's Me, Margaret*. New York: Dell Publishing, 1970. A wonderful adolescent novel with a positive attitude about menstruation.
Boston Women's Health Collective. *Menstruation*. A 1981 ten-page brochure including information on attitudes, examining your cycle, menstrual sponges, home remedies for menstrual problems and TSS.
Corinne, Tee. *Labiaflowers: A Coloring Book*. Tallahassee, FL: Naiad Press, Inc. (P.O. Box 10543, Tallahassee, FL 32302). Nice drawings of varied labia.
Dan, Alice, et al. *The Menstrual Cycle: Volume 1: A Synthesis of Interdisciplinary Research*. New York: Springer, 1980. Good research papers covering a variety of topics.
Delany, Janice, Mary Jane **Lupton** and Emily **Toth**. *The Curse: A Cultural History of Menstruation*. New York: Dutton, 1976. A wide-ranging exploration of attitudes.

Federation of Feminist Women's Health Centers. *A New View of a Woman's Body*. New York: Simon and Schuster, 1981. Excellent drawings and photos. Text sometimes confusing.
Friedman, Nancy. *Everything You Must Know About Tampons*. New York: Berkley Publishing, 1981. Just what it says.
Gardner-Loulan, J., B. **Lopez** and M. **Quackenbush**. *Period*. Burlingame, CA: My Mama's Press, 1979 (Box 2086, Burlingame, CA 94100, USA). A good book for girls. Shows all kinds of body types.
Golub, Sharon (ed.). 'Lifting the Curse of Menstruation: A Feminist Appraisal of the Influence of Menstruation on Women's Lives', *Women and Health* (special issue), vol. 8, nos. 2 and 3, 1983. (The Haworth Press, 28 E. 22 Street, New York, NY 10010, USA.)
Hubbard, Ruth, et al. (eds). *Women Look at Biology Looking at Women: A Collection of Feminist Critiques*. Cambridge, MA: Schenkman, 1979. Selections on menstruation and menopause.
Komnenich, Pauline, et al. (eds). *The Menstrual Cycle: Volume 2: Research and Implication for Women's Health*. New York: Springer, 1980. Another good group of research papers.
Laws, Sophie. *Down There – an Illustrated Guide to Self-examination*. London: Onlywomen Press, 1981.
Shuttle, Penelope, and Peter **Redgrove**. *The Wise Wound: Menstruation and Everywoman* (rev. ed.). London: Grafton Books, 1986. A psychoanalytic and provocative approach to menstruation and menstrual problems.
Sloane, Ethel. *Biology of Women*. New York: John Wiley, 1980. One of the few (only?) anatomy and physiology texts with a feminist perspective.
Weideger, Paula. *Female Cycles*. London: Women's Press, 1978.
Woman Spirit Magazine (Box 263, Wolf Creek, OR 97497, USA). Often has articles on menstruation.
See also Resources for Chapter 14 and Chapter 22.

ORGANIZATIONS

Wellwoman Information, 24 St Thomas Street, Bristol BS1 6JL. Tel: 0272–221925. Provides materials such as a poster on the menstrual cycle, books of charts and a booklet for ten- to sixteen-year-old girls.

FOOD

Rewritten by
ANGELA PHILLIPS

I can think of very few pleasures in life greater than the taste of summer fruit picked ripe from a tree. It beats anything even the greatest cook could achieve with sugar, butter and cream.

Many children brought up in Britain will never experience the taste of sun-ripened fruit or vegetables picked fresh from the ground. In our cities we may have a bewildering array of fruit and vegetables to choose from but most will have been picked early, ripened artificially, stored and transported many miles. In poorer suburbs, some inner-city areas and in the country during the winter months, poor distribution affects both choice and quality. Really fresh food is hard to find.

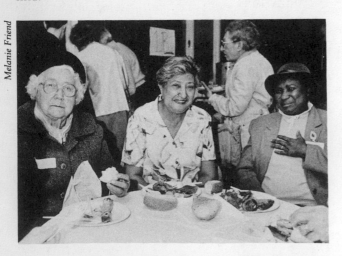

Melanie Friend

A hundred years ago, those who could afford a varied diet probably ate better, fresher food than we do today. However, many people were undernourished. Changes in food production and higher average earnings have improved access at the expense of quality. While most of us now eat well enough to keep the old deficiency diseases (such as scurvy) at bay and to resist infectious diseases,* we

*Though pockets of sub-clinical scurvy, anaemia and general failure to thrive due to malnourishment can still be found among the elderly and the poor.

now suffer from 'degenerative diseases' caused, at least in part, by dietary problems of a different kind.

WHAT HAS HAPPENED TO FOOD?

FOOD PRODUCTION

In Britain our connection with food as it is grown was severed earlier than in many other industrialized countries when compulsory enclosure of land, which started in the seventeenth century, drove peasant farmers into the towns. Displaced from the land, the growing urban communities gradually lost touch with their traditional diets. Patterns of eating have been wide open to manipulation by commercial interests ever since.

Our staple food, bread, has been refined and stripped of nutrients in order to make it cheaper to produce and extend its shelf-life. While the invention of rolling mills in the late nineteenth century increased production, it deprived those whose diets depended on bread for vital vitamins and minerals.

Sugar consumption in Britain rocketed during the nineteenth century in direct correlation to the colonial exploitation of the West Indies. This product satisfies hunger cheaply but contains virtually none of the micronutrients (vitamins and minerals) necessary for health. It was being produced at such low prices and in such large quantities that new products were invented to make use of it. Hence the invention of jam and syrup.

Between the beginning of the nineteenth century and the mid-1960s, the consumption of sugar, much of it hidden in manufactured goods, rose from less than 20 lb per head per year, peaking in the mid-1960s and settling at around 84 lb today. The British have the dubious distinction of being among the highest consumers of sugar in the world.

By the middle of the nineteenth century the increase in wheat imports turned the minds of British farmers to producing more meat. They concentrated on breeding fat animals and, in order to maximize profit, used the fat and offal to produce sausages and pies. These products arrived on the tables of working-class families because they were cheap and did not require preparation. They also increased the fat consumption of poorer families.

During this century, intensive farming methods have increased production while improved methods of packaging and preserving allow imports of even the most perishable foods (though storage, especially at high temperatures destroys some of the vitamin content). Since there is a limit to how much each person can consume, manufacturers now boost profits by producing novelty foods from extremely cheap and less nutritious ingredients. Much of this is 'play food' aimed at children and vast amounts of money (£313 million in 1984) are spent on advertising and packaging to increase demand. The sheer cost of marketing discriminates against small manufacturers. The control of what we eat has become concentrated in the hands of a few multinational corporations and, increasingly, large retail chains.

Not only have farmers and food manufacturers combined forces to exploit home markets to the full, they are also a very powerful political force. Subsidies paid through the EEC to farmers ensure high yields and high prices. We produce far more grain and milk than we need but the search for profit, which comes from high agricultural prices, results in the obscene situation whereby people in drought-stricken areas of the world may starve to death while we put uneaten food into storage, dump it in the sea or plough it back into the land.

OTHER INFLUENCES ON DIET

According to advertisements from the Canned Food Advisory Service:

> On average men spend 12 minutes a week washing up and 6 minutes a day cooking. Women, on the other hand, spend at least 2–3 hours on cooking and food preparation every day.

Throughout the world women have the prime responsibility for providing food. It is often an arduous and thankless task, particularly on top of a day's work outside the home. In industrialized countries much of the sheer labour has been taken out of the job but it has been replaced by other problems.

Isolation. A mobile labour force is an important advantage in an evolving industrial society. The inevitable break-up of extended families was encouraged by a growing ideology favouring privacy and individualism. Architecture has played its part by producing smaller and smaller units in which kitchens have become tiny cells separated from the rest of the living space where solitary women labour in isolation. Cooking and preparing food has become a chore, to be completed as quickly as possible. Manufacturers and their advertisers have seized gleefully on the notion that the busy working mum (or housewife) should avoid 'wasting' time preparing food and have come up with a vast range of 'convenience' foods. For them every process added to the basic product means more profit. For us, tired after a hard day working, opening a tin may seem a very seductive option.

Racism. For those of us who have come to live in Britain from other countries the erosion of traditional eating patterns is accelerated by a dual process of racism, acting as the stick, and advertising, acting as the carrot. Health-care personnel have caused real damage by criticizing traditional eating patterns in favour of a British food tradition which is in reality inferior. Asian children in schools are turned against their own food by taunts of 'curry-eater' and demand the hamburger-and-chip British alternative with its high fat content, vitamin and mineral poverty and low fibre.

Availability. While the supermarkets mop up the affluent car-driving customers with high disposable incomes, local shops are forced to restrict their supplies of fresh produce and raise their prices. While enormous stores can afford to cater for the growing middle-class interest in healthy food, as a minority interest, women with small children and dependent on public transport cannot choose to eat wholemeal bread or yoghurt without additives because so often it is simply not for sale in the most accessible local shops.

Poverty has a significant and growing part to play in malnutrition in Britain. The problem is made worse for those of us who have no nutritious staple food to fall back on except highly processed bread. In addition, past health-education campaigns have stressed the importance of meat. As a study of low-waged and unemployed people in the north of England illustrated, when money is tight people are inclined to give priority to meat (the most expensive dietary component) at the expense of fresh fruit and vegetables. Nearly 40 per cent of respondents did not eat fresh fruit or vegetables every day and 12 per cent hardly ever ate them. The researchers discovered that 25 per cent of unemployed people questioned did not have enough money to eat every day of the week.[1]

Unwaged or low-waged people, most of whom are women, cannot hope to meet their nutritional needs through a British-style diet because they simply cannot afford to buy all the different components. The Maternity Alliance in their study 'Poverty in Pregnancy' discovered that the cost of a diet conforming to standards set by the Department of Health represents 49 per cent of the entire income for a single woman on supplementary benefit. In larger households women do not gain from economy of scale because, as the Alliance points out:

> when income is insufficient to meet the competing demands of rent, fuel, food, and clothing, spending on food is often cut back and there is evidence to suggest that, in low income families, it is the women who go without an adequate diet.[2]

DIET AND DISEASE

One of the great paradoxes of the war years is that the overall health of the British people improved. The most likely reason for it is that food rationing ensured for the first time a relatively equal distribution between different sections of society, while, at the same time, sugar consumption was restricted and dropped by over 25 per cent. The National Loaf had to meet certain nutritional standards.

Since the war years people living in Britain have gradually consumed more sugar, and fewer unrefined, complex carbohydrates providing vitamins, minerals and fibre.

There is mounting evidence that the consumption of refined sugar in the sort of quantities considered 'average' in Britain affects our health. It causes tooth decay and possibly diabetes. It may play an important role in causing ill health generally because it satisfies hunger without providing any of the vitamins and minerals we need to function properly and fight disease. When we fill ourselves with sugar we are at the same time robbing ourselves of the food we need to keep healthy.

During this period our consumption of fats, as a proportion of the complete diet, has also risen, peaking in the early 1970s; a change which is thought by many nutritionists to be a major cause of our high level of heart disease (see p. 47). Some experts would add that a high-fat, low-fibre diet contributes to cancer (see p. 577), and there is clear evidence that people living on unrefined foods rarely suffer from bowel diseases.

When we are young the effects of poor nutrition may not be obvious, but long-term inadequate nutrition leads to illness in our middle years. Even in the short term a wholefood diet protects against bowel diseases (see p. 57), boosts our resistance, helps us to handle stress and simply makes us feel better. Reason enough, we feel, for a change.

One way to tackle nutritional deficiencies in a large population is to add micronutrients to popular, cheap, staple foods. Vitamins and minerals have been added to white bread partly to make up for those removed in the milling process but also to raise the consumption of certain nutrients such as calcium which is important for bone formation. The prevalence of rickets (a bone disease caused by lack of Vitamin D) among the children of the poor led to a policy of fortifying margarine with Vitamin D. As a result rickets virtually disappeared among English children.

One group which does not benefit from this policy is the Asian population. Few Asians eat margarine, but the problem is not, as health workers often imply, that Asians have an inadequate diet. Natural Vitamin D comes partly from fatty fish, eggs, offal and to a lesser extent dairy products, but it is mainly manufactured by the body from sunlight during the summer months. In India greater exposure to sunlight provides enough Vitamin D. The British sunlight is weaker and many Asian families (particularly women) derive little benefit from what there is because fear of racism and racial attacks keeps them inside their homes. Many black health workers have campaigned for legislation to fortify chappati flour with Vitamin D. So far

NUTRIENTS LOST IN MAKING WHOLEWHEAT INTO WHITE FLOUR	
Nutrients lost	**Nutrients replaced by enrichment**
88% of cobalt	iron
86% of Vitamin E	thiamine
85% of magnesium	calcium
85% of manganese	niacin
80% of riboflavin	
78% of sodium	
78% of zinc	
77% of potassium	
75% of iron	
71% of phosphorus	
70% of Vitamin B_6	
68% of copper	
66% of folic acid	
60% of calcium	
50% of pantothenic acid	
48% of molybdenum	
40% of chromium	
16% of selenium	
biotin (amount unknown)	
fibre (amount unknown)	
inositol (amount unknown)	
niacin (amount unknown)	
para-aminobenzoic acid (amount unknown)	
thiamine (amount unknown)	

this campaign has not met with success.

FOOD AND HEALTH EDUCATION

The previous nutritional advice in the UK to limit the intake of carbohydrates as a means of weight control now runs counter to current thinking and contrary to the present proposals for a nutritional education policy for the population as a whole. It is important therefore that a key feature of nutrition education should deal with *counteracting* the results of decades of teaching aimed at reducing carbohydrate intakes.[3] [our emphasis]

This is a quote from the National Advisory Committee on Nutritional Education (NACNE). It should perhaps be regarded as a warning to take nutritional advice cautiously rather than as a blueprint for nutritional progress.

Much health education tends to cast those of us who eat 'badly' as naughty children who are responsible for our own ill health. In fact, our nutritional problems lie not so much in our conservatism as in the fact that we listen too well to the experts and commercial interests who try between them to manipulate our diet. Large numbers of British women, for example, avoid eating bread and potatoes (which are for many people an important source of vitamins, minerals and dietary fibre) because the experts condemned these foods as fattening. They are often replaced by those foods, filled with sugar, salt and fats, which we are now being asked to avoid.

The most recent attempt at dietary manipulation is the COMA Report which attributes our rate of heart disease (among the highest in the world) to fat consumption.[4] While there is certainly a growing body of medical consensus in support of this view, the argument is far from closed (see Circulatory Diseases, p. 559). Indeed, studies which look at class and food consumption implicate lack of vegetables.[5] Lack of fibre has also been suggested as a contributory factor (as COMA recognizes). But it is simpler and less controversial for health propagandists to come up with a small adaptation to the average British diet (changing to skimmed milk and lean meat) than to encourage a return to a more complex wholefood diet which would lower fat consumption and increase fibre but might in the end expose poverty, food-manufacturing processes, and maldistribution of fresh foods as more important factors than individual ignorance or greed.

We can't afford lamb, poultry, fish or fruit. I buy four or six apples at a time and I find – I know it's wrong – if they have an apple during the day, that's thrown out the whole system because it means I haven't got enough for the pack-up [for school] the next day. So I tend to put them off which I feel very guilty about. I'd like to be able to encourage them to have an apple during the day.[6]

A GOOD DIET

In spite of these cautions there *is* such a thing as a good diet. You do not need to swallow a nutrient chart, much less learn the calorie content of every food, nor do you need to shop in expensive 'health-food' stores to eat well.

So, while we are cautious about blindly following the latest health education advice on diet, we would agree with the NACNE Report that most of us could usefully eat more unrefined carbohydrates such as wholemeal bread and flour, and increase our consumption of vegetables, fruit and pulses (such as beans and lentils). These unrefined and unprocessed foods are higher in vitamins, minerals and fibre. At the same time most of us would be better off

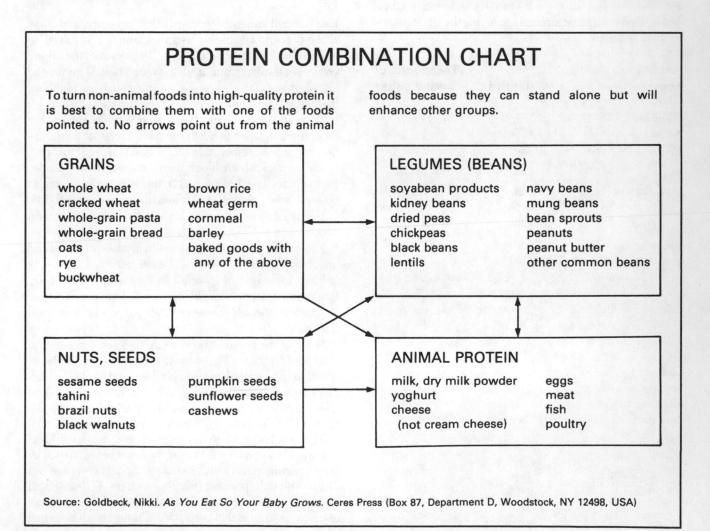

PROTEIN COMBINATION CHART

To turn non-animal foods into high-quality protein it is best to combine them with one of the foods pointed to. No arrows point out from the animal foods because they can stand alone but will enhance other groups.

GRAINS

whole wheat	brown rice
cracked wheat	wheat germ
whole-grain pasta	cornmeal
whole-grain bread	barley
oats	baked goods with
rye	any of the above
buckwheat	

LEGUMES (BEANS)

soyabean products	navy beans
kidney beans	mung beans
dried peas	bean sprouts
chickpeas	peanuts
black beans	peanut butter
lentils	other common beans

NUTS, SEEDS

sesame seeds	pumpkin seeds
tahini	sunflower seeds
brazil nuts	cashews
black walnuts	

ANIMAL PROTEIN

milk, dry milk powder	eggs
yoghurt	meat
cheese	fish
(not cream cheese)	poultry

Source: Goldbeck, Nikki. *As You Eat So Your Baby Grows*. Ceres Press (Box 87, Department D, Woodstock, NY 12498, USA)

reducing the amount of sugar, salt and fat we consume. How should this be done? The box on food groups (see p. 49) shows the rough proportions of different foods we need. But how do we know how to avoid eating hidden fat, sugars and salts added by manufacturers?

Sugar

Refined sugar is completely unnecessary to human beings young and old. NACNE suggests that we should halve our intake. We suggest you should:

- gradually decrease the amount of sugar you add to food;
- avoid adding any to food prepared for babies and young children;
- try not to buy manufactured foods with added sugars. Remember that 'glucose', 'fructose' and 'lactose' are all names for refined sugars. Beware of manufacturers who attempt to mislead by replacing sucrose with other sugars and claiming a reduced level of sugar.

The following list of 'hidden sugars' was taken from the City and Hackney Health Authority nutrition training pack. It suggests that you limit yourself to not more than 10 teaspoons (tsp) of sugar per day. However, when you look at the chart, remember that in some foods, such as cereal, the sugar is added to an otherwise useful product, while fruit gums, for example, provide nothing but sugar. Check labels – some manufacturers are reducing the sugar content of their products.

Food	Quantity	Teaspoons of added sugar
Biscuits:		
Rich Tea	1	$\frac{1}{4}$
Chocolate Digestive	1	2
Drinks:		
blackcurrant	1 glass	6
Coca-cola	1 can	7
lemonade	1 glass	2
Spreads: jam, etc.	2 tsp	2
Cereals:		
Shredded Wheat	1	0
Coco Pops	1 bowl	3
Shreddies	1 bowl	$\frac{1}{2}$
muesli	check labels	
Weetabix	1 bowl	$\frac{1}{4}$
Cakes:		
currant bun	1	1
doughnut	1	$1\frac{1}{2}$
fruit cake	1 slice	3
Desserts:		
fruit yoghurt	1 carton	3
creme caramel	2 tbsp	2
Instant Whip	1 packet	10
jelly	1 packet	19
tinned fruit	1 small tin	5

Food	Quantity	Teaspoons of added sugar
Soups, tomato:		
tinned	$\frac{1}{2}$ tin	1
packet	$\frac{1}{4}$ packet	2
Tinned veg:		
baked beans	$\frac{1}{2}$ medium tin	2
sweetcorn	$\frac{1}{3}$ medium tin	$1\frac{1}{2}$
Sweets:		
dolly mixture	1 small box	$20\frac{1}{2}$
fruit gums	1 tube	3

Sugar substitutes such as Aspartame and Saccharine are recommended by many health educators. While they do not cause tooth decay, obesity or the other diseases related to excess sugar consumption, they have no food value either. We would suggest that reducing your appetite for sweet foods is a better bet than substituting artificial sweeteners which may turn out to bring their own health problems in years to come.

Fat

Fats in small amounts are essential. They carry, and allow absorption of, fat-soluble vitamins and are involved in many other aspects of metabolism. Fat increases the calorie content of the diet without adding much bulk. This may be an advantage for very active people, such as children, manual workers and athletes, who need the extra energy, but it can cause problems. If the calories are not used up the fat is stored in layers beneath the skin. Excess fat consumption may also be responsible for the build up of fatty deposits inside arteries which block them, causing heart attacks. Fatty streaks have been found in the arteries of children as young as seven (they are not found in children who eat little fat). Fat consumption has also been linked to certain cancers (see p. 577).

Fats can be divided into two main groups: *saturated* and (*mono* or *poly*) *unsaturated*. The saturated fats are mostly animal in origin and tend to be solid when cool. Unsaturated fats are more likely to come from grains, fish or vegetables (though coconut and palm oils are both saturated).

Some of the polyunsaturated fats are known as *essential fatty acids (EFAs)*. These come in two groups: linol*enic*, found in fish and dark green vegetables, and linol*eic*, which comes from seeds. Both of them can be found in buds and sprouting shoots. If we eat enough EFAs we can make the other necessary fatty acids from them ourselves.

The problem underlying heart disease, we are told, is that we eat too much fat. We are therefore being advised by the Department of Health to reduce the fat content of our diet by about 25 per cent (the charts on pp. 47 and 48 will help you make your own calculations). However, some researchers suggest that the problem is too much saturated

WHERE DOES FAT COME FROM IN THE BRITISH DIET

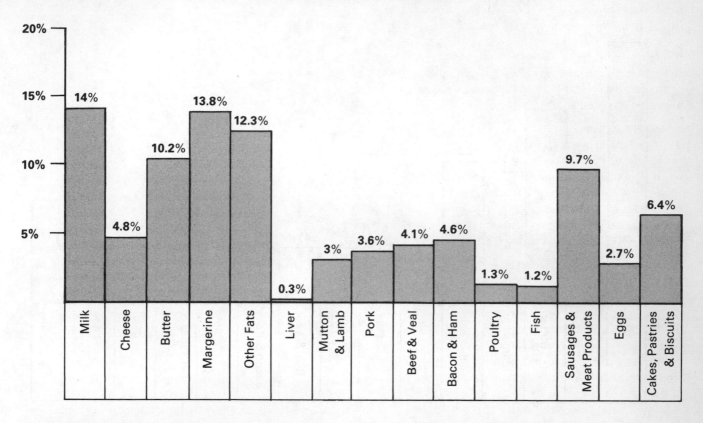

Source: *National Food Survey*, London: HMSO, 1984

fat and too few EFAs.[7] Indeed, we are beginning to learn that EFAs have many important functions which are not fully understood yet. Lack of EFAs may be associated with menstrual problems (see p. 511) and some cancer prevention diets stress their protective function. Unlike saturated fats, EFAs cannot be stored and should be consumed daily. They are also damaged in cooking, processing and even freezing and the enzyme which is needed to convert them into useful substances in the body is often used up by other saturated and hydrogenated fats consumed. If you reduce your 'solid' fat intake (including margarine) you should increase your body's use of EFAs.[8]

A diet which is high in whole, unrefined foods and low in manufactured foods with lean or no meat, will probably be at least 25 per cent lower in fat than that consumed in the 'average' British diet. It will also be much higher in EFAs, but if you want to make additional adjustments to reduce saturated fats and increase EFAs, you can:

- switch to polyunsaturated cooking oils (e.g. soya, sunflower or corn);
- avoid preserved meats and sausages;
- eat more chicken and fish;
- replace some meat meals with combinations of beans and grains (see Protein Combination Chart, p. 45) which are an ideal source of protein containing both essential fatty acids and fibre;

- eat sprouted seeds (see p. 50).

Health educators often advise switching to skimmed milk which will reduce the fat in your diet by 14 per cent (or semi-skimmed milk which will lop off 7 per cent) because it is the simplest way to decrease saturated fat without making more complex dietary changes. This probably doesn't matter if you eat a diet high in vegetables (particularly carrots which contain Vitamin A), grains and seeds. Otherwise, in reducing the fat content of your milk you will also be reducing your Vitamin A intake (about 20 per cent of the average intake of Vitamin A comes from dairy products), your calorie intake and you could also be missing out on some essential fatty acids. People who cannot afford a varied diet may well make up the missing calories with sugar. (Currently Department of Health advice excludes under-fives from the advice to drink skimmed or semi-skimmed milk.)

Salt

Salt is thought to contribute to high blood pressure (hypertension) which is associated with strokes. However, the link is not clear. Some people can eat as much as they like with no ill effects, others develop hypertension which can be controlled by a low salt diet. Since we eat far more salt than we need, it can do no harm to cut down.

WHERE DOES SATURATED FAT COME FROM IN THE BRITISH DIET

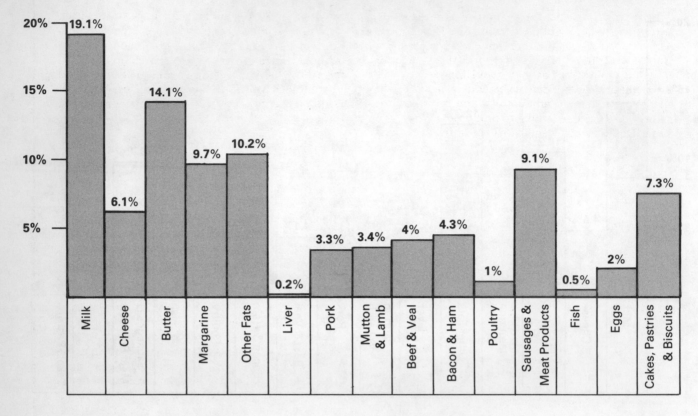

Source: *National Food Survey,* London: HMSO, 1984.

Approximately 80 per cent of the salt we eat is added by manufacturers. You can avoid it if you eat fresh foods and cut down on the salt you add during cooking.

Caffeine

Found in coffee, tea, chocolate, many soft drinks (particularly colas) and even in Lucozade and some herb teas, caffeine is a stimulant which is addictive and often causes jitters, insomnia, etcetera.

MAKING CHANGES

Don't try to alter your diet overnight. Start by adding new foods rather than trying to avoid foods which are 'bad'. If you start by depriving yourself of food you enjoy you will soon start to see the whole thing as a chore. Changing to a healthier diet should be a pleasure not a penance. Less money spent on meat will leave more to spend, for example, on fruit, but dropping the Sunday joint in favour of nut cutlets may be pushing things too fast. Keep favourite foods until they stop seeming so appealing.

- Try dishes with small amounts of meat mixed with pulses or vegetables.
- Buy a good vegetarian cookery book and try a few

dishes. You will probably surprise yourself by discovering how good it tastes. *
- When you are baking start by substituting wholemeal flour for part of the white flour and gradually experiment until you find a mixture which works for you. If you really do prefer white bread to wholemeal, try buying a wholemeal loaf once a week to start with. You will find that your tastes gradually begin to change and that a wholemeal loaf goes further.
- If you get wind, increasing the liquid content of your diet may help.
- A Chinese wok (a round-bottomed frying pan) allows you to stir-fry vegetables and meat very quickly in the absolute minimum quantity of oil.
- Involve other family members in food preparation so that you are not left in solitary confinement while you cook. Even pre-school children can cut up soft ingredients, help mix, lay the table and clear up. Adults can take turns at directing operations.
- Meals that take hours to prepare are a luxury to most of us. Many people assume that wholefoods always take a long time to prepare and manufacturers have done much to encourage that view. But good food does not

*See Resources, p. 61.

FOOD GROUPS

A good diet must include a variety of different foods from each of the groups listed below. They should be as far as possible unprocessed, or minimally processed. Raw foods (salads or fruit) provide more vitamins and enzymes than cooked foods so try to include some every day. If you cook vegetables, do so in the minimum amount of water or fat and for the shortest possible time to preserve vitamin content. Use the water elsewhere in the meal if you can.

CEREAL GROUP

At least four portions per day
These foods provide fibre, essential minerals (including iron, phosphorus, magnesium) and B vitamins. Since B vitamins are not stored they should be eaten daily. Depression and listlessness are some of the effects of Vitamin B deficiency.

Choose from wholegrain bread, chapatis, pitta, rice, breakfast cereals, pasta and potatoes.

FRUIT AND VEGETABLE GROUP

At least three portions daily
These foods provide vitamins, particularly vitamins C, A and folic acid, calcium (in greens), potassium and other minerals. They also allow the body to make use of minerals such as iron and calcium and they provide some fibre.

Include carrots (a major source of Vitamin A) several times a week and green vegetables (for folic acid) daily. Women often eat insufficient folic acid. This vitamin is important if you are considering pregnancy (see p. 341). Vegetables containing oxalic acid (spinach) reduce calcium absorption.

MEAT, NUTS AND PULSES GROUP

Two portions daily
These foods provide protein for body-building, hormones, antibodies (which fight infection) and enzymes, as well as essential minerals such as iron.

Combined nuts, pulses and grains (see Protein Combination Chart, p. 45) also provide essential fatty acids (see p. 47), calcium and other important minerals, vitamins and fibre. Fish provide EFAs and Vitamin D as well as calcium from bones. Red meat is a good source of iron but it also contains saturated fat (see p. 46).

MILK GROUP

Two portions per day
These foods are high in protein, provide most of our calcium and a large proportion of Vitamin A. They are also a major source of saturated fat (see p. 46). Milk is particularly important for women (because pregnancy and lactation depletes calcium supplies), growing children and the elderly who also have a particular need for calcium. Other groups can manage on one portion per day.

One portion is half a pint of milk, two small pots of yoghurt or 2 oz of cheese.

Since they provide most of our calcium in a Western diet, they are particularly important for women. Most of us don't get enough calcium anyway. Calcium deficiency leads to a variety of problems, including osteoporosis (see p. 469). If we cannot tolerate or do not like milk group foods, it is essential to get enough from other sources. This is not easy to do. Dark green vegetables, tinned fish, dried fruit, crushed or baked seeds (e.g. tahini or sesame spread) and soya (including tofu) are the major sources.

FLUID GROUP

6–7 glasses per day
Fluid is an essential part of body tissue. It should also supply important minerals and it is essential for digestion.

Water is as good as anything else. Avoid sugary bottled drinks and drinks with added colouring.

---

need to be a chore. Peeled raw carrots (unpeeled if they are organically grown), pieces of cheese, slices of fruit and a handful of nuts accompanied by a good slice of wholemeal bread take minutes to prepare, and save on washing up. In winter, a large jacket potato filled with baked beans or grated cheese can be on the table an hour after you open the front door.

• Some convenience foods are better than others. Frozen vegetables and fruit are on the whole more nutritious than tinned, and fish fingers are better value than most fancier prepared foods (look for brands which do not contain colouring or flavouring). However, tinned tomatoes are a good source of Vitamin C, tinned fish provides EFAs and Vitamin D and fruit is better in juice than in syrup. Baked beans, on wholemeal toast, in spite of the sugar content, are a good, cheap source of protein or, better still, you can buy canned beans which have no sugar added and cook them in a homemade tomato sauce. Start reading the labels before you buy.

FOOD AND CHILDREN

Children learn their taste in food by example. If you never have sweets, shop-bought biscuits or cakes in the house your children will learn not only to get by without them but also to prefer other foods. This does not mean they can have no snacks. Nuts (for older children), raisins, pieces of fruit,

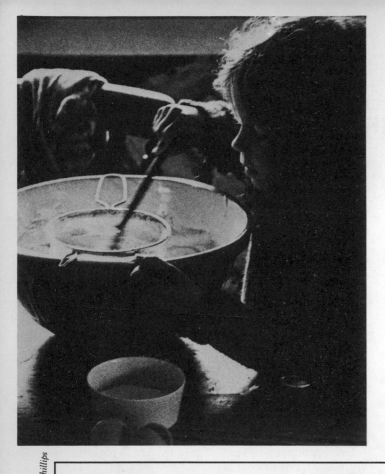

ice lollies made of frozen fruit juice, plain yoghurt mixed with banana or raisins are all very acceptable wholefoods providing the energy they need without being too sweet.

If you cannot cut out sweets completely, allow them once a week. Occasional indulgence is far less damaging to teeth than steady daily consumption.

When my five-year-old started school he refused to eat the cakes and custard which were standard puddings. I happily sent him off each day with an apple. After two terms he had adjusted to the sugar-filled school food and rejected the fruit. Five years of educating him away from sweet things undone in six months.

While your children are at home, or in a nursery with a healthy food policy, you have some control over their food consumption and education. Once at school many parents have seen years of careful training go down the drain. According to unpublished research by the Department of Health, school children live largely on crisps, chips and biscuits. Their intake of essential nutrients is 10 per cent

SPROUTING

Sprouting is a simple, cheap, way to provide yourself with first-class protein (equal to meat), vitamins and EFAs. Eaten raw, preferably while they are still growing, bean and seed sprouts are the richest source of nutrients you can get. What is more, they taste delicious. Most dried beans and seeds can be sprouted: mung, soya, pumpkin seeds and chickpeas are good (buy them in any health-food shop or good supermarket).* You can grow sprouts in a sprouter (available in health food shops) or simply

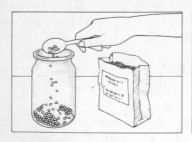 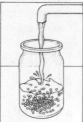 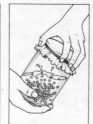 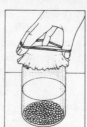 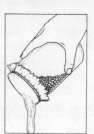

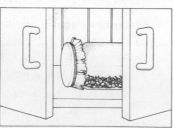 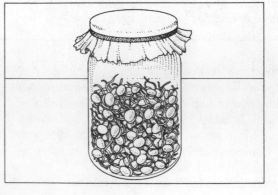

put a tablespoon of the beans into a clean jam jar. Cover the top with muslin tied on with string. Then fill the jar with lukewarm water, tip it over a few times and drain through the muslin. Do this twice a day, storing the jar in a relatively warm place. Within a few days the contents will germinate and sprout.

*There is some concern about the effects of alfalfa sprouts on the immune system.[9]

below recommended levels. Children on income support had even lower intakes than average and were significantly shorter. The survey was undertaken to show the results of the abolition of standards for school food in 1980. The results have (at the time of writing) been suppressed because they are extremely embarrassing to the government.[10]

Some education authorities are attempting to introduce the NACNE guidelines into schools. However, according to the Inner London Education Authority, this could take fifteen years. If you would like to see some faster progress:

- attend parent-teacher meetings to try and get backing for a good nutrition policy;
- approach your head teacher with suggestions for a combined educational and school-meal policy;
- contact the health authority dietician and health education department for support;
- talk to your divisional school meals organizer;
- approach the home economics inspector for your education authority;
- organize a meeting with the head of your school kitchen early on so that the kitchen staff become part of the process of change rather than having the changes imposed upon them.

Do not expect the school to change immediately to brown rice and beans; most of the children would find such foods unfamiliar and probably reject them. The school is responsible for ensuring that all children are fed and, since food tastes are hard to change and a child's system takes time to adjust to high-fibre foods, any change must be gradual.

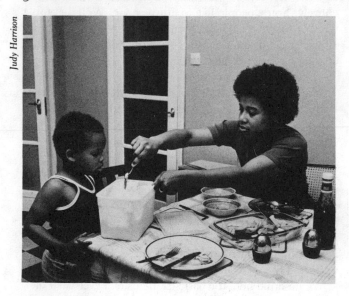

Judy Harrison

RECLAIMING TRADITIONAL FOODS

Much of the controversy over diet and health could be short-circuited by the simple advice to return as far as possible to eating traditional foods: stews containing barley and vegetables, rice 'n' peas, dal and rice. They are higher in fibre and richer in complex carbohydrates than most modern processed foods. For those of us who have no tradition of healthy eating to look back to, the newer communities may provide some useful models to follow.

The shops which are being drawn into inner cities filling the vacuum left by the superstores and catering for multi-cultural communities have much to offer those of us who have been brought up on convenience foods. Indian shops, for example, provide a variety of wholemeal, high-protein flours and dried beans (pulses) which are usually much cheaper than those in the health-food shops. The Turkish and Greek communities also provide a range of dried pulses, in addition to additive-free, natural yoghurt. Wholemeal Arab and pitta bread is a real favourite with children. We have a lot to learn from one another about good eating.

VEGETARIANISM

In Britain vegetarianism is still often considered cranky. It is assumed that a vegetarian diet is very boring – the veg without the meat. Yet in the rest of the world, meat-eating is a minority diet, or at least a small part of a mainly vegetarian diet.

For some people, avoiding meat is a matter of conscience. For others it is an ecological matter (feeding grain to cows in order to feed humans is a very expensive use of the world's food resources). In some cases it is simply a matter of preference. A mixed, balanced, vegetarian diet is not inferior nutritionally to a meat-eating diet; indeed, some people believe it is far superior. Many 'Get Well' diets are meat-free, at least to start with (e.g. Gerson and Bristol diets, see p. 52). However, it is important to eat a good combination of foods to ensure that you get enough protein. The Protein Combination Chart will show you how. (Vegans, who do not eat dairy products or eggs, may need to take supplements of Vitamin B12.) For more information and for exciting Indian, Chinese and Middle Eastern vegetarian cookery, see Resources, p. 61.

SHOULD WE TAKE SUPPLEMENTS?

Advertising campaigns aimed at women in various stages of their life – premenstrual, during pregnancy and during the menopause – suggest that we are all vitamin deficient and that, by swallowing a few pills, we will miraculously become healthy. Of course, vitamins and minerals are important for health but, if you eat a diet composed of mixed, fresh, whole foods, you should not need supplements. There may be many as yet unidentified micronutrients in the food we eat which we would not get at all from pills. In addition, foods interact: for example, iron cannot be properly absorbed without Vitamin C, and calcium absorption relies on Vitamin D.

However, many of us do not eat well, or are unable to get fresh foods easily. We may smoke, drink, live in a polluted inner city, take contraceptive pills or frequent courses of antibiotics. All these things affect the nutrients our bodies can absorb from food. For example, smokers need twice the normal amount of Vitamin C (i.e. the amount you would get in two oranges or 14oz of baked potato each day). Users of contraceptive pills may be deficient in B6 among other things. Pregnant women may need extra iron and/or folic acid. If we have been living on an inadequate diet for some time we may need extra vitamins and minerals for a while. When we are ill we may also need supplements.

If you decide to add supplements to the food you eat, do so with caution. Anything that has an effect on the body is theoretically capable of having an unwelcome effect. We know that it is possible to overdose with fat-soluble vitamins (A and D) and that large doses of Vitamin E should not be taken by anyone with circulatory diseases; large doses of Vitamin B6 have been found to cause neurological symptoms. Folic acid supplements may mask symptoms of pernicious anaemia. Vitamin C is usually thought to be safe in large quantities but there has been some evidence of an association with kidney stones (see also interactions with the Pill, p. 294). *Laurel's Kitchen* (Robertson, et al.), Michael Lesser's *Nutrition and Vitamin Therapy* and the *Bristol Recipe Book* (see Resources, p. 61) give extensive information about the nutrient value of foods as well as guidelines for supplementation.

GET WELL DIETS

Prepared with JILL RAKUSEN

A balanced wholefood diet may ensure that we get the nutrients we need when we are well, but when we are ill we need to maximize the nutritious and healing properties of food. There are several 'Get Well' diets devised to do just this. Naturopathic diets depend on fasting and particular food combinations, many other diets include the use of supplements and all suggest which foods to eliminate because they create an extra burden for the immune and excretory systems. Some seem rather bizarre but many who use them attest to their success. *

> With a radical change of diet to macrobiotics,† long-term depression went away and my general health improved considerably. I lost four stone in weight, could breathe better, asthma and hayfever virtually vanished and I went through the early winters bron-chitis-free.[11]

It was Hippocrates who said 'Let food be your medicine'. Unfortunately, it is not one of his closely-followed teachings (witness the appalling food served in most hospitals). However, some doctors are now taking an interest. If you want nutritional advice when you are ill you should contact a naturopath (see p. 96) or a doctor with a special interest in nutrition (see Resources for the Society for Nutritional

Medicine and the McCarrison Society). You may also wish to consider the following.

The Gerson Diet is an extremely strict diet which should be followed for at least eighteen months. It includes natural remedies, supplements and 'detoxification therapy' (see Cancer, p. 577). Though it is usually considered as a cancer diet it is suitable in a modified form for other conditions including heart disease, arthritis and diabetes. While still regarded with scepticism by most orthodox doctors, Gerson's work has never been systematically studied. However, a five-year controlled study in Austria[12] seems to be proving the value of Gerson's therapy for people with advanced cancer. *

The Bristol Diet is described in Alec Forbes' book of the same name. It is based on Gerson principles but is less strict. The book describes the diet which was used at the Bristol Cancer Help Centre. However, the centre has now modified its approach; they are now even less strict than the approach described by Alec Forbes. For more information on the current approach, see *The Bristol Recipe Book* by Sadhya Rippon and *The Bristol Programme* by Penny Brohn (both published by Century in 1987).

The current approach at Bristol is the easiest and you are more likely to find others following it for mutual support. We do not recommend that you try any strict Get Well diet without expert supervision (see Chapter 7 for self-healing techniques which can be used with diet therapy).

For curing short-term illness such as flu, ear infections and so on, diets need only be pursued for a few days. For chronic conditions longer periods of dieting may be necessary and it may be necessary to eliminate some foods entirely. Some people like to pursue a Get Well diet for a week or so every now and then just to pep themselves up. However, with some serious conditions you may require a complete change of lifestyle.

> How do you persuade your friends that it is not a disaster to serve you baked potato and salad while others gorge themselves! At home I was lucky because my partner offered to share my new eating habits.[13]

At the beginning of a Get Well diet you may feel a lot worse. You may go through a period known naturopathically as a 'healing crisis' in which you may feel sick, very tired and have bad headaches. However, this passes, and as your illness recedes you feel full of energy, quite unlike the low feeling following a course of antibiotics or a dose of untreated flu.

We describe here the basic elements of a Get Well diet while reminding you that it is always best to follow it with expert guidance.

---

*For more specific information on diet and cancer, see p. 577.
†Macrobiotics is a way of living centred round diet, brought to the West from Japan by Michio Kushi.

*For more about the Gerson diet, see Gerson in Resources. See also Beata Bishop's A *Time to Heal* in Cancer, p. 591 – an autobiographical account of a cure using the Gerson diet and transformational approaches.

1. *Whole* foods only, and the more *living* plant food the better (i.e. vegetables, fruit, sprouted seeds and grains). This food has the greatest ability to help the body to heal.

2. Food should be as *fresh* as possible and as much as possible eaten *raw* or freshly juiced. Essential vitamins, minerals and enzymes etc. deteriorate quickly through storage and cooking. Since fresh food is often difficult to get, an ideal and very cheap approach is to sprout your own grains and seeds (see box p. 50).

3. *Organic* food if possible: conventionally-grown food tends to be nutritionally deficient and contaminated (see box below). Contact the Organic Growers' Association for information about growers in your area. Alternatively, consult Alan Gear's *The Organic Food Guide*, available from health-food shops, or advertise in the local paper, along the lines of 'Desperately ill patient needs organic vegetables'.

4. If food is cooked, the least destructive method should be employed: i.e. vegetables should be cooked gently with little water or, better still, steamed. Over-cooking should be avoided, as should pressure cooking and microwaves which destroy all the important enzymes. Aluminium pans should also be avoided.

SOME USEFUL TIPS FOR GET WELL DIETS

- Avoid any plant foods that are mouldy or bruised (don't cut out the damaged parts and eat the rest, as the plant will be permeated with toxins).
- Store oil, flour, nuts, wheatgerm, etc. in the fridge to stop them going rancid (an oil is rancid if a white deposit forms when it is kept in the fridge).
- If you have cancer, preferably use ghee (clarified butter) rather than oil for cooking: it burns at a higher temperature and therefore avoids releasing carcinogens.
- Some people find that rye bread is easier to digest than wheat bread.
- Cider vinegar (available from health-food shops) aids digestion.
- Remember, it can take weeks before you begin to notice the benefits of healthy eating.

PESTICIDES
BY RIVA KLEIN

Pesticides – or agrochemicals as they are known in farmspeak – are big business in Britain. In 1986 over a billion gallons were used on crops, amounting to £300 million in sales, signifying a four-fold increase in the last ten years and representing over 400 different chemicals manufactured to destroy insects and rodents. Of these, according to the London Food Commission's report, *Pesticide Residues and Food – the Need for Real Control*, forty-nine are linked with cancer, thirty-one are linked with birth defects and sixty-one are associated with genetic mutation. By the time you bring your greengrocery home, some of the chemical residue will have gone; but some does remain. Out of 178 vegetables sampled in the market place by the Association of Public Analysts, one-third were still contaminated with pesticides. Among the contaminants found were significant levels of DDT, a substance so toxic that it is banned in Britain. DDT was also found in all samples of North Sea cod liver oil and halibut liver oil tested by the Ministry of Agriculture, Fisheries and Food.

The presence of DDT on such a scale points to the lack of firm government regulations on the use of agrochemicals generally, as well as a flagrant disregard for those regulations that do exist. Unfortunately, the passage of the Food and Environment Protection Act 1985 offers little comfort to the consumer. While it enables ministers to take measures such as setting maximum residue levels of pesticides in food and ordering tests on all pesticides, it doesn't actually require them to take any action. And so the existing situation, in which government inspectors may never visit a farm, or only call in once every five years, will persist, along with all the transgressions and abuses that such a system allows, if not invites.

What can we do to protect ourselves from pesticide residues? On a political level, Friends of the Earth and the London Food Commission (see Resources) need support for their research and campaigns for tighter regulations. On a practical level, eat organically-grown fruit, vegetables and grains – including bread – if you can afford to. Organic products are farmed without the use of toxic chemicals, and according to traditional, ecologically respectable methods of husbandry. They are more expensive than traditionally-grown produce and grains because of the extra time and labour that this system requires. When you prepare conventionally-grown produce, scrub and rinse it carefully in several changes of water. A mixture of vinegar and water (two caps of malt vinegar to a large bowl of water) is said to be a good cleansing agent. And eat a varied diet. Too much of one food, such as bread or dairy products or any one fruit or vegetable, can lead to a food sensitivity. And a possible culprit in such problems is chemical residue.

5. Eliminate meat if possible, plus salt, refined sugar, coffee, tea, preservatives, additives, all processed food and fried food. Meat should be avoided not only because of toxic residues but because, to digest it, enzymes are needed which could otherwise be used to fight disease.

6. Reduce fat intake and use only cold-pressed oils (available from health-food shops).

7. Avoid chemically-treated tap water.

8. Reduce dairy foods to a minimum. Buttermilk and yoghurt are often thought to be all right.

WARNING: No diet should be attempted except under experienced supervision, and then it's best to combine it with detoxification, counselling and self-healing techniques (see Chapter 7). Nor is any diet right for everybody. Some people cannot tolerate some of the requirements, particularly if their digestive system is affected. (For more about Get Well diets and cancer, see Chapter 25.)

PROBLEMS ASSOCIATED WITH EATING PATTERNS

Most of us at one time or another have used food to numb or deny our feelings, to comfort ourselves or to put some order into our lives. Who among us hasn't at one time either binged or felt nauseous when scared, angry, depressed, lonely or sad? However, when we let food become the *major* outlet for expressing our feelings, it becomes counterproductive and detrimental to our health. Unfortunately, this way of reacting is becoming more and more common for women, often starting in adolescence. 'Figure control is one of the few forms of control that women have been allowed to exercise.'[14]

Sadly, health educators have added their voices to the propaganda telling us to conform to a certain shape and size. We are told not only that fat is ugly but also that it is unhealthy. As a result women who may by nature be a different shape from the authorized 'norm' do damage to their health and their self-esteem by trying desperately to conform.

Actual weight or size is not often in itself a problem, though it can be a side-effect of an eating disorder. Compulsive eating, periodic starvation, actual self-starvation, while they have different effects on body weight, all stem from similar feelings of insecurity and lack of self-esteem. They are also all associated with distorted and inadequate eating patterns which may in themselves cause illness. Breaking the cycle is no easy task.

One ex-compulsive dieter remembers:

I was constantly pretending to diet but while I would deny myself proper meals I used to eat vast quantities of chocolate biscuits, pieces of bread and butter, anything I could find in fact. The most likely times were at parties, when I was trying to work, and when I was bored. My weight fluctuated wildly. It was many years later when I felt more

settled and confident and became interested in nutrition, rather than dieting, that I realized what I had been doing. The feeling of anxiety is quite like hunger. A kind of fluttery feeling in my tummy. I was eating to fill a gap inside. But of course food didn't fill it.

Problems with eating can take on more serious forms such as anorexia nervosa, a form of severe and deliberate self-starvation, sometimes leading to death. Another newly labelled syndrome is bulimia, which is bingeing and then purging with vomiting or laxatives. Women can seriously injure their intestines or oesophagus, develop severe tooth decay from regurgitated stomach acid and seriously upset their electrolyte balance, which can be life-threatening. You can have both anorexia and bulimia. Women with these problems often seem to be acting out the ultimate stereotype of the female role: extreme self-denial, repression of anger and conflict, the desire to remain childlike and conformity to the idea that a woman must be thin. These problems reflect graphically how little control women feel they have over their lives. Two former anorexics recount:

I remember I used to be desperately hungry – but by eating I would be in some way failing.[15]

Just as the worker's ultimate weapon in his negotiation with management is his labour and the threat of its withdrawal, so my body was my ultimate and, to me, only weapon in my bid for autonomy. It was the only thing I owned, the only thing which could not be taken away from me . . . I had discovered an area of my life over which others had no control . . . What was going on in my body was as unreal, as devoid of meaning, as were the events in the outside world. The two were part of one whole, a whole of which 'I' was no part. 'I' had shrunk to a nugget of pure and isolated will whose sole purpose was to triumph over the wills of others and over the chaos ensuing from their conflicting demands.[16]

One woman who has successfully helped many others out of this pattern has found that building self-esteem, developing a sense of control over one's life and receiving support from others are key factors for recovery.[17] In the words of a recovered bulimic:

I never 'mastered' the urge to binge. The urge to binge disappeared. I'm very glad of that, because fighting it was usually futile and took tremendous amounts of psychic energy which I can now devote to more constructive tasks.[18]

Some women find that by joining support groups (see Resources) they are able to resolve some of their guilt and fear of food and restore a normal eating pattern. Others see such groups as part of the problem and assert instead their right simply to be fat.

TOOTH AND GUM DECAY

The chief cause of tooth decay is the consumption of refined sugars. Experiments have shown that animals (and people) fed a sugar-free or low-sugar diet do not develop tooth decay or gum disease. The bacteria which cause dental diseases form a sticky coating on your teeth which you can feel if you haven't brushed them for a while. If you then eat sugar or foods containing sugar (honey and glucose are sugars too) the bacteria feed from it and produce an acid as a waste product which rots tooth enamel and causes gum inflammation.

The best way to cut down on tooth decay is to avoid refined sugars as much as possible (see p. 46) for sources of sugar). It is hard to cut sugar out of your diet completely but it helps if your teeth are not continually bathed in it. So eat sweets once a week rather than daily and look for foods which are sugar-free. Milk and peanuts* have a mildly protective effect against acid formation. It may help to give children a glass of milk after their weekly sweets.

Fluoride in toothpaste, tablets or the water supply is protective. Brushing does not itself prevent decay, but it does guard against gum inflammation. Brush thoroughly (not hard) daily, paying particular attention to the place where tooth and gum meet, and clean out the spaces between the teeth using dental floss once or twice a week.

*Peanuts should never be given to small children, who could choke on them. Nuts inhaled into the lung can cause very serious damage.

LOW-CALORIE DIETING

Full-blown anorexia nervosa is only the tip of an iceberg of nutritional problems associated with the developed world's obsession with slenderness. Aids to dieting have taken over as the major 'patent medicines' of our century. We spend millions of pounds on special foods, devices, magazines, slimming clubs, many of them medically endorsed, in an effort to 'cure' what we are brainwashed to see as unsightly fatness. (For more on the social consequences of fatness see Chapter 2.)

But low-calorie dieting doesn't 'cure' fatness. *Over a five-year period 98 to 99 per cent of the women who diet regain their weight.*[19] *In fact, 90 per cent regain more than they lost.*[20] *Dieting can make you fatter.* Most of us aren't aware that diets don't work in the long run and think that regaining weight is a personal failure rather than a physiological adaptation to stress that our bodies have made to help us survive. After repeated dieting, many of us begin to feel we can never control our eating.

Low-calorie dieting is debilitating, a form of self-starvation. The World Health Organization defines starvation as a calorie intake of less than 1,000 calories a day;

slimming diets commonly restrict calories to 700 to 1,000 a day. The recommended dietary allowance for calories for women ranges from 2,200 to 2,300 (fifteen to eighteen years) with 2,500 (for very active mature women), depending on size and physical activity. At calorie levels below this you can easily be lacking necessary nutrients, especially if you consume a quarter or more of your calories from alcoholic beverages, sweets and other low-nutrient snacks. When you don't eat enough, your body reacts in specific ways to help you survive. It doesn't matter if you deliberately choose to eat less or if you can't get enough food. Starvation is starvation. The longer you do it for and the greater the number of times you do it, the more likely you are to damage your body permanently, possibly causing bone problems (osteoporosis) among other things in later life (see p. 469).

Let's assume you are dieting and getting too few calories. (For some women the common 1,200-calorie diet is too few.) After a few days you are likely to feel physically listless. You may become apathetic, especially if you are on a low-carbohydrate diet. When fat from your body stores is broken down for energy, it doesn't provide any glucose, the fuel the brain normally uses. Your body must break down proteins from food and lean body tissues (muscles and organs, such as your heart) to provide this glucose. Processing the extra nitrogen from the proteins puts a strain on your kidneys. Fat metabolism without adequate carbohydrates leaves waste products called ketones in the blood. If the amount of ketones is too great, the critical acid-base balance of the blood can be upset. Extra blood ketones usually make you feel headachy, lethargic, dizzy, high or possibly lightheaded. Your breath will smell like acetone, somewhat sweet. After a couple of weeks the brain can adjust to using some of the ketones for fuel as a stopgap measure. You may feel irritable, partly because it is harder for you to control your blood-sugar levels without adequate food. You may also find yourself becoming depressed and less interested in sex. You may become obsessed with 'quick energy' foods, especially sweets, and devour them uncontrollably as a way of replacing missing calories and glucose for the brain, the most immediate deficits. 'High protein diets may actually generate cravings for carbohydrates and doom the dieter to periodic calorie-laden binges.'[21] One woman describes how she stopped bingeing (and didn't try to be thin).

I worked at ignoring the rules and eating whatever I wanted. In the first month of 'liberated eating' I craved only sweets. In effect, I was still binging [sic]. However, I chose not to berate myself for eating so much sugar. I reminded myself of all the sweets I'd been denied, and let feelings of nausea and hunger, rather than guilt, determine when I should eat again and what I should eat. At that point nausea and hunger were just about all I could be sure of. A month later, meat and dark green vegetables appealed to me very strongly. I chose a diet very high in protein and vitamins for a while. I think that

ALLERGIES

Allergies to common foods, as well as additives, are now thought to be responsible for a range of ills such as rashes, headaches, stomach pains and even depression. It is not easy to recognize food allergies. To be sure, you should cut out suspect foods for several weeks and reintroduce small quantities of the foods one by one to see if you have any reaction. If you suspect more than one or two food items, particularly if they are major items such as milk or wheat you will need specialist advice from a dietician or naturopath to ensure a balanced diet.

The most common allergies are to cows' milk, eggs, seafood, wheat, nuts, seeds, chocolate, oranges and tomatoes. Current advice suggests that many of these allergies may not develop if babies are not fed these foods until they are six months old when their digestive systems mature.

Migraines can be set off by foods containing non-essential amino acids such as tyramine, flavour-enhancers including monosodium glutamate and potentially carcinogenic preservatives such as sodium nitrate. They are found in chocolate, cheese, coffee, sour cream, red wine, pickled herrings, liver, pork, some nuts and seeds, avocados, ripe bananas, cured meats, many Oriental and prepared foods (read the labels). Children also react to certain foods with migraines or by becoming very excitable and wakeful. This behaviour is often labelled 'hyper-activity'. Foods to watch for are those containing azo dyes (especially the yellow colouring Tartrazine E102) commonly found in confectionery and soft drinks, and preservatives such as benzoates and sulphites.[35] A diet popularized by Dr Benjamin Feingold suggests also avoiding foods which are naturally high in salicylates such as almonds, peaches, green peppers, tea and grapes – though these foods have not shown up as problematic in controlled trials. The Hyperactive Children's Society provides information on this diet.

If you suspect food allergies, with help from a clinical nutritionist, a naturopath or a homoeopath (see chapter 7) it may be possible with careful diet control not only to cure a wide range of symptoms but also to desensitize yourself to some of these foods. (See Resources, p. 62, for more on allergies.)

during this period I was recovering from tissue damage due to previous years of dieting and binging [sic]. In the year that followed my cravings became more subtle and diverse. I ate smaller portions and greater varieties of food in one day.[22]

If you try to follow the often-cited rule that you'll lose one pound of body fat for every 3,500 calories you don't eat, you'll probably be disappointed. First of all, this calculation gives only average weight loss. For each month you continue eating the same low number of calories, your rate of weight loss is usually cut in half.[23] As a way of adjusting to a lower calorie intake, your body becomes more efficient at using and storing calories. Your basal metabolism (the calories you burn to keep your basic body functions going) can slow down by as much as 30 per cent.[24] When you stop starving yourself you will probably replace or even exceed your original weight quickly, and mostly in the form of fat.[25] Your body is more efficient now, burning off fewer calories immediately and storing more fat for later use.

Fat often replaces the lean tissue lost from muscles and organs, and you may have done permanent damage. You may have as much as 40 per cent more body fat than before you started.[26] On a total fast as much as two-thirds of the weight lost is a result of losing lean body tissue.[27] But usually muscle tissue can be developed again through vigorous exercise. If you continue dieting or adopt a pattern of repeat dieting, you risk amenorrhea, anaemia, liver impairment, kidney and gall-stones, vitamin and mineral imbalances, gout and elevated blood fats.[28] If you have diverticulitis, tuberculosis, gout, Addison's disease, ulcerative colitis or regional ileitis, weight loss will make you sicker.[29]

Your general body shape probably resembles your relatives', due perhaps to heredity or to learned eating patterns. If one of your parents was fat, you have a 40 per cent chance of being fat; if both were fat, you have an 80 per cent chance.[30] We don't really know why people are different shapes and sizes. We do know that people's basal metabolism rates are different and that vigorous exercise may increase the rate.

You may well be bigger than the advertised norm but, provided you adopt the healthy eating patterns suggested in this chapter, there is no reason why you should not be as healthy as anyone else.

OBESITY

The medical world considers fatness a disease. Certainly it is associated with heart disease, high blood pressure, gall-stones, diabetes and arthritis. However, studies do not show whether it is the weight itself which causes the problem. It could also be a poor diet, which often accompanies above-average weight, or indeed the frequent periods of 'dieting'* common among those who provide the data for research on

*Fat Liberation (see Resources) was probably the first group to speak about this. The 'Report on Obesity' from the *Journal of the Royal College of Physicians* (see note 33) raises the possibility in relation to gall-stones.

obesity in Western countries. (Africans who are considered obese by Western standards are no less healthy than their slimmer peers, a fact which adds credibility to the notion that it is what you eat, not how much you eat, that really matters.)[31] Few researchers consider these issues when drawing conclusions from their work. We have not been able to find any studies which show that, in the long run, thinned-down fat people avoid, or are cured of, diseases associated with fatness.[32] Slimming can improve high blood pressure and diabetes but repeated low-calorie dieting may make them worse.[33]

Even worse than starving are the various types of surgery medicine offers women labelled obese. They include carving fat off, jaw-wiring and various ways to make the stomach and intestines smaller, decreasing a person's ability to eat and thereby absorb nutrients. These operations are performed almost entirely on women, may have a death-rate as high as 10 per cent and are only moderately effective in achieving the stated goal of weight loss. Doctors performing them really believe they are improving the woman's health, but they actually impair her ability to nourish herself properly. After intestinal tract operations a woman often gets severe diarrhoea for several months and has a higher risk of getting gall-stones and arthritis, two problems supposedly 'cured' by weight loss.[34]

If You Choose to Lose Weight

Long-term bouts of low-calorie dieting are neither healthy nor effective. By changing to a healthy diet and becoming physically active you will, gradually, arrive at the body shape which is best for you. If you continue to eat well and stay fit there is no need for that shape to change; you will not need to diet. If you are determined to cut down your food intake, do not restrict yourself by more than 500 calories a day and concentrate on making every bit of food count nutritionally. On less than 1,200 calories you cannot get all the nutrients you need. These guidelines may help:

1. There are no magic foods or pills to help you lose weight. Diet pills, even medically prescribed, are harmful.
2. Keeping a food diary of exactly what you eat, when you eat it and why you eat it can give you insights into the psychological meanings food has for you, and can help you discover when you get hungry during the day. This can help you change your eating habits *if* they are undesirable.
3. Trust yourself and your body signals. Eat when you begin to get hungry. Don't wait until you are starved. If you feel ill, check what and when you are eating. You definitely should not have any severe symptoms, such as hair loss, shakiness, abnormally dry skin.
4. Don't weigh yourself more than once every one or two weeks if each pound is an obsession. Body water fluctuates daily.
5. Join with other women to discuss dieting, feelings about yourself and your body and societal issues, such as the way ideal body images, both sexual and medical, divert your attention from control over your life and from more productive work.

INTESTINAL PROBLEMS

Appendicitis and diverticulitis* are practically non-existent in cultures where unrefined food is the norm. It is probably the higher level of fibre which guards against these diseases. Unfortunately, many doctors have simply taken this as an indication to prescribe fibre additives such as bran without altering the rest of the diet. Like any other form of laxative, bran artificially stimulates the bowel. The muscle wall gets lazy and you may become constipated when you stop eating it. In addition, bran eaten as a supplement may reduce the absorption of minerals such as iron, calcium and zinc. It is far better to eat a diet rich in whole carbohydrates (grains such as rice, millet, vegetables) than to add bran to a refined diet.

Intestinal and stomach problems are a special problem for women with young children. The stress of irregular and inadequate meals combined with childcare, anxiety about care arrangements and often broken nights too, may lead to an over-production of acid which can cause gastritis (an inflammation of the stomach lining causing pain and often swelling) and ulcers. Hard though it may appear, it is necessary to sit down and eat calmly (not on the run) in the middle of the day. Organizing the space in your life to keep well should not be a luxury.

LABELLING AND FOOD REGULATIONS

A century ago, laws were passed to stop manufacturers adulterating food with poisonous and non-nutritious substances. Today we are still concerned about what goes into the food we buy. But our main concern is with additives put in to improve the flavour, colour or shelf-life of products. The use of additives has tripled in the last thirty years. On average we each consume 8 to 11lb per year. We know very little about the health effects of many of them (see Additives List in box). Of the nearly 4,000 additives in use, fewer than 350 are regulated. Of those which are regulated, a government/industry-funded research body was moved to comment that approximately 25 per cent deserve 'the highest priority for investigation because of the known toxicology associated with some of their component structures'.[36]

Many known poisonous substances are added to foods. The regulators say that levels in any one food are too low to cause problems. However, people eating large quantities of processed foods may accumulate enough to constitute a health threat. Since the additives are tested singly, not in the combinations used in products, no allowance is made

---

*A condition in which the gut lining is damaged, forming little pockets which can become seriously inflamed.

ADDITIVES LIST

Many of the most common additives cause health problems. Most in this list are known to cause allergic or intolerant responses – such as asthma, rashes, hay-fever, blurred vision and tummy upsets – in some people. Some are also irritant or corrosive and are known to cause problems like skin rashes, burns, and breathlessness in food workers (they probably cause problems to some consumers too).

At a Glance	Additive	Foodstuffs	Comments
ARTIFICIAL COLOURS			
E102	Tartrazine (yellow)	There are a total of 17 azo dyes used in every kind of processed food in Great Britain.	All the azo dyes are banned in Norway and highly restricted in Sweden, Finland, Austria, Greece and Japan.
E110	Sunset Yellow (yellow)		
E123	Amaranth (red)		E123 and E124 are also banned in the USA.
E124	Ponceau 4R (red)		
133	Brilliant Blue FCF (blue)		
155	Chocolate Brown HT (brown)		
NATURAL COLOUR			
E160(b)	Annatto (yellow/orange)	Used in dairy products and oil.	
PRESERVATIVES			
E210–E219	**Benzoic Acid and Benzoates**	Used in jams, fruit juice, desserts, tinned fruit, salad cream, yoghurt and sauces.	
E220–E227	**Sulphur Dioxide and Sulphites**	Used in jam, fruit juice, beer, wine, dried vegetables, sausage meat and dried fruit.	The use of sulphites is being reviewed in the USA.
E249–E252	**Nitrates and Nitrites**	Used in smoked sausages, bacon, ham, cooked meats, tinned meats and cheese.	Restricted in most European countries. Not permitted in baby food in the UK.
ANTI-OXIDANTS			
BHA and BHT E320 E321		Used widely in foods containing fats, such as butter, margarine, oils, crisps.	Not permitted in baby food in the UK. BHA is banned in Japan and restricted in Austria.
Gallates E310–E312		Used in breakfast cereals, margarine, oils, crisps, dried potato mash etc.	Not permitted in baby food in the UK.
EMULSIFIERS			
MDGs E471–E472		Widely used in food including margarine, chocolate drinks, desserts, custard, crisps, aerosol cream and cheese-cake.	
Polyoxyethylene Sorbates 432–436		Used in cakes, biscuits and packet cake mix	Banned by the EEC in 1984.

continues opposite

E407	Carrageenan	Used in ice-cream, cakes, desserts, frozen meals and cheese.	
Vegetable gums E410–416		Used in ice-cream, fruit pie fillings, sauces, scotch eggs and cheese.	Karaya gum (416) banned by the EEC.

FLAVOUR ENHANCERS

621–623	Monosodium Glutamate + Glutamates	Used in soup, snacks, sausages and frozen meals.	Not permitted in baby food in the UK.

SWEETENERS

	Saccharin	Used widely in soft and fizzy drinks, desserts, yoghurts and low calorie foods.	At one time banned in the USA – it now carries a health warning.

SUSPECTED CARCINOGENS

Over 55 approved food additives are suspected of causing or contributing to cancer. Some of the more common ones are listed below:

Colours
E123 Amaranth
E127 Erythrosine
 128 Red 2G
 133 Brilliant Blue FCF
E150 Caramels
 154 Brown FK
Preservatives
E230 Diphenyl
E249–E252 Nitrates and nitrites
Anti-oxidants
E320–E321 BHA and BHT

Emulsifiers and stabilizers
E407 Carrageenan
 430 and 435 Polyoxyethylene compounds
E466 Sodium carboxymethyl cellulose
Processing aids
 553 Silicates
 907 Mineral oils and waxes
Sweeteners
Saccharin
Solvents
Isopropyl alcohol
Ethyl acetate

for the combined effect (up to sixty different additives could be consumed in a single meal). Children, with lower body weights, are particularly at risk, a fact that the government has finally recognized. Artificial colouring has been banned in baby foods. Unfortunately, this does not extend to widely used weaning foods, such as yoghurts, which are not labelled specifically for babies.

Britain allows more additives than any other Western industrialized nation: seventeen artificial azo dyes are permitted while only twelve are allowed in the rest of the EEC, and the Norwegians do not allow any artificial colouring additives. The box, compiled by the London Food Commission, shows some of the additives used here which are banned in other countries.[37]

Labelling

If you look on the label of any packaged foods you can discover what the ingredients are. They are listed in order, the largest constituent first. So, for example, if sugar comes top of the list, it is the main ingredient. Packaged foods must also be date-stamped to give you some idea of how long they can be kept.

However, government regulation of nutritional labelling has done little to provide the consumer with more help. Manufacturers may use any of three forms of labelling. Category one lists only basic nutritional information: the amount of energy, protein, carbohydrate and fat. Category two provides a breakdown of fat to show the saturated fat content. Category three (which is voluntary) lists sugars and fibres.

As an article in the *Sunday Times* pointed out, since refined sugar can simply be included in the broad category 'carbohydrate', 'the result is that a bag of boiled sweets and a loaf of wholemeal bread could have similar labels showing a high carbohydrate content.'

Common Market regulations now ensure that additives approved for EEC use are listed under 'E' numbers (lists are available from the Ministry of Agriculture, Fisheries and Food). Additives without 'E' numbers are not EEC approved and though the broad category will be mentioned (emulsifier or preservative) the code number will not necessarily be used.

Don't take product names at face value. It may be called

'country fresh' and show a picture of green hills or fields of corn but it can still be filled with sugar, animal fat and additives. Laws specify that food names must not be misleading but manufacturers get away with a great deal. For examples, cheese *flavour* pizza contains some cheese but cheese *flavoured* pizza contains no cheese at all.

Controls

The Ministry of Agriculture, Fisheries and Food (MAFF) is the government department concerned with food. It is expected to balance the needs of consumers with those of farmers, retailers and manufacturers. The food producers and retailers form a more powerful lobby than the consumers. Their concern about profits and consumer acceptability tends to override health concerns. An imbalance which is not really surprising as consumers are not formally represented on the MAFF Food Advisory Committee (FAC). One member from the Consumers' Association sits in an 'expert' capacity. Like many other British committees the FAC meets in secret and its deliberations are covered by the Official Secrets Act.

Working with Additives

This seems to be even more dangerous than eating them. According to a report by Melanie Miller for the London Food Commission: 'large numbers of people working in the food industries are being needlessly exposed to harmful substances some of which are suspected of causing cancer.' Skin rashes or asthma are a common health effect from additives.[36]

SOME SUGGESTIONS FOR ACTION

What we eat is only partly our own business. Increased consumer understanding of the issues behind poor nutrition, and pressure applied on government, food producers and powerful institutions, will have a more far-reaching effect than individual attempts to change.

The establishment of the London Food Commission by the now abolished Greater London Council provided the first effective political lobby for food consumers in Britain. Working jointly with other consumer organizations it effectively halted the food manufacturers' attempts to legalize the irradiation of food. It was the LFC which alerted us to the dangers of irradiation, in particular the possibility that this technique could be used to 'launder' bad food which could then be sold to the unsuspecting public.

With the current wholesale destruction of local council democracy in Britain many of the recent tentative steps towards good food policies will be severely strained. The Inner London Education Authority, for example, had only recently moved towards using its purchasing power to improve school meals. ILEA bangers are low fat, the beans have reduced sugar and salt content, and recipes for cakes and pies are now based on a percentage of whole flour. As we go to press the ILEA is about to be abolished and there is discussion of the privatization of school meals. Without centralized buying, individual schools may not have the power to affect manufacturing policies. If meals are privatized, nutritional considerations will give way to profit.

However, there are still ways in which we can join together and make our voices heard:

- We can join with other people through political organizations, pressure groups, trade unions, mother and toddler groups, women's health groups, parent–teacher associations, etc. to push for wider representation on the Food Advisory Committee.
- Find out about the Food Additives Campaign Team (FACT), who are campaigning for better government controls (see Resources).
- Add our voice to the campaign for Freedom of Information (see p. 63) so that the FACT's findings become public.
- Pressurize local education authorities through the parent–teacher associations, and local hospitals through the Community Health Council, to establish good food policies and to use their buying power to influence commercial decision-making.
- Put the nutritional content of canteen meals firmly on the agenda for negotiation through unions.
- Write to food manufacturers and supermarket chains expressing a preference for additive-free foods.
- Those of us who live in an area where the choice of fresh food is restricted, can organize with others to establish a food co-op taking it in turns to buy in bulk from the nearest market.
- If we live alone, with or without children, we can get together regularly with others to pool resources and rotate cooking. It saves on fuel, enables us to buy a bigger variety of foods, and breaks down the cycle of isolation and depression which can so easily result in buying sugar-filled foods just for comfort.

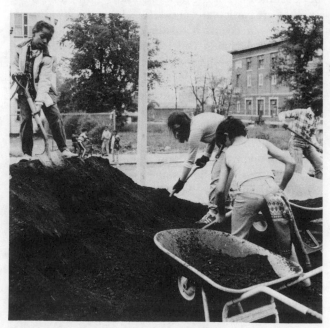

Read D. Brugg

NOTES

1. Tim Lang et al. *Jam Tomorrow?* Report by the Food Policy Advisory Unit, Manchester Polytechnic, 1984 (available from Food Policy Unit, Hollings Faculty, Manchester Polytechnic, Old Hall Lane, Manchester 14).

2. Maternity Alliance. *Poverty in Pregnancy*, 1984 (available from Maternity Alliance, see p. 638).

3. Health Education Council. National Advisory Committee on Nutritional Education (NACNE). Report. London: HEC, 1984.

4. Committee on Medical Aspects of Food Policy (COMA). *Diet and Cardiovascular Disease* (DHSS report). London: HMSO, 1984.

5. B. K. Armstrong, J. I. Mann, A. Adelstein and F. Eskin. 'Report on Commodity Consumption and Ischiemic Heart Disease', *Journal of Chronic Diseases*, no. 28, 1975, pp. 455–69.

6. A low-income mother quoted in Hilary Graham (ed.). *Caring for the Family*. Milton Keynes: Open University Press, 1985.

7. See, for example, D. A. Wood et al. 'Linoleic and Eicosapenpaenoic Acids in Adipose Tissue and Platelets and Risk of Coronary Heart Disease', *The Lancet*, 24 January 1987, p. 177.

8. Anne Nazaro et al. *The PMT Solution. Nutritional Approach*: Adamantine Press, 1986. For more information about EFAs, see Alec Forbes' *The Bristol Diet* (see Resources), which has a very clear explanation, and David Horrobin's *Clinical Uses of Essential Fatty Acids*: Eden (1982).

9. See, for example, *Journal of Alternative Medicine*, September 1986, p. 8, and February 1987, p. 4.

10. Andy Veitch. 'Survey on Chips and Biscuits Diet', *Guardian*, 4 April 1986.

11. Jo Spence. 'The Picture of Health?', *Spare Rib*, no. 163, February 1986.

12. Giuliano Dego. 'A Cancer Therapy that Refused to be Ignored', *Journal of Alternative Medicine*, October 1985, p. 8.

13. Spence, op. cit., note 11.

14. Vivian Mayer. 'The Fat Illusion', *Hagborn*, vol. 1, no. 4, 1980, pp. 3ff. (available through Fat Liberator Publications – see Resources).

15. Anonymous. *Spare Rib*, no. 83, June 1979, p. 43.

16. Sheila MacLeod. *The Art of Starvation*. London: Virago, 1980.

17. Marlene Boskind-White and William White. *The People Pleasers: Women Who Binge and Purge*. New York: W.W. Norton, 1983. (They have been working with bulimarexics for many years at 67 West Malloryville Road, Freeville, New York 13068, USA.)

18. Vivian Mayer. 'Why Liberated Eating?', pp. 14–15 (available through Fat Liberator Publications – see Resources).

19. Alvan Feinstein. 'How Do We Measure Accomplishment in Weight Reduction?' in Louis Lasagna (ed.). *Obesity: Causes, Consequences and Treatment*. New York: Medcom Press, 1974; see also Geoffrey Cannon and Hetty Einzig. *Dieting Makes You Fat*. London: Sphere, 1984.

20. Llewellyn Lauderback. *Fat Power*. New York: Hawthorn Books, 1970, p. 143, quoting Norman G. Joliffe of the New York City Department of Health: 'At least 90 percent of all the people who lose weight on a diet gain back more than they have lost.' This phenomenon is corroborated by the testimony of many dieters. See also Jane Rachel Kaplan. *A Woman's Conflict: the Special Relationship between Women and Food*. Englewood Cliffs, NJ: Prentice-Hall, 1980, pp. 50–1.

21. Judith Wurtman quoted in Jane Brody. 'Can Craving for Carbohydrates be Controlled? Chemical Studies of Brain Point to New Approach', *New York Times*, 29 September 1981.

22. Mayer, op. cit., note 18.

23. S. C. Wooley, O. A. Wooley and S. Dryenforth. 'Theoretical, Practical and Social Issues in Behaviour Treatment of Obesity', *Journal of Applied Behaviour Analysis*, vol. 12, no. 1, 1979, p. 9.

24. H. J. Roberts. 'Overlooked Dangers of Weight Reduction', *Medical Counterpoints*, September 1970, p. 15. See also J. S. Garrow. *Energy Balance and Obesity in Man* (2nd ed.). New York and Amsterdam: Elsevier, 1978, pp. 89–90; and Wooley et al., op. cit., note 23.

25. Kaplan, op. cit., note 20, p. 50.

26. Ibid.

27. Roberts, op. cit., note 24.

28. *Consumer Reports*, vol. 43, no. 2, February 1978.

29. See Roberts, op. cit., note 24; Garrow, op. cit., note 24, pp. 161–3; and Lauderback, op. cit., note 20, p. 171.

30. S. C. Wooley and O. A. Wooley. 'Obesity and Women – a Closer Look at the Facts', *Women's Studies International Quarterly*, vol. 2, 1979.

31. Douglas Black et al. 'Report on Obesity', *Journal of the Royal College of Physicians*, vol. 17, no. 1, January 1983.

32. See William Bennett and Joel Gurin. *The Dieter's Dilemma: Eating Less and Weighing More*. New York: Basic Books, 1982. Chapter 5 includes a summary of the literature on fatness and disease.

33. A few studies have shown *no* strong correlation between fatness and several diseases usually associated with it. See Bennett and Gurin, op. cit., note 32, as well as two of several studies of heart attacks in Roseato, Pennsylvania: C. Stout et al. 'Unusually Low Incidence of Death from Myocardial Infarction: Study of an Italian Community in Pennsylvania', *Journal of the American Medical Association*, no. 188, 8 June 1964, pp. 845–9; and S. Wolf et al. 'Roseato Revisited: Further Data on the Incidence of Myocardial Infarction in Roseato and Neighboring Pennsylvania Communities', *Transactions of the American Clinical and Climatological Association*, vol. 85, 1973, pp. 100–7.

34. See Garrow, op. cit., note 24, p. 180; and Teis Andersen, Erik Juhl and Flemming Quaade. 'Jejunoileal Bypass for Obesity: What Can You Learn from a Literature Study?', *American Journal of Clinical Nutrition*, vol. 33, February 1980, pp. 440–5.

35. J. Egger et al. 'Controlled Trial of Oligoantigenic Treatment in the Hyperkinetic Syndrome', *The Lancet*, 9 March 1985, pp. 540–56. This very carefully controlled trial showed definite reactions to tartrazine and benzoates (but not natural salicylates).

36. British Industrial Biological Research Association. *Annual Report*. Carshalton, 1983.

37. For more on this read Melanie Miller. 'Danger! Additives at Work', *A Report on Food Additives, Their Use and Control*. London Food Commission (available from PO Box 291, London N5 1DU), October 1985.

38. Ibid.

RESOURCES
PUBLICATIONS

NUTRITIONAL INFORMATION AND RECIPES

Brody, Jane. *Jane Brody's Nutrition Book*. London: Bantam, 1988.

Brohn, Penny. *The Bristol Programme*. London: Century, 1987.

Cannon, Geoffrey and Hetty **Einzig**. *Dieting Makes You Fat*. London: Sphere, 1984.

Chorley Well Women Centre. *Good Food Book* and *Summer Cook Book* (available from: 124 Clifford Street, Chorley, Lancs). Two very good examples of recipe books published by a women and health group based at a Well Women Centre. Simple, exciting recipes.

Committee on Medical Aspects of Food Policy (COMA). *Diet and Cardiovascular Disease* (DHSS Report). London: HMSO, 1984.

Cook, Richard and Elizabeth. *Sugar Off: Good Tooth Food Guide*. Cambridge: Great Ouse Press, 1983.

Cook, Richard and Elizabeth. *A Practical Guide to Sugar Free Living*. London: Pan, 1985.

Davis, Adelle. *Let's Eat Right to Keep Fit*. London: Unwin Paperbacks, 1979.

Davis, Stephen and Alan **Stewart**. *Nutritional Medicine: the Drug-free Guide to Better Family Health*. London: Pan, 1987.

Elliot, Rose. *Your Very Good Health*. London: Fontana, 1981.

Elliot, Rose. *Beanfeast*. London: Fontana, 1985.

Forbes, Alec. *The Bristol Diet*. London: Century, 1984. Has much useful information but has been superseded at Bristol as far as the actual diet is concerned.

Forsythe, Elizabeth. *High Fibre Gourmet*. London: Pelham, 1983.

Health Education Council. *Proposals for Nutritional Guidelines for Health Education in Britain*. 1984.

Health Education Council. *Food for Thought*. A short pamphlet produced to support the Channel 4 television series (available free from local health education units or from the Health Education Authority (see p. 74).

Health Education Council. 'Guide to Healthy Eating'. Booklet available from local health education departments.

Joint Advisory Committee on Nutritional Education. *Eating for a Healthier Heart*. London: HMSO, 1985.

Kenton, Leslie and Susannah. *Raw Energy*. London: Century, 1985. Includes many good recipes.

Lappe, Frances Moore. *Diet for a Small Planet*. New York: Ballantine, 1982. More than just a cookbook; a run-down on food economics and why global vegetarianism would alleviate world hunger. Useful nutritional tables.

London Food Commission. *Healthy Eating with Afro-Caribbean Foods*. Full colour poster (A2) illustrating traditional Afro-Caribbean foods, with accompanying leaflet showing how these fit into current nutritional guidelines.

Mellis, Sue and Maggi **Sikking**. *The Wholefood Express — High Speed Vegetarian Cooking*. Todmorden: Food & Futures, 1986.

Mellor, Constance. *Guide to Natural Health*. London: Granada, 1986. Low-priced general guide to healthy eating.

Mervyn, Leonard. *The Dictionary of Minerals*. Wellingborough, Northants: Thorsons, 1985.

Mervyn, Leonard. *The Dictionary of Vitamins*. Wellingborough, Northants: Thorsons, 1985.

Mumby, Keith. *The Food Allergy Plan*. London: Unwin, 1985.

NACNE Report 1983 (Available free from Health Education Authority, see p. 638). A report about the British diet with recommendations for healthier eating.

Open University in association with the Health Education Council and Scottish Health Education Group. *Healthy Eating Assessment Pack, Healthy Eating Study Pack*. For further information write to The Learning Materials Service Centre for Continuing Education, The Open University, P.O. Box 188, Milton Keynes, MK7 6DH. Tel: 0908 74066. A very detailed overview of the issues surrounding healthy eating.

O'Sullivan, Sue. *Turning the Tables — Recipes and Reflections from Women*. London: Sheba, 1987. If you find food a problem, read this — it should make you laugh.

Polunin, Miriam. *Fast Food Real Food*. Wellingborough, Northants: Thorsons, 1985.

Polunin, Miriam. *The Right Way to Eat — to Feel Good or Even Better*. London: Dent, 1986.

Rippon, Sadhya. *The Bristol Recipe Book*. London: Century, 1987.

Robertson, Laurel, Carol **Flinders** and Bronwen **Godfrey**. *Laurel's Kitchen*. London: Routledge and Kegan Paul, 1979. Detailed nutritional information with fairly simple recipes. Very American.

Robbins, Christopher. *Eating for Health*. London: Granada, 1985.

Santa Maria, Jack. *Indian Vegetarian Cookery*. London: Rider, 1973.

Scott, David. *Middle Eastern Vegetarian Cookery*. London: Rider, 1981.

Walker, Caroline, and Geoffrey **Cannon**. *The Food Scandal*. London: Century, 1984.

Westland, Pamela. *Recipes for Good Health*. London: Dunitz, 1982.

Westland, Pamela. *The High Fibre Cook Book*. London: Dunitz, 1982.

FOOD POLITICS

Cannon, Geoffrey. *The Politics of Food*. London: Century, 1987.

Erlichman, James. *Gluttons for Punishment*. London: Penguin Books 1986. About the politics of the food and chemical industries.

The FACT Manifesto (available, with large sae, from FACT, Room W, 25 Horsell Road, London N5 1XL).

George, Susan. *How the Other Half Dies: the Real Reasons for World Hunger*. London: Penguin Books, 1976. A well-documented look at how multinational corporations influence governments here and abroad to channel food to make themselves the most profit, not to feed the hungry.

George, Susan and Nigel **Paige**. *Food for Beginners*. London: Writers and Readers, 1982. A cartoon introduction to the politics of food.

Lang, Tim, Hazel **Andrews**, Caroline **Bedale** and Edward **Hannon**. *Jam Tomorrow*, 1984. A study of poverty and nutrition (available from the Food Policy Unit, Manchester Polytechnic, Hollings Faculty, Old Hall Lane, Manchester 14).

London Food Commission. *Foodfax*. LFC (see Organizations). A guide to the UK food system.

London Food Commission. *Report of the Food & Black and Ethnic Minorities Conference*. A compilation of the discussion and recommendations from the first conference on Food & Black and Ethnic Minorities held in London in November 1986.

London Food Commission. *Looking at 'Look After Your Heart'*. LFC briefing paper examines the government's £1.5m 'Look After Your Heart' campaign. It questions the effectiveness of a campaign that ignores the economic, social and psychological factors which shape our health. Includes recommendations and references.

Maternity Alliance. *Poverty and Pregnancy*. (Available from the Maternity Alliance, 15 Britannia Street, London WC1X 9JP).

Millar, Derek and Derek **Oddy** (eds). *Diet and Health in Britain*. London: Croom Helm, 1985.

Miller, Melanie. 'Danger! Additives at Work'. A Report on Food Additives, Their Use and Control. London Food Commission, October 1985 88 Old Street, London EC1V 9AR.

OPCS. *Report on Commodity Consumption and Heart Disease*. 1975.

Open University. *The Health of Nations*. Milton Keynes: Open University Press, 1985. Chapter 12, Nutrition and Health, gives a history of British dietary changes.

Politics of Health Group. *Food and Profit — It Makes You Sick*. (Available from 9 Poland Street, London W1.)

School Meals in Haringey. A Report by Haringey Women's Employment Project/London Food Commission (available from 88 Old Street, London EC1V 9AR.

EATING PROBLEMS

Bennett, William and Joel **Gurin**. *The Dieter's Dilemma: Eating Less and Weighing More*. New York: Basic Books, 1982. Shows role of exercise in weight reduction may be more important than how much you eat. Draws on many of the same sources as Fat Liberation. A more accessible book is Cannon and Einzig's *Dieting Makes You Fat* listed under 'Nutritional Information'.

Bruch, Hilde. *The Golden Cage — The Enigma of Anorexia Nervosa*. Shepton Mallet, Somerset: Open Books, 1980.

Bruch, Hilde. *Eating Disorders — Obesity, Anorexia Nervosa, and the Person Within*. London: Routledge and Kegan Paul, 1973.

Cataldo, Janine. 'Obesity: a New Perspective on an Old Problem', *Health Education Journal*, vol. 44, no. 4, 1985, pp. 213–17.

Chernin, Kim. *Womansize: the Tyranny of Slenderness*. London: Women's Press, 1981. A primarily theoretical analysis of women's image and society.

Chernin, Kim. *The Hungry Self — Women, Eating and Identity*. London: Virago Press, 1986.

Garrow, J. S. *Energy Balance and Obesity in Man* (2nd ed.). New York and Amsterdam: Elsevier; North Holland: Biomedical Press, 1978. A careful and critical overview of the scientific literature on obesity.

Kaplan, Jane Rachel. *A Woman's Conflict: the Special Relationship between Women and Food*. Englewood Cliffs, NJ: Prentice-Hall, 1980. An excellent anthology of issues vital to women. Good section on fatness.

Lauderback, Llewellyn. *Fat Power*. New York: Hawthorn Books, 1970.

Lawrence, Marilyn. *Anorexic Experience*. London: Women's Press, 1984.

Leghorn, Lisa and Mary **Roodknowsky**. *Who Really Starves? Women and World Hunger*. London: Routledge and Kegan Paul, 1984. (Available from Third World Publications, 151 Stratford Road, Birmingham.) Looks at international issues of women and food.

Macleod, Sheila. *The Art of Starvation: an Adolescence Observed*. London: Virago Press, 1981.

Orbach, Susie. *Fat is a Feminist Issue II*. London: Hamlyn, 1984.

Orbach, Susie. *Hunger Strike*. London: Faber & Faber, 1986. About anorexia nervosa.

Roth, Geneen. *Breaking Free From Compulsive Eating*. London: Grafton Books, 1986. Looks at the physical and emotional aspects of compulsive eating; and a variety of self-help approaches.

See also Resources for Chapter 2. For a more extensive listing of materials in all these areas send one US dollar with a self-addressed business-size envelope to Boston Women's Health Book Collective, 47 Nichols Avenue, Watertown, Massachusetts 02172, USA, tel: 0101 617 924 0271; closed on Mondays.

FOOD ADDITIVES

Ecoropa. *Food Additives – Are the Risks Worthwhile?* Ecoropa Information Sheet 12. (Available from Ecoropa, Crickhowell, Powys, Wales, NP8 1TA.)

Food and Drink Federation. *Food Additives*. (Available free from FDF, 6 Catherine Street, London, WC2B 5JJ.) Explains why additives are used.

Hanssen, Maurice. *The New E for Additives*. Wellingborough, Northants: Thorsons, 1987.

Lashford, Stephanie. *The Additive Checklist*. Bath: Ashgrove Press, 1986. Quick-reference shoppers' guide to natural additives and additive-free food.

Lawrence, Felicity (ed.). *Additives: Your Complete Survival Guide*. London: Century, 1986.

Look at the Label. Includes a list of additives and their serial numbers. (Available from: Ministry of Agriculture, Fisheries and Food, Publications Unit, Lion House, Willowburn Trading Estate, Alnwick, Northumberland, NE66 2PF.)

Millstone, Erik. *Food Additives: Taking the Lid off What We Really Eat*. London: Penguin Books, 1986. Includes a comprehensive overview of studies and supporting evidence behind the possible dangers of additives plus a good explanation concerning the controversy and politics of additives and the food industry.

Paterson, Barbara. *The Allergy Connection*. Wellingborough, Northants: Thorsons, 1985. An exploration of minor and major allergies and their links with food and chemicals. Includes self-help approaches.

Soil Association. *Look Again at the Label: Chemical Additives in Food*. (Available from the Soil Association, 86 Colston Street, Bristol, BS1 5BB.) A good booklet explaining the controversies surrounding additives, with an easy to use guide.

SLIDES, FILMS AND VIDEOS

Food for the Elderly. Tape/slide programme from Paddington and North Kensington/Victoria/Bloomsbury Health Education Depts.

Looking in the Fridge for Feelings. Film, UK, 1981, 30 mins. Groups of women talk with Susie Orbach about the problems of compulsive eating; distributed by the National Film School.

Picture of Health: Eat Your Heart Out. Film, Channel Four, 1983, 45 mins. Food and coronary heart disease.

Well Being: a Weight Off Your Mind. Film, Channel Four, 1982, 45 mins. The medical risks of obesity and whether fashion and fears about fatness do more damage than the extra pounds.

Well Being: Food Glorious Chips. Film, Channel Four, 1982, 45 mins. Junk foods, school meals, additives and their effect on children.

ORGANIZATIONS

AAA (Action Against Allergy), 43 The Downs, London SW20 8HG. Tel: 01–947 5082. Send large sae for information.

Anorexia Anonymous, 24 Westmoreland Road, Barnes, London SW13. Tel: 01–748 3994.

Anorexia Family Aid and National Information Centre, Sackville Place, 44 Magdalen Street, Norwich, Norfolk NR3 1JE. Tel: 0603–621414.

Anorexic Aid, The Priory Centre, 11 Priory Road, High Wycombe, Bucks. Tel: 0494–21431. Offers support and advice to sufferers of anorexia and bulimia and their families and friends. Network of voluntary self-help groups throughout the country.

Campaign for Freedom of Information, 3 Endsleigh Street, London WC1. Tel: 01–278 9686.

Compulsive Eating Groups, c/o Women's Therapy Centre, 6 Manor Gardens, London N7. Tel: 01–263 6200.

Compulsive Eating Groups, organized by Spare Tyre Theatre Company, 86–8 Holmleigh Road, London N16. Tel: 01–800 9099.

Coronary Prevention Group, 60 Great Ormond Street, London WC1N 3HR. Tel: 01–833 3687.

FACT (Food Additives Campaign Team), 25 Horsell Road, London N5 1XL. Campaigns for more stringent control of additives.

Fat Liberator Publications, PO Box 5227, Coralville, Indiana 52241, USA or c/o Judith Stein, 137 Tremont Street, Cambridge, MA 02139, USA. An extensive list of well-researched publications.

Fat Women's Group, c/o London Women's Centre, Wesley House, 4 Wild Court, London WC2B 5AU.

Food Allergies Association, c/o 27 Ferringham Lane, Ferring-by-Sea, West Sussex BN12 5NB. Tel: 0903–41178. Can help allergy sufferers through information leaflets and pamphlets.

Friends of the Earth, 26–28 Underwood Street, London N1 7JQ. Tel: 01–490 1555.

Health Education Authority, Hamilton House, Mabledon Place, London WC1H 9TX. Tel: 01–631 0930.

Hyperactive Children's Support Group, 71 Whyke Lane, Chichester, West Sussex PO19 2LD. Tel: 0903–725182. Send sae for information. If you would like their booklet DIET, please send £2 and mark the envelope 'Diet Please'.

London Food Commission, 88 Old Street, London EC1V 9AR. Tel: 01–253 9513.

McCarrison Society, 24 Paddington Street, London W1M 4DR. Tel: 01–935 3924. Organization for health professionals.

Ministry of Agriculture, Fisheries and Food, Whitehall Place, London SW1A 2HH. Tel: 01–270 3000.

National Society for Research into Allergy, c/o Mrs E. L. Rose, PO Box 45, Hinckley, Leicester LE10 1JE. Tel: 0455–635212. Offers diet sheets, practical advice and introductions to other allergy sufferers.

Nutrition Association, c/o ION, 5 Jerdan Place, London SW6 1BE. Tel: 01–385 7984.

Organic Growers' Association, Aeron Park, Langeitho, Dyfed, Wales.

Overeaters Anonymous, PO Box 19, Streatford, Manchester H32 9EB. Tel: 061–868 4109.

The Society for Nutritional Medicine, 126 Acomb Road, York YO2 4EY. Mostly for doctors.

Soil Association, 86 Colston Street, Bristol BS1 5BB. Tel: 0272–290661.

Vegan Society, 33–35 George Street, Oxford OX1 2AY. Tel: 0865–722166.

Vegetarian Society, Parkdale, Dunham Road, Altrincham, Cheshire WA14 4QG. Tel: 061–928 0793.

ALCOHOL, NICOTINE AND OTHER MOOD-ALTERING DRUGS

Rewritten by
SUE CLEMENTS AND JAN FULLER*

Virtually all of us at one time or another have taken a mood-altering drug. The reasons why we use drugs, including alcohol and tobacco, vary enormously. We may use them because we enjoy their effects, because it is expected behaviour in certain social situations or because we are seeking relief from stress or emotional pain. All drug use, however, carries with it potential risks which vary with the quantity and methods used, the situation in which it is used and the regularity of use. Some drug use, however moderate, is additionally risky because possession of the drug itself is illegal. Whichever drugs we use, tobacco, alcohol, tranquillizers or heroin, we owe it to ourselves to understand the risks involved.

ALCOHOL†

Over the last twenty-five years there has been a substantial increase in both the number of women who drink and the amount of alcohol consumed. Not only have we had more money to spend on drink but changes in the retail distribution of alcohol have made its purchase easier and more convenient. Moderate drinking by women is no longer socially unacceptable and the alcohol industry has been quick to take advantage of women's changing social and economic status with advertising campaigns geared to the 'female market'. Many millions of pounds each year are spent attempting to influence us to drink more.

There's a huge social pressure to drink, you've got to have one. It's really difficult to ask for an orange juice, especially with people from work, it's just not accepted.

*With help in the smoking section from Bobbie Jacobson.
†For alcohol in relation to pregnancy, see Chapter 18, p. 347, and concerning infertility, Chapter 21, p. 425.

The more alcohol we consume the more likely we are to experience alcohol-related problems. These may be problems associated with one-off intoxication, physical problems associated with regular excessive use or problems associated with alcohol dependence. Because alcohol is such a familiar ingredient of many of our lives it's easy to forget that it is a powerful, potentially addictive drug which acts as a central nervous system depressant. Taken in small quantities it has a pleasant, mildly relaxing effect. Taken in larger quantities it decreases muscle co-ordination, judgement and emotional control.

Drink is definitely a tool for me. I use it to get things out. The more pissed I get the less inhibited I am and I can express emotions that wouldn't be accepted normally. People say 'Oh, she's just pissed' – so it's not taken too seriously.

When we drink we can become intoxicated more quickly than men because we have a lower proportion of our total body weight in the form of water and so we reach higher blood alcohol levels more quickly. We also become intoxicated more quickly than usual during the premenstrual and ovulatory phases of our menstrual cycle. Alcohol levels are also considerably higher in women who take the Pill (see p. 294). If we want to get intoxicated occasionally, it's important to make sure we are in a safe environment where the risks of having an accident are minimized and where we are not vulnerable to the risk of sexual or physical abuse.

After going to the pub I usually have to go home on my own on the tube or the bus. For men it's OK, no one is going to bother them but for a woman it's bad enough at night anyway, and if your vision is blurred and you're a bit queasy then you're much more vulnerable to being attacked.

Drinking and driving is not only unsafe for us, it is also unsafe for others.
The amount of alcohol we consume is most commonly

measured in 'units'. A glass of wine, a small glass of sherry, a pub measure of spirits ($\frac{1}{6}$ gill) and half a pint of ordinary-strength beer or lager each contain one unit of alcohol. It is the amount of alcohol, not the type we drink, that's important. Those of us who drink approximately twenty-four units a week or more are putting ourselves at risk of developing physical problems as a result. Drinking at this level in the long-term increases the risk of liver disease, brain damage, heart attack, muscle disease, inflammation of the pancreas, stomach disorders and cancer (see Cancer, p. 569). Over the short term it can interfere with sleep, produce a feeling of being off-colour and permanently tired.

> *I just felt under par all the time, I thought perhaps I was just working too hard. I never thought it might be the drink.*

It is possible that as little as one unit a day can lead to cirrhosis of the liver in women, and this in turn can sometimes lead to liver cancer.

Women who drink regularly every day may become physically dependent upon alcohol, just as women who drink to try and cope with problems may become psychologically dependent. If we are physically dependent we will often continue to drink because we are afraid of experiencing withdrawal symptoms if we stop. Withdrawal symptoms may often be quite mild or they may be more severe and can range from dizziness and nausea to, much less frequently, fits and hallucinations (seeing things that aren't really there). Drugs such as heminevrin or diazepam (often prescribed as Valium) can be prescribed by your GP to help you cope with withdrawal symptoms. However, these drugs can themselves lead to dependence and should only be taken on a short-term basis on a reducing dosage.* Only a few women will need or be able to go into hospital to withdraw ('dry out') from alcohol. Most women can receive help, if it is necessary, at home. For those of us who have been physically or psychologically dependent, however, stopping or cutting down our drinking in the long term may be difficult unless we resolve the problems or change the situation which led to heavy drinking in the first place. There is a variety of services which can provide help and support in doing this. Even women who are not dependent but are regularly drinking more than approximately twenty-four units a week could consider cutting down because of the health risks involved. Some of the same services may be helpful if this proves to be difficult without support.

Many women who drink heavily will also experience anxiety and depression. Drinking itself may cause these feelings, so if you go to your GP for help, it is important to tell her/him that you want help with cutting down or stopping drinking first before you accept any treatment for these problems. Many women who have a problem with alcohol also become dependent on prescribed mood-altering drugs because their GPs have failed to recognize that heavy drinking is the underlying cause for their anxiety or depression. See also Chapter 8 for the different kinds of help and self-help.

GETTING HELP

There is a variety of places where you can get help and advice if you are concerned about your drinking. Services,

---

*Heminevrin will speed up the effects of alcohol if taken with it.

IF YOU DRINK

- It is a good idea to eat something before or while drinking. Sipping drinks rather than gulping them also slows down the rate at which alcohol enters the bloodstream. A woman weighing between 7 and 10 stones (44.5–63.5 kg) will take about two hours to metabolize, or 'burn up', one unit of alcohol. A woman weighing over 10 stones (63.5 kg) will take about one hour to metabolize each unit. (For a definition of 'unit' see above.)
- Sometimes the body is especially vulnerable to alcohol. When we're feeling sick or tired, for example, alcohol can affect our system more powerfully than usual. Women also become intoxicated more quickly than usual prior to menstruation and during ovulation. Try to pace your drinking throughout the evening, perhaps drink alternate soft and alcoholic drinks.
- It is illegal to drive with a blood alcohol level of more than 80 mg/100 ml. Most women will reach this level if they drink between three and four units in an hour. Between 1973 and 1983, convictions for drunk driving among women increased by over 300 per cent. Even at the legal limit you are more than four times as likely to have a crash because even small amounts of alcohol will interfere with judgement, co-ordination, vision and reaction time. The safest thing to do if you've been drinking at all is – don't drive.
- Don't use alcohol in combination with other drugs. It is particularly dangerous to drink if you are also taking sedatives (e.g. sleeping tablets, tranquillizers, narcotics, anti-depressants and antihistamines) as it can be lethal. Alcohol can also interfere with the action of other drugs, notably those used for the treatment of epilepsy, high blood pressure, diabetes and thrombosis. See also Flagyl, p. 491, and the Pill, p. 294.
- Avoid using alcohol as a problem-solver. Drinking to escape from stress keeps us from dealing with our underlying difficulties, often creates additional problems and can lead to us becoming dependent on alcohol.
- If you're planning to become pregnant or are already pregnant see Pregnancy, Chapter 18 and Miscarriage, p. 437. You may want to restrict your intake to zero.

however, vary in the extent to which they consider the special needs of women. Services oriented towards the needs of lesbian women and women from ethnic minorities are particularly scarce outside London. **Alcohol Concern** (see p. 74) operates a central information service about what is available throughout the UK. If you are concerned about the amount you are drinking but aren't experiencing major problems in other areas of your life, **Drink Watchers** may be helpful. They run groups which teach you how to monitor your drinking and will suggest strategies to help you cut down and provide support in doing so (mostly London-based but some regional groups). **Alcohol Advisory Centres** or **Councils on Alcoholism** are non-statutory (i.e. voluntary) agencies which provide more intensive counselling and advice about alcohol and associated problems. Some run women's groups. They also provide support to women who are experiencing problems because of the drinking of others. Their service is completely confidential. (Contact through Alcohol Concern or look in your phone book under Alcohol.) Within the NHS your GP may be able to offer you advice or may refer you to a general psychiatrist or to a **Regional Alcohol Treatment Unit**. Some Alcohol Treatment Units (ATUs) run women's groups and are very sensitive to the needs of women, others are very male dominated. All the above agencies can give you advice about whether you need to cut down or stop drinking totally. If you have already decided you want to stop drinking totally, you might find **Alcoholics Anonymous** (AA) helpful (look in your phone book for a contact number). AA does not run separate groups for women in this country. They do run affiliated groups if you need support in coping with a partner who is drinking (**Al-Anon**) or if one of your parents has a drinking problem (**Alateen**).

CIGARETTE SMOKING/ NICOTINE

Smoking is as much a problem for women as it is for men. We use cigarettes much like drink and other drugs to put the lid on the stresses we feel in our everyday lives. Smoking among women has risen inexorably since the Second World War, and women's and men's smoking rates are now virtually equal. Although smoking has been slowly falling among adult women in recent years – about one-third of women currently smoke – those of us who do use cigarettes are more likely to be heavy smokers than in the past. Teenage girls are beginning to smoke at younger ages than ever before, and have caught up with, and are beginning to overtake, boys for the first time.

Women depend on cigarettes for good reason. Like alcohol and other drugs, they offer only temporary solace from a society that neither supports nor acknowledges the contribution we make to it, nor the stresses it imposes upon

us. Hardly surprising then that we often have a poor image of ourselves. And the less we believe in ourselves, the more dependent we feel ourselves to be on cigarettes – or alcohol or tranquillizers. Cigarettes, however, are unique in some respects. Alcohol, and even tranquillizers, when used appropriately, do not necessarily threaten our health. Cigarettes, on the other hand, are dangerous under all circumstances. The only safe cigarette is the unsmoked one. And there is more to our reliance on cigarettes than straightforward chemical dependence on nicotine. We are subjected to powerful social and political forces that teach us we are helpless in general, and dependent on cigarettes in particular. Yet this dependence is as much a feature of a government which allows the tobacco companies to spend at least £100 million persuading us to smoke, at the same time as raising over £5,000 million from tobacco taxes each year.

Cigarette smoking is the single largest avoidable cause of death in the industrialized world and causes one-third of all deaths from cancers. Women who smoke have up to a three times greater likelihood of developing lung cancer than non-smoking women. In 1984, the female lung cancer death-rate in Scotland surpassed that for breast cancer (the chief cause of cancer deaths in women for many years) for the first time. Smoking also plays a part in other cancers too, particularly cancer of the cervix (see p. 525). This is especially important for young women who may also be on the Pill, and in whom rates of cervical cancer are rising.

Compared to non-smoking women, those who smoke cigarettes are more likely to suffer heart attacks and certain kinds of stroke. Women who use oral contraceptives and also smoke are ten times as likely as non-smoking women to suffer a heart attack. Women who smoke are also at greater risk of death from disabling lung disease, and are more likely than non-smokers to suffer from chronic bronchitis and emphysema. Smoking has also been linked with decreased fertility, and with a slightly earlier menopause, on average.

'Passive smoking' – that is, exposure to the cigarette smoke of others – is also a health risk. For example, non-smokers exposed to their spouses' cigarette smoke are more likely to develop lung cancer than non-smokers with non-smoking spouses. Other studies have shown that children of parents who smoke are more likely to develop colic and chest infections than children of non-smoking parents. For smoking in relation to pregnancy, see Chapter 18, and smoking in relation to infertility, Chapter 21.

KICKING THE HABIT

There is simply no 'safe way' to smoke. Although low-tar cigarettes may reduce the risk of lung cancer to some extent, there is no evidence that they lessen the risk of other lung diseases, heart attacks or damage to the unborn during pregnancy. And there are eight times as many deaths from heart attacks as from lung cancer among women. The safest and healthiest course is simply to stop smoking. Difficult as this may seem, more of us than ever – 3.5 million women in Britain – are successfully freeing ourselves from dependence on tobacco. Since 1976 the percentage of women who smoke has fallen from 38 to 32 per cent.

Even if you're a heavy smoker, after stopping, your risk of developing lung cancer drops gradually, equalling that of a non-smoker's after ten or fifteen years. Although some of us fear that when we stop smoking we will gain unwanted weight, research shows that up to half of those who stop smoking report no weight change, and some actually lose weight. Ironically, it is men who gain more weight than women when they stop. Women who stop report that they have never felt better.

It's a great feeling to be able to do so many of the things that were just out of the question while I was smoking – running around the park, dancing for hours at a time, little things like enjoying the fragrance of my own clean hair. Just knowing that I'm healthier and my kids are probably healthier.

There's a great sense of accomplishment and power that comes from stopping – power to get hold of your own life. But there's no way it's easy. I still identify with being a smoker. I still smoke in my dreams. If I thought I could go back to cigarettes and only smoke two or three a day, I'd do it in a minute. But I know I can't smoke that way. If I smoked one I'd smoke a pack, and won't do that to myself any more.

The ability to stop smoking successfully depends largely on a strong commitment to stop, the belief that we can stop. Nine out of ten people who stop do so without much more than supportive friends and relatives. Most who stop successfully have tried several times before. Trying to stop and going back to cigarettes is not a failure, but rather a practice run for success. And research shows that practice makes perfect.

GETTING HELP

There are a number of free programmes available. ASH UK (Action on Smoking and Health) will put you in touch with your nearest facility; or you can ring your local health education department.

While we can participate in a formal programme we can also ask a friend or relative to stop smoking with us. And if we swear off cigarettes but then 'slip' at some point along the way, we need to remember that nearly everyone does at one time or another. We need to try again – and again. It is not hard to stop smoking; what is hard is making the decision and sticking to it. But it is also possible – and it is one of the biggest favours we will ever do for ourselves and our health.

OTHER MOOD-ALTERING DRUGS

Every society has to decide about the extent to which it is prepared to integrate the use of various drugs into its cultural framework. In Western society, alcohol and tobacco have become the main drugs of choice and their use is powerfully reinforced by the multinational drinks and tobacco industries. In the UK all other psychotropic (mood-altering) drug use is illegal, with one or two exceptions such as solvents, unless the drug has been prescribed by a doctor to treat an 'illness'. Many prescribed psychotropics such as tranquillizers are also major drugs of 'street' misuse, i.e. they are bought and sold on the black market. Some 'street' drugs, such as heroin, also have legitimate medical uses (see p. 70). The distinction between a legal and illegal drug then is in many ways an artificial one. Any drug can become a drug of misuse, depending on the extent to which its use is pleasurable, the degree to which it is readily available and the need of the user to seek some kind of chemical relief from the stresses and strains of everyday life. Some drug use is socially sanctioned. Other drug use meets with social disapproval. Often the same drug can produce both kinds of reaction depending on the kind of user and the reason for use (e.g. the use of heroin for the control of pain in cases of terminal cancer versus its illegal use as a drug of 'pleasure').

The use of prescribed psychotropics remains the most 'socially accepted' way for women to obtain chemical relief. Of the 50 million prescriptions a year in the UK for psychotropic medication about two-thirds of these are given to women. Some women who suffer from a serious mental illness do benefit from some of these drugs and need to take them on a regular basis for extended periods. For other women, however, psychoactive drugs are all too often prescribed to 'treat' the ordinary stresses of daily life – relationship problems, loneliness, boredom at work, difficult children – because many doctors are unaware of or are too 'busy' to provide alternative forms of help. For older women the onset of menopause or their partner's death often becomes a reason to prescribe these drugs. (Adverts in medical and psychiatric journals often suggest that women are particularly unable to withstand the stresses of daily life without chemical relief.) Much of this 'medicalization' of normal life is encouraged by the drug industry, in the same way that the alcohol industry encourages women to drink more.

Although the following section gives information about the use of specific drugs, various common themes run throughout, regardless of the particular substances under discussion. The effects of any drug on the individual will tend to vary, for example according to the amount used, the situation in which it is used, the method of use (i.e. swallowed, injected, sniffed, smoked), the expectations of its effects which the user has and the mood s/he is in when s/he takes it. All of us who use any of these drugs need to be clear about the costs and benefits of using them and also about the reasons which underlie our use. Many women use a variety of different substances so it can often be much more important to examine why we need to take any drug (including alcohol) rather than focusing too narrowly on the actual substance used.

MINOR TRANQUILLIZERS/SLEEPING PILLS*

One in five women takes a tranquillizer at some time each year, usually for at least a month, compared with one in ten of all men. With one or two exceptions† the drugs prescribed as tranquillizers and those prescribed as sedatives (sleeping pills) belong to the same chemical group, the benzodiazepines. They are used to relieve anxiety symptoms or in slightly bigger doses to act as sleeping pills. Many also have the effect of relaxing the muscles and some also make convulsions less likely. They may sometimes be prescribed purely for these physical effects. The Department of Health has restricted the number of types of benzodiazepine which doctors can prescribe on the NHS. Those which remain available are chlordiazepoxide (Librium), chlor hydrochloride (Tropium), diazepam (Valium), lorazepam (Ativan), nitrazepam (Mogadon), oxazepam (Serenid D, Serenid Forte), temazepam (Euhypnos, Normison) and triazolam (Halcion).

While tranquillizers are certainly effective in helping people sleep and making them feel less anxious in the short term, they cannot do this indefinitely. There is little evidence that they are effective against anxiety for more

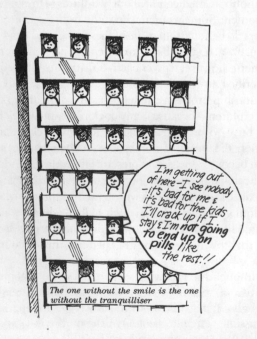

I'm getting out of here – I see nobody – it's bad for me & it's bad for the kids. I'll crack up if I stay & I'm not going to end up on pills like the rest!!

The one without the smile is the one without the tranquilliser

*The help of Release publications is gratefully acknowledged in the preparation of this section.
†Chloral hydrate, dichloralphenazone (Welldorm), triclofos, promethazine, chlormethiazole (Heminevrin), chlormezanone and barbiturates (used as sedatives).

than four months of continuous use. Used as sleeping tablets they can lose their effectiveness with three to fourteen days of continuous use. Unfortunately, it is not uncommon for women who were prescribed tranquillizers for some reason, such as a bereavement or even exam nerves, to be still taking them some ten or even twenty years later. There is good evidence that regular use for more than a few weeks can lead to both physical and psychological dependence, and that stopping use can lead to a definite drug withdrawal syndrome. This can often be interpreted as a recurrence of the original anxiety symptoms which precipitates continued usage. It has been estimated that more than 100,000 people in this country are dependent on tranquillizers.

Commonly reported side-effects of tranquillizers are dizziness, headaches and nausea, feeling drowsy, having blurred vision and slight loss of coordination. Taking tranquillizers increases your risk of having an accident while driving and if operating machinery because it slows your reaction times. If you are taking oral contraceptives your body may absorb these drugs less quickly which will make their effects more marked. Side-effects are also exacerbated by drinking alcohol, and they tend to be worse in old people, sometimes leading to confusion.

Very rarely, tranquillizers can have what doctors call paradoxical effects, which means that the person experiences very different feelings on taking the drug from those which would usually be expected. These have included becoming very excited and having aggressive outbursts. Taken over a long period benzodiazepines can lead to depression and blunted perception of pleasure and pain. They can also lead to a loss of concentration and memory lapses.

Taking tranquillizers does not 'cure' anxiety. The idea is simply that if a person gets so anxious that they cannot cope with their life then the drugs will help them calm down enough to cope again. It is assumed that the person will then, at some point, stop needing the drug to cope. Occasionally the drug may help the user to feel strong enough to tackle the cause of the problem itself. Unfortunately, the prescription of tranquillizers can actually stop us tackling the real problem or working through how we feel about it. This can happen in three ways. First, taking a pill for a problem can often make us feel that there is something wrong with us, that we are 'ill' rather than that there is something wrong happening in our lives. We come to feel that if we were well we would be able to cope – indeed, *should* be able to cope – and that the problem must be that we are inadequate; so we end up putting little energy into tackling the original problem for the simple reason that it is no longer seen as the problem. This feeling of inadequacy can become much stronger when we discover that we've become dependent on the tranquillizer. The second way in which tranquillizers can actually get in the way of tackling the problem is that they calm us down and make us feel much less miserable. Yet it's often realizing just how miserable we are that forces us to make changes in our situation. Finally, some problems need to be dealt with by 'working through' feelings about them, for example mourning the death of a relative or of a relationship. Tranquillizers can stop this happening and so actually prevent us getting over our grief.

If you want to stop taking tranquillizers it is advisable to wean yourself off gradually. Simply stopping suddenly may sometimes produce serious withdrawal symptoms which can be dangerous. A reduction of the dose every two to four weeks by approximately one-eighth of the previous dose has been suggested. Because some of these drugs have a shorter lasting action (a shorter 'half-life') than others you may need to switch to a drug with a longer half-life when you reach the lowest tolerable dose of your own drug. It is important to talk to a helpful doctor before attempting to cut down as you may need a new prescription at this point. Some areas may have self-help groups or other support groups to help you through coming off (contact your local health education department, or the Women's Health and Reproductive Rights Information Centre), or you can ask your doctor to refer you to a clinical psychologist or community psychiatric nurse who may be able to offer you alternative ways of dealing with any problems that you could still be encountering. The specialist drug agencies can offer help in coming off too (see Resources). See also Chapter 8 for ideas on helping yourself and getting help.

ANTI-DEPRESSANTS

There are two main groups of anti-depressant drugs, the tricyclics (the most commonly prescribed) and the monoamine oxidase inhibitors (MAOIs). Tricyclics and related anti-depressants are prescribed more often than MAOIs because they are generally more effective and do not show the dangerous interactions with some foods and drugs that are characteristic of MAOIs. The most commonly used tricyclics and related drugs are amitriptyline (Tryptizol), clomipramine (Anafranil), dothiepin (Prothiaden), imipramine (Tofranil), trimipramine (Surmontil), mianserin (Bolvidon, Norval) and nomifensine (Merital). It takes two to three weeks for these drugs to begin to work. Side-effects may include drowsiness, dry mouth, blurred vision, constipation and, less commonly, irregularity of the heartbeat. Tolerance to some of these side-effects will develop if drug use persists. Some doctors will try to prescribe more than one anti-depressant at a time to use in combination. This is *not* recommended by the Pharmaceutical Society. MAOIs will generally be prescribed if treatment with tricyclics has failed. These drugs may take up to six weeks to start working properly. If you are taking one of these drugs you must make sure to get a list of foods to avoid (such as cheese and Marmite). Any of these foods, most other medicines and alcohol may cause a dangerous rise in blood pressure when taken with any MAOI, the first sign of which may be a throbbing headache. Combining tricyclics with MAOIs is potentially lethal. The most commonly prescribed MAOIs are phenelzine (Nardil) and tranylcypromine (Parnate). There is a whole variety of nasty side-effects with these drugs.

They can, however, be very helpful to some women for whom no other form of support has been effective. Anti-depressants are far less dependence-producing than the benzodiazepines and barbiturates. If your GP prescribes one of these drugs you should always ask whether any other form of non-chemical help is available either instead of or in addition to the drug prescribed (see Chapter 8). Like all the other psychotropic drugs discussed so far, anti-depressants help only with symptoms, they will not resolve any underlying problems.

LITHIUM

Lithium salts are used for their mood-regulating action in the treatment of manic illness (when someone becomes overactive and unrealistically euphoric) and in the prevention of manic and depressive illness. If you have been prescribed this drug you should continue taking it unless the doctor prescribing it advises you otherwise or until you have obtained a second medical opinion. You should, however, have regular blood tests because the dose at which it works and the dose at which it can be dangerous are very close to each other and require careful monitoring. Toxic effects include blurred vision, vomiting, diarrhoea, tremor, unsteadiness, slurring of speech and fits. If you experience any of these while taking lithium you should see your doctor immediately. Brand names of lithium are Camcolit and Priadel.

There is some suggestion that taking lithium for longer than three to five years may cause a degree of kidney damage. If you have been taking it for this length of time you might want to talk to a psychiatrist about the costs and benefits of continued use.

ANTI-PSYCHOTIC DRUGS

Anti-psychotic drugs are also sometimes known as 'major tranquillizers'. They may be used in the short term to quieten down severely disturbed people or to alleviate severe anxiety. In the longer term they are mainly prescribed for schizophrenia and other psychotic illnesses. They are extremely helpful in relieving acute psychotic symptoms such as hallucinations and delusions and can be useful in preventing the recurrence of these symptoms in the long term. Stopping taking these drugs is generally unwise unless you do so under medical supervision, as it may lead to your symptoms reappearing, although this might not become apparent right away. The most commonly used anti-psychotic drugs taken by mouth (orally) are chlorpromazine (Largactil), thioridazine (Melleril) and haloperidol (Fortunan). If you find taking these drugs orally inconvenient or if you tend to forget to take them you may be offered long-acting (depot) injections at between one- to four-week intervals. Common depot anti-psychotics can impair fertility in women and have the same side-effects as drugs taken orally. Some of these side-effects can be involuntary—abnormal face and body movements (tardive dyskinesia), restlessness, drowsiness and parkinsonism-like symptoms (stiffness, decreased spontaneous movement). Parkinsonian effects can be modified by taking anti-cholinergic drugs, but you should not routinely take those unless you have already experienced these side-effects because they increase the risk of developing tardive dyskinesia. Once developed this can be irreversible even if you stop taking the medication. Although the side-effects of these drugs may be severe, not everyone experiences them. If you do you should talk to a psychiatrist about the costs and benefits of taking the drug before making any decision about discontinuing use.

HEROIN AND OTHER OPIATES

Heroin and morphine are drugs derived from the opium poppy which are used medically as pain-killers, cough suppressants and anti-diarrhoea treatments. Other opiates, which are synthetically produced, include pethidine, frequently used for pain in childbirth and after operations, dipipanone (Diconal), dihydrocodeine (DF-118), dextro-propoxyphene (Distalgesic), and methadone (Physeptone), usually used in the treatment of drug dependence.

Heroin and morphine can produce feelings of well-being, euphoria and indifference to unpleasant situations – hence their value in helping people with uncontrollable physical pain. It is only when prescribed in certain circumstances by a doctor that opiates can be used legally.

Powdered forms of heroin can be smoked ('chasing the dragon'), 'snorted' up the nose through a tube, or dissolved in water and injected. Intravenous injection maximizes the effects and produces a sudden burst of pleasurable sensations known as the 'rush'. On the first few occasions of use, nausea and vomiting commonly occur. These may be sufficiently unpleasant to deter further heroin use, although they do disappear with repeated doses. Your body gets used to the drug with repeated use, so that increasing the amount used or changing to a more efficient method of usage (such as injection – see box) becomes necessary in order to continue to experience the pleasurable effects. If after a break in drug use you immediately go back to using at the same level as before, there is a risk of overdosing (which could be fatal) because your body will no longer be used to coping with that amount of the drug.

There is a high risk of both physical and psychological dependence with all opiate drug use – although dependence is not inevitable. Some drug users believe they cannot become 'addicted' if they just smoke or snort rather than inject heroin. This is not true, but it is true that dependence is more likely with injection.

Suddenly stopping after a period of regular opiate use usually causes uncomfortable withdrawal effects which can vary from a mild flu-like illness to a more severe reaction including sweating, abdominal cramps, diarrhoea, irritability, goose-flesh, streaming eyes and nose, and mild fever. But getting over the physical withdrawal effects is often only a minor part of the battle in staying off. Psychological cravings and a powerful desire to re-experience the effects of the drug may well have to be overcome.

INJECTING DRUGS

Injecting drugs is the most hazardous way of using them. It increases the risks of health problems compared with other methods of drug use. The main dangers of injecting are:

- overdose;
- infections such as hepatitis B or AIDS (see p. 501) caused by sharing needles and syringes with other drug users;
- abscesses or septicaemia (blood-poisoning) from the use of dirty (unsterile) needles, or from impure drugs, or from injecting solutions made from crushed-up tablets;
- gangrene caused by hitting the artery not the vein.

The best way to cut down the risk of problems associated with drug use is to stop taking drugs (see p. 73).

There are no totally safe ways of using any drug. However, injecting drugs is very dangerous, so if you can't stop using drugs for the time being then you should stop injecting them (for example, change to smoking, snorting or swallowing the drug).

Coming off heroin wasn't too bad . . . but I know staying off is going to be much harder. (quote from a woman who had recently completed a detoxification programme)

If you are using opiates, it is possible to get yourself off without going to a doctor or specialist drug centre. The best way is steadily to reduce the dose you are using over a period of time, so that you don't get bad withdrawal effects. The advantage of asking a doctor to prescribe a substitute drug (such as methadone) in progressively reducing amounts is that s/he is helping you to avoid bad withdrawals that might make you want to go back to using again.

Using prescribed opiates in a hygienic and controlled fashion (e.g. for the treatment of severe pain) is unlikely to cause you any serious health problems. But injecting black-market heroin, which usually contains adulterants, may lead to serious problems. For the other dangers of injection, see box. Self-neglect, poor nutrition and other consequences of a drug-using lifestyle increase vulnerability to diseases generally.

Menstrual irregularities and reduced fertility are common with long-term heroin or opiate use, although many women still do become pregnant while they are using the drug. These changes are usually reversed after drug use has stopped.

BARBITURATES

The effects of barbiturates are similar to those of alcohol. They used to be commonly prescribed to treat insomnia but have now been almost totally replaced by benzodiazepines which are considered to be much safer. Barbiturates are the most inherently dangerous of the drugs widely misused in the UK and their medical use today tends to be restricted to the treatment of severe, intractable insomnia and epilepsy.

Most barbiturates are powders made up into coloured capsules or tablets. They are usually taken by mouth when prescribed for medical reasons. In illicit use they may be taken by mouth or the powder dissolved in solution and injected. Pentobarbitone sodium (Nembutal) and amylobarbitone sodium (Tuinal) are the two barbiturates found most often on the illicit market. Other barbiturate drugs are butobarbitone (Soneryl), glutethimide (Doriden), quinalbarbitone sodium (Seconal) and amylobarbitone sodium (Sodium Amytal). From 1 January 1985 many of the barbiturates were brought under the control of the Misuse of Drugs Act (1971). Accordingly, it is an offence to possess these drugs unless they have been prescribed for you by your doctor, or to supply (give) them to anyone else.

Using barbiturates usually produces feelings of pleasurable intoxication and/or sedation. They are particularly dangerous drugs because the normal dose is not much lower than that causing a lethal overdose. Taking alcohol with barbiturates is also highly dangerous. Regular barbiturate use can lead to physical and psychological dependence.

If you are taking barbiturates you must not stop them suddenly. Sudden withdrawal from a high dose can be fatal. You can come off barbiturates by reducing your dose very gradually, but we strongly urge you to consult your doctor or a specialist drug agency for help in doing this.

STIMULANT-TYPE DRUGS

Amphetamines

Amphetamines have a stimulant action – causing increased alertness and arousal. They commonly produce feelings of exhilaration, cheerfulness, increased confidence and loss of appetite. They are a major drug of illicit use and their medical uses are extremely limited.

Amphetamine and other amphetamine-like drugs produced in tablet or capsule form include Dexedrine, Durophet and Ritalin. They are taken by mouth, but misusers sometimes dissolve them in water and inject them. Illicitly produced powdered amphetamine ('speed', 'sulphate') is generally sniffed up the nose, but it can be smoked or injected.

Amphetamine use frequently leads to psychological dependence. After a 'run' of use lasting several days, the user may feel tired, hungry and depressed. Extended use, with the consequent lack of sleep, hyperactivity and little food consumption, leads to rapid physical debility. Heavy users may experience feelings of paranoia (feeling persecuted) and delusions (amphetamine psychosis). However, even after regular long-term use there are no dangerous withdrawal symptoms. So stopping them suddenly without medical supervision is all right, although it may be difficult

and advice and support from your doctor or a specialist drug agency could be useful.

Amphetamines were commonly prescribed during the 1950s and 1960s as anti-depressants and slimming pills. However, because of their high risk for psychological dependence, they have no place today in the treatment of depression or obesity. Slimming pills prescribed today such as diethylpropion (Apisate, Tenuate) act as appetite suppressants – they have less stimulant effects and rarely cause dependence, although abrupt withdrawal can produce depression. Slimming pills are not worth taking: apart from the risks of dependence and other adverse effects, weight loss is mostly regained once the pills are stopped.

Cocaine

Cocaine is a white powder derived from the leaves of the coca plant grown in South America. Its effects are very similar to those of amphetamines, although they only last a short time – about half an hour. It can be obtained only illegally. It can be injected or smoked, but more commonly it is 'snorted' up the nose.

Cocaine use does not lead to physical dependence, but its effect on moods and feelings may well lead to psychological dependence. Stopping the drug after a period of regular use may produce tiredness and depression, although these reactions are not as bad as those following regular amphetamine use. Long-term use of high doses of cocaine can cause feelings of paranoia or even development of paranoid psychosis. These feelings usually clear up after the drug has been stopped. Repeated 'snorting' of the drug through the nose can damage the nasal septum separating the nostrils. Overdose can cause death from respiratory arrest, but this is rare.

HALLUCINOGENIC DRUGS AND MUSHROOMS

In the UK the use of hallucinogenic drugs is rare compared to other psychoactive substances. LSD (lysergic acid diethylamide) is the most widely used of the hallucinogenic drugs. Very small amounts of LSD are required for a 'trip'. It is generally incorporated with other substances into tablets or capsules, or made into solution and spotted on to paper, stamps or sugar-cubes. A 'trip' generally lasts between four and twelve hours, depending on the amount of the drug used. LSD can produce striking visual effects including intensification of colours, distorted images and hallucinatory-type experiences (these are not true hallucinations as the drug user generally recognizes them as unreal). Distortions in hearing, taste and touch are commonly reported; also out-of-the-body experiences, heightened self-awareness, and altered thought processes. Unpleasant reactions to the drug can occur, especially if the user has been feeling upset, anxious or depressed beforehand. Friendly reassurance is the best help in the event of a 'bad trip'.

As yet, research has not shown that long-term use of LSD produces any physical damage. In the late 1960s there were some newspaper reports claiming that LSD can cause genetic damage. Scientific research has since found no reliable evidence to support this claim. Adverse psychological reactions can occur with LSD, although only rarely are these prolonged or serious. Physical dependence does not occur and psychological dependence is quite rare.

Other hallucinogenic drugs are mescaline, psilocybin, MDA, DMT and phencyclidine (PCP, Angel Dust). These are rarely to be found in the UK.

It is illegal to possess, supply or produce LSD or other hallucinogenic drugs. Hallucinogenic mushrooms containing psychoactive substances are to be found in many areas in the autumn months. The most commonly occurring are the Liberty Cap and Amanita muscaria species, both containing psilocybin. Their effects are somewhat similar to an LSD experience. The main danger of hallucinogenic mushrooms is picking a similar-looking poisonous variety by mistake, such as the Fly Agaric, a common mushroom which is deadly.

The possession of hallucinogenic mushrooms in their natural state is not an offence, but as soon as they are crushed, dried, boiled or otherwise prepared they become classified as a controlled substance which it is illegal to possess or supply to others.

CANNABIS

Cannabis is a drug derived from the plant cannabis sativa. Marijuana, pot, grass, hashish, resin, dope, draw and ganja are other names used to refer to preparations of the plant. Cannabis is most usually smoked together with tobacco rolled up into a cigarette or 'joint'. It can also be smoked in a pipe or put into drinks or food.

The effects of cannabis generally include relaxation, cheerfulness, talkativeness and heightened self-awareness. The majority of users describe their experiences as pleasurable, although psychological distress and confusion have been reported on occasion.

There is no firm evidence that occasional use of cannabis over a long period causes lasting physical or mental damage. However, it has been suggested that cannabis smoking can lead to bronchitis and lung cancer in long-term heavy use.

There is some evidence indicating that regular frequent use of cannabis during pregnancy can increase the risk of premature birth. Tobacco smoking is linked with the birth of smaller and less mature babies and cannabis smoking might have similar effects. Accordingly, it may be advisable not to use cannabis during pregnancy. Cannabis together with alcohol also seems to increase the chance of causing damage to the fetus compared with alcohol alone. For the possible effect of cannabis on fertility, see p. 425.

Cannabis does not produce physical dependence. Regular use can lead to psychological dependence involving desire to continue to use the drug for its pleasurable effects.

It is illegal to cultivate, produce, supply or possess cannabis, or to allow premises to be used for smoking, producing or supplying it.

SOLVENTS

Solvent-sniffing (glue-sniffing) is the inhalation of vapours from organic chemical substances. Those substances most commonly used include glue (contact adhesives), paint-thinners, petrol, dry-cleaning agents, nail varnish, lighter fuel, anti-freeze and propellant gases (in aerosols and fire extinguishers).

The early effects of solvent inhalation are similar to those of alcohol consumption or anaesthesia. Dizziness, confusion, slurring of speech, blurring of vision, and even visual or auditory hallucinations can occur. Repeated or deep inhalations can produce loss of control and unconsciousness. There may be headache and hangover afterwards and some loss of memory concerning what has taken place.

DRUG USE AND PREGNANCY

Please read Pregnancy chapter for information on smoking and alcohol.

If you are pregnant and have been taking any other drugs we strongly urge you to seek a specialist doctor's advice at the earliest opportunity. With opiates, barbiturates, tranquillizers or sedative-type drugs, it is extremely important not to stop taking them suddenly as this can cause fetal distress. Ask your GP to refer you to a doctor or consultant with some specialist knowledge of treatment of drug dependence in pregnancy. It is unwise to try coming off drugs on your own as drug withdrawal increases the risk of miscarriage during the first few months of pregnancy and premature labour in the later stages. Most doctors prefer to carry out drug withdrawal in hospital to allow for close monitoring in case of any adverse effects. A safer form of drug may be substituted for the one you were previously using and this will be reduced in dose at a slow rate (slower than might otherwise be used) to avoid risks to the fetus. If you continue to use opiates, tranquillizers, barbiturates or sedative-type drugs during the later stages of pregnancy, your baby is likely to develop withdrawal symptoms after birth. It is very important that you tell your doctor exactly what drugs you have been taking so that she can provide your baby with whatever treatment may be necessary. If you continue to take drugs after the birth you may be advised to avoid breastfeeding as many drugs can be passed on to the baby in breast milk.

Evidence suggests that there is no long-term damage, including brain-damage, in relation to glue. However, vapour inhalation in industrial situations, involving prolonged and repeated exposure to other solvents such as dry-cleaning agents, has caused liver or kidney damage.

The greatest danger with all solvent use is that of accidents occurring while intoxicated. Using solvents near canals, bridges, railway lines, roads or high places is especially risky. Death can result from passing out as a consequence of sniffing and then choking on vomit, or by squirting gases from aerosols directly into the mouth causing suffocation.

It is not illegal to possess or use solvents; however, it is an offence to sell them to people under eighteen years of age knowing that they intend to inhale them.

GETTING HELP

Information about local drug services can be obtained from **SCODA** (Standing Conference on Drug Abuse – see Resources). Send a large stamped addressed envelope with any request for information. Services offered by agencies range from telephone advice lines to residential treatment facilities and many can help with problems concerning prescribed drug use (such as tranquillizers) as well as illegal drugs.

Your GP may be able to help or can refer you to a psychiatrist or regional drug dependence unit. Community drug problems teams, offering advice and counselling, operate in a number of districts and your GP should know if there is one near you.

Narcotics Anonymous run self-help groups for people with illicit drug problems – along similar lines to Alcoholics Anonymous. Their London office (see Resources) can tell you where the nearest meeting is held or help you to start your own self-help group.

RELEASE offers advice on legal problems arising from drug misuse. They operate a twenty-four-hour emergency phone line.

Drug services have generally ignored the special needs of women. Until very recently residential therapeutic communities and in-patient drug dependence units did not accommodate women together with their children. Taking up this kind of treatment meant making alternative arrangements for the children or even putting them into care. There are now some places which will accommodate children, although these are still rare.

RESOURCES
PUBLICATIONS

ALCOHOL

Camberwell Council on Alcoholism. *Women and Alcohol*. London: Tavistock, 1980. Academic research papers.
Chick, J. and J. **Chick**. *Drinking Problems: Advice and Information for the Individual, Family and Friends*. Edinburgh: Churchill Livingstone, 1984. Practical advice and information for problem drinkers and those around them.
DAWN. *Women and Drinking* (available from DAWN – see Organizations).
McConville, Brigid. *Women Under the Influence*. London: Virago Press, 1983. Includes personal experiences.
MIND. *Women and Alcohol* (available from WHRRIC – see Organizations).
Swallow, Jean (ed.). *Out from Under, Sober Dykes and Our Friends*. San Francisco: Spinsters Ink, 1983. Excellent book, relevant to all women and to all types of addiction.

CIGARETTE SMOKING/NICOTINE

Health Education Council. *Women and Smoking: a Handbook for Action* (available from the Health Education Authority – see Organizations).
Jacobson, Bobbie. *Beating the Ladykillers: Women and Smoking*. London: Pluto Press, 1986.
Jacobson, Bobbie and Amanda **Amos**. 'When Smoke Gets in Your Eyes'. London: British Medical Association/Health Education Council, May 1985.
Seymour, Linda. *Women's Health and Smoking*. WHIC broadsheet, 1982 (available from WHRRIC).
US Department of Health and Human Services. *The Health Consequences of Smoking for Women: a Report of the Surgeon General*. Washington DC: US Government Printing Office, 1980. (Available from the Office on Smoking and Health, Park Building, Rockville, MD 20857, USA.)

MISCELLANEOUS

Blenheim Project. 'How to Help – a Practical Guide for the Friends and Relatives of Drug Users' (available from the Blenheim Project – see below).
Curran, Valerie and Susan **Golombok**. *Bottling it Up*. London: Faber & Faber, 1985.
DAWN. *Women and Heroin and Other Opiates* (available from DAWN – see Organizations).
DuQuesne, T. and J. **Reeves**. *A Handbook of Psychoactive Medicines*. London: Quartet Books, 1982.
Gossop, M. *Living with Drugs*. London: Maurice Temple Smith, 1982.
Institute for the Study of Drug Dependency (ISDD). 'Drug Abuse Briefing' (available from ISDD – see Organizations).
Mothner, Ira and Alan **Wetz**. *How to Get Off Drugs*. London: Penguin Books, 1986.
Parish, Peter. *Medicines – a Guide for Everybody*. 6th rev. ed. London: Penguin Books, 1987.
RELEASE. *Trouble with Tranquillizers* (available from RELEASE – see Organizations).
Women's National Commission. *Stress and Addiction among Women*. 1988 available from the Cabinet Office, London SW1.

SLIDES, FILMS AND VIDEOS

The Ladykillers. Video, 37 mins. Available from Concord Films Council Ltd, 201 Felixstowe Road, Ipswich, Suffolk. Tel: 0473–775754.
The Ladykillers. Video and tape/slide presentation, 12 mins. Available from ASH Scotland, Royal College of Physicians, 9 Queen Street, Edinburgh. Tel: 031–225 4725.
Women and Alcohol. Video, 35 mins. Available from Alcohol Counselling Service, 34 Electric Lane, London SW9 8JT. Tel: 01–737 3579.

ORGANIZATIONS

Al-Anon Family Groups, 61 Great Dover Street, London SE1 4YF. Tel: 01–403 0888.

Alcohol Concern, 305 Gray's Inn Road, London WC1X 8QF. Tel: 01–833 3471.

Alcoholics Anonymous, PO Box 1, Stonebow House, Stonebow, York YO1 2NJ. Tel: 0904–644026/7/8/9.

Alcoholics Anonymous, 11 Redcliffe Gardens, London SW10. Tel: 01–352 9779.

ASH UK (Action on Smoking and Health), Tower House, 5–11 Mortimer Street, London W1. Tel: 01–637 9843. ASH has a number of branches throughout the UK and will give advice on all aspects of smoking.

The Blenheim Project, 7 Thorpe Close, London W10 5XL. Tel: 01–960 5599.

DAWN (Drugs, Alcohol and Women Nationally), DAWN Omnibus Workspace, 39–41 North Road, London N7 9DP. Tel: 01–700 4653. A campaigning organization/pressure group which can give information about services for women in the London area.

Drinkwatchers, c/o Western Hospital, 200 Seagrove Road, London SW6 1RQ. Tel: 01–381 3157. Assessment service: 01–731 6598.

Families Anonymous. Tel: 01–731 8060. Helpline for families who have a member addicted to drugs.

Health Education Authority, Hamilton House, Mabledon Place, London WC1H 9TX. Tel: 01–631 0930.

ISDD (Institute for the Study of Drug Dependence), 1–4 Hatton Place, Hatton Garden, London EC1N 8ND. Tel: 01–430 1991. Library and information service: 01–430 1993.

Narcotics Anonymous, PO Box 417, London SW10 0RN. Tel: 01–351 6794/6066/7.

Northern Ireland Council on Alcohol, 40 Elmwood Avenue, Belfast BT9 6AZ. Tel: 0232–664434.

RELEASE, 169 Commercial Street, London E1 6BW. Tel: 01–377 5905 (during office hours); 01–603 8654 (answering service for emergencies outside office hours).

SCODA (The Standing Conference on Drug Abuse), 1–4 Hatton Place, Hatton Garden, London EC1N 8ND. Tel: 01–430 2341.

Scottish Council on Alcoholism, 147 Blythwood Road, Glasgow G2 4EN. Tel: 041–333 9677.

TRANX UK Ltd, 52a Masons Avenue, Wealdstone, Harrow, Middlesex, HA3 5AH. Tel: 01–427 2065/2827 (answering machine). For help with tranquillizer problems.

Women's Alcohol Centre, 254 St Paul's Road, London N1 2LJ. Tel: 01–226 4581.

Women's Health and Reproductive Rights Information Centre, 52–54 Featherstone Street, London EC1Y 8RT. Tel: 01–251 6580/6332.

WOMEN IN MOTION

Rewritten by
LIZ MERRICK
with help from Maggie Pether

More and more women are enjoying sports and exercise. We can be seen jogging, cycling, swimming, hiking and weight-lifting. We play netball, badminton, football, hockey, tennis and cricket. We take self-defence, keep fit, yoga and gymnastics classes. We are out in the world, becoming visible. Times are changing – women are in motion.

It is only fairly recently that women have started exercising for its own sake. For women in the nineteenth century working long hours in factories, mills and mines, in domestic service or on the land, life was so demanding physically that 'exercise' as such was meaningless. For the middle-class woman, exercise for the most part was considered unladylike – she was kept in idleness, expected to conserve her energies for the duties of being a wife and mother. Today only a few jobs are as physically demanding as those in the nineteenth century. Though many occupations are stressful and emotionally and physically demanding, almost none provides the kind of movement a healthy body and mind need.

Over the last decade we have grown more active, due to the combined effect of the fitness boom, our increasing awareness of the health benefits of exercise, and the way the women's movement has given us the confidence and assertiveness to be seen and heard.

Yet many of us are not taking regular exercise, for there are still obstacles for us to overcome, both internal and external.

EXERCISE, SPORTS – WHAT DO THEY DO FOR US?

Exercise is part of all our lives – whether we climb stairs, walk, carry shopping, or take exercise for pleasure. We move our limbs and use our muscles, for living is moving. Our well-being depends on our being able to get out and about in the world. But how many of us take our bodies for granted, how often do we accept that being out of breath, unable to lift or carry, or unable to stretch or bend is a fact of living? One of the most important reasons for exercising is that *you* can begin to ask your body to do what you want it to do, rather than accepting what your body allows you to do. A variety of regular exercise keeps our bodies in good working order, it increases the strength of our muscles, our stamina or endurance and the mobility of our joints – our suppleness. This means we are less likely to hurt our bodies when we need to do something a little more strenuous than

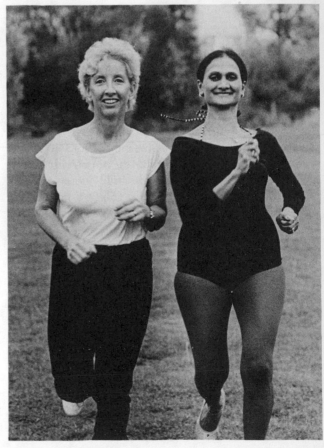

Maggie Murray

usual. There are fewer limitations on what we can do, and day-to-day activities become easier, leaving us feeling more energetic at the end of the day. Posture should improve as the muscles in our trunk strengthen to support the spine, which can prevent or alleviate lower back pain. Many women who take up sport find that they have lighter periods and less menstrual pain as their fitness improves. * Exercise will also help prevent the loss of fitness that so many people assume is an inevitable result of growing older. It may also slow or reverse the loss of minerals, especially calcium, from bones. This will help prevent brittle bones (osteoporosis – see p. 469), which becomes a serious problem for many elderly women. ** Regular exercise improves the efficiency of the circulation, which puts less strain on the heart. It keeps blood pressure down. Overall, exercise considerably improves the quality of our lives by increasing our confidence (especially when we do something we didn't think we could do) as well as making us feel good.

WHAT IS FITNESS?

There are three aspects to overall fitness: stamina, strength and suppleness. Fairly vigorous exercise taken regularly, like cycling or swimming, improves stamina; short and intense exercises, like lifting weights or quick sprints, improves the strength of the muscles we use; and stretching exercises like yoga improve suppleness. Improvement in any of these three areas will come quickly. In fact, the more unfit we are the more quickly we will notice an improvement.

Stamina

If you find yourself getting out of breath quickly and would like to be able to keep going for longer before you need to take a rest, then you need to increase your stamina. Stamina is the most important element of fitness, and the most likely to bring benefits to our lives. Improving stamina improves heart and circulation efficiency, which translated into day-to-day activity means we can exercise harder for longer before becoming out of breath. Stamina exercise is also called aerobic exercise because the muscles use oxygen for their movement. When we take fairly vigorous exercise for fifteen to twenty minutes at least three times a week,

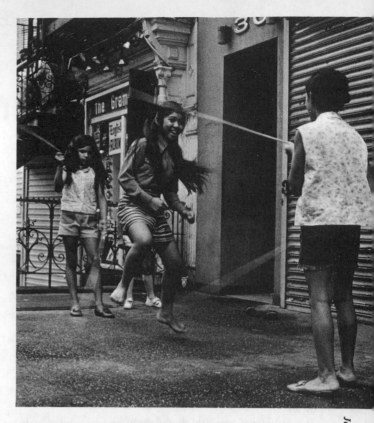

Jean Raisler

changes occur in our muscles which increase their capacity for taking up and using oxygen. In this way the oxygen we breathe is used more efficiently. The changes in muscle demand in turn affect the heart-rate – the beat rises much less, but the heart increases the amount it expels with each beat. The heart has less to do to achieve the same output and we keep going for longer.

The heart-rate or pulse is a good measure of stamina. By taking your pulse you can monitor your improvement; as you exercise you should find there is a reduction in the rate, which will continue as you train.

Strength

If you find you can't lift or carry, then it is muscle strength you need to develop. Strong biceps and triceps in the arms allow us to carry more and to perform everyday tasks with less effort and more independence. Sound leg muscles help us defend ourselves and get us where we want to go. For a muscle to increase in strength it needs to be exercised. If you ask muscles to lift heavy weights up and down you will increase the strength of those muscles. Short, sharp exercises are used to develop muscle strength. They are called anaerobic exercise because oxygen is not required for the muscle movement. Glycogen stored in the muscle is burned for energy. Strength training should be undertaken in short, intense bouts; the muscle contraction must be short or we can overdo it and raise our blood pressure too much. Briefly contracting a muscle between eight and ten times a day is enough to help strengthen it. Each exercise has an effect only on the muscle involved, so you need to do a range of strength exercises to keep your body in good condition.

*Lynn Fitzgerald, personal communication to Jill Rakusen. However, very intense training can adversely affect ovarian function. For example, about half the women who run more than 60 miles a week have amenorrhoea (no periods) for many months at a time; likewise half of professional ballet dancers (see Barbara Drinkwater, ed. *Female Endurance Athletes. Human Kinetics.* Illinois, 1986). Amenorrhoea also occurs in some swimmers, tennis players and cyclists, but the prevalence in relation to the intensity of training has not been examined. Normally, periods return once training is reduced.

**However, in the case of athletes or dancers who develop amenorrhoea as a result of their intense training, the effect on the bones could be the reverse, since decreased ovarian activity increases the risk of osteoporosis. Several studies have found reduced bone density in the spines of athletes with amenorrhoea. Dr Barbara Drinkwater, of the Pacific Medical Center, Seattle, Washington, has studied this problem and concludes: 'An awareness is needed among physicians and athletes that some amenorrheic athletes may have a decrease in bone density.'

Suppleness

If you find difficulty in stretching and bending then you may need to work on your suppleness. If we don't use our joints they stiffen up and everyday movements can become difficult and sometimes painful. Improvements to mobility can and should be done gradually – put all your joints through a full range of movement once a day. Don't push your joints to extremes, it is possible to make joints so flexible that they become liable to dislocate.

Mental Health

Getting fit is not just about the physical effects on our bodies but also about the tremendous effects it can have on our confidence and self-esteem. Doing things for ourselves gives us a sense of achievement, it is a way of taking control of our bodies. It feels good to be able to keep going when we want to, to lift and hold heavy things, to undo that jar lid which always gets stuck. Many of us have a low opinion of what we can do. We do not try things, sometimes because we have not considered exercise as anything to do with us, or because we are frightened we will 'make fools of ourselves'; sometimes we believe we just can't manage. But women who have taken the risk and started exercising or taken up sport report a sense of surprise that they were able to do so well. Their confidence has been boosted, not just in sport and exercise, but in all aspects of their lives.

> Now that I do run regularly, I notice that I have much more energy and generally feel alive. Being fit, healthy and feeling muscles develop is also important . . . The feeling of well-being becomes a way of life . . . I feel really happy after a run, calm inside and much more able to cope with my problems and the stresses of every-day life and relationships. I always have the same feeling after a good run: that I'm strong and OK, that I can cope with anything and I'll be alright no matter what happens. [1]

Far from being an extra drain on our energies, exercise can bring us alive. Regular exercise makes us feel refreshed, calmer and less tired to take on the demands of day-to-day living.

> *If I go out jogging or swimming, it seems somehow to restore my energy levels, it helps bring me alive so in the evenings I don't get so tired.*

Not only do we feel more energy and confidence, we may also find that exercise helps us to sleep better – maybe because we are finding an outlet for some of our tension. When our minds become tense our bodies do also. As a result we get headaches and stomach aches, our breathing becomes restricted and our heart beats faster. Our bodies express the tension that so often we cannot express to the world. Through exercise we connect the mind and body. In using our body we can begin to release some of the tension we have built up during the day.

You may not be 'flying' after a run or swim, lifting weights or whatever you choose to do, but you will invariably feel better than you did before, calmer, less tired and more refreshed.

GETTING STARTED

Now you've had the pep talk how do you decide on the exercise for you? The box overleaf rates popular activities for their effect on the three aspects of fitness. You may decide you want to work on one aspect in particular or you may want to work on all three aspects at once. Remember that stamina is one of the most important aspects of fitness, because of its effect on our circulation.

OPTIONS

- Pick an activity that gives you pleasure, or that you enjoy. If you don't find it fun, you'll end up giving up.
- Suit your exercise to your lifestyle. If you do a lot of sitting during the day pick an activity that gets you moving. If, on the other hand, you are a physically active person already, choose an exercise that will relax and stretch.
- Watch out for stereotypes – that certain races, body types or disabilities mean that we 'can't do this' or 'naturally excel at that'. Never restrict your options based on other people's say-so.
- Some of us find it reasonably easy to be motivated alone, we prefer performing only for ourselves. Others of us need the push and encouragement of a group to get going and stay at it. Some of us like team activities in which the social aspect – playing together – is very important.
- We can exercise in our own homes, it's cheaper and we can do it at the most convenient time. Stretching, strengthening exercises, yoga, dance, karate techniques, skipping, running on the spot can all be done in your home. Alternatively, you may want to be out and about. You can do this on your own or you could join classes, groups, or get together with friends. You could cycle, swim, jog, play badminton, football, go hiking or dancing. Other people may help keep you motivated and provide a social network. If you can't find the sort of group or class which suits you, you could start one yourself.
- Unfortunately, physical safety is always a concern for women. Walk, jog or run when possible with a friend or where there are a lot of people . . . or with the dog!
- Choose an exercise that isn't too demanding, one where you can set the pace. If you haven't taken regular exercise for a few years, it could take you several weeks to get your body to reasonable fitness. If you choose an exercise that you're not fit enough for you'll get disheartened or even give up.

VARIOUS FORMS OF EXERCISE: THEIR EFFECTS ON OUR BODIES

	Stamina	Suppleness	Strength		Stamina	Suppleness	Strength
Badminton	●●	●●●	●●	Hill walking	●●●	●	●●
Canoeing	●●●	●●	●●●	Jogging	●●●●	●●	●●
Climbing Stairs	●●●	●	●●	Judo	●●	●●●●	●●
Cricket	●	●●	●	Rowing	●●●●	●●	●●●●
Cycling (hard)	●●●●	●●	●●●	Sailing	●	●●	●
Dancing (ballroom)	●	●●●	●	Squash	●●●	●●●	●●
Dancing (disco)	●●●	●●●●	●	Swimming (hard)	●●●●	●●●●	●●●●
Digging (garden)	●●●	●●	●●●●	Tennis	●●	●●●	●●
Football	●●●	●●●	●●●	Walking (briskly)	●●	●	●
Golf	●	●●	●	Weight-lifting	●	●	●●●●
Gymnastics	●●	●●●●	●●●	Yoga	●	●●●●	●

● No real effect   ●● Beneficial effect   ●●● Very good effect   ●●●● Excellent effect

Source: 'Keeping Fit', *Which?*, February 1984.

Swimming

This is probably the most full-body and least physically stressful exercise going, once you know how to do it.* Non-swimmers may have to overcome fear of water, which is sometimes difficult, but the rewards are great. The water buoys you up, taking weight off aching backs, arthritic hips, bad knees, tired feet, weakened legs. Regular swimming exercises a wide variety of muscles and improves your circulation. Jean started swimming with a group of friends:

It's fun and I find the water very relaxing, yet I feel like I've had quite a lot of exercise without getting exhausted.

Walking

Walking is excellent for all women who can use their legs. It will improve the circulation, increase muscle and bone strength and is often a good time to think and calm the nerves. Climb stairs instead of taking lifts or escalators, go to the shops on foot, catch the bus two stops on from where you usually catch it. Start slowly and build up.

Cycling and Jogging

These are for those of us who are a little fitter. Combined with a few basic exercises for suppleness and strength, they are effective ways of reaching overall fitness.

Team Sports

Some team sports give your body a well-rounded work-out, some don't. Basketball, football, and hockey are great for

*However, it needs to be combined with weight-bearing exercise in order to maintain bone strength (see Osteoporosis, p. 469).

It is generally agreed that to improve our fitness we need to do fifteen minutes exercising at least three times a week. When you start this sort of programme you will see improvements quickly. But fitness can also be lost quickly; most improvements you make will be lost in a matter of weeks if you stop. If you have to stop for some reason, you just can't leap in where you left off. Ease yourself back in slowly.

general body strength and stamina; they are strenuous so you will need to build up to them. Volleyball and rounders (softball) are less vigorous. If you play a sport where you stand around waiting for the ball to come to you, combine this with some exercises that will improve your stamina.

EXERCISE AND WOMEN WITH DISABILITIES

For 'disabled' women to participate in sport and exercise we all need to change our ideas about the nature of sport and exercise and 'disability'. If we have a noticeable disability like being confined to a wheelchair, or if we lack sight or hearing, we are rarely accepted in daily life, never mind in the sports centre or exercise class.

Kim White is confined to a wheelchair but is a world-class athlete – she competed in the 1984 International Games for the Disabled in New York. She became interested in sport after becoming disabled and in spite of being successful at the events she tried she discovered what a struggle it was to be accepted:

> There are two battles – we're fighting the fact that we're women in sport, and the fact that we're disabled and have got wheelchairs.[2]

Differently-abled women are finding support from each other, working out their exercise needs together:

> I am very interested in sport, including canoeing, swimming, archery and various others. In my opinion not enough handicapped people know about the facilities that there are, or could be for this type of activity. Some people think that there is too much risk involved in such sports as canoeing and swimming, but providing that the disability is not too severe and correct coaching can be obtained there is no more risk for the disabled person than for the non-disabled.[3]

There are many organizations which exist for disabled people involved in sport and exercise at all levels (see Resources). Alongside this there is an increased emphasis on integration. Many public buildings, including sports centres and leisure facilities, are starting to provide full disabled access and some local authorities have paid advisers on disability issues to try to ensure that disabled people's views are represented. For many women who are disabled it is important to compete alongside able-bodied women:

> Not only do sports provide exercise, but also another way in which I can meet and compete with people as an equal. In canoeing I have the same advantages as able-bodied people as I only have to use my body above the waist and in some respects I have the added advantage of strength in my arms due to continued use of crutches and wheelchairs. I now attend an ordinary canoe club where I find my disability doesn't limit me at all. It becomes more of a challenge for me to do ambitious things.[4]

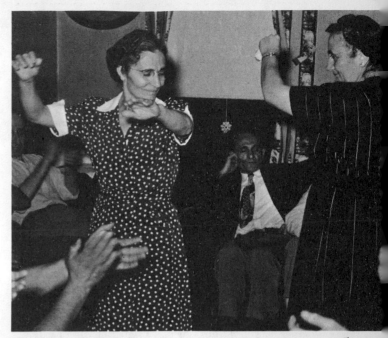

Varkey Sohigian

Many of us will lower our expectations of our bodies as we grow older, accepting stiffening muscles and joints as inevitable. 'What do you expect at your age?' How many times has that been said to you? It is important that we challenge these beliefs – many older women have taken up regular exercise with enthusiasm, to the benefit of their bodies and their confidence: Rose and a few friends set up a keep fit group in north London four years ago, and it's still going strong:

> *You should hear us sometimes, we've got a nice crowd, we have a laugh and a joke while we're exercising. I've had two artificial hip joints and I've found that going to the group once a week has been really beneficial to me, it's helped get the use of my limbs back again. I'm much more mobile than a few years ago. I've just started to play short tennis, it's like tennis with a soft ball and with a smaller court. Going to the group has given me a new lease of life – I swear by it!*

EXERCISE AND GROWING OLDER

Growing older does not mean we have to sit back and accept a loss in flexibility, muscle strength and aerobic power. Exercise can fend off many of the difficulties we associate with growing older. Typically, bones begin to lose their mass when we reach the age of forty. It has now been shown that exercise can help stop this decline and can therefore help 'brittle bones'. Being active will keep joints supple, although the first movements at the beginning of a workout may be more painful than in younger years. We can walk, swim, jog, lift weights, take up a new sport.

OVERCOMING OBSTACLES

For most of us, taking up exercise is not just a simple matter of choosing the sort of activity that suits us; there are real problems which keep us from becoming and staying physically active. It is surely significant that twice as many men play sport as women – it's women who create men's leisure.

Our attitude to sport and exercise is formed at a very early age. Even as babies we begin to learn that it's our role in life to be passive, docile and unadventurous, helping others rather than doing things for our own satisfaction. As young girls we quickly learn that it is OK to play hopscotch but not football, skipping but not running, hopping but not jumping: in short, grace and style, not strength and speed.

Some sports are just not considered 'natural' for us; we are no good at football because we are girls, not because we've never had a chance to acquire skills in this sport. Ted Croker, former Secretary of the Football Association sums it up:

We just don't like males and females playing together. I like feminine girls. Anyway, it's just not natural.[5]

These ideas about what is 'natural' are reinforced at school where particular sports and games are rigidly defined as either for girls or boys. School is the place where we gain our first experience of organized sport and exercise, and for many of us it is an experience we wish to forget:

Sport at school just made me feel uncomfortable with my body. For PE we had to wear navy blue knickers and T-shirts, which I hated because I was overweight. When we were in the gym the boys stood around and watched, making remarks about our bodies and our expertise. I hated it and did all I could to get out of it. It wasn't until many years later that I began to think of exercise as something I could do – and enjoy.

As we reach puberty we become increasingly aware of the tremendous pressure there is to conform to 'feminine' behaviour. Under this pressure, our interest in exercise declines and for many of us our participation is often reduced to being literally on the sidelines, watching TV or cheering others' efforts on the sports field.

In adult life we generally have much less time available for leisure than men. Those of us with child-care responsibilities are almost constantly 'on call'. Child-care doesn't fit into a conventional working day, making it difficult to plan any leisure time in advance. We earn less money than men, many of us cannot afford to join a club, or pay sporting facility charges. Those of us who are married or living with men may be financially dependent. Our leisure tends to be a low priority in the household budget (if it is one at all) whereas there is a much wider acceptance that men have a right to personal spending money. We do not all have cars (far from it), public transport is often infrequent and expensive and the streets at night are unsafe and badly lit.* Given these facts, a trip to the local sports centre or a jog through the streets may not be straightforward or easy.

When we get to the sports centre, swimming pool, weight rooms or wherever, we often find ourselves greeted by the overwhelming presence of men. Sports centres are still dominated by men both as managers and users. Many of us find this presence intimidating and would like more

space for women. Even the Sports Council has recognized that there is cause for concern:

Studies of sports centre users show women outnumbered 2 to 1 by men . . . several studies suggest that more women wish to take part and would do so if various constraints were overcome.[6]

It is important to remember that women are not a homogeneous group and older women, black women, disabled women and lesbians, for example, will have differing needs. However, these needs often go unrecognized:

In the sports I do, people sometimes treat me like I've got a double handicap – being disabled and a woman. You should hear some of the things people shout at me when I'm doing a marathon; they think it's alright for a woman to do sport in order to stay petite, or something, but not to do it for its own sake, and to train your body to do what you want it to. I was never really encouraged to do strength events when I was younger, probably because people thought it would be unfeminine. That's meant I've had a lot of ground to catch up.[7]

There is an argument used by sports providers which says that women are just not using what is provided for them. It is not enough to provide facilities if we can't get to them, can't get the children looked after, feel threatened or vulnerable in public places, or find the times inconvenient. When do we hear arguments about safe, cheap public transport, or street lighting as a way of helping us to use sports facilities? We need to make our voices heard – so let's tell them how it is!

WHAT WE CAN DO

Though what we have said so far indicates that there is a long way to go, things are beginning to change. We must make sure that we are actively involved in those changes, making our demands heard.

Throughout the country (though less in rural areas) there has been a general increase in sporting and exercise facilities and many sports centres now offer women-only sessions and a crèche facility, as well as sessions for those new to a particular sport. In 1985 the Greater London Council held a day for women only in centres throughout the Greater London area, and for some of us this proved to be a way back into sport and exercise we had enjoyed at school. This idea of being able to sample different sports in a non-threatening, social atmosphere is one which is being taken up by other local authorities. If your local centre hasn't taken such a step – suggest it. If they've already held a one-off women-only day suggest that they make it a regular event.

Our confidence in taking our own initiatives in sport and

*See Chapter 10 for ideas on how to make travelling safer for women.

exercise is also increasing. On a national level there is the **Women's Sports Foundation** (WSF), formed in 1984 to combat the dominance of men in sport and exercise and to recognize

> the needs of many women; we distinguish the special requirements that we all have because of differences in such areas as age, racial origins, class, sexuality, disability and religion.

The WSF (see Resources) is a rapidly growing voluntary network of women from all over the country; there is a monthly newsletter which encourages individual members to make suggestions and relate their experiences. They are particularly keen to monitor all cases of discrimination so you might find their support useful in any battles you have to fight in your area.

Another group for women whose emphasis is a bit different is **Outdoor Women** (see Resources), which produces a newsletter and contact sheet to keep women in touch with each other. The group enables women to experience some of the more unusual sports such as cross-country skiing and canoeing, as well as walking, cycling and mountaineering. Because the group has a stock of equipment for hire at nominal fees and a commitment to a sliding scale of charges according to income they hope to maximize the participation of all women in their events.

Locally, things are improving too. There are many ways as an individual or as a small group that we can get local councils or other statutory organizations to work for us, which is after all what they're supposed to do. If you don't feel up to taking on your local sports centre manager single-handed, to talk about women-only sessions or crèche facilities, then enlist some support. Many local authorities have funded women's centres or have their own women's units. These should provide a more supportive atmosphere in which to put your points across and get support for your demands. Adult education classes are another possibility. Usually, you can persuade your education authority to run a class if they think there is enough demand – so you'll need to collect names – but if you are successful it's a reasonably cheap way of exercising or learning a new sport, in a friendly, non-competitive atmosphere.

Exercise should also be a concern of your health authority, most of which will have a health education unit (see p. 627). If you can't get an adult education class together, ask your health education officer what they are doing to promote exercise for women: they'll probably be only too glad to hear your ideas. Community centres are interested in involving local people in local issues – if there's nowhere you can exercise that's easily accessible and cheap, talk to them about using their facilities. Women's sport often grows out of already existing groups of women who meet regularly for some other reason. In Northamptonshire members of the Kettering Mothers' Club decided to take up rounders. Seven years on there is the Kettering and District Rounders League, with a twenty-four-team membership.

TAKING CARE OF OURSELVES

- Always warm up before you start exercising. When we're cold, stiff or out of shape we can tear a ligament or tendon (which can take a long time to heal). Warm-up exercises can usually double as suppleness and strength routines. If you want to start an activity that puts a lot of strain on joints be sure that the surrounding muscles are strong (and co-ordinated) enough to support them; otherwise there will be trouble. Work up to exercising at least three times a week, for fifteen to twenty minutes. If you have decided to start jogging, begin with a mixture of walking and jogging. Walk briskly for five minutes, jog for thirty seconds, then carry on alternating walking and jogging for a total of ten minutes, ending up with a brisk five-minute walk. As you develop your routine, gradually shorten the first walk and extend the bouts of jogging. If you have just started swimming, begin by swimming widths. Swim until you feel a little puffed, then stop. Gradually increase the number of widths without a breather, then move to swimming lengths.
- Taper off any period of vigorous exercise slowly. Never flop down after an energetic run, you need time for your heartbeat, breathing and temperature to adjust; you need to keep your blood flowing well in order to remove the wastes that have accumulated in the muscles during the run and bring them fresh supplies of oxygen and glucose. Sudden relaxation may make you dizzy and nauseous.
- Don't linger outside if you have been exercising in the cold – that will cause undue stiffness. Put on something warm.
- Don't eat heavily before or after exercising. The stomach and intestines require a large blood supply to digest food, and exercise diverts blood from the digestive tract, to the muscles you are using. These organs' attempts to function actively with less blood than they need may cause pain.
- Wear clothes that are loose or flexible for full range of motion. For activities which make you sweat, cotton next to the skin is good because it is soft and absorbent.
- If you are walking, jogging or running, invest in a proper pair of running shoes with cushioned soles. You can hurt your calf muscles if you don't have shoes which absorb the shock.
- When exercising *stop* if you are uncomfortably breathless, you get chest or leg pains, your heart is racing or beating irregularly, you come out in a cold sweat, or you feel dizzy or faint.
- Expect some stiffness! If you're really pushing your muscles they are bound to hurt the following day(s). However, don't pamper yourself and stop, the best remedy is moderate exercise.
- If you are trying to recover from illness, moderate exercise together with wholesome food are an essential

part of any get-well programme. Do not go in for *excessive* training, though. As immunologist Dr Lynn Fitzgerald, herself an Olympic champion athlete, says:

> Moderate exercise appears to boost the immune system, but the extreme stress of excessive training appears to work the other way.[8]

REMEMBER

If you have or suspect any physical limitation, consider some kind of health check-up before beginning an exercise programme.

SO WHAT DO WE WANT?

We have talked a lot about the prejudices, problems and struggles faced by all of us if we want to take a full part in exercise and sport. That is only realistic but we must never let realism stop us from demanding our ideals. We want exercise and sports facilities in every area with equal access for all of us whether black, white, young, old, disabled, lesbian, heterosexual. We want safe areas, more leisure time, better pay, more and better childcare provision. We may not get everything we want today, or even tomorrow, but we owe it to ourselves to make sure that we are in there fighting, voicing our demands and refusing to be silent and inactive.

NOTES

1. Liz Sloan and Ann Kramer. *Running. The Women's Handbook.* London: Pandora Press, 1985, p. 6.
2. Ibid., p. 20.
3. Jo Campling (ed.). *Images of Ourselves: Women with Disabilities Talking.* London: Routledge and Kegan Paul, 1981, p. 6.
4. Ibid., p. 7.
5. Quoted by Lady Howe in 'A Little Too Strenuous for Women?' International Conference on Women in Sport, London, Central Council for Physical Recreation, 1978.
6. *Sport in the Community: the Next Ten Years*, Sports Council, 1982, p. 28.
7. Denise Smith quote in 'Women and Sport', *Sport and Leisure* (Sports Council Magazine), 1985.
8. Dr Fitzgerald, of St George's Hospital Medical School, London, is currently researching into this phenomenon further (*Immunology Today*, November 1988). Unfortunately we are not yet in a position to say precisely how much exercise might adversely affect the immune system. However, it is valuable to remember that intense stress (whether mental or physical) can have far-reaching effects on our immune system (see for example Cancer in Chapter 25). Again, the best approach is moderation.

RESOURCES
ORGANIZATIONS

BBS (British Blind Sport), Julie Whiting, 15B Bell Lane, Byfield, Northamptonshire. Tel: 0327–62214.
British Sports Association for the Disabled, 202 Glen House, 200–208 Tottenham Court Road, London W1P 9LA. Tel: 01–631 3735.
National Association of Swimming Clubs for the Handicapped, Rosemary Leeson, 84 Botley Road, Park Gate, Southampton S03 7BA. Tel: 04895–89185.
Outdoor Women, c/o London Women's Centre, Wesley House, 4 Wild Court, London WC2B 5AU
RADAR (Royal Association for Disability and Rehabilitation), 25 Mortimer Street, London W1N 8AB. Tel: 01–637 5400.
The Sports Council, 16 Upper Woburn Place, London WC1H 0QP. Tel: 01–388 1277.
Women's Sports Foundation, c/o London Women's Centre, Wesley House, 4 Wild Court, London WC2B 5AU. Tel: 01–831 7863 (answering machine).

ALTERNATIVE AND COMPLEMENTARY APPROACHES TO HEALTH AND HEALING*

Rewritten by
JILL RAKUSEN

MEDICINE

Grandma sleeps with
my sick
                grand-
pa so she
can get him
during the night
medicine
to stop
  the pain
    In
  the morning
    clumsily
      I
    wake
      them
Her eyes
look at me
from under-
            neath
        his withered
        arm
          The
        medicine
          is all
            in
        her long
          un-
              braided
                  hair.
© ALICE WALKER, 1968

Many women today are excited by a compelling range of healing methods which complement and challenge conventional medicine and broaden our options for health care. Some such methods, like massage, herbal medicine and visualization, are traditional female healing practices

in use for centuries. Women have used them in their simplest forms, soothing and caring for members of their families and communities, applying herb poultices to wounds, assisting one another during labour and birth, attending to people through long illnesses and handling this knowledge down from mother to daughter. In our culture a cool flannel for a headache, a massage for an aching back or a kiss to a child's bruised knee are simple examples of how we communicate positive healing energy; our confidence

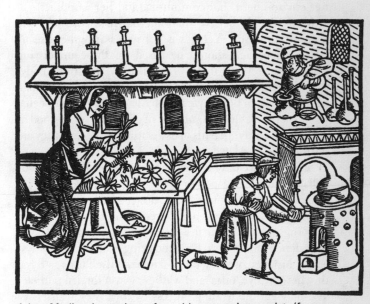

A late Medieval woodcut of an abbess as pharmacist. (from *A History of Women in Medicine*, K. C. Hurd-Mead)

*The term 'alternative' presents us with something of a problem, since it carries with it the implication that the norm is allopathy (the orthodox medicine of our Western culture) and anything else has to be seen as 'other' – and therefore somehow lesser. As feminists we are well aware of how such arrogant assumptions permeate our society: so often, for example, males are the norm, and females the 'other', with disastrous consequences for women (as Simone de Beauvoir so elegantly exposes in her classic book *The Second Sex*). By using the term 'alternative' it is not our intention to imply that orthodox medicine is necessarily better than other approaches. However, we are faced with the inescapable fact at present that in the UK it dominates health-care thinking and practice. We hope that this chapter might contribute to changes in that dynamic.

that we can make it better has a calming effect. The very fact that people think generously and kindly towards others is an important step in the healing process.

I think in terms of chicken soup and ice cubes. As a child I felt so reassured when my mother or grandmother cared for me. I felt so good lying in bed. The power of mother as healer, the oldest mode of care, can't be transformed into the setting of a doctor's surgery.

Some of us are using these methods alone, others in combination with (i.e. complementary to) conventional medicine. They can help us to stay healthy when we are well, cure some illnesses and enable us to live more comfortably with diseases for which there are no known cures. They have often helped where drugs and/or surgery could not. Finding and using these 'unorthodox' approaches has given us insights into their possibilities, powers and limitations.

HOLISM

Holistic health is based both on the idea that the body, mind, emotions and spirit form an integrated whole and on an understanding of the connectedness of the individual to her environment, her community and her world.

Many people believe that 'alternative medicine' is by definition holistic. Yet this is not necessarily the case. A holistic approach should be based on three underlying assumptions. First, that we are healthy when our body/mind/emotions/spirit exist in a dynamically balanced state of well-being. Though we are physically made up of cells, tissues, organs, etcetera, no part of us can be understood as an isolated entity; all parts of us are interconnected, they are harmoniously related.

Secondly, we have a great capacity for self-healing. Our cells are always engaged in the process of self-renewal, for our bodies continuously break down and build up structures, with tissues and organs replacing their cells in an ongoing process (with the exception of brain cells). We experience the physical body repairing itself in many ways, as, for instance, when scraped skin heals itself in a few days, or when the eye 'cries' and washes away a foreign particle. We may aid the healing process by means of a variety of approaches and techniques, some of which are discussed in this chapter.

Thirdly, in the broadest sense, our interactions with our family, community and world affect and shape our health. Positive, loving, supportive relationships with our family and friends help us keep healthy and give us opportunities to nurture and heal others and to receive love and nurturance which strengthen us. Our health also depends on our larger social, economic, political and ecological environment, which affects us through what we can afford to buy and live in, the nutritional content of our foods, the potential dangers of various products we are exposed to, the energy sources we use, the air we breathe and the educational resources available to us. It is as crucial to try to achieve a balance between the individual and her surroundings as it is to balance body, mind, emotions and spirit. *

The development of a truly holistic approach to health care is therefore in its infancy. In particular, the socio-political dimension remains unrecognized by most alternative and allopathic practitioners, while the mind/body/emotional/spirit connection is similarly lacking among most allopathic – and some alternative – practitioners. †

OUR ROLE IN BECOMING HEALED**

Healing comes from within. Every culture evolves a set of remedies that are given for dis-ease: some are thought to 'cure', while others comfort, take away pain, overcome dysfunction or disability. But no remedy, in and of itself, will restore good health. [2]

While all practitioners have the potential to bring healing qualities to the therapeutic relationship, and some have almost tangible healing powers, no practitioner is solely responsible for healing us. We ourselves play a significant role. We may have to change habits – the way we eat, the way we move, even the way we think. It is best to learn as much as we can about the method we choose. Understanding the terms the practitioner uses can make us more active participants in our care.

But while sound health practices can promote well-being and be a source of pleasure in their own right, they do not *guarantee* longevity or freedom from illness. The words 'heal' and 'cure' are not synonymous. Sometimes no cures exist for particular diseases, yet people feel 'healed', i.e. able to reconcile themselves to, accept and live with the effects of asthma, polio or even a terminal illness. Illness can provide opportunities for self-examination, growth and change.

I was in my forty-fourth year when I began experiencing what I called 'fatigue'. Weeks of good

---

*For example, Joanna Macy, a teacher, meditation instructor and organizer for social change, believes that deep despair about nuclear war keeps many of us from working effectively against it. [1] She runs workshops in which people go through the process of acknowledging this despair with each other and feeling it as fully as possible. As a result, many become re-energized, reconnect with others and are moved to greater commitment and social action. In the UK, an organization called Interhelp (see Resources for chapter 10) runs similar 'despair workshops'.

†The recently-formed British Holistic Medical Association (BHMA – see Resources) does, however, represent an attempt by some doctors to redress the balance, but the BHMA has yet to demonstrate its commitment to an understanding of socio-political considerations as a whole, and of feminist issues in particular.

**See also 'Self-healing', p. 87.

nights' rest did not change my stiffness and pain on arising. I had a three-year-old daughter, two teenage sons, a husband and a part-time job; I loved them all; I had no time to be ill or feel pain. When I found myself holding the wall as well as the bannister to creep down the stairs one step at a time, I had to admit to myself that something was wrong. My wrists and fingers hurt; my elbows, knees and ankles; my back, legs and neck. An orthopaedic surgeon told me that I had osteoarthritis.

Now I had to allow myself the luxury of time for exercise classes; a regime of exercise and aspirin soon made life more possible. I still only resentfully recognized that I probably would never be completely pain-free again, would never again feel that careless strength and flexibility which so informed my body in my first forty years. And for the last four years serious back problems have prevented my exercising as I used to; now I must more often live with pain. Some days the distance from car to shop or bed to bathroom seems the longest and most painful ten miles I could ever walk. Nevertheless, some days are better than others. I have learned to rest on the bad days, and to insist on some daily rest even on the good days. Good physical therapy is helping my back; I may be able to return soon to exercise.

Most important, in seeking to understand why I denied the pain so adamantly when I first felt it, I began psychotherapy and learned how forcefully I had been denying emotional pain. My life is qualitatively different now – and better, even though lived with pain – as a result of my re-evaluations of how I feel about myself, my goals, and my relations with others.

In the words of a woman who has since died of cancer:

A lot of people think dying suddenly in their sleep is a great blessing. I've realized that all I learn while I'm dying is important; dying suddenly would be like reading a good book and leaving out a very important part. I'm not for exaggerating: of course I do take pills to make myself more comfortable . . . but I don't feel pain is wrong. I don't feel it's out of the flow. It's hard – like childbirth.

Many alternative approaches present healing as taking place with the help of some form of *energy* coming from a source within ourselves; from both within and without; or from a god, goddess, or universal being, for example. See 'Healing' below.

The process of becoming healed is not necessarily easy: the shift in outlook that is often required can be quite painful, and it can seem a lot easier to become a 'patient' under doctor's orders and accept the antibiotics or whatever.

I went through a whole range of different therapies at first, and then gradually came to the idea that, although my relationship with the therapist was important, more important still was my relationship with my illness: it was part of me and I had to own it. Although ultimately this has been the key to my success, this process of owning – of integration – has at times been excruciatingly painful.

In addition, there is the possibility of 'healing crises', where you may get worse, or develop other symptoms, before you get better.*

Most of the many 'alternative' approaches to health care require our involvement in the healing process. We now examine a selection of them in turn, before discussing problems with alternative practitioners in general, and finding and choosing one.

First, we look at healing as such, not least because this is the most widely practised 'alternative medicine' in the UK,† but also because of its strong, female-dominated heritage, and because of what it can teach us about health, healing, ourselves, others and the world.

HEALING

There are many different approaches to healing. For example, it can involve contact ('contact healing', 'laying on of hands', 'therapeutic touch'), and/or prayer, meditation or visualization. The healer does not need to be present for healing (i.e. 'absent healing') to take place. The term 'faith healing', though commonly used, is misleading as it suggests that faith on the part of the person being healed is necessary. However, believing in its value, or being receptive to it is an advantage (this may be related to the 'placebo effect'), and many healers believe that the person's cooperation and commitment to getting better are essential.

There are many different theories about healing, too. However, most healers would attribute the 'energy' they use to something beyond themselves.** Most healers, too, emphasize the importance of 'compassionate, unconditional love' going from healer to person to be healed. This seems to create brainwave patterns in both healer and

---

*This concept can, of course, be a let-out for unscrupulous therapists, who can use it to justify their treatment whatever the outcome. See also 'Some Problems with Alternative Practitioners . . .', p. 101.

†It is estimated that there are over 20,000 healers in the UK, according to Fulder and Munro (see Resources).

**Though research is limited because of medicine's traditional antipathy towards healing, there is some tangible evidence for the apparent powers of healers. See, for example, books by Inglis and West, and MacManaway listed in Resources. It is also worth bearing in mind that the medical profession's ability to ascertain clearly the effects of its own methods is somewhat hampered by its historical lack of recognition of healers' activities, as is illustrated by the noted healer Harry Edwards.[3]

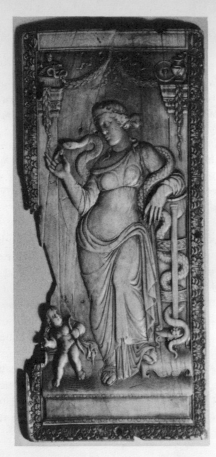

Ivory carving of Hygieia, ancient deity of health and healing.

recipient that are conducive to healing, e.g. see MacManaway in Resources. Healers can mobilize our own healing forces.

Healing is a worldwide, ancient tradition, in which women have played a highly significant part. Mary Chamberlain, for example, in *Old Wives' Tales* (see Resources), examines this history from a white European point of view. Black American women writers have recently been articulating their indebtedness to the crucial role of their female ancestors in ensuring the survival of the arts of healing and conjure . . . and hence of the spiritual well-being and survival of black people. Alice Walker's role in reviving general interest in the work of Zora Neale Hurston is of great importance in this connection.[4] Here, Uma speaks from the perspective of a black woman living in the UK:

> Unfortunately, when the colonizers/missionaries/ imperialist invaders came to our countries they brought with them their own medicines and most of them had contempt for any that were not their own. These invaders also had negative ideas about versions of the Supernatural other than their own Christian concepts. Since the medicines of Black people mostly included elements of traditional religious beliefs, they were condemned by the missionaries who quickly dominated the people of the land in many respects. Slowly, local culture and customs gave way to new teachings. Laws were often passed supporting Christian values, these laws quickly undermined the practice of traditional medicines (including traditional approaches to Healing).[5]

It is ironic that healing, practised by Jesus of Nazareth, was forced to go underground by the Christian Church. Many healers, the majority of whom were women, have been persecuted and burned as witches as a result. While healing is no longer illegal (though only since 1952), medicine has rendered it less and less acceptable – at least to the dominant culture – and the Christian establishment has continued to play a negative role in more recent years as well.* But healing remains a strong component of many people's lives, particularly in working-class communities.[6]

Some people, perhaps many, feel not only sceptical about healing, but possibly also angry and disgusted at the way that well-known spiritual healing centres such as Lourdes can leave people feeling beyond hope when the hoped-for miracle does not materialize.[7]

> *I'll never forget passing through Lourdes on a visit to the Pyrenees, and seeing shops making a mint out of 'pilgrims' – one, literally with a sign up selling 'Religion'. It just confirmed my antipathy towards religion, and made it all the harder to see what spirituality was, or could be, about for me.*

Yet healing, in responsible hands, is not about attracting pilgrims, as we discuss below. And sceptics may be reassured that healers are increasingly taking part in research projects, including a costly and ambitious project set up by the Confederation of Healing Organizations (CHO) to be run within the NHS (although the CHO has itself had to find the funds to do this).

SPIRITUAL HEALING

> Spiritual healing is the healing of the sick in body, mind or spirit by divine energy obtained by attunement through prayer and meditation.
> (NATIONAL FEDERATION OF SPIRITUAL HEALERS)

Spiritual healers believe that they act as a channel for a healing force from a spiritual source. Some healers call this source God, or *prana*, for example, others – spiritualists – heal through contact with God's agents in the spirit world, or spiritual 'guides'.† Spiritual healing does not require a religious framework to function; indeed, one such healer, Matthew Manning, is careful to debunk the idea that one can or should heal only through a church-based organization. Many spiritual healers believe that healing works by touching the soul and reaching aspects of ourselves that we may not even know exist. You don't need to be a believer to receive healing, but most spiritual healers see chronic ill health, particularly devastating diseases like cancer or

---

*The Churches' Council for Health and Healing provides a counterbalance to some extent, but as its latest *Report on Current Work* indicates, the approach of 'mainstream' churches is over-cautious, to say the least.

†Belief in life after death is a founding principle of the Spiritualist Church, for which there has been (suppressed) recognition by the Church of England, and increasing research evidence.[8]

multiple sclerosis as having an emotional and spiritual root, and their aim is not so much to effect a miraculous cure as to help the person grow through whatever traumas and spiritual difficulties have been unresolved, and hence be free to *live*. Spiritual healing is about enabling people to develop and to find peace. This may or may not involve 'getting better' in the usual sense. It may, for example, involve healing a part of ourselves that we did not know needed help, and it may involve helping us to approach life – and death – with equanimity and even joy.

Spiritual healing, therefore, can act as a catalyst for change. We can't expect to sit back and hope for a cure (though this does appear to happen very occasionally). What we can hope – and be open to – is that the healing will touch us in ways we haven't been touched, and help us to take the kinds of steps that will enable us to sustain ourselves without illness; steps that might involve anything from leaving a violent relationship, through changing our lifestyle, even just breathing more deeply, deciding to do yoga, psychotherapy and/or to attend to our spiritual needs. As Cynthia Evanson of White Eagle Lodge (see Resources) says:

> It takes time to learn/discover that quality of stillness. It is an enabling force – enabling the patient to make a link with God/light/infinite stillness. It involves almost a state of meditation.

'PSYCHIC' (OR 'MAGNETIC') HEALING

Some healers differentiate between psychic healing and spiritual healing, though they can appear to be exactly the same. The difference, they believe, is that psychic healers use their own psychic energy (and often get depleted as a result), and may not be able to reach us on a deep enough level. The effect of psychic healing is also said to dissipate relatively quickly. Some people teach that psychic healers should not work with people who have cancer, partly for this reason and also because they believe that psychic energy can stimulate the cancer. Dolores Krieger and Dora Kunz have studied and taught psychic healing very successfully in the form of laying on of hands, and they have generated considerable interest among allopathic practitioners (Dr Krieger is herself a nurse).[9] They call their approach 'Therapeutic Touch' (it is possible that the medical profession finds this label more 'acceptable', though it does not differ intrinsically from laying on of hands). Dr Krieger has demonstrated that anyone can learn this form of healing and has been teaching nurses in the USA for years.* As one of her pupils reports:

> A *woman had been to four or five doctors before she saw me. Her symptoms were back and leg pains with a lot of swelling on her ankles. She was told that she had no disc or circulatory problems, and was sent home with a diuretic for the swelling. 'Sometimes middle-aged women develop these problems,' one doctor said.*
>
> *I worked with this woman every three to four weeks for a year. With her energy back, she has returned to leading an active life with no physical restrictions. When she occasionally has pain, she returns for a single treatment.*

Increasing numbers of doctors recommend healing; some go themselves, or even do it. Dr Alec Forbes, for example, refers to a single parent in her forties with five children:

> . . . who had severe varicose veins with recurrent phlebitis and pulmonary emboli, who had been in congestive heart failure, but got very anaemic and had reactions to anticoagulants. After healing she changed completely, became cheerful, coped with her difficulties and stopped getting emboli. She no longer requires treatment, although she does get a little phlebitis from time to time.[10]

WHAT HAPPENS WHEN YOU GO TO A HEALER?*

This can vary enormously. Some healers like you to lie down; many prefer you to sit up. They may put their hands lightly on the body or just above it. Some healers simply say hello, ask you how you are, and get on with it. This can be discomfiting. Others like to prepare you by helping you to focus on your breathing, and possibly taking you on a guided meditation to a 'healing place'. Such healers often help you to protect yourself before you leave.

You may feel nothing at all, or heat, cold, pins and needles, a sense of deep relaxation or well-being, or other sensations, and you might even go into a light trance. It may require several sessions before you experience change (if any), though healing can appear to effect remarkable changes in a single session. Healing may be given over several years.

SELF-HEALING

We can consciously use the mind, e.g. through positive thought, prayer or visualization.†

> *As the acute stage of my asthma passes, I relax*

---

*Because of laws against healing in many parts of the US, training nurses to heal was one way of getting round the law – which of course carries with it the dangers of professionalizing healing.

*This is with regard to contact healing. For absent healing you may only need to give your name, although the Harry Edwards Sanctuary likes to maintain regular contact with people receiving absent healing.

†For visualization, see p. 108. For positive thought, all that may be necessary, according to Emile Coué, founder of 'Auto-suggestion', is to repeat in mantra-like fashion the phrase 'Every day in every way I'm getting better and better', or some such. We don't even need to consider the *words* of the mantra, it's the repetition reaching our unconscious selves which is important, according to Coué. See also Affirmations in the section on cancer, p. 574.

and further ease my breathing, reduce wheezing by feeling warmth and light flow through me, part of an energy I imagine to be universal energy of which we are all a part. As I am able to breathe fully again, I picture myself giving that energy back into the larger cosmos. In a concrete way this interchange enables me once again to be available to family, friends and co-workers.

I want to pray, but I don't believe in God. I'm going to pray 'To whom it may concern'!

When I need to take care of myself, I mentally cloak myself in a healing blue light from head to toe. I'm learning better to know when I need it.

We can pay attention to our environment and how we respond to it, learning, for example, to seek out people to be with who make us feel good and supported rather than negative and drained, and we can learn to fuse political awareness with subtle awarenesses. Sound and colour, for example, can affect us quite profoundly, as can the very shapes of the rooms in which we live and work.[11] Our overall environment has potential for healing or creating dis-ease. As we gain knowledge and confidence about how we are affected by, for example, damp housing, racist violence, open-plan offices, strip lighting, we can begin to take individual and collective action to make healthy living a reality (see Chapters 9 and 10). We can also use yoga, for example, t'ai chi chu'an, the Alexander Technique or pure sound to promote health and self-healing (see Appendix to this chapter for details about the first three approaches and Resources for details of music tapes). The healing process can be facilitated in countless ways, including through laughing, play, creativity (see p. 98), grieving, sharing and collective action. By paying attention to our own needs on a deep level, we can identify what is right for us.

Sharing with other women in my consciousness-raising group was my first experience of healing. Discovering that I could take political action – stand up and be counted – was another. Since then I've realized that I needed healing experiences on other levels too, particularly the expression of much grief and sadness, as well as rage.

See Cancer in Chapter 25, p. 574, for a detailed look at self-healing as applied to a particular illness.

LEARNING TO HEAL OTHERS

We are all capable of healing, and often share in this – consciously or unconsciously – with friends and family. Massage is a way of healing that we can easily explore (see Appendix, p. 105), and as Dolores Krieger discusses in her book, we can all learn to heal through 'therapeutic touch'. She points out:

Since Therapeutic Touch derives from a mode of healing that persons of all cultures since the dawn of documented history have been able to use, *you* too can learn to heal . . . there is little I have to teach you that you haven't done before at some point in your life.[12]

However, she also discusses that offering oneself as a healer is not something to enter into lightly. She asks the question, 'Do you want to do it to *be* loved or to *love*? Motivated by love, there is almost limitless power.' Love, compassion and empathy harness energy in a special way. Healing is a 'power tool' and the healer must be sure s/he works in the best interests of the person being treated. To do healing, like all therapy, requires self-knowledge and awareness at a deep level, otherwise the healer can wreak havoc, particularly on a psychological level.

Healers need to cultivate a healing presence. Our own consciousness is what is important. Unless we live it, we won't be much use. Most of us have a long way to go, not just in this lifetime. Who we are is the important thing. (Herthe Larive, College of Healing)

The development of our own healing abilities can be seen as a political act. For example, some women involved in anti-nuclear work are developing such healing abilities, whether living at nuclear bases or sending 'healing energies' there.

I have found laying on of hands, by myself or with others, to be one of the most powerful meditations I know. As I tune into the life-force of the universe, I physically feel it coursing through my body and direct it to unite with others. Mental, emotional and physical distractions recede, and the group truly becomes one whole being.[13]

Some go further, seeing female energy as the key. Jean Freer, a feminist healer, says:

At this time I believe that the creative power in the universe is female and that personal health and the future of life on earth are intimately connected. Female energy offers hope for the future, and our personal healing reflects and is reflected by the healing going on for the planet, and that vision is empowered by our feminist politic.

Healing, therefore, is deeply political, in the sense that we can effect change by changing ourselves.

FINDING A HEALER

To find a healer, you can go to a Spiritualist church (many large towns have several, and you don't need to be a

HEALING AND DYING

Allopathic medicine, being orientated towards curing rather than healing, often has little to offer us in our dying; indeed, its approach to death has obvious similarities to its approach to birth – preventing us from finding our own way.

One of the reasons why many of us are terrified of illness is because of the transient nature of health . . . and of life. If we can become more able to accept this transience, we can also become more healthy – freer to experience and to live life. And we can become more able to accept our dying too. Many alternative approaches to health and healing have a lot to offer us in our dying as well as in our living. Through meditation, visualization or spiritual healing, for example, we may find the solace, strength and courage that can help us – and our loved ones – face our own death, and to live through it with dignity, calm, peace and even joy. Few people have the opportunity to do this in our present-day society. However, as more of us clamour for the right to a 'good death' as well as a 'good birth', we can hope that care of the dying – and of their loved ones – will become literally more caring.

There is as much meaning in our dying as in our living. Discovering this is never easy and for some of us only begins to happen when we are jolted out of our 'everyday' consciousness by someone's death or maybe even the prospect of our own. We all need help to discover how to be in relation to death and dying. The help we need is within us and within our friends and loved ones if we can only dare to look. Jane Zorza, aged twenty-five, after a difficult struggle which we refer to in Chapter 25, found a way of dying that her parents describe thus:

> Happy? What a word to use in the circumstances. And yet that was the word Jane used herself, repeatedly, once her pain had been brought under control. She used it to describe her own state of mind – and she urged me to share it with her. I pretended that I did . . . Jane looked at me thoughtfully, with a small smile. 'Dad, you're just saying it. That's no good . . .' We had never before discussed my attitude to death. Now Jane was telling me something I had never fully reasoned out with myself. I *was* afraid of dying, Jane told me, and so long as I remained afraid for myself, I would be afraid for her. But, she said, she herself could only retain the state of happiness about her own dying if she could make me share in it. She could only be happy if she could make us happy too . . . if she could show us that it was possible to die with peace and in dignity when our time came – that, she said, would be a great thing to leave behind her. It would be the greatest gift she could bestow on us. And in the very act of accepting the gift, we would be returning it to her and making her own dying easy. And that is how it worked.[14]

believer), or contact one of the relevant organizations listed in Resources. These organizations attempt to maintain standards. Their members have been allowed into hospitals for many years (much to the BMA's fury) and they can be invited to visit you there. Furthermore, following a new ruling in 1977, the General Medical Council now allows doctors to recommend spiritual healing.

The most important thing is to find someone with whom you feel comfortable. If you don't like what they are doing, ask them to stop, try and discuss it, or find someone else.

Generally speaking a healer should focus on the whole person, rather than on just a particular part to be healed. Healing is unique among so-called 'alternatives' in that most healers do not charge for their services, seeing their work as a loving gift for humankind. Those that do charge are often looked down on by their colleagues, though this attitude is perhaps rightly open to some criticism, as making too many demands of healers (who, to be able to do their work well, need to spend much time – and money – developing their skills, keeping accurate records, let alone surviving financially). Nevertheless, there are some healers who exploit their clients, though not necessarily through money. They may promise a cure, or use tricks to reinforce belief in them. Healers, like doctors, have been known to touch women up.* (Touch, by the way, is not essential for healing to take place.)

Some time ago I went to a healer. He was always most courteous and kind. But one day, when his wife wasn't there to act as a chaperone, he suddenly bent down and kissed me on the mouth. I've never been to a healer since.

If you go to a healer, you can ask to see their membership card which denotes current membership of a professional body.

Legal Restrictions

Healers are not allowed to advertise concerning the treatment of certain diseases, including cancer (notwithstanding the fact that healing is being increasingly recommended for cancer patients specifically). An age-old law also forbids healers to treat people for VD (though the law does not define VD clearly enough to make this restriction workable). Healers are also liable to prosecution if they attend women in childbirth or within ten days of childbirth.

At present, healers in the UK enjoy more freedom than

---

*The major healing organizations recommend that healers should work with a chaperone at all times.

almost anywhere in the world, which is the main reason why the practice has taken root here to such an extent. However, there is a possibility that this might change, as EEC legislation is on the horizon which aims to 'rationalize' the laws of member countries. Unless there is a strong enough lobby for healing, therefore, we may find our current freedom eroded.

PLANTS AND HERBS

The use of plants for healing goes back thousands of years. Women have been in the forefront of their use, and the decline of herbalism is intimately connected with the rise of the (male) medical profession. Another major factor in the decline of herbalism was the discovery that money could be made out of 'patent medicines'. Thomas Beecham of 'Beecham's Powders', for example, began as a herbalist. He, together with Jesse Boot of Boots the Chemists, discovered that there was more money to be made out of patent medicines, often derived from plant extracts, than from herbs as used traditionally. Modern drug companies, anxious to maintain their monopoly of medicines, also play a strong part in preventing research into and promotion of herbalism.

But while herbalism declined in the nineteenth century, it has always managed to retain some kind of foothold among 'lay' people and, in an organized sense, through the extensive activities of Hilda Leyel who founded the Society of Herbalists. Now, in the latter half of the twentieth century, some thoughtful scientists are beginning to see that the value of herbs does not necessarily lie in their so-called 'active ingredients' (those that are usually isolated and standardized into drugs), but rather in the inherent qualities of the plants when used as a whole. While these qualities are not yet understood, many traditional herbalists would recognize them as forming each particular plant's 'vital force'.[15]

Most allopaths remain sceptical about herbs. Yet, increasingly, it is being recognized that they may be of equal, if not greater value than the wonders of 'modern medicine' – as in the case of Sphagnum moss, for example, a 'folk' healing remedy for treating wounds which appears to have better healing properties than conventional dressings.[16] The World Health Organization is also actively interested in herbs,[17] as are some nuclear war planners, although it would be ironic, to say the least, if we had to await a nuclear war before herbalism became acceptable. *

Many of us use plants, barely realizing their properties or their potency. Garlic, for example, has powerful anti-infective properties, it has been reported to be valuable in assuaging whooping cough, and many women can attest to treating vaginal infections, though inserting a (peeled) clove of garlic in the vagina can unnervingly affect the

breath as if one had eaten it. There is also evidence to suggest that garlic may be helpful in the prevention of heart disease.

My daughter loves garlic. I'm sure that's why she's never ill. We buy it in those long strips to make sure we never run out.

Using plants is appealing, not least because they are often easily accessible, either in our gardens, or in the form of various types of herbal remedies available in health-food shops, or even chemists; we can use them as self-help remedies. But if we are going to use herbal remedies as serious aids to health and disease, we must be wary of the promotional antics of many manufacturers, and we do need to be careful and responsible (see Safety and Side-effects, below). We cannot here give a guide to the use of herbs; what we can do is briefly describe some of the different approaches, give some suggestions for further reading, and also on how to find a practitioner.

MEDICAL HERBALISM

This is the most common form of treatment involving plants. As with many alternative approaches to medicine, herbs can be used either 'symptomatically' or 'holistically'. With the former approach, herbs are prescribed to alleviate specific symptoms, basing the diagnosis on what seems to be the main cause of the problem. A herbalist pursuing a holistic approach would aim to treat the whole person rather than the disease, if any. She would prepare or choose remedies specifically for the individual concerned, taking into account her total 'symptom picture', history and personality (in a similar way to a homoeopath, see p. 91) and would aim to enable the person to heal herself at her own pace. Most herbalists will combine both approaches, treating the immediate symptoms while aiming at the same time to consider our longer-term health needs.

A trained herbalist's approach will tend to involve taking a detailed history and examination. Selection of herbs is made on the basis of many, seemingly irrelevant, factors both to do with the person (e.g. aspects of lifestyle, such as favourite foods and habits), and to do with the plants, such as their habitat and botanical nature. (Herbalism has links with the homoeopathic concept of treating 'like with like'; indeed, homoeopathy can be seen at least in part as a refined form of herbalism.) Several plants may be selected. Trained herbalists should know about the potency and possible side-effects of all the plants they use. However, not all herbalists keep up with the medical and herbal literature, and some herbs have recently been found to be dangerous in certain circumstances (see below).

There is evidence which suggests that herbalism may be valuable for people with problems ranging from migraine to arthritis. However, how far herbs are effective is extremely difficult to say, as the medical monopoly on research has largely prevented serious investigation into herbalism.

---

*The East Anglian plan for defence against nuclear attack, for example, includes the use of herbal remedies.[18]

SAFETY AND SIDE-EFFECTS

While supporters of herbalism claim that unwelcome side-effects are rare, and no doubt they are in responsible hands, it is as well to bear in mind that they can occur, and can sometimes be dangerous. Herbal remedies can be contaminated by unwanted and sometimes toxic materials, particularly in countries (including the UK) where regulations are lax.[19] Also, there are herbs which, unless used for a limited time or in restricted amounts, can be toxic. These are mostly not common plants, but they can be bought over the counter at some shops. Care should be exercised when taking herbal remedies and none should be taken for longer than about two or three weeks without supervision, especially not if a condition worsens or does not improve.

Since even the consumption of large quantities of tea – herbal or otherwise – may cause problems,[20] perhaps as with most things, the operative word is moderation. However, many claims about the dangers of herbalism are based at least in part on biased reports and dubious research papers, often done by doctors. In one such report, a woman said to have suffered from the effects of mistletoe had in fact taken pills which contained no mistletoe at all,[21] and many herbalists feel that claims about the toxicity of certain plants are far from proven. There is little evidence at present that we can trust research into herbalism, whether by doctors or by herbalists.

FINDING HERBS AND A HERBALIST

Anyone can call themselves a herbalist. Members registered by the Institute of Medical Herbalists have all undergone a training that is at least recognized by the Department of Education. Some nurses are beginning to use herbs, and the occasional GP has also been known to prescribe herbs but their use within the NHS is very rare. Bear in mind there aren't many registered herbalists of any kind in this country. For information about practitioners, and for a list of herbal farms and suppliers, contact the Herb Society (see Resources). If you buy herbs, it's important to go to a reputable establishment which sells herbs that are properly cultivated, packed and stored.

HERBALISM AND THE LAW

The 1968 Medicines Act enables herbalists to exercise their own judgement when prescribing herbs. While the Act granted licences-of-right to most herbal products, these licences come up for renewal in 1990. Unless herbalists and manufacturers can come up with sufficient evidence concerning the safety and efficacy of each product (a tall order given the acute lack of help available from funding bodies), we may find that many products disappear. As Ruth West says:

> It must seem ironic . . . that the very reason for herbal medicine's popularity – the danger of synthetic drugs – also gave rise to the Act that is now threatening their existence.[22]

OTHER APPROACHES INVOLVING PLANTS

Aromatherapy

Aromatherapy uses 'essential oils' from plants that are either rubbed into the skin (in diluted form), or added to baths. They may also be used as inhalants, and sometimes they are taken by mouth, though these latter approaches are considered controversial by some aromatherapists. Unless used in the bath, essential oils should *always* be diluted with a mild oil such as almond oil. Otherwise they can burn the skin or internal membranes.

Bach Flower Remedies

These were developed by Dr Edward Bach, a doctor who left orthodox medicine in favour of homoeopathy and who subsequently devised his own remedies which owe a lot, in concept at least, to homoeopathy: they involve thirty-eight specially prepared remedies based on plant extracts that are taken by mouth in an extremely diluted form. His approach differs from homoeopathy in that the remedies are designed for people according to their underlying emotional state, on the basis that, by working on the emotional level, the person is able to find a way back to health. The types of emotional state that Bach categorizes are subtle and far-reaching. For example, he lists five different kinds of fear, each with its own remedy. One of his most famous remedies is the 'Rescue' remedy – for use at times of acute stress, emotional shock, panic or accident.

It is possible to use both Bach Flower Remedies and aromatherapy on ourselves and, though research into their value is negligible, they are, perhaps more than herbalism, unlikely to do harm to novices. There is a small but growing band of doctors practising within the NHS who admit to prescribing Bach Flower Remedies despite the lack of research. As one such doctor comments, 'I've been using them long enough to realize that they do have a real effect – it's not just placebo.' Exeter University's new Centre for Complementary Health Studies is currently researching into Bach Flower Remedies. For more information about the Remedies and about Aromatherapy, see Resources.

HOMOEOPATHY

Homoeopathy is the only 'alternative' system of medicine that is fully recognized by the NHS. It is widely used in many parts of the world, including Europe and India (the latter has about eighty schools of homoeopathy). It was conceived in the nineteenth century by Samuel Hahnemann, yet might not have survived had it not been for Melanie, an emancipated young woman who became his wife when he was seventy-nine, and whose energy ensured that it did not die with him.*

*The official history of homoeopathy is dominated exclusively by men. The full part played by Melanie Hahnemann in the history and development of homoeopathy has recently been unearthed by Rima Handley, and has yet to be published, though see her article listed in Resources for a taster.

Homoeopathy is based on the principle of 'what it can cause, it can cure'. There is nothing particularly odd about this idea: think of radiation therapy and cancer, or vaccinations. It was conceived as a 'whole person' system of medicine, looking at a person's symptoms (if any) plus their general 'constitution' (including their attitudes to life, to problems, etcetera), their overall history (including family history) and personality. The founding principles of homoeopathy are based on the belief that the remedies are able directly to influence the 'vital force' and thus enable the body to heal itself. Concerned with both the physical and spiritual causes of suffering, another principle of homoeopathy is that transformation, rather than cure, is the key to health.

Homoeopathic remedies can be made from any substance, though most are made from herbs and other natural substances which are so diluted as to be unmeasurable by orthodox means, and treated by 'succussion' (involving shaking the substance rapidly which appears to affect its physical state). There are some 6,000 remedies and each remedy can be made in many different potencies. They come in the form of pills, powders or liquids. *

To some people, particularly those immersed in the Western scientific tradition, the idea of succussion and using dilutions of substances that are not measurable by current technical means, seems utter nonsense. However, increasingly, research is providing more and more support for homoeopathic theories and practices, and increasing numbers of scientists from such disciplines as immunology and the new physics are becoming interested in the unanswered questions posed by homoeopathy.[23] One avenue of thought that is gaining increasing credence is that homoeopathy affects energy channels of some kind.[24] This fits in with the more esoteric theories – and Kirlian photography – which postulate the existence of a 'vital force', and of course with the founding principles of homoeopathy. Some people today translate this concept into the more modern phraseology of 'homoeostatic mechanisms' – which may or may not be the same thing.

There is still much prejudice against homoeopathy, despite the fact that it is recognized by the NHS (see box), and despite sharing with many aspects of allopathy an uncertainty about how it works, if at all. (It has also had royal patronage for years.) Much of this prejudice is based on inappropriate or misplaced concern about the relative lack of research into homoeopathy. For while homoeopathy might be recognized by the NHS, this recognition does not extend to the funding of research programmes, or of homoeopathic training of any kind. Allopathic doctors still call the tune and effectively hold the purse-strings: it is they who say that financial help isn't warranted until scientific proof of homoeopathy's effectiveness first exists. This not only represents a double standard, it also conveniently ignores the fact that it costs money to do the

research required to get funding for more research! In addition, good clinical trials in homoeopathy are far harder to perform than with drugs, and more costly.[25]

The situation is even further confused because there are several different schools of homoeopathy. Broadly, there are two types of homoeopath in this country: those who are medically trained and those who are not. Many homoeopathic doctors tend to look down on 'lay' homoeopaths, partly out of prejudice against anyone who isn't medically qualified, and partly because, to maintain their credibility with their medical colleagues and their foothold in the NHS, they feel the need to distance themselves from anything that might be construed as quackery. Needless to say, not all homoeopathic doctors share this attitude, and some are supportive of 'lay' homoeopaths – who have a longer homoeopathic training than doctors, but who, not being doctors, are not able to practise in the NHS. Some people would argue that a homoeopathic doctor is less qualified to practise homoeopathy than a registered 'lay' homoeopath, since a veneer of homoeopathic training can hardly be expected to eradicate years of seeing health and illness within an allopathic framework.

HOMOEOPATHY AND SAFETY

It would be surprising if something that can have such powerful beneficial effects is not also capable of harmful effects, and Hahnemann himself drew careful attention to this. The main power of homoeopathy to cause harm is probably through omission: cystitis treated badly for too long could lead to kidney damage, for instance, and some homoeopaths withdraw allopathic drugs too suddenly and completely, 'with disastrous results' according to one homoeopath. However, in untrained hands, homoeopathy can cause havoc in another way: for example, if someone had once had tuberculosis which was suppressed by orthodox treatment, an untrained person could inadvertently reactivate it. * It is wise, therefore, as with all practitioners, to seek out reputable ones, question them closely, and to consider carefully before embarking on self-help remedies.

HOMOEOPATHY IN PRACTICE

Homoeopathy can treat or prevent a wide variety of problems, ranging from acute conditions such as injuries or measles to chronic conditions such as migraine, skin conditions or rheumatoid arthritis. As one homoeopath says:

---

*Homoeopaths don't necessarily restrict themselves to remedies as such, but may also make dietary and other recommendations.

*Dr H. A. Roberts, who practised between the wars, drew attention to the need for particularly careful diagnosis in elderly people to ensure safe prescribing. There is a debate in homoeopathy about safe and unsafe practices. See, for example, Harris Coulter in the *Journal of Alternative Medicine*, November 1984.

All named disease conditions are regarded as expressions of a fundamental disturbance in the individual's balance of health, and treatment aims to restore that balance by removing layers of illness acquired through life and heredity. Thus an acute condition can be treated quickly and effectively as the most recent layer of illness in which the disturbance is clearly recognized, while more chronic conditions will need more extended treatment taking into account the person's unique history and character which co-exist with the appearance of particular pathological symptoms. Because homoeopathy recognizes patterns of imbalance before the appearance of pathological symptoms it is able to treat before gross pathology has taken too deep a hold, and therefore to act preventatively.

And a woman says:

When I was a child, I began to have hay fever, and then, when I was in my twenties, I started getting asthma as well, particularly during the summer months. It gradually got worse, and finally, the summer before last, when I couldn't breathe at all, I had to leave London and my kids, and spend the rest of the summer by the sea. Then I went to see a [lay] homoeopath. She's been treating me for nearly two years. It's been amazing the way everything's begun to fall into place. Last summer I hardly had any hay fever or asthma, and this summer I haven't had any. After nearly twenty years of misery, a mere two years' treatment to get rid of it completely seems pretty good going to me.

Homoeopathy may also be effective in ridding the system of overload from unwanted environmental toxins.[26]

Because of the way homoeopathy deals with our 'illness history', it can stimulate a kind of 'replay' of past ill health, but in reverse order: symptoms, traumas and even feelings that you've had before, possibly going back to childhood. This tends to happen more with treatment for chronic problems and is unlikely to happen with treatment for a sore throat or septic finger.

Homoeopathic remedies should always be kept in their containers and kept away from strong heat or light, and from exposure to strong odours. If you have more than one container, only one should be open at any one time, and for the shortest time possible to minimize contamination. Pills should be tipped into the mouth; powders should be tipped directly on to the tongue. If more pills are tipped out than needed, they should be thrown away, otherwise you risk contaminating the rest. All remedies should be put in a 'clean' mouth – i.e. not after food, drink, cigarettes or even toothpaste.

Some substances are thought to be antidotes to homoeopathic remedies. Many homoeopaths believe that coffee, peppermint and camphor, for example, affect all remedies and therefore have to be avoided throughout the treatment period. Similarly, some homoeopaths believe the Pill, and even acupuncture need to be avoided. (Yet increasing numbers of practitioners may even make a point of combining acupuncture with homoeopathy!) It is thought by some that dental treatment, including drilling, can antidote a remedy, though it does appear possible, at least in some circumstances, to combine homoeopathy with certain allopathic drugs, including antibiotics.

HOMOEOPATHY AND EQUALITY

There is a tradition among some 'lay' homoeopaths that, whatever the practitioner prescribes, it is none of the client's business. (Doctors who practise homoeopathy, curiously, do not usually seem to feel the need for such secretiveness.) While homoeopaths share the same sexist and patriarchal tendencies of all other practitioners, this tendency towards secretiveness is connected with the fact that homoeopathy involves assessments of clients' personalities. While a homoeopath may rationalize that s/he is protecting the client by not divulging diagnoses, this secretiveness has at least as much to do with the homoeopath's desire, conscious or not, for *self*-protection. Some homoeopaths are more secretive than others. A self-styled unconventional 'lay' homoeopath speaks:

I try to be as open as I can, feeding back observations at the time, though I don't tend to do it in homoeopathic *terms till the next session. It can be very difficult to reveal to people what your diagnosis is till they're ready to take it. After a remedy has been given, it's easier to tell them, and often easier for the patient to hear it – very often because the remedy has 'unlocked' them.*

Of course, not telling us what we're getting may not just be offensive to our politics:

When my homoeopath was away I had to see someone else as an emergency, when I developed cystitis. I couldn't tell him what I had been given so he had to work in the dark.

Feminist homoeopaths are challenging this secretive tradition, and other aspects of homoeopathy that are class-ridden, sexist or otherwise oppressive.[27] Many of these factors were introduced into homoeopathy not by Hahnemann, and certainly not by Melanie, but by James Tyler Kent, whose interpretations of Hahnemann's work have unfortunately come to dominate most homoeopathic teaching and practice.

HOMOEOPATHY AND SELF-HELP

It is now common to see homoeopathic preparations available over the counter in chemists and health-food shops. While few homoeopaths would quibble with the

HOMOEOPATHY AND THE NHS

Homoeopathy is practised in the NHS by some GPs (lists of such doctors are available from the British Homoeopathic Association) and by a handful of hospital doctors at the few remaining homoeopathic hospitals. Increasingly, chiropodists and some dentists are taking an interest in it as well, as are veterinary surgeons (see Resources for addresses).

However, although homoeopathy has always been recognized by the NHS, it has been in constant danger of being squeezed out – by a combination of uncompromising medical hostility on the one hand, and government and local health authority inactivity on the other.* This has been particularly apparent over the last few years because of the financial climate under which the NHS has had to work. In a letter to the Chairman of the Homoeopathic Trust, in April 1980, the then Health Minister referred to the 'considerable feeling in some places that homoeopathy should not be a priority call on NHS resources at a time of financial constraint'.[29] Community Health Councils in districts where homoeopathic hospitals exist (see Resources) may be ideal places to do campaigning work, but there is no reason why all health authorities should not be confronted with the lack of availability of homoeopathy in their areas, and be lobbied to do something about it.

Because of the appalling pressure homoeopathy is facing, there are long waiting lists at hospitals (at the time of writing, some new patients at the Royal London Homoeopathic Hospital [RLHH] have to wait a year) and few NHS doctors are able to devote adequate time to their consultations. At the RLHH, for example, a new patient gets fifteen minutes whereas most homoeopaths would consider that an hour or more was necessary. Since GPs are paid per patient, regardless of how much time they spend with them, homoeopathic GPs often feel they have to leave the NHS in order to give a decent service. Pressure should be put on the NHS to enable homoeopathic doctors to work within it. If you wish to go to a homoeopathic hospital (virtually all the work they do is on an outpatient basis), it is advisable to get a letter from your GP if possible; apart from anything else, this might cut down the waiting time.

*Perhaps one of the most telling stories about homoeopathy relates to the cholera epidemic in the mid-nineteenth century. While at the London Homoeopathic Hospital, the death-rate from cholera was less than 20 per cent, the death-rate in other hospitals was more than 50 per cent. However, because of strong opposition to homoeopathy, attempts were made by the medical authorities to suppress these figures (these attempts were defeated by the House of Lords and it was ordered that they be published in the official report).[28]

idea of self-help for acute problems, many are wary about the wisdom of self-help for chronic problems. Says one homoeopath:

Homoeopathic first aid is generally safe – e.g. for a cut or for shock. For chronic problems I certainly wouldn't recommend self-help, nor even for problems like cystitis, which can have very different whole-person symptom pictures: for some women, feeling the cold will be important, for others, grief, for yet others it may be connected with traumas like rape. Completely different treatment approaches are required for these different people.

It's wise, therefore, to treat homoeopathic self-help books with caution, at least aside from acute problems and first aid.

ACUPUNCTURE

Acupuncture is the healing art central to the practice of traditional Chinese medicine, developed and used over at least the last 2,000 years. It involves stimulating specific points on the body, for example by inserting needles, applying heat by burning a herb called moxa (like common mugwort), or pressing or massaging (acupressure, shiatsu or shen tao). The needles may hurt on insertion or removal, or you might feel only a slight prick, tingling, numbness or nothing at all.*

There are several different schools of acupuncture, but broadly they can be divided into two types: the traditional Chinese approach, and the 'symptomatic' approach. The former is mainly about maintaining 'wellness', while the latter is about treating the symptoms of 'illness'.

THE 'TRADITIONAL' APPROACH

Chinese medicine, intimately tied to the classical Chinese philosophy of Taoism, aims to maintain or restore balance in the body, mind and spirit to ensure health. Central to the beliefs of Taoism is the notion that we have the power to repair and regenerate ourselves and to restore our own

*Acupuncture is one of a variety of ancient systems of healing. As it is the most common such system in the UK, our discussion is confined to this. Another, Ayurveda, a traditional Hindu medicine from India, is based on similar principles, and is practised by a few practitioners in the UK (see Vasant Lad, listed in Resources; see also the Association of Ayurvedic Practitioners, p. 114).

equilibrium. Acupuncture is thought to stimulate or awaken these natural healing powers.

The concepts of Yin and Yang are important aspects of traditional Chinese acupuncture. These terms denote what the ancient Chinese saw as twin polarities that regulate humans and the universe. Taoism describes Yin as 'negative' (e.g. earth, moon, coolness, moisture, quiescence) and Yang as 'positive' (e.g. heaven, sun, warmth, dryness, movement). The terms are equivalent to modern physicists calling protons 'positive' and electrons 'negative'. A proton is not 'better' than an electron; they are equally powerful forces. Most practitioners refer to Yin as female and Yang as male – a misconception, as is argued by, for example, Capra.[30] Unfortunately, the use of this concept has led to misunderstanding and misuse, though many practitioners who adopt this approach would argue that it does not imply bias against the female. It remains to be seen, however, how far this concept affects their abilities to support women in lesbian relationships.

Chinese acupuncture focuses on how we function as a whole, rather than simply on the physiological or material structure of the body. In common with several other 'alternative' approaches, it recognizes the importance of a life force that keeps us alive and in healthful balance. This life force, or vital energy, is called *ch'i*. According to traditional Chinese medical theory, *ch'i* circulates throughout the body along precise pathways or channels, the acupuncture meridians. The *ch'i*, which controls the blood, nerves and all organs, must flow freely along the meridians and be of a certain strength and quality if we are to function correctly. When the flow of *ch'i* is impaired, we become susceptible to disease.

Trauma or shocks (even if they occurred long ago), improper nutrition, stress and many other factors can block or impair the flow of *ch'i*. In acupuncture, stimulating certain points along the meridians influences the flow of *ch'i* by attracting energy to a deficient area, dispersing an excess of energy or dissolving a blockage, thereby lessening distress or pain and strengthening our ability to maintain health.

A traditional acupuncturist diagnoses imbalances by taking a careful history, including family history, observing (e.g. facial colour, tongue, breathing, voice, etc.), and reading the pulses.*

I'd tried acupuncture before, but without any lasting improvement, for a viral illness now called Myalgic Encephalomylitis. Then I was recommended to someone else. My first

appointment lasted about two hours. I was asked all sorts of questions, some that initially seemed a lot more relevant than others. But by the end I began to see how relationships with my family, even from a very early age, were very relevant to what was happening to my body now. It felt very good having the opportunity to start making sense of my chronic illness historically, and at an emotional and spiritual level, as well as on a physical one. After the first few sessions I began to notice very gradual changes. And these changes lasted! It was like I had a petrol tank that was filling up: first my reserves, and then my main, deep, core tank that felt it had been empty for years. It happened slowly and surely over a period of about six months. I very much doubt if I could have got better any other way, unless I'd gone to another system of medicine that was practised on the same deep level.

If you go for help with a chronic ailment, you may experience relief straight away, or you may initially feel worse and begin to experience improvement only after many sessions.

I am sixty years old and have severe arthritis, especially in my hands, feet and hips. I had been pushing this pain out of my mind while I was taking care of my husband. He was very sick and if he knew I was in pain he would have wanted to go to the hospital. After he died I was very depressed, and when I went for psychological counselling the counsellor suggested that I try acupuncture for the arthritis. The first few treatments were very painful. I even screamed out. We went through hell together. The acupuncturist told me that chronic pain like mine was deep-seated and harder to take care of. I had to go twice a week for a long time. It was expensive for me, and when after eight treatments I didn't feel any better, I didn't know what to do. Meanwhile, I had been put on a special arthritis diet by a nutritionist who worked with the acupuncturist. I decided I would go on with the acupuncture treatment, and when I got to sixteen treatments I started to feel a little better. By twenty weeks I had found the acupuncture really helped me. Now the treatments have tapered off, one every two or three months, when I start getting sore. So it was definitely worth continuing with them. You either sink or swim, and I didn't feel like sinking.

*Reading the pulses is one of the primary diagnostic procedures. It can diagnose subtle fluctuations in the flow of energy along the meridian circuit. Pulses are taken at three finger positions on each wrist and at two depths for each finger position. Each of these twelve positions corresponds to one of the meridians. By feeling these pulses, an experienced practitioner can discover both the energy imbalances within the body at the time of diagnosis and some indication of past conditions as well as potential difficulties. Acupuncture therefore has a preventive aspect as well.

Because of its approach, restoring health and balance to the whole person, there is a wide variety of problems that traditional acupuncture can treat, including menstrual and conception problems, addictions, and sometimes also depression or anxiety. A World Health Organization seminar drew up a list of over forty diseases and conditions, including migraine, asthma and sinusitis.[31] Many acupuncturists would include considerably more conditions on the list. However, not everything is suitable for acupuncture: the Chinese used several approaches to medicine, of which acupuncture was only one. That is why a few traditional acupuncturists here use herbs as well as acupuncture, and describe themselves as practising traditional Chinese medicine rather than simply acupuncture.

THE 'SYMPTOMATIC' APPROACH

It can take years to master the art of taking pulses alone,[32] so it is not surprising that some acupuncturists try and take short cuts. Some courses in acupuncture are so short they can only hope to teach a very superficial approach. Courses for doctors can be the most superficial of all – some lasting for only a weekend. It is not therefore possible for people, largely doctors, who have attended such courses to practise anything but a very crude – 'symptomatic' – form of acupuncture. While this can help with relatively straightforward problems, lack of awareness of the subtle levels on which acupuncture functions can prevent effective treatment and even create more problems. In the case of addictions, for example, many 'symptomatic' acupuncturists simply favour a staple in the ear. This might work – but it's very much up to the person being treated, and if they're not helped with the deep-seated problem that led to the addiction, then failure or depression, for example, are possible. Perhaps the most widely acknowledged value of acupuncture, at least in medical circles, is its ability to act as an analgesic in the relief of pain either of a chronic nature or during and after operations or childbirth.

SAFETY, SIDE-EFFECTS AND SELF-HELP

As helpful as acupuncture can be, it can equally be harmful when not practised properly. In addition relief for chronic pain should be used wisely, as it can mask diagnosis of serious disease. Responses to treatment are not usually dramatic, but the effects can take us by surprise.

> The first major treatment I had really exhausted me the next day. Often if it's a strong treatment the energies are moving in a way that they haven't moved for a long time, so it can be very draining.[33]

> *I felt so euphoric afterwards I felt it was too risky to drive myself home!*

It is not a good idea to practise acupuncture on ourselves but we may wish to experiment with acupressure or shiatzu. These can be very helpful but it may be best to seek some guidance before embarking on them. As a feminist acupuncturist says:

> It's a very delicate balance and very important to make a correct diagnosis before giving treatment. That's why self-help manuals on acupressure,

Chinese herbs and shiatsu massage can be dangerous unless you have the guidance of someone who's skilled in these methods.[34]

FINDING AN ACUPUNCTURIST

Acupuncture is not commonly available on the NHS and, where it is, it tends to be only for symptomatic treatment and/or pain relief. Pain clinics are increasingly turning to acupuncture, and some women have managed to get acupuncture for pain relief during labour. It is usually only doctors who are allowed to practise acupuncture within the NHS, although some paramedics such as physiotherapists and nurses are beginning to do it too.

Outside the NHS you are more likely to find a traditional acupuncturist. As anyone can call themselves an acupuncturist, it is important to make sure that the person concerned is registered with a suitable organization (see Resources, p. 112).

NATUROPATHY*

Naturopathy can be considered the original holistic medicine of the West. Modern naturopathy traces itself back in essence to Hippocrates and his idea of the vital life force of the body. So does orthodox medicine but it is sometimes hard to see how the life force and 'intelligence' of the body are recognized by it, with the emphasis on the person as passive and being invaded by disease or attacked by microbes.

The philosophy underlying naturopathy is very important. It involves a complete turn around of many of our conventionally negative ways of viewing disruption in our experience of 'health'. It questions the meaning of health and suggests an experience far more dynamic than the mere absence of symptoms. A cough can be welcomed as the clearing out of debris from the bronchii and lungs, a spot may be seen as a channel for clearing the skin and the immediately underlying bloodstream, and so on. These ideas once thought cranky have gained support from occasional pieces of research. An example: the purpose of a fever has been recognized as raising the body's temperature sufficiently high to make a hostile environment for 'undesirable' viruses. In other words, the virus does not invade and 'cause' the fever: it is the body's intelligent perception of a potential takeover that initiates protective action. Fever, as long as it does not go uncontrollably high, becomes a friend, not an enemy.

Symptoms such as a cough, spots and fever may be signals to a naturopath of the existence of vitality and a drive to health in a person, rather than signposts to named diseases. In some ways it may be psychologically easier for

*This section is partly based on an article by Richenda Power that was published in *Self and Society* (vol. 12, no. 1, Jan./Feb. 1984). We are grateful to Richenda, and *Self and Society* for allowing us to use it.

someone to feel that they've 'got colitis' rather than to look at some of the factors that have predisposed them to get such a cluster of signs and symptoms which they have then maintained. If I have condition 'X' and I believe that drug 'Y' cures it (or merely controls it), then I can continue to operate within the same constraints that produce and maintain 'X'. In contrast, naturopathy aims to help us break out of these prescription-dependent ways of conceptualizing illness and cure.

Usually a naturopath will spend time with a person trying to understand how and why their body/mind is behaving in a particular way and recognizing predisposing factors, trying together to develop some overall approach to aid the situation. It is an educational process, involving the recognition of one's body as intelligent and trying to assist its natural efforts to heal itself.

WHAT DOES NATUROPATHY INVOLVE?

It may involve one or more of the following:

Dietetics: involving the prescription of a wholesome (much of it raw and preferably organic) natural diet, or possibly a specific, controlled diet for a time (e.g. involving nothing but fruit, salads or raw juice). *

Fasting: allowing the body to concentrate on dealing with the disease rather than focusing on digestion. (Fasting should only be done under supervision and it is contra-indicated for degenerative diseases such as cancer.)

Structural adjustments: such as osteopathy (see box) or neuro-muscular technique (NMT), which involves a particular type of slow, deep massaging over the body's connective tissue. A special type of NMT may be useful for heavy and/or painful periods.

Hydrotherapy (i.e. the use of water, in the form of mineral baths, packs, compresses, sprays or enemas): judiciously used it is thought that hydrotherapy can have anti-bacterial and anti-viral effects, as well as stimulate the immune mechanism.

> *I had been on antibiotics for a week with an ear infection. My longed-for holiday was coming up and I felt utterly miserable. When the condition started to get worse I rang a naturopath. I think I was looking for a miracle. She put me on a strict raw food diet plus a complicated regime of herbs, hot and cold packs and infusions. Four days later the infection had virtually gone.*

Some types are thought to be of particular value for gynaecological problems.[35] In addition, some naturopaths may employ a range of other techniques, ranging from iridology (a form of diagnosis involving the eye) to visualization (see Appendix to this chapter) or herbs (see p. 90).

Here is an example of how a naturopath might approach

*See also 'Get-Well Diets' in Chapter 4.

a woman who has a cluster of symptoms – high blood pressure, tense shoulders, stiff neck, sore throat.

> *Gradually we tease out the contributory factors. She types all day in a smoky office, drinks endless black coffee, feels she could be doing something more personally valuable, doesn't get on with the boss, grabs Kentucky fried for a quick supper on the way home to a demanding family life (etc.). We start by discovering the things that can be changed quite easily: maybe the coffee can be cut out, relaxation techniques and isometric exercises used at the typewriter, and a vitamin and mineral-rich diet started. Psychological work might be used to assist her assertiveness with the boss and the smokers surrounding her at work. It could be supporting her in a search for a more congenial job, or encouraging a fulfilling interest or activity during the lunch hour or after work.*

This particular naturopath is a feminist and clearly sees the relevance of politics to her practice.

> *As a naturopath I feel we need to engage in struggle with the 'manufacturers of illness' and that currently includes the tobacco industry, the sugar industry and the junk-food manufacturers as well as the government that produces huge inequalities in housing, education and recreational facilities, to name but the tip of the iceberg. I think it is useful to discuss these matters with patients as they arise naturally, say when discussing diet or a work situation.*

Of course, few practitioners, orthodox or 'alternative', approach health from this truly holistic standpoint.

Naturopathy is not appropriate in all situations. As Roger Newman-Turner says:

> A fibroid of the uterus . . . may well be contained healthily, or even reduced, by naturopathic treatment, but if it is too large to respond, or causes pressure on other structures such as the bladder, then surgical removal may be the best course of action.[36]

Naturopathy has impeccable scientific credentials in the form of Louis Pasteur who is reported to have said on his deathbed that his contemporary, Claude Bernard, was right: the body's ability to handle disease was paramount; 'germs' were of secondary importance. In Cancer, p. 577, we show in more detail how tackling this 'host response' can have a powerful effect on illness.

SAFETY AND SIDE-EFFECTS

Naturopathy like many other systems of medicine may involve 'healing crises' (see p. 85), and the return of old symptoms (usually in reverse order of their original

OSTEOPATHY

Osteopathy deals with the muscular–skeletal system – i.e. the bones, joints, muscles, ligaments and tendons – for treatment of this system *as well as* other tissues and organs of the body; treatment of the muscular–skeletal system can affect apparently unrelated symptoms such as migraine, asthma, uterine and circulatory problems, although its effects are not always predictable. It may help mobility problems such as those associated with arthritis, as well as postural difficulties associated with pregnancy. Central to osteopathy is the idea that structure and function are closely connected and interdependent. If there are problems in the structure (i.e. the skeleton), then the functioning of the body will be affected.

Some people visit an osteopath annually – somewhat like having an MOT. This can be especially useful before a physical trial or taking up any new physical activity. More often, people start when they have an immediate problem.

One day something happened to my neck and I could barely move it, and even then with difficulty. I managed to get someone to drive me to an osteopath, who freed my neck very quickly. I then carried on seeing him for a bit, so that he could work on my back, which seemed to be the cause of the problem.

Most naturopaths are trained osteopaths, though most osteopaths are not necessarily naturopaths. Some osteopaths have managed to find their way into the NHS, but very few; likewise, a few doctors practise osteopathy in the NHS. For how to find an osteopath, see Resources, p. 115. Members of reputable organizations cannot advertise.

appearance); the latter is particularly the case for symptoms that have been suppressed, e.g. with drugs. In some ways naturopathy parallels the freeing of blocks in an emotional sense as can be encouraged in psychotherapy. A facing up to and conscious exaggeration of the symptoms/distressing feelings so that the underlying disease/dis-ease may work itself out. It is as well to be prepared! Naturopaths may create problems by being insensitive or sexist – e.g. by fostering anxiety in us about food – and some have been known to make women feel guilty about having an abortion. Fasting can also be dangerous in unskilled hands, and hydrotherapy can have violent side-effects too if similarly ill-used.

FINDING A NATUROPATH

See Resources for organizations that register trained naturopaths. None of them can advertise.

PSYCHOTHERAPEUTIC AND CREATIVE APPROACHES

When I was at the Bristol Cancer Help Centre, I learnt how important my stopped-up creativity was in my illness. The counsellors there seemed to understand so much about what life – living and dying – is about. I learnt such a lot about myself, including new and exciting aspects to my life that I never dreamt of. It's helped me enormously.

My psychotherapist told me that my sessions were just as important when I was ill – if not more so.

It came as a shock to realize that being ill was relevant to my therapy, and vice versa.

While some therapists and counsellors recognize their healing role, psychotherapeutic approaches and creativity generally are not sufficiently recognized in terms of their value in healing and preventing illness of all kinds.* In Chapter 8 we give an idea of a range of psychotherapeutic approaches, and below we list some of the creative ones that can be valuable. Yet the boundaries between *psycho*therapy, *creative* therapy and *physical* therapy are becoming increasingly blurred as holistic ideas gain recognition. Indeed, there is a variety of approaches which embrace holism to such an extent that to categorize them as 'psycho-' or 'physical' or 'creative' therapy can seem inappropriate. Dance, movement generally, music or art, for example, can reach us simultaneously on the levels of mind, emotions, body and spirit, and some so-called psychotherapies such as psychosynthesis or transpersonal psychology (see p. 135) link these different dimensions of human existence in a subtle way. In addition, many of the practitioners of approaches already discussed in this chapter may use insights from various psychotherapeutic disciplines (though not necessarily with the care or skill that they require).

For those approaches that involve talking as a major component, see Chapter 8. A separate chapter is devoted to them because the context within which we need to understand psychotherapeutic interventions is complex and

---

*Unfortunately, many therapists fail to appreciate the subtle connection between mind, emotions and body, and they lack the awareness required to work with these subtleties. If we are looking for help with illness, therefore, we may need to shop around for someone who is skilled on several levels.

requires more discussion than is appropriate here. However, since so many practitioners of various kinds may use (or claim to use) some sort of counselling or psychotherapy in their work, please read the section on counselling and psychotherapy in conjunction with this chapter.

ART

All of us used images long before we learnt to speak, and continue to do so – in memories, dreams and fantasies. They continually affect and reflect our experiences in our lives and relationships.

Art therapy has become the most widely practised form of 'creative' therapies available in the NHS. There are, for example, art therapists in most psychiatric units. Their approaches vary enormously – from rather rigid interpretations of symbols to less directive approaches. Most see painting, drawing or clay-work as a form of communication between the client and the therapist, as well as a form of communication with the client herself. Rather than imposing their own interpretations, however, a skilled art therapist should focus on what the painting means to the person concerned.*

Mary Lynne Ellis, a feminist art therapist, believes art therapy is very useful for women:

The painting offers us a frame that is completely ours, enabling us to define ourselves. This is particularly important for women because so often we're defined only in relation to other people. Through art we may feel more able to express feelings that as women we're not supposed to have, such as feelings of neediness or anger, the frame of the paper containing them, allowing them to be less overwhelming. These may include less conscious feelings or feelings we don't have words for. In painting we discover our own language . . . Our artwork offers us our own mirror, a concrete reflection that we can return to and which offers us a source for exploration with the art therapist and the other women if in a group. In sharing what we create in our paintings, we can discover how to create changes in our lives.

Art can also be very helpful in working on physical ill health or disability, e.g. through visualization (see p. 108). However, the value of art in relation to physical health has yet to be developed in the NHS.

There are presently few art therapists working outside psychiatric units and day-centres, but there is no reason why they could not be asked to run sessions in women's or community centres. It may also be possible to see an art therapist on an outpatient basis if you ask for this. But the potential benefit of our own art is there for everyone: doing a painting a day, however crude, however quick, may unleash more energy and give us more insight into our health – or illness – than many more costly approaches (both in terms of time and money).

I remember when I became friends with an artist. I'd never ever felt able to create anything on paper (apart from words), but one day, when I was feeling very stuck – knowing I was angry but unable to feel it, unable to move on – she managed to persuade me to 'create' something on paper. At first it seemed totally impossible. Then I drew a line. Then another. Then I scribbled and scrabbled all over it. The relief! I tore into the paper. At last I could move on.

See Resources under Healing for more about art as therapy.

SOUND AND MUSIC

Music and rhythm find their way into the secret places of the soul. (Plato)

Music is the mediator between the life of the senses and the life of the spirit. (Ludwig van Beethoven)

It has been known for centuries that sound affects us very deeply, whether we are aware of it or not.[37] Certain types of sound can have healing or relaxing properties, and tapes are now available (see Resources) which are designed to promote healing and relaxation. Other types of sound can unleash energy in us . . .

You can coax them into a frenzy, you can make them sweat and sweat again, you can take them riding on one great wave of pleasure to one big communal orgasm.[38]

or stopped-up painful feelings . . .

Then I put on some Chopin by Alan Schiller . . . It made me cry . . . I couldn't stop, all this sadness and bitterness pouring out, and mixing in with the beauty of the music which had become painful.[39]

We can be affected not only by the sounds that we hear. The sounds that we make affect us too; they also reflect our inner world. We can use both sound that we hear and sound that we create for our growth and healing, for fun, relaxation, stimulation and liberation.

---

*The discussion in Chapter 8 on choosing a therapist applies as much to art therapists as to therapists who work primarily with words, although it is possible that a skilled art therapist without a feminist perspective is less potentially damaging for women than other types of psychotherapist, because whatever you've created is in *your* language, and it cannot be taken away from you.

For most of us, the most significant sound we make is with our voices, yet when young we were often taught to inhibit them. Learning how to reverse this can be an immensely liberating and joyful experience, releasing a lot of energy. Often we need someone to help us do it – and many women have found that voice workshops, pioneered by Frankie Armstrong in this country, have given them the help they needed.*

I started going to voice workshops and discovered a voice I didn't know I had. I had been able to sing in tune and softly and sweetly but this was strong and powerful and everyone was making a big NOISE. Everyone who came to these workshops had different reasons. Some felt they couldn't sing at all, others sang in tune in the bath but couldn't raise their voices anywhere else and others just wanted to sing together. It was supportive and encouraging and there was no pressure to perform and every chance to find mechanisms to liberate our voices.

Music or voice workshops for women are becoming increasingly popular in this country. If you want to find out more, contact *Spare Rib*, one of the women's therapy centres, or a local 'alternative' magazine such as *Cahoots* (see Resources). Some alternative practitioners use music in their work, to encourage us to be responsive with our bodies, emotions and souls. But music therapy as such is rarely available in the NHS, except for people with mental handicap. If you want to pursue this, try contacting the relevant associations listed on p. 114.

DANCE AND MOVEMENT

Dance and movement can have powerful therapeutic potential, as Rudolf Steiner's work with Eurythmy has shown.[40] Though rarely used as therapies in their own right in this country, some therapists involved with healing work with movement.[41]

At Bristol [Cancer Help Centre] I remember spending a whole morning just moving with my eyes closed. Though the music was wonderful, it still took me time to give myself permission to get into it – I'm so inhibited! But gradually I began to 'feel' my way in to moving, and that gave me a sense of how to connect up with myself, with the parts I deny, and which, not having any room or recognition, are dying. I've begun to give them life.

While movement and dance therapists are still rare in the

UK, many of us are discovering the power of the ancient art of circle dancing.

Within the Circle I transform myself and bring my inner journey to life. It's fun and I feel alive. When I experience a unity with others through the Circle I have hope for humanity and the future. I feel as though I am healing myself and the earth I dance upon. I am linked with all those who have danced in circles and spirals since the beginning of time. I dance as they did, to celebrate, to heal, to grieve and to prepare for battle and death. Primarily I dance the Circle because I enjoy it. For me, enjoyment is the best reason for doing anything and when I enjoy myself so much, I become so energized that it is like a tonic to myself and those around me. I feel united with the places in which I dance . . . Dancing joyfully in the Circle boosts the spirit of any place.[42]

All the approaches discussed here may be used on their own or in conjunction with visualization, meditation, etcetera. With the exception of circle dancing, they may be done individually as well as in groups.

SOME PROBLEMS FACING ALTERNATIVE MEDICINE AND ITS PRACTITIONERS

As doctors' power has increased, and particularly after the inception of the NHS, allopathy has had a stranglehold on our health care.* There are three major broadsides that the medical establishment regularly launches against alternative medicine:

- that 'alternatives' lack any scientific basis;
- that alternative medicine is another way of conning people;
- that only when the effectiveness of 'alternative medicine' can be demonstrated should it receive any official recognition.

Of course, there is a singular lack of any scientific basis for many allopathic practices,[43] and while there is some truth to the con-game argument,† it does not take into

---

*Frankie Armstrong worked with an anthropologist called Ethel Raim who had made field recordings of Balkan 'folk' songs. The sound that she encourages women to find is a raw-edged, open-throated, open-air voice that is very like a shout to start with, using energy not effort. Work-songs, sea-shanties, African songs and chants of slave gangs have similar qualities.

*This stranglehold varies in different countries. For example, homoeopathy has succeeded in maintaining a foothold in the UK, Naturecure likewise in Germany, but neither to any great extent in the USA.
†See, e.g., Martha Roth, 'Life among the Wellness People', *World Medicine*, 12 January 1980. The Festival of Mind and Body that now takes place annually in London may also be thought to represent the unacceptable face of the 'wellness' industry, in terms of the number of exhibitors who are clearly interested only in seducing people into spending money. Yet this exhibition also provides a platform for people concerned with true health and healing – not just of individuals, but of societies, and the world.

account the very powerful con-game that doctors themselves can be involved in. Since they so often marshal science in their support, this makes their own conning all the more difficult to spot, and to challenge. If similar criteria were applied to allopathic practices, few would clearly pass the efficacy test. As the report of The Netherlands Commission for Alternative Systems of Medicine concluded, disallowing a practice prior to its effectiveness being demonstrated is indefensible.[44]

The medical establishment acts as judge and jury of approaches for which its framework is inappropriate. The allopathic framework dominates the planning of our health service, and even research, so that the problem is perpetuated. Having established themselves where the power lies, doctors have consistently dictated the terms in which all alternative medicine is examined. The British Medical Association, for example, conscious of its appearance in the eyes of many people as a learned body (though it is no more than a somewhat self-important trade union representing doctors' interests), periodically emits dire warnings that we should avoid going to 'unqualified' practitioners. (The term 'unqualified' in this context means anyone who is not a doctor.) Recently, sensing change in the air, it initiated its own inquiry into alternative medicine. Yet an inquiry carried out by a monopolistic profession keen to protect its power and status from outsiders has to be seen in terms of the self-interest of that profession. It is in this context that the BMA report should be read.*

However, while doctors' power, roles and attitudes present a formidable problem, there are indications of change in some quarters. The General Medical Council, for example, which has statutory powers concerning doctors' behaviour, has reviewed its previous policy so that now a doctor is entitled to refer someone to an alternative therapist without fear of being struck off. More doctors are also beginning to recognize the complexity of human functioning, the nature of healing and of healing energies, and so on (see, for example, *Talking Health*, edited by Sir James Watt and Clive Wood, which is a report of eight meetings held at the Royal Society of Medicine between 1984 and 1987). Yet while many such doctors have joined the recently-formed British Holistic Medical Association, there is still a danger that self-interest will get the better of their more honourable motivations, and that the Association will end up shoring up doctors' power to the detriment of alternative practitioners and, ultimately, of the rest of us too.

Perhaps the major dilemma facing alternative practitioners today is how far they are willing to compromise in order to become accepted into the NHS. While there is undoubtedly growing pressure on the NHS to embrace alternatives, there is a grave danger that they will be incorporated only in so far as they do not threaten the power and status of doctors. One disturbing trend in response to this pressure is

that of doctors attending extremely short courses in alternatives, and then considering themselves proficient enough to practise them without further training.

Particularly insidious is the idea that alternative practitioners should be allowed into the NHS only if they are subordinate to doctors, and therefore do not see people independently in their own right. As one socialist practitioner says:

> *Even if I could practise within the NHS, I wouldn't. I'm simply not prepared for the ten minutes per patient routine. Nor am I prepared just to see bad backs – which as an osteopath that's all a doctor is likely to send me.*

For alternative practitioners to be brought into the NHS on an equal footing would require a government willing not only to have arguably the biggest confrontation with the medical profession yet, but also to foot the bill.

SOME PROBLEMS WITH ALTERNATIVE METHODS AND PRACTITIONERS

We have already discussed some of these in the introductions to this book (see discussion on 'Healthism', p. 19) and in this chapter (see Holism, p. 84), as well as under the specific practices examined. We must also emphasize the following.

Limited Availability

On the whole, most types of alternative medicine, with the singular exception of Healing, are not easily accessible. Most can be found only in large cities and/or in affluent areas and, as they are for the most part unavailable under the NHS, we have to go privately. Many private practitioners also support the values of private medicine.

Risks of Professionalization

Just as with conventional medicine, you can learn a lot from professionals who have crucial information you need to stay well. However, we live in a time of excessive dependence on experts, which means we often turn to professionals for things that they are not trained to do or that we could do better for ourselves. Some alternative practitioners, like conventional doctors, are setting themselves up as experts in such a way that they keep power for themselves, are unwilling to share their knowledge with you and try to get you to keep returning to them for additional services.

Lack of Social and Political Awareness

Implicit in the practice of much 'alternative' medicine is that you have a certain responsibility for keeping yourself healthy and for helping yourself get better. While trust in our capacity for self-healing is a welcome change from medicine's dependence on outside intervention, 'alternat-

*This report, published in 1986, though unfavourable to alternative medicine, does it a service by displaying a considerable amount of medical ignorance and prejudice.

ive' medicine sadly often falls into the same trap as conventional medicine by disregarding political and social factors – such as poverty and racism – as major sources of ill health. For instance, a practitioner might prescribe rest, exercise and change in diet, and not attend to the fact that the problem is caused by a dangerous on-the-job situation, or to the fact that, as a struggling single parent, your needs (and the possibility of fulfilling them) are far more complex and problematic. While alternative practitioners are well in advance of conventional medicine in appreciating the subtleties involved in health and disease, they have a long way to go before they can be considered to be truly holistic (i.e. incorporating social and political awareness into their practice). All too easily, they can end up 'blaming the victim', oblivious to the myriad ways in which our oppressive society affects us. And since, like conventional medicine, alternative medicine originated in male-dominated cultures, they can often be particularly sexist and homophobic.

'Heads I Win, Tails You Lose'

There are many ways in which human beings can and do affect the course of their illness or wellness, and we can all develop our understanding of ourselves in this respect. However, this does provide many a therapist with a cast-iron let-out which leaves their reputation intact if we remain ill: far from questioning the appropriateness of their own approach, some are far too ready to off-load any responsibility for the situation, claiming or suggesting, for example, that 'You haven't tried hard enough', 'It's not the right time for you to get better', or 'You don't want to get better'. This catch-22 is all the more problematic because there can also be some truth in these statements. To get the best out of any healing approach we use, we need to beware of this 'Heads I win, tails you lose' philosophy, while at the same time being open to considering the particular role we ourselves are playing in our dis-ease.[45]

Limited Controls

In the UK alternative practitioners have the freedom to practise under common law. This means that anyone, without any training at all, can set themselves up as an acupuncturist, osteopath or whatever. This state of affairs has enabled the development and practice of quite a strong alternative medicine movement, but leaves us vulnerable to poor standards and exploitation.* However, alternative practitioners are not allowed to claim that they can cure certain diseases, including cancer.

While membership of certain organizations does indicate a recognized training and qualification, most forms of alternative medicine are not officially recognized in any way. Of course, official recognition can be as meaningless as any trumped-up qualification, and while the current system is absurd, it does at least mean that alternative

practitioners can operate outside the stranglehold of allopathy's value-system. And as Robert Eagle says:

> There are vast areas of alternative medicine where therapy is largely intuitive and for which formal training is irrelevant . . . The pressure for control is coming from professional in-groups which, I argue, are more concerned with enhancing their own status than with broader public interests.

For ideas on how to choose an alternative practitioner, and how to avoid the worst quacks, see p. 103. See also Resources, p. 275, for details of bodies which can provide information on practitioners who have bona fide qualifications, such as they are. Check with organizations whether they are a recognized professional body and if so, in what way they are 'recognized'.

There are also limited controls concerning the production and preparation of alternative medicines, and on these grounds the pharmaceutical industry is currently pressing for the availability of such medicines to be limited by statute. So far, the government has resisted this pressure, but there will be a time very soon when all alternative medicines will have to be submitted to the kind of scrutiny which now applies only to allopathic medicines. The danger is that, unless an appropriate model can be developed for assessing such medicines and unless the assessing body comprises a wider membership than allopaths, it is possible that so-called 'natural' medicines may no longer be legally dispensable.

Lack of Research

There is little research that unequivocally demonstrates the success of alternative systems of medicine, partly because research in this area is so difficult to conduct, partly because the dominance of allopathy serves to prevent such research being conducted, and partly because of the complacent and to some extent irresponsible attitude of the alternative medicine establishment. (It is to be hoped that the Research Council for Complementary Medicine, founded in 1982, may have some effect in this respect.) While the vast majority of allopathic approaches have not been evaluated in terms of effectiveness and safety, this is even more true as far as alternative medicine is concerned. Sometimes alternatives provide little if any help, and they can also be harmful and even dangerous, particularly in unskilled and irresponsible hands. We need to choose practitioners carefully.

FINDING PEOPLE WHO PRACTISE ALTERNATIVE MEDICINE

The NHS

Although only in exceptional circumstances are you likely to find anyone, increasing numbers of NHS staff (not only doctors, but also physiotherapists, nurses, etcetera) are

---

*This situation is currently thought by some to be under threat due to proposed changes in EEC regulations, which could outlaw many alternative practices and practitioners.[46]

developing 'alternative' skills. A few doctors are beginning to work in conjunction with alternative practitioners and, increasingly, doctors are prepared to refer you to them. (From recent surveys, it seems that GPs are more knowledgeable and supportive of alternative medicine than the BMA's attitude would indicate.)[47]

There are also *ad hoc* and sometimes unofficial ways in which 'alternative' medicine is being integrated, and there is also the singular exception of homoeopathy (see p. 91). Unfortunately, progressive health workers sometimes have to operate in an extremely underhand way – which of course reinforces the status of allopathic medicine, and no doubt may even account for some of its 'success'. As a nurse said recently:

> I don't want it blazoned forth that alternative medicine [in this case, reflexology] is being practised at the —— Hospital because it could set things back before it's got a strong enough foothold. I know of numerous other hospitals where they're doing similar things to us. But we're all facing the problem of insurance, and one hospital stopped doing it for this reason: people are being inhibited by the law from broadening the approach within the NHS. And it's doctors who are responsible for that law.

It is possible, therefore, by keeping your eyes and ears open, asking around, and getting lists of membership from progressive organizations (see Resources, that you may be able to track down someone who can provide what you are looking for within the NHS. In the meantime, pressure via such organizations as CHCs and the BHMA (see Resources) may have a useful effect on the NHS in your locality, although, as we discuss on p. 100, the obstacles facing the integration of alternatives into the NHS are formidable.

Outside the NHS

Often there is more choice (if you can afford it). Local health-food shops can often tell you about practitioners, as can women's centres. While many advertise, bear in mind that most professional associations governing alternative practitioners do not allow their members to advertise. You will need to contact the associations or the Institute for Complementary Medicine (see Resources).

WHICH METHOD? WHICH PRACTITIONER?

Aside from the issues already mentioned, here are some guidelines for choosing and using alternative practitioners:

Investigate

- Speak to other people who have been helped by a certain practice. Make sure you ask about the particular practitioner they used. Ask about negative as well as positive experiences with both method and practitioner, including racist, heterosexist and sexist attitudes, for example.
- Seek out other women who are also interested in getting information about how to approach and heal a certain illness (you could put a notice in the local women's centre or health-food shop). Together you may be able to form a research or self-help group. Try and get your local library or health education department to stock relevant books, and subscribe to women's health and holistic health publications.
- Contact some of the organizations listed in the Resources. They may be able to tell you whether or not they think their approach might be effective for you, and/or suggest names of practitioners in your area.

Some possible questions to explore with a practitioner

- Do they have experience of treating someone with health problems similar to yours? Was the treatment successful? How do they know? How long did it take? What happened? Would they also be willing to ask on your behalf if someone who they have helped would be prepared to talk to you about the experience?
- What kind of training have they had? (While a qualification *may* indicate a certain amount of knowledge or standardized training, pieces of paper do not guarantee anything, and a practitioner can develop far better skills by becoming apprenticed to a particularly wise and experienced healer.)
- Do they consider themselves holistic and, if so, how far do they recognize that social and political considerations are part of a holistic approach?
- Are they willing to suggest ways in which you can help yourself? (Some may prefer you to keep visiting them so you can help pay their bills!)
- Do they think that their treatment is the best treatment, or do other therapies have something to offer? Would they be willing to refer you to other practitioners if necessary? (Beware of anyone who offers miraculous cures . . . even though you might want definite answers, they are rarely appropriate within any system of medicine.)
- Do they receive supervision? (As we indicate in Chapter 8, this is an essential prerequisite for practising responsibly though it happens rarely. A practitioner in training who is not receiving regular supervision should be avoided.)
- What are their weak spots? (Given the inadequacy of much training, they would be dishonest to indicate 'none'. The main purpose of this question is not necessarily so that you can avoid an ignorant practitioner, but rather so you can assess how far they're willing to acknowledge their fallibility, and the fallibility of their chosen approach.)
- You may want to combine the least invasive of allopathic diagnostic techniques with the best that a

healing method has to offer. Do they think that allopathic medicine has anything to offer and would they be willing to discuss things with your doctor?

- Do they operate on a sliding scale of fees, or provide any free consultations?
- Why have they taken up this line of work? (Many a good healer has done so after having gone through a serious illness/crisis of their own.)

Use all these questions, not simply to find out factual information but also so you can notice how you feel about the person, the *way* s/he is responding to you, whether you can communicate together, and so on. And since so many practitioners believe they are competent to practise psychotherapeutically, we recommend that you read the section in Chapter 8 on Choosing a Therapist.

Some Points to Bear in Mind

- When you first contact a practitioner, you may want to interview him/her before deciding if you want to go to him/her – in the same way as we suggest for a doctor on p. 628. No practitioner is used to this, even though it's an excellent idea, as you can *both* consider if you want to work together. After all, holistic health care involves a *partnership*. If they agree, make sure you've established that, as an interview, it is not something you will expect to be charged for.
- It is perhaps best not to set your heart on one particular therapy, particularly if you don't live in a large city. The practitioner is more important than the form of medicine they practise: if the form of medicine seems 'right' but the practitioner doesn't, it might well be better to explore other possibilities.
- Whatever methods we consider, we must bear in mind that a good practitioner can often help us get well *regardless* of what 'therapy' s/he practises. This is probably a lot to do with the placebo response – in allopathic terms a little understood phenomenon whereby people can get better apparently on the basis of no tangible or measurable intervention. It is very much promoted by a good relationship between therapist and client, and may have a lot to do with the therapist's ability to inspire us, or even with her/his own healing energy. Though scorned, particularly by many doctors and 'scientists', the placebo effect is not to be underestimated, and it is worth bearing in mind when assessing any therapy, including those offered by allopaths. The implications of the placebo response are far-reaching and do in fact challenge much medical research and practice . . . and, by implication, vindicate much 'alternative' practice. [48]
- Re-read Some Problems with Alternative Methods and Our Role in Becoming Healed, p. 101 and p. 84.

We need to keep talking with one another, checking out, evaluating and re-evaluating methods and practitioners.

I asked my friends for recommendations for a yoga teacher and several suggested one man. When I

went to meet him, a voice inside me told me this man was not the teacher for me. I said to myself, 'I really want to do yoga; this teacher has been highly recommended; perhaps it's because I don't get along well with men.' But that voice kept saying, 'I don't want to.' I contemplated the matter by sitting down, closing my eyes and just being quiet. The thought kept rolling through my mind, getting stronger and more persistent: This is not the right teacher for me. I dropped the idea of studying yoga with him.

In general, be as informed and assertive as you can. Balance the isolation of the one-on-one therapeutic encounter by joining or forming self-help groups of women who share your health problem or who want to learn more about the method. Work in whatever ways you can for changes which would make the alternative healing methods available to more people. There are many sincere, skilful, compassionate alternative practitioners. We must look for them, ask them to share their skills with us, tell our friends about them and find ways of using them without becoming unnecessarily dependent upon them.

APPENDIX

Here we look at a range of healing practices or techniques which can be learned relatively easily, and which we can practise either on our own, in our day-to-day lives, or with a partner. They are listed in alphabetical order.

THE ALEXANDER PRINCIPLE

This was originated by F. Matthias Alexander around the beginning of this century. It is based on the principle that by 'un-learning' the habitual ways we have developed of using ourselves (e.g. the way we think, feel, worry, stand, sit, walk, talk, breathe), we can achieve a better way of functioning. This can have far-reaching implications for our general health, both physical and mental. It can enable us to be and move more naturally and harmoniously, rather than being forced by habit and cultural conditioning into an alien mould. As a corollary, we can 'let go' of the ways in which our bodies take the strain of our emotions, although this of course may mean we have to face emotional pain we had previously managed to avoid.

The implications for women are particularly important, because we have been so pressurized over the years to misuse our bodies in the way we dress and move. The Alexander Principle can help us in childbirth as well as in other situations – from playing a musical instrument or bending over a desk to performing at a job interview or any other potentially anxiety-producing situation.

I started having Alexander lessons after I had almost permanent pain in my shoulder and back that no one could help except with short-term relief. Now I understand that no one was dealing with the cause of the problem, which was why it continued. Soon after I started having lessons, I realized I myself could make the pain disappear, by putting into practice what I had learnt. If I ever get those pains now, I know that it is because I am causing them by my reactions, and it is within my power to prevent them. But Alexander also made me feel more healthy generally and more competent to act in the world. I can deal with situations which I never dreamed I could and in a way I could never have done.

Learning Alexander can not only prevent – and sometimes heal – dis-ease,* but also enable us to be more freely creative. It is no accident that many musicians swear by it. But it is not necessarily easy, and, as with healing approaches in general, change is required – and that change can be threatening.

I didn't find it easy to let go of all the bodily ways I used to protect myself. My whole self-image had to go. I often felt very naked in the world without my usual 'props', though curiously free at the same time. Alexander confronted me with one of the paradoxes of life!

To learn Alexander you usually need to go to a teacher, for while it can be understood by reading about it, learning to practise it from books is as difficult – or impossible – as trying to psychoanalyse oneself. This is because our sensory awareness needs re-educating, and someone else is needed to guide us through the mass of what we think of as instinctive and unalterable habits.

Since we wrote our last edition, there are now many more Alexander teachers around, coming from several different training schools. Some teachers are beginning to run imaginative courses that involve applying the Alexander Principle to playing an instrument, running, singing, or (un)learning how (not) to be (un-)creative, etcetera. Other teachers are more traditional. To find a teacher, contact the organizations listed in Resources. While most work privately, some are beginning to find their way into educational establishments. Local education or health authorities could also be persuaded to engage teachers to run courses.

See Resources under Healing for further information.

MASSAGE

When done effectively, massage can relax the body, release muscle tension, improve joint flexibility, increase circulation and sensation and generally enhance our well-being.

*Wilfred Barlow, in his book *The Alexander Principle*, describes many instances of people becoming free of chronic problems following Alexander training, ranging from arthritis and asthma to headaches and stuttering.

We can use many massage techniques on ourselves as well as on others.

When you have the following conditions do not get a massage: phlebitis, skin disease, blood clots or infections. Skin that has become thin due to burn or injury should not be massaged either. Nor should skin which is red or bruised.

You don't need any special training to do general massage. Just get into a comfortable position and begin. Try holding your friend's foot, head, hand, back, neck, shoulders. Ask her where she wants pressure, whether you are applying too much pressure or not enough. Continue the communication as you progress, to make sure you are giving her what *she* wants. With your thumb or whole hand, find and rub tender areas or sore spots. Alternate gentle stroking with deep kneading; possibly using visualization, too, can be useful, although your partner may prefer a more consistent approach. Avoid direct pressure on the spinal column; instead, press on either side. Breathe regularly and deeply while giving the massage.

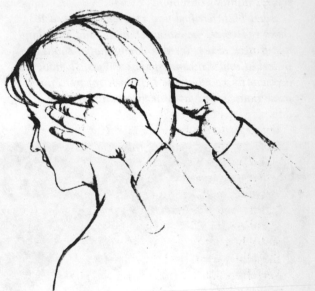

Christine Bondante

Many people who do massage see themselves as channelling energy through their bodies and hands to heal. There is a wide variety of massage methods, including shiatsu and acupressure (see p. 94). Most practitioners combine techniques from several methods. Some incorporate other techniques such as visualization (see below) or insights gained from bioenergetics or psychotherapy. See Resources under Healing for books about massage and related techniques. A masseuse said:

The way you touch someone is more important than the actual system you use. Whether you see yourself as channelling energy or are concerned with the muscle tone in your body and how you communicate it to someone else, you have to be rooted in your own body and pay attention to what is happening to you all the time you are giving the massage. While I give everyone the same massage in the order of things I attend to, my touch feels different to different people.

I had gone to see the masseuse (who worked at her home) because my body was filled with tension and I wanted some relief. When I arrived, she suggested to me that I might be storing old emotional wounds in my body, as indicated by my posture. I asked her what she meant, a bit defensively. After all, I was doing yoga, walking and eating well. I just had a lot of tension, that's all.

She didn't give a mental explanation. Instead, she asked me to lie down, and she began to massage the vertebrae in my neck. Massage, hold steady, massage, hold steady. At first I felt only the degree of tension in my neck; gradually I experienced a lump forming in my throat, my chest heaving and a bunch of old sensations returning to mind. I began to cry, small jerky sobs at first, like the opening of a faucet that has been shut off for a long time. Then a burst of tears, and finally several minutes of sobbing.

I was both terrified and relieved – terrified to think that there was so much deep emotion behind a stiff neck and relieved to know that it could be unlocked and soothed. At that moment I made a decision to see what else I could learn from this mysterious body that walked around with me all day.

Michelle Fiorenza

If at some point you decide you want a professional massage or want to take a course or apprentice yourself to someone, get names from friends, your local woman's (health) centre or from a holistic health centre or directory if one exists in your area. Carefully select the person you go to; recommendations from friends are often the best kind of referrals. Masseuses differ enormously. Some (very few) feel that pain is necessary! Some don't like to talk. Qualifications don't mean very much (training – such as it is – tends to be all about techniques). Look for someone whose approach is more that of a healer than of a manipulator, who uses techniques you like, and with whom you feel comfortable and can communicate well. Masseuses usually work in private practices, but some work as part of organizations like health clubs.

You may not know what you want or what to expect the first time you make an appointment for a massage.

Some people come in with specific physical complaints or problems with body alignment; others just want a chance to stretch and relax, and others want to do emotional 'work' along with the massage. Before we begin I work out an understanding with them about what they want.

MEDITATION

Meditation gives us the opportunity to be with ourselves. A simple definition of meditation is 'the intentional paying of attention from moment to moment'.

Meditation in its essence is different from every other human activity, but its essence is contained in every activity. Meditating, each one of us touches base with our deepest concerns, with the truth of our aliveness.

Meditating at its best doesn't remove us from living, numb us to stressful situations or stop us from acting effectively. It puts us in touch with the moment and helps us respond directly. If we have meditated recently we are more likely to be alert and resourceful when we are called upon to help someone.

People begin to meditate for different reasons – because it feels good in itself or because they want to feel calm, to diminish physical or mental stress or pain or to get through a spiritual crisis. You might approach meditation only for practical reasons – to relax or reduce stress – and then discover that something happens that makes you want to go deeper, to attain a different level of consciousness.

Although meditation practices have been directly or indirectly related to healing for millennia,[49] health practitioners in this country are only beginning to acknowledge its potential, and sadly, too few doctors are teaching people about it. Meditation helps us slow down breathing and heart rate, reduce oxygen consumption, lessen muscular tension, change brain-wave patterns and respond calmly to stressful situations, thereby lowering the risk of having a heart attack or a stroke.[50]

There are many ways to meditate. Though you can meditate while you stand, walk, dance or jog, many people sit or kneel in a quiet environment. You can sit on a cushion with your legs crossed or tucked under you or on a chair with your feet on the ground. Repeating a word or sound over and over again can calm your mind; concentrating on your breathing can help focus your attention. Praying is a form of meditation. You can meditate at home indoors or outdoors, or in formal settings – churches, synagogues and other places of worship. You can practise alone or with others in a common meeting place.

Like many women, I spent my whole life doing things for others, and looking to others for a definition of who I am. I've been successful in living this way but the price was high – constant anxiety over whether I would succeed or fail not only others but my own exacting standards as well. I turned to meditation as a way to help me feel good. It really helps to be with others in my meditation group who are committed to the same inner journey.

You might feel best learning meditation practice by yourself, or you might want a religious or secular teacher to guide you and discuss your progress and problems with you along the way. However, beware of teachers who provide answers or groups which offer prescriptions for living.

When practised consistently, meditation can help us pull our lives together.

My early-morning meditation is part silence, part chanting. Sometimes I actively pray while I sit looking at the rising sun. It's important for me to meditate every morning, if only for ten minutes, to touch base with myself. I am continually surprised at how I get upset more easily on the days I don't meditate. Sometimes during the day when I'm silent or alone I find myself automatically feeling the tranquillity I experience during meditation. This calmness helps me. Though usually my meditations are rather ordinary, on some days they are profound.

See Resources under Healing for further reading.

RELAXATION

Relaxation does not happen automatically the minute we want to relax. It doesn't even happen automatically in sleep. But it can be learnt, and it is deep relaxation particularly that promotes healing. (It has benefits similar to those discussed under Meditation.) A health visitor speaks from experience:

I do two relaxations a day, and, if I'm not feeling well, I'll do many, many more. I can even stop colds materializing if I follow this routine!

Amber Lloyd of Relaxation for Living says:

When you are tense and anxious, very little repair work is carried out, barely even the day-to-day maintenance, which is why nervous people tend to look old and worn before their time. The more often you can relax deeply, at odd moments as well as set-aside periods, the better will you feel and the better will you look.

Relaxation takes practice and is not necessarily easy. Learning in a group is ideal, but tapes and books can be very helpful too, as can advice from an experienced teacher.

There are probably more health professionals interested in relaxation than in any of the techniques mentioned in this Appendix. If you can't find a health visitor, health education officer or psychologist prepared to run a relaxation group, then you'll probably have to find a private teacher. Relaxation for Living (R for L), which has helped to pioneer the teaching of relaxation in this country, can provide you with a list of trained teachers. Private teachers may be prepared to charge reduced rates, and it may be possible to arrange for them to run classes as part of a local authority education or health education programme.

TRYING RELAXATION*

This is how you can practise relaxation from a sitting position, but it can also be done lying down (people often prefer their head slightly raised – either on a cushion or a book or two), and even standing.

First, take some fresh air, even if only from an open window. Make sure your weight is firmly on the bones beneath your bottom, so that your spine isn't taking unnecessary strain. Ideally, place your feet flat on the floor, with your legs apart the distance of your hips (the height of your chair should enable you to do this in comfort).

Then, check whether you have unnecessary muscle tensions as you are reading this: make sure your jaw is not clenched and that fingers not in use are uncurled; sit at the back of your chair so that your back is supported; let your shoulders drop and feel heavy; encourage your breathing to be low down, slow and slight, moving your tummy not your upper chest; wobble your head a little, to make certain it is balanced, centrally, on top of your spine; let your knees flop apart and uncurl your toes. Encourage your thoughts to be positive; realize that you are now comfortable and at ease; tell yourself these are sensible habits, and that to sit quietly relaxed is a very gainful way of spending time and will pay dividends; you are paying energy into your energy bank account. Stay like this for a few minutes.

*From Amber Lloyd's pamphlet, *A Relaxed Person*, available from Relaxation for Living (see Resources). Quoted with permission.

R for L also produces tapes and leaflets, for example on dealing with attacks of nervousness and panic, and runs a correspondence course. A list of recommended books can also be obtained from the organization (send large sae). See also Resources under Healing for further reading.

T'AI CHI
By LINDA CHASE BRODA

I saw a woman doing t'ai chi in the park. I was completely mesmerized and enchanted. I didn't even know what it was, but I knew that I wanted to do it myself. I wanted to be in that peaceful place she was creating for herself.

T'ai chi is a Chinese form of exercise which features a long slow sequence of moves based on martial art applications. Many films on China and Hong Kong show scenes of people (especially old people) practising t'ai chi in parks under the trees in the early morning. They are doing the 'solo' exercise, one aspect of t'ai chi practice.

Another aspect is pushing hands which is an exchange between two people based on pushing and yielding. The partners develop sensitivity, and the ability to respond.

At first, pushing hands seemed to be about punching and blocking. Now it seems to be about everything I can think of . . . an endless variety of possible actions, reactions and interactions. My friends say I've become better at listening before I respond. Pushing hands has taught me this.

Another aspect of t'ai chi is Chi Kung, or breathing exercises which coordinate the breath with repeated simple movements of the body. Chi Kung is a noted health practice as well as one which develops physical strength.

Individual teachers may emphasize a particular approach to t'ai chi, for instance, as a martial art, as a health practice or as a meditation. A martial art t'ai chi school would teach sparring, martial applications, uprooting and weapons as well as the solo form and exercises. The head of the school would be judged on his/her abilities as a fighter.

The first time we practised 'punching' [the air] in our women's t'ai chi class, I was so surprised at myself . . . I couldn't do it. I was afraid of my own power. I didn't really know what it was. Now, after long practice, it's getting much clearer. I like my power.

When t'ai chi is practised for health and healing, then relaxation and softness are stressed to keep the body responsive. Students are encouraged to improve their balance, breathing and physical coordination through their practice.

I started t'ai chi because I had such awful balance. I often felt as if the ground was pushing me away. The t'ai chi exercises for grounding, rooting,

walking and sinking have made me feel more connected and comfortable with my own stance.

T'ai chi as a meditation can be seen as a way of concentrating awareness of the body, mind and spirit through movement. Feelings of peace and harmony often accompany t'ai chi practice.

Styles of t'ai chi are named after the various founders of the original schools, e.g., Yang, Wu, Chen and Sun. Under each name are many more variations of styles which have developed as a result of the changes made by individual teachers within the larger schools.

Finding a Teacher

If you live in London, you'll have a great deal of choice. The two largest schools in London are the British T'ai Chi Chuan Association and the International T'ai Chi Chuan Association. However, both have misleading names. They are not really associations with a network throughout Britain (or the world), but rather names of private schools which network only with the teachers they have trained. There are many other teachers in London and elsewhere in Britain who are not attached to any school. To find them, consult newspapers, magazines, libraries and noticeboards in alternative bookshops and health-food shops. Ask if you can visit a class before making a commitment.

VISUALIZATION*

We all create images in our minds, sometimes consciously, sometimes without being aware of it. We picture how we would like a future event to turn out or how we want our relationships to change. Images fill our dreams; some of them last into the next day.

Positive images make us happy and carry us through difficult times.

Many women are finding that visualizing a certain symbol, scene or process has a positive healing effect on their bodies. Midwives have long used images and relaxation exercises to help women in labour relax, diminish fear or tension and open up. The earliest records of visualization techniques used in healing date back to Babylonia and Sumeria; other ancient peoples used these techniques as well.[51] In our day, Canadian Eskimos, Navajo Indians and some Hispanic peoples (to mention only a few) use forms of healing based on visualization.[52]

While visualization probably has a powerful placebo effect (see p. 104), it also works in a general way by helping people relax. We can also use visualization techniques to affect the involuntary systems of the body, increasing blood flow to one particular area or slowing down the heartbeat. And we can use visual images to help minimize or control pain. In the words of a scientist who had several operations for cancer:

---

*Though visualization can be used for everything from decreasing drug dependence to the improvement of athletic ability, we concentrate on visualization used in conjunction with meditation to help heal specific conditions.

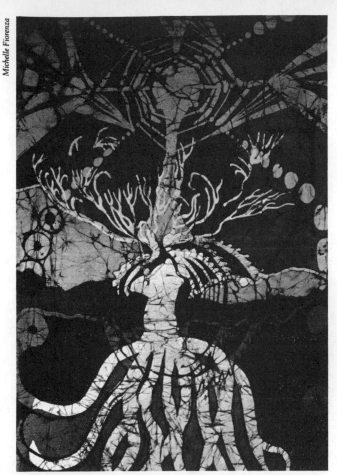

Michelle Fiorenza

Batik by Jane Pincus. One visual image: a strongly rooted tree

The two years since I've had the last operation have been the most productive of my life. I've had the opportunity to investigate healing in a way that I never did before. At first, when I felt the pain, I kept looking for an outside figure, a god figure to help me, to care for me, to make it better. Then I said to myself, 'Who's the most caring, best mother you know?' And I said, 'I am.' So I pictured myself cuddling myself. When the pain came, I went to it as a mother would to a child. I said, 'How can I help it? How can I go to it?' Now when it comes, I say, 'Poor baby.' I tried to treat myself in a loving way. The more loving I was to myself, the more healed I felt. Now the pain is mostly gone.

Visualization involves relaxing, feeling at one with the object, scene or process you imagine, letting it expand to fill your consciousness and become the only thing in your awareness. Hold your mind upon it. Sometimes it helps to have someone guide you. It often needs practice to be used effectively: it is a skill to be learned.

An example of a healing visualization:

Relax and let your attention go to the particular body part causing discomfort or pain, or which does not function as it should. Focus your attention on this place and let yourself experience what it feels like right now. Don't feel pressured to achieve a specific goal. After a while, allow an image related to that area to come to your mind. It may be a detailed picture of what you think that part looks like, or it may be more abstract. Keep your mind focused until you are content with your image. Change it whenever you want. Now begin to visualize something happening within that part of your body to make it work better or start to heal. You might see energy, light or colour flowing into it; imagine it becoming warm or cool. A powerful image could help you feel better right away.[53]

Autogenic training involves a specialized kind of visualization which is gaining a reputation in this country for its power and effectiveness for healing specific conditions. It involves the teaching of a series of powerful mental exercises. To learn it, you need guidance from a skilled practitioner. To find out more, contact the Centre for Autogenic Training (see Resources under Healing).

For visualization in relation to cancer, see p. 576.

YOGA

I get up in the morning and do the exercise 'Salute to the Sun' (actually a series of twelve postures). Whether I have a few minutes or a longer time to practise yoga, I benefit from the fullness of this exercise. I am cheered by the thought of saluting the sun. I am easily moved beyond the awkwardness of my body and the sleepy nature of my mind as I get into the movement of this exercise. After a while I am ready to welcome the day.

The aim of yoga is to renew the body, focus the mind and still the emotions. Yoga is a Sanskrit word which essentially means union. Underlying yoga practice is the belief that 'the body and mind are part of the continuum of existence, the mind merely being more subtle than the body.'[54] Studies show that yoga can cause physiological changes such as reduced blood pressure, lowered pulse rates, diminished stress, increased joint movement and improved hormonal functioning. The Yoga Biomedical Trust has collated information concerning the effects of yoga on a wide variety of health problems, ranging from back disorders to diabetes, and is hoping to obtain funding to investigate its value for menstrual and related problems (they have evidence from women who report being helped in a high proportion of cases). Having demonstrated from pilot studies the value of conducting further research,[55] it is disappointing but perhaps predictable that research bodies have been unwilling as yet to fund such research, preferring high-technology projects instead. Most research on the effects of yoga has been done in India.

The basic aspects of yoga practice include *asanas*, *pranayama* and *meditation*.

Asanas are physical postures which help stretch and limber the body.

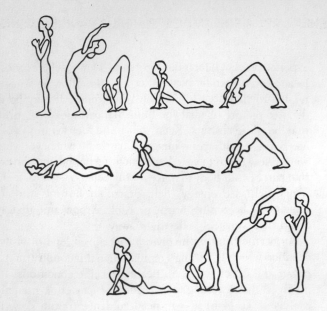

Jane Pincus

Before yoga my main experiences with exercise had been in gym or in modern dancing. These exercises were a variety of stretches to strengthen or loosen a particular part of my body and were usually done in short repetitive motions. In contrast, when doing yoga postures I was asked to move slowly into the posture, hold it still for some time, and then gradually release. This way of exercising has dramatic effects on my mind. I often begin in some turmoil, filled with the concerns of my day. As I focus my attention on my movements and my breathing, I experience my mind slowing down and relaxing. The practice gives me some distance from my problems. Doing the postures releases new energy, relaxes me and allows for another perspective to emerge.

Pranayama are breathing exercises which increase the flow of oxygen, thereby relaxing our whole being.

The first time I did yoga breathing exercises I was amazed at the capacity of my lungs. I watched my belly fill up, my chest expand, the air move into my shoulders. I realized I never had experienced a complete breath before – and I was in my thirties at the time!

Meditation. While the postures and breathing exercises are valuable in and of themselves, they also prepare us for meditation, or a practice of conscious relaxation that enables us to experience a coming together of the physical, mental, emotional and spiritual aspects of yoga. The breathing exercises and meditation are accessible to anyone, and no matter what our physical restrictions, we can do them.

We can learn yoga on our own (see Resources for useful books). However, there is no substitute for a good teacher. Yoga classes are taught in adult education classes, community and leisure centres, and church halls and private homes.* See Resources for organizations that have lists of qualified yoga teachers throughout the country. The Yoga Biomedical Trust can also help find suitable teachers for people with particular problems or disabilities. Whether you practise for fifteen minutes a day or for more extended times, it is important to practise regularly.

The problems with yoga are the problems of any healing method applied improperly. Don't push through the pain to complete the exercise no matter what. Proceed at your own pace, trusting your limits. Benefits come from your regular efforts rather than from reaching a specific goal.

NOTES

1. See Joanna Macy. 'Despair Work', *Evolutionary Blues*, no. 1 (available from Evolutionary Blues, Box 4448, Arcata, CA 95521, USA); also, *Despair. Personal Power in the Nuclear Age*. Philadelphia: New Society Publishers, 1983.
2. Mary Howell, MD, PhD. *Healing at Home*. Boston, MA: Beacon Press, 1979, p. 87.
3. See, e.g., Harry Edwards. *The Power of Spiritual Healing*. Harry Edwards Spiritual Healing Sanctuary Trust, 1978.
4. See, e.g., Alice Walker. *In Search of Our Mothers' Gardens*. London: Women's Press, 1984, especially pp. 83–116. For examples of how black women writers are incorporating this knowledge into their fiction and poetry, see Paule Marshall, Toni Morrison and Alice Walker in Mari Evans, (ed.). *Black Women Writers*. London: Pluto Press, 1985; and Marjorie Pryse. 'Zora Neale Hurston, Alice Walker, and the "Ancient Power" of Black Women' in M. Pryse and J. Hortense Spillers (eds). *Conjuring: Black Women, Fiction and Literary Tradition*. Indiana University Press, 1985, pp. 1–24.
5. Uma, 'Traditional Medicine is Our Ancestors' Gift for Life', in *Challenging the Racism that Harms Our Health*. Report of a conference sponsored by the Greater London Council, 1985. See p. 114 for Black Women Healers Group.
6. For an overview of how healing has reached its status – or lack of it – in the UK today, including the role of doctors in squashing the idea of healing via their trade union, the British Medical Association (BMA), see books by Inglis and West, and Harvey listed in Resources; see also Edwards, op. cit., note 3, on the role of the Christian Church in recent years.
7. Leslie Weatherhead discusses the Lourdes phenomenon in his book, *Psychology and Life*. London: A. James, 1985.
8. See, for example, Raymond Moody. *Life After Life*. New York: Bantam, 1976; and Elisabeth Kubler-Ross's work (see p. 581).
9. See Dolores Krieger, PhD, RN. *The Therapeutic Touch: How to Use Your Hands to Help or to Heal*. Englewood Cliffs, NJ: Prentice-Hall, 1979, for a detailed description of her method, philosophy and findings.
10. Alec Forbes. 'Healing Refreshes the Parts Other Therapies Cannot Reach', *General Practitioner*, 24 November 1978, p. 26.
11. See, e.g., Mary Anderson. *Colour Healing: Chromotherapy – How It Works*. New York: Aquarian Publishing Co., 1979; and Sarah Rossbach. *Feng Shui*. London: Hutchinson, 1984 (about the ancient Chinese wisdom which is based on recognition of the effects of our surroundings).
12. Krieger, op. cit., note 9, p. 17.
13. Hallie Iglehart. 'Expanding Personal Power through Meditation', in Charlene Spretnak (ed.). *The Politics of Women's Spirituality*. New York: Anchor Press, 1982.

*Unfortunately, because of education cuts, some free classes have been discontinued.

14. Rosemary and Victor Zorza. *A Way to Die: Living to the End*. London: Sphere, 1981.

15. See William Thomson. *Herbs that Heal*. London: Black, 1977.

16. Bryan Silcock. 'Medicines Moss Can Mend', *Sunday Times*, 11 August 1985.

17. See Chou Chien-Chung. 'Chinese Plant Medicine', *World Health*, July 1978.

18. Reported in 'The Arms Race', *The Lancet*, 30 January 1982, p. 290.

19. See Stephen Fulder. 'Ineffective Herbal Remedies in the UK Market', *Journal of Alternative Medicine*, February 1986, p. 4.

20. See, e.g., J. O. McGee et al. 'A Case of Veno-occlusive Disease of the Liver . . .', *Journal of Clinical Pathology*, vol. 29, 1976, p. 788; and Julia F. Morton. 'Is there a Safer Tea?', *Morris Arboretum Bulletin*, vol. 26, 1975, p. 24.

21. See Michael McIntyre. 'Exposed: the Inaccurate Reporting behind the Herbal Medicine Scare', *Journal of Alternative Medicine*, January 1984, p. 2. See also, Fred Fletcher Hyde. 'Herbs and Herbal Medicine Still Under Attack', *Journal of Alternative Medicine*, November 1985, p. 7.

22. Ruth West. *The College of Health Guide to Alternative Medicine*, London: College of Health, 1984.

23. In the 1950s Dr W. E. Boyd performed a number of experiments which suggested that substances which by conventional standards contained 'nothing' could in fact effect change in a biological situation (e.g. 'Action of Small Doses of Crataegus, Digitalis, Strophantus Gratus and S. Sarmentosus on the Heart Rate and ECG of an Exposed Frog Heart', *British Homoeopathic Journal*, vol. 43, 1953, p. 11); more recent research indicates that different numbers of succussions – as well as potencies – have a critical effect on the substance concerned (e.g. R. L. Jones and M. D. Jenkins. 'Effects of Hand and Machine Succussion on *in vitro* Activity of Potencies of Pulsatilla', *British Homoeopathic Journal*, vol. 72, no. 4, 1983, p. 217); for a double blind trial suggesting the value of homoeopathy for rheumatoid arthritis, see R. G. Gibson et al. *British Journal of Clinical Pharmacology*, vol. 9, 1980, p. 453; see also British Homoeopathic Research Group's journal *Communications*, which carries meeting reports and articles from a range of disciplines examining the effectiveness and mode of action of homoeopathy, and Professor Jacques Benviste's paper published in *Nature*, 30 June 1988, p. 816. Attempts have been made to discredit Benviste's paper; see paper by Maddox et al. in *Nature*, 28 July 1988. For an overview of the affair and the extraordinary lengths to which members of the establishment can go to maintain the scientific status quo, see Denis MacEoin, 'The Denaturing of Science' in *Journal of Alternative and Complementary Medicine*, September 1988, p. 14.

24. See, e.g., Dr R. Davey. 'Measurement Techniques with Special Reference to Immunology', Midlands Homoeopathy Research Group *Newsletter*, no. 6, August 1981.

25. See, e.g., R. Morris-Owen. 'On Controlled Trials in Homoeopathy', Midlands Homoeopathy Research Group *Newsletter*, February 1983. Perhaps because of the pressure to perform 'acceptable' trials, there have been times when homoeopathy has been distorted to fit in with trial requirements. The recent controlled trial by Shipley et al., investigating the treatment of osteoarthritis (*The Lancet*, 15 January 1983, p. 97) involved a single remedy, Rhus Tox, at a given dosage taken for fourteen days, compared with a placebo. It showed no significant difference from the placebo. But as Dr R. Morris-Owen says: 'In normal practice, unhampered by trial requirements, most patients presenting with osteoarthritis would receive an initial high potency treatment with a remedy chosen on personal detail, and the continuous treatment with low potency of Rhus Tox, or some other remedy, only in sequel to this' (*Communications*, no. 9, 1983). In other words, the trial was the equivalent of testing antibiotics in inappropriate doses for too short a time.

26. Such as lead, for example. This was referred to by Dr R. J. Pinsent at the Ninth Annual Symposium on Homoeopathy.

27. For an insight into homoeopathic sexism see Ellen Crowe. 'Women's Work? The Role of Women in Medicine', *The Homoeopathic Alternative*, Autumn 1984, p. 10.

28. For more information on the history of medical politicking in relation to homoeopathy see, for example, Michael Barraclough. 'Quis separabit?

– Some Reflections on Homoeopathy and Politics', *British Homoeopathic Journal*, vol. 69, no. 2, 1980, p. 57.

29. For more information about how NHS homoeopathy has suffered in more recent years see Jill Rakusen. 'Consumer Power in Action – That's What Homoeopathy Needs Now', *Homoeopathy Today*, Spring 1981, p. 6. Ironically, the wider use of homoeopathy is likely to *save* on the NHS drugs bill, not increase it.

30. Fritjof Capra. *The Turning Point*. New York: Simon and Schuster, 1982.

31. 'Acupuncture', *World Health*, December 1979 (available from WHO, CH-1211 Geneva 27, Switzerland).

32. See, e.g., Jack Worsley. *Talking About Acupuncture*. New York: Element Books, 1982.

33. Kim Smailes, quoted in Carole Spedding, 'Acupuncture, a Better Way of Healing', *Spare Rib*, no. 79, February 1979.

34. Quoted in Spedding, op. cit., note 33. An excellent system of health care for lay people is J. Thie and M. Marks. *Touch for Health*. Marina de Rey, CA: De Vorss Press, 1973.

35. See, e.g., Roger Newman Turner. *Naturopathic Medicine*. Wellingborough, Northants: Thorsons, 1984.

36. Ibid.

37. David Tame. *The Secret Power of Music*. Wellingborough, Northants: Turnstone Press, 1984.

38. Dave Haslam. 'The DJ and the Dancefloor', *Cahoots*, no. 20, 1987.

39. Jill Rakusen. 'A Musical Journey', *Cahoots*, no. 20, 1987.

40. This forms part of the Anthroposophical approach. See Francis X. King. *Rudolf Steiner and Holistic Medicine – an Introduction to the Revolutionary Ideas of the Founder of Anthroposophy*. London: Rider, 1986.

41. An inspiring account of what dance can do for people with heart problems is given in Arabella Melville and Colin Johnson. *The Long-life Heart: How to Avoid Heart Disease and Live a Longer Life*. London: Century, 1985.

42. Gerry Rowlands. 'Confessions of a Circle Dancer', *Cahoots*, no. 20, 1987.

43. See, e.g., US Congress OTA. *Assessing the Safety and Efficacy of Medical Technologies*. Washington DC: US Government Printing Office, 1978; and E. L. Cochrane. *Effectiveness and Efficiency*. London: Nuffield Provincial Hospitals Trust, 1972.

44. Dutch Ministry of Health and Environment Protection. *Report of the Commission for Alternative Systems of Medicine*. The Hague, 1981.

45. For further discussion of this tricky issue, see, for example, Jason Serinus, (ed.). *Psychoimmunity and the Healing Process – a Holistic Approach to Immunity*, Millbrae, CA: Celestial Arts, 1986; or Lawrence Le Shan. *You Can Fight for Your Life – Emotional Factors in the Treatment of Cancer*. Wellingborough, Northants: Thorsons, 1984.

46. See, e.g., Christine Eade. 'The Threat from Europe', *Journal of Alternative Medicine*, November 1986, p. 9.

47. See, for example, survey by Taylor Nelson Management Consultant Group, commissioned by *The Times* and the Koestler Foundation (Ruth West and Brian Inglis, *The Times*, 13 June 1985); and Eileen Anderson and Peter Anderson, *Journal of the Royal College of General Practitioners*, February 1987.

48. See, e.g., Linnie Price. 'Art, Science, Faith and Medicine: the Implications of the Placebo Effect', *Sociology of Health and Illness*, vol. 6, no. 1, 1984, p. 61.

49. Herbert Benson. *The Relaxation Response*. New York: Morrow, 1975.

50. Ibid., pp. 70–1, Table 2.

51. Mike Samuels MD and Nancy Samuels. *Seeing with the Mind's Eye*. New York: Random House, 1975.

52. See, e.g., Stanley Krippner and Alberto Villoldo. *Realm of Healing*. Millbrae, CA: Celestial Arts, 1976. See also Robert T. Trotter II and Juan Antonio Chavira. *Curanderismo: Mexican American Folk Healing*. Athens, GA: University of Georgia Press, 1981.

53. Paraphrased from Dennis T. Jaffe. *Healing from Within*. New York: Knopf, 1980, pp. 241–2.

54. Judith Hanson Lasath. 'Yoga: an Ancient Technique for Restoring

Health', in *The Holistic Health Handbook* compiled by the Berkeley Holistic Health Center, Berkeley, CA: And/Or Press, 1978, p. 36.
55. See, e.g., 'Yoga Survey Report', *Yoga Today*, vol. 9, no. 5/6, 1984.

RESOURCES

PUBLICATIONS (Material marked with an asterisk is specifically designed to be of practical value on a self-help basis.)

GENERAL

Association of Community Health Councils in England and Wales. *The State of Non-Conventional Medicine – The Consumer View*. London: ACHEW, 1988.
*****Berkeley Holistic Health Center**. *The Holistic Health Handbook*. Berkeley, CA: And/Or Press, 1978.
Capra, Fritjof. *The Turning Point*. New York: Simon and Schuster, 1982.
Chamberlain, Mary. *Old Wives' Tales, Their History, Remedies and Spells*. London: Virago Press, 1981.
Colegrave, Suki. *The Spirit of the Valley – Androgyny and Chinese Thought*. London: Virago Press, 1979.
Dossey, Larry. *Space, Time and Medicine*. London: Routledge and Kegan Paul, 1982.
Dossey, Larry. *Beyond Illness – Discovering the Experience of Health*. New Science Library, 1984.
Dutch Ministry of Health and Environmental Protection. *Report of the Commission for Alternative Systems of Medicine*. The Hague, 1981.
Eagle, Robert. *Alternative Medicine*. London: Futura, 1978.
Foulkes, Jane. *Institute of Complementary Medicine Yearbook*. Slough, Berks.: Foulsham, 1986. A directory of therapies and practices in the UK.
Fulder, Stephen. *The Handbook of Complementary Medicine*. Oxford: Oxford University Press, 1988. Not as comprehensive as Inglis and West (see below), but more thorough on the topics it does cover.
Fulder, Stephen and Robin **Monro**. *The Status of Complementary Medicine in the United Kingdom*. London: Threshold Foundation, 1981.
Inglis, Brian and Ruth **West**. *The Alternative Health Guide*. London: Mermaid, 1983.
Kidel, Mark and Susan **Rowe–Leete**. *The Meaning of Illness*. London: Routledge, 1988.
Pelletier, Kenneth. *Mind as Healer, Mind as Slayer*. London: Allen and Unwin, 1978.
Roth, Julius. *Health Purifiers and their Enemies: a study of the Natural Health Movement in the United States with a comparison to its counterpart in Germany*. London: Croom Helm, 1976.
West, Ruth. *The College of Health Guide to Alternative Medicine*. London: College of Health, 1984.

HEALING Including self-healing approaches ranging from music to yoga

Achterberg, Jeanne. *Imagery in Healing – Shamanism and Modern Medicine*. Boston: New Science Library, 1985. A somewhat academic discussion, but one that brings together strands from many cultures and practices.
*****Barker**, Sarah. *The Alexander Technique*. New York: Bantam, 1978. An attempt to explain how to learn it without a teacher.
Barlow, Wilfred. *The Alexander Principle*. London: Arrow, 1981.
Bek, Lilla and Philippa **Pullar**. *The Seven Levels of Healing*. London: Rider, 1986. Recommended by the National Federation of Spiritual Healers.
*****Benson**, Herbert. *The Relaxation Response*. London: Fontana, 1977.
Beresford-Cooke, Carola. *Massage for Healing and Relaxation*. London: Arlington Books/Thames TV, 1986.
*****Bokun**, Branko. *Humour Is Our Best Medicine*. London: Branko Bokun (26 Chelsea Square, London SW3), 1982.
*****Burns**, Echo Bodine. *Hands That Heal*. San Diego: ACS Publications, 1985. About healing yourself and others.
*****Chaitow**, Leon. *Your Complete Stress-Proofing Programme*. Wellingborough, Northants: Thorsons, 1983.
*****Cousins**, Norman. *Anatomy of an Illness – Reflections on Healing and Regeneration*. London: Corgi, 1981. A much-acclaimed personal ac-

count of the self-healing process, that focuses, among other things, on the importance of laughter.
Cowley, Elizabeth. 'Massage: Women and the Poverty of Touch', *Spare Rib*, no. 157, August 1985, p. 6.
Dalley, Tessa (ed.). *Art as Therapy*. London: Tavistock, 1984. Provides overall view of different approaches to art therapy in Britain.
*****Dickenson**, Donald. *How to Fortify Your Immune System*. London: Arlington Books, 1984.
*****Downing**, George. *The Massage Book*. London: Penguin Books, 1972.
*****Feldman**, E. B. *Becoming Human Through Art*. Englewood Cliffs, NJ: Prentice-Hall, 1970.
*****Fringe-Keyes**, M. *The Inward Journey: Art as Therapy for You*. Millbrae, CA: Celestial Arts, 1976.
Galante, Lawrence. *T'ai Chi: the Supreme Ultimate*. York Beach, ME: Weiser, 1982. Good all-round view.
Gardner, Adelaide. *Meditation – a Practical Study*. Beckenham, Kent: Quest, 1968.
*****Gawain**, Shakti. *Creative Visualization*. New York: Bantam, 1987.
*****Gelb**, Michael. *Body Learning: an Introduction to the Alexander Technique*. London: Anrum Press, 1981.
*****Hamel**, Peter M. *Through Music to the Self*. New York: Element Books, 1978.
*****Harrison**, John. *Love Your Disease – It Keeps You Healthy*. London: Angus and Robertson, 1986.
Harvey, David. *The Power to Heal – an Investigation of Healing and the Healing Experience*. Wellingborough, Northants: Aquarian Press, 1983.
*****Hay**, Louise. *You Can Heal Your Life*. Santa Monica, CA: Hay House, 1984 (available from Heaven on Earth Books, see Bookshops). About positive thought.
*****Hay**, Louise. *Heal Your Body – the Mental Causes for Physical Illnesses and the Metaphysical Way to Overcome Them* (pamphlet). London: Heaven on Earth Books, 1985. The above book is based on this.
*****Horn**, Sandra. *Relaxation: Modern Techniques for Stress Management*. Wellingborough, Northants: Thorsons, 1986.
Horstmann, Lorna. A *Handbook of Healing* (pamphlet). National Federation of Spiritual Healers (see Organizations), n.d.
Horwitz, Tem, et al. *T'ai Chi Chuan – the Technique of Power*. London: Rider, 1979. Excellent for beginners. Written from a Western point of view.
Inglehart, Hallie. 'The Unnatural Divorce of Spirituality and Politics', in Spretnak (see below).
*****Irwin**, Yukiko. *Shiatzu*. London: Routledge and Kegan Paul, 1977. Easy-to-follow self-help guide. (See Acupuncture, p. 94.)
Iyengar, B. K. S. *Light on Yoga*. London: Allen and Unwin, 1966.
*****Jampolsky**, Gerry. *Love is Letting Go of Fear*. Millbrae, CA: Celestial Arts, 1979 (available from Heaven on Earth Books, see Bookshops). A powerful book for self-healing.
*****Keleman**, Stanley. *Living Your Dying*. New York: Random House, 1974. An inspiring book that has much of relevance to healing.
*****Kent**, Howard. *Yoga for the Disabled*. Wellingborough, Northants: Thorsons, 1985.
King, Francis X. *Rudolf Steiner and Holistic Medicine – an Introduction to the Revolutionary Ideas of the Founder of Anthroposophy*. London: Rider, 1986.
Krieger, Dolores. *The Therapeutic Touch – How to Use Your Hands to Help or to Heal*. Englewood Cliffs, NJ: Prentice-Hall, 1979.
*****Lad**, Vasant. *Ayurveda – the Science of Self Healing – a Practical Guide*. Detroit: Lotus Press, 1984.
*****Le Shan**, Lawrence. *How to Meditate – a Guide to Self-Discovery*. Wellingborough, Northants: Turnstone Press, 1983.
*****Long**, Barry. *Meditation – a Foundation Course*. Barry Long Foundation (KBCM, Box 876, London WC1N 3XX).
MacManaway, Bruce, *Healing*. Wellingborough, Northants: Thorsons, 1983. Provides a useful overview, though it ignores women's involvement in history of healing. Includes chapters on developing healing ability and environmental factors.
*****Mariechild**, Diane. *Motherwit – a Feminist Guide to Psychic Development (Exercises for Healing, Growth and Spiritual Awareness)*. New York: Crossing Press, 1981.

Ornstein, Robert and David Sobel. *The Healing Brain*. London: Macmillan, 1988.

Ousely, S. G. J. *Colour Meditations*. Charleston: Fowler, 1949 (15th imp., 1983).

Pearce, Ian. *The Gate of Healing*. London: Neville Spearman, 1983. Written by a doctor.

*Pogson, Jose. *Healing Through Meditation* (pamphlet). National Federation of Spiritual Healers (see Organizations), 1983.

Rossbach, Sarah. *Feng Shui*. London: Hutchinson, 1984.

*Rush, Anne Kent. *Getting Clear: Body Work for Women*. London: Wildwood House, 1974.

*Schneider, Meir. *Self Healing*. London: Routledge and Kegan Paul, 1987.

*Segal, Jeanne. *Feeling Great! A Personal Program to Speed Healing and Enhance Wellness*. North Hollywood, CA: Newcastle Pub. Co., 1983. Goes further than most books with similar titles, drawing for example on music, movement and spiritual dimensions.

*Serinus, Jason (ed.). *Psychoimmunity and the Healing Process – a Holistic Approach to Immunity and Aids*. Millbrae, CA: Celestial Arts, 1986.

Sherman, Jill. 'The Laying on of Hands', *Nursing Times*, 20 November 1985, p. 18.

*Simonton, O. Carl et al. *Getting Well Again*. London: Corgi, 1986.

*Spence, Christopher. *Aids – Time to Reclaim Our Power*. London: Lifestory, 1986. Aids is spawning a powerful new awareness of how to live with the challenge of illness, and books such as this deserve a wide audience.

Spretnak, Charlene (ed.). *The Politics of Women's Spirituality*. New York: Anchor Press, 1982. Includes several chapters about healing.

*Struna, Monika with Connie Church. *Self-massage*. London: Hutchinson, 1984.

Tame, David. *The Secret Power of Music – The Transformation of Self and Society Through Musical Energy*. Wellingborough, Northants: Turnstone Press, 1984.

*Thie, J. and M. Marks. *Touch for Health*. Marina de Rey, CA: De Vorss Press, 1979.

Wadeson, Harriet. *Art Psychotherapy*. New York: John Wiley, 1980. Very expensive but worth trying to borrow from library. Includes a little discussion about art therapy with women.

*Wallace, Amy and Bill Henkin. *The Psychic Healing Book*. Wellingborough, Northants: Turnstone Press, 1981. A demystifying, practical (though not feminist) guide. Does not distinguish between psychic and spiritual healing.

Watt, Sir James and Clive Wood. *Talking Health: Conventional and Complementary Approaches*. London: Royal Society of Medicine, 1988.

White, Ruth and Mary Swainson. *The Healing Spectrum*. Saffron Walden, Essex: C.W. Daniel, 1986.

*Wilson, Annie and Lilla Bek. *What Colour Are You? – the Way to Health Through Colour*. Wellingborough, Northants: Turnstone Press, 1981.

Wood, Betty. *The Healing Power of Colour*. Wellingborough, Northants: Aquarian Press, 1984.

PLANTS AND HERBS

Bach, Edward. *The Twelve Healers and Other Remedies*. Saffron Walden, Essex: C.W. Daniel, 1933 (and still in print). An introduction to Bach Flower Remedies.

Dincin Buchman, Dian. *Herbal Medicine: the Natural Way to Get Well and Stay Well*. London: Herb Society/Hutchinson, 1979.

Grieve, M. *A Modern Herbal*. London: Penguin Books, 1980.

Griggs, Barbara. *Green Pharmacy: a History of Herbal Medicine*. London: Jill Norman, 1981. Surveys herbalism within historical context. Good, but fails to examine adequately women's role in history of herbalism.

Griggs, Barbara and Jill Norman. *The Home Herbal: a Handbook of Simple Remedies*. London: Pan, 1986.

*Mechtihld, Scheffer. *Bach Flower Therapy – Theory and Practice*. Wellingborough, Northants: Thorsons, 1986.

Mills, Simon. *The Dictionary of Modern Herbalism*. Hemel Hempstead: Herts: Argus, 1986.

*Potts, Billie. *Witches Heal – Lesbian Herbal Self-sufficiency*. USA: Hecuba's Daughters, 1981. The best book on herbs for women. Available from feminist bookshops.

Price, Shirley. *Practical Aromatherapy*. Wellingborough: Thorsons, 1987 (rev. ed.).

Tisserand, Maggie. *Aromatherapy for Women*. Wellingborough, Northants: Thorsons, 1985.

Vlamis, Gregory. *Flowers to the Rescue*. Wellingborough, Northants: Thorsons, 1986.

HOMOEOPATHY

Blackie, Margery. *The Patient, Not the Cure*. London: Macdonald and Jane's, 1976.

Boyd, Hamish. *Introduction to Homoeopathic Medicine*. Beaconsfield, Bucks: Beaconsfield, 1981.

*Clover, Anne. *Homoeopathy: a Patient's Guide*. Wellingborough, Northants: Thorsons, 1984.

*Cummings, S. and D. Ullman. *Everybody's Guide to Homoeopathic Medicines*. London: Gollancz, 1986.

Hahnemann, Samuel. *Organon of Medicine*. London: Gollancz, 1983. New translation of the definitive 6th edition.

Handley, Rima. 'Samuel Hahnemann's True Love: Melanie, the First Woman Homoeopath', *The Homoeopathic Alternative*, Summer 1984, p. 10.

*Speight, Phyllis. *Homoeopathy for Emergencies*. Saffron Walden, Essex: C.W. Daniel, 1984.

Vithoulkas, G. *The Science of Homoeopathy*. Encino, CA Gore Press, 1980.

ACUPUNCTURE

*Blate, Michael. *How to Heal Yourself Using Foot Acupressure* (Foot Reflexology). London: Routledge and Kegan Paul, 1983.

*Blate, Michael. *How to Heal Yourself Using Hand Acupressure* (Hand Reflexology). London: Routledge and Kegan Paul, 1983.

*Blate, Michael. *Natural Healer's Acupressure Handbook*. London: Routledge and Kegan Paul, 1978.

Lever, Ruth. *Acupuncture for Everyone*. London: Penguin Books, 1987.

Lewith, George. *Acupuncture: Its Place in Western Medical Science*. Wellingborough, Northants: Thorsons, 1982.

Robinson, Nicola and Monty Berman. *Acupuncture in General Practice – a Radical View*. London: East Asia Co., 1984.

Woollerton, H. and C. J. MacLean. *Acupuncture Energy in Health and Disease*. Wellingborough, Northants: Thorsons, 1983.

Worsley, J. R. *Talking About Acupuncture*. New York: Element Books, 1982. Beware sexist jokes.

Worsley, J. R. *Is Acupuncture for You?* New York: Element Books, 1985.

NATUROPATHY

Benjamin, H. *Everybody's Guide to Nature Cure*. Wellingborough, Northants: Thorsons, 1977.

Chaitow, L. *Osteopathy*. Wellingborough, Northants: Thorsons, 1982.

Cheraskin, Emanuel et al. *Diet and Disease*. New Canaan, CT: Keats Publishing, 1977.

Lindlahr, Victor. *Natural Therapeutics* (2 vols). Saffron Walden, Essex: C.W. Daniel, 1981. Classics.

Newman Turner, Roger. *Naturopathic Medicine*. Wellingborough, Northants: Thorsons, 1984. The author defines naturopathic medicine very broadly so he does not only discuss naturopathy.

Note: For more resources about dietary approaches, see Chapter 4.

MAGAZINES/JOURNALS

Cahoots, c/o 163 Palatine Road, Manchester M20 8GH. Excellent quarterly magazine, with listings of events in the north-west of England.

Human Potential Resources, 35 Station Road, London NW4. Listings of events nation-wide, plus articles.

Journal of Alternative [and Complementary] Medicine, Victory House, Leicester Place, London WC2H 7NB.

Out From the Core – a magazine about Radical Healing, c/o 23 Knowle Road, Leeds LS4 2EJ.

Panakaeia – 'a journal of feminist psychics and alternative healing' (on subscription from 1, Ravenstone Road, London N8). Contains articles ranging through mysticism, spiritual healing, therapies such as acupuncture, etc.

BOOKSHOPS AND DISTRIBUTORS

If you have difficulty obtaining any of the books listed in this chapter, the following bookshops are likely to be helpful:

Compendium, 234 Camden High Street, London NW1 8QS. Tel: 01–485 8944/01–267 1525.

Element Books, The Old Brewery, Tisbury, Salisbury, Wiltshire.

Heaven on Earth Books, 126 Elms Crescent, London SW4 8QR. Tel: 01–673 0962. Do mail order.

Waterstone's Booksellers, 193 Kensington High Street, London W8. Tel: 01–937 8432. Do mail order.

AUDIOTAPES

Healing and/or relaxation tapes can be obtained from the following organizations, which provide catalogues:

Matthew Manning Centre, 39 Abbeygate Street, Bury St Edmunds, Suffolk IP33 1LW. Tel: 0284–69502.

New World Cassettes, Freepost, Strawberry Vale, Twickenham TW1 1BR.

Relaxation for Living (see Organizations).

Slow Down, You're Going Too Fast, audiotape with *Stress and the Alexander Technique*, booklet, available from JDR Publications, 24 Cecil Park, Pinner, Middlesex HA5 5HH. Tel: 01–866 1262.

Women's Revolutions Per Minute, 62 Woodstock Road, Birmingham B13 9BN. Tel: 021–449 7041.

ORGANIZATIONS

GENERAL

British Holistic Medical Association, Gloucester Place, London NW1 6DX. Tel: 01–262 5299.

Campaign Against Health Fraud, Box CAHF, London WC1N 3XX. Tel: 01–673 4401. Started out as a campaign by orthodox practitioners against non-orthodox practitioners, but by the time you read this the campaign leadership and its policies may be more balanced.

Council for Complementary and Alternative Medicine, Suite 1, 19a Cavendish Square, London W1M 9AD. Tel: 01–409 1440. Set up in 1985 in an attempt to improve and maintain standards. Enjoys increasing support in some quarters but shys away from the spiritual component of alternative medicine.

Institute for Complementary Medicine, 21 Portland Place, London W1N 3AF. Tel: 01–636 9543. Information centre, with register of practitioners registered with some, but not all, professional associations.

Natural Health Network, West House, Salem Street, Gosberton, Spalding, Lincs. PE11 4NQ. Tel: 0775–840012.

Research Council for Complementary Medicine, Suite 1, 19a Cavendish Square, London W1M 9AD. Tel: 01–493 6930. A charity set up in 1983. Had a breakthrough in 1985 with some funding from the Medical Research Council, and another one in 1988 with some funding from the Department of Health.

HEALING

Association of Ayurvedic Practitioners (UK), 12 Agar Street, Leicester LE4 6ND.

Association of Professional Music Therapists in Great Britain, c/o The Administrator, The Meadow, 68 Pierce Lane, Fulbourn, Cambridge CB1 5DL. Tel: 0223–880377.

Black Women Healers Group, c/o London Women's Centre, 4 Wild Court, London WC2B 5AU. Tel: 01–405 0624/381 1159.

British Alliance of Healing Associations, Healing Secretary, Ms V. P. Hissey, 26 Highfields Ave., Herne Bay, Kent CT6 6LN. Tel: 0227–

373804. Registered charity; consists both of local associations, and of national bodies – ranging from the **Spiritualist Association of Great Britain** to the **Jewish Association of Spiritual Healers**. The Alliance is interdenominational.

British Association of Art Therapists, 13c Northwood Road, Highgate, London N6 5TL.

British School of Reflexology, The Holistic Healing Centre, 92 Sheening Road, Old Harlow, Essex CM17 0JW. Tel: 0279–29060.

British School for Reflex Zone Therapy of the Feet, Secretary, Ann Lett, 87 Oakington Avenue, Wembley Park, London HA9 8HY. Tel: 01–908 2201. Trains doctors and nurses and can supply addresses.

British Society for Music Therapy, The Administrator, Mrs Denize Christophers, 69 Avondale Avenue, East Barnet, Hertfordshire EN4 8NB. Tel: 01–368 8879.

British Wheel of Yoga, 1 Hamilton Place, Boston Road, Sleaford, Lincolnshire NG34 7ES. Tel: 0529–306851 (answering machine). Lists of qualified teachers throughout the country; runs teaching diploma courses.

Centre for Attitudinal Healing, PO Box 638, London SW3 4LN. Tel: 01–235 6733/200 7155. Runs workshops and meetings at St James's Centre, Piccadilly and at the Mary Ward Centre, London WC1. Also has contacts in other parts of the country.

Centre for Autogenic Training, 12 Milford House, 7 Queen Anne Street, London W1. Tel: 01–637 1586.

Churches' Council for Health and Healing, St Marylebone Parish Church, Marylebone Road, London NW1 5LT. Tel: 01–486 9644. Promotes healing within (Christian) churches, though does not recognize Christian Spiritualists who have a long-established healing tradition. Admits that 'official approach to Healing Ministry in the main-line churches often seems to be over-cautious'. Runs a healing centre at their premises, and can provide details of residential healing centres throughout the country.

The Circle Dance Network, c/o Nawall Gadalla and De Voce, 17 Vernon Road, Chester CH1 4JT. Tel: 0244–375945.

Confederation of Healing Organizations, General Secretary, 137 Cambridge road, West Wimbledon, London SW20 0PH.

Guild of Spiritualist Healers, 36 Newmarket, Otley, West Yorkshire LS21 3AE. Tel: 0943–2708.

Harry Edwards Spiritual Healing Sanctuary, Burrows Lea, Shere, Guildford, Surrey GU5 9Q6. Tel: 048–641 2054. Perhaps the best-known spiritual healing centre in Britain. Runs seminars as well as performing contact and absent healing.

National Federation of Spiritual Healers, Old Manor Farm Studio, Church Street, Sunbury-on-Thames, Middx TW16 6RG. Tel: 093–27 83164. Maintains a register of healer members and publishes a magazine, *Healing Review*. Membership does not require alignment with any particular religion or philosophy.

Relaxation for Living, Dunesk, 29 Burwood Park Road, Walton-on-Thames, Surrey KT12 5LH. Large sae for all details.

Shiatsu Society, 19 Langside Park, Kilbarchan, Renfrewshire PA10 2EP. Tel 05057–4657.

Society of Teachers of the Alexander Technique, 10 London House, 266 Fulham Road, London SW10 9EL. Tel: 01–351 0828.

Spiritualist Association of Great Britain, 33 Belgrave Square, London SW1X 8QB. Tel: 01–235 3351.

Touch for Health Foundation, Information Office, Adrian Voce, 8 Railey Mews, London NW5 2PA. Tel: 01–482 0698.

White Eagle Lodge, New Lands, Brewells Lane, Rake, Liss, Hampshire GU33 7HY. Tel: 0730–89 3300. London Centre at 9 St Mary Abbots Place, London W8 6LS. Tel: 01–603 7914. An independent Christian church, registered as a charity, with strong accent on spiritual healing (both for individuals and for the world), based on teachings of the spirit guide White Eagle. Has branches in several parts of the country, and individual healers in many more. All healers supervised. Welcomes and trains new healers.

Wrekin Trust, Runnings Park, Croft Bank, West Malvern, Worcestershire WR14 4BP. Tel: 0684–892898. Runs courses on a wide range of issues involving healing and spirituality.

Yoga Biomedical Trust, Director, Dr Robin Monro, PO Box 140,

Cambridge CB1 1PU. Tel: 0223–67301. Aims to promote research into effects of yoga and to publish results. Maintains a library, can supply references and reprints, maintains a register of qualified teachers, and aims to identify teachers suitable for people with special needs. Has set up 'Information Exchange Groups', e.g. for people over sixty-five, people with diabetes, where members with similar problems/disorders can compare notes and have access to research literature.

Yoga for Health Foundation, Ickwell Bury, Northill, Biggleswade, Bedfordshire SG18 9EF. Tel: 076–727 271. Runs courses, among other things, with reduced fees, e.g. for people of pensionable age.

PLACES TO GO

Burrswood, Groombridge, nr Tunbridge Wells, Kent TN3 9PY. Tel: 0892–863637: residential and healing centre.

Christian Fellowship of Healing, c/o The Holy Corner Church Centre, 15 Morningside Road, Edinburgh EH10 4OP. Tel: 031–447–9383: healing centre.

Divine Healing Mission, The Old Rectory, Crowhurst, Nr Battle, Sussex TN33 9AD. Tel: 042–483 204: healing centre.

Park Attwood Therapeutic Centre, Trimpley, Bewdley, Worcestershire DY12 1RE. Tel: 02997–444: a nursing and residential home staffed by doctors and therapists who practise Anthroposophical Medicine, after Rudolf Steiner (involving natural remedies and creativity). For more about Anthroposophy, see King under Publications, Healing.

Seekers Trust, Centre for Prayer and Spiritual Healing, The Close, Addington Park, Nr Maidstone, Kent ME19 5BL. Tel: 0732–843589: religious and healing centre.

PLANTS AND HERBS

British Herbal Medicine Association, PO Box 304, Bournemouth, Dorset BH7 6JX. Tel: 0202–435681.

Edward Bach Centre, Mount Vernon, Sotwell, Wallingford, Oxon OX10 0PZ. Tel: 0491 39489. For Bach Flower Remedies. Also provides postal consultation service and stocks books.

Herb Society (incorporating the Society of Herbalists), 77 Great Peter Street, London SW1P 2EZ. Tel: 01–222 3634. Membership open to anyone interested in herbs. Has a library, distributes books and publishes *The Herbal Review*.

National Institute of Medical Herbalists, The Secretary, 41 Hatherley Road, Winchester, Hampshire S022 6RR. Tel: 0962–68776. Recognized professional body. Send sae for list of registered practitioners (but there are only about 250 in the country). Members claim to take a holistic approach.

Natural Medicines Society, 95 Hagley Road, Edgbaston, Birmingham B16 8LA. Tel: 021–454 9390.

HOMOEOPATHY

British Association of Homoeopathic Chiropodists, 134 Montrose Avenue, Edgware, Middlesex HA8 0DR. Tel: 01–959 5421.

Faculty of Homoeopathy, c/o Royal London Homoeopathic Hospital, 60 Great Ormond Street, London WC1N 3HR. Tel: 01–837 3091: all members are doctors.

Homoeopathy Research Group, c/o Cadogan Gardens, London SW3 2RP. Tel: 01–730 4235.

NHS Hospitals

Bristol Homoeopathic Hospital, Cotham Road, Cotham, Bristol BS6 6JU. Tel: 0272–33068 (outpatients 0272–32007).

Glasgow Homoeopathic Hospital, 1000 Great Western Road, Glasgow G12 0NR. Tel: 041–339 0382. Outpatients Dept. Tel: 041–334 9800.

Liverpool Clinic, The Mossley Hill Hospital, Park Avenue, Liverpool L18 8BU. Tel: 051–724 23355.

Royal London Homoeopathic Hospital, 60 Great Ormond Street, London WC1N 3HR. Tel: 01–837 3091 (outpatients 01–837 7821).

Tunbridge Wells Homoeopathic Hospital, Church Road, Tunbridge Wells, Kent TN1 1JU. Tel: 0892–42977.

Society of Homoeopaths, c/o 2 Artizan Road, Northampton NN1 4HU. Tel: 0604–21400. Registers 'lay' homoeopaths.

ACUPUNCTURE

British Acupuncture Association, 34 Alderney Street, London SW1V 4EU. Tel: 01–834 1012. Publishes a register.

The Council for Acupuncture, Suite 1, 19A Cavendish Square, London W1M 9AD. Produces a register of the majority of qualified British acupuncturists.

Register of Traditional Chinese Medicine, 19 Trinity Road, London N2 8JJ. Tel: 01–883 8431. Publishes a register.

Traditional Acupuncture Society, 1 The Ridgeway, Stratford-upon-Avon, Warwickshire CV37 9JL. Tel: 0789–298798. Publishes a register.

NATUROPATHY

British Naturopathic and Osteopathic Association, Frazer House, 6 Netherhall Gardens, London NW3 5RR. Tel: 01–435 7320.

General Council and Register of Osteopaths, 21 Suffolk Street, London SW1Y 4HG. Tel: 01–839 2060.

Incorporated Society of Registered Naturopaths, 328 Harrogate Road, Leeds LS17 6PE. The oldest established naturopathic register.

Kingston Clinic, 291 Gilmerton Road, Liberton, Edinburgh EH16 5UQ. Tel: 031–664 3435. Produces quite a useful range of leaflets.

WOMEN AND MENTAL HEALTH

By
JILL RAKUSEN[*]

All chapters in this book touch on aspects of mental health. However, we feel it is important to devote a separate chapter to it in this new UK edition so that we can discuss some general issues, and also explore some specific ways in which women can find help.

WOMEN'S OPPRESSION AND MENTAL HEALTH

Circumstances and conditions that society has come to accept as normal or ordinary lead to profound unhappiness, anguish, and mental illness in women.[1]

Women's position in society affects our mental health. Those of us who are poor, black and/or lesbian face added socio-political, economic and environmental pressures that can take their toll on our resilience. Over the last fifteen years or so, many books have been produced which shed light on the mental strain that women's oppression causes. These include Sheila Rowbotham's *Woman's Consciousness, Man's World*, Jessie Barnard's *The Future of Marriage*, Ann Oakley's *Housewife*, Eva Figes' *Patriarchal Attitudes*, Jean Baker Miller's *Toward a New Psychology of Women*, Phyllis Chesler's *Women and Madness* and Luise Eichenbaum and Susie Orbach's *Understanding Women*.

Phyllis Chesler shows in *Women and Madness* how definitions of mental health are made in relation to men; for women this is always oppressive, and sometimes disastrous. Women are allotted the caring, sensitive role in our society. We therefore tend to be much more in touch with our feelings, and are often as a result able to find our way through impossible situations (sometimes too well). But this does present us with real problems. Often, for example, our experiences are invalidated and we are accused of being too sensitive; we can end up absorbing and taking on a lot of other people's problems, sometimes from an early age; and, as a corollary to our 'caring' role, we commonly end up perceiving our *own* need to be cared for as overwhelming, manipulative or just plain bad, despite the fact that this need is both unexpressed and unmet. Whatever our situation, the fact that we are socialized to be carers can challenge our emotional resilience to the utmost.[2]

For women with children, the major constraint involves responsibility for child care: we are expected to have sole responsibility for this, and to devote our lives to it. This leads to financial dependence – which militates against mental health and which frequently forces us to remain in unhealthy, or even violent, relationships.[*] It also can lead to a lack of stimulation and loneliness, pressures that can result in 'mental illness'. All these factors render us vulnerable – as well as affecting our children. While the importance of this issue is being increasingly recognized, the present Conservative government is firmly intent on reducing mothers' independence. As Patrick Jenkin, former Minister for Social Services, has stated:

Quite frankly, I don't think mothers have the same right to work as fathers. If the Lord had intended us to have equal rights to go to work, he wouldn't have created men and women. These are biological facts, young children depend on their mothers.

For many single as well as married women, loneliness is an issue. A *Woman's Realm* survey in 1978 found that one in four women aged between sixteen and sixty 'feels lonely or suffers symptoms of loneliness'. The survey didn't include women over sixty because it was felt this would

---

[*]Incorporating where possible material from the psychotherapy chapter in the US edition.

[*]Women's independence is being further reduced by the government's 'community care' programme for mentally ill people: 90 per cent of mentally ill people are already looked after in the community, mainly by women.

unbalance the survey as they can be *particularly* lonely. Women who were relatively well-off – e.g. who had the use of a car – were a lot less vulnerable. Not surprisingly, therefore, poor women may be particularly prone to mental ill health such as severe depression because of having less power over their lives, fewer choices, less money, and facing more hardship generally.*

When we try and break out of the constraints and stereotypes that confront us as women, this can lead to further problems. We may, for example, be labelled as deviant or even criminal. Young female 'criminals', for instance, have been shown to have committed far more trivial offences than boy criminals and, unlike boys, are far more likely to be given supervision orders for first offences. It has been suggested that the reason for this is that deviation from the sex stereotype is seen as in need of correction, whereas boys' 'delinquent' behaviour, far from being seen as maladjustment, need only be dealt with when it results in an actual criminal act.

Agoraphobia – where a woman has great difficulty leaving the house or being in crowds – is in many respects a logical response to societal attitudes which are at best ambivalent towards women being involved outside the home, particularly if we are mothers of young children. It can also be logical in another way: as our chapter on violence shows, the world isn't a safe place for women – though for many of us suffering from violent men, the home isn't a safe place either.

Depression, perhaps not surprisingly, is particularly common among women, and, as Kathy Nairne and Gerrilyn Smith show, our depression is connected to oppression.[4]

I was cooped up in a tiny flat with two toddlers, with my husband away a lot working, and my mother-in-law to look after. I stayed in hospital for about eight weeks and came right back to the same 'environmental' problems. These have increased with another baby, inflation and frequent illness in the family. The Samaritans have helped me keep sane.

Each new day is like the day before. You shop alone, eat alone, sit alone in despair until it is time to turn to your only friend, the sleeping pill. We are given plenty of good advice, like join some club, but we don't all have a club near, and we can't all face up to walking into a club alone.

I am not a women's lib member. I just feel very frustrated in a society where women are tolerated

rather than accepted as an equal – but perhaps this too is indicative of my personality disorder.

There are many reasons for women to feel depressed or overwhelmed. Sometimes the depression is transitory. But if nothing changes in our circumstances, it can continue to a greater or lesser extent for years.

For me, being married is like doing a life sentence of hard labour, literally in gaol and in an emotional desert; I hate being cooped up indoors and for the whole ten years of my marriage I have had a compressed, consumptive sort of churning emotion inside of me. I feel like a volcanically active pressure cooker and all the time the striving to simmer, rather than boil my own deadly brew, contrives to make me irritable, frustrated and desperate. This only being eased in the freedom of the 'great outdoors'. The irony of it all is that lately I am often unable to get myself out of the house to the shops. I seem to depend more and more on my daughter's arrival home from school for small sundries. With it being a main road area, I feel unprotected and extremely vulnerable and ache for the sort of anonymity and blending – which only seems to come from a communal atmosphere. I have become introverted to a frightening degree, and I'm sure my highly critical views of myself cannot be healthy . . . I tend to live in my highly active imagination more and more and in these fantasies I reap some, but little, satisfaction which I would get from a relationship with more depth. I

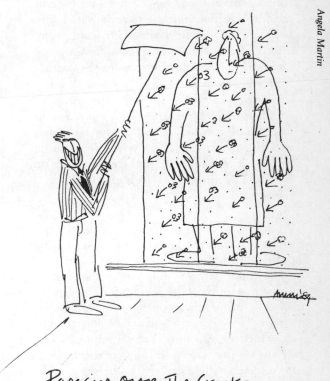

Angela Martin

Papering over the cracks . . . . .

---

*Brown and Harris have done some important research concerning women and depression. While they located various 'vulnerability' factors, they have been criticized for failing to make explicit links with poverty and class (and their conclusions are often used to confirm an individualistic approach to our problems rather than to support the need for social and political change which would tackle the causes of our isolation and poverty). See also Davies and Roche's critique of this study.[3]

think the worst aspect of the whole situation is that I do not 'give' to my children the time, love and affection of which I am capable. I was once absorbed (or as absorbed as a trapped person can be) in the older two, but I spend so much time gnawing over the impossible relationship with their father that the resulting feeling of failure, guilt and desolation is driving me to distraction. I have attempted to leave and wrote to four separate organizations inquiring about housing, but to no avail. Although I have been driven to the edge of despair where the only obvious solution has been to go, I could not *leave my children. I may be a bad-tempered, forever shouting mother, but I do have an empathy with their personal traumas, and my husband is simply far too inadequate a person to care for them. He is insensitive to anything on a personal level. But then if he had these qualities, I wouldn't be feeling this way, nor forever searching for a way out for us to become independent of him.* HOW DO I DO IT?

Depression can often be our own anger about the conditions of our lives, turned against ourselves. We can learn to direct our anger to our advantage, perhaps with the help of others (see p. 120 and p. 127). We can channel it creatively rather than destructively (e.g. putting it to good use in a tenants' association to campaign for improvements in housing, or joining a women's aid group). But to do so, we need support. Without it, we may remain trapped, unable to take the first step. As the woman quoted above said:

Any depression I may suffer has a tangible and removable reason, but how to remove it? I am a working-class woman. Even at my worst, I am always able to put on, or rather allow, my naturally happy nature to come to the fore, at least while out of the home environment. I am unable to even hint at the desperately panicky situation which is contained within my smiling face. It's all very well telling us to make friends with neighbours, etc. When you're depressed the problem is that you *don't feel capable of making friends. You just feel worthless and totally inadequate.*

While there are no simple answers to getting support when we're unable to take the necessary steps to find it, we hope that this chapter and the Resources section may be of use – at least in terms of discovering what is possible and realizing that much of the pain we suffer is similar to pain suffered by many other women, with similar causes and solutions. There is a variety of organizations and individuals to which we can turn. Yet we must first look at the problems we may face with the very people we go to for help; sometimes they can make our situation feel even more hopeless. If we are well informed, we are in a better

position, if necessary, to avoid or challenge such people and situations.

We hope that, if nothing else, this chapter will provide women with enough information to avoid destructive 'helpers' and to find people who have enough knowledge and imagination to enable us to begin to make the changes we need.

WOMEN'S OPPRESSION AND GETTING HELP

Most mental health professionals, especially male psychiatrists and psychologists, have distorted ideas about women. As three women professionals write:

Clinical theories of personality specify women's innate nature as passive, dependent, masochistic, and childlike, and psychological treatment has often aimed at reducing her complaints about the quality of her life and promoting adjustment to the existing order.[5]

A well-known study revealed that psychologists tended to see positive adult qualities and 'healthy' male qualities as *the same*, while they portray the 'healthy' woman in very different terms: for instance, as more submissive, suggestive, emotional and illogical.[6] The many professionals who hold such stereotypes are of little use to women, and can do a lot of harm.

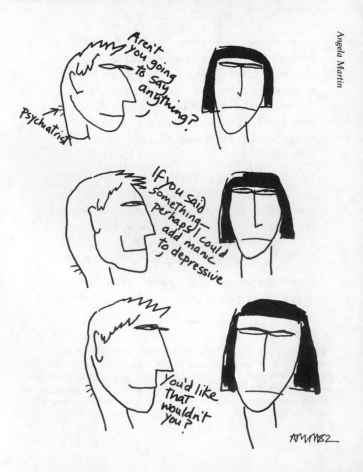

Angela Martin

Psychiatrist: Aren't you going to say anything?

If you said something – perhaps I could add manic to depressive

You'd like that wouldn't you?

Rarely do mental health professionals realize how women's disadvantaged status is directly damaging to our mental health. They are more likely to see women's emotional problems as internally caused (intra-psychic) than men's, and fail to look at the external reality and stress of women's lives. Consequently, they are more likely to prescribe mood-altering drugs to women than to men, and women are twice as likely as men to receive ECT (electric shock treatment). Practices like these draw many women into a web of inappropriate therapy, drug dependence and reduced self-esteem. Since most such professionals also hold negative – and therefore damaging – views about lesbianism, lesbians are particularly vulnerable when it comes to seeking help (see Lesbians and Mental Health, p. 136). So are women from ethnic minority groups, who have to suffer not only the racism of our society, but also the racism and racist practices of many health professionals (see box). The doctor-patient and therapist-client relationship carries a power imbalance which can work against women, especially when the practitioner is male and/or misuses this power.

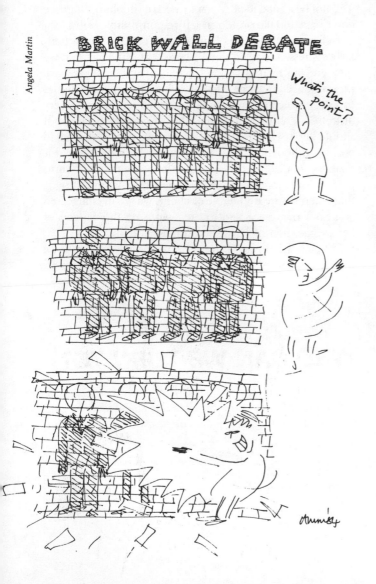

Angela Martin

Tragically, in the extreme, this power imbalance can lead practitioners psychologically and sometimes even physically to abuse women. Some have colluded with family members to lock us away in mental institutions (where women are the majority of patients) when we refuse to comply with society's norms for us. Some have molested and raped us in the name of 'therapy'. Most widely, they have used myths about women's supposedly passive, masochistic nature to keep us 'in our place'. Their underlying motivation is often a fear that we will gain and use our full powers. While extremes such as these by no means represent the majority of women's experiences, they illustrate the potential for the misuse of power which occurs with considerable frequency when women consult mental health professionals. The subtle ways in which we are encouraged to stay in positions of service to men rather than to realize our fullest potential are a permanent drain on our health and energy. Many health professionals' attitudes towards men reinforce our oppression as well. For some to consider, for example, that paedophiles could be shocked out of their love for children by turning them on to pin-ups instead[7] not only demeans us, but also sets us up for problems with men, culminating in rape and violence of all kinds.

Practitioners with a *feminist* approach (whether they name it this or not, because it is the attitude, not the label, that is most important) seek to help us find and use our strengths. They try to use respectfully the power they have. They are likely to recognize social, political and economic influences upon our emotional well-being. Often the first to raise mental health issues which others ignore – incest, rape, wife-battering – they are also likely to be more understanding of women. By no means is every woman practitioner a feminist, and a few men have a feminist approach. (For guidelines in choosing one, see p. 135.)

Partly because of the difficulties women have often had with the 'helping professions', many of us have turned to the concept of self-help, where we can participate in helping each other on an equal basis.

SELF-HELP

We can all develop ways of helping ourselves just as we can develop ways of hurting ourselves.

> I know just how to hurt myself, how to turn any
> event, any achievement, into a negative
> experience. It helps to remember that if I've learnt
> to do that so well, I should also be able to unlearn
> it – and to learn the opposite.

By eating well and taking regular exercise we are helping ourselves in two very important ways (see Chapters 4 and 6). As well as this, we need space where we can feel free enough to grow. Sometimes we need another, skilled person to help us find this space and claim it for ourselves (we discuss this in the next two sections). Sometimes we can do it on our own, for example by:

- going to a beautiful place;
- tapping into our creativity (see Creativity in Chapter 7);
- using visualization, ta'i chi, or many of the other techniques discussed in the Appendix to Chapter 7;
- using our dreams (books by Ann Faraday, Brenda Mallon and *The Dreamwork Manual* are excellent guides – see Resources);
- or through using some of the techniques described under Psychotherapeutic Approaches, p. 127.

In her book *Self Analysis*, first published in 1942, Karen Horney showed how even psychoanalysis can be used on a self-help basis; the more recent *In Our Own Hands*, by Sheila Ernst and Lucy Goodison, is full of a wide variety of ideas and suggestions for what we can do on our own.[8]

But there are aspects of self-help which require other women – our friends, our sisters – particularly since isolation and loneliness are major contributors to our feeling emotionally vulnerable. Since the second wave of feminism began, many of us have discovered the immense value of meeting together in groups for supportive action. Some of us might have ended up with some kind of psychiatric label if it weren't for our women's group and the support and clarity it gave us so that we could make changes for the better. Consciousness-raising (CR) groups have enabled many of us to see 'personal' problems in a new light. We have learnt, through sharing experiences, that what we thought of as problems stemming from our own inadequacies were in fact the logical result of our oppressed status and of the way our patriarchal and capitalist society is organized.*

Running alongside CR groups, or sometimes incorporating a consciousness-raising aspect, are women's groups that campaign around such issues as childcare and housing. They can enable us not only to take collective action on behalf of ourselves and other women, but also to develop a sense of solidarity and confidence that can give us a new perspective on what are often seen as 'personal' problems. Some of us have found that joining the Claimants' Union (for people on benefits), Depressives Anonymous, People Not Psychiatry, or the Carers' National Association, for example, have enabled us to break through our sense of isolation and self-blame. Others of us have found immersion in a cause, such as the miners' strike, has helped us overcome our difficulties.† Or we have formed groups on specific women's health issues. To find out about groups, see Resources at the end of this chapter and throughout the book. Alternatively, if you have a women's centre in your area, you can contact many such groups through that.

In addition, women have been pioneering the concept of self-help therapy groups, for, while CR is helpful, particularly in recognizing that 'the personal is political', it cannot pretend to enable us to deal with deep-rooted patterns formed in the unconscious. *In Our Own Hands* is an excellent guide for self-help therapy groups. Another potentially excellent self-help tool is co-counselling (see box on next page).

But while self-help is often invaluable, we need to be aware of some of the difficulties it can present us with. Under Groups on p. 134 we discuss where therapy groups as a whole might not be appropriate. As far as self-help therapy groups are concerned, we may need to be particularly careful to listen to our needs, as there will be no one person who has responsibility for running the group.

Even if we are severely distressed, self-help can sometimes still be valuable.

> It was like an adventure. There was a lot of warmth, even though some of us hardly knew each other, and I found it very supportive. All of which is amazing, since three of us were in a terrible state at the time, just keeping ourselves together and no more.[9]

However, if we are severely distressed or disturbed, or if our anxieties or our defences are increasing, self-help may well not be a good idea. We may need a situation where we don't have to take on too much responsibility – either for ourselves or anyone else. (And we don't need to be particularly distressed to need this.) There is also the fact that we may end up feeling very let down, or worse, if we have inexperienced helpers. Many self-help therapy techniques can stir up deep feelings very quickly, which, if we are very distressed, could be quite harmful. A competent therapist should know when to let us go at our own pace and when to push – although, as will be apparent by the end of this chapter, not all so-called professional helpers are competent. Since one of the basic tenets of co-counselling is that when we are in the role of client, we are in charge and go at our own pace and in our own way, the dangers of being inappropriately pushed should not apply.

When self-help isn't possible, appropriate or helpful, we may then need to find what we need from someone else.

WHO CAN WE TURN TO?

Theoretically, at least, there is an enormous range of possibilities, both within the NHS and social services, and outside (including charitable organizations and private

---

*To find a CR group, look through – or advertise in – the personal columns of *Spare Rib*.

†For an inspiring account of how Marsha Marshall overcame her agoraphobia through her involvement in the miners' strike, see Susan Aitken, 'The Case of the Agoraphobic Miner's Wife', *Changes*, vol. 3, no. 4, 1985. See also many other chapters in this book, e.g. 2, Body Image; 4, Food; 9, Occupational and Environmental Hazards; 10, Violence against Women, all of which are crucially relevant to our mental health, and which suggest self-help approaches.

CO-COUNSELLING

Co-counselling is based on the belief that human beings are born with a tremendous intellectual potential, natural zest and lovingness, but that these qualities have been blocked and obscured as a result of accumulated distressing experiences which begin early in life. One of the tenets of co-counselling is that we can recover from these hurtful experiences by the natural healing process of emotional discharge under controlled conditions, which can then lead to insight and re-evaluation of the hurtful experience, of what we want, and of our abilities to achieve it. People trained in co-counselling aim to assist each other in this process.

In co-counselling we are free from being prey to obvious power imbalances, partly because all co-counsellors participate as 'clients' and as 'helpers', and also because, when we take the role of 'client' it is we who are primarily in charge of what happens. Largely because of such principles, unique to co-counselling, there is enormous potential for reassessing any tendency we may have to see ourselves as powerless and passive. Co-counselling, particularly the approach of the Re-evaluation Co-counselling (RC) community (see p. 114), also embraces a broader political concept of equality, recognizing the oppression of women and members of all minority groups (including black and Jewish people, and people with disabilities). It is therefore also unique among psychotherapeutic theories (see p. 127) in recognizing both the importance of the myriad types of oppression in relation to people's mental health, as well as in placing emphasis on ways to fight it.

I find that co-counselling offers a victorious rather than victimized approach. It takes a stand very far outside the role of seeing people as victims. It's particularly good for women from that point of view alone. We've been through a long time of thinking/ seeing how awful it is for women and I think it's very important now to really appreciate how women are really wonderful and that there are lots of things about being women which are fantastic, and to appreciate our history and take pride in it: all of that is very much validated within co-counselling. It offers a way of seeing women's history and women's lives as a series of victories rather than as a series of horror stories. I think the horror stories are true, and I think the victories are true also – but so often the victories go unrecognized. The truth is, women have survived all those things.

Co-counselling gives us the opportunity to promote our mental health and develop our 'emotional education'. Since such education is rarely seen as important in our educational system, for many of us co-counselling can be a revelation, like learning to speak or to see for the first time. It can give us the opportunity to develop, and practise, 'emotional tools for living' – tools that we were in fact born with.*

There is a nation-wide network of co-counsellors, who are all trained to co-counsel – with anyone else who has undergone the training. Training courses (which are quite short) take place in many parts of the country. They are relatively cheap, and fees are usually charged on a sliding scale; the RC community makes money available for people who are under-represented in their co-counselling community which in many areas includes black people, single parents, young people and people on pensions. Anyone can apply for help with attending classes. The first free co-counselling course, organized by the author under the NHS in North Manchester, has just taken place as we go to press. We hope it will be the first of many.

Co-counselling can be an extremely effective and cheap way of helping yourself – and helping others. It offers a clear structure and theory that enable people to gain a great deal, without the risks that are involved in structureless self-help groups. However, it does require you to listen and respond to another person and it is not necessarily appropriate for everyone, nor all circumstances. To find out more, see Resources, under both publications (particularly by Button, Evison and Morrell) and organizations.

*For further discussion of the concept of emotional education and the promotion of mental health, see *The Promotion of Mental Health*, a paper presented by the author to the north-west branch of the Socialist Health Association, Summer 1988, and reprinted in the *Health Education Journal* (forthcoming).

counselling/therapy). How far they fit our needs varies greatly, depending on local policies, governmental pressure on finance, and/or individual practitioners' background, training and political awareness. What follows is an overview of what's available nationally. Please read it in conjunction with Women's Oppression and Getting Help, p. 118.

DOCTORS

Doctors are not often likely to be the best people to turn to for emotional help, and they can be the last people we can expect appropriate help from. But because of their position within the NHS, they may well be the first people we go to.

General practitioners can be helpful by referring you to

POSSIBLE PHYSICAL CAUSES OF OUR DISTRESS

There may, of course, be *physical causes* for fusion or depression, such as certain drugs or combinations of drugs (see, in particular, Chapter 22), or exposure to toxic substances at work or in the home. Lack of natural light may play a bigger part than we realize,[10] and diet is gradually becoming recognized as responsible for some mental distress, too. Dr Richard Mackarness in his book *Not All in the Mind* refers to one woman who was having dramatic mood swings ranging from elation to severe depression. She was hospitalized and given psychotherapy, and was considered to be a hopeless case after five weeks. However, she was later found to be allergic to certain foods (including white flour, sugar and egg white).

> The result was that I was discharged with no drugs, except ones as standby which I rarely need. As long as I stick to my diet, I'm fine.

'Orthomolecular psychiatry' is the term used for applying a nutritional approach to mental disturbance. Links have been made between low Vitamin C intake and manic depression, and caffeine has been strongly linked with anxiety.* Professor Dickerson of the Department of Human Nutrition, Surrey University, believes that the answer to many types of mental disorder, including autism, 'hyperactivity' and 'schizophrenia' lies in diet.

Often doctors will refer a woman for psychiatric treatment when they cannot identify a physical cause or treatment for a problem, or because they learned in medical training that many of our physical problems are 'all in our heads'. It makes sense to try and get your doctor to check for physical causes. See also Michael Lesser's book *Nutrition and Vitamin Therapy* (in Resources).

*Graham Naylor of Dundee University has conducted a double-blind placebo trial which strongly indicated the value of Vitamin C in this respect; the Canadian Medical Association has issued a strong editorial challenging hospitals to reduce patients' caffeine intake. It also asserted that caffeine intake should be considered an issue when drug treatment is being considered, as it can antagonize other drugs. It concludes, 'The widespread adoption of such changes will not come easily. In our experience it is the medical and professional staffs who oppose changes in caffeine consumption habits, not the patients.'[11]

---

appropriate individuals within or outside the NHS, and/or providing help themselves. However, in many cases they may well not think beyond the idea of psychiatric referral, or of prescribing tranquillizers or other drugs (see Chapter 5). GPs, like psychiatrists (see below), tend to be medically orientated.*

> I have been troubled with nerves and depression for years . . . when I first went to the doctor the cause was premenstrual tension, but since I had a hysterectomy five years ago, it is now my age.

However, you might hit on a good GP who can either give you counselling time her- or himself, or who is aware of the socio-political causes of women's problems.

> I went to my GP feeling ill and depressed, and totally unable to cope with the baby – who was also ill. All I was given was tranquillizers. I saw another GP who said, 'Of course you can't cope! You can't expect to feel well after so many bad nights.' She arranged help, and immediately things began to improve.

A few GPs employ counsellors in their surgeries, and one or two GPs are experimenting with working alongside a community worker (see below).

*The 'medicalization' of emotional issues leads some of us to see doctors as the only people who can help us, often with drugs to ease our anguish.

Psychiatrists. If you want more help through the NHS than your GP can offer, s/he can refer you to a psychiatrist. Psychiatrists are doctors who specialize in mental illness. They tend to set great store by trying to diagnose symptoms in people, and trying to fit them into categories that are medically-orientated and often of limited use. Their approach to providing help tends also to be medically-orientated (e.g. involving drugs and/or admission to hospital though they see most people on an outpatient basis). However, there are some exceptions who appreciate the subtleties and complexities of human experience,* but alas not enough who incorporate a feminist perspective into their work.

> The psychiatrist did his level best in every possible way to dissuade me from what I considered most healthy and right for me . . . He never really inquired as to what I thought was a fulfilling life, or to my own feelings and needs as a person.

> My psychiatrist spends ten minutes a month telling me how good my husband is and how lucky I am. My problems are real and I feel there is such a desperate need for something more imaginative. I don't want to bake cakes, join the PTA or stuff toys.

*R. D. Laing, for example, was a psychiatrist whose books (see Resources) have influenced a whole generation concerning the meaning of so-called mental illness and how it is produced, particularly within the family context.

Psychiatrists can refer you for psychotherapy (if they provide psychotherapy within their department) and some even do psychotherapy themselves (see p. 127).

A big problem many of us have about seeing a psychiatrist is the fear that this labels us as mentally ill. Our society does not look kindly on mental illness – perhaps precisely because so few people are mentally healthy anyway! We think it is important that the taboo about mental ill health is broken down. However, the fear of being labelled is still a very realistic fear.*

Psychiatrists have an enormous amount of power, which they sometimes abuse, reinforcing the sexism, homophobia or racism of the world at large, and/or acting with authoritarianism generally.

He never listened to what I had to say. He had his own ideas about what was wrong with me. He would make outright statements about what he believed was the matter with me, disregarding anything I said to the contrary. He threatened to discharge me 'if our relationship didn't improve sufficiently'. He blamed me for the failure of his methods, and said that I refused to comply with them. The nurses were sympathetic but said that I could not change to another doctor.

They can, however, be helpful, and we might choose to try and use their power to our advantage – for example, in asking to be referred to a therapist or counsellor, or to a crisis centre (see p. 126), or when negotiating with the council for better housing. Since the psychiatric profession is currently in a state of crisis itself (not least because of the burgeoning of other professions and the increasing recognition of the poverty of the 'medical model'), we can perhaps succeed in pushing for considerable improvements, and even major changes, concerning the role of psychiatrists in the years to come.

CLINICAL PSYCHOLOGISTS

Clinical psychologists often practise some form of therapy (see p. 127). Although they are now independent of psychiatrists, they often have a very uneasy relationship with them (not necessarily to our disadvantage!). They do not have a medical training, and their training will vary greatly, depending on which institution they attended and what further training they have decided to undergo. Some psychologists, for example, started off with quite mechanistic forms of 'behaviour therapy' but have developed to pursue a more 'humanistic' or 'analytic' approach (see pp. 127–135). Some simply administer and interpret psychological tests, which are not always of much use, are difficult to interpret, and may contain inherent value-judgements.

*For example, because of job discrimination, the possibility of mental hospital, loss of freedom, even loss of our children or repatriation to our country of birth.

Clinical psychologists are often based in hospitals but they are increasingly being located in health centres and GPs' surgeries. The main advantage of psychologists working in GPs' surgeries is that they are much more accessible than in a hospital. However, if psychological help remains within a medical setting, albeit in a GP's surgery instead of a hospital, there is still the danger that our problems may be medicalized.

To get referred to a clinical psychologist, the local clinical psychology department, usually based in the hospital, should be able to advise you. Some are only able to take referrals from doctors, others take them from social workers or health visitors, and some even take self-referrals.

NURSES AND HEALTH VISITORS

Although few nurses or health visitors have adequate training concerning mental health, some can be helpful as a listening ear, or for support or counselling, or for putting us in touch with self-help groups.

Health visitors. Your GP's or health clinic's receptionist should be able to tell you how to get in touch with a local health visitor. Alternatively, you can see a health visitor at any health centre or community-based (not hospital-based) clinic, either by making an appointment or by just turning up: health visitors are usually in their clinics from 9 A.M. to 10.30 A.M. and 4 P.M. to 5 P.M. Similarly, a *district nurse* might be a good person to talk to. Again, your doctor's receptionist can tell you how to contact her, or you can look in the phone book under 'Nurses', where all the district nurses should be listed by name.

Community psychiatric nurses (CPNs) are available in some districts though, as they are a relatively new type of nurse, only about 3,000 currently exist in the whole of the UK. The main part of their work involves helping people with the transition from hospital to home, but a growing part of it is concerned with helping people before they get to the point where hospitalization might be appropriate. They can provide help without the immediate threat of hospitalization, and can be contacted in an emergency – though most work on a 9 to 5 basis. CPNs can be very helpful in providing support, information and advice, and some may be good 'patient advocates'. But be prepared that a CPN may have a very limited training in – and understanding of – how to help people in distress, and many work solely within the medical model and perform the more traditional nursing tasks such as giving injections. Contrary to what their name implies, CPNs are often based in mental hospitals or psychiatric units of general hospitals. They report to consultant psychiatrists, from whom they take referrals; some also take referrals from district nurses or health visitors.

Nurse therapists are CPNs who have had further training. Few, if any, have undergone the type of rigorous training that a fully-fledged psychotherapist would undergo, but it would seem that they are expected to perform the same function – at a fraction of the cost to the NHS, as they are paid nursing rates. Most of them are

HOSPITALIZATION

If we are severely disturbed, hospital treatment can sometimes be useful, and occasionally can be just what we need. Drugs, electro-convulsive therapy ('shock treatment', ECT), and/or psychotherapy may be given.

However, hospitals have a poor reputation when it comes to helping 'psychiatric patients' in general, and women in particular – and with good reason (see, for example, Phyllis Chesler's *Women and Madness*). So often they represent simply another form of violence against us (see Chapter 10, p. 174). Drugs are frequently used, often in large quantities, to control our behaviour. And women can find it particularly difficult to stand up for what we want – and don't want. If you or a friend are given drugs, try and find out as much as you can about them, particularly their side-effects.[12] Likewise ECT – a controversial treatment with little clear evidence of value – is something else you may want to look into, particularly since it can result in long-lasting memory loss.[13] Women may be pushed into group therapy, regardless of whether we want it or can cope with it; conversely, we may be denied the opportunity and safety of regular, individual skilled help.

So often I've seen women sent out back to their families before they're ready; denied therapy with the platitude, 'Oh no, we don't want her to get too dependent on the hospital' . . . (they never say that about men) . . . even in a hospital where there is a lot of opportunity for people to stay until they're ready to leave.

Even worse is the possibility of sexual abuse.

I've seen a woman who'd just found out that she'd lost access to her son, so she was upset and started throwing things around. And out of nowhere were six male nurses, you know, big men. I couldn't believe it. They stripped her. Why they stripped her I don't know. I was absolutely stiff with fear. They injected her and were laughing because she passed out with fear before they got the syringe out of her bottom.[14]

Psychiatric wards, therefore, can be particularly oppressive places. They often provide little help or understanding, serving only to increase our isolation. Often, we have to be docile and compliant to 'earn' the goal of discharge – while our very compliance and passivity, socialized from birth, is a major contributory factor to our problems. Those of us who are neither white nor middle class are particularly vulnerable to oppressive and insensitive treatment.

Women who are, or have been, in psychiatric wards need all the support we can get. If you or a friend are in that position, we hope that this chapter, and the resources listed, will help you to find someone who can give you the support you need. In the meantime, we hope that in the not too distant future, women will have successfully fought for the type of mental health service that befits us all. (See What Some Women Are Doing, p. 140. See also Chapter 7.)

trained solely in behaviour therapy, although a few are beginning to train in psychodynamic or humanistic therapy (see p. 127) – often at their own expense. Nurse therapists can operate autonomously; they have their own case-load and take referrals from anywhere, including self-referrals (bear in mind there are far fewer nurse therapists than CPNs). They may be attached to a psychology or psychiatric unit, though some work in GPs' surgeries. Like CPNs, most nurse therapists are male.

SOCIAL WORKERS

Social workers can be helpful either as a support for ourselves or those who are caring for us. They may do home visits, provide counselling and practical help, and information about local facilities such as day-centres and clubs. A few do nothing but counselling or group work (see p. 134). A social worker should be available at any hospital or social services area offices. All psychiatric units have a psychiatric social work department. Around 1 per cent of social workers are attached to GPs' surgeries.

A major problem with social workers is that they have a statutory role, and women can quite justifiably feel 'policed' by them (for example, whether we are performing the child care role adequately). However, one of a social worker's duties under the new Mental Health Act is to inform us of our rights and to protect these rights.

Another major problem is that social workers are overworked and exploited. They are therefore often unable to give the time and emotional energy necessary to help in anything more than a superficial way. Yet good social work help can prevent us from becoming in severe need; it can also help us with the transition from hospital to the community.

COUNSELLORS AND PSYCHOTHERAPISTS

These are rarely available within the NHS, and though some of the professionals previously mentioned may consider that they offer counselling or psychotherapy, they are not necessarily equipped to do so. However, health districts are beginning to employ psychotherapists, and they are a resource that may be available if we push for them. See Psychotherapeutic Approaches, p. 127, for a discussion of counselling and psychotherapy. See also Art Therapy, p. 99.

COMMUNITY WORKERS

A community worker is often a good point of reference for knowing what groups/facilities are available, particularly for people interested in self-help or action groups (see Self-help, p. 119). Community workers often offer support for such groups, and some are particularly interested in women's health. They are often attached to community centres, but some work in community health projects or are employed by voluntary groups.

WELL WOMAN CENTRES

As we discuss on p. 649, many women's groups have set up, or are campaigning for well woman centres or clinics that serve women's needs. If there is one in your area (your local women's group or health council will know), the centre should be an excellent place for setting up a self-help group, e.g. for coming off tranquillizers or coping with hyster-ectomy – and it may also know of, or provide itself, suitable professional help. However, many well woman *clinics* (see p. 630), though set up as a result of feminist pressure, often offer only a medical screening service – though at some it may be possible to gain support for the setting up of self-help groups.

PHONE LINES

Phone lines exist in many parts of the country. They may be run by student unions, voluntary groups like MIND, the Samaritans, or by groups involved in a range of issues from poverty (such as Child Poverty Action Group) to violence (such as Rape Crisis, Women's Aid – see Chapter 10). Many people have found phone lines helpful.

To find your local Samaritans' number, look in the phone book. Look out for other local phone lines in newspapers, doctors' surgeries, libraries, etc.

MENTAL HEALTH DAY-CENTRES

These are quite commonly available as places where people can go who need support or help in adjusting after a crisis, or after a stay in hospital. Unfortunately, few are women-orientated, and many are more geared to *occupying* people with diversionary activities than seriously to directing themselves towards enabling us to become truly independent. Nevertheless, they can be helpful places for finding support and other people to identify with. Some of them offer preparation for work, too. You can be referred to a day-centre by a hospital, GP or social worker. MIND groups throughout the country often run their own centres or 'drop-in' clubs too.

PSYCHIATRIC DAY HOSPITALS

These are also widely available and differ from day-centres in that medical staff are present too. Referral is usually through a GP or social services, who arrange for you to see a psychiatrist on 'admission' or beforehand.

I have got a lot of support from both staff and 'patients' at my local day hospital for short periods of time. Either when I have been recovering from a crisis and needed to re-establish a sense of independence, i.e. an ability to manage on my own in my flat again, or when I was going through a mini-crisis and very much wanted to manage without going into hospital. As a woman who has experienced acute distress at times, it gives me a lot of strength being with other people, some of whom have had similar experiences to myself in the past, e.g. hallucinations, paranoia, overdosing, feeling suicidal (terrifying as it was). It's great to be able to sit and joke about such times and feel understood, instead of having to live with the everyday strain of denying such experiences and be a 'together' woman. The day is quite structured too – plenty of opportunity to take part in a range of activities such as carpentry, cookery, pottery, art, creative writing, discussion groups, etc., which has helped give me a sense of self-achievement at such times.

HALFWAY HOUSES

These are residential. There aren't many of them and they tend to be run by voluntary organizations such as MIND or the Richmond Fellowship.* Sometimes called 'therapeutic communities', halfway houses can be, and sometimes are, places to go for anyone who wants a supportive living place while they work on finding ways of changing their lives for the better. More often, they are somewhere to go to on leaving a psychiatric ward. They may be run quite dif-ferently: some may have staff on call or on duty round the clock, and have regular meetings and structured days, whereas others are like the Arbours centre:

We were all responsible for our lives there. We had no live-in staff. If the house couldn't support someone sufficiently, there was the possibility of extra support at the Crisis Centre. There was no imposed structure or routine. It was very helpful for me at the time, particularly because there wasn't a label around me saying 'mentally ill', and because I was living in a household where lots of different forms of behaviour were acceptable and not seen as illness, and because I was still able (allowed) to be in control of my own life: we all were.

*The Richmond Fellowship, however, runs houses for people of all ages with a wide variety of difficulties, nation-wide (see Resources).

IF YOU OR A FRIEND NEEDS URGENT HELP

Extreme mental disturbance can take many forms. As the disturbed person, we may be the last to know or accept that something is radically wrong. We may not realize, for example, that we are hallucinating or losing touch with reality. Or, knowing that something is very wrong, we may still feel too confused, desperate and/or frightened to seek help. Since our health and welfare services rarely respond adequately to women's needs at the best of times, we can be in an acutely vulnerable position when in need of help *in extremis*.

Nevertheless, *GPs*, *social workers*, or any of the professionals described above may be of some use, as can the *Samaritans*, who provide a nation-wide listening (and occasionally counselling) service for people who are depressed or suicidal; they also act as a referral agency, and can be very helpful – often a better bet than a doctor (see Resources, p. 144).

Often, psychiatric wards are considered to be the answer. While sometimes admission to such a ward can be helpful, at least for a short time, many of us have good reason to be wary of them – see for example p. 174. If admission to hospital is not what you or your friend want, *or* if neither a GP nor social worker is able to convince you or your friend of that particular ward's good practices, *or* if they cannot provide information about other options, see Resources (in particular MIND) for whom to contact: other organizations may be able to tell you about other possibilities in your area, or even offer help themselves.* While there are at the time of writing no facilities solely for women, or that acknowledge the particular needs that we have by virtue of living in a sexist society, other good options may include the following:

'*Crisis intervention teams*' exist in a few areas (run either by social services or by the health service). They tend to avoid falling into the trap of the 'medical model', usually visiting and supporting the person/family concerned at home. They also tend to make no assumptions about who is 'ill', if anyone. Some operate as an alternative to hospital admission, others simply try and avoid hospitalization if possible. As a member of one such team says:

> What we're after is to examine what the family wants or needs and what we, as a group of differently skilled professionals, can offer. Our aim is to be able to present a course of options for dealing with the crisis, which can range from treating one member of the family as mentally ill to working out a behavioural strategy for all.[15]

'*Crisis Centres*', though few and far between, can also offer the help we need to pull ourselves through a crisis, by providing us with a temporary home with support and psychotherapeutic help. Many are not without drawbacks, and at the time of writing there are none as yet specifically designed for women, but some are being planned – see p. 140 (see also Chapter 10 for refuges for women and girls experiencing domestic violence). Yet despite the

*See also Rights for Consumers of Psychiatric Services, p. 127.

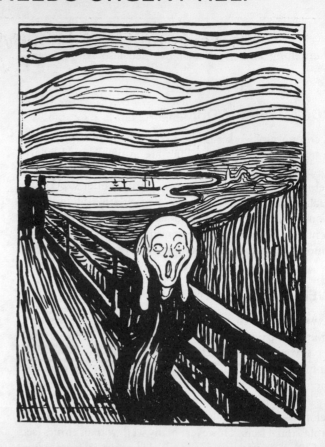

drawbacks of many centres, they may still be preferable to hospital.

> I would, given the appalling lack of choice at present, opt any day to go into the crisis centre instead of the mental hospital where I'd had to spend some time before. I was able to use the crisis centre to my advantage and managed to arrange that a rota of my women friends could stay with me there. At that time I was very needy, and felt particularly vulnerable as a lesbian, and knew that the centre was unable to offer any real twenty-four-hour attention. This set a precedent that I hope other women may benefit from in the future.

The dearth of suitable help available for women in crisis mirrors the limited help available at the best of times. Help in a crisis should involve recognition of the social causes of our pain – whether concerning housing (or lack of it), nursery facilities (or lack of them), or violent relationships. Emotional crises, though acutely painful, can provide a chance to learn and change – ourselves and our lives. We need the help and support to do this. Some women are trying to make that possible – see p. 140.

If a woman close to you needs help in a crisis, *The Radical Therapist* by The Radical Therapist Collective contains advice on how to help. See also *Asylum* magazine in Resources, in particular vol. 2, no. 3, 1988, 'What to Do if a Friend Goes Mad'. Books that can help us through crises include Pearlie MacNeill et al., *Through the Break – Women in Personal Struggle*.

RIGHTS FOR CONSUMERS OF PSYCHIATRIC SERVICES

Whoever we turn to, or wherever we find ourselves, knowing our rights is important. For example:

- we have a *legal right* to a second opinion from another psychiatrist;
- we cannot be forced to go into hospital unless it is in the interests of our health or safety, or in order to protect other people;
- we have the *right* to appeal against any decisions that might have been taken against our wishes;
- hospitals have a *duty* to inform us and our relatives of our rights.

We do not have the space to explore rights in any depth here, but MIND (the National Association for Mental Health) has been campaigning for people's rights for years, and it can provide anyone with information and help. See, for example, its series of leaflets on specific issues, including *Your Rights in Hospital* and *Mental Health Review Tribunals*. The Campaign Against Psychiatric Oppression and other groups concerned with our rights can also be of help (see Resources), as can CHCs (see p. 642), law centres and Citizens' Advice Bureaux.

As far as *benefits* are concerned, we need expert advice, as many of us don't know our rights and the system is so complicated. Many voluntary organizations such as MIND have excellent welfare rights officers and CABs can be very helpful. See also Catherine Grimshaw's *A to Z* published by MIND.

Halfway houses are not for people in crisis, though they may be useful for someone trying to avoid one, or emerging from one.

I went to an Arbours therapeutic community because I was quite depressed and wanted to explore what was going on in my relationships. The house seemed to offer a refuge for people with many different experiences of distress and the possibility of supporting each other through these.

For more information about Arbours, see p. 144.

While the government's policy is to reduce dramatically the numbers of people in mental hospital, there is as yet a derisory commitment to providing a decent community-based service to replace hospitalization.* As the Select Committee on Social Services pointed out in 1985, at least 90 per cent of people with mental health problems live in the community, but only 10 per cent of funding is directed at locally-based services. Only with political commitment at both governmental and local level can adequate mental health services be provided – either in hospitals or in the 'community'. Pressure groups such as MIND have still a long way to go as far as improving the level of mental health services generally is concerned. With regard to women specifically, we have even further to go. Many women, for example, end up in prison or in appalling accommodation and/or heavily drugged because of the dearth of help available. And, mentally healthy or not, many of us end up caring for psychologically disturbed relatives because current government policy, far from promoting community-orientated care, is simply expecting us to do it – for free.

For organizations concerned specifically with women and mental health, see Resources.

PSYCHOTHERAPEUTIC APPROACHES

I felt that therapy was a luxury and not something for the likes of me: an Asian woman born in the East End of London . . . I have been going to therapy for a year now and it has helped untangle the patterns that have formed the framework of my life, even though the process is slow and often painful.[16]

I saw a therapist on the National Health. With her, I have begun to have the kinds of dialogue about myself that I might have had years ago had I only known how. In a way, she has given me the gift of myself.[17]

Many of the individuals and organizations mentioned above may offer a variety of psychotherapeutic approaches. In this section we explore the major types. Knowing what they are and what they involve can help us choose what we want and be prepared for what they can and, perhaps more importantly, cannot offer. They cannot, for example, offer political solutions (and, let's face it, many of our problems have deep-seated political causes). And they have a tendency to individualize problems which are not really individual women's problems, as Phyllis Chesler has so

---

*For details of the many innovative community mental health projects, contact Good Practices in Mental Health or MIND – see Resources.

SURVIVORS SPEAK OUT*

CHARTER OF NEEDS AND DEMANDS

1. That mental health service providers recognize and use people's first-hand experience of emotional distress for the good of others.

2. Provision of refuge, planned and under the control of survivors of psychiatry.

3. Provision of free counselling for all.

4. Choice of services, including self-help alternatives.

5. A Government review of services, with recipients sharing their views.

6. Provision of resources to implement self-advocacy for all users.

7. Adequate funding for non-medical community services.

8. Facility for representation of users and ex-users of services on statutory bodies, including Community Health Councils, Mental Health Tribunals and the Mental Health Act Commission.

9. Full and free access to all personal medical records.

10. Legal protection and means of redress for all psychiatric patients.

11. Establishment of the democratic right of staff to refuse to administer any treatment without risk of sanction or prejudice.

12. The phasing out of electro-convulsive therapy and psycho-surgery.

13. Independent monitoring of drug use and its consequences.

14. Provision for all patients of full written and verbal information on treatments, including adverse research findings.

15. An end to discrimination against people who receive, or have received, psychiatric services: with particular regard to housing, employment, insurance etc.

*From SSO Conference, 1987 (see Organizations, p. 145).

---

graphically exposed – see, for example, her article in *The Radical Therapist*. Nor can they be much use if we are being given psychotropic drugs – since drugs are designed to dampen feelings, while psychotherapy and counselling aim to draw them out. But if used well, they can enable us to see the causes of our difficulties more clearly, to make any necessary changes and to take any necessary action – both on a personal and political level.

There are broadly three categories of psychotherapeutic approach. The first involves a *relationship* between therapist/counsellor and client: working on what happens in the therapeutic relationship as a mirror for what happens in the client's own relationships is an important aspect of this type of therapy. The term 'psychotherapy' is usually used for this type of approach. It may also involve *specific techniques* that tap the client's inner resources and enable understanding and change to take place. These techniques form the second broad category and are considered under the heading Humanistic Psychology. The third type of approach involves so-called *behavioural therapy*. This is mainly practised in the NHS and is much more problem-orientated: for example, working on a particular fear or symptom such as agoraphobia, not necessarily with reference to the general socio- and psycho-dynamic context of the person's life.

In addition, many of the various therapies can be conducted with individuals, with couples, with families or in groups. We now look at each of these approaches in turn, then we will examine the question of choosing a therapist. Bear in mind, however, that while many practitioners fit

easily into one of these categories, the boundaries are gradually becoming more blurred.

PSYCHOTHERAPY

The term 'psychotherapy' can be confusing, as sometimes any form of talking with a professional is referred to as psychotherapy. We are referring to it in the specific sense described here. The term 'therapy' is used instead to refer to any kind of therapeutic work.

Psychotherapy is, strictly speaking, analytically-based.* It usually involves working on a deep emotional level, and a psychotherapist should have a considerable amount of training to do this type of work (see Choosing a Therapist, p. 135). There are many different kinds of analytically-based psychotherapy, and many therapists of whatever kind operate along the lines of this approach in some, if not

---

*It is analytically based in the sense that it is based on psychoanalytic theory. Though classical psychoanalytic theory has been the cause of most of the distorted ideas about women that pervade much medical training, many people, including the following women, have done pioneering work on reshaping it so that it is relevant, and helpful, to women: Karen Horney in *Feminine Psychology*, Luise Eichenbaum and Susie Orbach in *Understanding Women*. There is still, however, a very long way to go: for example, virtually all training remains patriarchal in content, and even progressive theorists still base their ideas solely on heterosexual assumptions.

many, respects.* It involves regular sessions with the therapist, sometimes for a set period of time, but more often the time-scale is open-ended. It is not about 'help' in the sense that we have come to understand it through the 'medical model'. The emphasis is on the client talking with the therapist, and working out what she wants/needs, through exploring feelings and desires which she may as yet be unaware of. This can take a long time, as the client may have to 'work through' a need to be told what to do, for example.

The relationship between client and therapist is recognized as a crucial component of the therapy. In any therapeutic relationship, the client usually 'transfers' on to the therapist or counsellor feelings that are relevant to other, significant people in her life. Analytically-based psychotherapists recognize this phenomenon, which they call 'transference', and help the client to recognize where these feelings belong. A form of transference occurs in many of our relationships, and it can help enormously to be aware of this when it is happening. Perhaps even more important is that the therapist recognizes the phenomenon of 'counter-transference' – whereby she can transfer feelings about herself and her own life on to the client. While transference and counter-transference almost always occur unless the therapist takes steps to avoid it, many non-analytically-based therapists do not recognize this, and consequently misconstrue what is going on in the therapy. (The phenomenon of counter-transference is one reason why it is so important for a therapist to undergo therapy herself – see p. 137.)

The quality of the relationship we have with our therapist can significantly alter the quality of relationship we have with *ourselves*: much distress is about 'falling out' with ourselves – judging, hating or denying ourselves, as a result of absorbing negative and distorted messages about us. If we feel accepted by a therapist on a deep level, we 'internalize' that feeling, which can ultimately lead to self-acceptance and lasting change.

Psychotherapy, then, can help when we've become alienated from important parts of ourselves. We don't have to 'go mad' or 'break down' in order to benefit from it. Indeed, far from it: it can perhaps be most helpful if we undertake it when we are not in that type of situation, for then we have more resources to cope with the fears and uncertainties, sadnesses and grief that can come up. Often, however, we find ourselves looking for psychotherapy only

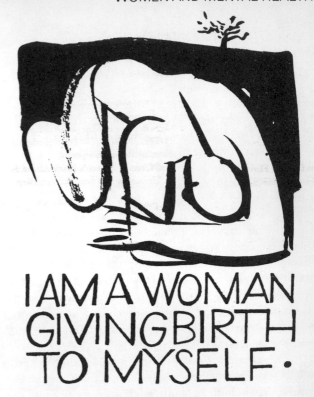

I AM A WOMAN GIVING BIRTH TO MYSELF.

when we feel we have reached an impasse, or our defences have broken down under stress. Then the therapy can help us uncover the underlying reasons for our difficulties which may appear to bear no obvious relation to them. In helping us discover more of who we are, psychotherapy can, in the words of the late Winifred Rushforth, 'liberate . . . valuable energy and long-forgotten creativity'.[18] It can also help us discover why we may seem to be propelled towards relationships and situations that don't nourish us, and learn how to avoid them.

Therapy has helped me focus on things I do over and over again in relationships, which result in my not getting what I need. For example, when I started therapy, I didn't realize how hard it was for me to ask for certain things. I didn't feel strong enough or confident enough to fight for myself. I found it hard to feel close, and I didn't understand how learning to get what I wanted would make me feel closer. It was a vicious circle. Now that I feel confident enough and aware enough of this pattern, it has changed.

Sometimes going to a therapist with a partner can help improve communication about painful issues.

He didn't feel totally comfortable with my handicap, and he would say so, and that made me terribly angry. I couldn't look at my anger at all, which made him very upset, and then he would clam up. I needed a place to feel safe to deal with all this. So we decided to go into couples' therapy. It helped for me to be able to relax and to hear what he was saying to me. He would say to me, 'I

---

*It may be based on the work of a variety of people – Freud, Jung, Adler, Guntrip, Fairbairn or Klein. Many psychotherapists are 'eclectic' – i.e. they use aspects of all these theoretical positions, and/or other techniques from 'humanistic psychology'. They all, however, recognize the importance of the unconscious and the need to work with it. For an introduction to these various approaches, see Joel Kovel, *A Complete Guide to Therapy*; Julia Segal, *Phantasy in Everyday Life*; Luise Eichenbaum and Susie Orbach, *Understanding Women*. (Psychoanalysts tend to work more intensively than psychotherapists; however, psychoanalysis as such is not discussed here, partly because it is so lengthy, with dubious additional benefit for the extra cost, and also because analysts often assume an authority about human relationships and the workings of the psyche that is highly debatable.)

love you, but I don't like how that part of your body looks.' And a lot of it was really my feeling, that I didn't like how it looked either.

But therapy for women in a heterosexual relationship can be a double-edged sword. Often the woman initiates the idea of seeing a therapist, while the man resists or refuses to go. If we accept the cultural conditioning which teaches us that our job is to maintain emotional relationships, to take care of and give to others, particularly our partners, to be sensitive and work out problems, then turning to a therapist may confront us with a sense of failure. Tragically, traditional therapy has often reinforced this perception. Women can also lose out in 'couples' therapy with a man if the therapist is not careful to avoid a common tendency to focus on the man to the detriment of the woman. If you go into therapy with a male partner it is particularly important to find a therapist who is aware of how our cultural conditioning affects us, and of feminist issues in general.

It is also possible for all the members of a family group to attend sessions together, with one or two therapists. This can be very helpful as family relationships can cause one person to 'carry' the brunt of everyone's emotional difficulties. However, 'family therapy' tends to be based on the concept of orthodox nuclear family groupings. It can thus be a risky venture if you don't conform to these norms, unless you can choose the therapists with care.

At times, psychotherapy can be very painful as deep and confusing emotions are uncovered. It can be helpful to know this in advance.

I went to a therapist when I was pretty depressed and angry. When it started to get extremely painful in ways I had not imagined, I felt cheated. I was extremely ignorant about what therapy involved, and all the therapist would say was, 'Well, I couldn't tell you in advance how you would feel.' I thought this missed the point. The therapy had involved only a short-term contract, so I ended up left with all these feelings stirred up and no help and support to deal with them. It took me some years to dare to begin trusting a therapist again.

HUMANISTIC PSYCHOLOGY

During the 1960s, psychology took a 'humanistic' turn, often making links between mind and body, and the 'growth' movement took off. In particular, many people who had hitherto practised a relatively traditional form of analytical psychotherapy became frustrated with its limitations and began to develop new ways of helping people. They saw that psychology could be harnessed, not simply to help people in severe distress or crisis but that all people could be helped towards fulfilling their potential as human beings. This led to the development of many innovative

ideas and techniques. In spite of the 'growth' movement's undoubted excesses,* it has also produced many ideas and practices which are of immense value, particularly if practised with care and sensitivity. We cannot possibly explore all the ideas of humanistic psychology here. We briefly look at three approaches concerned primarily with mental health which can be particularly useful for women, and list in Resources books and organizations where you can find out more.

Gestalt therapy focuses on the 'here and now' and, after the German word 'Gestalt', on integration. We often disown parts of ourselves, e.g. our creativity, our sexuality or our caring. By doing this, we not only remain fragmented, frustrated and/or lost, but we also lose energy. By facilitating integration, Gestalt therapy can enable a freeing of the spirit – and body – that may not be possible with straightforward 'talking' therapy. However, some Gestalt therapists have limited training in, and understanding of, the different levels of emotional patterning rooted in our pasts. Their approach can therefore be naive and clumsy, and we can end up feeling, perhaps yet again, that our experience is being invalidated. Gestalt therapy is quite confrontational, and perhaps it is particularly important therefore that you choose a Gestalt therapist with care (see p. 135). Yet Gestalt can be particularly valuable for women, for

Most of us have been thoroughly conditioned to feel intellectually inferior to men and put down by the (traditionally male) world of interpretation and theory. It is validating to work with a method which challenges the normal over-estimation of the intellect and focuses instead on the bread and butter (and jam) of what we feel from moment to moment. Our immediate experience is accessible to us all and cannot easily be mystified or taken from us.[19]

In addition, Gestalt encourages us to take – and see that we have the ability to take – responsibility for our own lives: as Ernst and Goodison say, this is also invaluable for women, as we often underestimate our own power to tackle the obstacles we face.

In working with the 'here and now', Gestalt therapy can often be used in conjunction with creative work on dreams, fantasies and art (see Creative Therapies in Chapter 7). It can be done in groups or individually with a therapist, or on one's own.

As an example of a Gestalt approach to therapy: you may start a session feeling nothing in particular, apart from a

---

*As Fritz Perls, the founder of Gestalt therapy, wrote: 'It took us a long time to debunk the whole Freudian crap, and now we are entering a new and more dangerous phase. We are entering the phase of turner-onners: turn on to instant cure, instant joy, instant sensory awareness. We are entering the phase of the quacks and the con-men, who think if you get some breakthrough, you are cured.' He went on to warn how such 'therapy' 'often becomes a dangerous substitute activity, another phoney therapy that *prevents* growth'.

COUNSELLING

Strictly speaking, 'counselling' means helping someone in a non-directive manner to explore and resolve personal issues, usually by meeting for regular (usually hourly) 'sessions'. It requires a considerable amount of skill and self-awareness on the part of the counsellor, and while some health professionals (ranging from GPs to health visitors) might claim to offer counselling, their training may not in fact have equipped them to do it (see Choosing a Therapist, p. 135). It is often assumed that counselling involves giving advice or encouraging people in prescribed directions, but most counsellors will not see it in these terms and will make clear their position, otherwise the client's freedom to discover her true feelings and wishes is endangered. However, while 'directing' or 'encouraging' people has its inherent dangers, it can be helpful, *providing* the client is in charge of the direction she's being encouraged in. The Pellin approach of 'Contribution Training', for example (see Resources), does attempt to safeguard the client's autonomy in this respect, and in addition, promotes equality on its training courses by enabling each person to work both as a client and as a counsellor. (It recognizes also, to some extent at least, the socio-political dimensions of our lives.)

Counselling may be indistinguishable from psychotherapy (see p. 128), but it often differs in not presuming to hold any theory about the client (after Carl Rogers's approach of 'non-directiveness'), and also in involving more direct engagement: if the counsellor does not know what's going on in someone, s/he is likely to ask you; a psychotherapist may wait – or even assume that s/he knows. For some of us, then, counselling may be a better bet because of this commitment to 'the client knows best'. Warmth, empathy and 'positive regard' are also part of most counsellors' approaches. However, since different counsellors may have a wide variety of perspectives, and not least because anyone can call themselves a counsellor, it is important to check them out. Here, a feminist counsellor speaks of her own experience of counselling and describes the process well:

Having trained in psychoanalysis, which I found limited, and then TA, which I found helpful, I then discovered an even more helpful approach in the work of Carl Rogers [whose books include Person to Person: the Problem of Being*]. For years I felt I had been searching for ways to become a person with all the implications involving growth, goals and values. I had already done in-depth work on my unconscious during my 'training analysis', but I had not experienced the deep, warm understanding and the positive regard from a therapist who was willing to help me find a meaning in my life, in my own experiencing. During a marital crisis, I decided I needed some help and went to a counsellor. I immediately felt the enormous benefit of talking about what I was experiencing. Through my counsellor's wisdom, I began to hear myself and learn to change what I found detrimental to my own growth. For years I had seen myself through the eyes of others; I looked through other people's windows, and saw none of my own truth. But now I felt understood by this counsellor, and I began to hear my own voice. He didn't say 'I know what's wrong with you'; he said, 'I understand how it feels.'*

I became aware of feelings in me that I had been suppressing for years. I learned to value what I was feeling. Because I accepted more of myself, I found it much easier to accept others. I stopped being so frightened of change and began to see change as a challenge, an opportunity to grow. I felt less like a helpless victim and more like an adult capable of decisive behaviour. I also was able during this process to leave an unhappy marriage and to find a deep, loving relationship with someone, a relationship which I was able to value strongly.

So although I had come to my counsellor for help in a crisis, I had as a fringe benefit begun to learn to live! And so I began in my work to change my approach to helping others who, like me, were suffering from life.

Some counsellors specialize in specific areas, as in the case of abortion counselling (see Chapter 17), or bereavement counselling. Sometimes counselling is available on the NHS (in GPs' surgeries or health centres) or from social services; sometimes, too, it is available at schools, colleges, universities and even at the workplace. Certain voluntary organizations offer counselling as well, such as some local MIND associations.

Relate, formerly the Marriage Guidance Council, offers relationship counselling in most towns in the UK, and some Relate counsellors work from GPs' practices (see Resources). You don't need to be married, nor do you need to be in a relationship. Although Relate does purport to offer counselling to *anyone* with relationship problems, lesbians would need to check whether it has any counsellors who are happy to work supportively with them (see Lesbians and Mental Health, p. 136).* While Relate's objectives hint that it is committed to keeping people married (no doubt in order to maintain financial support from government sources), it is perhaps fair to say that Relate counsellors are more committed than many to being non-directive and non-judgemental.

The British Association for Counselling (BAC) has recently introduced an 'accreditation' scheme for counsellors and can also act as a referral agency. While all practising BAC members are not accredited, membership of BAC might indicate a commitment to recognition of socio-political issues such as those involving race or unemployment

continues over

(both of which often figure in their publications). However, BAC as a whole has yet to demonstrate an unambiguous commitment to issues involving homosexuality and feminism. BAC publishes infor-

mation sheets, e.g. 'Guidelines for Those Seeking Counselling', and a referral directory; its Code of Ethics can serve as a useful guide on what to expect of a counsellor.

*Because of Relate's selection process for counsellors, which aims to weed out judgemental people, it is possible that Relate may in fact be a better bet for lesbians than many professionals.

vague feeling in your stomach. By starting a dialogue with your stomach – talking to it, and it talking to you – you can discover and integrate feelings that you may have been unaware of. Talking with parts of yourself, discovering what they represent, is an important component of Gestalt therapy. It can be particularly useful when we feel 'deadlocked' over an issue and feel unable to move. It can help us find ways of moving and changing. Co-counselling (see p. 121) uses some approaches from Gestalt therapy.

Bioenergetics recognizes the intimate, delicate and powerful way in which body and emotions are interconnected. It has a unique place in therapy; working with both, but in particular the body, in an attempt to free each from the constraints and constrictions of the other. Taking the example of the vague feeling in your stomach, bioenergetics can help you become more aware of it, e.g. by 'breathing' into it; the feeling may become stronger, or become transformed, often into something more powerful and more tangible. You may feel that you want to use your whole body to express this feeling – pounding a cushion, for example, stamping, shaking. This in turn may lead to both physical and emotional relief, a sense of liberation, and/or more insight and hence more integration.

Bioenergetics is based on the discoveries and theories of Wilhelm Reich – who is unique among theorists in recognizing for the first time the connections between the socio-political and the personal. (He was in fact a victim of politics and was eventually put in prison for his views – where he died.) Reich's ideas were developed by Alexander Lowen into bioenergetics therapy. Both Reich's and Lowen's ideas, recognizing the concept of a life-force based on energy, form an interesting link with Eastern-based philosophies and practices such as yoga, t'ai chi and acupuncture. Although neither Reich nor Lowen recognized the importance of sexual politics as feminists understand it (and Reich in particular had oppressive views about homosexuality), their ideas do have an enormous amount to offer women, particularly in enabling us to 'own' our bodies and our sexuality. Reichian and bioenergetics body-work can be practised with a therapist in groups or individually (e.g., through co-counselling) or, to a certain extent, on one's own. It can be very valuable both for those of us who find it difficult to express ourselves, as well as those of us who do not seem to experience such difficulties.

Transactional Analysis (TA) in the simplest definition is a method of looking at oneself – seeing the self divided into three parts:

Child – when we are expressing feelings/emotions;

Parent – when we are nurturing, judgemental, controlling;

Adult – when we are thoughtful/rational.

It can be an extremely useful means of helping us communicate, both with ourselves and with others. For example, at any time we may speak with a *child*, *adult* or *parent* voice, though we might hear them all inside our heads. On the whole, talking with the *child* voice will trigger off the *parent* in the person we are relating to, and vice versa. Such an interaction is characterized by crossed lines; there are several other types of 'crossed line' interactions. The clearest and most effective form of communication comes when we speak from the *adult* part of us (see illustration for how this part tends to be characterized by 'I' messages rather than 'You' messages): communication will be more straightforward, and the possibility of our needs being met is more likely.

Being able to 'own' all the voices and be aware which ones we're choosing to speak from can help us communicate more clearly and get what we want. Many of our inner and outer conflicts are between the child in us who 'wants' and the parent in us who says we 'ought'. The adult in us, if we can acknowledge her and use her can help us reach a compromise that is satisfactory to both parties. In the illustration over, the adult voices are most likely to lead to both parties feeling 'OK'.

A therapist, previously trained as an analyst, speaks:

I found in TA a more direct approach to the human condition than traditional psychoanalytic psychotherapy. It contains within it hints as to how to improve my life now.

For more about TA, see *I'm OK You're OK* by Thomas Harris.

Humanistic psychology can be gentle or powerful, liberating or, as Fritz Perls indicated, dangerous (comparing it to psychoanalysis, which he regarded as having little effect except to make people 'deader and deader'). Each therapy has its own strengths and weaknesses – many of which are discussed perceptively by Sheila Ernst and Lucy Goodison in *In Our Own Hands*.

Although the concept of humanistic psychology has become influential, it has infiltrated the NHS only in an *ad hoc* way, depending on the personal interests of particular psychologists (humanistic therapists trained, say, in Gestalt or bioenergetics are not employed as such in the NHS). As

Some examples of the different voices we may use in interactions
(see Transactional Analysis above)

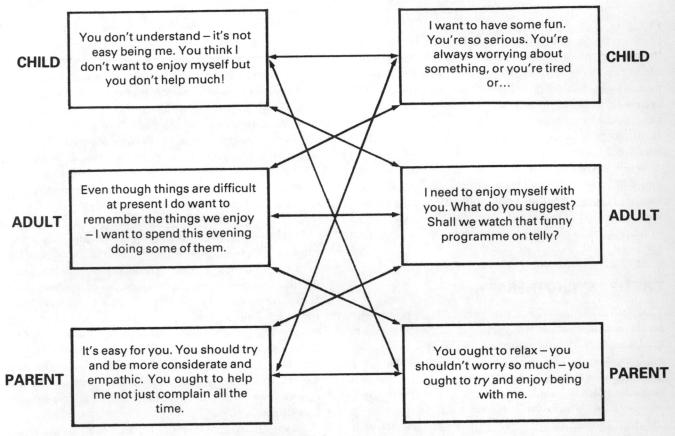

CHILD — You don't understand – it's not easy being me. You think I don't want to enjoy myself but you don't help much!

CHILD — I want to have some fun. You're so serious. You're always worrying about something, or you're tired or...

ADULT — Even though things are difficult at present I do want to remember the things we enjoy – I want to spend this evening doing some of them.

ADULT — I need to enjoy myself with you. What do you suggest? Shall we watch that funny programme on telly?

PARENT — It's easy for you. You should try and be more considerate and empathic. You ought to help me not just complain all the time.

PARENT — You ought to relax – you shouldn't worry so much – you ought to *try* and enjoy being with me.

*With thanks to Sue Dimond for help in devising this illustration.

with all other therapeutic approaches, it's crucially important to check out practitioners – whether within or outside the NHS – as much as you can. See Choosing a Therapist, p. 135. For more about these techniques and about which to choose, see Ernst and Goodison.

BEHAVIOURAL APPROACHES

Perhaps the most common types of therapy available on the NHS have a 'behavioural' orientation.* In other words, they are concerned simply with changing behaviour, and do not pretend to tackle the subtleties of experience either on an individual level, or the complexities of relationships. Nor can they deal with problems that have not already been defined. For some of us, the issue may be to *discover* what our real needs and goals are, and behavioural approaches, therefore, may not be appropriate or able to tackle this fundamental issue. But many of us might benefit from the

kind of clear-cut, practical and supportive help that they can offer.

Many behavioural therapists have increased in sophistication since the crude 'flooding' and 'desensitization' techniques of the 1960s. They may, for example, do 'goal planning': in the case of a woman who feels unable to get to the bus-stop, this becomes the 'goal' and is broken down into a number of components. Or they may take a 'constructional' approach – seeing things in terms of people's strengths instead of the traditional reward/punishment approach. They may also do 'skills training', e.g. teaching coping techniques, or assertion, or even 'listening skills'. Skills training, like behavioural approaches generally, is often used with so-called delinquents or people with varying disabilities. While skills training can in theory provide people with valuable tools for living, there is a great danger that it can also foster problems. As an ex-psychologist says:

It's the technological approach to human problems. It can help some people with some problems, but the long-term effect is dubious. You can end up simply being programmed to a stimulus, and unable to function from your inner self. It's therefore limited and, I think, short-sighted, for it's ultimately de-

*While some people consider that behavioural approaches are simply another form of psychotherapy, we have distinguished here between 'psychotherapy' which, strictly speaking, means a particular type of 'talking treatment' that derives from psychoanalytic theory, and all other approaches – or 'therapies'.

humanising – and most people's negative behaviour in fact comes from feeling dehumanised. I think the whole thing is politically suspect, at least unless it's handled very carefully, and with the necessary insight into people, with which 'skills trainers' aren't necessarily equipped. *

Some people involved in skills training have enough compassion and/or a sufficiently sophisticated understanding to cope with such problems. Some assertion training, for example, focuses on self-worth and the assertion that comes from inner confidence, well-being and caring. † Poor assertion training is literally skills training. It's the antithesis of relating to people and can actually set up conflicts. **

While behavioural approaches can lead to problems, they can be very useful. This is particularly the case when we are in charge of defining our problems, and the psychologist is able to be flexible, offering solidarity and friendship in helping us to change concrete problems in a practical way.

GROUP PSYCHOTHERAPY

This form of therapy is often easily available for people who are in-patients within the NHS. It is also sometimes available for NHS outpatients, and privately.

Group therapy can be short- or long-term – the latter meaning about eighteen months to two years – 'interaction'-orientated or 'problem'-orientated, or it may be based on one of the 'humanistic' therapies – see above.

In the *interactive* type, group members interact with each other and through this process learn how they are seen by others and how their actions and non-actions can affect their relationships. It requires an experienced group therapist to lead the group (usually someone whose training takes analytic theory into account – see above). Interactive group therapy can be a supportive experience.

I wanted to come off my drugs, but the psychiatrist told me that if I did I would go crazy. I found a group, which helped me a lot – in fact, it gave me the opportunity to go crazy, in that group. I could put the craziness away and let it rip at the next group.

It can be challenging too.

I have felt more in touch with all the different parts of me through analytic group therapy than through any other 'therapy' setting. I am a community of selves, and I speak in many voices – of anger, despair, happy child, teasing child, etcetera (the theatre of life in a way). I grew to feel safe, and familiar with the other group members – male and female. I didn't always feel comfortable. Far from it. I could spend a whole session in silence, brooding and locked in. But over time I felt accepted and part of this was my acceptance of the people I spent the time with; their voices were mine and I grew to tolerate and live with their discomfort and their irritating ways (as they did with mine) as well as their ability to survive and share. Through this process, I drew my selves to myself and began to emerge in the world as more present, more accepting and tolerant of all these selves and my – and others' – pain, however ugly it can at times appear.

Problem-orientated therapy groups are becoming increasingly common, not least because of the work of the Women's Therapy Centre in London, which has pioneered group work on a variety of issues ranging from compulsive eating to anger, 'mothers and daughters', 'dealing with abortion', 'ending a relationship' and so on. See, for example, Sue Krzowski and Pat Land's book *In Our Experience*. Some professionals within statutory services are taking up these ideas having attended training courses at the centre. A variety of other feminist-orientated therapy centres now exist too. For a far from exhaustive list, see Resources.

As with individual therapy, we need to assess the group leaders and listen to any doubts we may have.

I decided I wanted to attend an on-going group in order to work on some of my fears and difficulties in relating to other people. I decided I wanted a mixed-sex group, and found one. I quickly began to have doubts when one of the men began to get into some incredibly violent fantasies about women, and the co-leaders just left us women to deal with this as best we could, while they concentrated on this man. At first, I told myself that this provided me with something useful to work on, so I stuck it out for a few weeks (as sod's law would have it, I ended up being the woman in the group who was the butt of his fantasies). Then, after talking it over with some friends, including one who was a therapist, and who verbalized my shock at the sheer irresponsibility of the group leaders, I left. That group was one form of oppression I could do without.

You do need a certain amount of resilience to cope with a group, and group therapy can be particularly distressing or even overwhelming if you know that what you need is *individual* time with someone. While many women feel more comfortable in women-only groups, these can be

---

*In David Pilgrim's book *Psychology and Psychotherapy: Current Trends and Issues*, David Smail also discusses the dangers of focusing on 'appearances' and 'skills', and in particular the way they foster an erroneous sense of invulnerability.
†See Anne Dickson's book *A Woman in Your Own Right*, for example.
**A study involving one such approach to assertion training found that it often led to aggression and not to self-confidence.[20]

particularly difficult if any members are at some level needing the kind of nurturing that is only possible in a one-to-one therapeutic relationship.* If you have individual therapy/support *as well* as doing group therapy, this type of problem can be minimized.

PSYCHOTHERAPY AND HEALING

To end this section on therapeutic approaches, it is worth pointing out the links – often unrecognized – between psychotherapeutic work and healing. What often links the two is some kind of recognition of our spiritual selves. There is an increasing movement among therapists to recognize the importance of spirituality in therapy. Those who have trained in transpersonal psychology or psychosynthesis are easily recognizable as being in the forefront of that movement.

Transpersonal psychology fuses much that has been developed from psychoanalysis and, to a lesser extent, the 'growth' movement, with recognition of what Jung referred to as the craving for transcendence. Transpersonal psychology, therefore, recognizes the importance of the spiritual dimension, both for individuals and society.

Psychosynthesis was developed by Roberto Assagioli (see Resources) on the basis that 'nature is always trying to re-establish harmony, and within the psyche the principle of synthesis is dominant'. Working with the concept of this natural tendency, he devised a therapy to aid integration, including on a spiritual level. As the British Psychosynthesis and Education Trust says:

> It enables the individual to explore those regions full of mystery and wonder, beyond our ordinary aware-ness, which we call the superconscious, the well-spring of higher intuitions, inspirations, ethical imperatives, and states of illumination.

Psychosynthesis uses creativity and movement, among other approaches.

For more about psychotherapy and healing, see for example *Something is Happening* by Winifred Rushforth, who has inspired many therapists and helped them see the connection between psychotherapy and healing.

CHOOSING A THERAPIST†

While it should usually be possible to get access to a variety of professionals via the NHS or social services (see p. 120 above), this by no means guarantees a range of therapeutic options to choose from, nor is there any guarantee that they are aware of how the therapeutic relationship affects women, or of the overall effects of racism, sexism and homophobia. While clinical psychologists are employed through the NHS, psychotherapy and most other types of therapy are only available on a patchy basis. In addition, because the NHS is so underfunded, this means that, sometimes at least, we may have to exhibit severe problems before we can get help from that source. For anything less severe, or for more creative help, we will probably have to go outside the NHS.

While we may have more choice outside the NHS, this can still be limited outside London, particularly with regard to the therapist's commitment to a woman-centred approach. Money, of course, is a major constraint that prevents most of us seeing someone privately, but some practitioners do operate a 'sliding scale', reducing their charges to what you can afford. Some organizations, notably Relate (see p. 131), may not charge at all, though they do accept donations.

WHAT TO LOOK FOR

Despite the fact that many women do not have much choice, if any, it can still be useful to examine what to look for – not least because this can give us more confidence.

The particular title someone holds is no guarantee of their competence or attitudes. The most important thing is to try and take note of your perceptions: what do you feel about this person? This can be easier said than done if lack of confidence in your own perceptions is part of your problem; in which case, if you have any persistent doubts, it may be worth seeking help or advice from someone else.

I decided I needed psychotherapy in order to break through my appalling sense of paralysis following family traumas, and managed to get referred by my GP to a psychiatrist who I knew also provided psychotherapy. He offered me six months short-term therapy straight away, or long-term therapy when a vacancy came up with one of the psycho-therapists. Unfortunately he didn't offer me any guidance on the implications of these choices, and I opted for the immediate short course. It was with a very young man, who I sensed immediately was extremely inexperienced. However, I didn't follow my own perceptions and told myself 'If this guy is being recommended to me, he must be OK.' With hindsight I realized that he must have been doing his six-months psychiatry 'house job' (I might possibly even have been his first patient!). I also later realized that specific skills and awareness are required on the part of the therapist if they are doing short-term work, otherwise the ending can be extremely traumatic. I suspect that my 'ending' was unnecessarily so, and although I do not think he did me actual harm (everything, after all, is a potential learning experience), I can't say he actually helped, and it was some ten years before I

---

*For a discussion of women's nurturing needs, the reasons for our deprivation, and how to deal with this common sense of lack, see *Understanding Women* by Eichenbaum and Orbach.

†Many of the same criteria will apply to psychotherapists, social workers, counsellors, or other members of the 'helping professions'.

LESBIANS AND MENTAL HEALTH

Psychiatrists, therapists and other practitioners free from bias are quite rare. Many are likely to uphold any distorted views we have of ourselves, thereby reinforcing our internalized oppression (see Chapter 12). Most tend to believe in the existing 'norms', in which we as lesbians do not figure. It is important for all of us to realize that those from whom we seek help are often part of that very structure which oppresses gay people and women everywhere. Yet, as long as our society exists in its current form, many of us will need some form of therapeutic help.

Some of us have been lucky enough to find what we need, even from quite traditional therapists.

> I could have had a real disaster with a woman psychotherapist who wasn't what I needed. Mine was quite traditional, asked me questions that drove me crazy, but they were ones I wanted to have asked. She was just what I wanted. I wouldn't have stuck with her otherwise. I never felt an ounce of oppressive attitudes about lesbianism. There were certain challenges around it, but that's not the same thing. I felt her interpretation of a couple of dreams was very heterosexual, but she may have been right. And she still wasn't challenging my sexuality. She never ever made me feel guilty about it.
>
> When I went for the initial 'interview' I told her what I wanted and didn't want. She was noncommittal but I realized she would have been honest if she couldn't cope. I lay on a couch and she sat behind me. I found that a tremendous relief, not having to stare her in the face all the time. Much as I liked her I wasn't there to form a relationship of that sort with her. It was so relaxing.

However, many lesbians might prefer to seek out a feminist therapist if at all possible. Yet even (non-lesbian) feminist therapists are by no means always aware of their own homophobia. We do, therefore, need to be watchful. In her article 'Lesbians in Therapy',[21] Frances Rooney mentions the case of one such therapist who believed strongly in being open to everyone, and who urged her client to come out to her family, even though the client had felt it would be disastrous to do so. Having tried to get the therapist to drop the issue, the client reports:

> Finally, more I think to get her to shut up than for any other reason, I told them. My mother cried for days;

my father called me a pervert. He packed my suitcase and threw it down the stairs at me, saying he never wanted to see me again. That was four years ago. I've had a couple of hysterical phone calls from my mother since; nothing from my father. I sometimes write, but my letters usually come back. Thanks a lot, therapy.

Frances Rooney draws clear-cut conclusions for therapists:

> The limitations of our lives are facts of those lives. We can in therapy lessen the crippling effects; we cannot ignore the reality. Therapists must be willing to acknowledge this.

Practitioners who are lesbian do exist, but tend to be in the closet — with rare exceptions.

> I do therapeutic work with young people. There's no way I can come out without jeopardizing the work I'm doing — and even my job.

Sometimes it's important for us to see a lesbian, who may be more likely to understand our experiences from the 'inside'. However, as Frances Rooney found when interviewing for her article:

> All the women I spoke to had started out wanting a lesbian therapist. All had concluded that the therapist needn't be either a lesbian or a feminist or even, for some, a woman. Some thought it might even be easier to work with a man; a male therapist might try to convert a lesbian to heterosexuality, in which case it would be easy enough to walk out, but no male therapist will be personally challenged with the possibility of his own lesbianism. This is one of the major problems lesbians experience in therapy, and is often clouded and complex enough to remain hidden until serious damage has been done to the therapeutic relationship.

Whoever you consider going to, be wary of anyone who sees your sexual preference as the source of your problems, and therefore fails to take you seriously.

Aside from individual therapy, you may want to consider a lesbian support group, self-help therapy group or co-counselling.

dared to get involved in therapy again. By then I realized that the last thing I needed was to feel any doubts about my therapist. I took some time picking and choosing. It didn't involve any 'rational' choice: I just knew I was looking for some kind of connection. When I found it, I knew that that was what I'd been looking for.

A major clue is whether you feel the person concerned is acting authentically – in terms of their commitment to you. While many psychotherapists and counsellors would aim to do this (for sustaining an authentic relationship with the client is a crucial aspect of the therapy), it is not a prerequisite of the behaviourist model (though some behaviourists would consider being authentic was important too).

Recommendations from people you trust can be very useful. There may be a feminist therapy network in your area, or you could contact the London Women's Therapy Centre, who have lists of therapists in many parts of the country. Local branches of MIND or Relate may be able to recommend someone, but you still need to go on your instincts.

I was given the name of someone by the Women's Therapy Centre. I kept thinking she must be good, because they gave me her name. At the time, I couldn't explain what it was about her that I didn't like. I kept looking, until I found someone who 'felt' right. Then I knew what it was about the other woman's style that I didn't like.

You may feel more comfortable with a woman than a man, or vice versa. But often the sex of the therapist does not matter.

QUESTIONS TO ASK

No therapist can be perfect. What we have a right to expect is that they behave ethically, submit themselves to peer review ('supervision' – see below), and are aware of their limitations and biases.

Below we list some questions that you might consider important. At the end, we give some quotes from feminist therapists which provide some insight into the reasons for these questions.

1. *What is their training?* It's important to know what approach they take. If you ask what they felt was good – and bad – about their training, you can gauge their understanding of what a good therapist should be. The Royal College of Psychiatrists says that harm can result when therapy is carried out by unqualified practitioners. However, they miss the point, since qualified ones can cause harm too and, to the degree that they believe their training makes them infallible, they are more likely to! Many professionals have inadequate training. Psychologists and psychiatrists in particular can find their training of little use for the practice of psychotherapy.[22] As far as counsellors or psychotherap-

ists are concerned, four years' intensive training is not necessarily better than one year's feminist training, *and vice versa.* It may be necessary to bear in mind that in many parts of the country it is impossible to do formal therapy training.

2. *Has their training focused on women in particular, and have racism, sexism or homophobia been included in their focus?* Many training schools, particularly those that are psychoanalytically-based, are judgemental towards homosexuality, and it has been known for them to be actively antagonistic towards lesbians. Even if the professional training course has been inadequate in these respects, and most are, the way they respond to this question will give you a clear idea of how relevant they consider it, and how they would be prepared to deal with issues that concern you. You may want to ask specifically about their attitudes to violence against women, particularly in the home – i.e. are they aware of the extent of battering, rape and incest, and the mental effects such violence can have on women, or do they follow Freud's original teachings that such events are figments of our imagination, or that we were responsible for the attacks by inviting them?*

3. *Are they a member of a recognized body?* This can be some sort of guide, although it is no guarantee about the therapist's attitude – nor necessarily of their competence. While, in theory at least, professionals within the NHS can be more accountable for their actions, they can be the least equipped to help us. While some professionals outside the NHS can be unscrupulous (anyone can call themselves a therapist, regardless of their training), they can have higher standards than the NHS will allow them to operate within.

4. *Have they undergone therapy themselves?* This can be a reliable guide for choosing a therapist since no reputable therapist would consider themselves competent without it. Unfortunately, many professionals in the NHS, particularly psychiatrists, psychologists and nurses, do not receive adequate training on a personal level.

5. *What kind of supervision do they have, if any?* This too can be a reliable guide, for the same reason as given under (4) above. Doing therapeutic work requires help and support from a regular source, regardless of how long ago the therapist qualified. Asking the therapist about their training and supervision may give you a good idea of how omnipotent they think they are. Unfortunately, many professionals in the NHS, particularly those in *senior* positions, do not have supervision. However, Relate counsellors and accredited members of the British Association for Counselling all have regular supervision, as do many others who regard their work as a serious professional commitment. A counsellor/therapist who has well-

---

*This latter point is of particular relevance to professionals who have an analytically-based perspective. After the publication of his book *Freud: the Assault on Truth*, Masson received 'hundreds of letters' from women saying that their analysts refused to believe their stories of violence, or that it was relevant to their present state. Instead, they were asked what they did, for example, to seduce their fathers.

BLACK WOMEN AND MENTAL HEALTH*

Prepared together with

ROBINA SHAH,

MANCHESTER COUNCIL FOR COMMUNITY RELATIONS

The racism we encounter in society at large (e.g. see Chapter 10) shapes our lives and accentuates any ill-health we experience. It does nothing to foster our mental health.

> I learned to laugh at my Black skin and discovered later it was a way of dealing with the feelings of anger and rejection building up inside me.[23]

If our struggle to overcome these difficulties fails, we are then confronted with the institutional racism of the mental health services, which is primarily responsible for the creation of an alienated mental health service for black communities, and especially for black women. Because of institutionalized racism, many practitioners fail to recognize the real nature of our distress, its causes, and how to provide appropriate care for us. Fixed attitudes and assumptions about black women have been passed on through training and teaching of health workers – which perpetuates and reinforces professionals' ignorance. Their ignorance, therefore, creates an additional burden for us.

If mental health care for black women is to improve, training of staff has to include the opportunity to develop an understanding of racism and its effects on us. Unfortunately, many practitioners do not recognize that this sort of understanding and awareness is important in order to perform their job properly. Their training involves simplistic and stereotyped approaches which prevent recognition that women, and black women in particular, are individuals with varying needs.

> What I want is for someone to know me; to know where I am coming from, to know my history and to help me be myself. I feel that a white male doctor cannot help me. He cannot understand me as an Asian woman. It is important that someone does understand our needs. We Asian women will continue to suffer until our needs are recognized. And ultimately I think that it is only other Asian women who can help us to help each other.[24]

There are some hopeful signs, however. *Nafsiyat*, for example, the first 'inter-cultural therapy centre', was set up in London in 1983. It is doing pioneering work, helping individuals and their families from a variety of backgrounds, and developing a truly multi-cultural service. We hope it will be the first of many initiatives. Whether it is or not, black women are now challenging racist practices and will no longer accept the feeble excuses of the 'language barrier', or 'misunderstandings' of cultural or religious needs, to justify inappropriate and inadequate mental health care.

*Although in this chapter we have managed to present therapy within a feminist framework, we have been unable to incorporate a coherent anti-racist critique – partly because the author is white, but partly also because such a critique has yet to be developed. We hope that, despite its limitations, this chapter will be of some use to women from all cultural backgrounds, and that some of the Resources listed on p. 145 will provide further support and understanding.

supervised experience can be more reliable than someone who has had extensive training without supervision.

6. Good questions to ask are, *what do they consider to be a good outcome*, and *what do they like to foster in their clients?* Even quite 'progressive' professionals may consider a 'good' outcome to be the forming of a committed monogamous heterosexual relationship, and for the client to fit in socially in a general kind of way. If you don't see yourself as aiming for that kind of outcome, this question is particularly important.

7. *You may also wish to ask about confidentiality.* All therapists should have a clear policy that confidentiality between you is essential. However, it's worth checking them out on the issue. Most professionals, for example, need to make notes. The important thing is what happens to them. You may want an undertaking that the notes are for their eyes only. However, in the NHS, 'official' notes of some kind may need to be kept. If this is the case, you may want to establish their nature, whether you can see them, and who has access to them. Responsible practitioners also undertake supervision – where they discuss the people they're working with. You may wish to check out or negotiate exactly how you might be referred to, to protect your privacy. If you are considering going to a counsellor at your place of work, an important issue is not only confidentiality, but whether the counsellor may have divided loyalties.

8. If you have not already gained an impression of the therapist's values from the answers s/he has given, you could ask about them directly. All therapists hold values, and it is perfectly valid to expect a professional to talk about them.

This is what some feminist therapists have to say about their training:

In one job I had, the supervision was excellent. We had regular team meetings, as well as individual sessions, both weekly on the whole.

God knows what anyone in my training course would have done if they were a lesbian. I know a woman who's had to keep her lesbian self to herself in her counselling course.

I did a short course that was very good in many ways. It certainly tried to deal with sexism and homophobia. But I felt very worried about the lack of grounding in basic psychoanalytical concepts like transference, and the lack of discussion of pitfalls and of what was good practice. I dread to think what someone could do if that's the only training they had, and I'd think twice before recommending anyone from that course unless I knew them personally.

Some courses, like the one I'm doing at the moment, didn't offer individual therapy as part of their training. I'm one of the few students who's had therapy, and it worries me the way this isn't considered necessary. I know someone who's doing a twelve-month course in Gestalt. After only six months he's working as a therapist. I've done a lot of courses, and till I've completed this one I don't think I should really call myself one.

I'd always believed in the relevance of psychoanalytic theory for women, and the value of therapy, and after some years as a counsellor began training in one of the most respected psychotherapy training courses in London. I knew that as a lesbian it would be difficult, but gradually I became so concerned – and eventually appalled – at the value judgements and assumptions that remained unchallenged, that I left. I was put under considerable pressure to stay – as if my leaving would make the institution vulnerable. (Of course, they had every reason to fear that, for there were a lot of beans that could have been spilled.) I remember when I first began to feel worried, when the group I was training with all changed the way they dressed, and at the same time I was told by my training analyst and the lecturers that I needed to embrace a middle-class lifestyle (because my clients were all going to be middle class!). Then I noticed some of my fellow students becoming more certain, even arrogant. As time went on I realized I was being trained to become part of a secret cult, where we were actually being told we had power, but we mustn't disclose it. Clients were dissected in a manner that would cause raised eyebrows even in a medical school. They had no room to manoeuvre, and theory was constantly misapplied as a 'truth' rather than as a possible truth that needed to be tested with each client. The experience has challenged my

belief in psychotherapy to the utmost. In so far as it fosters therapists' belief in their own authority and infallibility, I think it is utterly unjustifiable. I am now far more respectful of other approaches. Although they have their failings, I believe that co-counselling or the Pellin-type approach, in attempting to be so respectful of individuals, and cognisant of political dimensions, can do less harm, and often a lot more good. They're also potentially far more accessible to most women.

In conclusion, there are many reasons why we need to be careful in choosing counsellors and therapists. They can be invaluable in helping us find our way through confusion and pain. Nevertheless, if you look for help, it's vital to take a consumerist approach and to shop around. While many professionals may not like this, they're the people you're unlikely to want to go to anyway. Someone who admits to being new to your ideas and threatened by your questions, *but who is prepared to talk honestly and at times openly,* may make an excellent therapist compared with someone who merely tries to appear confident or reassuring. As one therapist comments,

The growth movement has attracted many who like to perform, especially in the 'I'm a very open person' vein. In spite of years of analysis, there are also therapists who do more performing than skilful prompting in the wings. But no one has all the problems any more than all the answers. I wouldn't go to a counsellor or therapist who told me how they had dealt with their prejudices and were not at all homophobic, especially if they exuded a shiny, all-accepting glow. Much real growth always needs some darkness. I've gained most from a therapist who admitted to finding my lesbianism a problem, struggled within herself and, through 'my' therapy, learned quite a lot, even though we couldn't always see where we were going.

In choosing a therapist or counsellor, you can afford to be far more judgemental than in choosing a friend.

While therapy or counselling may be just right for us, sometimes, despite what others may tell us, they may not be what we need at all. Some of us may see them as serving simply to bolster up a sick society, by individualizing problems that are social and political. While there is a sense in which this can be true, it is also true that we cannot change society for the better if our good intentions are at the mercy of powerful unconscious – and therefore unknown – forces within us that so easily prevent us from achieving what we (thought we) wanted. The best type of therapist/counsellor guides you to yourself – to find your own way.

I don't think we necessarily have to be manipulated by psychology, we can use it for ourselves. The discovery of the unconscious and the recognition of

how it can be manipulated paradoxically provides us with the means to escape from socially imposed structures and to work towards new ones . . . Through the structure and process of psychotherapy I have been helped in resolving paralysing emotional problems. I have also learned to appreciate its value in examining the role of personality structure in political struggle.[25]

WHAT SOME WOMEN ARE DOING

Since the first **Women and Psychiatry** group was formed in the early 1970s (spawning the first national conference on women and mental health – coordinated by MIND), there has been a gradual increase in initiatives by women for women. The London **Women's Therapy Centre** is now one of several such centres in different parts of the country aiming to provide feminist therapy (see Resources). And since we began this new edition there has been another spate of initiatives.

Women Talking to Women is a counselling service, also based in Edinburgh, which grew out of a women's self-help group and offers a chance for women to talk to another woman, confidentially, as does a similar service in London: **Islington Women and Mental Health Project** grew out of discussions among local women about their experiences of isolation, depression and the psychiatric system. 'We have come together' they say, 'to fight the stigma attached to "mental illness", to give ourselves and other women in similar situations a voice, to end our isolation from each other, and to define "mental health" *our* way.' They hope that by coming together, women can share their pain and make the connection between the pain and their external oppression.

Our anger at the present mental health system continues to fuel our campaigning for better services. We maintain a precarious balance between providing services which, at the present rate of funding, are subsidized by women's unpaid labour, and trying to find secure sources of financial support.[26]

Womankind is a multi-racial women and mental health self-help project based in Bristol whose main work involves the setting up of self-help groups or personal support groups. They do this by putting women in touch with each other – 'networking' – or by forming a group if there are enough women in a particular locality or who are struggling with a similar emotional dilemma. They also keep a telephone line open as much as they can. As Pamela Trevithick says:

Seeing women struggling, and struggling ourselves, acts as a constant reminder that all oppression, mistreatment, injustice, deprivation, inequality – call it what you will – has an impact on our emotional lives that can interfere with our ability to trust, to feel

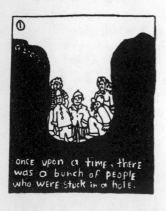

once upon a time, there was a bunch of people who were stuck in a hole.

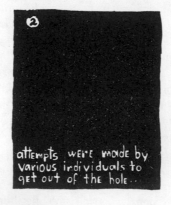

attempts were made by various individuals to get out of the hole..

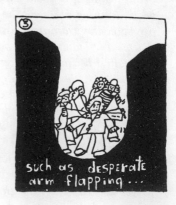

such as desperate arm flapping...

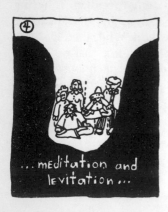

...meditation and levitation...

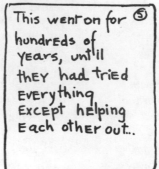

This went on for hundreds of years, until they had tried everything except helping each other out..

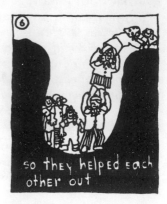

so they helped each other out

safe, to love and believe in ourselves, to act in our own interest.[27]

Women's Action for Mental Health is a neighbourhood counselling service provided by and for women living on or around the White City estate in London. It grew out of the White City Mental Health project, which works mainly with women and which offers counselling, brief psycho-therapy, problem-sharing groups and educational work-shops on mental health issues.

The objective . . . is to help the women develop an insight into their situations and an understanding of how to explore new possibilities for themselves. In theoretical terms, there is a potential progression from the psychic through the social to the political, a progression the women involved with Women's Action for Mental Health have followed right through.[28]

Following the establishment of the project, there has been a decrease in the number of women visiting a doctor for tranquillizers and anti-depressants.

By the time you read this, we hope that these projects – and many more – will be flourishing and that our demands for mental health care appropriate for our needs gain in strength and power. As Islington Women and Mental Health Project says:

We believe that a mental health care system should be an integral part of our lives. Psychiatry, with its present philosophy and organization, does not have the ability to give us better mental health since . . . our mental health depends on how much love and respect we get, how we relate to each other as well as on satisfactory housing, fulfilling work, decent wages and the absence of racism and sexism. Mental health services must be involved in struggles and campaigns to improve our lives . . .

We demand the demedicalization of our health and the setting up of clinics within the NHS where 'alternative therapies' which take a holistic approach to our health are available. We see the need for a whole range of mental health facilities such as advice and counselling centres and counsellors employed in schools, workplaces, leisure centres and community centres. Supportive women's centres with counsel-ling/therapy and educational facilities, safe asylums and women's crisis centres with twenty-four-hour intensive support are all necessary to respond to women's needs. All of these must have a comprehen-sive child-care service, workers from relevant ethnic groups and translating provision, and facilities for disabled women, ensuring accessibility to all women.

NOTES

1. From Report of Subpanel on Women to the US President's Commission on Mental Health, 1978.
2. For a discussion of the overall effects and implications of society's expectations in this respect, see Luise Eichenbaum and Susie Orbach. *Understanding Women*. London: Penguin Books, 1985.
3. George Brown and Tyrril Harris. *The Social Origins of Depression. A Study of Psychiatric Disorder in Women*. London: Tavistock, 1978; Celia Davies and Sheila Roche. 'The Place of Methodology: a Critique of Brown and Harris', *Sociological Review*, vol. 28, no. 3, 1980, p. 641.
4. Kathy Nairne and Gerrilyn Smith. *Dealing with Depression*. London: Women's Press, 1984.
5. Elaine Hilberman Carmen MD, Nancy Filipe Russo PhD and Jean Baker Miller MD. 'Inequality and Women's Mental Health: an Overview', *American Journal of Psychiatry*, vol. 138, no. 10, October 1981, p. 1324.
6. I. K. Broverman, D. M. Broverman, F. E. Clarkson, P. S. Rosenkrantz and S. R. Vogel. 'Sex Role Stereotypes and Clinical Judgments of Mental Health', *Journal of Consulting and Clinical Psychology*, no. 34, 1970, pp. 1–7. While this study might be considered too old to be relevant today, more recent research sadly indicates little change in mental health professionals' attitudes. See Kathleen O'Malley and Susan Richardson, *Journal of Counselling and Development*, vol. 63, no. 5, 1985, p. 294.
7. Lynda Birke et al. *Spare Rib*, no. 84, July 1979.
8. Karen Horney. *Self-Analysis*. New York: Norton Library, 1968; Sheila Ernst and Lucy Goodison. *In Our Own Hands: a Book of Self-help Therapy*. London: Women's Press, 1981. The Institute of Self Analysis, set up in January 1987, aims to develop the work of Horney and Alice Miller – see Resources.
9. Fiona McKay. 'Self-help Therapy', *Spare Rib*, no. 48, June 1976. Also published in Sue O'Sullivan (ed.). *Women's Health – a Spare Rib Reader*. London: Pandora, 1987.

10. See, e.g., Austin Mitchell. 'Getting Wound Up by the Winds of Winter', *Sunday Times*, 12 October 1986; and Jill Collings. 'Seeing the Light', *Guardian*, 18 February 1988.
11. K. Z. Bezchlibnyk and J. J. Jeffries. 'Should Psychiatric Patients Drink Coffee?', *Journal of the Canadian Medical Association*, vol. 124, no. 4, 15 February 1981, pp. 357–8.
12. See, e.g., Terence DuQuesne and Julian Reeves. *A Handbook of Psychoactive Medicines*. London: Quartet Books, 1982; Peter Parish. *Medicines: a Guide for Everybody*. London: Penguin Books, 1984; and the various MIND publications about drugs. See also Chapter 5.
13. For two opposing viewpoints on ECT, see Frank Roy. 'Shock Tactics', *Open Mind*, no. 15, June–July 1985; and Arthur McDowall. 'The Case for ECT', *Open Mind*, no. 16, August–September 1985. See also the subsequent correspondence in *Open Mind* and the MIND factsheet no. 10 on ECT.
14. Quoted in WHIC broadsheet on women and mental health.
15. Quoted in David Berry and Mandy Williams. 'First Aid in Mental Health', *Open Mind*, no. 6, December 1983–January 1984.
16. Sunna quoted in Pearlie MacNeill et al. (eds). *Through the Break – Women in Personal Struggle*. London: Sheba, 1986.
17. Val Johnson in MacNeill et al., ibid.
18. Winifred Rushforth. *Something is Happening – Spiritual Awareness and Depth Psychology in the New Age*. London: Gateway, 1983.
19. Ernst and Goodison, op. cit., note 8, pp. 58–9.
20. M. Fagan. *Small Group Behaviour*, vol. 10, no. 1, p. 136.
21. Frances Rooney. 'Lesbians in Therapy' in 'Women and Therapy' issue of *HealthSharing*, Winter 1982.
22. See, for example, David Pilgrim (ed.). *Psychology and Psychotherapy: Current Trends and Issues*. London: Routledge and Kegan Paul, 1983.
23. Isha McKenzie-Mavinga. 'Smiling Anger', in MacNeill et al., op. cit., note 16.
24. Saroj. 'Did it Really Happen?', in MacNeill et al., ibid.

25. Frances Seton. 'Opening Myself to Change', *Spare Rib*, no. 44, February 1976.

26. Jan Wallcraft. *Finding Our Own Solutions*, Women in MIND booklet. MIND, 1986. For more about women's initiatives, see this booklet.

27. Pamela Trevithick. 'Womankind – a Women and Mental Health Self-help Project', *Radical Health Promotion*, no. 6, 1987, p. 16.

28. Sue Holland in Wallcraft, op. cit., note 26.

RESOURCES

Note: See also other relevant sections of the book for Resources concerning specific issues such as food, menopause, miscarriage, relationships, violence, etc. Information about tranquillizers is given in Chapter 5. Materials concerned solely or mainly with self-help are marked with an asterisk.

PUBLICATIONS

GENERAL

All-Party Parliamentary Social Services Select Committee. *Community Care*. London: HMSO, 1985. Endorses concept of a comprehensive mental health service within the community and heavily criticizes current policies. Contains over 100 recommendations. Useful campaigning material (though doesn't direct itself to women's issues specifically).

Assagioli, Roberto. *Psychosynthesis*. Wellingborough, Northants: Turnstone, 1975. See text for short description of psychosynthesis.

*Assagioli, Roberto. *The Act of Will – a Guide to Self-Actualization and Self-Realization*. Wellingborough, Northants: Turnstone, 1984. Self-help sequel to the above.

Aveline, Mark. 'What Price Psychiatry without Psychotherapy?', *The Lancet*, 13 October 1984, p. 856.

Banton, Ragnhild et al. *The Politics of Mental Health*. London: Macmillan, 1985.

Barnard, Jessie. *The Future of Marriage*. London: Souvenir Press, 1973.

Beardshaw, Virginia. *Conscientious Objectors at Work*. London: Social Audit, 1981. About ill-treatment of mental patients, and includes suggestions for trades union and management action that would allow nurses to become more effective advocates for in-patients.

Berke, J. *I Haven't Had to Go Mad Here*. London: Penguin Books, 1979.

Berne, Eric. *Games People Play – the Psychology of Human Relationships*. London: Penguin Books, 1967. Based on transactional analysis (see text).

Boadella, David. *Wilhelm Reich: The Evolution of His Work*. London: Arkana, 1985. By the author of one of the foremost therapists practising bioenergetics (see text).

Brent Irish Mental Health Group. *The Irish Experience of Mental Ill-health in London*. London, 1988 (available from the group – see Organizations).

*Button, John. *Making Love Work – a Radical Approach*. Wellingborough, Northants: Turnstone, 1985. Based on co-counselling principles (see text).

Dryden, Windy. *Individual Therapy in Britain*. New York: Harper & Row, 1984.

*Evison, Rose and Richard Horobin. *How to Change Yourself and Your World – a Manual of Co-Counselling Theory and Practice*. Sheffield, 1983 (available from Co-counselling Phoenix, 5 Victoria Road, Sheffield).

*Faraday, Ann. *Dream Power – the Use of Dreams in Everyday Life*. London: Pan, 1973.

*Faraday, Ann. *The Dream Game*. New York: Harper & Row, 1976.

Forty-Second Street. Reflected Images – Self Portraits of Stress. Manchester Youth Development Trust, 1983. Eleven people, mainly young, discuss their experiences and search for understanding and support.

Gale, Derek. *What is Psychotherapy? A Personal and Practical Guide*. London: Gale Centre, 1987. A clear and thoughtful booklet, available from The Gale Centre, Freepost, Loughton, Essex IG10 1BR (Tel: 01–508 9344).

Gale, Derek. *A Therapist's Bibliography*. London: Gale Centre, 1987. Has some valuable annotations which can provide insight into a wide range of psychotherapeutic approaches.

GLC Women's Committee. *Challenging the Racism that Harms our Health!* London, 1985.

*Harris, Thomas A. *I'm OK – You're OK*. London: Pan, 1973. A self-help therapy book, based on transactional analysis (see text).

*Horney, Karen. *Self-Analysis*. New York: W. W. Norton, 1942 and 1968. A pioneering book, way ahead of its time in terms of recognizing the possibility of self-help. Also unusual, even by today's standards, in coming from an analyst.

*Howard, Alex. *Finding a Way*. London: Gateway, 1985.

Ingleby, David. *Critical Psychiatry – the Politics of Mental Health*. London: Penguin Books, 1981. Includes a chapter by Franco Basaglia on the pioneering community mental health service he set up in Trieste.

*James, Muriel et al. *Born to Win*. Wokingham, Berkshire: Addison—Wesley, 1971. An inspiring book.

*Jeffs, Martin (revisions by Sandy Merritt). *Manual for Action – Techniques to enable groups engaged in action for change to increase their effectiveness*. Action Resources Group, 1982 (c/o 13 Mornington Grove, London E3 4NS).

*Jennings, Sue (ed.). *Creative Therapy*. Banbury, Oxfordshire: Kemble Press, 1983.

*Kaplan Williams, Strephon. *The Dreamwork Manual*. Wellingborough, Northants: Aquarian Press, 1984.

Kennard, David. *An Introduction to Therapeutic Communities*. London: Routledge and Kegan Paul, 1983.

Kovel, Joel. *A Complete Guide to Therapy*. London: Penguin Books, 1978.

Laing, R. D. *The Divided Self; Self and Others; Sanity, Madness and the Family* (with Aaron Esterson), etc. All Laing's books published in the 1960s (by Penguin Books) raised important issues about so-called sanity and so-called madness, providing for the first time a framework and a language for understanding them. For his current ideas, see his latest book, *Wisdom, Madness and Folly – The Making of a Psychiatrist*. London: Macmillan, 1985.

Lesser, Michael. *Nutrition and Vitamin Therapy – the Dietary Treatment of Mental and Emotional Ill-Health*. Wellingborough, Northants: Thorsons, 1985.

Littlewood, R. and M. **Lipsedge**. *Aliens and Alienists: Ethnic Minorities and Psychiatry*. London: Penguin Books, 1982.

Lowen, Alexander. *Bioenergetics*. London: Penguin Books, 1976 (see text).

Masson, Jeffrey M. *Freud: The Assault on Truth*. London: Faber & Faber, 1984. This book took Freudian psychoanalysts by storm. Particularly interesting for what Masson has exposed concerning Freud's attitude to women, especially for unearthing facts concerning the reality of women's experience of incest, which Freud transformed into mere fantasy.

*Melville, Joy. *First Aid in Mental Health*. London: Unwin, 1980.

MIND. *Common Concern*. London: MIND, 1983. MIND's manifesto for a new mental health service. Advocates among other things the establishment of 'community mental health workers'.

Morrell, Carol. 'With a Little Help from Ourselves', in Marsha **Rowe** (ed.), *Spare Rib Reader*. London: Penguin Books, 1982. About co-counselling (see text).

*Parish, Peter. *Medicines: a Guide for Everybody* (rev. 5th ed.). London: Penguin Books, 1984.

Perls, Fritz. *Gestalt Therapy Verbatim*. New York: Bantam, 1971.

Pilgrim, David (ed.). *Psychology and Psychotherapy: Current Trends and Issues*. London: Routledge and Kegan Paul, 1983. Critical look, particularly at behaviourally-trained psychologists. Also has chapter on social class issues.

Rack, Philip. *Race, Culture and Mental Disorder*. London: Tavistock, 1982.

Radical Therapist Collective. *The Radical Therapist*. London: Penguin Books, 1974. Collection of papers by therapists who disagree with 'deviance' concept among other things. Somewhat dated in parts, but useful chapters on dealing with emergencies.

*Rainwater, Janette. *You're in Charge! A Guide to Becoming Your Own Therapist*. Wellingborough, Northants: Turnstone, 1981.

Reich, Wilhelm. (see text) His books include *The Mass Psychology of Fascism*. London: Penguin Books, 1975 and *The Function of the*

Orgasm. London: Souvenir, 1983. See also Boadella and Lowen listed above.

Release. *The Trouble with Tranquillisers* (pamphlet). London: Release Publications, 1982.

Richmond Fellowship. *Report of the Richmond Fellowship Enquiry into Community Approaches to the Mentally Ill*. London: Richmond Fellowship Press, 1983.

Rigge, Marianne. *Hello, Can I Help You? The Growth of Telephone Advice Services*. London: Mutual Aid Press, 1980.

Rogers, Carl R. *On Personal Power – Inner Strength and its Revolutionary Impact*. London: Constable, 1978.

*****Rogers**, Carl R. and Barry **Stevens**. *Person to Person: the Problem of Being Human*. London: Souvenir Press, 1973.

Rowan, John. *The Reality Game: a Guide to Humanistic Counselling and Therapy*. London: Routledge and Kegan Paul, 1983.

Rowan, John. *Ordinary Ecstasy: Humanistic Psychology in Action* (rev. ed.). London: Routledge and Kegan Paul, 1988.

*****Rowe**, Dorothy. *Depression: the Way Out of Your Prison*. London: Routledge and Kegan Paul, 1983. Not just about depression: about negative thinking in general. Deservedly the MIND Book of the Year in 1983.

Rushforth, Winifred. *Something is Happening – Spiritual Awareness and Depth Psychology in the New Age*. London: Gateway, 1983.

Ryan, Joanna and Frank **Thomas**. *The Politics of Mental Handicap*. London: Penguin Books, 1980. Critique of institutionalization of mentally handicapped people. Relevant to mental health of our society as a whole.

*****Schiffman**, Muriel. *Gestalt Self Therapy*. Berkeley, CA: Wingbow Press, 1971. Distributed by Element Books.

Sedgwick, Peter. *PsychoPolitics*. London: Pluto Press, 1982. An attempt to reassess many of the radical ideas from the 1960s, including Laing's (see above).

Segal, Julia. *Phantasy in Everyday Life*. London: Penguin Books, 1985. An impressive book which manages to be extremely accessible while tackling complex issues involving the unconscious (see text).

*****Sheehy**, Gail. *Passages*. New York: Bantam, 1976.

Shepherd, Michael. 'What Price Psychotherapy?', *British Medical Journal*, 17 March 1984.

*****Shohet**, Robin. *Dream Sharing*. Wellingborough, Northants: Turnstone, 1985.

Smail, David. *Illusion and Reality – the Meaning of Anxiety*. London: Dent, 1984.

*****Southgate**, John. *The Barefoot Psychoanalyst*. London, 1976.

Steiner, Claude (ed.). *Readings in Radical Psychiatry*. New York: Grove Press, 1975.

Szasz, Thomas. *The Manufacture of Madness*. London: Paladin, 1973. Traces links between persecution of heretics and witches and society's use of homosexuals as scapegoats; labels of 'madness' and 'eccentricity' seen as control instruments of the dominant ideology.

*****Watzlawick**, Pail. *The Situation is Hopeless But Not Serious – The Pursuit of Happiness*. New York: W. W. Norton, 1984.

Woodman, Natalie and Harry R. **Lenon**. *Counselling with Gay Men and Women: a Guide to Facilitating Positive Lifestyles*. New York: Jossey-Bass, 1980. Phenomenally expensive but included here as a prerequisite for professional reading.

ON OR SPECIFICALLY FOR WOMEN

Alexandra. *I Speak for the Silent*. Enfield: Alexandra Press, 1984 (196 Great Cambridge Road, Enfield, Middx). The experience of psychiatric hospital and a plea for action. As relevant today as when the events happened.

Baker Miller, Jean. *Toward a New Psychology of Women*. London: Penguin Books, 1978.

Chesler, Phyllis. *Women and Madness*. London: Allen Lane, 1974. Passionate book that dispels many myths about 'female psychology'.

*****Dickson**, Anne. *A Woman in Your Own Right*. London: Quartet Books, 1982.

Dinnerstein, Dorothy. *The Mermaid and the Minotaur: Sexual Arrangements and Human Malaise*. New York: Harper & Row, 1976.

Dowling, Colette. *The Cinderella Complex*. London: Fontana, 1982. Explores women's struggle between wanting independence versus dependence.

Eichenbaum, Luise and Susie **Orbach**. *Outside In Inside Out – Women's Psychology: a Feminist Psychoanalytic Approach*. London: Penguin Books, 1982. (An expanded version of this, entitled *Understanding Women*, was published in 1985 by Penguin.) A significant book (see text).

Eichenbaum, Luise and Susie **Orbach**. *What Do Women Want?* London: Michael Joseph, 1983.

*****Ernst**, Sheila and Lucy **Goodison**. *In Our Own Hands – a Book of Self-Help Therapy*. London: Women's Press, 1981. About self-help therapy and therapy in general, within an overall feminist perspective.

Ernst, Sheila and Marie **Maguire** (eds). *Living with the Sphinx – Papers from the Women's Therapy Centre*. London: Women's Press, 1987.

Feminist Therapy Study/Support Group. 'Women and Therapy', in *HealthSharing*, Winter 1982 (Canadian women's health magazine on file at WHRRIC).

Field, Joanna. *A Life of One's Own*. London: Penguin Books, 1934, reissued by Virago Press, 1987. Illustrates the value of diary-writing as a vehicle for self-discovery.

Figes, Eva. *Patriarchal Attitudes*. London: Panther, 1970.

Friar Williams, Elizabeth. *Notes of a Feminist Therapist*. New York: Dell, 1976.

Friday, Nancy. *My Mother Myself*. Fontana, 1979.

Friedan, Betty. *The Feminine Mystique*. London: Penguin Books, 1965. Classic, though dated.

Gilman, Charlotte Perkins. *The Yellow Wallpaper*. A short novel, reprinted in *The Charlotte Perkins Gilman Reader*. London: Women's Press, 1981.

'Guidelines for Therapy with Women' in *American Psychologist*, December 1978, p. 1122. Available from WHRRIC.

Hare-Mustin, Rachel. 'An appraisal of the Relationship between Women and Psychotherapy', *American Psychologist*, May 1983, p. 593.

Harpwood, Diane. *Tea and Tranquillisers*. London: Virago Press, 1981. A novel.

Horney, Karen. *Feminine Psychology*. New York: W. W. Norton, 1967.

Krzowski, Sue and Pat **Land** (eds). *In Our Experience: Workshops at the Women's Therapy Centre*. London: Women's Press, 1988.

Lipshitz, Susan. 'The Personal is Political: the Problem of Feminist Therapy', *M/F* 2, 1978, p. 22.

London Women and Mental Health Group. *Women's Health and Mental Illness*. Broadsheet about the politics of mental illness in relation to women. Women's Health Information Centre, 1985 (available from WHRRIC).

MacNeill, Pearlie et al. (eds). *Through the Break – Women in Personal Struggle*. London: Sheba, 1986. Contains chapters by many black and/or working-class women.

*****Mallon**, Brenda. *Women Dreaming*. London: Fontana, 1987.

Mitchell, Juliet. *Psychoanalysis and Feminism*. London: Penguin Books, 1974.

*****Nairne**, Kathy and Gerrilyn **Smith**. *Dealing with Depression*. London: Women's Press, 1984.

Norwood, Robin. *Women Who Love Too Much*. London: Arrow, 1986.

Oakley, Ann. *Housewife*. London: Allen Lane, 1974.

Oakley, Ann. 'The Family, Marriage and its Relationship to Illness', in D. **Tuckett** (ed.), *An Introduction to Medical Sociology*. London: Tavistock, 1976.

Penfold, Susan and Gillian **Walker**. *Women and the Psychiatric Paradox*. Oxford: Oxford University Press, 1985.

Plath, Sylvia. *The Bell Jar*. London: Faber & Faber, 1963. A novel.

Repetti, Ren L. and Faye **Crosby**. 'Gender and Depression: Exploring the Adult-Role Explanation', *Journal of Social and Clinical Psychology*, vol. 2, no. 1, 1984, p. 57.

Robbins, Joan and Rachel **Siegel**. *Women Changing Therapy*. New York: Haworth Press, 1983. Contains many thoughtful chapters, including chapters by and about black women.

Rowbotham, Sheila. *Woman's Consciousness, Man's World*. London: Penguin Books, 1973.

*Rush, Ann Kent. *Getting Clear: Body Work for Women*. London: Wildwood House, 1974.

Scott, Sara and Tracy Payne. 'Underneath We're all Lovable', *Trouble and Strife – a Radical Feminist Magazine*, no. 3, Summer 1984. An article critical of therapy for women.

Smith, Dorothy E. and Sara J. David. *Women Look at Psychiatry*. Vancouver: Press Gang Publishers, 1975.

Strouse, Jean (ed.). *Women and Analysis – Dialogues on Psychoanalytic Views of Femininity*. New York: Dell, 1974.

Whyte, Judith. *Beyond the Wendy House: Sex Role Stereotyping in Primary Schools*. London: Longman, 1983.

Women in MIND. *Finding Our Own Solutions – Women's Experience of Mental Health Care*. MIND, 1986.

Women in MIND Directory./MIND, 1989.

PERIODICALS

Asylum – a Magazine for Democratic Psychiatry. 'Offers the freest possible non-partisan forum for debate for anyone in any way involved in mental health matters.' Available on subscription from Prof. F. A. Jenner, Royal Hallamshire Hospital, Sheffield S10 2JF. Free to inmates.

Changes. Psychology and psychotherapy journal available on subscription. Though written for professionals, contains many valuable articles, e.g. Gill Edwards, 'Helping and Hindering', in vol. 3, no. 1, 1984. Available from Ms Rohays Perry, Lawrence Erlbaum, 116 Pentonville Road, London N1 9JB.

Open Mind (formerly Mind Out). Magazine of MIND and available from them (see below).

Self and Society – European Journal of Humanistic Psychology. Available on subscription from 62 Southwark Bridge Road, London SE1 0AS. Tel: 01-928 8253/4.

ORGANIZATIONS

Action on Phobias, 8/9 The Avenue, Eastbourne, Sussex BN21 3YA. Self-help groups in many parts of UK.

Arbours Association (see text), 41a Weston Park, London N8. Tel: 01-340 7646. Provides short-term crisis accommodation and long-term supportive accommodation.

Association for Analytic and BodyMind Therapy and Training, 8 Princes Avenue, Muswell Hill, London N10 3LR. Tel: 01-883 5418. Clinic specializing in anxiety, depression, psychosomatic and relationship problems. Group therapy and hypnotherapy available.

Association of Humanistic Psychology, 62 Southwark Bridge Road, London SE1. Tel: 01-928 8253.

Association of Humanistic Psychology Practitioners, c/o Judith Dell, 45 Lichfield Way, London NW11 6NU. Tel: 01-455 8737. Has statement of standards and ethics, and provides information and referral service.

Brent Irish Mental Health Group, 76 Salisbury Road, London NW6 6NY.

British Association for Counselling, 37a Sheep Street, Rugby, Warwickshire CV21 3BX. Tel: 0788-78328/9. Has statement of standards and ethics and a referral directory. Also publishes newsletter, information sheets, e.g. 'What is Counselling', and other publications.

The British Network for Alternatives to Psychiatry, 158 Rivermead Court, Hurlingham, London SW6.

Campaign Against Psychiatric Oppression (CAPO), c/o Frank Bangay, 28a Edgar House, Kingsmead Estate, Homerton Road, London E9.

Co-counselling (see text). For 'Co-counselling International', contact Jean Trewick, Westerly, Prestwick Lane, Chiddingfold, Surrey GU8 4XW. Tel: 042-879 2882. For 'Re-evaluation Co-counselling' write to Sue Edwards, 7 Kemble Road, London SE23 1DH, putting your address on the back, so your letter can be forwarded unopened to your nearest contact.

Fellowship of Depressives Anonymous, 36 Chestnut Avenue, Beverley, N. Humberside, HU17 9QU. Tel: 0482-860619. 'A national association of people with personal experience of depression, who believe that by joining together they can help themselves and others.' Has some local groups, publishes newsletter and runs a pen-friend scheme.

Good Practices in Mental Health, 67 Kentish Town Road, London NW1. Aims to promote good practices in the NHS and health services.

Institute of Psychosynthesis, 310 Finchley Road, London NW3 7AG. Tel: 01-486 2588. Runs counselling service for individuals, couples or groups, plus offers weekend courses and professional training in their version of transpersonal psychology (see text).

Institute for Self Analysis, 12 Nassington Road, London NW3. Tel: 01-794 4306.

Irish Mental Health Forum, c/o Camden IBRG, 112 Camden High Street, London NW1 0LU.

Mental After Care Association, Bainbridge House, Bainbridge Street, London WC1A 1HP. Tel: 01-436 6194. Provides accommodation for people recovering from mental illness, through statutory agencies.

Mental Health Review Tribunals (look up the address in the phone book and write to the one nearest the hospital).

Hepburn House, Marsham Street, London SW1P 4HW. Tel: 01-211 7325;

2nd Floor, New Crown Buildings, Cathays Park, Cardiff CF1 3NQ. Tel: 0222-825111;

Cressington House, 249 St Mary's Road, Garston, Liverpool L19 0PZ. Tel: 051-494 0095.

Government Buildings, Spur A, Block 5, Chalfont Drive, Western Boulevard, Nottingham NG8 3RZ. Tel: 0602-294222.

Mental Welfare Commission for Scotland, 22 Drumsbeugh Gardens, Edinburgh EH3 7RB. Tel: 031-225 7034.

MIND – *National Association for Mental Health*, 22 Harley Street, London W1N 2ED. Tel: 01-637 0741. Acts as a pressure group, provides an advice service, publishes a magazine, and has a number of local associations throughout England and Wales. Leaflets range from *Bereavement – What to Expect and How to be Helpful* to ECT and information about the rights of mental health service consumers. Local associations vary in what they do. Some have set up mental health projects, self-help groups or counselling services, others do educational and campaigning work. MIND has recently set up a new policy group on women.

National Association of Young People's Counselling and Advisory Services, National Youth Bureau, 17–23 Albion Street, Leicester LE1 6GD. Tel: 0533-558763. Produces referral directory.

National Schizophrenia Fellowship, 78–9 Victoria Road, Surbiton, Surrey KT6 4NS. Tel: 01-390 3651/2/3. Organization mainly for carers. Runs groups and national advisory service. Disease-orientated.

Northern Ireland Association for Mental Health, Beacon House, University Street, Belfast BT7 1HE. Tel: 0232-228474.

Nurses Association for Psychodynamic Psychotherapy, c/o Harry Wright, Gwinllan, Y Maes, Rhayader, Powys LD6 5DE. Tel: 0597-2951 (messages).

Open Door, 447 Pensby Road, Heswell, Merseyside LG1 9PQ. Information service for people with phobias. Send sae for information.

Pellin Training Courses for Men and Women (see text), 15 Killyon Road, London SW8 2XS. Tel: 01-720 4499.

Phobic Trust, 25a The Grove, Coulsdon, Surrey CR3 2BH. Tel: 01-660 0332.

*Phobics Society, 4 Cheltenham Road, Chorlton cum Hardy, Manchester M21 1QN. Tel: 061-881 1937.

Psychiatric Rehabilitation Association, 21a Kingsland High Street, London E8 2JS. Tel: 01-254 9753. Aims to help prepare people for leaving psychiatric wards, and afterwards.

Relate: National Marriage Guidance, Herbert Gray College, Little Church Street, Rugby CV21 3AP. Tel: 0788-73241. Or see telephone directory under Relate or Marriage Guidance for local branch (see text).

Richmond Fellowship, 8 Addison Road, London W14 8DL. Tel: 01-603 6373. Runs houses for ex-psychiatric patients and others in need of help with transition back to 'normal' life. Some houses might have a more feminist perspective than others. Also runs training courses.

Samaritans, 17 Uxbridge Road, Slough, Berkshire SL1 1SN (see telephone directory for local branch).

Sanity, c/o Chairman, Mrs Margery Hall, Robina, The Chase, Ashley, near Ringwood, Dorset BH24 2AN. Funds research into nutritional and biochemical factors in mental illness. Send sae for information. Local groups: Mrs Shirley Ward, 132 Langley Hall Road, Olton, Solihull, West Midlands B92 7HD. Tel: 021-076 8046; Mrs Dora Whitlock, 1 Belgrave

Avenue, Penwortham, Preston, Lancashire PR1 6BH. Tel: 0772–744500.

Schizophrenia Association of Great Britain, International Schizophrenia Centre, Bryn Hyfryd, The Crescent, Bangor, Gwynedd LLS7 2AG. Tel: 0248–354048.

Scottish Association for Counselling, Queen Margaret College, 36 Clarewood Terrace, Edinburgh EH12 8TZ. Tel: 031–339 8111 (Tuesdays and Thursday mornings only).

Scottish Association for Mental Health, 40 Shandwick Place, Edinburgh EH2 4RT. Tel: 031–225 4446.

*Survivors Speak Out, c/o Lorraine Bell, 8 Nile Road, Southampton SO2 1PF. A coalition of people from many different mental health service 'consumer' groups.

ORGANIZATIONS SPECIFICALLY FOR WOMEN

Note: At the time of going to press there are still no women-orientated centres where we can go in a crisis. But by the time you read this, we hope this situation may have begun to change.

Birmingham Women's Counselling and Therapy Centre, Coordinator: Margaret Meredith, 43 Ladywood, Middleway, Birmingham B16 H8A. Tel: 021–455 8677.

Bristol Crisis Service for Women, c/o Bristol Women's Centre, 44 The Grove, Bristol 1. Tel: 0272–293575/522248.

Bristol. Womankind – a Women and Mental Health Self Help Project, Bristol Settlement, 43 Ducie Road, Barton Hill, Bristol BS5 0AX. Tel: 0272–556164.

Leeds Women's Counselling and Therapy Service, Oxford Chambers, Oxford Place, Leeds LS1 3AX. Tel: 0532–455725.

London. Camden Women with Disabilities Telephone Contact. Coordinator: Rhaune O'Brien. Tel: 01–722 3982.

London. Islington Women and Mental Health, Caxton House, 129 St John's Way, London N19. Tel: 01–281 2673.

London. Pellin Feminist Therapy Centre, 43 Killyon Road, London SW8 2XS. Tel: 01–622 0148 (answering machine). See also Pellin Training Courses above.

London Women and Mental Health, Caxton House, 129 St John's Way, London N19. Tel: 01–281 2673. Discussion group; also produces a newsletter.

London. Women's Action for Mental Health, 131 Bloemfontein Road, London W12. Tel: 01–749 9446.

London. Women's Therapy Centre, 6 Manor Gardens, London N7 6LA. Tel: 01–263 6200.

Oxford. Women's Counselling Centre, 9 Hayward Road, Oxford OX2 8LN. Tel: 0865–58068.

Redwood Women's Training Association, Invergarry, Kitlings Lane, Walton-on-the-Hill, Stafford ST17 0LE. Tel: 0785–662823. Runs courses on assertiveness and sexuality, as do most of the organizations listed in this section.

Southampton Counselling and Therapy Service (CATS), c/o Well Women Centre, Mayfield Road, Southampton SO2 3SW. Tel: 0703–557578. Mondays 6–8 p.m., Tuesdays 1–3 p.m.

In addition, MIND has a Women and Mental Health Group.

ORGANIZATIONS SPECIFICALLY FOR BLACK PEOPLE

Afro-Caribbean Mental Health Association, 35–37 Electric Avenue, London SW2. Tel: 01–737 3603.

Asha – Asian Women's Resource Centre, 279 Santley Street, London SW4 7QF. Tel: 01–274 8854/737 5901.

Association of Black Counsellors, Ms E. Gentle, Secretary, 4 Alexander Avenue, Sutton, Surrey SH1 2NZ. Tel: 01–644 5479.

Birmingham Asian Women's Project, Community Psychiatric Nursing Department, Highcroft Hospital, Eddington, Birmingham 23. Tel: 021–378 2211, × 4129.

Black and Ethnic Minority Mental Health Development Team, East MIND Office, 4th Floor 24/32 Stephenson Way, London NW1 2HD. Tel: 01–387 9070.

Black Health Workers and Patients Group, Annexe B, Tottenham Town Hall, 259a High Road, London N15. Tel: 01–809 0774.

Black Women and Mental Health Group, c/o Peckham Black Women's Group, St Giles Parish Hall, Benhill Road, London SE5.

Brent Black Mental Health Project, c/o Clare Lancaster, 25 High Street, Harlesden, London NW10 4NE. Tel: 01–965 0524.

Caribbean House Group, Caribbean House, 75–8 Bridport Place, London N1. Tel: 01–729 0988.

Fanon Project, 33 Effra Road, London SW2 1BZ. Tel: 01–737 2888.

Haringey Greek Cypriot Women's Health Group, Cypriot Community Centre, Earlham Grove, Wood Green, London N22. Tel: 01–881 2329.

London Black Women's Health Action Project, Wickham House, 10 Cleveland Way, London E1 4TZ. Tel: 01–790 2424.

Nafsiyat, Inter-Cultural Therapy Centre, 278 Seven Sisters Road, Finsbury Park, London N4 2HY. Tel: 01–263 4130.

Woolwich Simba Project, 48–50 Artillery Place, London SE18. Tel: 01–317 0451.

In addition, many of the women-orientated organizations listed above are becoming more sensitive to black and ethnic minority issues and some are not necessarily white-dominated.

CHAPTER

9

OCCUPATIONAL AND ENVIRONMENTAL HEALTH

Rewritten by
ANGELA PHILLIPS

ENVIRONMENTAL HEALTH*

The environment affects our health in ways which are not always obvious. High percentages of all cancers and of lung, heart, nerve and kidney diseases, as well as birth defects and behavioural disorders, are now thought to be caused by our environment (including our diet and living habits).

While toxic chemicals and radioactive substances add to the risks of living in the twentieth century for the majority of us, unfit housing and the effects of unemployment are a more immediate source of ill health and, like most causes of ill health, they are heavily class biased.

> The lack of insulation means that no matter how much heat you pump into the flats you can neither keep them warm nor dry – you know your children wake up crying from the cold even though you keep a heater on overnight in their bedroom and then you've got the worry of those enormously high electricity bills.[1]

A government report published in September 1984, showed that unemployment among men increases the death-rate for them, and their wives, by 20 per cent.[2] According to the 1980 Black Report, 'Inequalities in Health' (which was commissioned by a Labour government and then suppressed by a Conservative one):†

> We have shown that the inequalities in health tend to arise from the cumulative deprivation of a life-time. The length as well as the fact of exposure to bad housing, poor working and environmental condi-

tions, activities inimical to health (like smoking) and low income will be associated with the incidence and severity of chronic ill-health and disability as well as premature death.[3]

HOUSING

According to the national Anti-dampness Campaign, there are 6 million damp homes, many of them system-built during the last twenty years using untried methods and inadequate materials. The government's own statistics, which do not include these newer homes suffering from condensation, record that over a million occupied dwellings are 'unfit for human habitation'.[4]

In a survey of the system-built 'Baloon Wood' flats in Nottingham, three-quarters were found to be damp and two out of every five tenants complained of ill health including chest trouble, continual colds and depression. The death-rate for babies was one-third higher on this estate than the Nottingham average.

It is not only dampness which makes housing conditions a leading cause of ill health. The accident rate among children in high-rise flats is significantly higher than among other children; isolation, which is endemic among high-rise dwellers, contributes to depression; and over-crowding (an almost entirely class-based problem) is known to be a major contributor to childhood respiratory disease which, as the Black Report points out: 'if inadequately treated can lead to disability at age 15. Sometimes due to permanent damage caused to the respiratory tract.'

While working-class people, black and white, share these problems there is evidence to show that black people suffer disproportionately. An investigation by the Council for Racial Equality into housing policy in Hackney, east London, discovered that institutionalized racism caused systematic discrimination against ethnic minorities in the allocation of housing.

Over the last few years tenants' action groups have brought these problems to public attention. Most of these groups draw their main support and most active

---

*With special thanks to Claire Holman, who provided much of the information in this section.
†This is now published together with 'The Health Divide' under the title *Inequalities in Health*; see Townsend et al. in Resources.

THE HEALTH EFFECT OF ENVIRONMENTAL HAZARDS

To understand environmental health, we must understand that *everything* is connected – our body systems and organs, our life habits, our work and our wider environment. Environmental hazards can attack a particular organ or body system, directly damaging it and/or leading to further complications. While scientists generally test substances in labs one at a time, in real life our bodies always deal with more than one hazard at once. The combined interaction of two or more hazards to produce an effect greater than that of either one alone is called *synergism*. The amount of exposure, route of exposure and the toxic substance(s) we are exposed to determine whether we will feel acute or chronic effects.

An *acute effect* is a severe immediate reaction, usually after a single, large exposure – like the nausea and dizziness of pesticide poisoning or the pulmonary oedema (a blistering of the air sacs in the lungs) from the burns of toxic gases like ammonia or chlorine. A *chronic effect* is a recurrent or constant reaction usually after repeated smaller exposures. Chronic effects can take years – the *latency period*– to develop. For instance, exposure to asbestos causes lung disease years later, and most cancers and progressive liver diseases develop only after fifteen to forty years. Many scientists think we will see more and more problems as the toxins introduced after the Second World War 'come of age'.

We can absorb toxic substances in three ways: through the skin, through the digestive system (eating or drinking) or through the lungs. Often, toxins cause damage on first contact – burns, rashes, stomach pain, for example. Once in the bloodstream, they can damage many internal organs and systems.

In general, toxins affect women and men in the same ways: anyone can have an allergic reaction or liver damage, chronic headaches or respiratory problems, mental retardation or lung cancer. Environmental hazards put extra stress on our bodies and compound any other health problems that we might have.

ENVIRONMENTAL HEALTH TERMS

Carcinogen (car-*sin*-o-jen)
A substance or agent that causes cancer, a condition characterized by usually rapidly spreading abnormal cell growth.

Mutagen (*mew*-ta-jen)
A substance or agent that causes changes (mutations) in the genetic material of living cells. When a mutation occurs in the egg or sperm (germ cells), it can be passed on to future generations. Recent research suggests that since genetic material controls the growth of cells, mutagens may either immediately or after a latency period cause abnormal cell growth, which becomes cancer.

Teratogen (teh-*ra*-to-jen)
A substance or agent that can cause a spontaneous abortion or birth defects and developmental abnormalities in the fetus.

---

campaigners from among the working-class women who have to contend daily with the cold, the damp and the bills. With support from the nationally-based organizations such as SCAT (Services to Community Action and Trade Unions) these groups have often won significant concessions from local councils such as rate reductions or special heating subsidies; removal and replacement of an entire electrically-powered heating system; and in Newcastle, for example, whole blocks of system-built flats have been demolished to make way for healthier accommodation. More recently, concern about the health effects of asbestos used in building construction has added another dimension to these campaigns.

The quality of housing is yearly undermined by lack of spending on repairs, and privatization of council housing will reap a bitter harvest of decay in years to come. But spending cuts have bitten even deeper into our environment.

EXPENDITURE CUTS

Chronic under-spending by government on the infrastructure of our cities is in itself becoming a health hazard. Women on an estate in Bootle, Merseyside, became suspicious about high levels of gastroenteritis and diarrhoea. They formed an action group and commissioned a full survey which revealed extensive problems of sewage flooding. In fact, the incidence of dysentery (an epidemic disease associated with water pollution) is rising dramatically. In Hull, between 1982 and 1983 860 cases were confirmed, 38 per cent among the under-fives.

Indirectly, cuts in nursery provision, day-centres, old people's homes and the complicated web of the welfare state leave women ever more vulnerable to the cycle of isolation, overwork, stress and depression as we individually shoulder the load of caring.

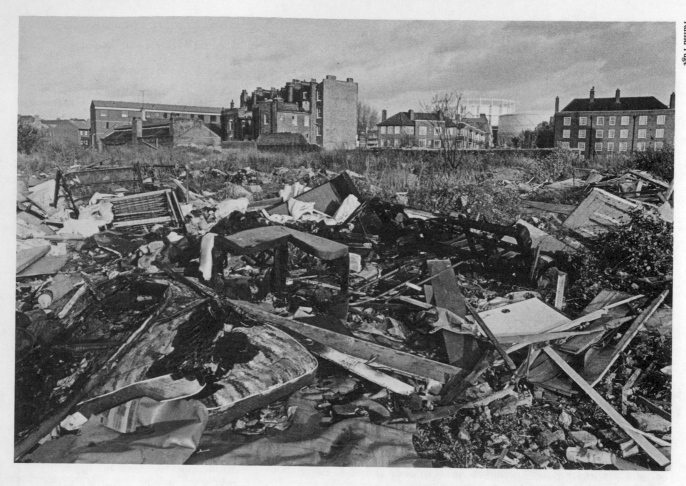

Raissa Page

CHEMICALS

There are between 50,000 and 75,000 chemical substances in common commercial use. About 1,000 new chemicals appear each year in the USA. The vast majority have not been tested for their potential ill-effects and industry spills them into our water, food, air, clothing, homes and workplaces every day.

Pesticides are one of the most common toxic substances in regular use. According to a report from the London Food Commission, of the 426 pesticides and rodenticides cleared for use in 1985, forty-nine are linked with cancer, thirty-one with birth defects and sixty-one with genetic mutation.[5] The report states that 30 per cent of foods sampled had detectable pesticide residues. The Commission is highly critical of the standard of surveillance of pesticide residues in food. Friends of the Earth (FOE) comment:

All too often it is not safe to walk in the countryside, even along public footpaths, nor sometimes venture into your own back garden, nor may it be advisable to take a deep breath of country air, in case it contains pesticides.[6]

The Transport and General Workers Union has been campaigning for several years against the use of pesticides containing 2,4,5-T which is contaminated by dioxin (a lethal chemical which poisoned thousands of people living near an Italian factory in Seveso after a chemical explosion in 1976 and is linked with miscarriages and birth defects). Yet traces of this deadly substance are still sprayed in parks and gardens, in forests and fields. The T&G along with FOE and other groups have succeeded in restricting its use by many local authorities. But there is still no total ban. Nor is 2,4,5-T the only suspicious pesticide, nor are agricultural workers the only people at risk.

I took my cat to the vet for tapeworm which I wanted treated before my baby was born. He told me also to treat it for fleas and gave me an aerosol containing dichlovos. I looked it up and found that it is classified as 'highly hazardous', acutely toxic and possibly teratogenic by the World Health Organization. American researchers suggest that it should be 'handled with caution by women of childbearing age'. I was clearly pregnant but I wasn't even warned.

Pesticides can also be found in new carpets. Used in a wood preservative they are a serious hazard to babies and young children who should never be allowed into an enclosed space while these products are being applied. Many household cleaners give off toxic fumes and dust. Even foam used in insulation and gas used for cooking can give off fumes which may cause headaches and impair mental abilities.

CHEMICALS WHICH PROTECT PROPERTY BUT MAKE HUMANS ILL[7]

All the chemicals used in timber treatment are chosen to be toxic and 'persistent'. They cannot be harmless to humans at the same time. Many can poison through the skin as well as through the lungs and digestive system. People can become ill after handling treated timber, or by breathing spray mist, vapour, contaminated dust or sawdust, or by eating food that has been in contact with wood preservatives.

Several of the most commonly used chemicals cause cancer, allergy, nerve damage or birth defects. Some have killed. Effects may take some time to develop and as they are not always obvious, sufferers and doctors may not relate them to chemical exposure.

Victims include workers in pre-treatment plants, remedial work and building, people whose homes and workplaces have been treated and children exposed at their schools. Hundreds of cases have come to light since the London Hazards Centre began to publicize the issue. They include a child who has contracted aplastic anaemia and is not allowed to live in his own home; two adults who have contracted epilepsy and several who now have cancer and other serious illnesses.

As the dangers of traditional poisons become clearer the industry uses chemicals more recently developed whose effects are even less known. Among the treatments that seem the least hazardous are those accepted by the Nature Conservancy Council for use on bat roosts; for example, Permethrin, an insecticide that belongs to the synthetic pyrethroid family (all ending '-thrin') and boron compounds (e.g. borax). However, even these chemicals can be hazardous and should be used with great care.

ACTION

Use chemicals only as a last resort:
- Damaged wood can be replaced and preventing damp conditions stops wet rot. Woodworm may be long gone. New wood, properly installed, only needs treatment in exposed locations (e.g. roof battens). Woodworm rarely attacks planed, painted and varnished wood. Dry rot is more serious: ask a competent surveyor or builder.

If chemicals must be used:
- Only do small outdoor jobs yourself; wear protective clothing.

- Before contracting work check that the company is registered with a trade association – British Wood Preserving Association or Nationwide Association of Preserving Specialists.
- Get an exact written specification of the work to be done, the reasons for it, the methods and chemicals (full names and safety data sheets).
- Only allow the least hazardous chemicals in water-based formulations to be used by drill-and-plug, paste or brushing.
- Don't treat unaffected areas.
- Don't use dual purpose chemicals if there is only one kind of attack.
- Keep away from treated areas for as long as possible. The standard forty-eight hours is too short. PCP and dieldrin can stay at dangerous levels for years, and lindane for weeks. The period for new chemicals is not known.
- Ensure that treated areas are well ventilated.

If you are exposed to wood preservatives at work:
- The best safeguards against hazards of timber treatment chemicals have been won where workers have organized in trade unions, such as UCATT.
- Use your health and safety representatives to get the relevant information such as manufacturer's data sheets, work system specifications etc., to which they are entitled under the *Health and Safety at Work Act* and the *Regulations on Safety Representatives and Safety Committees*.
- Ensure your employer is meeting duties to provide safe systems of work, supervision, training, and protective equipment.
- Report any incidents, accidents, or work-related illness.
- Call the Health and Safety Executive (HSE), or local authority Environmental Health Department, to get the law enforced.

If you are exposed to an already treated structure:
- Find out when it was treated so you can assess the hazard.
- Ventilate well especially if there is a smell.
- Seal treated wood and masonry to avoid touching and breathing the chemicals. Ordinary decorating sealants and paints can reduce the risk.

With thanks to the London Hazards Centre.

It is hard to measure the overall effects of chemicals in general use. However, even the snow in Antarctica carries residues of polychlorinated biphenyls (PCBs), DDT and lead. Accidental spillage or explosions can cause irreversible damage on a vast scale as we have been warned by the tragedies of Seveso and Minamata (where mercury poisoning caused hundreds of deaths and an epidemic of fetal damage) and Bhopal (where over 2,000 people were killed and thousands more maimed by a gas explosion at a Union Carbide plant).

If we think it cannot happen here we need only look to the poisoning of the river Dee in 1984 when water contaminated with phenol was pumped into millions of homes. Over 40 per cent of those drinking the water suffered from effects including vomiting, diarrhoea and headaches. Although 2 million people were involved it took the water authorities five days to inform local health officials of the contamination. Accidental pollution does not always come to public notice as water authorities in Britain usually meet in secret and do not have to reveal details of their proceedings to the public.* However, local groups can monitor water independently. Tower Hamlets Tenants' Federation and Tower Hamlets Health Campaign won an important victory when they sent samples of local water to the European Commission in April 1986. High nitrate levels were confirmed and the EEC started proceedings against the UK for failing to comply with the directive on drinking water standards. Since then, Thames Water Authority has been forced to take action on lower nitrate levels. The campaign will continue to monitor their water independently.

LEAD

The effects of lead poisoning have been common knowledge for very many years. Plumbism, as it used to be called, is known to contribute to miscarriage and birth defect rates and to affect the IQ of children at a level far below that which causes symptoms of lead poisoning in adults. As a result of this knowledge, lead in the working environment is controlled, although there is some concern that the permitted levels are too high, particularly for men whose contribution to childbearing (and vulnerability to sperm damage) is not legally recognized. However, lead is by no means confined to the working environment. Its use in petrol, paint and even in pipes carrying the domestic water supply is acknowledged to cause levels too high for the safety of children. Sir Henry Yellowlees, the then Chief Medical Officer at the DHSS had this to say in 1981:

> There is a strong likelihood that lead in petrol is permanently reducing the IQ of many of our children. Although the reduction amounts to only a few percentage points, some hundreds of thousands of

children are affected and, as Chief Medical Officer, I have advised the Secretary of State that action should be taken to reduce markedly the lead content of petrol in use in the United Kingdom.[8]

Lead-free petrol has now been introduced, but we are still waiting for the government to set a date by which all new cars should be manufactured to run on it. Until then, as lead from petrol is poured on to the soil and liberally sprinkled on vegetation, any question of cultivating fresh vegetables in the inner cities must be considered potentially hazardous to health. After a sustained campaign by the Campaign for Lead-free Air (CLEAR), new controls are to be brought in lowering the levels of lead in paint to the US standard level. Yet, according to a report from the Royal Commission on Environmental Pollution, 45 per cent of British households drink water that has passed through lead pipes. Many people are taking in six times the EEC recommended maximum from their water supply.

RADIATION

The threat of radiation is probably the greatest hazard we face. Even supposedly safe nuclear plants yield a regular supply of accident, near-miss and low-level contamination stories. After the disaster at Chernobyl in the USSR (in 1986) no one can again be complacent about the safety of harnessing nuclear energy to peaceful uses, and the possibility of nuclear war continues to loom (see p. 183 for more on the peace campaigns).

Available evidence suggests that low-level radiation from the nuclear industry, and in particular nuclear fuel reprocessing plants, contaminates our environment and our bodies in slow stages. Radioactive waste which is currently spilled into the sea is now known to be washed back on to beaches creating radiation 'hot spots'. Nobody really knows how such hot spots will affect people; however, independent researchers have been able to pinpoint clusters of childhood cancers around nuclear plants. The Yorkshire TV programme on nuclear reprocessing at Sellafield ('Windscale, the Nuclear Laundry', November 1983) discovered a ten-fold increase in childhood cancers in the area.

> No one with children is using the beaches any more, and I can't see a time when people will feel that it is safe to return.

Official sources deny the existence of cancer clusters. However, the dearth of published research material on the issue is a source of suspicion in itself. According to the *Guardian*'s science correspondent Anthony Tucker:

> Systematic censorship operated by government departments in conjunction with industry, has already corrupted British science to unprecedented levels and is specially active in such 'sensitive' areas as industrial pollution and environmental radiation.[9]

---

*The privatization of the water industry is unlikely to improve the situation though more stringent regulations are to be built in to privatization plans. However, it remains to be seen whether or not performance will be adequately monitored.

REPRODUCTIVE HEALTH HAZARDS

A reproductive hazard is any agent that has harmful effects on the male or female reproductive system and/or the development of a fetus. These hazards can be chemicals (like pesticides), physical agents (like X-rays) or work practices (like heavy lifting).

Reproductive health hazards are probably the most controversial issues in environmental health. Because women bear children, reproductive hazards are too often considered 'a woman's problem' involving pregnancy alone. This view ignores two important facts: that men are also affected by reproductive hazards, and that reproductive health means more than having healthy babies. All through life, men and women need healthy sexual and reproductive systems. As it is, reproductive hazards are often used as excuses to penalize women workers and permit management to avoid cleaning up the workplace.

Infertility in either sex, a spontaneous abortion early in pregnancy or a baby with birth defects can all be early signs of a toxic environment. These can be important signals that something is wrong, since other signs like cancer can take a fifteen- to forty-year latency period to develop.

HOW REPRODUCTIVE HAZARDS AFFECT MEN

A recent US government study found PCBs* in every human sperm sample tested.[11] Environmental toxics can disrupt the production of male hormones in the testes, causing loss of sex drive and impotence. They can also cause problems with sperm production. A toxic agent can disturb sperm cells at any one of several stages of rapid growth, causing problems with fertility through a total lack of sperm, low sperm production or malformed sperm. Toxins may be causing an overall decline in sperm counts.

In addition, some reproductive hazards are mutagens. When a mutation occurs in sperm cells, men can pass damaged genes on to future generations, which can result in spontaneous abortions or inherited birth defects.

- Men exposed to lead have decreased fertility and malformed sperm.[12]
- Higher rates of birth defects are showing up in the children of agricultural workers, possibly due to pesticide exposure.[13]
- DBCP (dibromochloropropane), a pesticide, was found to cause dramatically decreased sperm counts in men who work with it or in its manufacture. The men in one California factory noticed that none of them had fathered children since they started working there, and demanded fertility tests. Many were found to be sterile.[14]

HOW REPRODUCTIVE HAZARDS AFFECT WOMEN

When toxic substances disrupt the reproductive hormones, they can cause menstrual disorders, sterility or loss of sexual drive.[15] Toxic substances may also directly damage the ovaries, eventually resulting in early menopause or ovarian disease. And, as with sperm cells, environmental mutagens can damage the genetic material in a woman's eggs, with the same effects – spontaneous abortion or birth defects. Recent animal studies show ovary damage from polycyclic hydrocarbons (used in the petrochemical industry), alkylating agents (used in cancer treatment) and ionizing radiation. Exposure to lead, PCBs and vinyl chloride can cause menstrual changes.

THE DEVELOPING FETUS AND YOUNG CHILDREN

The fertilized egg and the fetus can react to toxins that do not apparently harm an adult.

Teratogens (see p. 147) are particularly dangerous during the first three months of pregnancy, so early that the woman may not be aware she is pregnant. During the first two weeks, the fertilized egg is so sensitive that an environmental hazard powerful enough to damage it will also destroy it. From the fifteenth to the sixtieth day of a pregnancy, the cells of the fetus multiply and differentiate into specific organs and systems. A toxin can disrupt this process, and there is no second chance for the system to establish itself. If the teratogen is very strong, the pregnancy often ends in a spontaneous abortion (miscarriage). If the fetus survives, the child may have a low birth weight or physical, developmental or behavioural defects, some of which may not show up until years later.

The most common way that a fetus is exposed to toxins in the environment or workplace is through the mother's direct exposure. However, since semen is one place where toxins accumulate, having intercourse during pregnancy may expose a fetus to concentrations of toxins that can cause birth defects.[16] (Men exposed to environmental hazards can use condoms or you could consider other ways of making love during pregnancy.)

The developing fetus and young children are particularly susceptible to environmental hazards because their cells are dividing and growing rapidly. Yet governments still set standards for 'safety' levels of toxins based on effects on adults.

Certain toxins concentrate in human breast milk, to be passed along to newborns. According to one study, 99 per cent of all American women have enough PCBs in their breast milk to show up in

continues over

tests.[17] (A study by the Environmental Defense Fund concluded that breastfeeding infants get almost a hundred times the amount of toxins ingested by adults in proportion to body weight.) Yet breastfeeding is so beneficial to babies that unless you live in an area where there's known excessive pollution, the benefits outweigh the risks.[18]

OTHER EFFECTS

Environmental mutagens also pose dangers for the entire human species. Damaged genetic material, whether it causes visible damage or not, contributes its permanent changes to the total human gene pool. A mutation rate increased by the effects of chemical and radioactive toxins could not only produce a general decline in human health, it could threaten human existence.

*Polychlorinated biphenyls, once widely used in adhesives, paints, lubricants, electric insulators and printing inks, can cause everything from skin discoloration to liver disorders to cancer.

We in Britain have very special cause for concern as our reactors emit the highest levels of radiation in the West and the level of radiation that our government considers safe for the general public (0.5 milliSieverts) is higher than that set in Germany and three times higher than the US limit. Even these levels are considered by some to be higher than they should be. This means that when, for example, Scottish cattle consumed grass affected by the radiation from Chernobyl, no official action was taken and no official advice was given out, although the detectable rise in the radiation level in milk was higher than that which would have been considered safe in other countries. Attempts to check radiation levels in children's thyroids were abandoned on the spurious grounds that parents would be alarmed.[10]

Waste from reactors remains radioactive for as long as 250 centuries and yet British companies, with government encouragement, are actually importing waste from other countries for reprocessing plants at Sellafield and now, it is planned, at Dounreay in Scotland. These reprocessing plants are capable of producing weapons-grade plutonium.

In spite of the worries about safety at Sellafield and the concern of the Norwegian government (just across the sea from Dounreay) the British government would not even allow a parliamentary debate about Dounreay on the grounds that it is a 'local' issue. One thing that we have learned from the Chernobyl accident is that no nuclear facility is a 'local' issue. Nuclear clouds do not respect national boundaries let alone local ones. Nor is it only an issue for today: we are lumbering our children and our children's children with an environmental problem which we have no means of controlling.

TACKLING ENVIRONMENTAL ISSUES

Environmental issues are community issues and it is through organized community action that they can best be tackled. We do not need to be 'experts'. Armed with the knowledge that our own health is important and supported by organizations locally and nationally, we can insist on our right to involvement in decisions which could affect the maintenance of a healthy environment.

Residents in Livingston, Scotland, have shown how potentially dangerous chemical processes can be curbed. Union Carbide, the company responsible for the Bhopal disaster, had just received outline planning permission to set up a factory locally when the Livingston Action Committee (LACE) was established. It has successfully called for a full programme of public consultation before planning permission could be confirmed.

We really have a right to know how much of the poisonous gas will be stored at the plant. We have a right to know how it will be transported to Livingston and we have a right to know what kind of safety measures the company will be taking. If we don't find out exactly what Union Carbide intends doing here, and force a process of consultation, then we will have betrayed the people of Bhopal. (Helen MacKenzie)

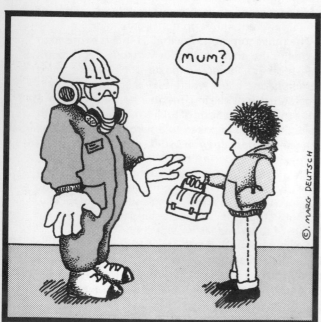

Marg Deutsch

In this country we have a great many obstacles to overcome, the greatest of which is a government mania for secrecy.

SECRECY

Government agencies which should be protecting our interests as citizens are restricted by laws aimed at protecting business interests. Even trade unionists who have a right to know what substances they are working with are prohibited by law from providing this information to people outside the workplace.

When chemicals are screened for use on the UK market (and not all are screened), the evidence on which decisions are taken remains secret. New regulations governing the use of pesticides are likely to include a public 'right to know clause' not because of any change in attitudes here but because most products are available in the USA where freedom of information legislation gives the public access to information banned in the UK. It would be inconsistent if campaigners in the UK could get information from the US which local officials were barred by law from revealing.

The Industrial Air Pollution Inspectorate has the job of inspecting and regulating the level of air pollution from certain 'registered works'. However, the inspectorate is prohibited from disclosing information on these discharges. In 1974 the Control of Pollution Act was passed, giving local authorities the right to disclose some information. However, they do not take advantage of it; for example, in 1981 only one piece of information was disclosed under the terms of this Act.

The Water Act recently introduced more secrecy by allowing water authorities to meet in private. All the water authorities have taken up this right to keep the public out and measures for greater public information about water pollution have been repeatedly delayed.

We do not even have the automatic right to know where the 2,000 sites handling dangerous chemicals in Britain are located. If local Livingston residents had not heard about Union Carbide's involvement in the Bhopal disaster, no questions would have been asked and no information given about the deadly poisons being used there. From 1989, companies operating the 200 most dangerous plants are required to inform local people of the hazards. The lists will not, however, be available nationally.

Campaigns for a Freedom of Information Act such as that in force in America have so far met with little interest from governments. Each party, when out of power, pretends to be the party for 'open government' and democracy. Once in power they usually allow the public's right to know to slip very far down the agenda while protecting the government's right to keep things from us.

OBSTRUCTION

According to the *Guardian* newspaper, local people trying to organize against the Dounreay reprocessing plant

. . . believe that their phones are tapped, say their jobs have been threatened unless they give up the campaign, and that people have been told they will lose their rights to a council house if they join.[19]

On a broader level, the government is able to control the flow of information in our supposedly free society by judicious use of its spending power. Anthony Tucker, writing in the *Guardian*, bitterly attacked the 'government asset-stripping' which by privatizing public research institutes makes them dependent on piecemeal grants and, therefore, more vulnerable to governmental displeasure than they ever were as state-funded institutions:

Scientists and research directors trapped in the censorship system are reluctant to discuss what is happening because they know that, if they blow the whistle on the departments [i.e. the Department of the Environment], then neither they nor their institutes are likely to get another penny of contract research money from the government.[20]

In 1988 the government announced plans to tighten up copyright provisions for research carried out by government-funded researchers. Researchers are now being prevented from publishing their findings without permission from their funders. The fear is that information which does not support government policy will be suppressed.

STRATEGIES

1. We can *talk to other people*. Parent-teacher associations at local schools, community and political groups, trades councils (where representatives of local trade unions meet), our community health council. All these provide opportunities to share information about local hazards and can form the basis of a group to fight them.

2. *Write letters* to local papers expressing concern about particular environmental issues. Many campaigns have been established this way.

3. *Inform ourselves*. National campaigning groups will provide background information and speakers (see Resources). Local information can be gathered through local surveys.

4. *Pressurize local councils* to make information about pollution publicly available under the terms of the Control of Pollution Act.

5. *Contact local doctors* who may be aware through their own day-to-day work of changing health problems. Enlist their help.

6. If specific problems are discovered, we can *contact MPs* and *lobby local councillors* to ensure that the issue is raised publicly.

7. We can *keep our MPs informed* about environmental issues and put pressure on them to support Bills for Freedom of Information in Britain.

WORK CAN BE HAZARDOUS TO OUR HEALTH

The work we do affects us not only while we are at our place of work but also at home, during holidays and for the rest of our lives. There were 468 deaths and 388,000 industrial accidents officially reported in Britain in 1982. However, much of the injury suffered by women at work goes unreported because most of us do not work in the recognized high-risk occupations such as mining, heavy industry and construction.

Many of the risks we face are not recognized as industrial injuries but seen as individual 'problems': back strain, debilitating pains in the hands and arms from repetition strain, headaches and dermatitis from chemicals. These are usually combined with the effects of sexism, which confines us to the lowest paid and most repetitive jobs, and ensures that we do two days' work in one (houseworker and employee); and, if we are mothers, we do most of the worrying about childcare arrangements too. For those of us who are black, there is the additional problem of racism. If we work alongside men (particularly in jobs previously considered male preserves), or if our jobs make us subordinate to male managers, we suffer the additional stress of sexual harassment (see p. 164) which is now recognized by many trade unions as a health hazard which should be dealt with by collective organization (see p. 167).

Working at home, paid or unpaid, can also be hazardous. Accidents in the home are very common. Those of us who are doing paid work at home suffer the combined risks of household accidents and the specific risks attached to the work we do. Chemicals, paints, solvents and solder give off fumes; fabrics give off fibres which can be inhaled; close work, for long hours with insufficient lighting causes eye-strain; and homeworkers, paid or unpaid, share the debilitating effects of isolation, exploitation and poverty.

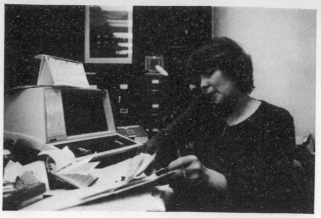

Ellen Shub

At home your work becomes your life, it takes over, nothing else is important. In my case it took up a great deal of room in the living-room. I couldn't put it anywhere else and even when I stopped working, which I rarely did, it was there defying me not to start again. All the paraphernalia attached to the job, the varnish and its smell, the glue that wouldn't wash out, the problem of having razor blades around, the dust from the cork butts and the metal filings from the rings were all extra problems. I scraped my knuckles so often with the file, smoothing the edges of often as many as 500 rings that even the prospect of having to do it brought me near to tears. The nylon thread had to be pulled very tight and cut my fingers – deep cuts which took ages to heal and often reopened. Force sprained my wrist turning a rod, but on I had to go. The close work in artificial light to make sure the intricate patterns of thread were accurate has damaged my already none too good eyesight. I seem to work all the hours god sent, from morning till late at night, often it's early hours, and sometimes through the night to meet deadlines. I worked when I was ill, I wasn't entitled to sick pay.[21]

The combination of these factors may lead to stress which in itself may cause physical problems. In the short term it can lead to a general lowering of resistance to infection, indigestion, muscle tension causing aches and pains and, in the long term, an increase in ulcers and heart disease (see Heart Disease, p. 559).

In the clothing factory where I work, a lot of us who've been sewing there for a while have been having pains in our hands or our legs. The union is collecting information to see if some jobs are worse than others (like hemming or making linings). We're hoping that we can find out whether there are any changes that would help, like changing the height of the tables or the angle of the machines. Anything that would make the job more comfortable would help my general level of tension! Between the noise from the steam pressers, working fast enough to make a good rate and bending over the machine all day without enough light, I'm lucky if I get out of there without my shoulders all bunched up and a splitting headache at the end of the day.

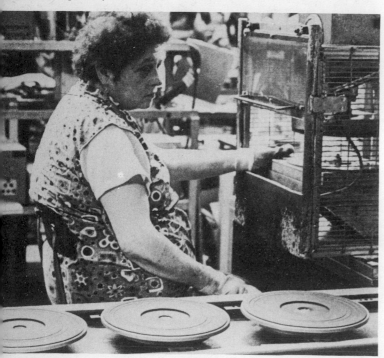

Angela Phillips

WHERE WOMEN WORK

Professional	1%
Teaching, medical and other	19%
Clerical	30%
Sales	9%
Skilled manual	7%
Semi-skilled (inc. domestic)	25%
Unskilled	9%

Women can rarely afford to take evasive action and leave a job when confronted with health hazards. Black women, who have to deal with racial harassment in addition to a much higher level of unemployment due to discrimination, are even more vulnerable. Women migrants, who work long hours for low pay in catering and cleaning, are particularly powerless because work permits depend on jobs. And it is a tragic irony that the new technologies which are causing anxiety about health hazards among women in Western industrialized countries have been built at the expense of the health of women in South-East Asia:

Young women are employed to test the silicon chips. Caustic chemicals, all poisonous and many suspected of causing cancer, sit in open containers giving off fumes. Eye ailments are another serious hazard. 'After a time we cannot see very clearly; it's blurred. We'll have to work with these gold wires, very thin like our hair.'[22]

ORGANIZING IN THE WORKPLACE

Women are responding through workplace organization. The level of female participation in trade unions, now around 41 per cent, has risen by over 25 per cent in the past ten years. Who controls the workplace is an important, if unstated, issue in workplace health and safety struggles. When workers become more knowledgeable about work practices and processes in order to make them safer, we are more likely to question other aspects of the relationship between workers and managements. Issues of work

organization have often been more potent in breaking down barriers between women workers than the traditional wage issues which have united men:

The heat continued, and the women complained of discomfort, headaches, tiredness, etc. . . . With the temperature at 92° F we stopped work. The non-members all joined the union. Emergency measures were agreed and the Maintenance and Minor Works committee met and agreed to find a permanent solution.[23]

The Health and Safety at Work Act gives workplace-elected health and safety representatives the right to represent union members on health and safety committees, and access to information about workplace hazards and safety. These representatives have the right to be consulted before any changes are made in working practices which could affect the health and safety of workers. The box on page 158 outlines the rights of safety reps.

Women who are not organized in trade unions (home-workers, sweatshop workers and large numbers of shop workers), will have more difficulty in organizing to protect themselves. However, by getting together, sharing information, contacting the appropriate union for your kind of work and approaching management as a group you should have more effect. If you are dismissed for protesting against unsafe working conditions you have the right to take an unfair dismissal case to an employment tribunal. (Contact a Citizens' Advice Bureau [CAB] for help if you are not in a union.)

RECOGNIZING HAZARDS IN THE WORKPLACE

Under the Health and Safety at Work Act, your trade-union representative or health and safety representative has

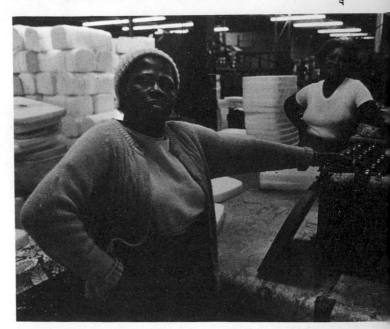

Earl Dotter

a legal right to see and read the safety data sheets which should accompany all new and existing chemical products listing the contents, effects and handling procedures necessary as well as other information on workplace hazards.

Unfortunately, managements may not be very well informed themselves about product safety. Research at Glasgow University draws attention to the fact that only 13 per cent of companies questioned regularly received manufacturers' data and less than half received information from the Health and Safety Executive (the government body dealing with safety at work), or from their employers' federation.[24]

Clearly, health and safety reps should be putting pressure on managements to improve the flow of information but, at the same time, they can pressurize their own unions to put more emphasis on health research and training courses for members so that they are not totally dependent on managements for information.

Hazards Bulletin, a bi-monthly publication produced by trade unionists at the British Society for Social Responsibility in Science (BSSRS; see p. 160) is a must for any safety representative. The *Office Workers Survival Handbook* by Marianne Craig (see Resources) is an excellent guide to identifying and dealing with many of the hazards faced by women workers.

While written information is a useful back-up, the most essential weapon is vigilance on the part of workers. Use your own eyes and ears to spot obvious hazards, and compare notes with colleagues to identify illnesses which stem from workplace organization and procedure. If you suspect that a new process is causing discomfort or disease, circulate a simple questionnaire to discover if the symptoms are widespread and can be traced to the process.

COMMON HAZARDS AND WHAT TO DO

- **Noise** may be responsible for stress, headaches and permanent hearing loss. Legal noise limits are equivalent to working within twenty yards of a pneumatic drill. Hearing damage may occur at one-tenth of this limit. Try to negotiate a 75-decibel limit. Most machines can be muffled. Agree to personal safety equipment only as a last resort.

- **Inadequate lighting** can cause eye-strain and headaches; good lighting is what is comfortable to work with. Special care should be taken to light areas where Visual Display Units (VDUs) are in use to minimize glare and reflections which contribute to eye-strain.

- **Seating** may be responsible for backaches or even permanent spinal deformities; you have a legal right to sit down at work and to an adjustable chair with a back support and adequate footrests. It must be suitable for you, and for the job you do.

- **Heating.** Overheating can cause a variety of problems such as dizziness, muscle cramps, weakness and sickness. Heating in an office cannot legally drop below 60° F but there is no upper limit (except in the pot-

teries). Under the Offices, Shops and Railway Premises Act you have a right to 'adequate ventilation' but this is not defined.

- **Ventilation** systems with humidifiers can pipe bacteria into offices causing 'flu' epidemics and even Legionnaire's Disease, which caused deaths at the BBC in London in 1988. Monitor for flu symptoms which start on Monday night and insist that ventilation systems are regularly cleaned and maintained.

- **Tools** designed for 'average' men are unsuitable for 'average' women who are smaller. Badly designed tools can increase the risk of accidents as well as adding to stress. Machinery should be designed for people. Workers should not be discriminated against on grounds of size.

- **Safety equipment and protective clothing** designed for men may be dangerously ill-fitting for women.

- **Lifting** heavy loads (such as patients in hospitals and laundry bundles) is a particular hazard for women because of our more flexible pelvic structure. Staffing levels should ensure that workers do not have to lift heavy loads without assistance. Wherever possible mechanical hoists should be introduced. The Factories Act lays down the maximum weight you can lift.

- **Dust** can cause permanent lung damage such as byssinosis (from cotton dust), silicosis (in the potteries), asbestosis and cancer (suffered by people working with asbestos). Dust levels should be controlled by extractors and ventilation. Only where this is impossible should safety equipment be introduced. Factory inspectors are empowered to check dust levels and enforce them; they can be contacted through your area health and safety executive.

- **Chemicals and fumes** are a hazard not only to the workers producing them but also to a growing section of the workforce who use them. Office workers can be affected by the ozone given off by photocopiers and the chemicals in correction fluids; cleaners cope with a variety of toxic and corrosive materials; nurses work with anti-cancer drugs which are highly toxic; hairdressers handle wet hair and chemicals which cause dermatitis; laundry workers breathe in solvent fumes. Exposure level guidelines have been laid down for some 500 substances but there are many thousands of others which we know little about. You have a right to information about chemical hazards (see p. 148). For more information see Resources.

- **Visual Display Units** can be a source of eye-strain, postural pains and stress, if the pace of work is dictated by the machine rather than the operator. Correct lighting, seating, and frequent rest breaks should be negotiated. Many unions have produced model health and safety claims for VDU operation.

- **Repetition** of tasks can cause Repetition Strain Injury (RSI). The commonest form is Tenosynovitis, a recognized industrial disease. Word-processing, egg packaging and textile work have all been known to cause RSI because of the long bouts of rapid, repeated movements. RSI can cause bad pain which does not stop when you stop work. It can only be treated by extended rest and often redesign of the job. When rapid repetition cannot be avoided, unions should be negotiating for frequent rest breaks to guard against strain.

- **Infection** is a particular risk for hospital workers and for anyone working in a close, caring role (such as nursery workers, care attendants). The health service unions have produced guidelines for dealing with particular virus infections (such as HIV and Hepatitis B). Safety standards for dealing with soiled linen need to be rigorously monitored. Staff cuts and privatization (with an inevitable drop in the level of union organization) militate against proper maintenance of safety standards.

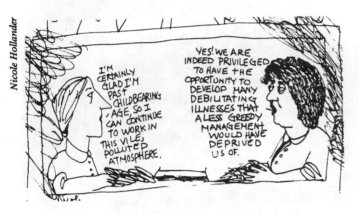

Aside from all these hazards, workers must be aware of possible accidents from untidy workplaces, unsafe electrical wiring, old and under-maintained equipment, unguarded or inadequately guarded machinery and a pace of work which is too fast to be compatible with safety. Piece-work and bonus payments are in themselves a major contributor to accidents because they put the onus for maximizing income on speed of work.

PROTECTIVE LEGISLATION

There used to be several separate laws designed to give protection to women workers and, in particular, pregnant women workers. Many of them have recently been repealed or amended. The 1975 Employment Protection Act, for example, gave most pregnant women the right to ask for a transfer to a safe area of work (without loss of employment rights). Since changes to the law in 1985 only 25–33 per cent of unskilled and semi-skilled women workers now qualify for job transfers. Specific laws regulating the working hours, night and shift work have gone. The only protective laws which remain set safety levels for working with lead and radiation, or substances harmful to fertility.

These protective laws can also be used against women. In one recent case a lorry driver who was banned from carrying loads containing the chemical DMF lost her claim of sex discrimination because, as a woman who could become pregnant, health and safety considerations in respect of any possible pregnancy were deemed to override the conditions of the Sex Discrimination Act.* Concern for male fertility has not led to a reduction in lead levels for male workers, in spite of growing international evidence that lead affects sperm.

The answer to protective legislation should not have been to level women down so that they can compete with men for more hazardous jobs. Legislation could have been extended to men to ensure that no workers are expected to work unsocial hours (unless the job has a real social value); be exposed to levels of toxins which may damage either developing sperm or a developing fetus; to supplement an inadequate basic wage with regular overtime; or lift loads beyond their physical capacity.

Your Legal Rights to a Safe Workplace

Under the 1974 Health and Safety at Work Act, employers have a duty to ensure, as far as is reasonably practicable, the health, safety and welfare of workers. If you are organized in a recognized trade union you also have the right to elect safety representatives and a health and safety committee. If you suspect that there are hazards where you work you can call in an inspector from the Health and Safety Executive, or a local authority environmental health inspector. Their job is to enforce the law but they are overworked and under pressure to persuade rather than enforce.

Cuts in government expenditure since 1980 have led to a massive 15 per cent staff cut for the H&SE, so they are even less able to monitor working conditions. Cuts are also affecting the university departments researching occupational health.

Compensation and Benefit

If you suffer from an injury at work or are suffering from one of a number of specified industrial injuries, then you may be able to claim industrial injuries benefit or disablement benefit. If you are not eligible for these you can claim statutory sickness benefit. You can also sue your employer for compensation for work-related injury or disease but you will need help and backing from your trade union, a CAB or a law centre.

WOMEN TAKING ACTION

The matchgirls are probably the most famous symbol of the industrial exploitation of women. Forced to work in appalling conditions, many suffered from 'phossy jaw' from handling phosphorus. In 1888 they struck and, backed by suffragist Annie Besant who whipped up unprecedented public support for their cause, won many of their demands. A few years later, the laundresses, backed by the Women's Trade Union League, started to campaign for hours of work legislation to cut their fourteen- to sixteen-hour day.

Women clerks and secretaries organized their own union in 1912 and campaigned alongside the male National

*Employment Tribunal: Ms J. D. Page v Freighthire (Tank Haulage) Ltd.

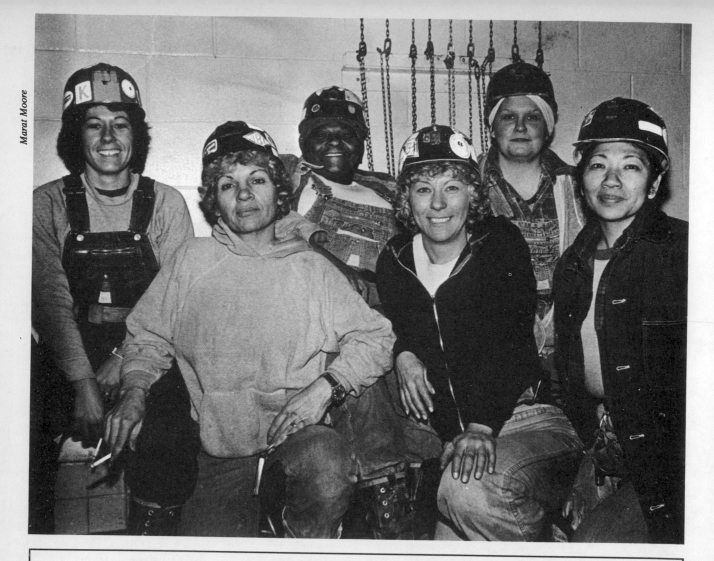

RIGHTS OF SAFETY REPRESENTATIVES[25]

1. You can investigate any complaints made by one or more of your members. This can mean going to her machine/part of the workplace and having a private conversation with her. Your employer must, by law, give you paid time off and any facilities you require to carry out this and other Safety Rep functions.

2. You can investigate a part of the workplace at your own initiative. In other words, if you have a feeling that something is going on there that may be hazardous to any of your members, you have the right to go and take a look.

3. You can investigate any accidents, 'near misses', or dangerous occurrences, whether or not any of your members have been hurt.

4. You can investigate the outbreak of any disease or other health problem that you feel may be caused by work, such as dermatitis, rashes, itching, headaches, dizziness, stomach aches, heart disease, cancer, etc.

5. You can investigate the workplace following any substantial change in working conditions, such as introduction of a new chemical, a new machine, or piece of equipment, a new method of working, an extension to the workplace, etc.

6. You have the right to be consulted *before* any of the above changes are brought about.

7. You have the right to any information relevant to health, safety or welfare from your employers, and from the manufacturers, suppliers, importers or distributors of any chemicals or equipment your members work with.

8. You have the right to inspect the workplace if any relevant new information is published by the Health and Safety Commission.

9. Your employer must make available detailed information on the hazards of any machinery, substances or processes you work with and the precautions to eliminate or minimize these dangers.

10. Your employer must provide information on any environmental hazards, including measurement of temperature, noise, dust, fumes, etc. taken at your workplace.

11. You have the right to call in the Factory Inspector, to be informed of any hazards they discover, results of any measurements they take, and what they have asked management to do.

12. You have a right to 'stop the job' if hazards are evident.

13. You are entitled to time off *with pay* to train as a Safety Rep.

Union of Clerks for the extension of the protection offered by the Factories Acts to offices. Clerks in the nineteenth century had a lower life expectation than miners; the main killer being tuberculosis which spread rapidly through badly ventilated, damp and insanitary offices. Regulations covering offices were not finally introduced until 1963.

More recently, women trades unionists like the T and G's Sylvia Greenwood, have taken broader issues of health care and health and safety into factories. Writing in the *T and G Record* she recalls her campaign for bringing cervical screening to women in an engineering factory.

The personnel officer instructed me with a very serious face that he could not contemplate having cervical cytology for women as that would be discrimination.

I informed him rather strongly that it is a well-known fact that amongst Jewish women there is less cancer of the cervix because of the religious requirement that all male children are circumcised at birth. So he had an option – we either had cervical cytology on site or all the males circumcised. He granted the facility with a rather blushing face.

Perhaps one of the bravest latter-day fighters for workplace safety was Alice Jefferson whose fight both for compensation and more public awareness of the killer cancers associated with asbestos was filmed by Yorkshire TV in 'Alice: a Fight for Life'. Said Alice:

You've got to keep on fighting, and when they knock you down, you've got to get up.

NOTES

1. Marilyn Steane. *Damp, Defective, and Dangerous*. London: Services to Community Action and Trades Unions (SCAT) (27 Clerkenwell Close, London EC1).
2. Nuffield Centre for Health Service Studies. *Unemployment, Health and Social Policy*. Leeds University, 1984.
3. Peter Townsend et al. *Inequalities in Health*. London: Penguin Books, 1988.
4. *English House Condition Survey*. London: Department of the Environment, 1981.
5. Nicol Snell. *Pesticide Residues in Food: the Need for Real Control*. London Food Commission, 1986.
6. Friends of the Earth. *Pesticides, the First Incident Report*. FOE, 1985.
7. London Hazards Centre. Adapted from *The Daily Hazard*, vol. 16, March 1988.
8. Letter, March 1981, leaked to *The Times*.
9. Anthony Tucker. 'Why Shouldn't We be Scared When They Won't Tell Us the Truth?', *Guardian*, 1 March 1986.
10. Anthony Tucker. 'Fears of Parents Dash Thyroid Test Plan', *Guardian*, 14 May 1986.
11. Robert Richter. *A Plague on Our Children*. Boston, MA: WGBH Educational Foundation 1979, p. 39 (transcript of a television documentary).
12. Vilma Hunt. *Work and the Health of Women*. Boca Raton, FL: CRC Press, 1979, p. 155.
13. *The Lancet*, 14 May 1983.
14. Ben-Horin, David. 'The Sterility Scandal', *Mother Jones*, May 1979, p. 61.
15. M. Donald Whorton et al. 'Reproductive hazards', in Barry S. Levy and David H. Wegman (eds), *Occupational Health: Recognizing and Preventing Work-related Disease*. Boston, MA: Little, Brown, 1983.
16. Jane E Brody. 'Sperm Found Especially Vulnerable to Environment', *New York Times*, 10 March 1981.
17. Deborah Baldwin. 'The All-Natural Diet Isn't', *Environmental Action*, vol. 9, no. 15, December 1977.
18. Mason Barr, Jr. 'Environmental Contamination of Human Breastmilk', *American Journal of Public Health*, vol. 71, no. 2, February 1981.
19. *Guardian*, 10 June 1985.
20. Tucker, op. cit., see note 9.
21. Valda's Report in Field, F. *70 Years On; a New Report on Homeworking*. London: British Society for Social Responsibility in Science (BSSRS), 1981.
22. Marianne Craig. *The Office Workers' Survival Handbook*. London: British Society for Social Responsibility in Science (BSSRS), 1981.
23. Ibid.
24. John Leopold and Rob Coyle. *Report on Health and Safety Committees* (available from John Leopold, Dept of Social and Economic Research, University of Glasgow).
25. From Women and Work Hazards Group. *Danger, Women at Work*. London: BSSRS, 1983.

RESOURCES
PUBLICATIONS

Barlow, S. M. and F. M. **Sullivan**. *Reproductive Hazards of Industrial Chemicals*. London: Academic Press, 1982.
Bertell, Rosalie. *No Immediate Danger: Prognosis for a Radioactive Earth*. London: Women's Press, 1985.
Bond, Meg. *Stress and Self-Awareness*. London: Heinemann, 1986. A book for nurses on coping with the stress of the job; much of it is suitable for anyone.
Cavendish, Ruth. *Women on the Line*. London: Routledge and Kegan Paul, 1982.
Cook, Judith. *Red Alert*. London: Hodder and Stoughton, 1986.
Cooper, Cary and Marilyn **Davidson**. *High Pressure: Working Lives of Women Managers*. London: Fontana, 1982.
Craig, Marianne. *Office Workers' Survival Handbook*. London: British Society for Social Responsibility in Science (BSSRS), 1981.
Dalton, A. *Asbestos: Killer Dust*. London: BSSRS, 1979.
Doyal, Lesley et al. *Cancer in Britain: the Politics of Prevention*. London: Pluto Press, 1983.
Elkington, J. *The Poisoned Womb*. London: Viking, 1985.
Fox, J. and D. **Gee**. *Reproductive Hazards at Work, Cancer and Work*. London (GMBATU, 1984).
Frankel, Maurice. *Chemical Risk: a Workers' Guide to Chemical Hazards and Data Sheets*. London: Pluto Press, 1982.
General and Municipal Workers Union. *Risks à la carte: safety representative's guide to catering hazards*. London: GMWU, 1981.
Hadjinicolaou, Nicole. *Sexual Harassment at Work*. London: Pluto Press, 1984.
The Hazards Bulletin (BSSRS), bi-monthly from PO Box 148, Sheffield S1 1FB.
Health and Safety at Work: Safety Representatives and Safety Committees. London: HMSO, 1978.
Huws, Ursula. *Your Job in the Eighties: A Woman's Guide to New Technology*. London: Pluto Press, 1982.
Kinnersley, Patrick. *The Hazards of Work: How to Fight Them*. London: Pluto Press, 1977.

Labour Research Department. *The LRD Guide to the Health and Safety at Work Act*. (Available from LRD, 78 Blackfriars Road, London SE1 8HF.)

London Hazards Centre. *Repetition Strain Injuries: Hidden Harm from Overuse*.

VDU Hazards Handbook: A Worker's Guide to the Effects of New Technology.

Fluorescent Lighting: A Health Hazard Overhead.

Southwark Health and Safety at Work. Available from the London Hazards Centre (see Organizations).

London Homeworking Campaign and the Women and Work Hazards Group, *Health Hazards and Homework* (available from BSSRS, see Organizations).

McVeigh, Elizabeth. 'Women's Work, Women's Ill-Health', Workers Educational Association, vol. 7, no. 25, May 1981 (available from WEA, 9 Upper Berkeley St, London W1H 8BY).

Massachusetts Coalition for Occupational Safety and Health and the Boston Women's Health Book Collective. *Our Jobs, Our Health: a Woman's Guide to Occupational Health and Safety*. Boston, MA, 1983.

Stellman, Jeanne and Susan **Daum**. *Work Is Dangerous to Your Health*. New York: Pantheon, 1973.

Stellman, Jeanne. *Women's Work, Women's Health: Myths and Realities*. New York: Pantheon Books, 1977.

Townsend, Peter and Nick Davidson. *Inequalities in Health*. London: Penguin Books, 1988.

Women and Work Hazards Group. *Danger, Women at Work* (available from BSSRS, see Organizations), 1983.

Women's Health, Work and Stress, available from the Women's Health and Reproductive Rights Information Centre, 52–59 Featherstone Street, London EC1Y 8RT.

SLIDES, FILMS AND VIDEOS

Bitter Wages. UK. Available from Women and Work Hazards Group, see Organizations.

Picture of Health: the Dyeing Industry, Channel Four, 1984. Dye workers and cancer, and a look at the Sheffield Occupational Health Project which involves cooperation between workers and GPs to prevent illness. Distributed by Concord Films Council Ltd, 201 Felixstowe Road, Ipswich, Suffolk IP3 9BJ. Tel: 0473–726012.

Picture of Health: Just Like Rain, Channel Four, 1983, 45 mins. Looks at the relationship between ill health and the use of pesticides. Distributed by Concord Films Council Ltd. (see above).

Picture of Health: Who Cares? Channel Four, 1983, 45 mins. How the health of hospital workers is put at risk. Distributed by Concord Films Council Ltd. (see above).

Risky Business. Video, UK, 1980, 15 mins. A cartoon video on health and safety at work from the point of view of a woman worker. Leeds Animation Workshop; available from Cinema of Women, see Organizations.

Windscale: The Nuclear Laundry. Yorkshire TV, 1983.

Working for Your Life. Film, USA, 1980, 57 mins. Looks at health and safety hazards in a wide variety of women's jobs; available from Cinema of Women, see Organizations.

EXHIBITION

Women, Work and Health. Sixteen coloured boards illustrating the double burden of paid employment and unpaid work for the family, rural women's work, industrial hazards, service sector mirroring domestic roles, unemployment and the fights to change women's status, work and health worldwide. Available for hire from War on Want, 37–9 Great Guildford Street, London SE1. Tel: 01–620 1111.

ORGANIZATIONS

ALARM, 47 Roderick Road, London NW3 2NP. Tel: 01–485 6495/4144. Monitors and campaigns against the transport of nuclear waste through London.

British Society for Social Responsibility in Science (BSSRS), 25 Horsell Road, London N5 1XL. Tel: 01–607 9615.

Campaign for Lead-Free Air (CLEAR), 3 Endsleigh Street, London WC1H 0DD. Tel: 01–278 9686. Campaigns to reduce levels of lead from all sources in the environment.

Chemical Cancer Hazards Information Service, Department of Cancer Studies, University Medical School, Birmingham B15 2TJ. Tel: 021–472 1010.

Cinema of Women, Unit 313, 31 Clerkenwell Close, London EC1 0AT. Tel: 01–251 4978.

Earth Resources Research (ERR), 258 Pentonville Road, London N1. Tel: 01–278 3833.

Friends of the Earth, 26–8 Underwood Street, London N1 7JQ. Tel: 01–490 1555.

Greater Manchester Hazards Centre, Room 36, Cavendish Building, Manchester Polytechnic, Manchester M15 6BG.

Greenpeace, 30–31 Islington Green, London N1 8KE. Tel: 01–354 5100. Presently campaigning on the civil nuclear industry, effects of nuclear weapons testing, titanium dioxide, North Sea pollution and preservation of the Antarctic.

Health and Safety Executive, Secretariat, Baynards House, 1 Chepstow Place, Westbourne Grove, London W2 4TF. Tel: 01–243 6000.

London Hazards Centre, 3rd floor, Headland House, 308 Gray's Inn Road, London WC1X 8DS. Tel: 01–837 5605.

Marine Conservation Society, incorporating the **Coastal Anti-pollution League**, 4 Gloucester Road, Ross-on-Wye, Herefordshire HR9 5BU. Tel: 0989–66017.

National Society for Clean Air, 136 North Street, Brighton BN1 1RG. Tel: 0273–26313.

Nature Conservancy Council, Northminster House, Peterborough PE1 1UA. Tel: 0733–40345

Scottish Campaign to Resist the Atomic Menace (SCRAM), 11 Forth Street, Edinburgh EH1 3LE. Tel: 031–557 4283.

Services to Community Action and Tenants (SCAT), 27 Clerkenwell Close, London EC1. Tel: 01–253 3627. Produces *Public Service Action* magazine.

Socialist Environment and Resources Association (SERA), 26–28 Underwood Street, London N1 7JQ. Tel: 01–490 0240.

Soil Association, 86 Colston Street, Bristol BS1 5BB, Avon. Tel: 0272–290661.

The Trades Union Congress, Congress House, Great Russell Street, London WC1B 3LS. Tel: 01–636 4030. Has some officials working on health and safety; they run courses for trade unionists and publish *The TUC Handbook on Health and Safety at Work*. They also publish a range of booklets on hazards such as asbestos, noise, solvents, dust and office hazards, and on safety representatives' rights.

Women and Work Hazards Group, BSSRS, see above.

Work Hazards Group, c/o A Woman's Place, Hungerford House, Victoria Embankment, London WC2.

GOVERNMENT AGENCIES

Consumer Safety Unit, Department of Trade and Industry, Millbank Towers, Millbank, London SW1. Tel: 01–211 3000. Safety of consumer goods.

Department of the Environment, 2 Marsham Street, London SW1. Tel: 01–212 3434. Environmental pollution.

Department of Health, Alexander Fleming House, London SE1. Tel: 01–407 5522. General health inquiries, effects of chemicals.

Ministry of Agriculture, Fisheries and Food, Great Westminster House, Horseferry Road, London SW1. Tel: 01–216 6311.

VIOLENCE AGAINST WOMEN

Rewritten by
JILL RAKUSEN

SMILE

'Smile' they said
the men on building sites
the boys at school
strangers on the street
'Give us Give us
Give us a smile'

I learnt to smile
and was their love
their duck, their chick
their oh so happy little flower

I learnt it like an animal
who needs its owner's food and warmth
I learnt it as a girl
searching out the ways to please, succeed
And when I grew
I learnt to carry it around
a handy little, deadly little, smile

Now, when they jeer at me
for wearing out-of-fashion clothes
and when they leer at bits of me
as though my breasts and legs
did not belong to me
I bare my teeth and spread my lips
give them a smile.

© PENNY WINDSOR

Every day we see real and fantasy violence against women in the news, on TV shows, in films, in advertising, in our homes and workplaces. The abuse of women, whether physical or mental, occurs with shocking frequency, as will become clear in the following pages. Much of it is so much a part of our male-dominated culture that it is seen as 'normal' except in extreme cases. We absorb it so readily that we ourselves may not even see it for what it is.

Until about twenty years ago, most forms of violence against women were hidden under a cloak of silence or tacit acceptance and guilt on the part of many women. As more and more women talked to each other in the recent wave of the women's movement, it became apparent that violence against us occurs on a massive scale, and that no woman is immune.

Public institutions, by their very nature, have consistently failed to respond adequately – either by doing nothing or by being openly judgemental, dismissive or even punitive towards women. Sometimes the very people we look to for support don't want to know – perhaps because they and/or their relationships are threatened when confronted with reality. Even our families can be directly implicated: indeed, the family can be one of the most dangerous places for a woman to be (see 'Domestic Violence', below).

Over the past fifteen years, women throughout the UK have been building a network to provide services for those of us who encounter violence, to educate people about the range and nature of violence against women, and to develop strategies for resistance. This chapter attempts to reflect the important work of such women.

THE CONTINUUM OF VIOLENCE

Many of us feel that violence against women is on a continuum. 'Social' harassment of women ('just good fun'), expecting us to smile all the time ('Cheer up, it may never happen') are at one end of the spectrum where our integrity is violated. Physical harassment, rape, vicious assaults and other extreme forms of degradation are at the other. All forms of harassment and violence against women serve as a tool to subdue and control us. Sexual violence is particularly confusing because sexual acts are ordinarily considered a source of pleasure and communication. It may even be unclear whether a sexual violation was done out of sexual desire or violent intent, or whether these motivations are even distinguishable, since violence itself has become eroticized in this culture.*

WHY?

One man's violence against one woman may *seem* to result from his individual psychological problems,† sexual frustration, unbearable life pressures or some innate urge towards aggression. Each of these 'reasons' has been used to explain and even justify male violence. *Yet male violence against women is a means of exerting and maintaining power and control over us.* When a battering husband uses beatings to confine his wife to the home and prevent her from seeing friends and family or pursuing outside work, he exerts dominance, hostility and control. When men harass, assault or rape women, they act out of a wish to dominate or punish, a desire that is often eroticized.

Whether or not an individual man who commits an act of violence views it as an expression of power is not the point. The power men hold as a group over women as a group is shown by the assumption of so many *individual* men that they have the right to express their anger and frustration in violence to individual women.

Thousands of daily acts of violence throughout the country create a climate of fear and powerlessness which limits women's freedom of action and controls many of the movements of our lives.[2]

> *I learned not to walk on dark streets, not to talk to strangers or get into strange cars, to lock doors and to be modest.*

The threat of male violence continues to keep us from stepping out from behind traditional roles and boundaries. It literally 'keeps us in our place'.

---

*'Hard core' pornography underpins the eroticism of violence in our culture. We do not have the space to address the complex role that pornography plays, nor do we all necessarily agree with each other on all aspects of the issues that pornography confronts us with. Indeed, many people disagree about pornography: some for example would claim that parts of this book are pornographic, and likewise any book that seeks to provide women with information about our sexuality in an affirming way. However, we do agree on the following:

- we abhor all pornography which we find violent or degrading to women;
- we believe it important to campaign against the existence of this type of pornography, though we would not seek government censorship;
- we deplore the fact that a huge pornography industry is making a fortune by objectifying, degrading and dehumanizing women, children and sometimes men. The work women are doing to expose this industry is central to our understanding of violence against women in cultures throughout the world.

We recognize that some of us will find offensive what others view as erotica, and vice versa; that not all pornography represents 'violence against women'. But this need not keep us from speaking out against what we believe is degrading to women, and, ultimately, everyone.

We are not happy about leaving discussion about pornography out of the book, particularly because of the cases, such as that of George Tyler (see p. 175) where we know it has played a part in unleashing brutality on women; however, we cannot do justice to the issues here, but hope that the range of reading given in Resources will be a help for those trying to confront them.

†For example, one researcher, Nicholas Groth, reports that 80 per cent of rapists in the USA were themselves sexually abused as children.[1]

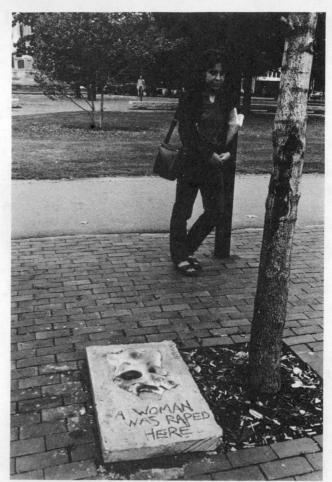

Ellen Shub

A common myth about male violence towards women is that the men involved are somehow 'abnormal' or 'sick'. The media bill rapists as monsters, as pathological. Yet as Diana Scully and Joseph Marolla found,[3] rapists are much more 'normal' than is generally assumed. What they have in common with many men is a view of women as sexual commodities – a view that our society as yet does nothing to dispel. The objectification of women in the media and the portrayal of women as constantly available to men reinforces men's fantasies about women.

BLAMING THE VICTIM

We too may get erotically caught up in the male dominance/female submission fantasy, through our past patterns of distress and hurt. It is crucial we learn about this without *ever* feeling this makes us responsible for male violence. It is a separate but significant issue – in terms of our contribution to the culture we have to change.

Women who have been raped, battered, sexually harassed or sexually assaulted in childhood often report feeling guilt and shame. The guilt is fostered by a society which tells us that we brought it on ourselves in some way – a clear case of blaming the victim. Most of us heard from our parents, 'Boys will be boys, so girls must take care,' the message being that we can avoid unwanted male attention provided *we* are careful enough. If anything goes wrong, it's *our* fault.* Blaming the victim releases the man who commits violence from the responsibility for what *he* has done.** By making us feel guilty, it discourages us from fighting back. NO WOMAN IS GUILTY FOR VIOLENCE COMMITTED BY MEN ON HER BODY, MIND AND SPIRIT. THIS VIOLENCE HAPPENS BECAUSE OF MEN'S GREATER POWER IN OUR SOCIETY AND THEIR MISUSE OF THAT POWER.

Yet the causes of male violence towards women – and of violence in general – are far more complex even than recognizing the social and political dimensions addressed so briefly above. Our own violent feelings – whether we manage to avoid acting on them or not – may give us some insight into other people's violence, including men's violence against women.

> I'm doing therapy now but I wish I'd had the opportunity a long time ago to be able to express my feelings and to feel where they came from so that I didn't continually punish my children.[5]
> I loved her more than any other human being (apart from my daughters) and I was more violent with her than with any other human being. Love and violence. Love and violence.[6]

Few of us can deny violent behaviour to our own kids, or deny how close to the edge we can sometimes get. And it can be easy to recognize what pushes us there – not just the kids. As social worker Cosis Brown wrote:

> With the structure of child care, division of labour within the home, class, poverty, housing, racism and sexism, to me it is staggering that the numbers of abusing parents, particularly women, are so low, not so high.[7]*

Equally, we can abuse demanding elderly or bedridden parents, and white women can express violence through racism too.

Some of us may fear our own violence to such an extent that we can't even seek help. It is our responsibility to recognize that we too can be violent. We must also guard against playing into the victim philosophy which ultimately leaves us feeling more powerless, while at the same time obscuring our own violence – potential or actual.

Nevertheless, the overriding problem with male violence is that it is condoned, excused, justified. One way this is done is by putting the woman on trial. It happens in court when a rape victim – the chief prosecution witness – finds herself at the receiving end of the defence lawyer's accusations and insinuations. It can also happen out of court: doctors, neighbours or whoever may subtly or not-so-subtly suggest that 'she asked for it' (in the case of a battered

woman, for example) or 'she led him on' (even applying this to cases of child abuse when the child in question is eight years old or younger).

One of the most shocking of recent cases occurred in 1982 when Peter Wood, killer of Mary Bristow, was put on trial. Mary, who happened to be a happy, generous person, had taken pity on the man who subsequently killed her, and given him support and shelter when he needed it. His trial turned out to be an outrageous assassination attempt on Mary's character, the defence seeking by doing this to 'prove' provocation and therefore reduce the crime to manslaughter rather than murder. The jury was persuaded, and returned a verdict of manslaughter. Jill Radford wrote in *New Society*:[8]

> In this case, the alleged provocation was simply Mary's disinclination to enter an exclusive sexual relationship with Peter Wood. And it was, according to Winchester Crown Court, enough. Thus, any reasonable man might be provoked into killing a woman if she has the temerity to refuse to marry him.

She goes on to show how psychiatrists played a role in excusing Wood's actions:

> . . . the psychiatrists agreed that the cause of Peter Wood's stressful life was Mary Bristow's determination to live her own life in preference to one prescribed by Wood. Both psychiatrists agreed, too, that when they met Wood after the murder he was not then, in their opinion, suffering from depression – because the cause of his stress (Mary) had been removed. This was enough to persuade the jury to accept a plea of diminished responsibility – implying again that, if a woman's lifestyle, independence and refusal to be ruled by a man is stressful to him, she is deemed to be responsible for any violent reaction on his part.

Finally, the judge, in his summing up, reinforced the view that Mary was responsible for her own death:

> Mary Bristow, with an IQ of 182, was a rebel from her middle-class background. She was unorthodox in her relationships, so proving that the cleverest people aren't always very wise. Those who engage in sexual relationships should realize that sex is one of the deepest and most powerful human emotions, and if you're playing with sex you're playing with fire. And it might be, members of the jury, that the conventions which surround sex, which some people think are 'old hat' are there to prevent people if possible from burning themselves.

Male violence, being institutionalized, is endemic. It pervades our entire culture. While individual men have to change, the culture has to change too. All of us have a responsibility to deinstitutionalize violence against women.

---

*The rape victim likely to get most sympathetic response in court is white, young, middle-class, 'respectable' and sexually inexperienced. If she is not any one of these things the blame tends to shift slowly towards the victim.
**Research has shown that an appallingly high proportion of 'sex' offenders do not consider they were responsible for the offence – blaming not only alcohol or drugs, but also the women themselves.[4]

RACE, CLASS AND VIOLENCE AGAINST WOMEN

White men often use violence as a means of asserting *racial* dominance. A married black woman who was fired for refusing to sleep with her supervisor said:

On many occasions, he said to me, 'For a coloured girl, you are intelligent.' I told him that if he has to refer to a colour or race concerning me, I considered myself 'black'. He replied, 'I don't believe in black or all that stuff. To me you're coloured, and that's it.' One day he made a comment concerning my, as he called it, 'voluptuous' shape. When I asked him politely to discontinue making such comments that include sexual overtures, he replied, 'Why not? For a coloured, you're very stacked, light-skinned and pretty.'

It can be difficult for a black woman to tell whether violence or harassment is prompted by her sex or race or both. In rape, the double jeopardy is even worse.

The man who raped me was white, and the cops here are all white. I didn't report it. I just told a few people I trusted. It helped, but I still feel scared, knowing he's out there and that nobody would do anything about it.

People in positions of power (usually white, affluent men) dismiss violence done to black women as insignificant.[9] In addition, a black woman faces a heightened vulnerability if she is not fluent in English or does not have citizenship here, because it is easier for men to take advantage of her and harder for her to get help.

Other forms of discrimination create other special vulnerabilities. People rarely take acts of violence as seriously if the woman is poor, a prostitute, a lesbian, a woman with physical or intellectual limitations or is institutionalized. This is true for all women whose 'male protectors' are non-existent, invisible or socially less powerful than other men. Open lesbians have been raped by men or groups of men angry at their social independence or 'denial' of men. ('All she needs is a good fuck.') Older women have less freedom to fight sexual harassment at their jobs or to leave a battering husband, because age discrimination means they won't easily find other ways of supporting themselves. Older women and disabled women are as, or more, vulnerable to rape as any other groups.

HARASSMENT

Harassment of women may or may not be sexual, it may or may not be racial; it may occur 'out of the blue' or when a woman becomes 'uppity' – i.e. steps out of line in some way. It may also occur when we play the traditionally feminine role.

Harassment can involve men who have some form of 'authority' over us – for example, as welfare workers, doctors or teachers.* It can happen at work or on the streets. If we cannot afford to own and run a car, we may feel unable to go out at night. Women have less access to cars than men,** and Dial-a-Ride services for people with disabilities are used mainly by women (for example, 70 to 80 per cent in Brent, London). In 1985, Southwark Women's Committee (London) commissioned a survey of women in their locality and found that half felt curfewed and would not go out at night because they did not feel safe.

*In 1984, the Women's Committee of the Oxford Students' Union carried out the first study of sexual harassment at a British university. Of 361 women who completed questionnaires, sixty-three incidents were reported. Over half involved tutors, supervisors, doctors or visiting academics; the incidents included two rapes, five assaults and two attempted rapes. The report was dismissed by the authorities.[10]

**The GLC Women's Committee survey of women's transport needs in London (1985) found that women use public transport far more than men because they have less access to cars. Only one quarter of women in the survey had a car available for their use all the time.

One-third of the sample had been physically attacked or threatened. Ethnic minority women are particularly vulnerable to harassment and attacks.

If I'm with a white boy, say just on the way home from college, they shout in the street, 'What's it like to fuck a Paki?' or if I'm on my own or with other girls it's, 'Here comes the Paki whore, come and fuck us Paki whores, we've heard you're really horny.' Or maybe they'll put it the other way round, saying that I'm dirty, that no one could possibly want to go to bed with a Paki. I can't tell you how degrading that gets to be, even when you've learnt to steel yourself, to stand up to them and not cross the road when you see a group of white guys coming towards you. I don't think any white person can possibly identify with what it's like . . .

All the time they were shouting, 'Get the Paki whore, we're going to have a gang bang.' I have never been so scared. I was convinced I was going to be raped.[11]

Racist harassment of women and children is growing, not only in the street but in our homes. The murder of Sharmira Kassam and her three children in an arson attack on their home in July 1985 was a horrifying instance of what black people face from white society.

PLEASE DON'T LOOK!*

In the dark, my footsteps quicken.
My eyes dart everywhere furtively.
The park railings look like
The bars of a prison.
The empty shopping centre
Enclosed the worst of the
Nightmares.
The key in the lock
Home safe at last.

Shopping, the next morning
Unnoticing, in daylight.
The fears of the night before.
My eyes contact unseeingly
A man who winks.
I look the other way
Men stare out from a cafe.
I look ahead, straight.

Forever I am looking at
The yellow parking lines.
The drains.
The lamp-posts.
The road-signs.
At anything, but a somebody.
Closed in,
My head bent.
Cat-calls, rent the air
From the site, nearby.
Passing youths stare
At breasts or crotch.

I glare at the
Next man.
With a look
Full of contempt
He glances away.
Can I win?
Whether 'gutter-gazing'
Or 'man-fazing'.
My look is
Veiled.
Indistinct
Blurred objects
Pass by.
Buildings, cars, people.
Fear of the threat
Of violence,
From men.
Meant, I was not
Free to look.

© ABIDA PARVEEN

---

*First published in the newsletter of the Feminist Library. Thanks to Abida and to Feminist Library for allowing us to use it.

WHAT CAN WE DO?

Racism and sexism are at the core of harassment. We need to challenge them wherever possible, and support each other when faced with them. Ethnic minority women are owed particular support from white women.

Workers Against Racism is a political organization of over 2,000 people that has developed a relatively successful anti-racist strategy. It could be learnt from – and emulated – elsewhere. On one East London estate, for example, by canvassing every home, it has managed to organize support for people suffering from racist violence, which has led to a complete change in the climate so that people are no longer subject to racist attacks. *

Some progressive local authorities have begun to take the problem of harassment seriously, and we can pressure more to do so. Camden Women's Committee in London recently funded a new community transport scheme for black and ethnic minority women's groups in the borough. The Greater London Council, before its demise in 1986, instituted a survey of women's transport needs, mindful of the safety issues that affect women, and it also instituted restrictions on sexist advertising on buses and undergrounds. The GLC also contributed funds to the Stockwell Women's Lift Service, a pioneering venture set up in 1982. Due to this service, some women, particularly elderly women, have started to go out after dark for the first time in years. †

Some of us have worked against sexual harassment – whether in the form of adding graffiti or stickers to offensive ads, or handing out leaflets in the streets. Many of us have found that 'Reclaim the Night' marches have been a turning point in our understanding of the threat of male violence on the streets. Here are some reports from *Spare Rib*[13] on a series of marches that took place nation-wide:

130 women congregating in City Square, torchlit figures shouting in the windy darkness, and suddenly we're in a big circle holding hands. Voices hoarse from singing rise again in memory of the walk down to town from Woodhouse, where rapists lurk on the moor, or Chapeltown, Ripper '77 territory. Strong knowing our sisters all over Britain are marching tonight too. [Leeds]

The best thing was the constant warmth and support we got from other women. There was no arguing about us being 'extreme' or 'crazy' or 'anti-men'. They knew exactly what we were shouting about and shouted their support back. [Lancaster]

Hundreds of women wailing and dancing through the streets of Soho. 'Sexist crap, sexist crap, SEXIST

---

*See, for example, Yvonne Roberts and Keith Tompson in Resources.
†As we go to press, we have learned of the first controlled survey of the effect of lighting on the rate of assaults on women.[12] It gives proof to the theory that bad lighting plays an important role in making us vulnerable, and is available from Middlesex Polytechnic Department of Criminology. Use it to campaign for safe streets.

Val Wilmer

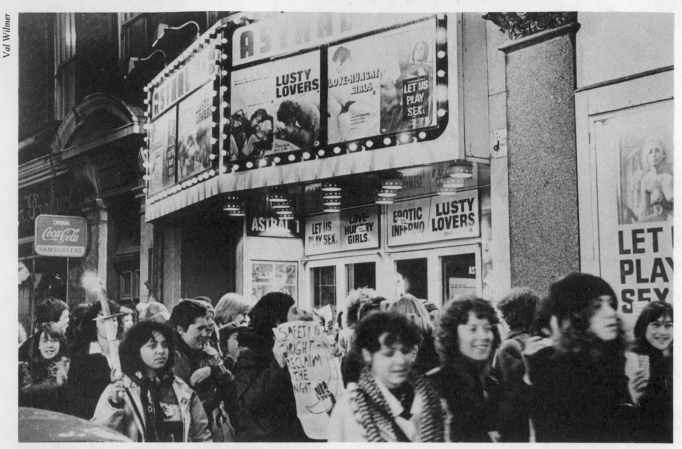

First London "Reclaim The Night" demonstration, Soho 1977

CRAP!' . . . The manager of The Pussy Parlour tight-jawed, face flesh quivering as he scrapes stickers off his windows. 'What does this mean?' he hisses at me as I take his picture. 'Can't you read?' I say. THIS DEGRADES WOMEN, THIS EXPLOITS WOMEN. One woman is running ahead squirting windows with water, followed by others slapping stickers on with such exuberant violence you think the windows must break, and hope they will. A man steps out of a fluorescent-lit doorway and gets his chest squirted then slapped with a sticker. [London]

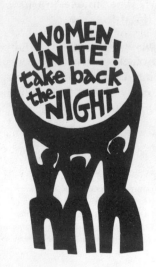

In the summer of 1986, about two thousand women marched through London protesting against harassment and all forms of male violence. They included women from women's centres, lesbian groups, Women's Aid, Rape Crisis groups, Incest Survivor groups, black women's groups.

As we marched from Hyde Park singing and chanting, we handed leaflets to bystanders, whose reactions ranged from support to amusement. I saw none of the harassment I had expected from men; we must have looked so strong, marching together. At Trafalgar Square we exchanged shouts of support with the vigil outside South Africa House.[14]

See also Self-protection, p. 171.

RAPE AND SEXUAL ASSAULT

In English law, rape is defined as sexual intercourse without a woman's consent.* The law does not require

*The one exception to this is that a woman cannot be raped by her husband, although legal separation might allow for this possibility in law. In Scotland, a husband *can* be accused of raping his wife usually only if they are legally separated, although this could change following a recent High Court decision by Lord Mayfield.

SEXUAL HARASSMENT AT WORK

Sexual harassment at work has been hidden until recently – like domestic violence in the early 1970s. It is still seen as acceptable by the majority of men and a surprising number of women. The harasser may be an employer, supervisor, co-worker, client or customer. Women who challenge or object to men's behaviour are often thought to be making a fuss about nothing, or lacking a sense of humour.

Sexual harassment occurs on broadly two levels. It is least easy to define when it is in the form of repeated, unreciprocated and unwelcome comments, looks, jokes, suggestions or physical contact.

> *Jokes are the worst because they are not as obvious as someone pinching your backside, but just as humiliating. You have to respond in a particular way or you are a social outcast. But if you do laugh, you end up hating yourself.*

At the other level, physical contact may take the form of physical attack, including attempted or actual rape.

Recent surveys in the USA reveal that the majority of women will experience workplace sexual harassment at some point during their working lives. Similar work in Britain has yet to be done, but limited research confirms that the problem is as great here.[15]

> *Joan is a forty-three-year-old waitress. She likes her job because it's close to home and it gives her a steady income to support her children. She often feels isolated, though, as many of her co-workers are white and have racist attitudes.*
>
> *A customer who comes in every day begins to flirt with Joan, making suggestive comments about her clothing and physical appearance. Unnerved by his comments, she tries not to show it because she doesn't want to lose any tip money. Often he grabs at her and touches her when she walks by.*
>
> *After several weeks of this treatment, Joan can't take it any more. She feels so anxious at work that her stomach hurts, and she starts to be off sick more and more. She knows she needs to work something out or she'll eventually lose her job. She's afraid if she complains she'll get blamed because she's friendly and attractive-looking.*

Ms T worked as a secretary in the headquarters of a well-known multinational company in London. Ms T had to endure all the usual suggestions, innuendoes and remarks. After it was made clear that she did not welcome these advances, two men started rumours about her sleeping with one of the managers. During this time she received several letters from the manager saying that he would like to have sex with her. She complained to the personnel officer but was told that 'this sort of thing goes on all the time'. On her doctor's orders she took sick leave and during that time received several 'heavy breathing' phone calls forcing her to change her number. In the end, Ms T had a nervous breakdown and was eventually sacked.[16]

Firewoman Lynn Gunning, one of only five women in the London fire brigade, was posted to Soho fire station in 1984. After only a short time there she was subject to sexual harassment which a GLC official described to me as 'verging on rape'. At one point she was stripped, hung upside down and urinated on. Yet she was reluctant to make a complaint.[17]

Sexual harassment at work is another powerful way for men to undermine and control us. It can drive women out of a particular job or out of the workplace altogether.

IF YOU ARE SEXUALLY HARASSED*

Note: It's crucial to realize that every situation is different. What kind of strategy you choose will depend on many factors, including how much you can afford to risk losing your job and whether you feel you can get support from your co-workers. (Race and class differences sometimes isolate workers from each other, for instance.)

1. Remember that you are not to blame.

2. Document what happens. Keep a diary; save any notes or pictures from the harasser.

3. *Generate support for yourself before you take action:* break the silence, talk with other women – they might well be having the same experience. If you ask for help from colleagues in working out a response, they may feel more committed to backing you up if your response to the harasser fails. Collective action and joint complaints strengthen your position. Some who have not been harassed may join in collective action.

4. Consider writing to the harasser, explaining exactly what is offensive about his behaviour. Some women have found this very effective. (Contact NCCL for further information.)

5. Consider talking to your union shop steward. If he is your harasser, contact your district official. Some unions, notably NALGO and the SCPS, have taken up the issue seriously, and a number of other unions have recently followed suit.

6. Evaluate your options. What do you want from any action you take? What are your primary concerns and goals? What courses of action are available to you? What are the possible outcomes, including the risks of each course of action?

7. First consider taking actions *within* your workplace, planning with others to be as creative as possible; using the law is difficult, though it has been done. You may wish to consider, for example, going to an industrial tribunal.

For more information on sexual harassment at work and how to fight it, including using trade unions and/or the law, see the NCCL pamphlet; *Sexual Harassment at Work*, 1984; you can also contact WASH (see Resources).

*Based on guidelines formulated by the National Council for Civil Liberties (NCCL).

CHILDREN

Rape and sexual abuse of young girls is most often committed by family friends who have access to children within their family setting. Abuse is also perpetrated by people normally in a position of trust – by doctors, dentists, teachers, babysitters and of course, parents (usually fathers).

> For a period of three years, between the ages of seven and nine, [M] was sexually abused by the seventeen-year-old youth who babysat for her mother. The abuse involved a lot of violence and threats of death if she told anyone. As a result, her family never found out and she had to cope with the mental injuries inflicted on her own.
>
> M is now twenty and, at the beginning of this year, told her mother for the first time. This was traumatic as her mother tried to dismiss what happened as M's imagination saying that he could not have tried to rape her because she – her mother – would have known if he had and even made an excuse for the youth, 'Oh, boys go through such a difficult and confusing time at that age.'[19]

Despite popular myths, 'stranger danger' poses much less threat to children. Yet parents teach children to expect danger from strangers, not from trusted authority figures, and the violation of this trust is often frightening and confusing.

Sexual abuse of children may include sexually suggestive language; prolonged kissing, looking and petting; vaginal and/or anal intercourse and oral sex. Signs of physical abuse do not always show. Some of us become pregnant or contract a sexually transmitted disease.

Another form of abuse involves child prostitution, often in the form of child sex rings. Girls involved in child prostitution, whether as organizers of sex rings or whatever, may themselves have been victims of incest or other forms of child abuse.[20]

As parents, we face the difficulty of warning our children against sexual danger without making them frightened of sex. For a discussion of the sexual abuse of children, within the family see p. 177.

---

ejaculation to take place, nor is physical violence necessary. Other forms of sexual attack, however violent they may be, do not constitute rape in legal terms, but rather 'indecent assault'. Thus, penetration of a woman's body by, for example, bottles, sticks, knives or screwdrivers does not count as rape. Nor does any form of forced oral or anal sex.* In some parts of the world the law regards these forms of violation as rape. We use this broader definition in this chapter, and look forward to the time when our legal system recognizes the true meaning of 'mere' sexual assault on women.

Rape may or may not involve force, threats or blackmail. It may involve one man or many. It is always traumatic. When we are raped, survival is our primary instinct and we protect ourselves as best we can. Some women choose to fight back; others do not feel it is an option. If you were raped and are now reading this chapter, you did the 'right' thing because you are alive.

Here are several facts which disprove common myths about rape. Rape is more likely to be committed by someone we know than by a stranger ('acquaintance' rape and marital rape). Two-thirds of reported rapes are planned and more than half occur indoors, usually in the woman's own home. Nine out of ten rapes occur between members of the same racial group. Most rapists lead everyday lives, go to school, work, have family and friends.

Children as young as six months and women as old as ninety-three have been raped. Rape can happen to any woman – rich, poor, young, old, of any racial or ethnic background. Even the 'good girl' (a destructive stereotype in our society) can be raped. As, of course, can prostitutes: women looked on aghast during the trial of Peter Sutcliffe (the so-called Yorkshire Ripper) as the media and the court (including the prosecution) suggested, implied or asserted that the rapes and killings of prostitutes were somehow 'lesser' crimes than those of women who were 'just in the wrong place at the wrong time'.

The woman is a nineteen-year-old student at university. It is about two o'clock in the afternoon and she is in an isolated part of one of the buildings. Her attacker is a young married man who is a lecturer at the university.

The woman is seventeen, a school student. It is about four o'clock in the afternoon. Her boyfriend's father has picked her up in his car after school to take her to meet his son. He stops by his house and says she should wait for him in the car. When he has pulled the car into the garage, this thirty-seven-year-old father of six rapes her.

The woman is thirty-nine, separated from her husband, the mother of five children. Her attacker breaks into the house in the middle of the night. He turns out to be a friend's husband, the father of several children.

The woman is twenty and has recently got a new job. The boss asks her to come in on a holiday to help with the inventory. When she arrives, there is no one else there. Her boss, a man of about thirty, rapes her.

The woman is sixteen, still at school. She has a

---

*Until 1985 the maximum sentence for rape was life imprisonment. The maximum sentence for a sexual assault on a man by a man was ten years, but for a sexual assault on a woman was two years. The latter has now been changed to ten years; it is still a lesser crime than 'rape'.

date with a student she knows fairly well. He drives her to an isolated area and rapes her.[18]

The number of rapes (using the current English legal definition) recorded by police in England and Wales was 1,225 in 1980 – an increase of 30 per cent since 1970. Yet it is widely acknowledged that most rapes still go unreported. Only about a quarter of women who contact rape crisis centres go to the police.* In one study, 25 per cent of a sample of over 400 young women reported having been raped.[21] Since police procedures in some areas have begun to improve, it is possible that women's willingness to go to the police has further increased. Any increased willingness to report rape may also be connected with suggestions by the police that rapes are 'getting nastier' – as Detective Chief Superintendent Thelma Wagstaff told a Howard League for Penal Reform conference in 1985.

WHAT TO DO IF YOU HAVE BEEN RAPED

The first thing you may want to do is to have a shower or bath and try to forget what happened. Do whatever feels most comfortable, but consider two things. First, it is very important, both physically and emotionally, that you receive medical attention as soon as possible, even if you have no obvious injuries. Second, don't bathe or shower if you think you may later decide to prosecute, as you will wash away evidence that may be crucial to your case.

If possible, call a friend, relative or local rape crisis number if there is one (see p. 187): they can give comfort, support and go with you to the police and/or to a hospital. It really helps to confide in someone and to talk over what to do next.

Should You Report the Rape to the Police?

You are under no obligation to do so, but your evidence could protect others, and, if the man can be caught immediately, he is more likely to confess and spare you the misery of cross-questioning in court. If you know the man/men involved, this may make you unwilling to report it, either because they are pressuring you, and/or because you expect to be disbelieved, and/or because you feel responsible for what happened in some way. NO WOMAN IS RESPONSIBLE FOR BEING RAPED.

It is never easy to decide whether to prosecute a rapist. Of the few rapes that are reported, fewer still are prosecuted. Whether you report it or not, write down everything that you can remember, so that if you do report or prosecute later your statement will be accurate.

While you are deciding whether to prosecute, here are several things to keep in mind:

- The police and the legal system very often make prosecuting a rapist a more difficult, painful experience for the woman than it should be, even during the initial visit to the police. It will help tremendously to have a

friend or rape crisis counsellor with you *throughout* the process, and to talk to other women who have been through a prosecution and know what to expect. Doing a 'role-play' with an experienced rape crisis worker can be helpful in preparing yourself for the cross-questioning.*

- The legal process can last for as long as two years, so you need to be prepared to continue thinking and talking about the rape for a long time, including giving an account of the event over and over while people judge whether you are telling the truth.
- You will be a witness for the prosecution. You will not have a lawyer to represent you in court.
- You may not be able to claim compensation if you do not prosecute.

If You Decide to Report the Rape

Go to the police as soon as you can. If necessary go there first and ring from the police station to get a friend to come down and help you. Speed is important because your behaviour and appearance immediately after the rape could be used by the police as '*corroborating evidence*'. As rapes are rarely witnessed, evidence of distress, disarrayed clothing, etcetera, can be important, and the police are more likely to be considered impartial observers of your condition than your mother or husband.

You will be questioned by the police, often for hours and not always with tact and sympathy. You are under no obligation to answer any question and if you find the whole process too much, you can at any stage insist on going home.

The police will arrange for you to be examined by a doctor and your clothes may be taken away for forensic examination (you may wish to take a change of clothes with you if you can). This is to establish whether intercourse has actually taken place and to gather evidence for a possible prosecution. The examination may also be a humiliating experience. The doctor has often to be called out late at night, he may be asked to examine you in a place which is not suitable, and he may not be kind or sympathetic. You can ask for a woman doctor, and you can ask for your own GP to be called.

Medical Attention

Whether or not you report the rape, see a doctor as soon as possible to be checked for STDs (see p. 486). Obviously it is impossible to find out if you are pregnant immediately. You might be offered a 'morning-after' pill, which can stop

---

*For each rape reported to the police, it is estimated that between ten and twenty-five go unreported. This does not include rapes within marriage, nor sexual assaults.[22]

*As a result of strong protests from women, some changes have taken place, e.g. in the form of the Sexual Offences Act 1976. This aims to ensure anonymity for women who go to the police, and that in court we may not be questioned about our private lives. While the Act does give us some protection, in many cases a woman can still be treated as if *she's* on trial, and the man's lawyer can apply for leave to introduce 'evidence' about her at the trial. In some areas, police procedures are improving in response to pressure, e.g. some forces now ensure that *women* police officers take initial statements, some have initiated training programmes for their staff in the facts of rape, and concerning women's needs – including asking you if you want a rape crisis centre representative to be present while you are at the police station.

pregnancy if taken within seventy-two hours of the rape (see p. 295). A 'morning-after' IUD is not advisable, for the rapist(s) might have given you an infection which could then spread very easily to your womb. You might prefer to wait until you can get a pregnancy test (see p. 309) and decide whether or not to have an abortion. Few doctors would refuse an abortion in these circumstances. Contact WHRRIC (see p. 638) if you have any problems.

An additional check-up six weeks later is also advisable. The doctor should examine you for any tearing, bruising or general damage both internally and externally.

If you have no obvious signs that force has been used, you might find the doctor somewhat sceptical about rape. When one woman we know reported a rape to her GP he angrily told her not to try to cover up an illicit affair with a story like that. If you have a friend with you it is less likely that the doctor can behave in this way.

EMOTIONAL REACTIONS TO RAPE

Immediate responses to rape can range from numbness and disbelief, causing us to appear calm and rational, to extreme anxiety, fear and disorientation.

We deserve support however we respond to rape. We need supportive friends and/or counsellors to talk to about our feelings. We may feel too embarrassed or humiliated at first but it is a difficult burden to carry alone. Women who have been raped and have talked about it afterwards are apt to feel less guilty and ashamed, because they were able to express their anger and discuss the crime as something that happens to many women. We must remember that rape is *not our fault*. Because rape violates our self-respect, anger is a most appropriate response. We need to help one another to feel and express our anger about rape, since we can suffer a lot from turning these feelings inwards. Relationships can break down, we may be unable to continue working, or we may even try suicide. One woman who was raped was severely depressed for six months, until she finally expressed her rage at what had been done to her. Many women have joined anti-rape groups to use their angry energy in positive ways.

Humiliation, embarrassment, guilt, disgust, horror and anxiety – these are all possible reactions to rape. Sometimes a close friend has the skills and ability to help us express and work through our feelings, but in some cases we may need help from a counsellor (see Chapter 8), ideally someone who is experienced in the needs of women who have been raped. Co-counselling (see p. 121) can also be very helpful for women who have been raped – even if it occurred many years ago. Groups organized by local rape crisis centres can be a good way for us to share their experiences and support one another. If we have had the opportunity to work through our feelings we can be especially helpful to others.

Many fathers, boyfriends, husbands and lovers feel violent anger towards the rapist, often because they see the rape as a personal violation of themselves (this is especially true of men who view women as their 'property'). When this reaction to rape is not accompanied by sympathy and support, it can be demoralizing for us. Other men are more casual and insensitive to the seriousness of the act ('Why are you so upset? After all, he didn't hurt you'). Fortunately, more men (and women) are beginning to understand the serious consequences of rape and are learning to be supportive and sensitive regardless of their own reactions.

Children who have been raped have special needs. A little girl may not understand what has happened to her or that the rape was somehow a 'bad thing'. Her reactions depend largely on the reactions of those around her: if everyone gets very upset, then she will be very upset; if others express strong anger towards the rapist, she may feel that this anger is directed towards her or is somehow her fault – this response to anger is common in children.

If we have been raped as children or teenagers, we often feel tremendously guilty, and may keep the rape a secret for many years.

The experience of courts and the functioning of the law can still be a further agony for most women, although the law does now protect us to some degree from having our past sexual histories dragged through the court. But the law does not protect us from male violence. If women are to be protected we must set about changing society's view of us and we must learn to defend ourselves.

LEGALLY-ENFORCED VIOLENCE AGAINST WOMEN: WOMEN IN PRISON

When women come under the jurisdiction of courts we are exposed to many kinds of violence, largely, it seems, *because* we are women. Contrary to popular belief, women tend to receive harsher sentences than men who have committed similar offences. In 1975, of people with no previous convictions, five times as many women as men were jailed. (Male offenders are twice as likely as women to receive 'community services orders' instead of prison sentences.) Between 1979 and 1984, although there was a decrease of about 3 per cent in the number of women sentenced by the courts, there was an increase of 50 per cent in those receiving immediate custody.

Sentencing reflects traditional assumptions about women. As Baroness Seear and Elaine Player found:

> Women and girls who have engaged in what is described as 'inappropriate sex-role behaviour' receive particularly severe sentences.[23]

Thus, according to radical lawyer Helena Kennedy, a very disturbed lesbian who, after a long period of misery, murdered her lover in a classic case of '*crime passionnel*' got a life sentence, while a man who murdered his three daughters to punish his wife for running off with another man got six years.[24] Even if women's actions are clearly in self-defence and the result of torture and severe provoca-

SELF-PROTECTION

One of the best forms of self-protection is to learn self-defence (see p. 181), particularly self-defence involving assertion training – for then we can often pre-empt problems. Self-defence and assertion training (see Chapter 8) can be helpful in relation to all forms of attack and harassment. With regard to attacks from strangers or unwelcome visitors, here are some tips.

Writing this list reminds us how angry we are that we have to protect ourselves from men's actions. Yet if we want to hitch-hike, to live alone, to walk home alone at night, to enjoy the solitary freedom of city parks, to do things that most men take for granted, we must learn to protect ourselves against unwelcome attention from men, violent or otherwise.

When possible, *the most effective protection comes from being with other women.* Arrange to walk home together, set up a safe-house pro-gramme in your area, get to know each other on your street or in your block of flats.

Where you Live

Keep the windows locked and in place; have strong locks on every door; be aware of places where men might hide; don't put your full name on your door and list only your initials in the phone book; know which neighbours you can trust in an emergency; find out who is at your door before opening; say, 'I'll get the door, Bill!' when going to the door. Door-ways and landings should be well lit; pressure landlords to do so if it is their responsibility, and badger the local council to do the same for dark alleyways and secluded streets. Avoid fumbling for keys at the door – have them in your hand as you arrive.

On the Street

Be aware of what is going on around you. Walk with a steady pace; look as if you know where you are going; don't carry a lot of stuff; dress so you can move and run easily; walk in the middle of the street; don't go near a car at night if the driver stops and asks for directions; don't walk through dark places or a group of men; if you fear danger yell 'Fire' not 'Help' or 'Rape'; carry a whistle around your wrist.

Travelling

If you have a car, check the back seat before getting in; while driving, keep doors locked; don't stand near groups of men on station platforms; try and sit on an aisle seat; look aware and don't fall asleep; if you don't know where you are going on a bus, ask the conductor/driver and sit near the exit.

'Legal Weapons' as Protection

In the UK it is illegal to carry anything that could be called an 'offensive weapon', no matter how much you may have good reason to protect yourself. However, a cheap heavy ring worn on the inside of your hand, keys, an umbrella are all useful. So are hatpins.

Hitch-hiking

When hitching (particularly alone), avoid taking lifts if there is more than one man in the car. Never sit in the back of a two-door car. Check that you can open the door from the inside. Try to make a note of the registration number and make of the car and whenever possible take lifts from lorries or vans rather than private cars. A professional driver has a schedule to follow, a reputation to keep and is easier to identify. Try to avoid hitching at night. Some of us feel that *all* hitching should now be avoided.

These tactics can help you but they are not fool-proof. Practise tactics for the situations in which you feel most at risk and least powerful. Try to remain calm and to act as confident and strong as you can. A purposeful and confident air is our best protection when walking alone. If you are followed, walk up to a house and if necessary break a window to attract attention.

tion, sentencing is often harsher than for men. For exam-ple, in the case of the Maw sisters, each received a three-year sentence for killing her father.

The Maw sisters, Annette and Charlene, had suf-fered years of violence from their drunken father. In court Mrs Maw, their mother, described how Mr Maw attacked Charlene: 'I pleaded with him to stop. I heard screaming and shouting. I went upstairs and saw him attacking Annette. Her forehead was bleed-ing and blood streaming down her face. I pushed him on the mattress and he screamed abusively. He said he was going to kill the girls. I have never been as frightened in my life.' The fight continued and Annette stabbed her father with a weapon passed to her by Charlene.[25]

The case of Guardsman Thomas Holdsworth is in marked contrast: he brutally attacked a young woman in a park after she had refused to have sex. (He had not met her before.) The attack included rape by his whole, ringed, hand causing her to pass out with the pain, biting her nipples and ripping her earrings off. Holdsworth's initial sentence of three years was quashed on appeal and replaced by a six-months' suspended sentence. As Polly Pattullo says: 'Their Lordships agreed that Holdsworth was an asset to the

British Army and should be allowed to continue serving.' In fact, he was subsequently thrown out of the army.

In her book *Women on Trial*, Susan Edwards argues that women are judged twice over: 'They are on trial as offenders, and also as women – and the kind of justice they get is concentrated or diluted according to that.'[26]

The vast majority of women prisoners have been convicted of petty theft or failure to pay fines, including for prostitution 'offences'.[27] And proportionately more women than men (over 3,000 per year) have not been convicted of any offences at all. Of these 'remand' prisoners, only a minority eventually get prison sentences (less than a third in 1984). The average time on remand is three to four *months*. For a description of the punitive and degrading remand system as it affects women, see Audrey Peckham's *A Woman in Custody* (details in Resources).

Once legitimately imprisoned, women's treatment is harsher than men's. We are punished for disciplinary offences twice as often as men[28] and women are constantly punished over and beyond the 'legal' punishment of deprivation of liberty. One of the assessors visiting women's prisons wrote for Baroness Seear's report:

The rattle of keys, the locking and unlocking of doors, the internal escorting of prisoners by prison officers creates an atmosphere that must continuously reinforce the fact of imprisonment and must for some people have a claustrophobic effect.

As Seear comments in her report, 'This seems to come very close to being punishment applied to prison, *contrary to declared policy*' (our italics). Locked doors also mean that attendance at education and training classes or at recreation is severely restricted, and that women are locked up *all* day because of lack of 'available' staff to perform escorting and warder functions. There are no maximum security prisoners in women's prisons. As Seear and Player indicate there is no justification for constant locking and unlocking of internal doors.

STRIP-SEARCHING AND SEXUAL VIOLENCE IN PRISON

Enforced stripping is often used on women in prison. It first came to public attention because of its widespread and continuing use on Republican women political prisoners remanded in custody in Northern Ireland.

They've no regard for you. They use your body as a weapon against you.

The searches have been described by a professor of psychiatry at University College, Dublin, as 'a very powerful way of breaking down a personality'.

There's no way you can tell people the anguish and trauma that you actually go through. You can't describe the way they look at you. You can't describe the atmosphere, the oppressive atmosphere.

In a typical strip-search which can last from five to twenty minutes, you are taken from the wing and

---

AN OPEN LETTER FROM HOLLOWAY PRISON, LONDON*

We, the prisoners of Holloway Prison,

Would like, **once again**, to make a formal complaint against the conditions and abuse we are subjected to by the prison authorities. In December 1984 a protest was made, in the form of an **unrecognized** riot, whereby 31 women were forcibly dragged from their units and segregated. Each woman was adjudicated and as a result spent 4–5 days in solitary confinement, lost the privilege of receiving meals etc, from outside, for 14 days, and lost 14 days' remission pending sentence. This was for protesting about the conditions that we, as human beings and unconvicted prisoners are subjected to.

Yesterday – one such woman was removed, with unnecessary brute force, and placed in the punishment block, where her and other women's screams were heard as she was beaten. This was because she refused, as an unconvicted prisoner, to be placed on a convicted unit. The said woman has been, on more than one occasion, subjected to unfair discrimination and has been held in solitary confinement for unqualified reasons. Most women feel very strongly about this and as a result, 15 women have been forcibly removed from their units and have been subjected to questionable violence.

Violence within the prison system is a direct contravention of the judicial system, yet it is allowed to continue without retribution or recrimination. This must be stopped before another 'Winsom Green' tragedy arises, where an inmate was found, in a locked cell, beaten to death.

We the prisoners demand that an immediate enquiry is satisfactorily conducted or will not be held responsible for our further subversive action.

16.6.85

*Signed by forty-four women prisoners.

a screw accompanies you to reception. You pass these male warders on the way in. You are told to strip and all of your clothes must be removed. These are taken from you. If you have a period your sanitary towel or tampon is taken from you as well. It doesn't matter to them that you are actually bleeding.

Strip-searching has been systematic throughout the UK for years. It is also sometimes used in police cells, and can even involve male police officers. It is possible that strip-searching in police cells may have increased since the Police and Criminal Evidence Act of 1984 came into force in January 1986, giving police increased powers to carry out strip-searches, in particular intimate body searches, at police stations. Body orifice searches may even be carried out by a police officer, authorized by a superintendent, if a dangerous item is suspected. And although rules also say they must be carried out by, and in the presence of, officers of the same sex as detainees, this is not always the case, certainly for 'simple' strip-searches. Black women and political demonstrators may be at particular risk of being strip-searched by police. For example, in 1983, nine people were arrested at a vigil outside the South African embassy following the hanging of three black men in Pretoria. The women – not the men – were forcibly strip-searched. The same year, the Sari Squad went along to Leon Brittan's house to protest against the deportation of Afia Begum. It was a very quiet protest, but they were all taken to Rochester Row police station and told to strip. As Pam, one of their members said:

They didn't say why. We don't go to public bathing places or anything like that. Ghazala and another woman refused. They were taken to another room, their saris removed and dragged back in front of the male officers in just an underskirt and a very thin piece of material on top. I took off my own sari and then properly stripped. They felt us up. They used their hands. It was quite a horrible experience.

The case against them was thrown out of court.

Peace demonstrators seem to be particularly liable to strip-searching. In 1985, following a demonstration at Faslane in Scotland, six women demonstrators (again, no men), were strip-searched. No reason was given nor charges made. One of them described the ordeal to Cynthia Kee of the *Observer*:

They unzipped my trousers and pulled them down and searched in between my legs. The woman put her hands inside my pants and pulled them down so you could see and they searched up my jumper. There were all these policemen standing round and they stared. I couldn't understand it. All these men could be my father. How could they allow this to happen to me? . . . Then they took me into a

---

BLACK WOMEN IN PRISON*

Black women represent a disproportionate number of the female prison population, not least because of discrimination suffered through immigration laws, police and courts, and endemic racism in our society. Accurate figures do not exist. It is widely recognized that black women represent more than 35 per cent of the female prison population, and visitors to Holloway prison in London have reported that 50–60 per cent of prisoners are black.

Those in prison are often cut off from their children, subdued with drugs, subjected to racism from other prisoners and staff, and also ostracized by their own communities. Many of their offences have been committed out of need, reflecting the difficult circumstances black women are forced to live in. They tend to be stereotyped as 'aggressive' or violent, because white society tends to interpret the slightest show of assertion in this way. Prison staff therefore can treat black women particularly roughly.

There is a lot of racism from prison officers, teachers, the lot, but mainly from prison officers.

But the attitude has come down from the Home Office. About two-thirds of the black women prisoners are drugged. In prison, there's a system, and if you don't play it, they beat you up and attack you, and if you're black you get more pressure, because you are not only fighting for your prisoners' rights, you're fighting for your black rights. The treatment of prisoners is so bad, I think on the whole the way women are treated there is a reflection of society.

Recently, black women prisoners and their supporters have started to organize. The London-based Black Female Prisoners Scheme aims to increase awareness of the racial and social problems experienced by black women prisoners. Its four workers visit all prisons detaining women from the London area, and they organize educational and social activities, as well as arranging legal advice and community support. They have recently set up a group for deportees in one prison. The scheme also operates a building society account to provide extra money for women in gaol. Donations are welcome. For their address, see Resources.

*This box is based on information contained in a report of the first ever conference on black women in prison, held in 1985 and sponsored by the now defunct Greater London Council.

cell with two other women and I realized I had taken my period. They called for a sanitary towel, which was then brought.

Twelve hours later, she was released, soaked in blood. They had ignored repeated calls for another sanitary towel.

The real purpose of strip-searches would seem to be harassment. Says Lynette Edwell who was arrested at Greenham Common on Good Friday 1984 while reading the Passion:

I had to remind them to look inside my boots and my handbag.

Other forms of harassment of women prisoners include verbal abuse by male police officers or warders, as well as actual assault. An anti-apartheid demonstrator, who was arrested and strip-searched in 1986, had her arms lacerated by a male officer while standing naked.[29] One woman was awarded an out of court settlement for loss of virginity while under interrogation.[30]

These violent practices in Northern Ireland and on the mainland are still a long way from the degree of violence experienced by women prisoners in other parts of the world such as Chile (where mice were put in women's vaginas and dogs trained to rape women), or Iran (where women may be raped and then forced into marrying their attackers). Yet *all* of the practices we have mentioned contravene the European Convention on Human Rights.

LABELLED 'MAD' AS WELL AS BAD

Women are also more likely to be labelled 'mad' as well as bad when in prison. Many prisoners appear to be given cocktails of drugs 'as a matter of routine',[31] and women's prisons are highest on the league table of drug use – whether the drugs be valium, stelazine, largactil, modecate, etcetera. In Holloway in 1979, mood-altering drugs were issued to women at an average rate of three doses per prisoner per day. The drug regimes often mean that normal functioning is impossible. By 1981, not least because of the public outcry, the average daily dose of these drugs was reduced to one. By 1983, the annual average drug dosage was 228 per prisoner per year, though individual prisons' averages were close to the 1981 figure. Women held in open prisons and borstals are more likely to be prescribed drugs than men detained in maximum security prisons. While many women may ask for drugs, many are forced to take them.

I was in the medicine queue and as soon as the sister gave me my medicine I spat it out into my tea mug. I

MEDICAL AND IN PARTICULAR PSYCHIATRIC VIOLENCE AGAINST WOMEN

Feminists have long recognized the violence done to women under the guise of medical 'care'. The history of medicine's violence against women is as old as medicine itself and has been amply documented (e.g. by Phyllis Chesler in *Women and Madness*, by Barbara Ehrenreich and Deirdre English in *For Her Own Good*, by Dorothy Smith and Sara David in their collection of articles entitled *Women Look at Psychiatry* and, more recently, by Susan Penfold and Gillian Walker in *Women and the Psychiatric Paradox*).*

Such violence includes possible sexual assault by male doctors and nurses. In the words of one woman psychiatrist:

I reported a psychiatrist who had had sex with two of his patients to the medical society. I called back two months later to find out what had been done. They told me the doctor denied everything, and it was his word against the patients'; so they were dropping the matter.

It also includes more prevalent and insidious forms of social control meted out to us – whether through drugs, ECT, surgery, sanctions or whatever – to render us compliant, passive and unthreatening. Black and lesbian women are particularly vulnerable to medicine's oppressive view of women.

In fact, the whole notion of 'mental illness' has been used against us, so that whenever we step outside the 'norm', we run the risk of being defined as mad – or bad. Not that long ago, women were incarcerated in mental hospitals for having an illegitimate child – often to remain there for the rest of their lives, certainly until the 1970s. Committal to mental hospital has also been forced on some Greenham protestors for peace.

So, while mental hospital may be an appropriate asylum at times (as we discuss in Chapter 8), for many of us it can represent the epitome of social and medical violence against women.**

We hope that this book gives an indication of the collective strength of women against the oppressiveness of what often passes for health care. Please see Resources in Chapter 8 for information about consumer- and/or women-orientated groups organizing around mental health issues and the psychiatric system.

*See Resources in Chapter 8 for details of these publications.
**See WHIC Broadsheet, 'Women's Health and Mental Illness' for more discussion on this. Details in Resources in Chapter 8.

was caught and put on report. The next morning I saw the deputy governor and I was given loss of pay and privileges – so I never refused again.[32]

Yet it is universally acknowledged that help given to truly disturbed women is appallingly inadequate, and that such women should never be imprisoned in the first place. Prue Stevenson, an ex-member of staff at Holloway prison, commented that 'you'd hesitate to keep animals in there', referring to the psychiatric wing. She resigned in protest at the conditions. Prisoners are often locked up in their cells twenty-three hours a day, with minimum light, inadequate food and limited exercise. This wing has an appallingly high incidence of stress-induced self-mutilation, and has been responsible for at least two such incidents which led to death in two years. With the old mental institutions vanishing, more women in need of help will end up in such inappropriate institutions unless big changes take place. While the Home Office recognizes that the psychiatric wing should be closed, there is as yet no commensurate commitment to ensuring that adequate care will be forthcoming elsewhere. For more information about women in prison, see Resources, p. 186.

WOMEN'S DEMANDS

Women's organizations, including Women in Prison which campaigns on behalf of women prisoners, are demanding changes in the way women are treated by the prison and court system, including:

- an end to strip-searching;
- decriminalization of prostitution;
- improved safety conditions, particularly in Holloway Prison where women have burned to death in their cells;
- the introduction of a range of facilities aimed both at reducing tension and, subsequently, the number of drugs prescribed for behaviour and mood control rather than the benefit of prisoners;
- improved education and training facilities;
- improved training and supervision of prison officers, aimed at reducing their present discriminatory practices against women from ethnic minorities and lesbian, disabled or mentally or emotionally disturbed women;
- improvement of childcare facilities in prisons;
- improved medical facilities in general and specialized facilities for women during pregnancy,
- dismantling of the punitive disciplinary structure coupled with the development of official recognition of prisoner participation in the organization of the prison;
- non-discriminatory sentencing of women;
- unrestricted access to the Boards of Visitors for representatives from women's organizations, community, ethnic minority and other minority (e.g. lesbian) organizations.

For details of organizations which campaign and/or offer help for women in prison, see Resources, p. 187.

DOMESTIC VIOLENCE

BATTERING

Any woman living with a man can be battered. She might be any woman we know – our sister, our daughter, our mother, our friend, our neighbour . . . or ourselves. It doesn't matter where we are, how many children we have, whether we're married or not, how much money we've got, or what race or nationality we are. While women with children and without jobs *may* be more vulnerable to prolonged battering, because being economically dependent means that escape is very problematic,[33] this does *not* mean that financially secure, independent, childless women are necessarily any better protected.

Women are physically and mentally battered by husbands, boyfriends, and even sons and other relatives. It has been estimated that in one in a hundred marriages, the women suffer *severe* violence – in other words, 140,000 women in the UK; 25 per cent of *reported* violent crime is that of men abusing the women they live with; and less than 3 per cent of women in refuges for battered women have reported the assaults to the police.[34]

These are three examples we quoted in the last UK edition of this book.

A woman awakens and tugs at a blanket on the bed; the next thing she knows her husband is attempting to suffocate her with a pillow. A husband finds a photograph in his wife's wallet; five minutes later he places a hot iron on her arm in an attempt to make her confess to having an affair. A man complains of his wife's untidiness and they have an argument; he goes and works all day, but when he returns the argument continues, he beats his wife and throws her and the children out into the cold.[35]

Ten years later, the stories continue:

He punched me and broke my arm after picking an argument. I ran and locked myself in the bathroom but he kicked the door in and beat me again. It was only when he produced the shotgun that he used for killing ducks that his cousin intervened.[36]

Battering often has links with sexual violence.

I just let him get on with it. I didn't really think about rape. I just thought, well, it'll save another beating.

Kathleen Tyler, whose husband George terrorized her whole family, reports how things changed after he began to rent porn videos:

He'd sit down in front of them, make me watch them, then he'd say, 'You watch carefully, my girl; you're going to do that in a minute.' And he meant it. I dreaded him coming home from the pub, and most of all I dreaded going to bed. *[37]

Other forms of brutality include mental torture and humiliation, attempted strangulation, repeated punching, kicking, the use of weapons, boiling water, etcetera.

The physical beatings are bad. But the torture of not being allowed to be me is pushing me, driving me mad. [38]

Battering is not a new phenomenon – a pamphlet on 'Wife Torture' (by Frances Power Cobbe) appeared in the 1870s. But battering did not become a recognized 'problem' until the first refuge was set up in Chiswick in 1971, when women kept on arriving in order to escape 'home'.

Refuges are essential for many women, in order to escape battering. In many marriages, the home is in the husband's name. If a woman wants to leave home, she faces the prospect of being homeless, she has worries about the children and, of course, money. She may not be considered eligible for a council home if she left 'of her own free will' – the reasoning being that she still has a home with her husband. Even if a woman is in the fortunate position

Often, women finally leave only when they fear that their children are in physical or mental danger from their fathers.

I have left my husband in desperation five times but have had to return for my children's sake as he didn't take care of them in my absence. [39]

If a woman does have a job, or if she manages to find one if and when she leaves the home, the pay is unlikely to be much. The average female wage is less than 75 per cent of the average man's; the lowest-paid jobs are done by women; many women have to work part-time and consequently for little money because they are expected to have full responsibility for children; facilities for children – provided by the state or by employers – are getting fewer; maternity pay and maternity leave are rarely adequate.

Then there's the total loss of confidence, fear, feelings of helplessness, and the belief in what *he's* said of her; this keeps her trapped without an escape route . . . and perpetually vulnerable to the abuse. If we believe that we're useless, ugly, it's our fault anyway, and that he'll find us and kill us if we leave, there's not much incentive to go. In addition, we rarely get adequate protection from clergy, courts or police, who often do not take us seriously.*

I went early in our marriage to a clergyman, who after a few visits told me that my husband meant

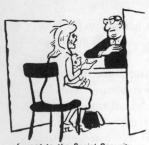

I went to the Social Security but they said I had a husband to support me.

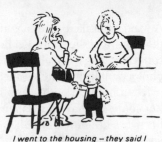

I went to the housing – they said I already had a house.

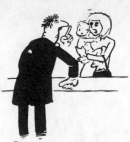

The police told me they couldn't get involved in domestic disputes.

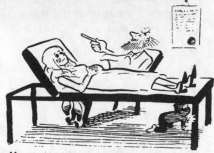

My psychiatrist thinks I'm a masochist as I keep going back.

of being able to put the man out of the home (and, even harder, keep him out), she can still be held liable for her husband's rent arrears. So many battered women don't leave home because they can't.

Another reason some women put up with battering for so long is because of concern about how to cope with bringing up the children.

When Mum was alive, I'd go there. But it's hard when you've got three children. Sometimes I'd stay away for three or four weeks, sometimes just two days. I'd go back because it's not easy on your own with three kids and it's upsetting people's lives.

no real harm, he was just confused and felt insecure. Things continued. I turned this time to a doctor. I was given little pills to relax me and told to take things easier. I was 'just too nervous'. I turned to a friend, and when her husband found out, he accused me of either making things up or exaggerating the situation. She was told to stay away from me.

Indeed, fear of being killed if we leave is by no means an unwarranted fear for some women: women will continue to

*George Tyler was eventually killed by his daughter Karen; evidence of the man's brutality had little effect, initially, on the legal system's response to Karen's action, the result of extreme provocation.

*Male upholders of the established 'order' are not immune to violent behaviour themselves, as we have already seen (p. 171). Roger Graef vividly dramatized policemen's violence against their wives in 'Closing Ranks' (Central Television, 1988). Clergy can also be violent, as Martin Roe reported in *The Independent* (see Resources). Wives of violent ministers of religion can contact a new counselling service run by Elaine Stokey called Men, Women and God (see Resources).

suffer and die at the hands of husbands – estranged or otherwise – until law enforcement agencies regard 'domestic violence' as the crime that it is.

Refuges – a safe place to stay

> I had visions of a cold, empty room with a couple of beds to put us up for maybe a night or two if we were lucky. Instead, there was a furnished sitting room with a roaring fire, two other rooms – a kitchen and bathroom – all fully equipped. They said – stay as long as need be, call us if you need us, we'll be there.[40]

While many women are working to eliminate the causes of battering, it is still essential that enough refuges are provided to enable women to escape and to start making a new life. Women's Aid (WA) believes that there should be at least one refuge in each town. Such refuges must operate not only as a sanctuary but also as a means by which women can discover their strength and recognize that battering is not a personal but a political problem. Throughout the UK, WA coordinates refuges. Contact them to find out about refuges in your area and for help in setting up new ones. Some refuges specialize in providing help solely for Asian women. WA can also give advice to women who don't want to go to a refuge.* (See Resources, p. 188.)

Refuges are for children too, and, although the conditions can be cramped and difficult, children can discover advantages of living in a communal setting and the relief of not having to witness any more beatings.

> I like being in a refuge 'cause it keeps my daddy from battering my mum. They are kind in a refuge. They help my mum forget about everything.[41]

If you are being battered, try to remember that there are ways out.

> I used to be terrified at the idea of coping alone but I've come to realize I always *was* a single parent when I was with my husband. What I've left behind is the violence, intimidation and abuse and I've found new strengths I never knew I had.[42]

> It's a big wrench having to give it all up and start again, but it's worth it.[43]

Contact one of the organizations listed on p. 188. They can give you expert advice and/or put you in touch with local women who can help.

More and more women are leaving men who batter, and finding help in making a new life despite economic hardships. Over the last decade, women throughout the UK have been organizing to help women leave abusive situations, to provide refuge and a more responsive legal system (see p. 181). Women have found the courage to tell their stories publicly. *We are not helpless, and we are not alone.*

*As we go to press, new social security regulations to cut housing benefit are coming into force that threaten the very existence of WA.

SEXUAL ABUSE OF CHILDREN WITHIN THE FAMILY

Most sexual abuse of children within the family is incestuous and involves older male relatives and younger female children, in families of every class and colour. A trusted family member or person in authority uses their power – as well as the child's love and dependence – to initiate sexual contact, and to ensure also that the relationship continues and remains secret. The child is rendered powerless.

> I was told so often that my husband was good to his daughters – look how they cling to him – that I was incapable of telling anyone directly that he sexually abused one of them. When I hinted at this to a very good friend she merely replied that I should be grateful he did not beat me. He did, but I kept this hidden too because I was so ashamed.
>
> I upped and left that expensive Surrey home five years ago; my eldest daughter still cannot talk about her experiences, and is still liable to collapse when she sees her father. She has learned, through careful training by my new husband, not to touch certain parts of his body, and not to allow herself to be touched. Her father still manages to upset her by punishing her 'neglect'.
>
> I have been ignored by my relatives since I left the father, while he enjoys regular visits from them. They include a nurse and a retired magistrate – all would have preferred two damaged children to grow up rather than have the disgrace which I have brought on the family by walking out of my home.
>
> If I had to do the same thing again I do not think I would be more capable of denouncing him. His power was so strong that my mind was paralysed, only my instinct to care for my children remained intact.[44]

> I live with my dad . . . I'm sixteen. He called me into his room to keep him company. He pushed me on to the bed and took his clothes off then mine. Then he made love to me in all sorts of ways. He has done it five times since then. It is becoming a sort of habit. I am disgusted and frightened to death. I want to run away. I can't tell my mum because he said it will be a secret between the two of us till we die.[45]

> I am just sixteen and feel like committing suicide . . . eight months ago I was raped by my father. I did not tell anyone but shut myself away . . . as much as I could . . . I was a virgin when it happened. Now I am eight months pregnant. About three months ago I told my mother I was pregnant. But I could never tell her who the father is. She was very shocked and would not speak to me. She forbade me to have an abortion.[46]

It is difficult to talk about sexual abuse within the family.

SOME IDEAS ABOUT HOW YOU CAN HELP YOURSELF

- Apply to the court for interim custody so that the man involved cannot legally take the children from you.
- Apply to the court to have him put out of the house (even if he owns it or it is in his name).
- Apply to the court for an injunction in England and Wales, interdict in Scotland, to stop him beating, harassing or frightening you or your children.
- Apply for a new house from the council if you are planning to leave or have had to leave home as a result of the violence.
- Claim social security money for you and your children if you have no job or are on a low income. You will also get free legal help.

SOME IDEAS FOR EMERGENCIES

- Think about how you would escape. Get the help of your neighbours or friends if you can.
- Put money aside for taxis, bus fares, telephone calls.
- Try to have your child benefit book, your rent book and if possible other certificates (e.g. marriage and birth certificates) handy to take with you.
- You might need to leave quickly – keep some clothes ready for you and the children (perhaps at a friend's house). Your children might also want to bring a small, favourite toy.
- Keep a key to your home.
- Keep the telephone numbers of your nearest Women's Aid group, the police, Samaritans and social worker handy. Have a pen and paper for the phone.
- Call the police immediately. If there were any witnesses ask if they'll make a statement.
- Get medical attention even if the injuries or bruising appear slight.
- Contact Women's Aid.

Some of us may never have told anyone, though the abuse may have continued for years. We never mentioned how we dreaded family gatherings, where a particular uncle would come after us. Every survivor has her own story. Many of us have kept our stories secret for years. This may be because of threats, feelings of guilt or responsibility – particularly if we enjoyed the sexual contact in any way – and also because it may have been the only physical warmth, or warmth of any kind, that we received as a child. We may also fear not being believed, in many cases with good reason,* as well as fearing the *results* of being believed, such as feeling 'responsible' for our father ending up in prison and/or the break-up of our parents' marriage.

My mother blamed me for the loss of her husband and bringing shame on the family. I've lost my family.

Feminist Insights

For many years 'experts' blamed mothers for 'abandoning' their children to sexually deprived husbands and accused young girls of being 'seductive' or of fantasizing about a sexual relationship with a male relative.** Feminists have challenged these victim-blaming views: sexual abuse in the family occurs primarily because men have power and women and children do not. Fathers, uncles and significant family contacts take advantage of the powerlessness of children because family structures allow them to misuse their power.

The worst thing . . . was not being able to tell anyone . . . It was not only that my father threatened to kill any of my family who talked, but also the fear that no one would believe us if we did.

[Noreen Winchester – who was convicted in 1976 for killing her father who had been raping her for years. She was released in 1978 following a concerted feminist campaign.]

Survivors

I am *not* a VICTIM of incest, but a SURVIVOR from incest.

I do not care for the term VICTIM because it too easily makes the woman believe that giving in is her function.

For a VICTIM is someone who has been struck down and accepts themselves as victim, and by staying down she signals that she can still be humiliated and will offer no protest.

A SURVIVOR from incest, on the other hand, is someone who has risen in protest and fought, and by this signals that she will not tolerate further abuse, be it from others or from herself through the self-oppression induced by the way in which girls are brought up.

To be a SURVIVOR from incest is the victorious conclusion.[47]

Those of us who have survived incest know that the effects of this abuse are life-long.* We often blame our-

---

*Professor Donald West's research confirms this (see Resources).

**Freud's betrayal of women's early memories of incest – insisting they were fantasies rather than reality – is a legacy that we still have to live with. See, for example, Alice Miller's *Thou Shalt Not Be Aware, Society's Betrayal of the Child* (see Resources).

*Kinsey suggested that incest as such had little long-term effect, but feminists have been contradicting this view for years. Now research is beginning to validate what we have always known.

selves long after the abuse has ended – for not saying no, for not fighting back, for telling or not telling, for having been 'seductive', for having trusted the abuser. Often there was no one to confirm that someone treated us cruelly and that this abuse was truly terrible.

Many of us have difficulty with sexual relationships because of the memories they revive. Many of us desire sexual intimacy yet have difficulty trusting. Some incest survivors feel comfortable with sex yet know that something is vaguely wrong.

It's been really hard to work out how this has affected me with men. I've had a hard time sorting out who is safe and who isn't. Now the only way I will sleep with someone is if I can have complete control. I need permission to feel uncomfortable with certain sexual acts.

Sometimes blaming ourselves takes other forms. Many teenagers with a history of abuse 'sleep around' to feel accepted, or run away. Many teenage and adult survivors feel depressed and don't know why, and/or turn to drugs and alcohol to mask the pain.

I often feel hopeless and suicidal. My father treated me with such violence that this is the only way I know to treat myself. I'm learning better ways now, but it's difficult.

I have been a drug addict. I have been anorexic. I have been a compulsive eater. Food was the only thing I could control and trust when people in my life failed me.*

To heal the emotional scars, we need to tell our stories to people who understand deeply what we have experienced.** Increasingly, women are setting up counselling or support groups for women who have been abused as children where they can break the silence, gain perspective and know they are not alone. Women who have been lucky enough to find this kind of help feel healthier and stronger.

I now have a lot of compassion for myself, because I know the implications of the abuse that occurred in my life. I owe myself all the understanding, patience and acceptance I can find.

Some women find that they need to confront the family members who abused them. This is a frightening task, but may also be rewarding:

I feel empowered by letting him know I am aware that the incest occurred. I feel empowered by the fact that I didn't ask him if he remembered, I just told him I knew he would deny it. I just wanted to say, 'This happened.' I did not expect results. Telling him was the total opposite of all that happened – what was invisible is now out in the open.

Those of us who have been sexually abused within our family need to know that whatever we do or don't do, we have done OK because we have survived a childhood that wasn't like a childhood at all.

See Resources for where incest survivors can find help. If you have suffered sexual abuse, however long ago, contact your nearest incest survivors' group.

PROSTITUTION

Contrary to the ugly stereotypes of prostitutes as fallen women, dope addicts or disease carriers,* prostitutes are women at work – supporting children as single parents, surviving economically in a job market which underpays women at every economic level. Many are housewives or secretaries moonlighting as prostitutes to make ends meet.

Once politically voiceless and isolated from other women, over the past ten years prostitutes have organized for support and political action.† As they speak out and write about their lives, they expose the many forms of violence which prostitutes experience:

1. The poverty which forces women – especially poor women, black women and runaway teenagers – into work as hookers (many women have no access to other jobs); the sexist job discrimination which means that even middle- and upper-class women can earn more in prostitution than in other jobs available to them; the fact that a great number of incest victims become prostitutes.

2. Police harassment.

3. Intimidation and beatings by pimps, to whom many prostitutes must give their earnings in return for protection. Many of them fear for their lives.

4. Lack of police protection: prostitutes without jobs in safer massage parlours or houses are often raped, beaten and left unpaid.

5. The arrest and prosecution of prostitutes while clients (most of whom are white, middle-aged, middle-class married men) go free.**

6. The racism and class bias which leads to the harass-

---

*In an eating disorders clinic in Leicester, of seventy-eight women, 64 per cent had been sexually abused, *80 per cent of whom had been abused as children*. In all cases, the anorexia continued until the scars had been healed. In a pilot study of women psychiatric patients, a very high level of sexual abuse in childhood was also reported.[48] Incest survivors may also find it difficult to be close to their own children.

**There is now increasing recognition both of the prevalence of abuse and of the degree of sensitivity required by people attempting to help incest survivors. We hope that increasingly, incest survivors and currently abused children will get the help they need.

*Only a tiny percentage of sexually transmitted disease is spread by prostitutes.
†Examples of such groups in Britain are PLAN (Prostitution Laws Are Nonsense) and ECP (English Collective of Prostitutes).
**Since 1982, imprisonment was abolished for the offence of street soliciting, but many prostitutes are still imprisoned because they cannot pay the hefty fines now being imposed.

ment of a disproportionate number of black women and poor women (whether prostitutes or not).

> As a middle-class white woman, trained as a registered nurse, I could work in a private call business instead of hitting the streets. I was arrested but never did time in prison; the system isn't aimed at putting me in jail. Women of colour have less easy access to places like upper-class hotels, where if you're black and alone you're automatically tagged as a hooker.

Some feminists have been critical of prostitutes for 'reinforcing sex-role stereotypes' by allowing themselves to be sex objects. Prostitutes point out that they are no different from most women in having to sell their services to men. In the words of an ex-prostitute:

> I've worked in straight jobs where I've felt more like I was prostituting my being than in prostitution. I had less control over my life, and the powerlessness wasn't even up front. People didn't see me as selling myself, but with the minimum wage so little and my boss so insulting, I felt I was selling my soul.

In a world where women have so little power, nearly all women depend in some way on men's money, protection, favour. Many who are not hookers, for example, feel they must have sex when their man wants to because he provides financial or emotional security. From feminist Karen Lindsey:

> The question of whether or not to sell ourselves to men is a false one: the real question is how to sell ourselves in the way that is least destructive to ourselves and our sisters. That is not a decision any one of us can make for any of the others. . . . Prostitutes don't need our condescension. What they need is our alliance. And we need theirs.[49]

Prostitutes have organized in this country and abroad (including the famous French prostitutes' strike in 1975) to demand *decriminalization*, the abolition of all laws against prostitution.* With decriminalization, prostitutes would have more control over their work and the money they earn. Most of all, they would no longer be prosecuted for providing a service which society itself puts in such high demand, and for choosing the highest-paying work available to them. (Legalizing prostitution isn't enough. In West Germany, where women work in government-run houses, prostitutes feel they have traded illegal pimps for a legal one: they have little control over their working conditions and still turn over a big part of their income in fees.) A longer-

*This campaign has been supported most notably by Tory Baroness Joan Vickers and by Maureen Colquhoun when a Labour MP. Ms Colquhoun's Protection of Prostitutes Bill was passed at its first reading, but never became law as a general election intervened and she lost her seat.

range goal is, in the words of one prostitute, that 'No woman should have to be a prostitute because she has no alternatives' and from another: 'The end of women's poverty is the end of prostitution.'[50]

WHAT ELSE CAN WE DO?

We need to find ways of protecting ourselves, while resisting the commonly-held view that *women* are responsible for whatever violence happens to us. As Golda Meir said, when legislators proposed a curfew on women in an attempt to lower the incidence of rape: 'It is the *men* who are attacking women. If there is to be a curfew, let the *men* stay home.'

We particularly need to learn better how to avoid violence *from a position of strength*. We need to cease trying to control men and limiting our own freedom.

> When he gets jealous, he can't control himself and that's when I'm scared because he usually hits out. He got so jealous of the few friends I had that it seemed best to stop seeing them. He had me to himself, and as long as I kept the house tidy and the kids quiet, and there was no one else around, he didn't hit me. The trouble is, you can't keep it up . . . and I had to talk to somebody.

Instead, we need to reframe our responsibility to ourselves, and clarify men's responsibility for their own actions. While we can be powerless against men's violence, we can also be powerful in deterring it. We need to believe in our power to change the course of male violence. This is different from believing we are responsible for the violence. But we will be able to do so from a position of strength only if we maintain full awareness that the true responsibility for male violence belongs to men. *Men must stop committing violence against women, stop each other from doing it, stop condoning it in others, and stop blaming women for it*. The problem must be *owned* by men. Women are not the problem.

In the meantime, we need to examine what may attract us, for example, to a man whose emotional vocabulary is so limited, or to a relationship that does not acknowledge either partner as a full human being. There are very many complex ways in which we can collude in our own oppression and one of these can be unconsciously to seek out relationships that make us feel comfortable by virtue of the fact that they demean us. We also need to examine our own violence.

> Those who stand up against violence should be honest about their own violence and their struggle with it. In that way, we, I, can be seen as ordinary and human like everyone else, but with a firm resolve to heal and stop the things within me that damage me and hurt people I love, because it is with people I love that I am most likely to feel the need to hurt.[51]

Our own knowledge about ourselves is an important key – but again only as long as we rigorously maintain our awareness that the responsibility for male violence is men's and our society's, which sustains them in their violent roles and behaviour.

Over the past fifteen years, we have directed our collective anger into many kinds of action opposing violence against women.*

- We organized consciousness-raising groups and discovered that our experiences of dominance by men were common and shared.
- We have taken on particular offenders. Women Against Violence Against Women (WAVAW), formed in 1980, has instituted a campaign against sex shops and has sought to have films banned that depict brutal violence against women. †
- Women have supported each other through the process of taking offenders to court.
- As a result of pressure from feminists, the laws relating to rape and domestic violence have been amended (although unless the attitudes of society generally and of judges and police change, legal reforms cannot be effective).
- The 1976 Tribunal of Crimes Against Women, held in Brussels and attended by women from all over the world, expanded the definition of violence against women to include dowry murders and genital mutilation.
- Some men have begun to work with other men on dealing with their violence. For groups we know about as we go to press see p. 188. Other men have worked for legislation, written articles or leaflets or made films. Some men have begun to hold each other accountable, legally and socially, for their violence, recognizing that men who do not take action support the system which promotes violence against women. They talk about their socialization in relation to women, question the extent and consequences of male dominance, listen to and respect the women around them.

Yet funding of projects and developments that protect women is becoming increasingly hard to get. Many refuges and other services are suffering from lack of funding.

We must continue to express our outrage loud and clear by keeping alive and expanding all the services to women, and by continuing to speak out. We will continue to teach our daughters to demand equality for themselves and others, and our sons to question sexism and violence, to respect women as equals and fight all forms of dominance.

*Throughout history women have protected themselves and each other from men's violence by fighting back, offering shelter, nursing and caring for each other. Unfortunately this chapter has no room for this proud history. Please see Resources.

†In the US, WAVAW organized a national boycott of Warner-Atlantic-Electra (a record company) and created a slide-show to educate teenagers and adults about ways in which companies profit from depicting violence towards women. After years of sustained pressure, WAVAW won an agreement from Warner to adopt guidelines on the depiction of violence against women and children on record sleeves.

We will continue to support one another in protecting ourselves with ingenuity, strength and pride. We applaud women who say no to male violence, who offer support to a friend, who protect each other, who fight back, who survive.

NO WOMAN IS SAFE UNTIL ALL OF US ARE SAFE

SELF-DEFENCE

Self defence is not a sport, it's a necessity! In Lewisham black and Vietnamese girls and women are taking classes because of the frequency of racial attacks on a particular estate.[52]

Many of us are reared in protective environments where fighting among girls is discouraged. As a result, we feel helpless and vulnerable and even go so far as to question our right to defend ourselves. We believe it's essential that women begin to take self-defence seriously. We need to build up and maintain strength and endurance to accomplish this (see Chapter 6). That strength alone, however, will not equip us to fight. Most women are afraid of pain and violence, and we have little sense of the potential power of our bodies. The physical and mental togetherness that comes from exercise and self-defence training not only teaches us this but also gives us added confidence in all areas of our lives.

'I used to feel as though I became public property whenever I walked in the city. Now I feel a private space around myself.' 'My fantasies are changing since I joined the class. When I think about situations that make me angry, I visualize the kinds of things we've learned to do, not just a vague blur of wanting to struggle.' 'It's especially mind-blowing for a short person like me. I've always felt totally helpless and walked around as if waiting to be victimized. Not any more.'[53]

Any activity which promotes self-confidence, self-knowledge or self-reliance is a form of self-defence. Learning self-defence, therefore, can include assertiveness training, exercise and/or sports, as well as 'self-defence' as such.

I have experienced such profound changes in my self-image and in the way that I see the world and relate to people that I really can't separate my study of self-defence from the rest of my life.

Inner and Outer Obstacles

Several myths can prevent us from defending ourselves effectively against a physical assault: that the assailant is invulnerable, that greater physical strength will decide who is to win, that we don't know how to defend ourselves. Yet we *can* defend ourselves against attack. One woman frightened off three adolescent males who were following

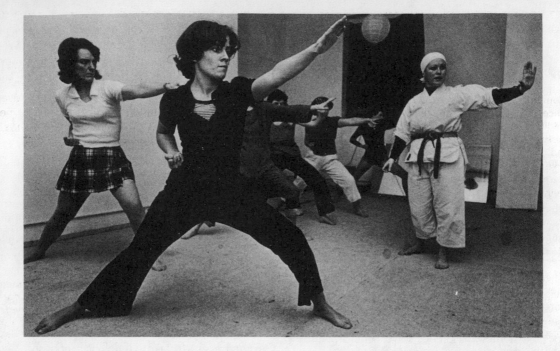

her along a city street by turning quickly and letting out a blood-curdling yell. Another stopped a would-be assailant with a kick. A young girl sitting on the train found a wayward hand on her knee. She took the man's wrist in her grasp, raised his hand high in the air and said loudly enough for the entire carriage to hear, 'Who does this belong to?' He got off at the next stop. There are hundreds of such stories. We don't see them on TV, we don't read them in the newspapers, but stop in at any self-defence class run by and for women and you'll hear them. We often attribute such escapes to luck or good fortune, not crediting our own courage and resourcefulness. It is important to our self-confidence to reclaim those successes.

There are people around us, particularly the men in our lives, who may consciously or unconsciously seek to discourage us from learning self-defence. As we begin to learn physical techniques, we begin to feel our confidence growing. We know how to break a hold, to avoid a grasp, to stay on our feet and keep our emotional and physical balance. Yet when we practise these techniques on men we know, we often fail, both because we have eliminated the element of surprise and because their resistance to our new skills undermines us. It is important to practise with people who support our efforts to become stronger.

We need to be on guard against the ideas that 'a little learning is a dangerous thing', and that fighting back only makes matters worse. Although compliance is sometimes a prudent response to assault (and self-defence classes can teach us when this is the case), it does not guarantee that a situation will not get worse. *In fact, studies have shown that women who use active resistance and who act quickly are more likely to avoid rape than those who use passive or no resistance.*

Classes

Teachers of judo, aikido and karate can all train us in fighting techniques. Jujitsu and some other martial-art styles train you to do combinations of the above in confrontation situations. But rather than recommending any one particular style, we suggest that you pick the school or class with the best attitude towards its students. Ideally, the instructor should take a really complete approach to women's safety, involving discussion, sharing, psychological aspects of self-defence, and role play. A good self-defence class teaches us to shift our self-awareness so that we remember that we are the sources of our own energy and the initiators of our own actions. Instead of freezing in the face of assault, we learn to mobilize our thoughts, assess the situation, make a judgement about the level of danger, choose the response we wish to make and then make it.

In some areas, special schools exist, for example in judo or karate. You can look them up in the phone book under the relevant technique. If no classes exist in your area, or you do not like the ones that do, you could ask your local authority to provide you with classes as long as there are at least ten people interested. It's also worth approaching your local branch of the workers' educational association, colleges of further education, university extra-mural departments or even your union. Try to find an instructor who takes women seriously.* If at all possible classes should be taught for women by women. A useful way to begin physical training is in a supportive atmosphere – to begin building your confidence. Ideally, a women's group can join a class or start a class together. Differently-abled women will have a greater chance of developing their own unique strengths in a supportive atmosphere.

Many male instructors give women a watered-down version of karate that allows no body contact. It could be helpful to arrange extra women's classes to work on techniques that are particularly hard or useful to the women

---

*Try to observe a class and if possible talk to the instructor; try to assess whether the students are learning what *you'd* like to learn.

LESSONS FROM GREENHAM

In December 1982:

> Women turned on their televisions and saw the fence, the baby clothes, and thirty thousand women holding hands around a nuclear base. The image spoke to them in a way that a hundred CND marches had failed to do ... Then came the blockades and base invasions, and the day at Halloween when men in uniform watched helpless as women cut down their fence.[54]

Since then, hundreds of women have cut down the fence, and countless forays have been made inside the base. By 1984:

> Lately, women have cut the fence and entered the cruise missile base almost every day and night. On Good Friday a large crucifix was planted inside, and a service completed before women were escorted out. On April 30th two women gained access to the control tower, again, and on May 1 twenty women cycled and roller-skated towards the air-strip.[55]

In 1985:

> Two women gave themselves up to the Ministry of Defence police yesterday after spending three days and nights living in a tent next to the runway inside Greenham Common Cruise missile base. Faye Johnson ... and Paula Yates ... were demonstrating, they said, that it is impossible to make the nine-mile perimeter of the US base secure against the determined protester or terrorist.[56]

> In 1986 two women entered the air base's vehicle compound on June 8th, for long enough to paint 50 vehicles; since the bombing of Libya, hangar doors have been painted every couple of days.[57]

The Greenham Women's Peace Camp brought home to many of us our strength and potential in the face of enormous opposition. Greenham shows us that we can *take action* – take the initiative – for our own peace and freedom. It stands as an inspiration for all women in relation to male violence as a whole.

For Greenham is not only about nuclear war, but also about exposing the nature of a society which endorses nuclear war, which is itself underpinned by the culture of male violence. 'Which side are you on?' goes the song sung in the film *Carry Greenham Home* by Sue, Ceri and Sally to some police as they busy themselves trying to get the women out of the way. Verse follows verse, with no hesitation, no letting up. The tenacity, the sense of purpose, the sheer power are almost tangible. The song begins with the violence of Cruise missiles and ends with the day-to-day violence of life on earth:

> Which side are you on?
> Are you on the side of death or life?
> Are you on the side that batters your wife?

Actions at Greenham like the above are non-violent, strong, courageous. They are often witty, colourful, dramatic and fun too. As Jean Freer says:

> *I believe Greenham has been an inspiration to the world because of the underlying appreciation of fun. As a woman from Belfast said recently, 'It's good to see happy people.' Being happy is a political act.*

Feminists in the anti-nuclear movement have made links with a broad range of issues, including imperialism and oppression worldwide (see Chapter 29), the campaign for a nuclear-free Pacific, and supported the miners' wives' movement.

Nuclear war is only the *ultimate* result of our patriarchal society. Peace is not merely the absence of war, but the absence of all forms of injustice.

In January 1984 *Jane's Defence Weekly* quoted Pentagon sources saying that the US and UK governments were concerned about the impact of the Greenham Women's Peace Camp, and that they couldn't carry out full exercises. The activity of Greenham women and other groups that have followed suit continues to disrupt deployment of Cruise missiles, despite a news blackout. Documents taken from inside the base indicate that they have continued to prevent 'nuclear alert exercises'.[58]

The 1987 Gorbachev/Reagan peace initiative must also be seen as a response to women's activities at Greenham and elsewhere. But perhaps more than this material effect on a handful of rulers, Greenham has ignited people's imagination throughout the world. Greenham is dynamite politically, morally, spiritually.

To find out about Greenham, other women's peace initiatives and the anti-nuclear movement generally, see p. 188.

there and to discuss ways of coping with the day-to-day sexism you face in the school. There are, of course, advantages in a mixed class: you learn how to fight men and see that they have weaknesses, too. A lot of male instructors know useful stuff about how women can effectively fight men, and if it's a good school they should teach it to you in a decent way as fast as you want to absorb it.

While self-defence cannot be learned from reading alone, Kaleghl Quinn's book *Stand Your Ground* is an excellent guide if we can't get to a class.

THINGS YOU CAN DO *NOW*

Strengthen your body with good nutrition and regular exercise, preferably with some combination of aerobics and weight training.

Work with friends to give feedback or in front of a mirror:

1. practise walking with strong, even strides, looking as if you know where you're going;

2. practise loud yelling, accompanied by ferocious facial expressions;

3. tell someone to take his hands off you, giving a coherent message through a combination of words, tone of voice and facial expression;

4. act out 'what if' situations, discuss various responses and drill the best ones.

ASIAN GIRL IN BRITAIN

My stomach tightens
Sickeningly,
As I read of the
Murder of the Sikhs.
Of the women, who cry
'That they have no family left'.
Not mentioning their
Daughters.
Raped and Invisible.
My mind protests
At the momentary Insanity
Of my people.
The Hindus, Sikhs
Muslims and Tamils.
My colour betrayed
My womb, Violated.
The killing and dying
A reflection of the
White man's maxim
'Divide and Rule'.
As I am called
Names in the streets,
My body flinches
And my Anger appears.
Wondering, if it is

Racist or Sexist abuse.
If it's my lucky day
It's both!
Age is no barrier
In this game called
'Keeping a coloured girl down'.
As a little old white woman
Attacks.
As a Four-year-old throws
A Stone.
And the white youth of my age
Gang up!
And I realize
'Self-defence becomes no offence'.

However my fighting spirit
Is suddenly submerged
As I mentally laugh and cry
On hearing yet another
'Right-on' Black man
Listing on the
'Political Agenda'.
The Woman's Question
To be dealt with
Last.
And feeling Ignored
And Distanced.
As I hear yet another
Young Asian boy saying
'I will never let my sister
Come to a function like this!'
As he walks out with his
White girl friend . . .
My voice is then silenced
Into a Whisper.
But soon, gaining in
Strength.
You will hear me
Shout, loud.
For a new place
In this world
For me.

© ABIDA PARVEEN

NOTES

1. 'Rapists' Aid', *New Society*, 8 November 1985, p. 228.

2. A US study revealed in 1981 that women far more than men report that fear curtails their daily activities. The most fearful women are the elderly, the poor and members of racial/ethnic minorities. See Stephanie Riger and Margaret Gordon. 'The Fear of Rape: A Study of Social Control', *Journal of Social Issues*, no. 37, 1981, pp. 71–92.

3. Diana Scully and Joseph Marolla. *Social Problems*, vol. 31, no. 5, 1984, p. 530.

4. See, e.g., ibid.; and *New Society*, op. cit., note 1.

5. From a letter to *Spare Rib*, no. 170, September 1986.

6. Gillian Booth quoted in Barbara Harford and Sarah Hopkins. *Greenham Common: Women at the Wire*. London: Women's Press, 1984.

7. Cosis Brown. 'Child Abuse – a Failure of Social Work Practice?' *Spare Rib*, no. 161, January 1986.

8. Jill Radford. 'Retrospect on Trial', *New Society*, 9 September 1982, p. 423.

9. A US study in 1980 found that black women were less likely to have their cases come to trial and to result in conviction than white women. See G. D. LaFree. 'Variables Affecting Guilty Pleas and Convictions in Rape Cases – Towards a Social Theory of Rape Processing', *Social Forces*, no. 58, 1980, pp. 833–50.

10. Leonie Abrahamson. 'Dodgy Dons', *Spare Rib*, no. 144, July 1984.

11. Reported in the *Guardian*, 5 September 1985.

12. *The Independent*, 20 May 1988.

13. *Spare Rib*, no. 71, June 1978.

14. Linda in *Peace News*, August 1986.

15. See Anne Sedley and Melissa Benn. *Sexual Harassment at Work* (pamphlet). London: NCCL, 1984; Elizabeth Wilson. *What is to be Done About Violence Against Women?* London: Penguin Books, 1983.

16. From NCCL, op. cit., note 12.

17. Melissa Benn. *Spare Rib*, no. 156, July 1985.

18. Medea, Andra and Kathleen Thompson. *Against Rape*. USA: Noonday Press, 1975.

19. From a letter to *Spare Rib*, no. 150, January 1985.
20. See, for example, N. J. Wild, 'Sexual Abuse of Children in Leeds', *British Medical Journal*, 26 April 1986, p. 1113; and Gitta Sereny, *The Invisible Children*. London: Pan, 1986.
21. Fern Mims and Audrey Chang. 'Unwanted Sexual Experiences', *Journal of Psychosocial Nursing*, vol. 22, no. 6, p. 7.
22. Lorenne Clark and Debra Lewis. *Rape: the Price of Coercive Sexuality*. London: Women's Press, 1987.
23. The Baroness Seear and Elaine Player. *Women in the Legal System*. Report for the Howard League for Penal Reform, 1986.
24. Angela Neustatter. 'Defence Tactics', *Guardian*, 13 February 1985.
25. Polly Pattullo. *Judging Women – a Study of Attitudes that Rule Our Legal System* (pamphlet). London: NCCL, 1983.
26. Susan Edwards. *Women on Trial*. Manchester: Manchester University Press, 1984.
27. See, for example, Seear and Player, op. cit., note 21.
28. NACRO. 'Offences Against Discipline in Women's Prisons', 1986.
29. As reported in the *Guardian*, 19 January 1988, p. 3.
30. London Armagh Group. 'Strip Searches in Armagh Jail'. *Women Behind the Wire*, no. 2, 1984, p 14. Available from Stop the Strip Searches Campaign (see p. 188).
31. Chris Shaw. 'Crisis in Holloway Prison', *Openmind*, no. 12, December 1984–January 1985.
32. Quoted in ibid.
33. H. Saville et al. 'Spouse Abuse: Economic and Psychological Factors', *Australian and New Zealand Journal of Sociology*, vol. 17., no. 1, 1982, p. 83.
34. R. E. Dobash and R. Dobash. *Violence Against Wives*. Shepton Mallet: Open Books, 1980.
35. D. Marsden and D. Owens. 'The Jekyll and Hyde Marriages', *New Society*, 8 May 1975, p. 333.
36. Scottish Women's Aid, *Newsletter*, December 1984.
37. Polly Toynbee. 'Shocking Sentence', *Guardian*, 17 March 1987.
38. Scottish Women's Aid, *Annual Report*, 1983.
39. From Erin Pizzey. *Scream Quietly or the Neighbours Will Hear*. London: Penguin Books, 1974.
40. Scottish Women's Aid, op. cit., note 3.
41. Ibid.
42. Scottish Women's Aid, op. cit., note 34.
43. Scottish Women's Aid, op. cit., note 3.
44. Anonymous letter to the *Guardian*, 8 October 1985.
45. Anonymous letter to *Just Seventeen* magazine, 1985.
46. Anonymous letter to ibid.
47. Inge Halles. *Spare Rib*, no. 144, July 1984, p. 6.
48. Michael Levin. 'A Major New Factor in Mental Illness Say Doctors', *The Times*, 30 November 1984.
49. Karen Lindsey. 'Beginning to Demystify the Oldest Profession', *The Second Wave*, Summer 1976.
50. Claude Jager (ed.). *Prostitutes: Our Life*. Bristol: Falling Wall Press, 1986, p. 31.
51. Gillian Booth quoted in Harford and Hopkins op. cit., note 5.
52. GLC Women's Bulletin, January–February 1984.
53. Sarita Cordell. 'Self-Confidence/Defence', *The Second Wave*, vol. 2, no. 4, 1973.
54. Rachel Lever. *Spare Rib*, no. 142, May 1984.
55. Diana McKenzie. 'Bigger Gates', *Guardian*, 25 May 1984.
56. Paul Brown. 'Two Women Camp Inside Greenham Base', *Guardian*, 6 September 1985.
57. 'Greenham Common', *Peace News*, 20 June 1986.
58. Susan Thomas. 'Why They Break the Law in Order to Keep the Peace', *Guardian*, 26 January 1985.

RESOURCES
PUBLICATIONS

GENERAL

Barry, Kathleen. *Female Sexual Slavery*. Englewood Cliffs, NJ: Prentice Hall, 1979.
Brownmiller, Susan. *Against Our Will*. London: Penguin Books, 1977.
Coveney, L. et al. *The Sexuality Papers – Male Sexuality and the Social Control of Women*. London: Hutchinson/Explorations in Feminism Collective, 1984.
GLC Women's Committee. *Women on the Move*, Women's Committee Bulletin, special issue on transport, August–September 1985.
GLC Women's Committee. *Racial Harassment on Lincoln Estate*. Report, 1984.
Gus, John. 'The Trials of Jackie Berkeley', *Race Today*, May–June 1985, pp. 8–10. About a young black woman's conviction for 'wasting police time' for alleging that she had been raped by police officers in a Manchester police station.
Hanmer, Jalna. *Violence Against Women*. Unit 15 of Open University Course 'The Changing Experience of Women'. Milton Keynes: Open University Press, 1983.
Hanmer, Jalna and Sheila **Saunders**. *Well-founded Fear: a Community Study of Violence to Women*. London: Hutchinson, 1984.
Hanmer, Jalna and Mary **Maynard** (eds). *Women, Violence and Social Control*. London: Macmillan, 1987.
Hollway, Wendy. '"I Just Wanted to Kill a Woman" – Why? The Ripper and Male Sexuality', *Feminist Review*, no. 9, Autumn 1981.
Jaget, Claude (ed.). *Prostitutes: Our Life*. Bristol: Falling Wall Press, 1986.
James, Selma. 'Hookers in the House of Lords', in Joy Holland (ed.). *Feminist Action I*. London: Battle Axe Books (distributed by J. M. Dent), 1984.
Lamplugh, Diana. *Beating Aggression*. London: Weidenfeld and Nicolson, 1988.
Levine, June. *Lyn, A Story of Prostitution*. London: Women's Press, 1988.
Lobel, Kerry (ed.). *Naming the Violence – Speaking Out About Lesbian Battering*. Seattle: The Seal Press, 1986.
London Rape Crisis Centre. *Sexual Violence – the Reality for Women*. London: Women's Press, 1984.
Manchester Police Monitoring Unit. *Breaking the Silence: Manchester Women Speak Out*. Manchester, 1988. (Available from PMU, St James' Building, 4th Floor, 89 Oxford Street, Manchester M1 6FQ.) Based on the experiences of nearly 2,000 women, and includes recommendations.
Miller, Alice. *For Your Own Good. Hidden Cruelty in Childrearing and the Roots of Violence*. London: Faber and Faber, 1983. Chilling overview of the roots of violence, from a psychoanalytic perspective.
Quinn, Kaleghl. *Stand Your Ground*. London: Macdonald Optima, 1988. Comprehensive and outstanding book on self-defence. Also a Channel Four series.
Rhodes, Dusty and Sandra **McNeill**. *Women against Violence against Women*. London: Onlywomen Press, 1985.
Roberts, Yvonne. 'Tackling Racism by Doorstep Canvassing', *The Independent*, 2 October 1988.
Sedley, Anne and Melissa **Benn**. *Sexual Harassment at Work* (pamphlet). London: NCCL, 1984.
Sereny, Gitta. *The Invisible Children*. London: Pan, 1986.
Smart, Carol and Barry **Smart**. *Women, Sexuality and Social Control*. London: Routledge and Kegan Paul, 1978.
Thornhill, Teresa. 'Other People's Revolutions', in *Trouble and Strife*, no. 6, Summer 1985. A thoughtful article which, among other things, makes links between violence against women generally and the way this is viciously played out in wartime.
Tompson, Keith. *Under Siege: Racial Violence in Britain Today*. London: Penguin Books, 1988.
Wilson, Elizabeth. *What is to be Done about Violence Against Women?* London: Penguin Books, 1983.
Women's Health Information Centre. 'Women and Violence'. Special edition of *The Newsletter*, No. 9, Autumn 1987. Available from WHRRIC (see p. 638).

PORNOGRAPHY

Brown, Beverley. 'A Feminist Interest in Pornography – Some Modest Proposals', *m/f*, nos 5–6, 1981.
Campbell, Beatrix. 'A Feminist Sexual Politics: Now You See It, Now You Don't', *Feminist Review*, Summer 1980.
Coward, Ros. 'What is Pornography? Two opposing feminist viewpoints', *Spare Rib*, no. 119, June 1982.
Delacoste, Frédérique and Priscilla **Alexander**. *Sex Work: Writings by*

Women in the Sex Industry. London: Virago Press, 1988.

Dworkin, Andrea. *Pornography: Men Possessing Women*. London: Women's Press, 1981.

Everywoman Magazine. *Pornography and Sexual Violence: Evidence of the Links*. London: Everywoman, 1988.

Griffin, Susan. *Pornography and Silence*. London: Women's Press, 1981.

Kappeler, Susanne. *The Pornography of Representation*. Oxford: Polity Press, 1986.

Lederer, L. (ed.). *Take Back the Night: Women on Pornography*. New York: Morrow, 1980.

Lovelace, Linda. *Ordeal: an Autobiography*. London: W. H. Allen, 1981. A horrifying account of what Linda Lovelace's life was really like and the horrendous abuse she suffered.

Rich, B. Ruby. 'Anti-Porn: Soft Issue, Hard World', *Feminist Review*, no. 13, Spring 1983.

Seaton, Jean. 'Pornography and Feminism', *New Socialist*, no. 8, November–December 1982.

Snitow, Ann et al. *Desire: the Politics of Sexuality*. London: Virago Press, 1984.

Tomkinson, M. *The Pornbrokers: the Rise of the Soho Sex Barons*. London: Virgin Books, 1982.

Women Against Violence Against Women. 'Pornography: Two Opposing Feminist Viewpoints', *Spare Rib*, no. 119, June 1982.

See also books in other sections, e.g. Brownmiller, Hanmer, Wilson.

RAPE

Box-Grainger, Jill. *Sentencing Rapists*. London: Radical Alternatives to Prison, 1982.

Clark, Lorenne and Debra **Lewis**. *Rape: the Price of Coercive Sexuality*. London: Women's Press, 1987.

Hall, Ruth E. et al. *The Rapist Who Pays the Rent*: Evidence submitted to the Criminal Law Revision Committee on Changing the Law on Rape. Bristol: Falling Wall Press, 1984.

Hall, Ruth E. et al. *Ask Any Woman. A London Inquiry into Rape and Sexual Assault*. Bristol: Falling Wall Press, 1985.

Medea, Andra and Kathleen **Thompson**. *Against Rape: a Survival Manual for Women*. USA: Noonday Press, 1975.

Smart, Carol. 'Investigating Rape', *New Society*, 24 January 1985.

Warren-Holland, Diana et al. *Self-defence for Women*. London: Hamlyn, 1987.

WOMEN IN PRISON

Black Women in Prison. GLC Conference Report 1985.

Carlen, Pat. *Women's Imprisonment: a Study in Social Control*. London: Routledge and Kegan Paul, 1984.

Carlen, Pat (ed.). *Criminal Women*. Oxford: Polity Press, 1985.

D'Arcy, Margaretta. *Tell Them Everything*. London: Pluto Press, 1984.

Edwards, Susan. *Women on Trial*. Manchester: Manchester University Press, 1984.

GLC Women's Committee. *Women's Imprisonment: Breaking the Silence*, 1986 (available from Women's Equality Group, London Strategic Policy Unit, Room 401, Middlesex House, 20 Vauxhall Bridge Road, London SW1V 2SB).

Kee, Cynthia. 'Strip Search', *Observer*, 17 July 1986, p. 41.

Murphy, Pat and Nell **McCafferty**. *Women in Focus: Contemporary Irish Women's Lives*. Dublin: Attic Press, 1987.

NACRO (see Organizations). *Offences Against Discipline in Women's Prisons*. London: NACRO, 1986. *Mothers and Babies in Prison*, 1986.

NCCL. *Strip Searching – an inquiry into the strip searching of women remand prisoners at Armagh Prison between 1982 and 1985*. London: NCCL, 1986.

Pattullo, Polly. *Judging Women – a Study of Attitudes that Rule our Legal System* (pamphlet). London: NCCL, 1983.

Peckham, Audrey. *A Woman in Custody*. London: Fontana, 1985.

Seear, The Baroness and Elaine **Player**. *Women in the Penal System*. Howard League (see Organizations), January 1986.

Shaw, Chris. 'Inside Dope', *Openmind*, no. 4, August–September 1983.

Shaw, Chris. 'Crisis in Holloway Prison', *Openmind*, no. 12, December 1984–January 1985.

BATTERING

Battered Women Need Refuges. Booklet available from Women's Aid Federation, see Organizations.

Binney, Val et al. *Leaving Violent Men – a Study of Refuges and Housing for Battered Women*. Women's Aid Federation (England), 1981.

Borkowski, Margaret et al. *Marital Violence – the Community Response*. London: Tavistock, 1983.

Clout! – The Story behind the Bruises. Manchester: Commonword, 1980 (available from feminist bookshops or Scottish Women's Aid).

Dobash, R. E. and R. **Dobash**. *Violence Against Wives*. Shepton Mallet: Open Books, 1980.

Evason, Eileen. *Hidden Violence*. Belfast: Farset Coop Press, 1982. About battering in Northern Ireland.

Horley, Sandra. *Love and Pain: How Women Can Survive Destructive Relationships*. London: Bedford Square Press, 1988.

Kennedy, Stanislaus. *But Where Can I Go? Homeless Women in Dublin*. Dublin: Arlen House, 1985.

London Strategic Monitoring Service. *Police Response to Domestic Violence*. Police Monitoring and Research Group Briefing Paper, no. 1, London, 1986.

Pahl, Jan (ed.). *Private Violence and Public Policy. The Needs of Battered Women and the Response of the Public Services*. London: Routledge and Kegan Paul, 1985.

Pizzey, Erin. *Scream Quietly or the Neighbours Will Hear*. London: Penguin Books, 1974.

Robertson, Sue. *Shared Housing for Women Who Have Left a Violent Relationship*. Edinburgh: Culdion Housing Association, 1984. Available from SWA (see below).

Turner, Janine. *Behind Closed Doors*. Wellingborough, Northants: Thorsons, 1988.

Welsh Women's Aid. *Don't Break Down – Break Out*. Report from Women and Mental Health Conference, 1982.

Women's Aid Federation (England). *You Can't Beat a Woman – Women and Children in Refuges*, 1985. Personal histories by battered women and their children.

Wroe, Martin. 'The Violent Chauvinism that Lies behind the Church', *The Independent*, 24 August 1988, p 19.

SEXUAL ABUSE OF CHILDREN

Baker, Anthony. *Survey of Sexual Experiences in Childhood of Cross Section of British Population*, MORI and Channel Four, 1984.

Campbell, Bea. *Unofficial Secrets – Child Sexual Abuse: the Cleveland Case*. London: Virago Press, 1988.

Elliot, Michele. *Preventing Child Sexual Assault: a practical guide to talking with children* (pamphlet). London: Bedford Square Press, 1985.

Feminist Review. *Family Secrets: Child Sexual Abuse Today*. Special Issue 28 March 1988.

Fitzgerald, Kitty. *Marge*. London: Sheba, 1984. A novel, about incest among other things.

Forward, Susan and Craig **Buck**. *Betrayal of Innocence: Incest and its Devastation*. London: Penguin Books, 1981. This book includes a chapter on mother–daughter incest.

Fraser, Sylvia. *My Father's House: A Memoir of Incest and Healing*. London: Virago Press, 1989. A personal testament to the extent to which a child's horrific experiences can be completely buried, and then uncovered in adult life and ultimately, through forgiveness, healed.

Herman, Judith. *Father–Daughter Incest*. Cambridge, MA: Harvard University Press, 1981.

Kraizer, Sherryll Kerns. *The Safe Child*. New York: Delacorte, 1985.

MacFadyean, Melanie. 'I is for Incest', *New Society*, 24 January 1986, p. 140.

Miller, Alice. *Thou Shalt Not Be Aware: Society's Betrayal of the Child*. London: Pluto Press, 1985.

National Society for Prevention of Cruelty to Children, South West Region Working Party. *Report: Developing a Child-centred Response to Sexual Abuse*. London: NSPCC, 1984.

Nelson, Sarah. *Incest: Fact and Myth*. Edinburgh: Stramullion, 1982. Gives an excellent overview of the issues.

Porter, Ruth (ed.). *Child Sexual Abuse Within the Family*. London: Tavistock, 1984.

Rush, Florence. *The Best Kept Secret: Sexual Abuse of Children*. Englewood Cliffs, NJ: Prentice-Hall, 1980. Documents the history of the sexual abuse of children by reviewing the Bible, myths, fairy tales and popular literature. Looks at the role of legal institutions, psychology and 'kiddie porn' in perpetuating the victimization of children.

Scottish Women's Aid. *Information Pack on Incest*. Available from SWA, DASS, 1 High Street, Dundee. Tel: 0382–24422.

Spring, Jacqueline. *Cry Hard and Swim: the Story of an Incest Survivor*. London: Virago Press, 1987.

Ward, Elizabeth. *Father Daughter Rape*. London: Women's Press, 1984.

West, Donald (ed.). *Sexual Victimisation*. London: Gower, 1985.

GREENHAM AND THE PEACE MOVEMENT

Brown, Wilmette. *Black Women and the Peace Movement*. Bristol: Falling Water Press, 1984 (pamphlet, available from King's Cross Women's Centre, 71 Tonbridge Street, London WC1).

Caldicott, Helen. *Nuclear Madness*. London: Bantam, 1981.

Cambridge Women's Peace Collective. *My Country is the Whole World*. London: Pandora, 1984.

Cook, Alice and Gwyn **Kirk**. *Greenham Women Everywhere*. London: Pluto Press, 1983.

Harford, Barbara and Sarah **Hopkins**. *Greenham Common: Women at the Wire*. London: Women's Press, 1984.

Jones, Lynne. *Keeping the Peace: Women's Peace Handbook*. London: Women's Press, 1983.

McKenzie, Diana. 'Bigger Gates', *Guardian*, 25 May 1984.

Radical Statistics. *The Nuclear Numbers Game: Understanding the Statistics behind the Bomb*, 1982 (available from BSSRS, 9 Poland Street, London W1).

Rowe, Dorothy. *Living with the Bomb*. London: Routledge and Kegan Paul, 1985.

Thompson, Dorothy (ed.). *Over Our Dead Bodies – Women Against the Bomb*. London: Virago Press, 1983.

Women Working for a Nuclear Free and Independent Pacific. *Pacific Women Speak: Why Haven't You Known?* Oxford, 1988. (Available from Green Line, 34 Cowley Road, Oxford OX4 1HZ.)

ORGANIZATIONS

GENERAL

Campaign Against Pornography, c/o 9 Poland Street, London W1V 3DG. Tel: 01–287 0519.

Campaign against Pornography and Censorship. PO Box 844, London SE5 9QP. Tel: 01–908 7093.

Criminal Injuries Compensation Board, Whittington House, 19–30 Alfred Place. Chenies Street, London WC1E 7LG. Tel: 01–636 2812/9501.

English Collective of Prostitutes, King's Cross Women's Centre, 71 Tonbridge Street, London WC1 9DZ. Tel: 01–837 7509.

Interhelp, 4a High Tenterfell, Kendal, Cumbria LA9 4PG. Tel: 0539–29256. A growing network aiming to provide people with the opportunity to share their deepest responses to planetary dangers such as the nuclear threat, in order to move beyond feelings of powerlessness and numbness into action. Based on the 'Despair and Empowerment' work of Joanna Macy.

Men, Women and God, c/o St Peter's Church, Vere Street, London W1. Aims to counter the oppressive attitudes towards women by members of the Church of England, and to help women who are suffering from violent men in the Church.

National Children's Homes Careline (formerly **Family Network**), Cardinal Heenan Centre, 326 High Road, Ilford, Essex IG1 1QP. Tel: 01–514 1177. For your nearest number, ring this number or the Samaritans or look in the phone book. Provides confidential help for parents under stress.

National Council for Civil Liberties, 21 Tabard Street, London SE1 4LA.

Safe Women's Transport, c/o London Women's Centre, Wesley House, 4 Wild Court, London WC2B 5AU.

Suzy Lamplugh Trust, 14 East Sheen Avenue, London SW14 8AS. Tel: 01–876 1838. Set up to increase awareness of aggression at work.

Women Against Sexual Harassment (WASH), 242 Pentonville Road, London N1 9UN.

Women Against Violence Against Women (WAVAW), c/o London Women's Centre, Wesley House, 4 Wild Court, London WC2B 5AU.

Women's Media Action, c/o London Women's Centre, Wesley House, 4 Wild Court, London WC2B 5AU.

Workers Against Racism, BM WAR London WC1N 3XX. Tel: 01–729 0414 (24-hour answering service).

RAPE

Rape Crisis Centres. Tel: 01–837 1600. *Spare Rib* magazine (see p. 637) publishes up-to-date lists of rape crisis centres and phone lines throughout the UK (see also p. 188). Alternatively, ring the Samaritans for your nearest contact, or try looking under 'Rape' in the phone book.

WOMEN IN PRISON

Belfast Strip Search Campaign, c/o The Women's Centre, Falls Road, Belfast 12.

Black Female Prisoners Scheme, Brixton Enterprise Centre, 444 Brixton Road, London SW9. Tel: 01–733 5520.

Christian Response to Strip Searching Group, 224 Lisburn Road, Belfast. Publishes a booklet, *The Christian Response to Strip Searching*, 1987.

Howard League for Penal Reform, 320–22 Kennington Park Road, London SE11 4PP. Tel: 01–735 3317: campaigns for reform and takes up individual cases.

National Association for the Care and Resettlement of Offenders (NACRO), 169 Clapham Road, London SW9 0PU. Tel: 01–582 6500: sponsored by the Home Office but has an excellent information service and runs many valuable projects, e.g. on housing and employment.

PROP (National Prisoners Movement), BM-PROP, London WC1N 3XX. Tel: 01–542 3744: organized by and for prisoners/ex-prisoners. Campaigns for prisoners' rights and also helps individuals.

Radical Alternatives to Prison, BMC Box 4842, London WC1N 3XX. Publishes a quarterly journal, *The Abolitionist*.

Stop the Strip Searches Campaign, 52–4 Featherstone Street, London EC1 8RT. Tel: 01–251 6538/253 2033.

Women in Prison, Unit 3, Cockpit Yard, Northington Street, London WC1 2NP. Tel: 01–609 7463. Campaigning group of women ex-prisoners. Practical help to prisoners and ex-prisoners.

Women Prisoners' Resource Centre, 1 Thorpe Close, Ladbroke Grove, London W10 5XL. Tel: 01–968 3121: offers practical help to prisoners and ex-prisoners, not only in London.

BATTERING

International Working Group on Women and the Family, c/o London Women's Centre, Wesley House, 4 Wild Court, London WC2B 5AU.

Women's Aid Federations can put you in touch with your nearest women's aid refuge:

England: PO Box 391, Bristol BS99 7WS. Tel: 0272–420611 (admin)/428368 (helpline).

Scotland: 11 St Colme Street, Edinburgh EH3 6AA. Tel: 031–225 8011.

Wales: 38–48 Crwys Road, Cardiff CF2 4NN. Tel: 0222–462291/390874.

Northern Ireland: 129 University Street, Belfast BT7 1HP. Tel: 0232–249041/249358.

The above organizations also distribute a wide variety of materials, including videos.

Asian women needing help can contact WAF addresses above, or **Brent Asian Women's Resource Centre** (134 Minet Avenue, London NW10. Tel: 01–961 6549/5701) can put you in touch with Asian women's refuges direct. **Asha Women's Resource Centre** (27 Santley Street, London SW4 7QF. Tel: 01–274 8854 or 737 5901) also runs a refuge for single girls and young women, and can put you in touch with other, similar refuges. **Shakti Women's Aid** (PO Box 21, Edinburgh EH1 3JY. Tel: 031–557 4010) provides support and refuge for black and Asian women.

CHILD SEXUAL ABUSE

Black Women's Campaign against Rape and Sexual Abuse, c/o 241 Albion Road, London N16 9JT.

Bristol S.A.I.L., (Sex Abuse and Incest Lifeline): 0272–555578.

Childline 0800–1111. Telephone counselling service.

Incest Crisis Line, 66 Marriott Close, Bedfont, Feltham, Middlesex. Tel: 01–890 4732/01–422 5100. Aims to help anyone in any way involved with incest.

Irish Society for the Prevention of Cruelty to Children. Tel: 0001–760423/4/5 or 760452.

Kidscape, Campaign for the Prevention of Sexual Assault on Children, 82 Brook Street, London W1Y 1YG. Tel: 01–493 9845.

Mothers of Abused Children. Tel: 0965–31432.

National Society for Prevention of Cruelty to Children (head office), 67 Saffron Hill, London EC1N 8RS. Tel: 01–242 1626.

Royal Scottish Society for the Prevention of Cruelty to Children. Tel: 031–337 8539/8530.

Scottish Sexual Abuse Liaison Group, c/o Women's Support Project, Newlands Centre, 871 Springfield Road, Glasgow G31 4HQ. Tel: 041–554 5669.

Spectrum Incest Intervention Project, 7 Endymion Road, London N4 1EE. Tel: 01–348 0196. Registered charity providing counselling for anyone who has experience of incest in any way, as well as training and education for those working with sexual abuse. No person is turned away for lack of funds.

Taboo, PO Box 38, Manchester M60 1HG. For survivors of sexual abuse. Crisis Line number: 061–236 1712.

Touchline. Tel: 0532–457777. Telephone counselling service.

GREENHAM AND THE PEACE MOVEMENT

Campaign against the Arms Trade (CATT), 11 Goodwin Street, London N4 3HQ. Tel: 01–281 0297.

Campaign for the Demilitarization of the Indian Ocean, c/o Jaya, 30 Stonedene Close, Forest Row, East Sussex RH18 5DB. Tel: 034282–4603.

Campaign for Nuclear Disarmament (CND), 22–4 Underwood Street, London N1 7JQ. Tel: 01–250 4010.

Greenham Women Support Group, c/o Lynette Rees, 10 Northcote Road, Southsea, Portsmouth. Tel: 0705–829390.

Women Opposed to the Nuclear Threat (WONT), 40 Thornhill Square, London N1.

Women's Peace Alliance, c/o Sue Scott, 18 Bromley Gardens, Codsall, Wolverhampton WV8 1BE.

Women's Peace Camp, Wood Gate, Greenham Common, Northside, Burys Bank Road, Newbury, Berkshire.

GROUPS THAT WORK WITH VIOLENT MEN WHO WANT TO CHANGE

Change, c/o Russell Dobash, Stirling University, Stirling, Scotland.

Men Overcoming Violence (MOVE). Many men from MOVE are prepared to answer calls from anywhere. These are the MOVE groups we know about: **Bolton**, PO Box 25, South PDO, Manchester M14 6ND. Tel: 0204–364550; **Bristol**, c/o 1 Mark Lane, Bristol BS1 4XR, Tel: 0272–710763; **Manchester**, address as for Bolton, Tel: 061–227 9931.

By the time you read this, there will also be a project in London. Contact Adam Jukes, c/o 7 Hylda Court, St Albans Road, London NW5 1RE. Tel: 01–267 8713.

RAPE CRISIS CENTRES

Many rape crisis centres now have 24 hr ansaphones on which you can leave a message at any time.

ENGLAND

Birmingham (02–233 2122) 24 hr counselling: PO Box 558, Birmingham B3 2HL. **Bradford** (0274–308270 Mon 1–5pm/Thur 6–10pm): c/o 31 Manor Row, Bradford BD1 4PS. **Brighton** (0273–203773 Tue 6–9pm/Fri 3–9pm/Sat 10–1pm): PO Box 332 Hove, East Sussex. **Bristol** also contact for incest survivors group (0272–428311 Mon–Fri 10.30–2.30pm): 39 Jamaica St, Stokes Croft, Bristol B2. **Cambridge** (0223–358314 Wed 6–9pm/Sat 11–5pm): Box R. 12 Mill Rd, Cambridge. **Carlisle** (0228–36500 Mon 1.30–4.30pm/Wed 7–10pm): (PO Box 34 CA 112 Kendal, Cumbria. **Chelmsford** (0245–467076 Fri 7.30–9.30pm): PO Box 566, Chelmsford. **Cleveland** (0642–225787 Mon–Wed 10.30pm/Thur 10–30pm and 7–10pm): PO Box 31, Middlesbrough, Cleveland. **Coventry** (0203–77229 Mon 11–3pm and 7–10pm/Tue–Fri 11–3pm): PO Box 176, Bishop St, Coventry CV1 2OS. **Croydon** (01–656 5362 Sat 3–6pm/Tue 7–10): c/o 13 Woodside Green, London SE25. **Derby** (0332–372545 Thur 7.30–9.30pm): c/o Women's Centre, The Guildhall, Derby. **Dorset** (0305–772295): c/o 34 Charles St, Weymouth. **Exeter** (039–90871) 24 hr counselling: c/o Exeter Women's Centre, 94 Sidwell St, Exeter. **Gloucester** (0452–26770 Mon/Tue/Wed/Fri 7.30–8.30pm/Thur 11.30–2pm): Russett House, Russett Close, Tuffley, Gloucester. **Grays Thurrock** (0375–380609 Mon 6–9pm/Wed 1–5pm/Thur 12–4pm 0375 381322 office line): Bridgehouse, Bridge Rd, Grays Thurrock. **Halton** (051–423 4192 Tue 7–9pm/Thur 11–2pm and 4pm–12am/Sun 4–7pm/office line 051 423 4251): PO Box 13, Widness, Cheshire WA8 7UJ. **Hull** (0482–29990 Thur 4–12pm): PO Box 40, Hull, Humberside. **Lancaster** (0524–

382595 Tue 7.30–9.30pm/Fri 1–3pm): PO Box 2, Lancaster. **Leamington Spa** (0926–39936 Mon 1–3pm and 7–9pm): PO Box 27, Wellington St, Leeds LS2 7EG. **Leicester** (0533–666666 Tue 7–9pm/Sat 2–5pm): 70 High St, Leicester. **Littlehampton** (0903–726411 Mon–Thur 7–10pm 24 hr ansaphone). **Liverpool** (051–727 7599 Mon 7–9pm/Thur and Sat 2–5pm): PO Box 64, Liverpool LG9 8AT. **London** (01–837 1600 24 hr counselling/01 278 3956 Mon–Fri 10–6pm): PO Box 69, London WC1X 9NJ. **Luton** (helpline 0582–33426 Mon–Fri 9–5pm): c/o 12 Oxford Rd, Luton (office line 0582–33592 Mon/Wed 7–10pm). **Manchester** (061–228 3602 Tue/Fri 2–5pm Wed/Thur/Sun 6–9pm): PO Box 336, Manchester M60 2BS. **Medway** (063–472 6311): 69 Woodstock Rd, Stroud, Rochester, Kent ME4 2DJ. **Milton Keynes** (0908–670 333 Mon 7–9pm/office 0908–670 312): The Bakehouse, 6 Church St, Wolverton, Milton Keynes. **Northampton** (0604–250721 Mon–Thur 7–9pm/Fri 10–2pm/office 0604–232635): PO Box 206, Northampton NN1 1NF. **North Staffordshire** (0782–414288) Mon–Fri 11–3pm: PO Box 254, Stoke-on-Trent, North Staffs, ST4 4DE. **Norwich** (0603–667687 Mon 6–8pm/Thur 8–10pm/Fri 11–2pm/Sat 4–6pm): PO Box 47, Norwich NR1 2BU. **Nottingham** (0602–410440 Tue–Fri 10–4pm/Sat 10–1pm): c/o 37a Mansfield Rd, Nottingham. **Oxford** (0865–726295 Mon and Tue 7–9pm/Wed 2–10pm): PO Box 20, Oxford OX3. **Peterborough** (0733–40515 Thur and Fri 2–4pm/Tue 7.30–10pm/Sat 10–12pm): c/o PCVS, 51 Broadway, Peterborough PE1 1SQ. **Plymouth** (0752–23584 Thur 7.30–10pm): c/o Box A, Virginia House, Palace St, Plymouth. **Portsmouth** (0705–669511 Wed/Fri 7–10pm/Sun 3–6pm): PO Box 3, Southsea, Portsmouth. **Rochdale** (0706–526279 Mon 7–10pm): PO Box 9, Rochdale OL16 1UT. **Scunthorpe** (0724–853953 Mon 7–9pm): PO Box 38, Scunthorpe. **Sheffield** (0742–755255 Mon–Fri 10–5pm/Sat 12–3pm/office 0742–757130): PO Box 34, Sheffield S1 1UD. **Shropshire** (0952–504666 Mon 12–3pm/Wed/Fri 7–10pm): PO Box 98, Wellington, Telford. **Southampton** (0703–701213 Mon 7–10pm/Tue 10–1pm/Thur 1–4pm): PO Box 50, Head Post Office, Southampton, Hants. **Southwark** (01–639 1106 Tue 7–10pm/Thur 2–5pm): PO Box 815, London SE15. **Swindon** (0793–616511 Wed 10–4pm/7–10pm 24 hr ansaphone): PO Box 57, Swindon SN5 8AZ. **Tyneside** (0632–615317 Mon/Fri 10–5pm/Sat/Sun 6.30–10pm/office 0632–329 858): PO Box 13, Gosforth, Newcastle upon Tyne. **Wirral** (051–666 1392 Thur 7–9pm/Sun 2–5pm): PO Box 20, Wallasey, Merseyside LH4 9HE. **York Rape Crisis** (0904–610917 Thur 6.30–10pm): PO Box 265, York.

IRELAND

Belfast (0232–249696 Mon–Fri 10–6pm/Sat 11–5pm): PO Box 46, Belfast BT2 7AR. **Clomer** (010–353 522 4111 Mon/Wed/Fri/Sat 10–4pm). **Clonmel** (052–24111 Mon/Wed/Fri 10–4pm/Mon 8–10.30pm/Sat 10–1pm 24 hr ansaphone): 14 Wellington St Clonmel, Co. Tipperary. **Cork** (021–0002 968 086 Mon 7.30–10pm/Wed 2–5pm/Fri 10–1pm/Sat 1–4pm): PO Box 42, Brian Born St, Cork, Eire. **Dublin** (01–0001 614911 Mon–Fri 8am–8pm/Sat–Sun 24 hrs): 70 Lower Leeson St, Dublin 2. **Galway** (010–35391 64983 Mon–Fri 9–5.30pm/24 hr ansaphone): 15a Mary St, Galway. **Letterkenny** (010–353 74 23 067 Mon 10–12pm/Sat 12–4pm). **Limerick** (0103–5361 311511 Mon–Fri 10–4pm/emergency counselling available after 8pm/24 hr ansaphone): PO Box 128, Limerick. **Waterford:** PO Box 57, Waterford, Eire.

SCOTLAND

Aberdeen (0224–575 560 Mon 6–8pm/Thur 7–9pm 24 hr ansaphone): PO Box 123, Aberdeen. **Dundee** (0382–201 2291 Wed/Sat 7–9pm): PO Box 83, Dundee. **Edinburgh** (031–556 9437 Mon/Wed 1–2pm and 6–8pm/Thur 7–10pm/Fri 6–8pm): PO Box 120, Edinburgh EH1 3ND. **Falkirk** (0324–38433 Mon/Thur 7–9pm): PO Box 4, Falkirk, Central Scotland. **Glasgow** (041–221 8448 Mon/Wed/Fri 7–10pm/Thur 11–1pm): PO Box 53, Glasgow G2 1YR. **Highland Rape Crisis and Incest Survivors Line** (0463–233089 24 hr ansaphone provides details): PO Box 58, Inverness. **Strathclyde** (041–221 8448 Mon/Wed/Fri 7–10pm/Thur 11–1pm): PO Box 53, Glasgow G2 1YR.

WALES

Bangor (0248–354885 Wed 7–9pm): The Abbey Road Centre, 9 Abbey Rd, Bangor. **Cardiff** (0222–373181 Mon 7–10pm/Wed 11–2pm/Thur 7–10pm 24 hr ansaphone). **South Wales** (0222–373181 Mon/Thur 7–10pm/Wed 11–12pm): c/o 2 Coburn St, Cathays, Cardiff. **Swansea** (0792–475243 Tue 7–9pm/Fri 10–12pm): 58 Alexander Rd, Swansea.

PART II

RELATIONSHIPS AND SEXUALITY

RELATIONSHIPS: SOME ISSUES FOR US ALL

Prepared by
JILL RAKUSEN

NEW FACE

I have learned not to worry about love;
but to honour its coming
with all my heart.
To examine the dark mysteries
of the blood
with headless heed and
swirl,
to know the rush of feelings
swift and flowing
as water.
The source appears to be
some inexhaustible
spring
within our twin and triple
selves;
the new face I turn up
to you
no one else on earth
has ever
seen.

© ALICE WALKER

Loving is essential to our lives. Most of the people we love we are not sexually involved with; some we are. Sexual relationships are intense, puzzling, frustrating, energizing, potentially oppressive and potentially freeing. They enable us to learn about ourselves and our lovers and to get close in ways we never expected. They raise issues of power and vulnerability, commitment and risk. Sexual relationships can be painful; a long-time union breaks up or turns abusive, a love affair promises much and then fizzles out, a lover dies. Yet most of us want and need intimacy, so we usually recover from the hurt and try again.

Part II looks closely at our sexual relationships. What do they give us? How can we make them more what we want? What is unique to sexual relationships with women? With men? How can we understand our sexuality better and enjoy it more? How can we change the social structures and attitudes – about age, disability, sex roles, sexual preference – which keep us from freely loving others and ourselves?

RETHINKING SEXUAL PREFERENCE

It is a myth that every woman is 'innately heterosexual'. More than twenty years ago, research by Kinsey showed that most people have both heterosexual and homosexual feelings. A woman might have played around sexually with girls and boys in her childhood or fallen in love with her best girlfriend at school, then married. Another who had been involved with men for thirty years may then find herself relating sexually to women. Some women are sexually and emotionally intimate with both women and men through their lives.

As we come to understand that most people have some homosexual feelings, we begin to accept a lot of things we were taught to fear. In our families and schools people either didn't mention lesbians or gay men at all, or joked cruelly about them; they made us feel hesitant about some of our closest female friendships.

When I was seven or eight, I had this best friend, Susan. We loved each other and walked around with our arms around each other. Her older sister told us not to do that any more because we looked like lesies. So we held hands instead.

Society penalizes lesbians through job discrimination and violence. Our culture teaches us a fear and hatred of homosexuality in ourselves and others (*homophobia*). Homophobia insults those of us who are lesbian and bisexual and makes our lives unnecessarily difficult and painful. It also hurts those of us who are heterosexual. Fear and prejudice turn us against lesbian friends and family members, depriving us of important relationships. Homophobia makes us fear and dislike aspects of our own personality and looks which are not 'feminine' enough (assertiveness, muscular build, body hair, deep voice). It causes us to deny attractions which are natural to us and may prevent us from choosing the sexual partners who are right for us. And it divides us from each other as women. Homophobia is politically useful for those who want to preserve the traditional forms of family life and to suppress any alternatives. In the late 1980s it has developed a new lease of life, symbolized perhaps by the notorious Section 28 which seeks to ban the 'promotion' of homosexuality.

With time, familiarity and friendship we can unlearn homophobia, and discover our right as lesbians and our responsibility as heterosexuals to fight against it.

> *The main thing that finally helped me start letting go of my homophobia was getting to know a few lesbian women. I found out to my amazement – and my shame – that they were as different from each other as I am from my heterosexual friends.*

> *Once I admitted to myself that I do have sexual feelings for women, I didn't feel so alarmed by lesbians any more. It was as if they had represented something in myself I was scared of.*

> *Even after I became a lesbian at thirty-five, I found that I had big doses of homophobia inside me. Sometimes I'd wake up after having sex with a woman I loved and have an attack of thinking that the wonderful thing we'd done was 'queer'. Or I'd get upset when other dykes seemed 'too obvious' in public. Slowly I've become prouder and more deeply affirming of lesbians and lesbianism – that is, of myself.*

Many heterosexual women believe they know no lesbians personally. However, only very courageous lesbians feel safe about being completely open with all their friends and acquaintances. By not being supportive of lesbian and gay rights movements, and not challenging homophobia whenever we meet it, those among us who are heterosexual prevent lesbians from having the rights that we have, including the right fearlessly to walk down the street holding hands, or to show their joy at being in love, or grief at the death of a relationship or a partner.

Fear of Lesbians and Our unity as Women

Some women hesitate to join feminist projects because friends and family assume that being a feminist means one is a lesbian. Ultra-conservative political and religious groups play on these fears by portraying all feminists as man-haters and actual or would-be lesbians. Using homophobia as a tool to divide us and turn us against each other, they rob us of our energy and unity as a movement of women trying to build a more just society for everyone. On the other hand, some lesbians struggling for legitimacy and acceptance suggest that 'straight' women are less feminist

than lesbians or that 'true' feminists wouldn't ally themselves with men in any way. As a collective of heterosexual and lesbian women, we hope all women will feel safe enough in this society to become less condemning of each others' choices. We urge more heterosexual women who share feminist goals and visions to identify themselves openly as feminists. The women's movement will become a stronger force for social change when women of all sexual orientations can find friendship, growth and power within it.

Questioning 'Heterosexuality'

Can heterosexuality be a free choice when we are taught such a deep fear of loving women? Can we comfortably assume that women are 'naturally' drawn to men when we consider the many reasons why we can be driven to seek protection from men? – fear of being alone, rape, harassment, poor pay and pension schemes for women, the fact that prostitution is often the only available work which pays enough to support a family, the derision of 'old maids' and lesbians, and so on. If it is *unsafe* to be a woman without a man, then heterosexuality is not so much natural as compulsory.*

Compulsory heterosexuality may make us feel desperate when we're not with a man, and cause us to jump into the arms of men who are available but not good for us. It means we never have a chance to make a real choice, to ask ourselves whether we would be happier with a man, a woman, with several relationships, or none.

Bisexuality

Today many women are entering or at least thinking about sexual, intimate relationships with both men and women.

> *I ask myself: is it possible to be bisexual, or is it some kind of new-age fantasy that I can have a man lover and a woman lover?*

> *I've been in lesbian relationships for ages. Then suddenly last year I fell in love with a man. A total surprise!*

> *When I first started getting involved with women as well as men, I wanted to be more intimate with them as an extension of being friends.*

Sometimes thinking of ourselves as bisexual is a safe stopping place in a transition from one identity to another.

> *For years I said to myself and my friends, 'I think maybe I'm bisexual,' meaning, 'I'm probably a lesbian but I'm scared to death to admit it.'*

Yet for many of us bisexuality is not transitional at all.

> *I've tried to define myself using labels of lesbian, straight, bisexual, and I didn't feel that any of*

---

*See Adrienne Rich's important and challenging article, 'Compulsory Heterosexuality and Lesbian Existence'.[1]

*them were mine. I think of it in terms of people I
could love, not sexes I could love.*

Being lovers with people of both sexes opens our eyes to
social and political realities which may be new to us. If we
were sexually intimate only with men before, a relationship
with a woman may introduce us to the world of lesbian
experience, with its particular satisfactions and
oppressions.

If we have been exclusively lesbian, being lovers with a
man puts us temporarily into the dominant heterosexual
culture: we have the privilege of 'fitting in', of being able to
show our love freely in public. There also may be more
struggles with sex-role stereotypes than we are used to and,
before menopause, the unfamiliar need for birth control.

Invisibility is a problem. Few people know we exist,
because we don't 'fit' into either the heterosexual or the
lesbian world. When we are open, both worlds judge us.

*I'm cautious about talking about it, fear being
judged, being told, 'Your sexuality is wrong!'*

Heterosexual friends may be shocked and scared when
we have a woman lover. (See chapter on lesbian relationships.) Lesbian friends may be mistrustful, too, afraid that
we may in the future slip back into the 'safer' heterosexual
role and hurt lesbians who have fallen in love with us. If we
as lesbians become lovers with men as well, other lesbians
often see us as disloyal.

*When I'm having troubles with a man and tell a
lesbian friend, she usually gets a look in her eye
which means, 'What did you expect, being with a
man?'*

All these judgements isolate us. And we may feel pressured to choose. As more women feel comfortable and safe
in being open about bisexuality, we will create more of a
community for ourselves, and we will further challenge
assumptions about who and how women can love.

PRESSURE TO BE IN A COUPLE

There are powerful social pressures to 'be in a couple',
especially one kind of couple – married, heterosexual,
racially alike. The pressure starts early. Storybooks and
films of our girlhoods ended with romantic marriage and
perpetual bliss. Relatives asked us at three or four who our
boyfriends were and, at twenty, when we were going to
marry and have children. Recently it has become more
socially acceptable not to marry and not to have children,
but the pressure to be part of a couple can still be very
strong. Indeed, the idea of the 'relationship' has taken on
some of the mystique formerly reserved for marriage and
the nuclear family. Even after separation or the death of a

partner, friends assume we are seeking another relationship. Lesbians and heterosexual women alike can feel
powerful pressure to be in a couple.

*We're so conditioned to think we're only half a
person without somebody else.*

*The only thing that we have in our heads is: you
meet someone, you feel for them, you enter into a
relationship, you relate only to them. It's been the
downfall of many intimacies.*

*When I'm around couples for any length of time I
feel this sense of creeping desperation, like
something's wrong with me because I'm not in a
relationship. The pressure makes you latch on to
anybody instead of thinking the thing through.*

*When I think of the hours I've spent in discos and
at parties trying to meet someone, I am bitter
about such wasted energy. I could have started my
own business or got a degree in that time.*

There are economic pressures to be in a couple. Women
experience severe pay discrimination and are often
financially insecure and overworked.

*I am part of a circle of friends who have been
single for most of the past ten years. We moved
fairly easily in and out of relationships or were
involved in several at a time. Now all of a sudden
everyone is coupling off. You know, I think it's the
economy and the state of the world. Many of my
friends are being laid off and losing their pensions.
When people are scared they want to be with
someone else.*

It can be hard to imagine being older and single.

*I love my life the way it is now – the freedom to be
with different partners or not with any, living by
my own rhythms, feeling strong and happy with
myself. But sometimes when I wake up in the
middle of the night I see myself old and alone, and
it is terribly scary and empty.*

Ageism (see p. 447) makes us fear growing older, because
we assume that old people don't have friends or community, that someone who's not with a partner will be
totally alone. For many of us it is literally dangerous to be
alone because of violence and sexual harassment.

It is important to acknowledge that single, and particularly lesbian women, are oppressed in our society. Lesbian
women, whether seeking refuge in a homophobic society or
not, need particular support, which is why we have devoted
a large chapter to lesbian relationships. For all of us as
single women, lesbian or heterosexual, we need to give one
another support both for our lives as single women and for
our efforts to find a partner. While we don't want to be
pressured to find someone or get married, neither do we

want friends to assume that we love being single. It is up to us to let people know if we *are* interested in meeting someone. By loving ourselves more when our community values us, we are more likely, when and if we go looking for a partner, to find a suitable one. Surrounded by the affection and caring of friends and family, we become less vulnerable to exploitative relationships, more able to resist the emphasis on being or becoming part of a couple.

When I broke up with my lover I luckily had a circle of warm affectionate friends who would give me a hug or a pat on the back. Yet I felt the lack of that very intimate whole-body contact. I didn't want to rush precipitously into a new relationship just because I felt so hungry to be touched. One answer was to get a massage every other week for several months.

When my younger sister got engaged my parents bought each of us a beautiful set of cookware. They said they loved us both and wanted to support the life choices that each of us was making by getting us each something for our homes. I felt so affirmed because I understood they were saying, 'This is your life, and we value you and your choices.'

MONOGAMY/ NON-MONOGAMY

Some of us are excited by the possibility of relationships which are free of sexual exclusivity, and we explored this in our last book. However, some of us are less interested in the idea than before, and not necessarily because we have found non-monogamy difficult.

I have always known at some level that, for me, being non-monogamous suited me because I was frightened of loving. I also knew that the fact that non-monogamy was politically acceptable also suited me. I didn't need to face the truth if I could hide behind this cloak. Damn it, I could even be proud of the ease with which I related to different people. Thinking about all this now makes me cringe with shame and embarrassment. As I struggled towards gaining the courage for self-knowledge, I gradually became more aware of the motives behind my supposedly acceptable behaviour. Now I regard anyone's motivation towards non-monogamy as suspect until proved otherwise. I distrust heterosexual men who are into non-monogamy because I find it tends to sustain them in one of their most oppressive modes – an inability truly to love and be vulnerable. They hide behind the same smokescreen that I did. I know it well! I also distrust women who, from the safety and comfort of a socially acceptable relationship

with a man (the power of which they always underestimate), get involved with a single woman. She becomes the 'adventure', the 'frisson', and often ends up experiencing a lot of pain due to the gross inequality of the relationship (despite its apparent political acceptability in terms of not being exclusive). However, its very existence is based on the heterosexual woman's security through her man. Living in real social security, the heterosexual woman has no idea of the oppressiveness of her role and behaviour. She may even, as I have witnessed, add insult to injury by labelling her lesbian lover's pain as being due solely to her personal difficulties. It makes me very angry to see lesbians treated like this, and all under the guise of political acceptability.

Clearly, we can feel pressure not to be in a couple. This can be difficult to resist.

Being lesbian gives me a chance to do things differently from heterosexual couples I've seen. I'd like to be less possessive than they often are. But when it comes down to my lover being sexually involved with someone else, it hurts. It could even split us up. I've decided I've got to be up front about my need for sexual dependability; while it may not in some circles be 'politically correct', it is very human.

Some of us are clear that we do or do not want to be monogamous. Some of us are split between what our head tells us and what our guts tell us. Some of us wrestle with the issue over and over again. Perhaps many of us at times find being single or celibate a welcome relief. Fear of the spread of AIDS has also made many of us stop and think more carefully about multiple relationships (see Chapter 23 for how we can protect ourselves).

BEING SINGLE

NOW ALONE IS A BED PARTNER

Now *Alone* is a bed partner, is a
precious gem,
is a bandit she wants, is a woman with
silver hair,
is better than a man.

Alone was a gift she didn't recognize
when it first
arrived. She locked it in the bedroom
and stayed
downstairs. She wouldn't let it come
to meals.

She knew the sweet faces of her friends,
she didn't

trust *Alone* who slept in her mirror, in
her voice,
in the hollow where her hands covered
her eyes.

Alone was patient and when she took its
hand, it gave her
songs and poems, drawings and slow
breath, a peace
larger than sunset. Everyone felt it.
The children

drew around her as if she were the
hearth.
Alone moved in as no one else could,
unpossessive,
leaving space for women and men to
interact with her. Now

Alone is there in the morning and
welcomes her home
and wants nothing from her and gives all
of itself
to her and never turns her away.

©JUDITH W. STEINBERGH

Being single means either fitting lovers into our lives without living with them and settling down together, or living with no romantic attachments at all. Here some lesbian and heterosexual women affirm not being in a major relationship.

Being on my own lets me find out what my needs are, and find out who I am and just get a better sense of myself.

I like not being answerable to anybody. One reason to be single or celibate is to have clarity about what you want in your life. You make emotional and physical space. What you want is not dependent on what somebody else wants.

When I was in a couple we had to spend so much time hassling out all the little details of everything. Everything had to be a compromise – everything, from the most minute detail to the biggest thing – and it seemed like such a waste of energy most of the time.

When I'm on my own, my security comes from myself and the connections I have with different people. In a relationship, my security depends so much on that relationship and on that one other woman.

I simply don't plan my life around a man even when I am in love. There are so many other things that I want to do, too. I've had two husbands. I also have three grown kids. Naturally I still think about them, but not like when they were little. I can really focus on what I want to do now.

It's amazing how much energy it frees up for me. I feel great; I feel a real surge of power!

Not being in a relationship has given me time to reconnect with my friends in a really intimate way.

There are so many more women in my life now, so much room for so many more women.

I found I can get a good deal more work done and am more creative.

I like the feeling of trying to create something new.

In choosing not to be in a couple, we do not necessarily distance ourselves from others. We still want intimate friendships. Some are sexually intimate with friends.

It's very hard for me to draw the line between friends and lovers, so I sleep with some of my very close friends. I find that really satisfying. A lot of the time I sleep with very close friends without having sex, which I find equally satisfying.

We may choose this kind of intimacy without sex because we like our friendships as they are and don't want to change them.

The lesbian community has completely copied the heterosexual community in thinking that relationships, to be really intimate, to be really close and to supply the affection that's needed in a person's life, have to be sexual. I don't think that's true. I think you can have really good relationships, intimate and the most binding, without sex. Bringing sex into a relationship does not necessarily improve it.

The experience of being single depends on how we respond to the pressure, subtle and unsubtle, to be in a couple (see p. 193 above). How well being single works for us depends on our ability to avoid slipping into becoming dependent on particular people for our sense of well-being. We often rely on the happiness of somebody else liking and valuing us; and we would do well to find that satisfaction in liking ourselves.

Being single can be hard because in our society, couples are the norm.

A single woman . . . is not buttressed by a family and the responsibilities of a family . . . She has made a choice that cuts her off from a lot of things most people consider life, for the sake of something else, something both chancy and intangible. No wonder anxiety is the constant attendant of such a one![2]

Being a single parent can be particularly hard, not just because of social norms, but because we can so easily end up being financially deprived.

Community, therefore, is especially important to us as

single women. We can develop strong and supportive friendships and grow old with them.

I hope I'll be growing old together with Dan, but since he is considerably older [eighteen years] than me it is possible that he will die before me. Then I imagine growing old with Margie, who has been my best friend for the past fifteen years. I like thinking of us as old women together.

A NEW UNDERSTANDING OF CELIBACY

Traditionally, 'celibacy' meant choosing not to marry. Today many people use it to mean not having sex for a certain period of time. It can mean no sex with someone else, or no masturbation as well. Sometimes we choose celibacy in response to our culture's overemphasis on sex, as a break from feeling we must relate to others sexually all the time: 'I was tired of having to say yes or no.'

Or it's a personal adventure.

I'm exploring myself as a sexual person but in a different way. My sensitivity to my body is heightened. I am more aware of what arouses my sensual interests. I am free to be myself. I have more energy for work and friends. My spirituality feels more intense and clear.

As part of a religious commitment (for nuns, priests and others) celibacy offers a freedom to use one's energy for other people, not so much because love-making drains energy but because sexual relationships necessitate commitment, time and attention. Yet religious celibacy has often been misunderstood or ridiculed. A nun wrote to the collective as follows:

For many religious women sex means so much that we use it as a gift of our life in the service of all people. Not to engage in an active sex life or to marry is for the purpose of being free to be of service. It is painful and depressing when others speak of this gift as though to have made this decision is necessarily to have a warped personality.

When we choose celibacy, we can experiment with any form that offers what we want.

I spend part of each day in yoga and meditation. Sometimes I go for days without thinking about my sexual identity at all. I masturbate only when inspired, which is seldom these days. Yet in meditation last week I found myself having an orgasm. It was ecstasy!

In couple relationships, we may choose celibacy when we want some distance or solitude, or when we just don't want to have sex for a while. This can be awkward and requires careful communication if a partner isn't feeling the same way.

I say to my lover, 'I don't feel like making love this month, and I may not next month.' Now, who does that? Is it OK? Am I allowed to? The last thing we were ever taught was that it was OK to try what we want.

Some couples choose celibacy together, which allows both people to explore other dimensions of loving. It can help us get out of old sexual patterns, expand our sensual/ sexual focus beyond genital sex and make us feel more self-sufficient and independent.

Sometimes we can feel obliged to be sexual when we'd rather have no relationships at all. Lesbians in particular can find this difficult.

It can be quite taboo to be on your own – lesbians can feel obliged to be sexual – which is partly a result of feeling ruled by our sexual identity. Heterosexuals don't have to be sexually active; nor do lesbians!

Sometimes we are faced with celibacy when we *don't* choose it – after a break-up or divorce, or when a lover dies. Sometimes being a parent to a new baby enforces a time of virtual celibacy. Painful if we don't want it, celibacy sometimes surprises us with its own satisfactions.

WORKING TOWARDS MUTUALITY: HAVING ONE PRIMARY LOVER*

Although we might sleep with someone else from time to time, many of us are in monogamous relationships. What do we value about them? Here are some women's voices, both lesbian and heterosexual, aged between mid-twenties and mid-sixties.

I have someone in my life who I can get to know really deeply over a long period of time, who can get to know me and who I can be the best and worst of myself with.

The quality of our intimacy is exquisite. It's like a river that runs between us, and we can tap into it

---

*In earlier editions of *Our Bodies, Ourselves* we focused on alternatives to couple relationships. In this edition we have tried to redress the balance, focusing in depth on mutuality for the first time – both for heterosexual and lesbian relationships. This section explores issues that tend to affect all couple relationships, and the following two chapters explore issues relating solely to loving women and men respectively.

whenever we want. To me it's a rich and wonderful thing that someone can be intimate with you in so many ways . . . as a lover, as a friend.

The best thing is that we have a long, intimate history together and still feel connected to and admiring and turned on to each other. I consider it a minor miracle as I look around me. I have learned that my husband has many of the same weak feelings – fragile feelings – that I used to think were female – just as he has learned that I have certain kinds of strengths that he doesn't have. The crucial thing is to take time to build up confidence and trust and comfort and kindness.

I like being with someone who follows all the threads of my life, even the most mundane.

It's like having my childhood magical playmate come to life – my best friend who is family to me.

I've never been so close, so close to someone who can release and relieve me of light and dark according to the rhythm of the days . . . I know I kick against it, long to hide, pretend I'm not here and even dress up as someone else (occasionally) but I value and specially treasure her more than anyone else I've known in my life. We are both explorers, sometimes deep in pot holes, sometimes glimpsing beauty from the heights – but always moving, even when we don't feel it, towards each other and greater love.

Even with all my wonderful friends and my job, which I love, and my dancing and my cat and everything else, life used to be very lonely. Simple little details could suddenly seem so hard . . . like finding someone to go to the launderette with. Now I really don't live much differently than I did before, but life feels quite different. We are committed to each other in a way that transcends the little daily ups and downs. Having him there, even with all the fights and issues we have yet to resolve, is like a big, soft cushion between me and the roughness of life.

The hard thing about widowhood is that I have lost the person I held hands with in life. I was extremely important to my husband . . . When I was unhappy I could always go to him and talk to him, and when I was happy he had a smile from ear to ear. He gave me unlimited support throughout my whole married life. I don't have that any more. That's a very, very important loss. I've made up for it by relying more on other close people in my life. I have a close friend that I can call at the drop of a hat and say, 'Something is bothering me and I have to talk to you about it,' and I'm extremely close with my children. I need about a dozen close people to fill in for the loss of that one special relationship.

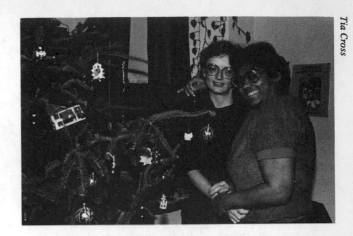

Tia Cross

He has a deep, keen interest in what I do, in my work and my interests, that no other man I've been involved with has ever had. The mutuality, the give and take and the constant questioning of gender stereotype is critical. And it's not just on an intellectual plane, either; it's also about the mundane stuff like taking care of the house and doing the dishes, not just who does things but who thinks about what has to be done.

The best thing about my relationship is that I have a real friend. When you've done a lot of things together you have a commonality of ethics, a way of looking at the world which is terribly important, so I trust my partner a lot.

There are many different facets to knowing each other well and communicating on a deep level, letting our vulnerabilities show and our secrets be known, trusting enough to depend on someone and to allow them to depend on us.

Commitment means working on the relationship even when the early passion and urgency have evolved into a deeper if less dramatic kind of loving, and sticking through the hard, awful, painful, lousy and deadening times (which can be dramatic in their own way!).

I'm still drawn to that rush of passion that I get early in a relationship, but now I'm old enough and I've been through enough with lovers to know that the rush doesn't last. We can rekindle it; there are times when I feel that passion that always exists at the beginning, but I certainly don't feel it twenty-four hours a day every day. It takes a lot of work and creativity to keep things sparking in a relationship. Sometimes I'm attracted to other people, but I think this has mostly to do with my fears about intimacy and with wanting the rush . . . and trying to disperse some of the intensity of being with one person. As I get older, I'm more interested in whether this person is going to be with me. If the passion isn't there every night, it's OK.

We both need to keep our eyes and hearts on what we are aiming for – more. We both need to remember more, and not pursue our irritations with searchlights on: such interrogation deprives us of such energy and we cease to focus on where we are going. I always thought I was humble, but the shadow side is my pride, my difficulty in learning, in not owning up to what I don't know. I am also tired of being a complainer, so next year I shall try and unlearn this pointless activity. We have to accept and live and learn from our horrid dark places and transform ourselves by constantly remembering how we really want to live – with love and gentleness and peace – with courage and creativity and care for others.

Somewhere, somehow, I have this vision of us being together in love, creating something I cannot name . . . but it is beautiful and strong and shiny like most visionary things – to do with what lies behind this huge curtain of conflict/terror and tension that confronts us. I feel we are near to where we want to be, but it feels so far because we're so close we can't see where we are.

In any long-term relationship, problems and painful issues come up regardless of how 'right' we are for each other, of how hard we have worked to build the relationship and even of how stable and solid we feel together. It can be frightening to look squarely at what is difficult and hurtful, for we want to believe that we chose a good partner, that we have made wise decisions; to become aware of aspects we were afraid to face, to admit deep conflicts may mean that we have made a major error. Sometimes, as we begin to get angry, we fear that if we do not immediately squelch this anger it will rage out of control and lead us inevitably to the end of the relationship.

Yet avoiding confrontation is more likely to result in stagnation and resentment than in keeping the peace or making things better. *Conflict can be part of a creative process of working things out.* As a start we can identify the social aspects of our conflicts and avoid the common pitfall of blaming one another or blaming ourselves for everything that goes wrong. Below we look briefly at making long-term relationships work, and then at knowing when to leave. We discuss those crucial social and political factors that influence lesbian and heterosexual relationships in the respective chapters which follow.

CONSTANTLY QUESTIONING OUR ASSUMPTIONS

We need to make a conscious and continuing effort to articulate what we really want in our intimate relationships, particularly with men, or the conventions of society will inevitably take over. One way to begin changing our relationships is to reconsider the kind of partner we (think we) are looking for and our patterns of relating to them when we first meet them. Making changes at the beginning of a relationship may help us to shift the balance that gets set up in our future relationships.

My wish was to marry a Marlboro man. I grew up in a family of Marlboro men. But I worked out eventually that I didn't want that any more. Max is very intense and verbal. He is about my height and weight. From the back we even look alike. He's very emotionally accessible – and vulnerable. We have a great deal of fun together. And it's very easy to talk to him. But sometimes I look at him and think, You're so much a friend and a peer . . . I wonder if you are strong enough for me to lean on.

I thought I was marrying this very exciting man, and I didn't see that his dynamism was an expression of the control he needed to have. I just saw the excitement, the energy. I didn't realize that it would make me feel smaller in the process. I learned that it's not just how 'wonderful' the other person is but how they make you feel. Now I pay a lot of attention to how I feel with someone at the beginning of a relationship. If I feel distinctly less wonderful in a man's presence, I don't care how sparkling or brilliant he is – I'm not interested.

But many of us didn't question our behaviour until years after patterns were set. We may be scared to change or for our partners to change. If we become more assertive, for example, our partners, even though they might welcome it, may have to make some adjustments because we will have overturned the status quo. Perhaps he or she has got used to being deferred to, or to doing all the cooking, or not doing all the cooking. Or perhaps our partner has finally begun to take more responsibility in the home or for the children, and we find that although this pleases us, it also threatens us in a way we hadn't expected.

After fifteen years of being a full-time housewife, I decided to go to college. My husband and I divided up all the jobs and responsibilities so I could finish college and work at a fairly demanding job full time. Everything was working out fine, I thought, until one day Jim made some passing remark about one of our daughters and some problem she was having with her boyfriend. I was shocked to realize that something was going on I knew nothing about. I was no longer the 'nerve centre' of the family. That was a loss, because for many years knowing all those details had been my source of power within the family. Yet on balance the change has been good for all of us. Being the nerve centre was holding me back from developing other parts of myself, and as I moved out into the world, Jim grew a great deal closer to the kids.

Often, we need to renegotiate arrangements time and again.

We need to ask for what we want, earlier, more clearly and repeat this, with the insistence of authority. I have the authority to demand from my lover, and she from me, and I hurt if I do not act on this strength. There is no way I wish to be allowed to break up what I really value and love. I need help from her sometimes!

By now we have struggled through the business about making dinner five or six times – different times at which decisions were made and they're acted on for a time, then something happens like he goes away for three weeks, and when he comes back he's tired and he doesn't take the thing up again. So we have to negotiate the whole thing over again. At one point he said, 'You know, the truth is I'm just lazy. It's just so much more comfortable not to have to do it.' He can recognize that, but it doesn't prevent it from happening again. But the thing that makes it work is that he's open to being challenged about it. And from what I've heard and read about it, an awful lot of men are not.

OUR CHILDREN/OUR PARTNER'S CHILDREN

While children can bring us closer, often their presence distracts us, or just cuts into the time we have alone together.

One of the hardest things for us since having kids is just getting enough time alone together. When I can't get a sitter he feels neglected, and I'm sure I've failed, even though I know there's no reason why it should just be up to me to arrange our time alone. When we do have a sitter, the kids complain. Both of us come from working-class families where the kids were always included in everything, so it's easy for us to feel guilty when we do something by ourselves.

Children can also make one of us feel jealous or left out, and this can become a major issue in the relationship.

Sometimes he falls completely apart. He drags around the house in his bathrobe, doesn't shave, feels sick and talks endlessly about it and generally comes unglued. This almost invariably happens when I am under the most pressure at work, or when the kids are in shreds and demanding extra attention. I get so enraged at him for getting weak just when I need him that I yell and scream and berate him . . . just what he doesn't need – to be kicked when he's down.

This can be particularly so if they're not our 'own' kids: if our partner already had children before we started our relationship, and we haven't had any ourselves, it can take quite a time to work out how we're going to live together; whether and how we will take on a 'step-parenting' role will be a major issue. If we're in a lesbian relationship, it can be particularly hard working out a 'step-parenting' role as it usually has to be such a private function. While many of us in this position have to remain private for the security of ourselves and our children, some lesbians are making their parenting role public, and as more lesbians have children together, we will gain courage and strength from each other.

When I became a parent to my lover's children, we decided to be open from the start. So when she and her kids came to live with me, and the kids had to attend a new school, we both went to meet the head together. We made it clear that we were both equally responsible for the kids, that we were both parents to them. It helped because I knew the head through my work. But it was a risk . . . and the risk paid off.

Some lesbians are developing a new concept of relating to children: co-parenting (see p. 218). Though not without its difficulties, it is a much more egalitarian approach to parenting than the traditional 'step-parenting' role.[3]

I think heterosexuals could benefit a lot from thinking in terms of co-parenting: co-parenting to me means trying to be an equal partner in parenting a child; it means two people agreeing to share 50:50 the emotional and financial commitment to a child.

PAYING ATTENTION TO EACH OTHER

So many things vie for our attention apart from children: work, friends, our various activities and chores. A new love eclipses almost everything else, but before too long the balance changes and it gets squeezed in between the children's needs, the washing, the leaking roof and evening meetings.

An intimate relationship, while often background and sustenance to the rest of our lives, must at times have our full attention.

Several evenings a week since we married eleven years ago, we sit in the living-room, each of us in our own favourite chair, and we have a glass of wine after the kids are in bed. And we talk . . . about the day, about ridiculous details of what happened at work, about some problem we've been having, or whatever. Sometimes it's hard to take the time . . . the dishes need washing or there is a good show on TV or I just don't feel like it. But this, more than any other single thing, has kept us from getting too far apart without touching base.

We've been through a lot of upheavals since the beginning of our relationship, and it feels like

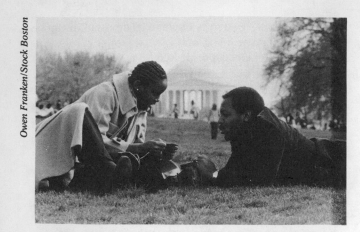

Owen Franken/Stock Boston

they're all taking their toll. We've moved jobs and houses, started to live with each other for the first time, and in another town, plus I'm learning to cope in a pseudo-parental role, and the devastating experience of my partner's therapist turning out to be so homophobic that she actually rejected my partner when told that she had no intention of leaving our relationship. In short, a lot to deal with. Sometimes it feels like both of us have so much sheer surviving to do that we can't, either of us, give the kind of attention each of us needs. While women are better at giving attention, it doesn't necessarily work out that we can do it when we're feeling so needy ourselves. I feel angry knowing how much I can give, and how much Sophie can give, and how all our energy is dissipated into just coping. We both want to give attention but to survive we can't. Yet the relationship can't survive without it. Aaargh.

What we do when we want to be alone together is go for long drives and talk. That's a way that we can relax, something we enjoyed doing even when we were eighteen years old. But we have to work at it. The kids take up an enormous amount of time and energy that we used to have just for ourselves. Both of us realize that now that I have a career, too, it would be easy for us to drift into our careers as the kids leave home, and to have nothing left between the two of us. It's a danger that we have to pay attention to. In thinking about our future years together, we have considered buying a shack or a beachhouse, something that we could afford, and we would go there on weekends and work on it together. It's relaxing, it's being outdoors and it's doing something we enjoy doing together. And we know from past experience that this is how we can stay close.

Sometimes, particularly if we are experiencing a lot of demands in our lives, we lose sight of our relationship with ourselves, making it very difficult to pay attention to another person.

I don't want my relationship with myself to get between us and I don't want your relationship with yourself to exclude me so we have to live and work and care for the whole group of us . . . In the beginning it was more simple, there was me and you, two women together. The nearer we get to each other the more we become aware of and need to get to know the dormant selves, the primary relationships of which we are made . . . we don't just find one, but many . . . (I think I always liked Hinduism because the god-head is crowded out with selves, not just one).

Some couples have an annual celebration to affirm their commitment, to review their contract and renew their vows. It can be particularly important for those of us who are lesbians to create our own rituals and celebrations as we are denied the opportunity of significant social events to which our heterosexual sisters have access, however much they might rail against them.

There is no one 'right' way to nurture a relationship; we must all find what works best for us.

HAVING OTHER FRIENDSHIPS

Having just talked about the importance of paying attention to each other, it may seem contradictory to stress the importance of other friendships. However, couples can sometimes close in on themselves and let other friendships drop. Yet it is unrealistic to expect that one person can meet all our needs. Other friendships are crucial to our emotional well-being, our happiness, our growth.

Having deep friendships with other people creates a garden in which our whole self can grow and flourish. We get a broader idea about who we are or can be, and call upon different strengths. We are richer, more complex. What we learn through our intense friendships with others – about how to be close, how we seem to other people, how to fight constructively, what we enjoy – we can then weave back into our lives with our partners. By expanding our intimate circles we relieve some of the pressure on our main relationships, and when times are hard other people can then give us support, nurturance and understanding. We don't have to depend only on our partners.

Many women have developed strong friendships with other women in the support and consciousness-raising groups which have proliferated over the past fourteen years. Women have always got together to talk with each other about the details of their personal lives. Though both women and men have considered these gatherings to be idle and unimportant, trivial 'chatting', what we are really talking about is the fabric of our lives. By spending time with other women, we see the potential power of articulating and clarifying what is going on in our lives. We learn that many of the issues we struggle with are not unique to us.

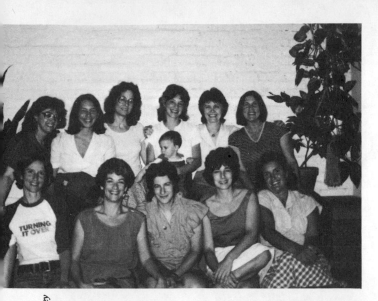

Gina Hawley

The six of us have been meeting every week, or sometimes every other week, for almost five years. Many times I've gone to a meeting with one perspective and come out with another . . . we talk about work, children, lovers, husbands, friendships, parents and anything else that is important to us. My husband said once that he thought he owed the fact that our marriage was still in existence to my group, even though this goes directly against the stereotype some people have that the main activity of women's groups is to go around busting up marriages. Our group helped me work for what I really wanted.

Some men, seeing the value of these groups, have set up their own.* Other support groups include lesbian groups, single-parent, post-divorce and widow/widower groups, and groups which deal with a particular problem, such as alcoholism or drug abuse.

Support groups are helpful at all ages. Sheila is sixty years old and has been married for thirty-seven years.

I've been a member of a women's group for seven years now, and I think we came together out of a feeling that here we were, middle-aged. We didn't really fit into the women's movement totally. And yet there were things we wanted to talk about, and that was the only place they were getting talked about. We could recognize many of the things these women were talking about. And we looked at our lives and how not *having a women's movement when we were younger had made an impact on our lives.*

KNOWING WHEN TO LEAVE A RELATIONSHIP

Many of us struggle along for years in relationships that are

*See Resources in Chapter 10 for information about men's groups.

not rewarding or affirming, wanting to make them better but not succeeding, and not yet convinced that we would be better off if we left. We may come again and again to the brink of leaving, and then back off, not necessarily because things are not quite 'bad enough' (see, for example, discussion of violence in Chapter 10). What holds us back? We may, even with all the problems, still love our partners and be reluctant to lose them; we may feel loyal to them and perhaps not want to hurt them. Perhaps we think that breaking our commitment is a great personal failure, that we will be harshly judged by friends and family. If our partner is a woman, we may wish to avoid being told what a relief it is for our family. We may try to stay together 'for the good of the children' or may dread the prospect of being alone. And there is often the very real fear that we will not be able to support ourselves, and perhaps our children, financially. Yet many women do ultimately decide that they want to end their relationships.

At first Phil seemed to revel in my accomplishments, my growing self-confidence. But I also grew more able to challenge him where he didn't want to be challenged. I have wanted more from him: more involvement with the children, more sharing of paid jobs and housework. I want him to value my strength as I have come to value myself more. His response has been to have a string of affairs, all with women who are much younger than I am and, as you might guess, totally undemanding, unthreatening, willing to accept him precisely as he is.

It lingered for months and months – the relationship I mean. I meant to end it and somehow we drifted from crisis to crisis, becalmed by boredom in between. She and I had sworn undying love and in some ways I still felt it was alive but day-to-day life bulldozed it under. Also I felt, as I have since, that ending a lesbian relationship can be particularly painful. There was no marriage to dissolve, and in our case no parents to inform (they knew but refused to know), no ritual to end it. Because we purposely didn't live together, we had no property to split. Yet our lives were all tangled up. The habit of telling all, the intimacy of daily contact. I still can't 'see' her in my mind as I can other friends – her presence looms as if she were still a part of my senses.

When I was first thinking about getting out of my marriage, I would think, Well, I get a lot of satisfaction out of being a parent and I'm very close to my kids. I get a lot of satisfaction from my friendships and I have a really good work situation. My relationship isn't so good, but maybe you just can't have everything. My husband had some serious problems, so I felt I couldn't blame him or just leave him. I never stopped to consider what it was doing to me to be spending years of my life with someone who was giving me so little. After a while I built up so much resentment that I just wasn't able to treat him in a loving way. And I began to be afraid that I would lose my capacity to love someone. I knew that I had a potential for loving that wasn't getting expressed. Yet it was a leap to assume that getting out of our marriage meant that I would have a good relationship again.

If you wind up just accommodating your partner to prevent fights rather than having some hope that it's worth sitting down and trying to work things out; if your relationship is based on evasiveness, deception and withholding; if it is characterized by stagnation and a lack of room for change and growth; or if it just doesn't seem that your life is better in the relationship than it would be out of it, then it is time to consider the options, including ending it. You don't need to do this in isolation. There are good books on the subject (see Resources, below and in Chapter 8). Turning to friends, particularly ones who are willing to talk openly about their hard times with their partners, can be an excellent source of support and insight. Co-counselling or therapy (see Chapter 8) can help as can support groups.

Far too often, heterosexual women don't get the help they need to leave a non-life-affirming relationship; lesbians equally don't get the support they need to find ways of maintaining a relationship through difficulties; this is partly due to homophobia within the 'caring' professions, but also partly due to inability on their part to understand the pressures. For how to get help, see Chapter 8.

NOTES

1. Adrienne Rich. *Compulsory Heterosexuality and Lesbian Existence*. London: Onlywomen Press, 1980.
2. Sarton, May. *Plant Dreaming Deep*. New York: W. W. Norton, 1983, p. 91.
3. For more about shared parenthood, see Boston Women's Health Book Collective. *Ourselves and Our Children: a Book by and for Parents*. UK edition edited by Michele Cohen and Tina Reid. London: Penguin Books, 1981. For a discussion of some issues facing collective child care, see Marsha Rowe, 'Changing Childcare', in Marsha Rowe (ed.). *The Spare Rib Reader*. London: Penguin Books, 1982.

RESOURCES
PUBLICATIONS

Below are listed some books of general interest; for books more specifically concerned with either lesbian or heterosexual relationships, see the relevant chapters.

Boston Women's Health Book Collective. *Ourselves and Our Children: a Book by and for Parents*. UK edition Michele Cohen and Tina Reid (eds.). London: Penguin Books, 1981. Includes discussion of 'considering parenthood', 'sharing parenthood', 'step-parenting' and lesbian mothers.
Cartledge, Sue and Joanna **Ryan**. *Sex and Love*. London: Women's Press, 1983. A must. Very thoughtful and wide-ranging.
Clark, Clara. *Coping Alone*. Eire: Arlen House Women's Press, 1982. Written for women living in Eire and Northern Ireland.
Dick, Kay. *The Shelf*. London: GMP, 1986. A novel about a relationship between women, from a bisexual perspective.
Federation of Claimants' Union (FCU). *Women and Social Security*, 1985. Available from FCU, 296 Bethnal Green Road, London E2 0AG, tel: 01-739 4173. A straightforward, practical guide.
Garner, Lesley. *How to Survive as a Working Mother*. London: Penguin Books, 1982.
Gilligan, Carol. *In a Different Voice*. Cambridge, MA: Harvard University Press, 1982.
Haddon, Celia. *The Powers of Love*. London: Michael Joseph, 1985. Discusses the relative importance of love – rather than sex – in relationships.
Hailey, Elizabeth Forsythe. *A Woman of Independent Means*. London: Pan, 1987. Fictionalized account of a strong woman told through her letters.
Hodgkinson, Liz. *Sex is not Compulsory*. London: Sphere, 1986.
Kitzinger, Sheila. *Women as Mothers*. London: Fontana, 1978.
Lindsey, Karen. *Friends as Family*. Boston, MA: Beacon Press, 1981.
Maddox, Brenda. *Step-parenting*. London: Allen and Unwin, 1980.
Malos, Ellen (ed.). *The Politics of Housework*. New York: Schoken, 1980. Anthology includes the ground-breaking article of that same title by Pat Mainardi.
Peterson, Nancy L. *Our Lives for Ourselves: Women Who Have Never Married*. New York: Putnams, 1981.
Rich, Adrienne. *On Lies, Secrets and Silence*. London: Virago Press, 1980.
Rich, Adrienne. *Compulsory Heterosexuality and Lesbian Existence*. London: Onlywomen Press, 1980.
Rights of Women. The *Cohabitation Handbook*. London: Pluto Press, 1984.
Segal, Lynne (ed.). *What is to be Done about the Family?* London: Penguin Books ('Crisis in the Eighties' series), 1983. Good as far as it goes, but doesn't have much to say about lesbian families, despite contributions by lesbians.
Sharpe, Sue. *Double Identity – the Lives of Working Mothers*. London: Penguin Books, 1984. Based on interviews; section on single mothers but no mention of lesbian mothers.
Singer, June. *Androgyny – Towards a New Theory of Sexuality*. London: Routledge and Kegan Paul, 1977.
Stack, Carol B. *All Our Kin: Strategies for Survival in a Black Community*. New York: Harper and Row, 1974.
Von Sommers, Peter. *Jealousy: What It Is and Who Feels It*. London: Penguin Books, 1988.
Wolff, Charlotte. *Bisexuality – a Study*. London: Quartet Books, 1979.

Bi Monthly. Newsletter for bisexuals. Available by post from London Bisexual Group, BM B1, London WC1N 3XX. Send sae for subscription details.

ORGANIZATIONS

OPUS. For parents under stress. Tel: 01-263 5672, 01-645 0469.
The Parent Network, 44–46 Caversham Road, London NW5 2DS. Tel: 01-485 8535. Organizes a national network of support groups for anyone in a parenting role.

LOVING WOMEN: LESBIAN LIFE AND RELATIONSHIPS*

Prepared by
JILL RAKUSEN

Being a lesbian for me is about the joy and wonder of loving women. It means being woman-identified, making women my priority. It is a way of life, so much more than a matter of who I want to sleep with.

Sometimes when I talk positively about being a lesbian, heterosexual friends say they hear me criticizing their choice to be with men. That's not true. For me, part of what's essential in being a lesbian is caring for other women, and this includes women who have made choices other than mine.

In this chapter, we aim to reach out with information and support to women who are newly exploring their lesbian identity and to lesbians who find themselves isolated from other lesbians, geographically or otherwise, and to give heterosexual women a clearer picture of our lives.

Lesbians are numerous in every ethnic group, economic class and political persuasion. We are factory workers, teachers, doctors, school and college students, clergy, shopkeepers, politicians, trade unionists, athletes. Some of us have physical disabilities, some have or plan to have children, some are sure we don't want children, some have relationships which last a lifetime, some are disappointed in love, some are celibate. Some of us are married to men and cannot easily leave our marriages, yet we identify ourselves as lesbian and even make primary commitments to women.

All of us, by our very existence, challenge patriarchy. Aware of this challenge, patriarchy responds with prejudice

*The quotes in this chapter involve lesbians from diverse backgrounds and experiences, ranging in age from twenty-four to seventy-six. The chapter is quite different in focus and tone from the original which contained several long, detailed and powerful personal stories. This time briefer stories are used so as to make room for more topics. Readers are referred to the previous UK edition, where the chapter was written by a socialist feminist collective, for more detailed description of lesbians' lives.

and oppression which are a daily part of our lives. This means that a major part of our conscious and unconscious energy has to be taken up simply with coping with this oppression.

LESBIAN OPPRESSION

Heterosexuals can hold hands in public, go anywhere together, be welcomed as a couple by their families and at religious services, celebrate their relationships openly, make decisions for each other in times of sickness and provide for each other's material well-being in case of death. Lesbians can take none of these commonplace things for granted.

'Coming out' is a major issue for us. Coming out is the process of coming to accept and affirm our lesbian identity and choosing how open we want to be about it. It can involve many stages – admitting to ourselves that we are lesbian, getting to know other lesbians, telling friends and family, marching in a gay-rights demonstration, being open at school or work. Many of us will never be free to do all these. We spend a lot of energy deciding whether, when, how and to whom we want to come out. When/if our society one day freely accepts lesbians, we will be able to use that energy in many other ways.

COMING OUT TO OURSELVES

Each of us has her own story of growing lesbian awareness. Since we grow up in a culture which assumes everyone to be heterosexual, becoming aware of our lesbian identity and accepting it is often a gradual process.

I think I was always gay, but it took me seventy years to realize it.

I didn't think about becoming a lesbian until at twenty-five I just fell in love with a woman and had to deal with it. As long as I was with her it was pretty simple, but when we broke up three years later, I finally had to ask myself, 'Am I really a lesbian?'

After my divorce I went out with men and even slept with a few, but something was missing. I was celibate on and off for five years, mostly glad of the clear space and solitude, but at times in despair that I'd never let anyone really close. I felt a strong political and personal commitment to women and a fascination for lesbians, but it scared me to think that maybe I wanted to love a woman – my parents would explode, my ex-husband would try to get custody of our kids, my friends might think I was out to seduce them. I was also afraid it would be a choice against men instead of for women. Slowly I worked through all this and finally one day I said to myself, 'For now, I am a lesbian,' and some important piece of my identity clicked into place. I'm glad I chose to be a lesbian before I had a woman lover.

There were only two other black students at college, and they came from comfortable middle-class families. I felt as out of place with them as I did with the middle-class white students. It was about this time that I began to become aware of an attraction to women, which I kept trying to suppress.

Since I was out of my element socially, I always came on as tough and aggressive to cover up, and people started accusing me of being a dyke. I was terrified that my fantasies were showing in some way, and I began going out with men to show that I wasn't 'like that'. Now I realize that the accusations were intended to bring me into line and make me behave 'like a lady', and it worked. I knew that being a black woman gave everyone the right to walk on me (or try to, anyway), and I thought that being a black lesbian was some sort of capital crime. It was this more than anything else that made me steer clear of women who showed an interest in me.

The women's movement came along about the time I finished college. The movement gave me support because I could see other women having the courage to change their lives. Their example gave me the courage to see that I was cheating myself by pretending to be straight. I finally did come out sexually with a black woman I met at work. I reasoned that if a racist society wanted my head they'd get it because I was black, and being gay wasn't going to make all that much difference. My life has been much fuller since then and a lot happier.

Many of us try to deny our lesbianism at first. It contradicts all the expectations our families and society have for us – and, often, the expectations we have had for ourselves. All we've ever heard about lesbians is negative, and stereotypes of lesbians may scare us away.

I was fascinated by the idea of loving a woman, but totally turned off by what I thought lesbians were supposed to be like. I didn't want to be a man or look like one.

We may want to reject our lesbianism because our upbringing has taught us that women are inferior, or because we know life will be hard or complicated for us as lesbians in certain ways.

I was afraid that if I touched other girls I would like it and keep on touching them. So I became repulsed at the idea. I'm angry that I held the feelings down for so long that now I have a hard time just relaxing and touching someone I love.

Coming out to ourselves means primarily letting go of the guilt, self-hatred and fear learned from living in a homophobic society. Coming out means loving ourselves as women and as lesbians.

When you first come out, it's like you're telling yourself something you don't want to believe. 'You kissed that girl, didn't you? It felt good, didn't it? So what's wrong with it?' You finally begin to be honest with yourself. After that the rest of your life opens up.

When I came out, I didn't know any Asian lesbians in my city. After I realized my sexual preference was for women, despite all the traditional Chinese expectations and the extreme homophobia of Chinese culture, I tried to maintain

Norma Pitfield

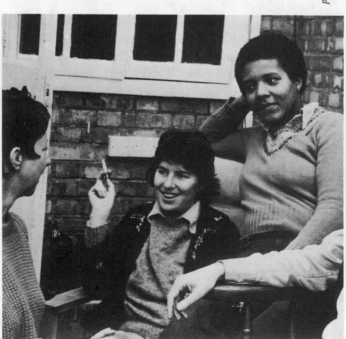

my Chinese identity and to integrate that with feeling strong as a woman, tracing it basically through feelings of closeness with my grandmother, who was the matriarch of the family. I tried to pick out strong women in my personal past and to combine the traditions there that could help me to be strong as a woman and help me be able to feel strong about being a lesbian. So although I am not out to my family, I don't feel as if I'm going to be put out on the mountain to die.

COMING OUT TO FRIENDS AND FAMILY

Letting other people know we are lesbians is usually even more problematic. If we decide to be openly lesbian we become visible targets for physical and psychological harassment. We may be labelled sick, kept away from children, fired from our jobs. Yet if we keep our lesbianism hidden we face insults and embarrassment when people assume we are heterosexual: friends want to 'fix us up' with men, men make passes at us. We live with the fear that others will find out. We feel cut off from many of the people we love.

I want my family and friends to know I'm a lesbian because I want to be honest with them. I don't want to be hiding something from them, especially something so central to my life, something I'm glad about and proud of.

Many of us come out to friends first, choosing the ones who seem likely to be the most accepting.

One friend I came out to said, 'I'm happy that you're in love. But I also feel that it's wrong, that you should have those feelings for a man.' Once she said the negative part she seemed to let it go. From then on I asked my friends for their negative as well as positive responses, so they wouldn't try to be good 'liberal' friends and hide the homophobic feelings that most people have somewhere.

My best friend for thirteen years broke off our friendship several months after I told her, and I haven't heard from her in ten years. No matter how well you know someone, you can never know exactly what to expect from them when you come out.

Not being out to family is often particularly painful.

It's hard at family events when everyone is very heterosexual and brings their families and I'm not able to bring my lover. My aunts all ask when I'm going to marry.

Most parents have a hard time with the news.

I look at my parents as being totally isolated. Who can they talk to about their daughter being lesbian? In this society people make very harsh judgements about gay people, and a judgement about a kid is taken as a judgement about the parents. My parents feel that they are responsible for the person I am, and they can feel guilty about what they 'did wrong'.

Believing lesbianism is 'not right', many parents see themselves as part of both the 'cause' and the 'cure'. Their reactions can be very destructive: therapy can be used, either in an attempt to change our orientation or, more subtly, to help us 'for our own good'. Invalidation is common, and a daughter's choice is rarely taken seriously; they keep hoping we'll meet a nice man and fall in love. Sometimes parents' attempts to control and change us can lead to severe disorientation or even breakdown. Some parents are more accepting, however.

My mother's reaction was exceptional. She said, 'I don't understand it at all, but I'm glad you're happy.'

Coming out to family is usually a process which takes several years. Some parents do come to an understanding, even if they refuse any contact at first; some do not. Coming out can make family relationships more honest and sometimes more close than they were. We may even be pleasantly surprised, as a lesbian grandmother reported:

One of my nineteen grandchildren said, 'I love telling my friends about my gay granny.'*

BEYOND FRIENDS AND FAMILY

Once we were moderately content to restrict our expression of our lesbianism to our leisure time, perhaps because we assumed that heterosexuals expressed *their* sexuality only in their 'own' time. But we have come to realize that heterosexuals express their sexuality at every moment; any dismissal of our openness about declaring our lesbianism at work and in public as 'ramming it down their throats' is quite unjust, for their sexuality confronts us at every turn, whether or not they are acting in a specifically sexual way. The endless assumptions by heterosexuals that they are the 'normal' people have constantly to be challenged. Lesbianism is not a spare-time private activity that waits until the lights are low.

Yet coming out publicly is risky. Job discrimination, a problem for all women, hits lesbians hard. If we are openly lesbian, we are likely to be the last hired and the first fired. And if we hide our lesbianism in order to find a job, we fear being found out. Many lesbians keep totally 'closeted' in

*For a discussion of coming out to our children, see p. 216.

the public eye, living a scrupulously careful double life. Teaching, nursing and some areas of social work contain their own special prejudices against gays who might 'contaminate' children or dependent people. However, teachers and, even more actively, social workers are in the vanguard of those organizing to make sexuality a political issue in the workplace and some unions, such as NALGO are becoming increasingly supportive.

If we are working-class, the situation is usually especially difficult. On the factory floor or in the normal office situation the conversation is predominantly about heterosexual relationships, and any references to homosexuality will almost invariably be in the form of 'jokes' or derogatory gibes. Overall, we don't think that there is any type of work where being a lesbian can be easily and openly evident without, at best, a painful period of 'explanation' and 'acceptance'.

Coming out while still at school can be more of a problem. Adolescent lesbians have to resist constant propaganda that they are just 'going through a phase'. The pressures on every adolescent girl to become the object of a boy's desire are tremendous. The idea that a relationship with a woman can be mutually beneficial and supportive is never advanced, so that the young lesbian may have to wait several years to find the support she needs to establish her identity.*

Over 600 women marched from Holland Park to Trafalgar Square on Saturday 23 June 1984 for the national Lesbian Strength march. Despite a late start, there was a carnival mood with singing and chanting amongst the many groups represented.

The march continued without incident until Trafalgar Square where police arrested Andy Smart, a gay man who had been supporting the march until he was harassed by two passers-by. Jill Posener, one of the photographers, was then arrested as she recorded the incident. Two women who went to assist Jill were also taken away. In a show of solidarity the women marching sat down in the road and refused to move until all four were released.

The situation became tense as the stewards near the police operations van heard that extra police were being brought in, and deployed in the back streets around the square. Despite pressure from his superiors, the officer-in-charge stopped his reinforcements from arresting the marchers for obstruction, and negotiated with the stewards. After about half an hour, all four were released and the women brought back to the march, which then continued in good humour, and high spirits to the evening celebration.

Julie Walkling, *Spare Rib*, no. 145, August 1984

---

*The situation is even more damaging and isolating now that the 'promotion' of homosexuality is disallowed by the notorious Section 28 of the Local Government Act (1988).

Too often we don't feel comfortable or safe seeking health care when we need it (until an emergency arises) because of the ignorance, anti-woman and anti-lesbian attitudes we encounter in most of the medical system. This is a serious health problem for lesbians. Most of us are dependent on medical care providers who know little about our special issues, such as which sexually transmitted diseases (STDs) we are most likely to catch.

I went to the clinic haemorrhaging badly. The doctor, who knew I was a lesbian and not trying to get pregnant, insisted I was having a miscarriage.

Practitioners who don't know we are lesbian can put us into all kinds of uncomfortable situations, asking questions about our home life, sex, 'intercourse' and what kind of birth control we want. Yet if we tell them we are lesbian we may get lectures, snide remarks and voyeuristic questions. ('What do lesbians do in bed anyway?') Our lesbianism may become the focus of the visit, and our medical problems may never be seriously addressed. We also risk having our lesbianism documented on our medical records, which are supposed to be confidential but are not always kept that way.

I would not come out in a medical situation unless there were compelling reasons to do so, because in the 'patient' role I have so little power and am especially vulnerable to harassment. So I practise in advance how to maintain my privacy and still get the care I need – ways of refusing to answer offensive or unnecessary inquiries, and of asking direct, specific questions about what I need to know. For instance, if a practitioner says, 'No sex for a month', I can ask whether I should avoid sexual arousal itself or just vaginal penetration. The book Lesbian Health Matters! *[see Resources] has helped me invaluably in dealing with medical visits.*

The more we are able to be visible, the more we can contradict the lesbian stereotypes – which are partly caused by the constraints we are subjected to. Our mutual support gives us strength, and our increasing visibility in numbers enables us to work more effectively against job discrimination, stereotypes and other kinds of oppression which have distorted our lives.

However, despite and perhaps even because of our increased visibility, attacks upon us and efforts to silence us continue. In July 1982, arson destroyed the offices of a major American weekly newspaper, *Gay Community News*. This attack was mirrored in Britain by an arson attack which burned down *Capital Gay*, a London newspaper, in 1987. As Polly Toynbee reported in the *Guardian*: 'Elaine Kellett Bowman, [a Tory] MP, supported the action in Parliament when she shouted about the incident: "There *should* be intolerance of evil!" and was made a Dame in the New Year Honours List.'[1]

Increasingly, gay and lesbian individuals, groups and organizations are becoming subject to more violent harassment, which is partly connected with heterosexuals' fear of AIDS (fanned for political reasons by the 'family' lobby in government circles and the community at large, and supported by the Anglican church hierarchy) and which many use as an opportunity to unleash their bigotry and hatred. Lesbians of course are the least high risk of any sexual grouping.

I don't think I'm an alarmist when I say that I find it is more often not safe to be obviously out. In my experience homophobia is as intense and pervasive as racial and sexual prejudice, plus it is still legally and socially reinforced. I don't think the answer is to act closeted. I think it is to be aware of the risks, evaluate them, prepare for them and then take them.

SUPPORT AND SOLIDARITY

Contact with other lesbians is crucial and all the more so when as a group we are under such constant attack.

Where I work, I hear the other teachers talking about their relationships . . . nothing heavy, but they do give each other a lot of support. Since being out to them would mean losing my job, I can't let off steam all day; if she's ill and I'm worried about her I can't get any comfort at work. If we have a big decision to make, I can't ask for help in sorting it out. All this makes our lesbian friends terribly important, especially the ones who talk with us about our relationship.

Lesbians can be extremely isolated from each other.

My friend and I have been together for five years. We have not 'come out' as gay. We have always felt that all we need is each other, but now we are beginning to feel very alone and isolated. When you constantly live a secret, you begin to feel as if you are not real. *We need contact with other gays so we can say to someone, 'Look! We love each other and we* do *exist!'*

I didn't think there were any older lesbians in the whole city. Then two friends of mine gave a party and invited all the lesbians they knew over forty years old. It made me feel entirely different to look around that room and see how many we were. Now we meet every month.

However, thanks to the many lesbians and gay men who have struggled for our rights to live and love openly and with pride, we now have growing networks for reaching out to one another. Although pubs, clubs and discos offer a

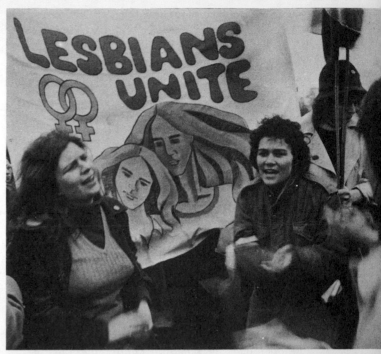

Angela Phillips

place for some lesbians to meet openly and relax together, it has been important to create gathering places which are not built around alcohol and night life, and which reflect all the different interests lesbians have. Increasingly, we now have groups for young lesbians and gays, for black lesbians, for older lesbians, for lesbians with disabilities and for lesbian mothers. (See Resources organizations, including Lesbian Line, a phone line that operates throughout the country.)*

Many of us have felt shy or hesitant about walking into a lesbian gathering for the first time.

The first time I headed for the lesbian support group at the Women's Centre I walked around the block four times and went home. I was scared to come out to a whole new group of people. The next month my need for friendship and support won out over my fears, and I went in.

While support and solidarity can put us in touch with our courage and strength, we need to be realistic about what we can get from our friends.

While we choose our friends, the irony is that the act of choosing is problematic, because it carries with it the corollary that you can choose not to have them too – and they you. When it comes down to it, the people I turn to are my blood family (I don't even like my brothers, but they or other family members would be there to give to me if I really needed something), or my ex-lovers.

*As we go to press we have yet to see the full effect of the Local Government Act 1988 on our meeting places.

Nor can our solidarity as lesbians be expected to span the myriad differences we may have. We may be oppressed in other ways as well as being lesbians; if, say, two women of different colour or different background form a relationship, additional oppression will be present and will have to be worked on *within* that relationship.

Our need for support and solidarity can be problematic in other ways too. Sometimes women 'become' lesbian, and become part of a mutual support network, only to return later to a man.

God, I find this very threatening, particularly as they so often become 'born-again' heterosexuals.

This is particularly threatening because, in order to feel strong as a lesbian in this alien society, we have to embrace the label and affirm ourselves, and to do this we need to be connected with a network of other lesbians. For some of us this presents no problem.

I love the label of lesbian! The reason I like it (which I think reveals how immature I am!) is that I like the rebelliousness that being lesbian represents.

But for others of us, any label is alien, and we're therefore caught in a trap of hating the label but needing to embrace it.[3]

I've never liked labels. I identify myself as a lesbian in certain situations, though not necessarily publicly. Politically, I think it is important to identify as a lesbian if you're in a relationship with a woman. Even though you might not rule out relationships with men, either in the past or the future. However, I feel strongly that the fact that I love my lover is because of who she is, and though this may seem odd, or paradoxical, I feel it demeans and dismisses the depth of our relationship by giving us labels: the unspoken sentence is, 'Well, if they're lesbians, I suppose then it's OK.' WELL, IT'S NOT OK!! It's fantastic and wonderful being so close and so loving and so loved, to and by this wonderful person who is also a woman. The fact that she might well not be so wonderful if she weren't a woman may well be true. But I love her first and foremost as a person.

Yet however problematic our support and solidarity is, we need to pay attention to the range of needs that we and our friends have. In simple daily ways we can ask our friends how their relationships are going, give each other a chance to talk about fights, commitment, jealousy, work, housework and all the other things people need to talk about. We can create our own rituals, where friends and family (sometimes blood relatives, sometimes alternative families) come together to celebrate important events: to affirm our identities as women and lesbians, to honour commitments between women, to mark our children's comings and goings or the endings as well as beginnings of relationships.

Loving each other – as friends, lovers and family – is potentially a source of power, joy, struggle and growth.

ISSUES IN LESBIAN RELATIONSHIPS

Some of us want a relationship but don't really know how to go about it. As women we've had our share of being trained to be passive, which doesn't help at all. Nor does it help if we don't fit the young, able-bodied norm. Or we find someone, but we don't know how to create the loving and committed relationship we would like. We can feel like a bundle of love, wanting to give to someone, and not knowing how to get someone to accept it. And if we've never had sex with a woman before, or with a man either, we can feel very vulnerable (see Virginity, p. 244).

'Do I deserve to be loved?' is an inner doubt that many of us can really suffer from. While heterosexual women can suffer from this too, we have a double dose of it, mainly because of homophobia.

We may also have the problem of wondering how to find women interested in forming relationships.

I started going around with a group of gay men, hoping they would lead me to places where I could meet other lesbians. Usually this was not the case, as the clubs and bars which we frequented were ghettoized and yet another facet of male-dominated culture both in form and attitude. Gradually, however, I got to know other lesbians and began to know other women whom I could relate to politically, socially, emotionally and sexually.

Listed at the end of this chapter are a variety of organizations and publications that can be helpful to us if we need to find out how to meet other lesbians.

Knowing that we love women and acting on that is usually an exhilarating experience. Being outside the dominant culture can give lesbians a certain freedom in shaping the kinds of relationships we want. However, there can be a 'flip' side to this freedom – the sense of confusion that can come from not having clear roles or models to follow.

When I was married at nineteen, I knew exactly what I was supposed to do for ever. I didn't have to think about it. When I entered into my first lesbian relationship I didn't have any idea. It's scary. I don't know where I'm going half the time; there's no one to turn to and ask, 'Is this right?' because nobody knows – there isn't any 'right'. Without role models, how we live has to come from our gut, and mostly I like it that way.

INTIMACY

Many of the issues in lesbian friendships and sexual relationships have more to do with our personal history of intimate relationships than with the fact that we are lesbians.

Family Patterns

Even though we may want different lifestyles from our families', we may find that we have tendencies towards familiar patterns.

In my family no one ever got outwardly angry. There were no fights, only 'discussions'. So when a lover or close friend blows up at me my first reaction is panic. I know I want to fight more openly and not get so quiet with my anger, but it's hard.

My parents lived and worked together twenty-four hours a day until they died. My lover Lou's family was more traditional; her father was away all day working or being with his male friends and his wife spent a lot of time with her sisters. Lou saw her parents enjoying separate time, and she needed that. I had trouble accepting that she wanted to be without me sometimes. We struggled over these differences until we could help each other feel safe doing things differently from how our families did.

Separateness

Every one of us who loves another woman has grown up in a sexist society which devalues women and fails to give us a strong sense of identity. Women's 'role' in relationships has traditionally been to give in, give over, bend, care for our loved ones. While there are endless differences between any two women, there is a certain closeness that comes from being the same sex. We can slip into being so close that there isn't enough breathing room.

It's critical that my lover and I really understand our boundaries, where we want to say no and where we want to say yes. If I don't build my own privacy right away into a relationship, then the next thing I know I'm either spacing out or leaving.

At the moment, I'm obsessed with the need for space. I just have to have the space in a safe place – that's at home – and if I don't I die. To have more long-lasting wonderful times, I must have more time by myself in this safe place. I must discipline myself and go away, not just for my sake, but for my lover's sake as well. We both can retreat and come forward as if it were a dance – over time – different steps – where we keep meeting and touching and sun shines as we join up and then we let go and turn away and we keep the rhythm going – the ebb and the flow – so we don't keep stopping and feeling lost and anxious, and my needs for being safe and close and merged, don't end up in total conflict with the need for my own precious time and space by myself to look at it all, to reflect, to write and, God, to express it. I shall never do it unless I take more time away from her and it's because I love her I must do it.

If you get involved with a woman who lives far away or has to move for a job, you can't either of you assume the other is going to give up her home, friends or job so you can be together. You both know how important all these are. My lover right now lives in another city. I hate the separation but I value her independence as I value my own.

When we are secure in our identity, and feel sure of our boundaries between ourselves and our lover, we can choose the closeness of merging.

It's such a wonderful feeling, leaving the enclosure of my own space to really arrive and be with her.

But there may be many times when we, or our lover, resist this, and the reason may be because it feels like a fight for survival.

I felt something shift last night when she said maybe her passivity and lack of interest in sex were a last-ditch attempt to stay separate. I think this is so true, I'd forgotten the fear of merging.

We may have to work hard to find a healthy balance between closeness and distance, to define ourselves assertively and to encourage each other to grow as individuals.

Butch-Femme

Partly in an attempt to deal with the problem of separateness, many lesbians in the past followed a strict dress and behaviour code, especially in social situations; they chose either a butch role (masculine, aggressive) or a femme role (feminine, receptive). Butches were supposed to initiate sexual relationships, and femmes were supposed to continue their passivity even in bed, allowing butches to make love to them but not reciprocating, though often the reverse would be the case. Butch-femme relationships can become dangerously close to perpetuating sexism and oppressive heterosexual models.

I went from a mother who spoiled me to a classic butch role where I had no responsibility for any housework. About ten years into living with my lover Roz I realized I had a lot of growing up to do. I saw I was no different from any male if Roz was the one who did all the work around the house.

However, in one way or another many lesbians continue to explore the butch-femme evocation of assertiveness and receptivity, either choosing to play roles occasionally, or living out particular roles.

I think the major plus about lesbian sexuality is the never knowing from moment to moment who's being assertive and who's lying back and enjoying it . . . or being active and enjoying it.

I was a femme, a woman who loved and wanted to nurture the butch strength in other women. Although I have been a lesbian for over twenty years and embrace feminism as a world view, I can spot a butch fifty feet away and still feel the thrill of her power. Contrary to belief, this power is not bought at the expense of the femme's identity. Butch-femme relationships, as I experienced them, were complex erotic statements, not phoney heterosexual replicas. They were filled with a deeply lesbian language of stance, dress, gesture, loving, courage and autonomy . . . Butch-femme was an erotic partnership, serving both as a conspicuous flag of rebellion and as an intimate exploration of women's sexuality.[3]

SUSTAINING RELATIONSHIPS

Because there is no social support for our relationships, it can be very difficult to affirm them continually. A crucial factor is how far our relationships are accepted by people who are significant to us.

Our relationship needs validation. It needs a mirror from the outside world to reflect its value back to us. Mere 'acceptance' (whatever that means) is not enough. We need tangible recognition – that most heterosexual relationships get without knowing it. My family is significant to me. Ergo I need them to see me (and that includes my relationship) as significant. Likewise my therapist.

The negativity of 'significant others' can destroy a lesbian relationship very easily, without either party necessarily being aware of it.

Searching for ways to protect and preserve our relationships, we can often end up seeming like a heterosexual married couple. Some of us may like this, some of us may not.

As far as I am concerned, we're married. At the moment it feels essential to me to see our relationship like this. I really need the feeling of commitment and security. I crave it – I think because I find the aloneness of being in a lesbian relationship in an alien world unbearable otherwise. Unfortunately, my partner hates the

married feeling – it's what she's always hated about heterosexuality.

We joke about it all the time. My partner desperately wants to 'get married'. She wants that 'total commitment', exchanging rings, etc. (Ironically, I think it's because then she really thinks she could do what she wanted!) I refuse. I just don't want to be 'married' . . . I've been married – for fifteen years. I don't want to live with someone. I prize, adore and luxuriate in my being independent and on my own at last. It's been very hard to acknowledge that and fully own it, and not flirt with my lover saying 'Well, maybe we might live together some day.' And it's taken her over two years to finally accept that I mean what I'm saying.

Sometimes, fear of old age affects our attitudes to couple relationships.

I think there's something that drives us towards wanting the 'security' of a 'married' relationship. Heterosexuals have it, but I think we have it worse, because we are so alone in this homophobic world. I think there's a lot of difference between being 'free' when young (though I think this is often an illusion anyway), and the sudden fear that can hit you when you're a bit older. I think most lesbians get hit with this fear sooner or later. The fear of a lonely old age. Either it's taking in the accusations from society out there that that's our true fate, or it's a natural sense of insecurity about the future, about being on our own.

I think most lesbians want to have some form of security at a certain point, like a home base. There used to be a lot of communal households but it didn't seem to work out too well, and now there are a lot more couples on their own. And a lot more lesbians having babies. The same sort of thing has happened with heterosexuals too.

Because of the difficulties our society creates for lesbians, perhaps there is some inevitability about the way our long-term relationships can mirror those of heterosexuals. And who is to say whether that is a bad thing? However, in lesbian relationships, it may be harder to fall into a rut.

Even in my worst times, it's never totally predictable how I should negotiate with my lover, and that can be a help (though it can also be a hindrance too!).

It is difficult to overestimate the impact of our oppression on our relationships. At the beginning of this chapter we talked about external oppression. Here we talk about how this oppression can be internalized.

INTERNALIZED OPPRESSION

The ageing issue for me is somehow tied up with the idea that haunts me – that being a lesbian is immature. I don't know where I've absorbed this idea from. I didn't feel it from my therapist (and in any case, it pre-dates therapy). But I know it's part of orthodox psychoanalytic theory, which of course our society has embraced. It backfires on you: you end up feeling immature – and being immature, because that's what you're supposed to be. I find it very hard to scotch this one. But I'm not surprised that so few lesbian relationships seem to last. And this is only one form of oppression that we have to face! I really want our relationship to last, and I know that one of our problems is about acting enough from our adult selves (particularly me).

It is easy to feel that being heterosexual is so much easier – because of the internalized oppression that we have to fight against, the burden of being 'unacceptable', and the fact that our relationships go unrecognized. When the slightest thing goes wrong in our relationships or even when we find ourselves unable to solve big issues with a lover, we can also feel that this simply confirms that our relationship cannot survive.

Every single woman alive knows in her heart that nothing is simple and clear-cut: we need this but we can't stand it, we want independence but we want security, we love our kids but we hate them, we hate them but we love them. We need to be honest about this. So much is stacked against us, the temptation is to say everything is wonderful and to hide all the things that might go wrong.

We need to be aware of just how powerful internalized oppression can be. And also how other forms of internalized oppression can affect us and our relationships – for example, because of our colour, class or religious background. If we can do this, we can sustain our relationships and give and gain the strength, joy and love that is our birthright.

I feel so encouraged by J. to live, to realize myself, to do and be what I can do for myself and other people. I don't think I've ever been so encouraged over time in such a sustained and deeply caring way. It's like being loved all over, all through, very profoundly understood. It must have been difficult and will be in the future to go on believing so much in me but I feel at last I really do believe in what I can do. How it isn't enough to just be together and love each other. I feel a great release because of this; it's like balancing on the waves while surfing (I've only done it once but J. says I'm very good at that!). Now as she is touching my

hair and holding me I feel all those lovely melting feelings and how I never want to be living with anyone else and how strong and wonderful this relationship is. I always thought we came together to grow and it's at moments like this that I know it to be true, and that this is what 'love' is really about. We need to work at it though: always expressing our positive feelings (we always make plenty of room for the negative ones!), remembering to enjoy ourselves, and the many times we enjoy being together, endlessly linking all the happy times so that the circle of all these good feelings can overcome the straight, coldly narrow lines of the past on which someone had written 'Thou shalt not enjoy thyself. You have no right to be happy'.

SEXUALITY*

Part of loving women is feeling sexually attracted to women. What we do with this attraction is as varied as we are. Through sex we may express love, friendship, lust, nurturance, need, a sense of adventure, delight in our own bodies. We may kiss and hug a lot, caress our lover's body for hours or have a 'quickie'. We may play with her nipples or clitoris, explore her vagina with our fingers or our tongues, touch our own bodies, too. We may have orgasms, not have orgasms, use erotic pictures, share fantasies, play sex games, laugh while making love, sleep together without genital sex. There is no one way to be sexual as a lesbian, and no 'right' way.

Books and films always show men and women being sexual together, with certain roles that everyone expects. For lesbians, what 'having sex' means isn't so clearly defined. For me and my lovers it's always been teaching each other, learning together, making it up as we go along. That's how I like it. I feel anything is possible.

Sex with my male lovers was always OK. But with Paula I'm amazed at the intensity. I want to touch and be touched, make love all the time, be rough, be gentle, penetrate her, feel her moving on me. I think I'm finally feeling the fullness and depth of my sexuality. I had always suspected there must be more to it.

In finding out what turns my lover on, exploring her body, tasting her, learning her odours and textures, I am growing to love myself more, too.

It's wonderful not having to think about birth control!

There are also problems, of course.

With lesbian sex there's so much choice. That's

---

*Please read this section in conjunction with Chapter 14, which covers more of the specifics about women and sex.

great. But it can be frightening being confronted with having to choose what you're going to do.

One problem is the myth that lesbian sex is problem-free. We can run into trouble by expecting sex with women to be 'blissful, intuitive, spontaneous, and never dull'.[4]

Making love with a woman for the first time usually involves a lot more than what happens sexually (see Virginity, p. 244). We may feel suddenly freed as sexual beings. We may feel exhilarated and joyful and terrified out of our skins. It can take months and even years to learn about our shifting patterns in sex, what we like and what our particular stumbling blocks are.

The more women I sleep with, the more I realize you can't assume what you like is what she likes. There are tremendous differences. All kinds of stuff needs to be talked about and often isn't.

I have a hard time getting started in sex, but once I'm started I have an easy time coming. My lover loves to get started but has a hard time coming and gets really frustrated. We have trouble talking about it.

We had a wildly passionate sex life for a year and a half. When we moved in together, sexuality suddenly became an issue. It turned out our patterns were very different. My lover needs to talk, to feel intimate in conversation, to relax completely before she can feel sexual. I need to touch and to make a physical connection first before I feel relaxed enough to talk intimately. I'd reach out for her as we went into the bedroom and she'd freeze. We battled it out for months, both feeling terrible, before we worked out what was going on.

Because women are so deeply socialized not to be sexually assertive or to seek pleasure openly, it can be a revelation to learn with a lesbian lover how to talk freely about what you both want in sex.

When I make love with a woman, the challenge is to be honest more often; to say what I am really feeling; to explore when I'm not feeling present instead of pretending that I am; if I am spacing out, to ask what's the fear.

We can come to lesbian sex with . . . a legacy of heterosexual role models harmful to women. Whether we have been heterosexual or not, those ideas creep in anyway.[5]

We may bring to love-making:

- the belief that we don't like sex much and are perhaps 'under-sexed' or 'frigid';
- the feeling that sex is OK but not very profound;
- the assumption that we owe it to our lovers to have sex when they want to;
- distrust of our sexual responses – the conviction that we can't have an orgasm with a partner;
- little experience in being assertive or taking the lead in sex;
- shyness about touching ourselves in sex because we think (or we think our partner thinks) she should do it all;
- a focus on performance in love-making, including orgasm as a goal every time;
- emotional scars from having had our bodies used or abused sexually.

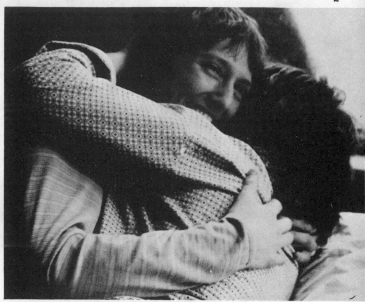

Joy Schneider Kendra

Some of us may suspect our own impulses and preferences when they seem to follow a male model. We may feel uncomfortable with lust, for instance, or with acting aggressively, having fantasies of dominance or using erotic materials. Yet these may be aspects of sexuality which we would enjoy, and commonly the experience with a woman bears no relation to heterosexual sex.

With men I felt I could take it or leave it. But with women I cannot believe the different emotional response I get – so intense that I could never have with a man. Why is it? I think it's because fucking with a man is tied up with giving in or something. Perhaps because I grew up in the fifties and had a very clear sense of differences between men and women. They were out for one thing and I had to put up with it. Fucking was always about giving in, not giving in, letting them have their way, etc. It had nothing to do with pleasure and I never had an orgasm fucking. I wanted to fuck . . . but only until I started to. Then it was ohmygod this is going to go on for ever. With women I am so much freer about fucking. I like fucking with women – using our fingers. (I've never used a dildo though I'd love to try!) I don't like fucking with men.

Fingers can produce feelings in my vagina that no penis has been able to. Fingers can push up, with a strength that a penis can't seem to do.

Some of us have fantasies about fucking with men. This can make us feel confused or worried about whether we're not 'really' lesbian. The issue can be far more fraught than if heterosexual women fantasize about making love with a woman. But as we discuss in Chapter 14, our fantasies can be as weird as we like. They're not things to be ashamed of.

I have fantasies in the shower – where I love to masturbate! They always involve a male image. This may seem surprising given how I love being a lesbian, particularly since the fantasies can involve all sorts of non-women-orientated things like fellatio and anal rape (neither of which I've ever liked!). Sometimes I even turn the fantasy round so that I'm being the sadist – which is even more disturbing. It's such a ritualized thing for me. I can almost get into the shower, wash my hair and stand there just for two seconds. I don't have to have fantasies when I masturbate, I just like it.

When I want a quick wank, I usually go into fantasies about men – I choose that rather than past women lovers because I don't feel that's fair on my current lover.

As lesbians we have a chance to move away from male-defined sexuality, and to reclaim all the dimensions of sexuality which deepen our intimacy, pleasure and love.

If you or you and your lover(s) have problems with sex, you may want to join a lesbian discussion group or seek counselling. (See Chapter 8 and the Appendix in Chapter 14.) Most important, we can probably help each other as friends a lot more than we do now, by bringing sexual problems and issues into our conversations. 'How's your sex life?' may be a timely, kind and enormously helpful question to ask.

LEGAL AND POLICY ISSUES

Prepared by members of RIGHTS OF WOMEN LESBIAN CUSTODY GROUP, *and the* NORTH LONDON LESBIAN MOTHERS' GROUP.

During the past few years there have been some improvements with regard to law and policy. A few local authorities (e.g. Camden and Islington in London, the Greater London and Greater Manchester councils) have adopted policies of non-discrimination towards homosexuals in relation to employment and housing allocation. Sadly, the latter two are now defunct, as is the Inner London Educa-

tion Authority, which adopted a policy of non-discrimination towards lesbian teachers. In child custody cases, there has been a slight shift away from the totally negative attitudes of judges towards lesbian mothers. Also, the law no longer classifies our sexuality as a 'mental disorder'.

However, as is discussed elsewhere in this chapter, it is still the social and legal norm to discriminate against lesbians. In addition, police harassment of lesbians has been made easier by the Police and Criminal Evidence Act 1984, which enables the police to arrest for an 'affront to public decency' (e.g. kissing or holding hands in the street). This will make the situation even worse for black and ethnic minority lesbians who already suffer racist treatment and abuse from the police; there are also many other legal issues which we are unable to deal with here, such as protection of lesbians' rights in prisons and mental hospitals, and the full implications of Section 28 of the Local Government Act (1988), which arrived on the statute book as we go to press and which is a major setback for lesbian and gay rights generally. (See p. 223 for resources which may be helpful on legal issues.)

RELATIONSHIP RIGHTS

There are many legal and financial benefits not available to

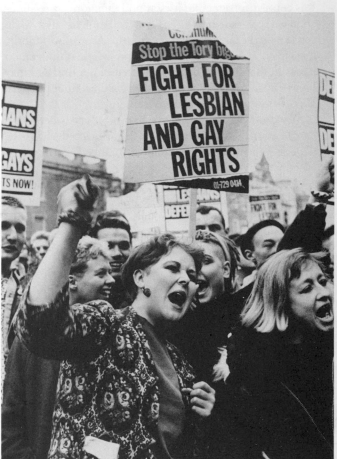

Demonstration protesting against Clause 28 of proposed Local government bill banning 'promotion' of homosexuality, January 1988

Brenda Prince

us because our relationships don't have any legal status. For example, on the death of your lover, you have no automatic legal rights unless she has made a will. If there is no will, all her property passes to her nearest blood relatives who can make all the decisions about her funeral and the disposal of her property. You may have a claim over money/property, but only if your lover contributed towards your maintenance immediately before her death. To guarantee control, you should both make wills so that you choose who deals with your property and to whom it goes. Also, if before her death you were living in rented accommodation, and your lover was the 'protected' or 'secure' tenant, you won't be able to succeed to her tenancy as a 'member of the family'. If you rent, you should try to get a tenancy in joint names. If you own a home, make sure it is held in joint names.

In time of sickness, the law again automatically entrusts all decisions about you to your nearest blood relative. You can give a lover control in medical situations by giving her a Power of Attorney (you can get a form for this from a law stationer's – see Resources), but this will cease to have effect if you become mentally ill. In this case, she will count as your 'relative' only if you've been living together for five years.

Racist and sexist immigration laws also discriminate against lesbians. For instance, a lesbian who is admitted to this country for a temporary stay and then forms a relationship with a lesbian UK resident will not be allowed to remain on the basis of that relationship. An ethnic minority lesbian who has been married and whose immigration status in this country depends on that of her husband may be in danger of deportation if she separates from him (see Resources for where to get advice/help).

We can't claim various non-contributory benefits nor can we claim a full state retirement pension on the basis of a deceased lover/friend's national insurance contributions. Occupational pension schemes often cater only for married couples; if you want to provide for a lover/friend, try checking with your union rep and employer about the scheme and nominate whom you want as your dependant(s). As regards insurance, you can't take out a policy on your lover's life; if you want to insure your own life, you should make sure that you assign (by trust deed) the benefit of the policy to whomever you want.

Lesbians today are beginning to explore ways of establishing and protecting their relationships. If you wish to define your rights and responsibilities within a relationship, you could try to protect yourselves by working out a formal agreement about matters such as expenses, purchases, childcare, maintenance of children. While accepted by American courts, it is uncertain whether courts here would uphold or enforce them (see *The Cohabitation Handbook* for more details). You should also bear in mind that agreements are easily broken and that court proceedings can be painful and costly (if you're not eligible for legal aid). In any case, you may not wish to involve a racist, sexist, anti-lesbian legal system in any stage of your relationship. If you wish to separate and cannot resolve prop-

erty disputes, couples therapy (see p. 131) or mediation may be an option, as this can help you to continue to treat each other more decently. Some lesbian lawyers in America encourage women to draw up contracts that agree to 'community arbitration' in the event of a dispute, in order to avoid the sexist, homophobic legal system. Lesbians in this country have yet to set up such 'arbitration' procedures.

LESBIAN MOTHERS AND THE LAW

Lesbians who have had children through alternative insemination, or a casual encounter with a man, in general do not stand in any risk that the law will take them away, since the father is not around to claim custody. Some social service departments still take a dim view, however, of lesbians bringing up children, and it is not wise to let them know that you are a lesbian, unless they have a policy of non-discrimination against lesbians.

Child Custody

If the children have had some relationship with the father, the situation is very different. In cases where the mother is

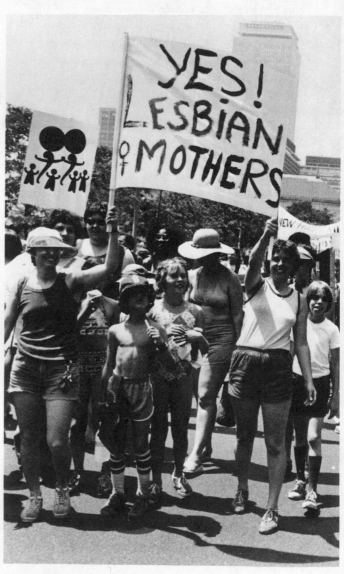

Susan D. Fleischmann

SEEKING CUSTODY

Try to find a sympathetic solicitor even if you don't expect that your lesbianism will be an issue. Make sure that your solicitor accepts your lesbianism, has experience in custody (preferably lesbian custody) cases and is prepared to consult you fully at all stages (see Resources for finding a solicitor). If your income and capital don't exceed certain limits, you'll be able to receive free legal advice and legal aid.

Even if you think your children's father will agree to your having custody, you should try to keep the children with you (if you leave the 'matrimonial home', take them with you) in order to be in a stronger position if he subsequently disputes custody.

If the custody is disputed, there will eventually be a full court hearing at which a judge makes the final decision, supposedly on the basis of the best interests of the child. Prepare for the case with great care. Your behaviour and lifestyle will be under close scrutiny. A 'court welfare officer' will prepare a report for the court on you and your circumstances, and on the father, so try to make sure that you're friendly and cooperative with them. They should show you the report. Whoever you are living with will also be under scrutiny. You can call witnesses in support of your case, such as friends and lovers; you may consider calling 'expert' witnesses, like child psychologists, especially if the father is bring-ing one in. Recent research shows that the only differences between lesbian and heterosexual mothers are the discrimination and oppression experienced by the former,[6] and children of lesbian mothers are no more likely to develop 'problems' than those of heterosexual women. In fact, in one study the evidence points the other way, if anything.[7] It is also worth pointing out that it is for the most part heterosexual males who sexually abuse children, and one in ten girls experience some form of father/daughter abuse (see Chapter 10).

Living through a custody case is likely to be a great strain. You will need a lot of support (there may be a lesbian mothers' group in your area – see Resources); your lover may need support too.

If you lose custody or don't want to live with your children, you have a right to access, i.e. to see them at weekends, and/or in the holidays. If you don't think the father will agree to the access you want, make sure that the court defines your access. Get your solicitor to resist any conditions being put on your access, for example, not seeing the children in the presence of a lover. Once a custody and access order is made, it is not fixed for all time. Either parent can go back to court to ask for a variation of the order if there is a change in circumstances. There is also the possibility of appealing against the order.

---

heterosexual, the majority of fathers are usually content to let her have care and control of the children.* This is not the case for lesbian mothers, where the majority of fathers seem to want to fight for custody – either because they want to get revenge on the mother, or because they do not want *their* children brought up by lesbians. Many of us, therefore, find ourselves in a dispute over custody.

On divorce, arrangements have to be made about the children before the divorce can be finalized, and these have to be approved by a judge. If the parents cannot come to any agreement, the court will decide who shall have custody, care and control.

Lesbian mothers often avoid contesting custody in court either because we believe we have little chance of winning, or because that has been our legal advice. Lesbianism alone is not supposed to prevent a mother winning custody, and in a recent case the judge gave a woman custody, stating that the mother's lesbianism was 'irrelevant'. The courts are meant to do whatever is in the best interests of the child, but of course they operate from a biased standpoint. In some cases, it is clear that the only reason for not giving a mother custody is her lesbianism. (See Box and Resources for further information.)

Sharing Motherhood with a Woman

It is not legally possible to appoint anyone a guardian of your child while you are still alive and caring for them. However, you could name your lover/friend as guardian by deed, which would at least show whom you wish to care for your child if, for example, you become ill. If you wish to appoint her as guardian after your death, you can do this by

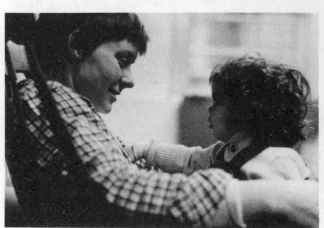
Susan Butler

*The English courts distinguish between 'care and control' (i.e. who has the day-to-day care), and 'custody' (i.e. the right to make major decisions in a child's life); in Scotland, 'custody' means the same as 'care and control'.

will. She will then become legal guardian of your child on your death, unless you were legally married to the child's father, in which case she will become joint guardian with him. Although there is no guarantee that this would not be overturned by a court on the application of a father or grandparent, it is the best you can do.

For adoption and fostering, and alternative insemination, see Chapter 21.

HOUSING

Lesbians do not figure high on local authority housing lists because we're classed as single people – whether we're in relationships or not; housing policies do not favour single people, and accommodation that is offered can often be substandard or hard to let.

We can feel very vulnerable living in such accommodation. And racism in housing policies makes it very difficult for black women to find suitable and secure accommodation. It's particularly important, therefore, that housing policies recognize the needs of women who don't have the 'protection' of men, and the additional needs of those of us who are black or physically challenged. A report on single homeless women[8] showed that of single people housed by a sample of local authorities in 1981, only about half as many women as men were granted tenancies.

Lesbians and gay rights groups have had some successes on the housing front, and a few local authorities now have policies that do not discriminate against us. For information about lesbian housing co-operatives and housing trusts, contact ROW or the Older Lesbian Network which is actively concerned about housing for older women, see p. 219.

LESBIAN PARENTHOOD

Many of us were mothers before we knew we were lesbians. Some of us have become mothers since. Others of us have become co-parents to lovers' or friends' children. While the main issues we face are shared by most mothers in our society, being a lesbian parent adds some unique satisfactions and special difficulties.

The heterosexual world of school meetings, visits to doctors and birthday parties rarely recognizes that we are both lesbians and parents. Even within the lesbian community we often feel like an invisible minority. While our need to come out of isolation and make ourselves known has sometimes brought us loss and pain, it has also created experiences of joy and understanding in support groups and in many friendships.

COMING OUT

Coming out to our children depends very much on our custody situation, as well as our own feelings, and circumstances.

My children are all under eight, and their father has 'access' to them while I have custody. He does not know I am a lesbian so I feel that I have to stay firmly in the closet to my children.

Where there are no problems around custody, then it may be easier to tell our children, depending on their ages and understanding. But being out to our children may bring problems. Children may feel they have to hide our lesbianism, and resent it.

If they [other kids] knew about my mum I'm afraid they wouldn't like me. Sometimes I feel I'm in the closet, too, and I'm not even gay.

My daughter's father doesn't know I am a lesbian, and I don't know what his attitude would be (and I'm not going to ask him), but the fear of what he could do controls a lot of my life and her life too. She goes to stay with him regularly and has to keep a careful silence on my lifestyle.

Our sons may feel that our choice of women implies a rejection of them. A seventeen-year-old remembers:

My mother told me she was gay when I was twelve. It made me feel very different from everyone else. I thought that if you were a lesbian then you didn't want boys around. My mother said that wasn't true, but about six months later I went to live with my father. Now that I'm older, I view it differently and I've also proved to myself that it didn't matter as much as I thought. I'm moving back home now.

Or we may simply not know how our children feel.

The emotional dynamics and the political implications of women living together, particularly with a child who is female, are as yet totally unexplored. With the inept and inappropriate language of our culture, we try to understand the relationships, but it's like trying to map-read on the moon with an A–Z of London. Who models what, how does my pre-adolescent daughter really see what's happening, how can we all make it easier for children of this age to speak and tell us what they feel? Are we brave enough to do so and strong enough to hear their own needs, and inspire as well as comfort them along the way?

Whatever the problems, it's important to keep them in perspective. Sometimes we can be pleasantly surprised by people's responses.

At the school medical, I explained that I wasn't his biological mother, and the doctor asked outright whether I was in a lesbian relationship. I was really pleased that she asked; I said yes, and I

*didn't want it written down. I came out feeling
ten feet high – simply because I was able to be
direct at last. I think people should ask.*

For many of us, the rewards of coming out to our
children outweigh the problems.

*A lot of women in my lesbian mothers group have
said that their kids were relieved to know instead of
thinking it anyway and wondering why it couldn't
be said.*

*I heard my four-year-old daughter telling a
communal sister that girls could fall in love with
girls and it was OK for boys to fall in love with
boys. Where is the revolution? Sometimes it's right
in our own backyards.*

*I think because we make ourselves open to our kids
in this one area we are open to them in a lot of
ways. We dare to be different, and sometimes it
hurts to be different. That we share that with them
creates a very special relationship.*

*We told the school that we both parent Jack. We
felt it was the best way to do it. His teacher, and
the head, have been fine. On Mothering Sunday,
he came home with two cards. He had to make two
while everyone else had only one, and he was very
pleased about it!*

We all need support during the process of coming out,
and often afterwards too, so that we can develop and sustain
a strong identity as a lesbian and a mother or co-parent. The
better we can feel about ourselves and our choices, the
more we have to share with our kids and each other. (See
Support and Co-parenting below.)

RESISTING GUILT

All mothers are made to feel guilty about not being 'good
enough'. Lesbians can carry an extra burden of guilt.
Sometimes it seems as if we can't do anything right. If our
children live with us, we're accused of making their lives
unnecessarily difficult, or even of contaminating them. If
we decide not to live with them, we're the epitome of the
rejecting mother. Yet it can be because of the cost to our
children, e.g. in going through a custody case, that we may
decide not to live with them. Nevertheless, not living with
our children may be what we need or want, though in this
society it can be hard to admit, particularly for lesbians.
Other mothers who have made the same decision are often
the best women to talk to about this. Our self-doubt about
our worth as mothers, or guilt about abandoning our
children needs to be talked through, so that we can feel
positive about resisting the institution of motherhood.

If we are divorcing, we have to remember that our
children would be hurt, sad and angry at this time even if
we weren't lesbians. All children, especially teenagers,
have problems, because that is the nature of growing up. It
is difficult to let go of the guilt because society's disapproving view of lesbians supports and reinforces it. It helps to
look at our heterosexual friends: their children have nightmares, stay at home 'sick' from school, fight with their
friends, get depressed, get furious at their parents, think
they have the worst luck a child has ever had – just like our
children do.

SUPPORT

One of the best ways to get the support we need for us and
our children is through other lesbian parents. (See
Resources for how to find a group.)

*My main support comes from my lesbian mothers'
group, both from our monthly meetings and from
the informal network it has given me access to. I
have also derived enormous strength from the
occasional national conferences of lesbian mothers.*

*Some of my daughter's closest friends are daughters
of other lesbians that she has met through the
lesbian mothers' network. Because they know each
other, they don't find it that 'unusual' to have
mothers who are lesbians.*

*I do babysitting swaps once or twice a week with a
lesbian mother who lives nearby. This is possible
because the boys are close in age and attend the
same school. We moved to live near each other
with this specifically in mind.*

However, the support we often need may be at a more
profound level.

*As an invisible female child constantly being
'looked at', I became male-identified and
heterosexually conditioned, before choosing to have
a baby (which earned me the label of 'mother'),
and then living with the woman I love (which gave
me the title 'lesbian'). Both these terms come from
a society I share little with, and I find the label of
'lesbian mother' and the concept of 'lesbian
mothers' groups' alien to me. I can share
experiences with friends, and this is essential. But
the support I need comes both from seeing my child
valued, and my relationship being seen as
significant, by those I love.* It is not surprising
therefore that I get more support from my mother
than I do from the lesbian parents who live down
the road.*

CO-PARENTING

Co-parenting can mean that women you live with or who
live nearby take some responsibility for your child (and
perhaps vice versa).

---

*See the importance of Significant Others, p. 210.

In my communal lesbian house, the other women were co-mothers to my daughter. Everyone did one night of childcare a week. Everyone also took on part of the child's rent so I didn't have to pay double.

I co-parent my daughter with two friends. They pick her up from school, and attend parents' evenings and school functions. She also goes away with them on weekends and holidays sometimes. At first I had some difficulty getting the school to accept them as co-parents, but now they do and it's OK.

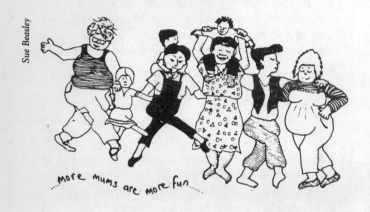

...more mums are more fun...

Co-parenting can also involve a mother who already has a child being joined by another woman who becomes a co-parent as well as her lover.

When we moved in together, I became a co-parent overnight. Up until then, I'd been involved with Sophie's daughter, but it was nothing like what I would call real *co-parenting.*

Or it can involve a joint decision by a lesbian couple to become parents together (see AI etc. in Chapter 21).

I had had lots of stable heterosexual unions before, but I didn't decide I wanted a child till I started my first lesbian relationship. Ten years and two kids later (one each), we're still together. We're part of a lesbian mothers' group where all the members are women who decided to have children as lesbians – though not all of us are in couples.

Co-parenting can be extremely rewarding and supportive for everyone concerned.

It gives me permission as a surrogate parent to enjoy childish things: ET, funfairs, etcetera. It gives me access to ordinary things like community life that childless lesbians often feel excluded from.

As a childless lesbian I felt much more segregated from society and the community: we had no access to their world and vice versa. The world is very child-centred: one is a far greater oddity being a lesbian without children than a lesbian with children. My own family can suddenly talk to me now – through and about the kids. And the kids love this third set of grandparents.

With us there's a real sharing of the load. It's different from being with a man, where things tend to be assumed. We have the freedom to think about roles, what the hell you want. There isn't a father's role and a mother's role. Instead, there are roles for two people to share out, to really negotiate.

However, it does require careful thought, sensitivity and hard work, that many of us are not prepared for. Here are some quotes from women in a variety of co-parenting situations.

Having seen my daughter hurt by women showing interest in her, and then fading out of her life, I think twice before encouraging anyone now in a co-parenting role.

The only women who share childcare successfully are sisters (they know they won't go away), and couples: not friends. I myself have had very bad experiences with caring for other women's kids.

I lived as a heterosexual until about three years ago, and now I experience a real separation from families and parents of the children's friends that I never felt before. It's a different feeling from when I was a single parent. Now, when I go to the PTA etcetera, I feel a complete fish out of water. I never did before, and it's not to do with the school: there's no awkwardness there. It's to do with other kids' parents.

I had problems at first because of his marked preference for Jane when she was breastfeeding. Now we spend very equal amounts of time with him. Damn it, I put the bloody sperm in. I organized all the donors, did all the planning!

I am co-parenting the child of my lover, who I first met when she was eight (the child, not the lover!). I'm finding that lesbian co-parenting in a couple has all the pitfalls of step-parenting, but magnified and multiplied. It's pioneering stuff, trying to forge your own ways of relating without the constraints of the heterosexual world. But most of the time, I crave for the knowledge of some ground-rules, for the security of a clear role. And since we both had problematic relationships with our own mothers, we both worry about giving 'our' daughter two problematic mothers to contend with! So I'm trying to be a parent who is neither a mother nor not-a-mother.

This brings us to the question of roles and labels. What do we call ourselves? How do we define our roles?

I see myself as a parent, when I see myself as a parent. When I don't, I see myself as living with three other people in the same house where I have a major financial responsibility for two of them. In heterosexual couples where one of them already has a child, the couple often try and produce another one, to fuse the relationship. This gives the man a 'proper' role. I can understand why this seems to happen in the majority of heterosexual cases, as sorting out roles can be very difficult otherwise. I know of lesbians who are planning to do the same thing, but I know it wouldn't be right for me.

Perhaps more urgently, what do the children call co-parents? Kids can feel acutely embarrassed or uncomfortable by not being able to refer to us with a suitable label. Perhaps the most suitable ones – 'surrogate mother' or 'surrogate parent' – have been denied us by a society that has defined these terms differently (see p. 436), and, as it happens, incorrectly.

But while lesbian parenthood can be tough, other types of parenthood can be tougher.

My sister has a terrible deal. Her husband's out seven days a week. She's worse off than a single parent. At least then she could just be responsible for herself and her kids. But she's got to be responsible for him too. Wash his socks and everything.

Whatever kind of parenting we do, whether we're mothers, co-parents or mothers' lovers, we need to develop and maintain support systems which can help us cope with the challenges of our roles. For more about parenting, see Chapters 11 and Chapter 21.

WE ARE EVERYWHERE

OLDER LESBIANS*

I have a whole different feeling about ageing since I met Ruth. Partly it's loving her and feeling so loved and so fully known for the first time. Also, as she and other lesbians teach me about being strong, being your own person, I feel more optimistic about growing older. (Forty-five-year-old woman in her first lesbian relationship.)

Many women have a false security. A woman will say, 'I'll always have my husband to take care of me.' No, she won't. There's no security for any

*See also Chapter 22, which considers ageing in general, both for heterosexual and for lesbian women.

animal, any organism in the natural world. But lesbians are accustomed to the reality of life. That keeps them flexible and more prepared for the later years. It's partly the rigidity that people nurture within themselves that makes their old age hard for them. Most lesbians don't have the luxury of being rigid. (Seventy-year-old woman.)

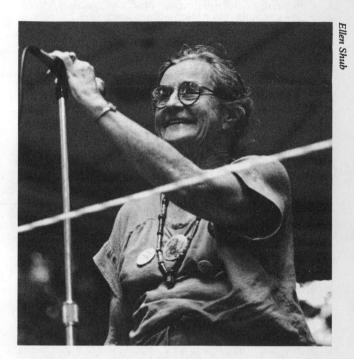

Ellen Shub

While the term 'older lesbian' covers a huge range of life experience, all of us to a certain extent share the same oppression. No longer young, we experience ageism from younger lesbians as well as from society as a whole.

Why is an ageing body thought to be less desirable, and ageing flesh disgusting?

It can be particularly difficult to assert our sexuality as older lesbians, because of society's twin antipathy to women who are either lesbian or deemed 'too old' for sex. To be both can be too much. It is not surprising, therefore, that older women unattracted to men are so easily stereotyped as 'dried-up spinsters' or 'predatory' lesbians. However, when asked about the disadvantages of being lesbian and old, the second woman quoted above said:

You've asked the wrong person. For me there are no negative aspects to it at all.

Any older woman can find herself isolated and unable to find satisfying, sustaining work. This is even more true for older lesbians, because homophobia operates in addition to ageism and sexism. Therefore, it's necessary for us to find and develop a family – if not our own, a family of friends,

THE OLDER LESBIAN NETWORK

The Older Lesbian Network (OLN) has been in existence since March 1984. We hold monthly meetings (in wheelchair-accessible places), and although we are currently still London-based, some women travel from as far afield as Northampton and Bath to attend. We produce a newsletter which is available on tape and has nationwide coverage.

The OLN welcomes all older lesbians regardless of class, creed, colour, physical ability or political perspective. There is no artificial age limit; the range covered so far is probably from thirty-six to somewhere in the seventies. The network also aims to be of help to those women who are struggling/ feeling their way towards a lesbian identity.

The OLN's aims are both political and social: we hope to continue to voice the needs of older lesbians in our society and to give each other strength and support. Our meetings and newsletter have an important social function, since many of us are very isolated, and we have all made many new friends through the network. Meetings usually start at midday and time is set aside for socializing, sharing food, discussion of topics of interest (usually in small groups) and a general 'business' meeting. The OLN has spawned smaller sub-groups, and the following are some of the issues that we have been examining on both a personal and political level: housing, bereavement, transport, legal and medical advice, caring for adolescent children. OLN occasionally holds socials and discos and of course smaller groups can be organized for other outings (theatres, restaurants, picnics, etc.).

To contact the network, write to BM OLN, London WC1N 3XX, enclosing a stamped addressed envelope.

---

homosexual and heterosexual, old and young, with whom we can share, care, love and encourage. This is especially important for older lesbians who are single, have lost a lover or live in remote areas where it's hard to find support.

For some single older lesbians who feel that there isn't much time left, a scary question is 'Can I ever find a lover?' It takes courage and initiative. If a lover is considerably younger, age difference can be an issue. Some women feel that wide age differences are inappropriate ('I should act my age' or 'I won't be able to keep up with her'); others feel that age doesn't matter.

Alice and I grew up in different worlds – she in the fifties and I in the twenties. So much has changed, especially for women. What she wants for her life is not what I ever wanted or expected for mine. As long as both of us notice, respect and understand these differences, we do well together. In a way, the age span is good – it makes us see that we can't be everything for each other, that we need friends of our own age.

Older lesbian couples need to be prepared for some special situations. See 'Legal and Policy Issues' (p. 213) for strategies to make sure that close relationships are honoured in times of sickness or death, and Chapter 22, for more on ageing in general.

An older lesbian who is out, strong, independent and unafraid, can find support from younger women who may welcome such a role model. But we also need support for our fears, dependencies and weaknesses.

It's good to mix older and younger lesbians. When younger people get together more often with older lesbians and see that they're not doddering and so on, they'll be aware that there's not that much difference, and perhaps it will make it easier for them as they grow older.

While we need support for our fears, dependencies and weaknesses, we need to recognize our strengths. As the report of the first Older Lesbian Conference concluded:

Older lesbians have always made a huge contribution to society: teaching, civil service, nursing, etc., would no doubt collapse if we all suddenly retired! We are here to stay, our numbers are increasing, and gradually, we are confident, as we make our voices heard, and take our rightful place in society, everyone will be better off, and we will live in a more healthy and a more truthful society.

LESBIANS WITH PHYSICAL DISABILITIES

Disabled lesbians are a growing group which the lesbian community is beginning to acknowledge. We are all colours and races, all cultures, shapes, sizes and ages. Some of our disabilities are hidden, some are very visible. Some of us are born differently-abled; some of us acquire a disability suddenly and unexpectedly, or over time.

For a long time we have been isolated from each other in our dual identity as lesbians and disabled women.

From my perceptions and from other disabled dykes I've talked to, there are lots of reasons differently-abled dykes hesitate to come out as lesbians. Being someone who is physically different in appearance leaves me already open to ridicule and stares. Lesbians are attacked all the time for being different. Why choose to get hurt twice if you can avoid it? Also, people think disabled women are sexless. If I came out at work I don't know if they'd be upset or just laugh. They'd say, 'How can you be a lesbian if you have no sex?'

Today more and more of us are coming out, e.g. becoming involved in groups such as GEMMA (a group of disabled and able-bodied lesbians) and SAD (Sisters Against Disablement) – see Resources.

Loving women is sometimes part of coming to accept ourselves as women, which can be hard to do if we don't fit the description of what a woman is 'supposed' to look like.

I was disabled by an accident before I became a lesbian. As a woman in a wheelchair I felt something less than a person. But my nurse, who is a lesbian, told me I could have a strong self-image. She said that we are taught to hate ourselves because we are women, and that we can love ourselves instead. I started spending time with lesbians. The closer I came to lesbianism the more I began to like myself.

Lesbians are often more accepting of us and our bodies than men are. But even lesbians often hold us at a distance.

Some women are uncomfortable just being around a disabled woman; others are comfortable with being a friend but can't consider a sexual relationship. I feel like my sexuality is taboo.

Sexually we are often stereotyped as sexless or overtly needy.

When I tell people Janet is my lover they look at her like they're thinking, Poor thing! or, She must be a nurse! or, Maybe she's a pervert who gets off on sex with a disabled woman. They can't imagine that she loves me and the disability is only one thing about me.

Though it is common for those of us who spend time in institutions or hospitals or with daily attendants to have sexual relationships with our primary caretakers, it isn't necessarily a 'nursing' relationship. Our lovers take care of us no more than we take care of them. We may have to make special arrangements for sex or give our lover certain information about our sexuality, but every sexual relationship in the world is shaped by both individuals' wants, needs and capabilities.

I felt weird because I had to explain what my sexual needs were to anyone I wanted to sleep with until I realized that everyone has to explain what their needs are in order to get them met. I don't have sensation in my pubic area, but since there is no set standard to what lesbian love-making is, it leaves a whole world of sexuality and sensuality open to explore.

Once we have accepted our dual identity, we would like to be able to live it more easily. But many people we meet have a hard time with it.

People on the street will deal with my disability sometimes, but no matter how butch I am or what badges I have on, they won't deal with me as a lesbian.

In health care, heterosexual doctors will look at our disability but are rarely sensitive about lesbianism and thus do not see us as whole people. We wind up most of the time being seen as either lesbian or disabled but not both.

The lesbian community is committed at a certain level to including all kinds of women. Lesbians usually look for wheelchair-accessible spaces in which to hold concerts and community events, and offer signing there for the deaf and hearing-impaired. Yet this risks being tokenism if a tremendous amount more is not done.

It is time for the lesbian community to hear our voices. Don't segregate us from our other sisters. We all need each other.

BLACK LESBIANS
by PRATIBHA PARMAR

Over the last few years black lesbians have become more visible than ever before. This is not to say that black lesbians were not around before, but it is an indication that more and more black women have the confidence to come out. The growth of the black feminist movement in this country has provided the political and emotional context for black women to come out to each other.

The first black lesbian group was formed at the third OWAAD (Organization of Women of African and Asian Descent) conference in 1981. Asian and African–Caribbean women came together at a workshop at this conference and history was made. It was the first time that such a meeting had taken place and the large turnout was a wonderful affirmation for many women who had been isolated. Becoming visible was difficult for many women but also very exhilarating. For many women this was their first opportunity to meet and talk with other black lesbians.

The group continued to meet for a number of years. Women from outside London used to travel great distances to come to group meetings, and the support and friendship networks that such a group provided were invaluable. Today there exists the Black Lesbian Support Network, which was formed in 1984 to provide support, advice, information and counselling to women who 'are questioning their "hetero" sexuality'.

The Women of Our Tradition

Black lesbians have a long and rich history of being women-identified women in our countries of origin. Increasingly,

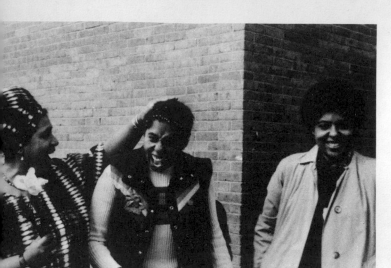

Tia Cross

more and more such women are being rescued from the hidden closets of history, providing us with a sense of continuity of our existence and also highlighting the deep-rooted and ancient oppression of lesbians in our communities. The silence that has veiled their lives obscures our heritage as black lesbians.

Coming Out

The whole notion of 'coming out' is different for black lesbians than it is for our white counterparts. Racism as much as homophobia controls how many come out and in what circumstances. Many black lesbians do not want to take the risk of total rejection by families relied on for many other different kinds of strength and support. The emotional involvements, the ties and roots our families embody in a fundamentally racist society are enormously strong. This is not to say that the family is not oppressive for black women, because in many ways it is: witness the number of women in refuges as a result of experiencing domestic violence, and many black women are severely and rightly critical of the black family even while acknowledging its important supportive role. However, this is in complete contrast to the attacks made by many white feminists on the family, especially black families, since for black women it is always done with an awareness of the attempts to break up and separate black families.

> *The family is very contradictory for us. There are emotional involvements, there are ties, the roots that it represents for us all as individuals in a racist/sexist society . . . We have to recognize that not coming out can exact a terrible toll, in the sense of living this huge personal/political lie.*

As the numbers of visible black lesbians grow so does the strength of the black lesbian community, which provides a base and a core from which both the racism of white lesbians and the homophobia of the black communities can be challenged. Black lesbians have gained support from each other to come out, and define their own sexuality and

to some extent provide the alternative source of emotional and personal support.

Our Particular Oppression

Challenging racist myths about black lesbians is a continual struggle for many of us. Within the white lesbian community the idea that black communities and cultures are more anti-lesbian than the white communities is often expressed. This comes directly from the racist stereotype of black cultures being more repressive and backward than white, European cultures. Lesbianism has existed all over the world throughout history yet many black people believe that it is a white 'problem'. Black lesbians are seen to be part and parcel of a 'conspiracy' against the black family and communities. So black lesbians don't only have to deal with the racism of the white society and white lesbians but they also have to challenge the homophobia within the black communities.

Many black lesbians are involved in all areas of political action and don't necessarily organize around issues of sexuality alone. Many are aware of the simultaneous and multi-faceted nature of our oppression, and are active against racism, sexism and state repression as much as against threats to the right to define our own sexuality.

Creating Ourselves

In a society which actively works against the interests of all minority groups, we come under attack as women, as black people and as lesbians. In the face of such constant opposition and threat to our very beings, we are creating our own communities and networks where there is relative safety from hostile forces. Black lesbians incorporate women from many different cultural and national communities and we are constantly exploring our diverse cultures and draw from each other not only points of common identity but also strength through our differences.

NOTES

1. 'Freedom's Roadblock', *Guardian*, 14 January 1988, p.13.
2. For more on the effects of adopting labels concerning our sexuality, see Sue Cartledge and Joanna Ryan. *Sex and Love*. London: Women's Press, 1983, p. 198.
3. Joan Nestle. 'Butch-Fem Relationships: Sexual Courage in the 1950s', *Heresies*, Sex Issue, vol. 3, no. 4, issue 12, May 1981, p. 21.
4. Tacie Dejanikis in *Off Our Backs*, November 1980, p. 25.
5. Ibid.
6. E. Lewin, et al. 'Lesbian and Single Heterosexual Mothers, Con-

tinuity and Difference in Family Organization', paper presented to American Psychological Association, 1979 (available on file at ROW – see Organizations).

7. Susan Golombok, et al. 'Children in Lesbian and Single Parent Households', *Journal of Child Psychology and Psychiatry*, vol. 24, no. 4, 1983, pp. 551–72.

8. Helen Austerberry, and Sophie Watson. *Women on the Margins*. (On file at ROW.)

RESOURCES
PUBLICATIONS

The following is a selective guide. Check out feminist bookshops and publishers (see p. 638) for other books including more recent material. All of the material listed below is available in the UK, though for American publications, it would be best to go to a feminist bookshop. We are grateful to Sisterwrite Bookshop for helping us to compile this list.

AN OVERVIEW

Abbot, Sidney and Barbara **Love**. *Sappho was a Right-on Woman*. New York: Stein and Day, 1973. Descriptions of various lifestyles and personal histories in the context of gay liberation, and a section on how the growing lesbian struggle influenced the American women's movement.

Athey, Phyllis and Mary Jo **Osterman**. *The Lesbian Relationship Handbook*. USA: PUSH, 1984. An American import, fiendishly expensive (for what it is – a booklet), but because of the dearth of help available, can be very useful. Discusses issues like communication, boundaries, addiction.

Beck, Evelyn Torton (ed.). *Nice Jewish Girls: A Lesbian Anthology*. Watertown, MA: Persephone Press, 1982.

Berzon, Betty and Robert **Leighton** (eds). *Positively Gay: New Approaches to Gay Life*. Millbrae, CA: Celestial Arts, 1979. A collection of topical articles dealing with coming out, relationships, lesbian mothers, older lesbians, parents of lesbians and more.

Bethel, Lorraine and Barbara **Smith** (eds). *Conditions: Five*, The Black Women's Issue (Autumn 1979).

Cant, Bob and Susan **Hemmings** (eds). *Radical Records: 30 years of Lesbian and Gay History*. London: Routledge, 1988.

Cassidy, Jules and Angela **Stewart-Park**. *We're Here: Conversations with Lesbian Women*. London: Quartet Books, 1977.

Dublin Lesbians and Gay Men Collective. *Out for Ourselves – the Lives of Lesbians and Gay Men*. Dublin: DLGMC, 1986.

Ettorre, Betsy. *Lesbians, Women and Society*. London: Routledge and Kegan Paul, 1980.

Faderman, Lillian. *Surpassing the Love of Men*. London: Women's Press, 1985.

Hanscombe, Gillian and Martin **Humphries** (eds). *Heterosexuality*. London: GMP, 1987. Lesbians and gay men challenge the assumed 'naturalness' of heterosexuality. A tonic!

Hart, John. *So You Think You're Attracted to the Same Sex?* London: Penguin Books, 1984. Written for young people.

Irish Women's Community Press. *Out for Ourselves*. Dublin 1986. Banned from most bookshops in Ireland but available from the press at 44 East Sussex Street, Dublin 2.

Kaufman, Phyllis A. et al. 'Distancing for Intimacy in Lesbian Relationships', *American Journal of Psychiatry*, vol. 141, no. 4, April 1984. Demonstrates awareness of some of the problems that lesbians can face in monogomous relationships, and offers therapeutic solutions.

Kitzinger, Celia. *The Social Construction of Lesbianism*. London: Sage, 1987.

Lesbian and Gay Media Advocates. *Talk Back! The Gay Person's Guide to Media Action*. Boston: Alyson Publications, 1982.

London Lesbian Line. *Women Talking*. Booklet about being a lesbian. Available free from LLL, BM Box 1514, London WC1V 3XX (also on tape).

Martin, Del and Phyllis **Lyon**. *Lesbian/Woman*. New York: Bantam, 1972. Personal account by a lesbian couple who founded first lesbian movement in USA. Enlightening account of how older lesbians have struggled to get lesbianism incorporated into the women's movement, with other case histories.

Masters, William H. and Virginia **Johnson**. *Homosexuality in Perspective*

London: Bantam, 1982. A study that documents, among other things, the fact that gays are more sexually secure than heterosexuals, but never once mentions the effects of our oppression on our sexuality. Also contains some questionable assertions. Should be read in conjunction with a critical review, by John C. **Gonsiorek**, in *Journal of Homosexuality*, vol. 6, no. 3, Spring 1981.

Moraga, Cherrie and Gloria **Anzaldua** (eds). *The Bridge Called My Back: Writings by Radical Women of Color*. Watertown, MA: Persephone Press, 1981. A highly recommended anthology of essays, poetry and conversations by Asian, Afro-American, Latin and American Indian women, many of whom are lesbians.

Noda, Barbara, Kitty **Tsui** and Z. **Wong**. 'Coming Out: We Are Here in the Asian Community: A Dialogue with Three Asian Women', *Bridge: An Asian Perspective*, 7, Spring 1979.

O'Donnell, Mary, et al. *Lesbian Health Matters!: A Resource Book about Lesbian Health*. Santa Cruz, CA: Santa Cruz Women's Health Collective, 1979. (Order from Santa Cruz Women's Health Center, 250 Locust Street, Santa Cruz, CA 95060.) An indispensable handbook. Discussions include problems of the current health-care system in relation to lesbians, gynaecological examination, alternative treatments, etc.

Older Lesbians Conference Report, 1984.

Rich, Adrienne. *Compulsory Heterosexuality and Lesbian Existence*. London: Onlywomen Press, 1980. A now classic and often cited article.

Roberts, J. R. *Black Lesbians: An Annotated Bibliography*, first ed. Tallahassee, FL: Naiad Press, 1981. A generously annotated and carefully researched guide to over 300 references to writings by and about black lesbian women.

Smith, Barbara (ed.). *Home Girls: Black Women's Anthology*. Kitchen Table Press, 1983. Contains section on black lesbians.

Vida, Ginny (ed.). *Our Right to Love: a Lesbian Resource Book*. Englewood Cliffs, NJ: Prentice–Hall, 1978. An inclusive survey of lesbian life, including personal testimonies. A major resource produced by the National Gay Task Force.

LESBIAN YOUTH

Alyson, Sasha. *Young, Gay and Proud!* Boston: Alyson Publications, 1980. A supportive guide covering many concerns of lesbian and gay youths. Includes a clear chapter on special health concerns.

Fairchild, Betty and Nancy **Hayward**. *Now That You Know: What Every Parent Should Know About Homosexuality*. London: Harcourt Brace, 1982.

Trenchard, Lorraine and Hugh **Warren**. *Something to Tell You: the Experiences and Needs of Young Lesbians and Gay Men in London*. London Gay Teenage Group (6–9 Manor Gardens, London N7), 1984.

Trenchard, Lorraine (ed.). *Talking About Young Lesbians*. London Gay Teenage Group, 1984.

Veronica & Rose. Cinema of Women, 1982, 60 mins. A video in which young lesbians talk about coming out, relationships and sexuality. Made for Channel 4.

Warnette, Tim. 'Exploring Sex with Someone of your Own Sex', in Ruth **Bell** (ed.), *Changing Bodies, Changing Lives: a Book for Teens on Sex and Relationships*. New York: Random House, 1980. The voices of many lesbian and gay youths are heard in this informative chapter.

LEGAL ISSUES

Crane, Paul. *Gays and The Law*. London: Pluto Press, 1982.

Rights of Women. *The Cohabitation Handbook*. London: Pluto Press, 1984.

OYEZ Law Stationers can be found in most main cities (for forms for Power of Attorney and Wills).

(See also under Lesbian Mothers and Organizations)

LESBIAN MOTHERS

Golombok, Susan et al. 'Children in Lesbian and Single Parent Households', *Journal of Child Psychology and Psychiatry*, vol. 24, no. 4, pp. 551–72: can be useful for fighting custody cases and suchlike, as it is a sound study that provides no evidence in support of the belief that lesbians are bad mothers. In fact, lesbians turned out to be rather better at producing psychologically healthy children than the other mothers studied.

Hanscombe, Gillian E. and Jackie Forster. *Rocking the Cradle: Lesbian Mothers – a Challenge in Family Living*. London: Sheba, 1982.

Lesbian Rights Project. *Lesbian Mothers and their Children. An Annotated Bibliography of Legal and Psychological Materials*. Lesbian Rights Project (1370 Mission Street, 4th Floor, San Francisco, California 94103, USA), 1983. (Available from Sisterwrite.)

Lorde, Audre. 'Man Child: A Black Lesbian Feminist's Response' *Conditions: Four* (1979). A sensitive article about raising a son within the lesbian community; important reading for non-mothers as well.

Our Lives: *Lesbian Mothers Talk to Lesbian Mothers*. 1984. Available from 'Our Lives', c/o Gay Centre Ltd, Sidney Street, All Saints, Manchester.

Pollard, Ingrid and Caroline Halliday. *Everybody's Different*. Dalston Children's Centre (112 Greenwood Road, London E8), 1984. Children's book about having lesbian mothers.

Rights of Women. *Lesbian Mothers on Trial: A Report on Lesbian Mothers and Child Custody*. Rights of Women (available from 52/54 Featherstone Street, London EC1), 1984.

Rights of Women. *Lesbian Mothers' Legal Handbook*. London: Women's Press, 1986.

(See also Organizations)

SEXUALITY*

Califia, Pat. *Sapphistry: The Book of Lesbian Sexuality*. Tallahassee, FL: Naiad Press, 1980.

Corinne, Tee, Jacqueline Lapidus and Margaret Sloan-Hunter. *Yantras of Womanlove*. Tallahassee, FL: Naiad Press, 1982. Erotic photographs and text.

Lootens, Tricia. 'Lovers who don't make love' in Love/Sex issue of *Off Our Backs*, vol. 14, no. 2, February 1984.

Loulan, Jo Ann. *Lesbian Sex*. San Francisco: Spinsters Ink, 1985. Though expensive, arguably the best book around on lesbian sex. Has a good section on lesbian mothers and relationships.

Loulan, Jo Ann. *Lesbian Passion – Loving Ourselves and Each Other*. San Francisco: Spinsters Ink, 1987.

Nomadic Sisters. *Loving Women*. Sonora, CA: Nomadic Sisters, 1976.

Yarborough, Susan L. 'Lesbian Celibacy', *Sinister Wisdom*, issue 11 (Fall 1979). Celibacy considered as a self-affirming choice. (See 'Magazines' below.)

FICTION AND POETRY

Below is a very inadequate list which does not do justice to the wealth of lesbian fiction now available. Consult feminist bookshops and catalogues for up-to-date information. Many of these authors have also published several novels.

Arnold, June. *Sister Gin*. London: Women's Press, 1979.

Bradshaw, Jan and Mary Hemmings (eds). *Girls Next Door*. London: Women's Press, 1985.

Bulkin, Elly (ed). *Lesbian Fiction: An Anthology*. Watertown, MA: Persephone Press, 1980.

Bulkin, Elly and Joan Larkin (eds). *Lesbian Poetry: An Anthology*. Watertown, MA: Persephone Press, 1981.

We have not listed many poetry books – for lack of space. Many fine poets are currently in print, such as Paula Gunn Allen, Gloria Anzaldua, Robin Becker, Olga Broumas, Stephanie Byrd, Jan Clausen, Michelle Cliff, Sandra Maria Esteves, Elsa Gidlow, Judy Grahn, June Jordan, Willyce Kim, Irena Klepfisz, Audre Lorde, Adrienne Rich. Watch out also for Only Women poetry – e.g. by Caroline Halliday and Mary Dorcey.

Duffy, Maureen. *That's How it Was*. London: Virago Press, 1983.

Galford, Ellen. *Moll Cutpurse*. Edinburgh: Stramullion, 1984.

Gearhart, Sally Miller. *The Wanderground: Stories of the Hill Women*. Watertown, MA: Persephone Press, 1980.

Gilbert, Harriet. *The Riding Mistress*. London: Methuen, 1984.

Guy, Rosa. *Ruby*. New York: The Viking Press, 1976.

Hall, Radcliffe. *The Well of Loneliness*. Virago, 1986 (re-published version of this classic lesbian novel first published in 1928).

Hanscombe, Gillian E. *Between Friends*. London: Sheba, 1983.

Harris, Bertha. *Lover*. Plainfield, VT: Daughters, Inc., 1976.

Jin, Meiling. *The Shape of Fear*. London: Sheba, 1986. Poetry by Chinese lesbian feminist living in Britain.

Jones, Jo. *Come, Come*. London: Sheba, 1983.

Livia, Anna. *Relatively Norma*. London: Onlywomen Press, 1982.

Lorde, Audre. *Zami: a New Spelling of My Name*. London: Women's Press, 1984.

McEwan, Christine and Sue O'Sullivan. *Out The Other Side: Contemporary Lesbian Writing*. London: Virago Press, 1988.

Mohin, Lilian and Sheila Strulman. *The Reach, and Other Stories*. London: Onlywomen Press, 1984.

Namjoshi, Suniti. *The Conversations of Cow*. London: Women's Press, 1985.

Okoro, Elaine. *Thoughts, Feelings and Lovers*. Tightfisted Poets, 1985. Poems by a black lesbian living in Britain, distributed by Common Word, 61 Bloom Street, Manchester M1 3LY. Common Word books aim to 'speak for the working class, blacks, gays and women – all of us who are normally ridiculed or unheard in published work'.

Rule, Jane. *Outlander*. Tallahassee, FL: Naiad Press, 1981.

Russ, Joanna. *On Strike Against God*. New York: Out and Out Books, 1980.

Sarton, May. *Mrs. Stevens Hears the Mermaids Singing*. New York: W. W. Norton and Co., 1975.

Sarton, May. *As We Are Now*. London: Women's Press, 1983. Older lesbians' novel.

Scoppettone, Sandra. *Happy Endings Are All Alike*. New York: Dell Publishing Co., 1978. (Young adult novel.)

Shockley, Ann. *The Black and White of It*. Tallahassee, FL: Naiad Press, 1981.

Shockley, Ann. *Loving Her*. New York: Avon Books, 1978.

Taylor, Valerie. *Prism*. Tallahassee, FL: Naiad Press, 1981.

Walker, Alice. *The Color Purple*. London: Women's Press, 1983.

Wilson, Anna. *Cactus*. London: Onlywomen Press, 1980.

Also look for the reissues of the 1950s novels by Ann Bannon and Paula Christian. Other writers to look for: Sarah Aldridge, Maureen Brady, Rita Mae Brown, Jane Chambers, Rosamund Lehmann, Gail Pass and Monique Wittig.

MAGAZINES*

Artemis. For women who love women, available from BM Perfect, London WC1N 3XX.

Mukti. Asian women's magazine, available from 213 Eversholt Street, London NW1.

Sinister Wisdom. Excellent American lesbian magazine, available from some feminist bookshops, such as Sisterwrite, which also stocks several other American lesbian journals.

Spare Rib. Feminist magazine that recognizes throughout that lesbians exist, available from all good magazine stores and on subscription. Further information from 27 Clerkenwell Close, London EC1R 0AT.

Trouble and Strife. A radical feminist quarterly magazine, available on subscription from The Women's Centre, 34 Exchange Street, Norwich NR2 1AX.

We Are Here. By and for black women only, 94 Belgrave Gate, Leicester LE1 3GR.

ORGANIZATIONS

Black and Ethnic Minority Lesbian Group, c/o London Women's Centre, Wesley House, 4 Wild Court, London WC2B 5AU.

Black Lesbian and Gay Centre Project, BM 4390, London WC1N 3XX. Tel: 01-885 3543.

Black Lesbian and Gay People of Faith. Support network, BM Box 4390, London WC1N 3XX.

Campaign for Homosexual Equality, PO Box 342, London WC1X 0DU. Tel: 01-833 3912.

Campaign for Press and Broadcasting Freedom: Lesbian and Gay Group, 9 Poland Street, London W1V 3DG. Tel: 01-437 2795.

Catholic Lesbian Sisterhood, BM Reconciliation, London WC1N 3XX.

*See also Resources in Chapter 14.

*All these publications are available from feminist bookshops.

LESBIAN LINE

BM BOX 1514, LONDON WC1N 3XX. TEL: 01-251 6911.
MON.–THURS. 7–10 P.M.; FRI. 2–10 P.M.
ALL TIMES PM UNLESS OTHERWISE STATED

Aberdeen Lesbian Line 0224–586869 Wed. 7–10
Bangor Lesbian Line 0248–315263, Tues. 6–8
Belfast Lesbian Line 0232–222023. 8–10, 1st & 3rd Thurs. of every month
Birmingham Lesbian Line 021–359 3192 M–F 7.30–9.30, Tues. 4–6
Bradford Lesbian Line 0274–305525 Thur. 7–9
Brighton Lesbian Line 0273–603298 Tues. 8–10, Fri. 2–5 & 8–10 or PO Box 449, Ship Street.
Cambridge Lesbian Line 0223–246113 Fri. 6–10
Cardiff 0222–374051 Thur. 8–10
Colchester Lesbian Line 0206–870051 Wed. 8–10
Coventry Friend Women's Line 0203–25991 Tues. 7–10
Coventry & Leamington Lesbian Line 0203–77105 Wed. 7–10
Dundee Friend Women's Line 0382–21843 Tues. 7–10
Edinburgh Friend Women's Line 031–5564049 Thur. 7.30–10 (Always a woman on duty; should a man answer please ask for a woman to come to the phone.)
Glasgow Lesbian Line 041–248 4596 Mon. 7–10
Lancaster Women's Line 0524–63021 Wed. 6–9
Leeds 0532–453588 Tues. 7.30–9.30
Leicester (Friend) 0533–826299 Tues. 7.30–10.30

Liverpool Women's Line 051–708 0234 Tues. & Thur. 7–10
London Lesbian Line 01–251 6911 (see times at top of box)
Manchester Lesbian Line 061–236 6205 Mon.–Fri. 7–10
Merseyside Friend Lesbian Line 051–708 0234 Tues. & Thur. 7–10
IGRM Munster Cork 010–353 505394 Tues. 8–10
Newcastle Lesbian Line 091–261 2277
North Staffordshire Lesbian Support Group 0782–266998 Fri. 8–10
Nottingham Lesbian Line 0602–410652 Mon. & Wed. 7–9.30
Oxford Lesbian Line 0865–242333 Wed. 7–10
Peterborough (GPG) 0733–238005/265181 nightly before 10
Plymouth Lesbian Line 0752–261251 Tues. 7.30–9.30
Preston Lesbian Line 0772–51122 Mon. & Wed. 7.30–9.30
St Andrews Lesbian Line 0334–72604 Mon. 7–10
Sheffield Lesbian Line 0742–581238 Thur. 7–10
Swansea Lesbian Line 0792–467365 Fri. 7–9
Eire Dublin (NFG) – Switchboard 0001–710608 Thur. 8–10

Edinburgh Lesbian and Gay Community Centre, 58A Broughton Street, Edinburgh EH1 35A. Tel: 031-557 2625.

Family Rights Group, 6-9 Manor Gardens, Holloway Road, London N7 GLA. Tel: 01-263 4016/9724. Telephone advice sessions 9.30-12.30 Mon., Wed., Fri.: 01-272 7308.
For rights of parents with children in care.

Friend, National network advice and counselling service. London number 01–337 3337, 7–10 p.m. Women only: 01-837 2782 Sunday 7–10 p.m. will advise on your nearest service.

GEMMA, BM Box 5700, London WC1N 3XX A friendship, information and support group of lesbians with/without disabilities. Publishes a quarterly newsletter in print or on tape. Inquiries welcome in braille or on cassette with sae.

Glad (Gay Legal Problems). Tel: 01-821 7672, 7 to 10 p.m.

Jewish Gay and Lesbian Helpline, BM Jewish Helpline, London WC1N 3XX.

Jewish Lesbian Groups, can be contacted via the Jewish Feminist Newsletter, PO Box 39, c/o Sisterwrite, 190 Upper Street, London N1.

KENRIC, BM Kenric, London WC1N 3XX. 'Non-political social group' for lesbians in London. Monthly newsletter, social events, correspondence circle and 'phone a friend' scheme.

Lesbian and Gay Christian Movement, BM 6914, London WC1N 3XX. Tel: 01-283 5165 (answering machine).

Lesbian and Gay Youth Movement, BM GCM, London WC1N 3XX. Tel: 01-317 9690.

Lesbian Archive, London Women's Centre, Wesley House, 4 Wild Court, London WC2B 5AU.

Lesbians at London Friend, 86 Caledonian Road, London N1. (Telephone line and social group: 01-837 2782.)

Lesbian Employment Rights, Room 203, Southbank House, Black Prince Road, London SE1 7SJ. Tel: 01-587 1636. Supports lesbians where discrimination at work is taking place, and campaigns against anti-lesbian discrimination in un/employment.

Lesbian Health Workers, c/o Women's Centre, The Plough, Moor Lane, Lancaster.

Lesbian Line, A network of phone lines now operating in many parts of the country (see Box below) and run by lesbians. Check the phone directory or ring the London number for up-to-date numbers (some may have changed, and there might be more).

LESPOP (Lesbian and Policing Project), Wesley House, 4 Wild Court, London WC2 5AU. Tel: 01-404 4318 or 01-833 4996. Offers support and advice to lesbians having dealings with the police.

London Lesbian and Gay Centre, 67–9 Cowcross Street, off Farringdon Road, London EC1M 6BP. Tel: 01-608 1471.

London Lesbian and Gay Switchboard. Tel: 01-837 7324. Free 24-hour service: what's on, flats, flatshares and information about women's groups, advice centres, etc. They will tell you whether there is a switchboard near you if you do not live near London.

Manchester Gay Centre Ltd, Sidney Street, All Saints, Manchester. Tel: 061-274 3814.

Mothers Apart from Their Children MATCH, (Mothers Apart from Their Children) c/o BM Problems, London WC 1N 3XX. Support group for mothers who are living apart from their children for any reason.

Older Lesbian Network, BMOLN, London WC1N 3XX.

ROW (Rights Of Women), 52–4 Featherstone Street, London EC1. Tel: 01-251 6577. Legal advice phone line open Tuesday, Wednesday and Thursday, 7 to 9 p.m.

ROW Lesbian Custody Project. See address above. Tel: 01-251 6576 – available daytime only.

Scottish Homosexual Rights Group, 58A Broughton Street, Edinburgh EH1 35A. Tel: 031-556 1279.

SIGMA, BM Sigma, London WC1N 3XX. Tel: 01-837 7324. Ask for the Sigma contact number. There is a country-wide network of members. For non-gay partners of gay/straight/bisexual marriage.

MAJOR AREAS OF TENSION IN HETEROSEXUAL RELATIONSHIPS: THE PERSONAL IS POLITICAL

Prepared by
JILL RAKUSEN

Most women seek to fulfil much of their need for closeness through intimate sexual relationships with men. As we grew up, we learned one pattern or model for these relationships:[1] our families and communities expected us to marry and have children. This was the way things had to be, and when our lives fitted this pattern we would automatically be happy.

But during the recent wave of the feminist movement, we began to question these assumptions and affirm one of the basic principles of the feminist movement – that our lives, work, ideas, perceptions and wishes are important, as important as those of men, and that society should be reorganized to reflect and support this belief. We saw that most heterosexual relationships in this culture reflect those old assumptions about women and men. In talking with each other about our lives, our dissatisfactions, frustrations and sometimes anger began to crystallize and became newly articulated feelings which affected each of our lives differently: some of us worked with our husbands or lovers at changing what went on between us; long-standing relationships which just couldn't change in response to our new visions broke up. Some of us lived communally, decided not to marry or chose to live only with women. Our examination of male–female relationships led to a variety of 'solutions', some women came to equate feminism with hating men and rejecting marriage and family, and many of these women became reluctant to identify with the women's movement. However, many of us were committed to finding ways to live out our feminist beliefs without having to give up intimate relationships with men. Frustration and anger don't mean that we want to end these relationships; instead, they make us determined to change them.

While there may be many other sources of tension between a woman and a man – personality differences, family history, ethnic and class differences, education, illness, economic hardship – this chapter focuses on the tension which comes from living in a culture based on inequality and limiting role definitions between the sexes.

When we work towards an equal relationship we are, in effect, swimming against the tide.

Our culture stresses the importance of the individual rather than of the group, and teaches us to believe that our personal circumstances and problems arise from qualities within us, from our own individual histories, our personalities and our conscious choices. As a result, most of us tend not to see the ways in which gender, race and class affect personal 'choices'. The feminist insight that 'the personal is political' expresses our belief – that what seem like 'personal' problems are often symptoms of larger social problems.

TOWARDS SHARED POWER

Women and men belong to groups which have different degrees of power. The resulting imbalance inevitably influences the way we think, act and relate to each other. How people perceive and treat us outside our relationships inevitably affects how we feel within them. The conventional heterosexual relationship has been a marriage in which a man agrees to support a woman economically and share his status with her. In return she is responsible for the personal and household services which enable him to perform his role in society without such 'menial' distractions.* In the relationship we envisage, each partner supports the other, so both play a role in the world outside the home as well as in the home, and one partner does not gain power at the expense of the other.

---

*Women do 80 per cent of household chores, whether we work outside the home or not.[2]

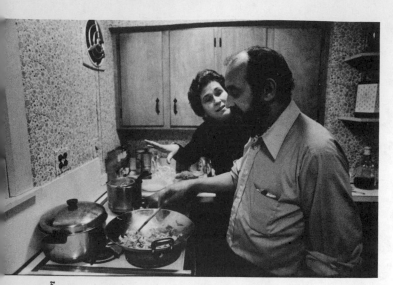

SOCIAL AND ECONOMIC POWER

Politics is not just to do with power relationships among large-scale groups and nations; there is a politics of intimate relationships as well. However strong our commitment to each other and to treating one another as equals may be, it is naive to think that widely-held social attitudes and pervasive institutional practices will not affect what goes on between us. For example, a conflict within a heterosexual relationship is not simply a conflict between two persons who are everywhere regarded as social equals, but between two people who have different standing before the law (especially if married) and different rights and privileges. Most societal institutions are thoroughly permeated with the assumption that the rights of men should take precedence over the rights of women. Since money is the most common source of power in this society and frequently symbolizes social power, it is not surprising that the person who brings economic resources into a family or a relationship has increased power.*

This society values and rewards men's work a great deal more than women's work. Most women cannot bring in an equal amount of money, for we earn on average far less than men earn.

Men's power in relationships is partly based on the fact that they usually earn more money. If a man abuses this power imbalance, he may show it during the early stages of a relationship by making a woman feel indebted to him and implying that she should 'repay' him with sexual favours. If he does this, watch out. In the words of a forty-year-old divorced woman:

> A man took me out, and on the second or third date he wanted to sleep with me. So I told him I

*In a study of married couples, wives who worked in paid employment were found to have greater power in family decision-making than non-earning wives.[3]

didn't want to be that intimate on so short an acquaintance. And he grumbled and said, 'I just want to know if there's a pot of gold at the end of the rainbow.'

Some men imply that paying for dates is burdensome, but may be reluctant to give up the control that goes with paying when offered a chance to share expenses. Others may be more flexible. A single woman in her twenties told us:

> I believe in paying my share when I go out with a man. The man I'm involved with now earns a lot more money than I do, and he enjoys spending it on things that are fun. We often end up arguing about what kinds of things both of us can afford, which he feels limits us to what I can afford. Sometimes we compromise and he treats so we can do something special.

Economic independence is crucial for women, as any battered woman will testify (see Chapter 10). Yet we are socialized to see paid work as secondary to our job as wives and mothers, and believe that work and parenting are mutually exclusive choices. Or often we may only find work which we can balance with childcare, usually 'women's occupations', e.g. primary school teaching, nursing, secretarial work, waitressing, which pay far less than 'men's' jobs. When a woman is not able to earn as much as a man she (and he) are more likely to see her work as less important, more dispensable when children come, less important when a move is contemplated, less worth disrupting the family routine for. Even in couples which start out with egalitarian ideals and plans, the woman usually adapts more and more to the man. Because of this economic imbalance, a man may simply assume that it is his right to take charge. If a woman wants to make changes, she has to change his ideas as well as this conventional pattern. From a woman in her thirties:

> When I buy something, even if it's for the house, I'm often afraid to tell him. He gets upset and says, 'We can't afford it.' But what he really means is that I shouldn't have bought it without consulting him. I get afraid to tell him because I think that since he earned the money, it's not really mine, even though he couldn't be out earning it if I weren't here running the house and taking care of the kids.
> Sometimes I think getting a job and earning some money myself is the only thing that will resolve the conflict. But I get a strong message from him that he doesn't want me to work even though we could use the extra income. He's afraid that then he would have to deal with me differently.

This is not a simple disagreement about *how* to spend

money, but raises the issue of decision-making power within the family.

When we were first married, I earned much less than my husband but enough to support myself. But from the time when our first child was born seven years ago, I have worked only part time and my salary is very low. We could not find part-time work for both of us that paid well enough to support us. Neither of us wanted to have the children in full-time day-care when they were young. Now that the children are both at school, I want to earn a living again. All along, he has regarded my work as equally important to his own but, in truth, I have more often left work to stay at home with a sick child than he has, and while his identity comes largely from work, mine comes primarily from being a mother. I want to change this now and get on an equal footing.

It's going to be a long time before we can unlearn our powerlessness, and a long time before we get equal pay* or a real sharing of responsibilities within the home. The best we can do is to begin to insist that the contribution of both partners is equally valid.

OUR PERSONAL POWER

By 'personal power' we mean self-reliance, assertiveness, the ability to earn a living, independence, self-confidence; many of us were taught to find a man with these qualities and literally attach ourselves to him ('If you can't be one, marry one'). In this way, we would become complete. Creating an intimate relationship with a man was not to be simply a way to enrich our lives but the foundation of our identities as whole adult people. Who we are close to became confused with who we are. And so we faced a paradox: to feel stronger, many of us followed the best-travelled route and found a man, yet we were stepping into a role which only served to undermine our inner strength.

And what of physical strength? Many women have been taught that to be physically strong is 'unfeminine', and a man's greater physical strength can pose an unspoken threat of intimidation which causes all sorts of problems, from feeling overpowered in a sexual encounter to being intimidated in an argument. Because we live in a society where violence or the threat of violence is ever present, it is not surprising that we have such feelings. When we refuse to accept the cultural image of women as lacking in physical strength and competence, learn new skills and become physically stronger, our self-esteem grows.

*In fact, any progress that occurred when the Equal Pay Act came into force has been lost, and since 1978 women's wages have been falling even further behind those of men.

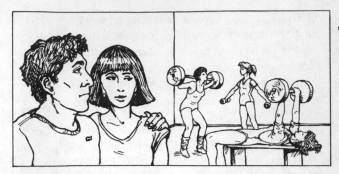

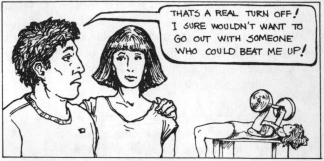

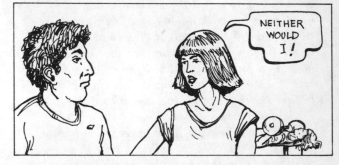

One of the things I plunged myself into at age fifty-four was to take Tae Kwon Do [a Korean martial art]. I had always been fascinated by martial arts but never had enough nerve to try it. I was stirring up long years of status quo; one more unorthodoxy didn't matter, I reasoned. All through our marriage I was never able to stand up to my husband, and I felt taking a martial art might perhaps help me to become more assertive. My husband was totally put off by my taking up such a 'masculine' activity. But I have persisted.

Women are often tentative, prefacing statements with a little laugh and apologies about how little we know about the subject under discussion, while men learn to present their strongest points and to remain silent about their reservations.

One of the hardest things for me to do is to hold my own at points when we really disagree about something. I might start out knowing just what I think but then, the more I listen to him argue his point (he is always so sure of himself), the less sure I feel of mine and the more confused I get about what is true. Sometimes I wind up crying when what I really want to do is fight for myself. Then, later on, I feel angry; a sort of smouldering resentment sets in, and I don't even want to sleep with him at those times. It's because I still feel angry about not being able to hold my own in the fight and I know I can hurt him by withholding sex.

While 'experts', including some doctors, often 'scold' women for withholding sex when we are angry about something else, they fail to recognize that is is often the best indirect way of exercising power when more direct ways are blocked.

Women are taught to be uncomfortable with the idea of having power. (It is as unladylike as being physically strong!) Often when we 'do what is expected of us' we abdicate our power almost entirely.

I always arranged my life around him. When we were first together I was beginning a career in teaching. But soon he got a job offer in another city, and so we moved there. Then he wanted to have children, which I didn't really care about. But he wanted them badly, so it seemed all right to me. Then we moved again, this time to a fancy house in a fancy suburb, but I had no car – he took it – and I was quite lonely. The children became the centre of my life, and I loved them and my husband deeply. Several times I thought of returning to college part time to get my certificate. But my husband was not willing for me to do that; he did not want the responsibilities for the house and the children to fall on his shoulders. And he said he was glad to support us, which I think he really was. Then, one day when the children were still quite young (our son was not even a year old), I learned something that terrified me . . . that for more than a year my husband had been having

affairs with other women. They were all women whom he met in his job as a supervisor, professional women, very bright and competent and unattached and ten years younger than I was.

When I confronted him, he said that he found me dull, always talking about the house and the children – of course, since that was my world! – and that these other women were far more interesting, as they had professional lives and were more worldly and more knowledgeable than I was about things which interested him in his work. He did not say, but I think it is true, that he also hated my asking him to be more involved with the children and the house. He ran to these women whenever I criticized him, looking for the things in them which he discouraged me from developing in myself. When I was younger, I did not see any problem with my shaping my life around him. Now I know I have paid a very high price.

When I started my degree I was ambitious to become really well known in my field. Then I got involved with Dave and began to spend more and more time with him. He wanted total support for his work and since we were in the same field I could help him a lot and be learning at the same time. But I definitely put my own ambitions in the background for about two years. I began to be more attached to the idea of staying in the city when I finished so I wouldn't have to leave Dave, and I even began to fantasize about a less demanding job, maybe even just three days a week.

When we broke up all my options opened up again and I could reconsider my early ambitions. It was scary to consider the possibility of being as successful as my original fantasies.

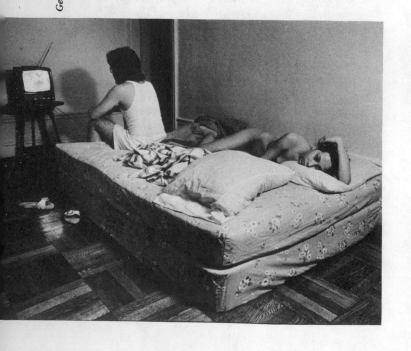

George Malave/Stock Boston

TRADITIONAL ROLES AND GETTING BEYOND THEM

Roles are like parts in a play. We learn how to be a sexual partner, a wife or a mother by following scripts that we learned as children. The scripts save us the trouble of creating our lives from scratch each and every day, but they may also lead us to drift into rigid roles without questioning them.

Certain qualities are usually reinforced as being appropriate to women or to men. When our behaviour varies from the stereotype we may be punished: while a male's assertive behaviour is called 'leadership', in a female it is called 'aggressiveness'. Nurturing may be labelled 'warmth' in a woman and 'weakness' in a man. One US study of mental-health professionals' attitudes found that when they were asked to list the traits of a healthy adult, a healthy man and a healthy woman, they equated traits

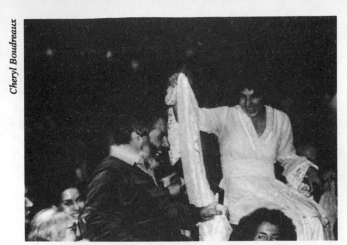

Cheryl Boudreaux

tion of one parent, war or a period of unemployment occurred and roles had to be shared or varied in non-conventional ways.

When I was growing up my father was away fighting in the war, and so my mother and I moved in with my grandmother and aunts. I grew up seeing women managing by themselves without men for years at a time.

Some parents mistakenly believed they were teaching us that we could do everything boys could do, but they really gave us a mixed message.

I grew up in a household where we believed there were no distinctions between boys and girls. We were always told that girls were equal and the five of us had exciting, far-reaching discussions and no-holds-barred, stimulating, intellectual arguments over dinner. But later I realized that while my father held court with us, my mother was clearing the table. At some point he would call for his coffee to be brought to him. This affected my marriage. I feel intellectually equal or superior to Steven, but it's hard for me to feel OK about doing anything for my own work which demands or requires any adaptation by my family.

listed for males with those for healthy adults; but the traits for a 'healthy' woman differed from and often contradicted those for a healthy adult.[4] No wonder that women experience so much role conflict and difficulty reconciling contradictory expectations.

Each partner begins a relationship with a set of experiences and beliefs which shape her/his notions about masculine and feminine roles. Many of us grew up in families which followed conventional patterns. Others of us may have grown up in situations where death, divorce, emigra-

SOME CONSEQUENCES OF ACCEPTING TRADITIONAL ROLES

The conventional role structure, in which the woman functions as a support system for the man, while receiving no support to earn a living and/or to develop herself, leaves us extremely vulnerable emotionally and economically. Thousands of displaced homemakers,[5] after nurturing others most of their lives, are then left without resources or marketable skills. (Most do have skills, unrecognized because of a combination of age and sex discrimination, and because household skills are devalued when in fact they are similar to professional and management skills.) In the West today, where the divorce rate is high, where women outlive their male partners, often by a decade or two (80 per cent of surviving spouses are women) and where the inflation rate makes the old pattern of one salary supporting two adults and children an alternative available only to a small elite, the traditional role of woman as support system to the man exists only at great risk to women.

From a very first meeting with a man, we may play roles. If we want to pursue the relationship, continue to see one another and spend time together, live together or get married and have children together,

each step towards permanence, commitment and formalization of the relationship increases the pressures to assume conventional roles. It requires hard work to stay friends and lovers as we become parents.

If we leave our paid work, we lose not only our independent income but our status as a paid worker and our community of work friends. We lose our source of validation in the world (whatever anyone says, motherhood, though worshipped, is *not* valued); we may feel less competent and respected, and become almost completely dependent on our partner and our child(ren). Even when we want to share work and childcare equally, the shortage of good childcare services, the lack of well-paid part-time work and the severe sex discrimination limiting our earning power as women all contribute to a gradual drift back towards conventional arrangements during the early parenting years.

We believe that as long as women do most of the childcare, this will have a fundamental impact on our lives and opportunities and thus influence subsequent generations and *their* choices.

We are not taught gender roles simply out of sentiment and tradition, but because they fit us into existing social forms. As we struggle to change our relationships we must at the same time work to end sex discrimination at our workplaces, establish childcare in our communities and end the legal inequities women still face. In this transitional time we have the task of fitting the kinds of relationships we want into a society which may not only fail to support our vision but often actively opposes it.

MAKING CHANGES

We can begin to take small steps to change fixed roles. We can devise an 'affirmative action' plan, taking time for ourselves to build up our work skills, to work on something which interests us and which brings in some income. We don't have to say no automatically to opportunities that require travel. We can leave an unsatisfactory relationship or work hard towards changing our partner's attitudes and the structure of the relationship.

The change began for me as I prepared for a full-time job when all the kids were finally old enough to take some responsibility. I knew then I had to have Matthew as an active partner, though he preferred being passive and having everything done for him. My therapist told me to make a list of all the jobs that a family required in order to run. It was pages long; it just grew and grew. When I got it all written out after several weeks, it was clear that I did about 95 per cent of it. And then I got very angry that I was the only one who kept everything working around here. I basically decided I was going to go on strike. We began slowly and painfully to work out a more equitable system in the distribution of housework and cooking and parenting. Matt . . . felt that he 'couldn't' do things that he didn't want to do, so it was painful. But I told myself it was worth it because it was the beginning. I was getting ready to start college.

In the six months before term started, I determined that I would teach the kids how to run the washer and dryer, to cook simple meals, to scrub the kitchen floor, to clean a bathroom. We set up job lists and everybody had to do one thing a week: they would cook, and I would just be here if they needed help. And then I started college full time, and I was immediately overwhelmed. I was struggling. It was far more competitive than I had thought it was going to be . . . I wasn't home after school, I had study groups late at night and on Saturday and Sunday. Things started to fall apart. Nobody liked it. The kids would grumble because other mothers didn't make their children do so much. We all need order in our lives, and it was chaotic for a while. By the time the first year had gone by, our job system was pretty well in place. This is really my break away from the

house. I am no longer going to be here the way I have always been.

To create mutually supportive relationships rather than one in which one partner functions only as the support system for the other, we must realize that there is a difference between sharing *tasks* (taking turns calling for babysitters or paying the bills) and sharing planning (the 'overview' – being *aware* of when sitters are needed, when a child needs to go to the doctor and what the long-term financial plans are).

Even when a woman and man both work, they fall into the pattern of the man doing long-term planning, because women until recently have not been in the habit of doing so and believe that men are better at it. Women develop skill at saving small amounts of money day by day, but often do not deal with the larger question of their future economic security. Middle-class women are often brought up with the assumption that there will always be someone there to take care of us, while women from working-class backgrounds often learn to be more self-sufficient, providing for ourselves. But most women's incomes are so marginal that we can't put any money aside for the future. Middle-class women often find it hard to assume responsibility for planning because we can't envisage a time when the coffers may be empty, and it is tempting to let someone else worry, just as our parents once did. When we try to take more responsibility, some in-laws, parents – perhaps even therapists – may accuse of us being emasculating. But many of us have found that when we take more responsibility for money matters, not only do our partners appreciate it but we have more control over our lives.

FEARING INTIMACY

Intimacy can not only make us feel good, but it can enrich other parts of our lives and contribute to our energy and creativity. However, we are all too often *expected* to merge our identities with our men's, taking *their* names, moving to where *their* jobs are, and so on. We may fear too much closeness if in previous relationships we merged our own wishes, aspirations and identities with those of our partners to such an extent that we lost sight of what we wanted for ourselves.

I wanted to be a satellite to him, revolving around him in his world . . . to let his life, his work, his friends, his energy pull me along. I was so relieved not to have to work any more to build my own identity. This is what ultimately suffocated him and me and the marriage.

Often we experience conflicts between dependency and self-sufficiency, between the security of being in a good relationship and our need to remain separate.

One thing that's clear about my second marriage is that, because I'm older and because of who he is, I am much closer to him than I was to my first husband. I am able to care for him much more deeply. And there are moments when he's away even overnight that are very painful to me. It's not 'Oh, my God, I couldn't take care of myself', because I have and I can – but it's deeply, passionately missing somebody. And it's ironic because I had so strongly identified with the women's movement's 'superwoman agenda' of being self-sufficient. Yet it's come home to me just how painful it would be if something were to happen to him, how empty life would be. Not because my life isn't full in addition to him, but because I risked having a certain depth of commitment and feeling.

This society, which assigns active and dominant roles to men and passive or subordinate roles to women, exaggerates these conflicts. When we become conscious of men's greater power and prestige, we may fear the vulnerability that naturally comes with intimacy.

My work is lecturing and writing about pornography, child sexual abuse in battering situations and other areas of female sexual slavery. I live two truths all the time: I live in a male-supremist culture, yet I have a relationship with a man who is not a sexist. I used to feel that to be a totally strong woman and a feminist I should be alone, and I would feel guilty for having this real partner who loves me and helps me, whom I love and trust and depend on. But now I think, Why not just enjoy the special life I have and not worry about how I 'should' be?

The stronger and more confident I feel about myself, the more able I am to be close to someone without fearing I'll lose myself.

WE LEARN DIFFERENT STYLES OF INTIMACY

Traditionally, women have tended to value talking as a way of being close, while many men express intimacy mainly through physical activity or sexual closeness, without the same need for words.

My idea of being intimate, more than making love, is having long, deep conversations. My fantasies of love affairs are about conversations like that. You just keep on talking and every once in a while something important or interesting will get said. John's idea is that you don't talk until you have something to say. I want to talk about everything from every possible angle. He considers that gossipy, repetitious and intrusive. He's not secretive, but he wants to work things out for himself. His idea of intimacy is doing something together, like camping or canoeing. I sometimes

think that John does not really know the part of me that I cherish most, and vice versa.

Society holds up 'the strong, silent type' as a masculine ideal. Many men find self-disclosure very threatening;[6] showing one's softer side is not considered masculine. While over the past several years some men have been trying to be more emotionally open, the male world continues to expect them to be goal-oriented and to keep feelings concealed, and does not reward openness. Since our sexist culture does not value a personal, 'feminine' style of relating to others, most men are not motivated to learn it.

A man I almost married said to me, 'I'll bring home the money and you can do the rest', by which he meant all the childcare, the housework, the endless small tasks and, most importantly, I came to understand, all the emotional work.

Men, therefore, are often emotionally impoverished. Women who turn to them for intimacy can find them seriously lacking. Very often women end up being responsible for the emotional climate in which a couple exists and also, since many men have no or few intimate friends except for the women they are involved with, we end up having to give them a huge amount of emotional support. Again, a woman winds up doing 'invisible' work. Her energy is sometimes so taken up with maintaining a relationship that she is diverted from her own personal aims and development.

Most men have not yet caught up with women in terms of personal growth, knowing how to work on a relationship or knowing how to be a good friend. Some men have begun to meet together in groups to talk about these issues, to develop the skills necessary for intimate personal relationships and to learn how to pay more attention to their relationships with children, wives or lovers and friends, even though little in our society encourages them to do so.*

As a relationship develops we must continue to be aware of our assumptions. The danger in taking small things for granted is that they are often attached to larger issues. A seemingly small gesture, like choosing a last name when we decide to get married, can serve as a statement right from the start that we want to have a different kind of connection to a husband than that implied when a woman automatically takes his last name as her own.

---

*Some men, either individually or in groups, having begun to develop an awareness of feminist issues, are beginning to see the need to take their share of responsibility for effecting change. A Sheffield group, for example, has produced a booklet for schools concerning violence against women; Manchester Men Against Pornography and Sexual Harassment have written a leaflet which they distribute outside violent film shows; and some adult education centres have set up 'men's awareness groups' or run courses such as 'Thinking About Men'. Men's groups in several parts of the country run crèches in an attempt to redress the imbalance in child-care responsibilities between men and women. Men's groups can be contacted via the *Men's Anti-Sexist Newsletter* (see Resources).

I had been married once before, had changed my name and then changed it back, and I knew I didn't want to go through that again. I gave up an important part of myself, which didn't feel like a comfortable way to begin a relationship of equals. When Sam and I decided to get married, we wanted a new beginning. We thought about somehow combining our last names, but we couldn't come up with one that we liked. The decision to choose an entirely new name has had a lot of meaning for both of us. The name itself is rich in meaning for me . . . It is from the language that our grandparents spoke, and it means 'rebirth' or 'renewal' . . . The process of choosing it was very moving. I didn't stop using my original name. I still use it as a middle name, and I like it to be very visible. People often ask about our name, and when I tell them how and why we did it, it's like offering them a new option, a new way to deal with old assumptions. This name is a gift.

ENJOYING SEPARATENESS

When we go on separate holidays or see separate friends, other people often take it as a sign that something is wrong. Sometimes one member of a couple may be threatened when a partner's life excludes him or her in some way.

I have been seeing a man for almost a year now. I like him a great deal, but he is unable to understand my way of life. He is retired and enjoys just sitting with his feet up for the first time in his life. But I have a new volunteer job, and so I have a number of activities which to me are really stimulating. And these very things, which I've always wanted to do, make it seem to him as if I can't stay at home and am always running around.

I remember years ago wanting so badly to go to a party we were invited to. But Carl really couldn't stand those people; he refused to go. What I really wanted was to go alone, and I would have had a grand old time, but in those days if you did such a thing people would surely have gossiped that you were on the brink of divorce! Several years ago our college-age daughter said to me, 'Well, why don't you just tell them next time that Daddy really doesn't enjoy parties very much, but that you'd love to come!' I have done this several times now; recently I even went out to dinner alone with a couple I particularly like. It's so much better than missing the parties and resenting Carl, or dragging him along and having him sulk and then having to leave earlier than I want to. I resent it far less now when he watches sport on TV, which I dislike. I think that I wasted many years not doing what I

enjoyed because sometimes it was different from what we enjoyed.

Martin and I have been together for thirteen years. By together I don't mean married; it has always seemed sort of ridiculous to me to have the state involved in what is really a personal contract. And beyond that, I think that when you get married you begin to make a lot of assumptions and you don't even realize you're doing it. I use my relationship with Martin as a solid base to move out from . . . I have a very active life independent of him . . . work and political meetings and seeing my friends. He and they are equally important to me – neither alone would be as good.

While some women think that avoiding legal marriage is a safeguard against falling into conventional roles, most want the commitment that marriage symbolizes.

Sometimes when we are involved with a man we fail to develop certain of our abilities. We may be lulled into

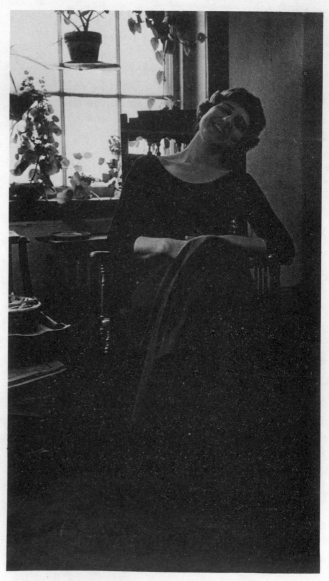

Vaughn Sills

thinking that there will always be a man to take care of us. We avoid learning skills like money management, home repairs, strenuous physical tasks.* As a result we may think of ourselves as weaker or less competent than we really are.

I know that I've got through the worst times as a single parent, and I've survived and flourished. Being alone and having to learn certain skills, like putting up a Christmas tree alone when your husband used to do it, wasn't something that gave me so much pleasure, but the fact that I did it was another small incident that showed I could manage, and there's a certain satisfaction in just being able to manage your life. Being able to manage with the house and kids and work – it's a sense of accomplishment. Learning new skills, like putting up shelves, taking the car to the mechanic and negotiating with him, managing your finances, deciding where you're going to go on holiday and with whom – it's all just learning to rely on your own strengths.

Keeping some distinct turf for ourselves, whether it's separate cheque-books or separate holidays, separate friends or not rushing into living together, does not have to threaten our relationship. In fact, it can be renewing to us and contribute to the vitality and growth of what goes on between us.

One of the reasons we have lasted together is that we have always lived in places where each of us could really build a whole life for ourselves – in terms of friends, work, interests – and not have to depend on each other for more than the other could give.

We are not proposing any fixed model of 'The Ideal Couple Relationship' with a man. How we talk together, how we play and fight and work and make love, grow not from any external prescription but from who we are. We do propose that the cost of the intimacy we build together should not be our own richness as individuals; that we see each other not simply as two halves of a whole, each with our own immutable territory, but as two separate, whole people who have chosen to touch closely, to build something together, to intertwine – enriching one another, rather than detracting from the potential ways that each may grow. Working towards an egalitarian relationship with a man is not a matter of creating a one-time 'grand design' that will guide us for years to come, but a slow and

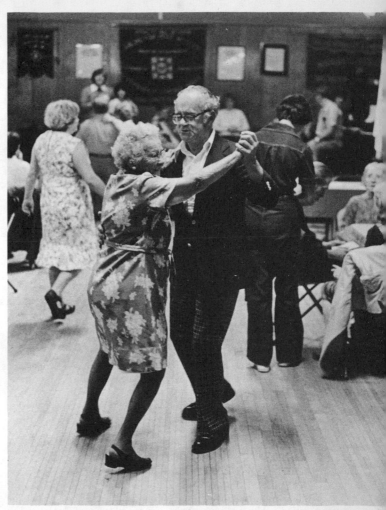

Patricia Hollander Gross/Stock Boston

continuing process of negotiation, compromise and renegotiation.

Changes will occur, for the most part, slowly and in very small steps. In an efficiency-minded, goal-orientated culture heavily influenced by technology, these small, slow processes of fixing and adjusting are neither taught nor valued. We live in a disposable age: when it breaks, throw it out and get a new one. When *we* speak of commitment, we don't mean the traditional pressure to be 'committed' to a relationship at all costs, which has often meant letting go of our needs or putting up with an empty or abusive relationship. We have in mind a true commitment to a process of working on the relationship, which may make things harder for a time as we attempt to make them better. It involves risk-taking, constant questioning and not always waiting for the 'right' moment to bring up a problem. It also means being willing to change as we are asking our men to change.

*Many men in turn look to women for the kinds of caretaking they may associate with mothering, like the provision of balanced meals, day-to-day household management and the maintenance of general emotional well-being. The difficulty men have in coping without a woman to take care of them in these ways is suggested by their much higher and earlier remarriage rate after divorce or widowhood, and also by their higher death and illness rates after these same life crises.

NOTES

1. See, for example, Sue Sharpe. *Just Like a Girl: How Girls Learn to be Women*. London: Penguin Books, 1976; and Elena Gianini Belotti. *Little Girls*. London: Writers and Readers, 1975.
2. Department of Employment. *Manpower Paper*, no. 11. London: DOE, 1982.

3. R. O. Blood and D. M. Wolfe. *Husbands and Wives: the Dynamics of Married Living*. New York: Free Press, 1960.

4. I. K. Broverman et al. 'Sex-role Stereotypes and Clinical Judgments of Mental Health', *Journal of Consulting and Clinical Psychology*, vol. 34, 1970, pp. 1–7.

5. The term is used by Laurie Shields in *Displaced Homemakers*. New York: McGraw-Hill, 1981.

6. See, for example, Sidney Jourard. *The Transparent Self: Self-disclosure and Well-being* (2nd ed.). New York: Van Nostrand, 1971.

RESOURCES
PUBLICATIONS

Belotti, Elena Gianini. *Little Girls*. London: Writers and Readers, 1975.

Bernard, Jessie. *The Future of Marriage*. London: Penguin Books, 1976.

Brown, Rosemary. *Breaking Up: a Practical Guide to Separation and Divorce*. London: Arrow, 1980.

Burgoyne, Jacqueline. *Breaking Even: Divorce, Your Children and You*. London: Penguin Books, 1984. Includes chapter on 'Thinking about splitting up'. Written for both sexes.

Dowling, Colette. *The Cinderella Complex*. London: Michael Joseph, 1982. About our fear of independence.

Franks, Helen. *Remarriage: What Makes It, What Breaks It*. London: Bodley Head, 1988.

Friedman, Scarlet and Elizabeth **Sarah** (eds). *On the Problem of Men*. London: Women's Press, 1982.

Hanscombe, Gillian and Martin **Humphries**. *Heterosexuality*. London: GMP, 1987. Written by gay people which highlights the way heterosexuals talk about homosexuality.

Hooper, Anne. *Divorce and Your Children*. London: Allen and Unwin, 1983. Excellent chapter on children's questions.

Lear, Martha W. *Heartsounds*. New York: Pocket Books, 1980. Autobiographical account of a woman's relationship with a husband who is suffering from a serious and eventually fatal heart condition.

Mansfield, Penny and Jean **Collard**, *The Beginning of the Rest of Your Life*? London: Macmillan, 1988.

McNichols, Anne. *Going It Alone*. London: SHAC, 1987. Written for women cohabiting who are splitting up. Available from SHAC (London Housing Aid Centre), 189a Old Brompton Road, London SW5 0AR.

Metcalf, Andy and Martin **Humphries**. *The Sexuality of Men*. London: Pluto Press, 1985.

Miller, Stuart. *Men and Friendship*. Boston, MA: Houghton Mifflin, 1983.

Norwood, Robin. *Women who Love Too Much*. London: Arrow, 1986. A constructive book which speaks to many women.

Oakley, Ann. *Housewife*. London: Penguin Books, 1976.

Open University. *The Changing Experience of Women*. Open University course, 1983. Many of the accompanying booklets for this course give a useful overview of women's situation in the family to date. See especially Unit 9, 'The Family – Daughters, Wives and Mothers', and Unit 12, 'Economic Dependence and the State'.

Rubin, Lillian. *Intimate Strangers: What Goes Wrong in Relationships and Why*. London: Fontana, 1985.

Sanders, Diedre and Jane **Reed**. *Kitchen Sink, or Swim?* London: Penguin Books, 1982.

Sharpe, Sue. *Just Like a Girl: How Girls Learn to be Women*. London: Penguin Books, 1976. Includes sections on Asian and West Indian girls.

Spender, Dale and Elizabeth **Sarah**. *Learning to Lose*. London: Women's Press, 1980.

Sternburgh, Judith W. *Lillian Bloom: a Separation*. Green Harbor, MA: 1980. Fine poems chronicling a woman's separation from her husband, her pain and anger, and her growing sense of competence and joy as a woman and a mother.

Triere, Lynette with Richard **Peacock**. *Learning to Leave: A Woman's Guide*. New York: Warner Books, 1982.

Walczak, Yvette. *He and She*, London: Routledge, 1988.

Which? *Divorce – Legal Procedures and Financial Facts*. London: Consumers' Association, 1984. Although not particularly women-oriented, can be useful.

Wise, S. and L. **Stanley** (eds). *Men and Sex*. Women's Studies International Forum, vol. 7, no. 1. Oxford: Pergamon Press, 1984.

Witherspoon, Sue. *A Woman's Place*. London: SHAC, 1987. A clear guide for married women facing divorce. Available from SHAC (London Housing Aid Centre), 189a Old Brompton Road, London SW5 0AR.

Zilbergeld, Bernie. *Men and Sex*. London: Fontana, 1986.

Men's Anti-sexist Newsletter, from 60 Rhymey Street, Cathays, Cardiff CF2 4D6.

SEXUALITY

Prepared by
JILL RAKUSEN

Our powers to express ourselves sexually last a lifetime – from birth to death. Whether or not we are in a sexual relationship with another person, we can explore our fantasies, feel good in our bodies, appreciate sensual pleasures, learn what turns us on, give ourselves sexual pleasure through masturbation. Taught to be embarrassed about or ashamed of our sexual feelings, we have spent a lot of energy denying them or feeling guilty. We are learning to experience our sexuality without judging it and to accept it as part of ourselves.

We are all sexual – young, old, married, single, with or without physical disability, sexually active or not, heterosexual or lesbian. As we change, our sexuality changes. Learning about sex is a lifelong process.

When we have relationships with other people, sexuality is pleasure we want to give and get, communication that is fun and playful, serious and passionate. It can be a tender reaching out or an intense and compelling force which takes us over. It can get us into situations that delight us and ones we wish we could get out of. Sex can open us to new levels of loving and knowing with someone we love and trust. It can be a source of vital energy. Misused, it can hurt us tremendously.

At times, sexual awareness and desires are quiet and other parts of our lives take centre stage. Then, after a month or a year or ten years, the sexual tide may come flowing in.

SOCIAL INFLUENCES

Society shapes and limits our experiences of sexuality. We learn, for instance, that if our looks don't conform to the ideal – if we are fat, old or disabled – then we have no 'right' to be sexual. If we are women of colour, stereotypes often picture us as being more sexually available and active than we are or want to be.

The so-called 'sexual revolution' has had mixed results. While it did encourage people to be less restricted about sex, it has also made many women feel we *ought* to be available to men at all times. And the double standard still prevails. Women are not really 'free', sexually or otherwise, as long as we remain socially and economically unequal to men. (A dramatic example of this is the way men continue to use sexual violence as a weapon against women.)

Finally, we do not have full access to services crucial to our enjoyment of sex – sex education, protection from unwanted pregnancy and sexually transmitted disease, abortion when we need it. Current efforts by conservative political groups threaten to limit our access even further, in an attempt to squeeze *all* our sexuality back into the confines of marriage and motherhood.

BREAKING THE SILENCE

When the women's movement surfaced again in the late sixties, women began speaking in small groups about sexual experiences and feelings. Talking more openly about sex with our friends or in small groups is not always easy at first, and shyness comes and goes, but we have much to learn from each other. Such discussions can be funny, painful and healing. We can affirm each other's feelings, help each other challenge society's distortions of our sexuality, encourage each other in our sexual adventures and learn together to be more assertive about our own sexual needs and desires.

Over the past fifteen years, we have begun to redefine women's sexuality according to our own experiences and not what 'experts' (usually male) have defined it as. Wanting to do more than merely react to sexist patterns that we don't like, we ask: what do *we* want? What images, fantasies, practices unlock the powerful erotic forces within us? We are delving deep into our own sexual imaginations and our satisfying sexual experiences with men and/or women for a fuller vision of what sex can be. We are working for a society free of male/female inequalities, sexual violence, homophobia and media misuse of sex, so that our sexuality

can be a source of refreshment, play, passion, connection
and energy.

GROWING UP

*I watch my daughter. From morning to night her
body is her home. She lives in it and with it.
When she runs around the kitchen she uses all of
herself. Every muscle in her body moves when she
laughs, when she cries. When she rubs her vulva,
there is no awkwardness, no feeling that what she
is doing is wrong. She feels pleasure and expresses
it without hesitation. She knows when she wants
to be touched and when she wants to be left alone.
It's so hard to get back that sense of body as home.*

We are born loving our bodies. But it is rare for us to be
allowed to continue doing so. From family embarrassment,
what *isn't* said, the 'don'ts' that come as our fingers start to
explore vulva, vagina and clitoris, we learn to think of sex as
forbidden, dirty and shameful.

When we become teenagers our developing bodies are
usually a mystery to us. * We discover that what the media,
and most people, consider beautiful falls into a narrow
range. We lose respect for our uniqueness, our own smells
and shapes. We judge ourselves in relation to others. We
come to feel isolated ('Could anyone else be as ugly, dull,
miserable as I?'). An advertisement for sanitary towels
reinforces our aloneness and shame: 'When you have your
period, you should be the only one who knows.'

It takes time – sometimes years and years – and positive
experiences to get rid of these shameful, negative feelings.
Many of us with young children want to help them grow up
feeling good about their bodies and their sexuality, though
sometimes it is hard to move beyond our own upbringing.

*The other day I was taking a bath with my almost-
three-year-old daughter. I was lying down and she
was sitting between my legs, which were spread
apart. She said, 'Mummy, you don't have a
penis.' I said, 'That's right, men have penises and
women have clitorises.' All calm and fine – then,
'Mummy, where is your clitoris?' OK, now what
was I going to do? I took a deep breath (for
courage or something), tried not to blush, spread
my vulva apart and showed her my clitoris. It
didn't feel so bad. 'Do you want to see yours?' I
asked. 'Yes.' That was quite a trick to get her to
look over her fat stomach and see hers, especially
when she started laughing as I first put my finger
and then hers on her clitoris.*

*For more on teenagers' experiences, see *Changing Bodies, Changing Lives. A
Book for Teens on Sex and Relationships*, also by the Boston Women's Health
Book Collective.

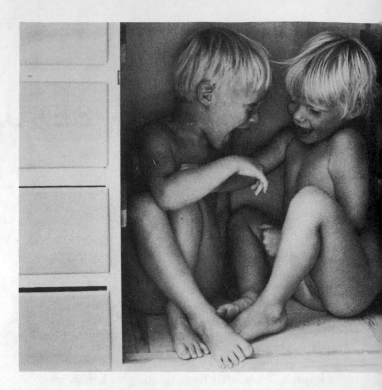

It took us time to develop bad feelings about our sexuality, and we must allow ourselves more time to undo those
feelings and develop new and healthier ones. Thanks in
part to the women's movement, many of us with grown
children and grandchildren talk with them more freely
about sex now than we once would have. 'Growing up'
sexually never ends.

It is a freedom and openness that we must defend. Public
discussion of AIDS and of child sexual abuse is currently
contributing to a renewed climate of sexual hysteria. If our
children are not to absorb these messages – that sex is about
misery and disease – we must find ways of discussing such
issues openly and honestly while at the same time affirming
our right to sexual pleasure and intimacy.

FANTASIES

*Sometimes when I'm making love with myself or
someone else, I think about the ocean roar and feel
the waves swirling about me. Perhaps this means
that I'd rather be floating in the sea than be in my
bed. But it's also a way of heightening the
experience for me. The fantasy makes me feel loose,
easy, fluid. It makes me more relaxed. I usually
have the fantasy just before orgasm, and it helps
me let go.*

*A fantasy before I made love to a plumber I know:
I was entertaining myself one night by imagining I
was dancing with a Stillson wrench (the most
enormous wrench I ever saw, very businesslike!),
and it turned into the plumber. He said, 'Well,
men are still good for something!' We were fixing*

the pipe while we were dancing, and the scene changed. We were swimming in a sea of rubber doughnuts (the connector between the tank and the bottom parts of the toilet), and the doughnuts got stuck over our arms and legs. The scene changed again, to the beach, where we fell asleep.

I used to have a fantasy that I was a gym teacher and I had a classful of girls standing in front of me, nude. I went up and down the rows feeling all their breasts and getting a lot of pleasure out of it. When I first had this fantasy at thirteen I was ashamed. I thought something was wrong with me. Now I can enjoy it, because I feel it's OK to enjoy other women's bodies.

I had the fantasy of making love with two men at once. I pictured myself sandwiched between them. I acted on this one, with an old friend and a casual friend who both liked the idea. It was fun.

Nearly everyone has fantasies, in the form of fleeting images or detailed stories. They express depths within us to learn about and explore. In fantasy we can be whatever we imagine. Yet it can be difficult to accept sexual fantasies.

I was scared they would take me by surprise, tell me things about myself that I didn't know, especially bad things.

I imagined I was sitting in a room. The walls were all white. There was nothing in it, and I was naked. There was a large window at one end, and anyone who wanted to could look in and see me. There was no place to hide. There was something arousing about being so exposed. I masturbated while having this fantasy, and afterward I felt very sad. I thought I must be so sick, so distorted inside, if this image of myself could give me such intense sexual pleasure.

We have been brought up to think that sex should be 'one way'. We often decide we are bad or sick for imagining something different, or feel disloyal when we fantasize about someone other than the man or woman we are with. Yet our fantasies treat us to *all kinds* of erotic experiences. It takes a while to learn that this is OK, and that we can enjoy these stories and images without having to act on them.

What about rape fantasies? Some people say that if we fantasize about having sex forced on us, that means we 'want' to be raped. This is untrue: totally unlike actual rape, fantasizing about rape is voluntary, and does not bring us physical pain or violation. For those of us who grew up learning that 'good girls' don't want sex, a fantasy of being forced to have sex frees us of responsibility and can be highly erotic. It can allow us the feeling of being desired uncontrollably.

In one of my juiciest fantasies a woman and a man tie me up and make love to me and to each other. There is something extremely erotic in

imagining being that powerless. In real life my lover and I do at times feel totally vulnerable to what the other does or wants. This fantasy lets me play around with the power dynamics that are sometimes so intense between us.

We may distrust fantasies which seem to play into male pornographic images of women as submissive or masochistic, and imagine that in a less sexist future fantasies of dominance would come to us less often. Yet this is difficult to predict. For now it seems important to accept that all kinds of fantasies may be erotic for us and free our vital sexual energies. *

SEX WITH OURSELVES: MASTURBATION

Masturbation is a special way of enjoying ourselves.

As infants, touching and playing with our bodies, sometimes our genitals, felt good. Then many of us learned that we were not supposed to touch ourselves sexually. Some of us continued to masturbate, but guiltily, some of us 'forgot' it, and some of us never discovered masturbation at all.

I never even knew about masturbation. When I was twenty-one, a man-friend touched me 'down there', bringing me to orgasm (I didn't know that word either). Then I had a brilliant thought – if he could do it to me, I could do it to me, too. So I did, though it was a long time before I could feel a lot of pleasure and orgasm.

Masturbation allows us the time and space to enjoy and experiment with our own bodies. We can learn what fantasies and touch turn us on. We can learn our own patterns of sexual response without having to think about a partner's needs and opinions. Then, if and when we choose, we can tell our partners what we've learned or show them by guiding their hands to the places we want touched. As women, who have been taught to 'wait for a man to turn us on', knowing how to give ourselves sexual pleasure brings us freedom.

I used to think masturbating was OK only if I didn't have a lover, and only for a quick release. Now I see it's part of my relationship with myself, giving myself pleasure. My rhythms change. Sometimes I masturbate more when I have a lover. Sometimes I'll go for weeks without doing it.

For me at seventy-three, masturbation is better

---

*If you repeatedly have fantasies which disturb or scare you, they may be a sign that you need help. Talk about them with a friend whom you trust to be wise and empathetic, or a trained counsellor or therapist (see p. 135).

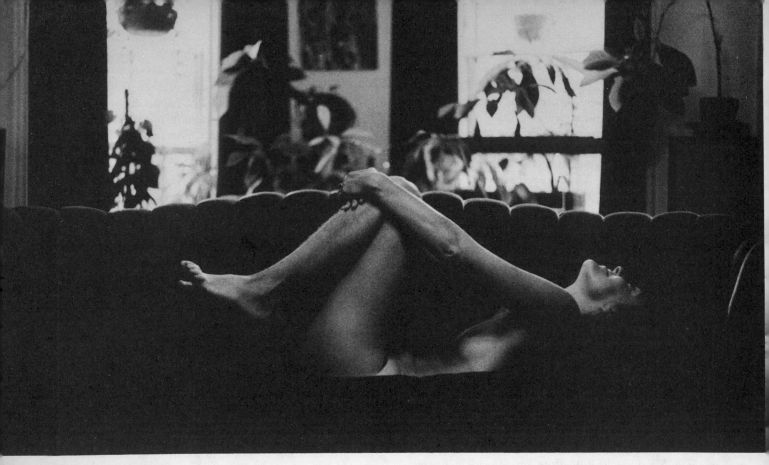

Ann Popki

*than a sexual relationship, as most of the time I'm
more interested in non-sexual pursuits. Sustaining
a relationship with all the time and thought
involved would be a nuisance.*

We can enter a sexual relationship knowing more about
what we want. We aren't totally dependent on our partners
to satisfy us, which can be a freedom for them, too. After
menopause, masturbating also helps us avoid the drying up
of vaginal tissues which can come with age.

Not everyone enjoys masturbating.

*I have tried masturbating because I learned about
it, not out of natural desire. Sometimes it seems
like a chore. I feel I should take the time to explore
my body but I quit after a few minutes because,
quite frankly, I'm bored. It just doesn't seem to
have the effect another person would.*

If masturbating doesn't bring you pleasure, trust your
own preferences and don't do it.

LEARNING TO MASTURBATE[1]

If you have never masturbated and want to, you may feel
awkward, self-conscious, even a bit scared at first. You may
have to contend with voices within you that repeat, 'Nice
girls don't . . .' or 'A happily married woman wouldn't want
to . . .' You may fear losing control of yourself or you may
feel shy or guilty about giving yourself sexual pleasure.
Many of us have these feelings, but they change in time.

Some suggestions: find a quiet time when you can be by
yourself without interruption. Make yourself as comfort-

able as possible: you are expecting a lover, and that lover is
you! Take a relaxing bath or shower. Rub your body all over
with cream, lotion, oil or anything else that feels good.
Slowly explore the shape of your body with your eyes and
your hands. Touch yourself in different ways. Put on music
you like, keep the lights soft, light a candle if you want.
Think about the people or situations you find sexually
arousing. Let your mind flow freely into fantasy. Let your
body relax. *

Women have many ways of masturbating. We can
moisten our fingers (with either saliva or fluid from the
vagina) and rub them around and over the clitoris. We can
gently rub or pull the clitoris itself; we can rub the hood or a
larger area around the clitoris. We can use one finger or
several. We can rub up and down and around and around,
and try different kinds of pressure and timing. Some of us
masturbate by crossing our legs and exerting steady and
rhythmic pressure on the whole genital area. We may insert
something into the vagina – a finger, peeled cucumber,
dildo. We may rub our breasts or other parts of our bodies.
Some of us have learned to develop muscular tension
throughout our bodies.

*At sixteen I gave up masturbation for Lent. Since
I defined masturbation only as touching my
genitals in a sexual way, in those six weeks I
learned that I could have wonderful orgasms
through a mixture of fantasy and quietly tensing*

---

*Such a relaxed and special atmosphere isn't always possible – or necessary!
Desire can overtake us at the most unexpected moments. We can find ourselves
sexually aroused and masturbate while cooking a meal, working at a desk,
riding a horse or bicycle, climbing a tree.

*up and relaxing the muscles around my vagina
and vulva.*

Still other ways of masturbating include using a pillow instead of our hands, a stream of water, an electric vibrator.*

*I can direct our shower nozzle so the water hits my
clitoris in a steady stream. I have a real
relationship with that shower! I wouldn't give it up
for anything! It's nice when I get up for work and
don't have time for sex with my lover but do have
a little time for the shower. Those few minutes are
really important for me.*

As you get sexually aroused, your vagina will become moist. Experiment with what you can do to feel even more. Open your mouth, breathe faster, make noise if you want or move your pelvis rhythmically to your breathing and voice.

As you are getting more aroused you may feel your muscles tighten. Your pelvic area will feel warm and full.

*For me the most pleasurable part is just before
orgasm. I feel I am no longer consciously
controlling my body. I know there is no way I will
not reach orgasm now. I stop trying. I like to
savour this rare moment of true letting go!*

It's this letting go of control that enables us to have orgasms. If you do not reach orgasm when you first try masturbating, don't worry. Simply enjoy the sensations you have. Try again some other time.

*Masturbating opens me to what is happening in
my body and makes me feel good about myself. I
like following the impulse of the moment.
Sometimes I have many orgasms, sometimes I don't
have any. The greatest source of pleasure is to be
able to do whatever feels good to me at that
particular time. I rarely have such complete
freedom in other aspects of my life.*

PHYSICAL ASPECTS OF OUR SEXUALITY

Sounds, sights, smells and touch can arouse our sexual feeling, as do fantasies, a baby sucking at the breast, the smell of a familiar body, a sexy picture, a dream, touching our own bodies, a lover's breathing in our ear, brushing against someone or hearing the person we love say, 'I love you'.

*Vibrators are sold at many chemists and department stores, often as body or neck massagers.

*When I'm feeling turned on, either alone or with
someone I'm attracted to, my heart beats faster,
my face gets red, my eyes are bright. My whole
vulva feels wet and full. My breasts hum. When
I'm standing up I feel a rush of weakness in my
thighs. When I'm lying down I may feel like doing
a big stretch, arching my back, feeling the
sensations go out to my fingers and toes.*

No matter what arouses our sexual feelings or how we express them, if we continue to receive sexual stimulation our bodies go through a series of physical changes, sometimes called 'sexual response'. While these changes may feel different each time, they follow certain basic patterns which are helpful to know about.*

Early on in sexual excitement, veins in the pelvis, vulva and clitoris begin to dilate (open) and fill with blood, gradually making the whole area feel full. (This is called *vasocongestion.*) In the vagina this swelling creates a 'sweating' reaction, producing the fluid which makes the vaginal lips get wet – often an early sign that we are sexually excited. At the same time, sexual tension rises throughout the body as muscles begin to tense up or contract (*myotonia*). We may breathe more quickly, nipples may become erect and hard, the whole body feels alive to touch.

ORGASM

Enough stimulation of or around the clitoris and (for some women) pressure on the cervix or other sensitive areas cause pelvic fullness and body tension to build up to a peak. Orgasm is the point at which all the tension is suddenly released in a series of involuntary and pleasurable muscular contractions which expel blood from the pelvic tissues. We may feel contractions in the vagina, uterus and rectum. Some women describe orgasms without contractions.

Orgasm can be mild like a hiccup, a sneeze, a ripple or a peaceful sigh; it can be a sensuous experience, as the body

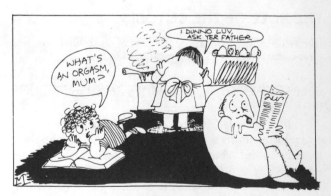

*The following description comes primarily from the ground-breaking laboratory research of William Masters and Virginia Johnson in the 1960s, with a number of modifications in response to more recent findings and especially to women's criticisms and additions to the Masters and Johnson model. For more details, see Sexual Arousal and Orgasm in the Appendix to this chapter.

glows with warmth; it can be intense or ecstatic, as we lose awareness of ourselves for a time.

Orgasm may feel different with a finger, penis, dildo or vibrator in your vagina, and different when you masturbate from when you make love with another person. It may feel totally different at different times even with the same person.

Often we become aroused at times when we can't get additional stimulation and reach orgasm. Although sexual tension subsides eventually without orgasm, it takes longer. When we get sufficiently aroused and don't have an orgasm, our genitals and/or uterus may ache for a while.

Quite a number of women have never had an orgasm. With all the publicity about orgasms in the past ten years, many of us who don't orgasm* believe we're missing something pleasurable. We can try to orgasm by masturbating, reading books about it,† asking a partner to help, joining what is sometimes called a 'pre-orgasmic women's group'. A fifty-three-year-old woman wrote to our collective that after reading an earlier edition of this book she had masturbated and reached orgasm for the first time in her life. Yet it's important that orgasm doesn't become one more 'performance' pressure.

> When I try too hard to have an orgasm it usually doesn't work and I end up frustrated and bored. For me it's best if I relax and let it happen if it's going to.

Some women can orgasm twice or more in quick succession (which men cannot do). Knowing that 'multiple orgasms' are possible has made some of us feel we 'ought' to have them, that we are sexually inadequate if we don't. Men may expect it, too; one woman wrote that a man she knew was considering a divorce because the woman he was married to didn't have multiple orgasms. Yet one orgasm can be plenty, and sometimes sex without orgasm is pleasurable. Seek whatever feels best to *you*.

THE ROLE OF THE CLITORIS

It may be arousing to stroke any part of our bodies, exciting to have our thighs caressed or our necks nibbled or our breasts sucked. However, the clitoris – the organ that is the most sensitive to stimulation – has a central role in elevating feelings of sexual tension.

Until the mid-1960s, most women didn't know how crucial the clitoris was. Even if we knew it for ourselves, nobody talked about it. Medical texts and marriage manuals (written by men) followed Freud's famous pronouncement that the 'mature' woman has orgasms only when her vagina, not her clitoris, is stimulated. This theory made the penis very important to a woman's sexual satisfaction (what brought a *man* sexual release supposedly satisfied women, too). Following Freud, psychoanalytic theories belittled women's enjoyment of masturbation as 'immature', and labelled lesbian sex as a pale imitation of the 'real thing'. In the sixties, sex researchers found that for women *all* orgasms depend at least in part on clitoral stimulation, although some women respond to internal pressure as well.

Learning about the clitoris increased sexual enjoyment for countless women and freed many of us from years of thinking we were 'frigid'. Our ability to give ourselves orgasms and to show our lovers how to please us has been one of the cornerstones of a new self-respect and autonomy, and has therefore been politically as well as personally important for women.

The clitoris is not a button. It has several parts to it. The glans (or tip, the part you can see) attaches to the shaft, which runs along internally from the glans towards the vaginal opening. The clitoris connects to a branching interior system of erectile tissue that runs through your genital area. (Erectile tissue responds to sexual arousal by filling with blood, becoming erect and hard. A penis also contains erectile tissue.) During sexual excitement, the clitoris swells and changes position. (See Chapter 3 for a fuller description of the clitoris.)

You or your lover can stimulate your clitoris in many different ways – by rubbing, sucking, body pressure, using a vibrator. Any rubbing or pressure in the pubic-hair-covered mons area or the lips (even on the lower abdomen and inner thighs) can move the clitoris, and may also press it up against the pubic bone. Although some women touch the glans to become aroused, it is often so sensitive that direct touching hurts, even with lubrication. Also, focusing directly on the clitoris for a long time may cause the pleasurable sensations to disappear. As women grow older the hood of skin covering the clitoris may pull back permanently, so that if you are past menopause you may need extra lubrication in order to enjoy having your clitoris rubbed.

Vagina-to-penis intercourse gives only indirect clitoral stimulation. As the penis moves in and out of the vagina it moves the inner lips which are connected to the clitoral hood, and therefore may move the hood back and forth over the glans. When the inner lips become swollen and firm they can act as an extension of the vagina, hugging the penis as it moves back and forth and further increasing clitoral friction.* To reach orgasm during vagina-to-penis intercourse, many of us need *direct* and sometimes prolonged clitoral stimulation both before and during intercourse.

Many women making love to other women focus less exclusively on vaginal penetration and give more (and longer) stimulation to the clitoris. Many women who make

---

*Writer/researcher Shere Hite suggests we use orgasm as a verb, to highlight the fact that it is something women *do* and not just something which happens *to* us. We have decided to use it occasionally, along with other more familiar forms.
†See books by Dodson, Barbach, Hite, Meulenbelt and Hooper listed in Resources.

*Some feminists criticize this Masters and Johnson theory as an attempt to justify penis-in-vagina intercourse as the norm for love-making. See, for example, *The Hite Report*.

MAJOR AREAS OF CHANGE DURING SEXUAL AROUSAL AND ORGASM

- The blood vessels through the whole pelvic area swell, causing 'engorgement' and creating a feeling of fullness and sexual sensitivity.
- The clitoris (glans, shaft and crura) swells and becomes erect.
- The inner lips swell and change shape.
- The urethral sponge and the bulbs of the vestibule enlarge.
- The vagina balloons upward.
- The uterus shifts position.

See the diagrams in Chapter 3 for other views.

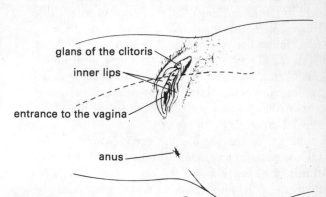

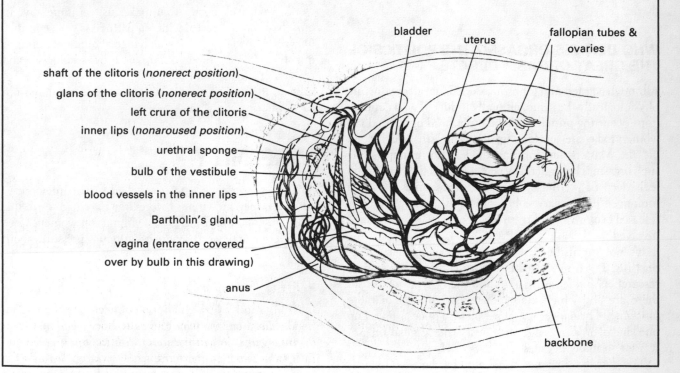

love with men in their sixties and older (when erections happen less frequently) find that sexual pleasure increases, partly because penetration by the penis is no longer the focus of love-making.

THE ROLE OF THE VAGINA, UTERUS AND CERVIX

Women have the potential to respond to sexual arousal throughout the entire pelvic region. When we are aroused, the erectile tissue around the outer third of the vagina becomes full, and nerves in that area become more sensitive to stimulation and pressure. When the muscles around this part of the vagina (pubococcygeus muscles) are strong and well exercised, many women find they orgasm more easily. (See Pelvic Floor Exercises, p. 347.) Childbearing increases the venous system in the pelvis, often making arousal quicker and stronger.

Two researchers have recently identified what they call the 'Grafenberg spot' ('G-spot'), a sensitive area just behind the front wall of the vagina between the back of the pubic bone and the cervix. They say that when this spot is stimulated during sex through vaginal penetration of some kind, some women orgasm with a gush of fluid from the urethra which is not urine. This is at present a controversial theory among sex researchers. It's a relief for those women who feel a urethral gushing of liquid during orgasm to find an explanation for this apparent 'ejaculation', and for some others to find what may be another source of pleasure. However, if a G-spot orgasm becomes a new 'ideal' for the sexually liberated woman, or is used to reinstate so-called 'vaginal' orgasms as superior, it will become a new source of pressure, making us feel inadequate or unaccepting of our own sexual experiences.

Further up in the vagina, the cervix and uterus are crucial to orgasm for a number of women. While the inner two-thirds of the vagina and the cervix itself have little sensitivity, a penis, finger or dildo pressing repeatedly on the cervix 'jostles' the uterus and indeed the whole lining of the abdominal cavity (peritoneum). This can create a different kind of feeling internally before and during orgasm. If we have had a hysterectomy we may have to learn to focus on different kinds of sexual stimulation and feelings, because the cervix and uterus are no longer there.*

WHO DEFINES ORGASM? THE POLITICS OF THE GREAT ORGASM DEBATE

Although Masters and Johnson asserted that all orgasms are physiologically the same (clitorally induced, with contractions occurring primarily in the outer third of the vagina), women today are speaking up about orgasms which don't 'fit' the Masters and Johnson model. For example, one such orgasm is brought on by penetration of the vagina, and feels 'deep' or 'uterine'. The build-up sometimes involves a prolonged involuntary holding in of the breath, which is released explosively at orgasm. No contractions seem to be involved.

It's not surprising that women experience a range of orgasms. But a new debate is stirring among sexologists, researchers and feminists as to how many 'types' of orgasm there are and which kind is better or stronger or more satisfying. The danger is that people will once again set up one kind of orgasm as the norm, just as the 'vaginal' orgasm was for so many decades.

The debate on women's sexuality has become increasingly professionalized: a number of researchers, many of them women, have claimed this as their field of 'expertise', wielding studies, scientific language and statistics to make their points. In modern society professionals have enormous power to shape our understanding of ourselves. Much so-called scientific debate ends up defining women for society's purposes rather than enabling us to arrive at our own chosen development. Women doing sex research must constantly ask what people are going to do with the results, and whether their efforts may be used against women in a society where women do not have adequate social or political power.

It is crucial that women have accurate information about our sexuality, and some form of research is necessary. We believe that the information we need comes most usefully and powerfully from women talking about our experiences in settings of our own making.

The female orgasm has been the subject of intense – and often prejudiced – debate for decades. There has been no such concern about definitions of the male orgasm. Yet few men who are honest will deny that they themselves experience a range of orgasms, and some men even acknowledge that orgiastic feelings do not necessarily require ejaculation. Our ideas and attitudes to our own sexuality therefore are not only affected by male-orientated debate about our own sexual response, but also assumptions about the limitations of male sexuality: for it is still the norm for female sexuality to be discussed within the context of so-called 'normal' heterosexual sex, which is of course dominated by assumptions concerning male sexuality in general, and the male orgasm in particular.

There is no one 'right' pattern of sexual response. What works, what feels good, what makes us feel more alive in ourselves and connected with our partners is what counts.* Our sexual patterns, too, will change at different points in our life. If the 'models' proposed by sexologists and researchers (or feminists) don't fit our experiences of orgasm, then we must trust ourselves and learn more from each other.

VIRGINITY

A virgin is someone who hasn't had sexual intercourse. Although men are virgins before they have had sex in this sense, the main pressure to *be* a virgin is on women. If we are heterosexual, we experience conflicting pressures about virginity.

My mother told me it's a gift I can give only once, so I'd better hold on to it.

The day I left the Church was the day I had an argument in the confessional with the priest about whether having intercourse with my fiancé was a sin. I maintained it wasn't; he said I would never be a faithful wife if I had intercourse before marriage. He refused me absolution and I never went back.

I've done everything else I can do – even oral sex, which personally seems to me as close as you can

---

*See Hysterectomy, p. 597.

*Many women with spinal cord injuries have no feeling in the pelvic area yet report experiencing orgasm and its sensations elsewhere in their bodies. Clearly we all have lots more to learn about sexual responses.

get to someone. But I feel I'll be 'dirty' if I lose my virginity. Why does that one act make such a difference?

Among my girlfriends in my last year at school, I was the only virgin. This caused me embarrassment and teasing from my friends. I was branded as a nice girl, chicken, weird, etc., even though I did all the same things they did except have sex.

The idea of virginity is an old one. People in early Greece and Rome used it to refer to a woman (or a goddess) who was autonomous, on her own, not 'owned' by any man. Later it came to mean only sexual virginity and, ironically, to reflect the prevailing view of women as man's property. Remaining a virgin until she married guaranteed that a woman would uphold the family 'honour' by passing from father to husband like unspoiled goods. Since there was no dependable birth control, it guaranteed also that babies would be born only to married couples.

Many parents today are less concerned about preserving their daughters' actual virginity than about how soon or with whom they have intercourse. Some parents respect and encourage a daughter's decisions about sex. But in many other families, the message is still 'Stay a virgin!' We may 'do everything but' have intercourse and feel confused – though 'technically' virgin, we may have become as emotionally and physically involved as we would have with intercourse. If we start having intercourse, we may feel troubled, guilty or ashamed about having 'lost' our virginity. This may keep us from enjoying sex then or later, from asking for what we want or from feeling free to say no later on if we want to. It may keep us from finding out about birth control and using it.

Meanwhile, schoolmates and the media may pressure us to be sexually available, a pressure that can be as strong as the more traditional pressure to remain a virgin.

If we want to have sex with a man we must be free to have it as we think best. Sex usually brings many changes in the relationship and in our life. Since it is often a big decision, it makes sense to think about it, talk it over with friends and the person we're involved with, choose a method of birth control if necessary. We may well want to say no to someone who is pushing us to have sex when we don't want to.*

If we decide to have intercourse we can be disappointed at first. Intercourse like many other things gets better with time and practice.

For lesbians the first experience of sex can be even more confusing; social attitudes and inhibitions combine with inexperience and often deep feelings of guilt.

After hanging around for about three months, one night we managed to get it together. We were sitting

in front of the fire, seeming to get closer and closer, talking about anything but the situation we were in. She eventually took over and made love to me fully clothed. I didn't touch her at all – I couldn't, I was too caught up in my own feelings as to what was actually happening.[2]

Clearly, for those of us who are lesbian, there is still a sense in which we are virgins until we have had sex with a woman. For *all* women, it would be helpful to think of 'virginity' differently. Instead of virginity being something we 'lose' or have to 'save' for someone, it could mean our physical, spiritual and emotional wholeness, our self-respect and bodily integrity, our freedom to make a choice. When we make choices about sex out of this feeling of self-respect and 'virginity', we will more likely put ourselves into situations we can be glad about. We are virgins with each new lover, whichever sex they are, sometimes even with the same lover, and in each new phase of our lives.

SEX IN A RELATIONSHIP

Currents of sexual attraction and passion criss-cross our lives and pull us into new relationships, deepen the ones we're in, teach us about ourselves. We may act on them with a look, smile, touch, kiss, or we may not want to. When we make love with someone familiar or new, woman or man, we are often at our most open, most vulnerable and also our most powerful. Sex can be dramatic, dull, comforting, scary, friendly, funny, passionate, frustrating, satisfying.

Sex doesn't take place in a vacuum. We take struggles about other things – power, money, mutuality, competition – into bed with us.

Sex in relationships can vary in meaning and intensity.

Sometimes I make love to get care and cuddling. Sometimes I am so absorbed in the sensations of touch and taste and smell and sight and sound that I feel I've returned to that childhood time when feeling good was all that mattered. Sometimes we tumble and tease. Sometimes sex is spiritual – High Mass could not be more sacred. Sometimes I make love to get away from the tightness and seriousness in myself. Sometimes I want to come and feel the ripples of orgasm through my body. Sometimes tears mix with juices mix with sweat, and I am one with another. Sometimes through sex I unite with the stream of love that flows among us all. Sex can be most anything and everything for me. How good that feels!

I enjoy sex with Mike more than I have with anyone. When we get aroused, we make the most beautiful music together! Still, sex often feels difficult to me. When I feel good about myself and

---

*For more on virginity and first intercourse, see books by Bell et al. and Cousins–Mills listed in Resources.

close to him, when the pressures of our children and my work and friends are not demanding a lot of my energy, our sex is very fluid and strong. When I feel angry, sad, depressed or very childlike and needy, or any combination, or busy with other people in my life, I have a hard time being sexually open with Mike. We've talked about this, and he experiences a lot of the same ups and downs and distractions as I do.

Sometimes a brief encounter can be intensely exciting and can free us to try things we wouldn't with someone we were in a certain pattern with. On the other hand, a brief encounter or an affair we know will end can be unsatisfactory if we don't want or trust our partner well enough to ask for what we want. In a long-term relationship there is an opportunity to learn about each other's bodies over time; to explore different sexual techniques, roles and fantasies; to express deeply our many and varied feelings through sex.

I couldn't bear the thought of getting really involved with someone so that I would have to give up faking [orgasms] and worst of all, really face up to the possibility of a less than satisfactory sex life stretching ahead of me for years. One-night stands became the norm. The excitement of a new encounter was enough in itself . . . eventually I realized that my inability to achieve orgasm was becoming a major issue in my life, I knew that everything would not suddenly 'come right' outside a totally trusting relationship.[3]

Yet some long-term couples get into sexual patterns that fail to satisfy either or both partners. Some of us have had short-term relationships and have been able to use what we've learned in them to get out of unsatisfying patterns with a long-term partner.

Whatever kind of relationship we have, good sexual sharing requires trust, clear communication, appropriate technique, a sense of humour, time and privacy. We want

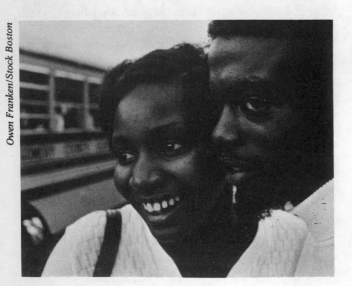

Owen Franken/Stock Boston

relationships based on mutual respect and equality. We want relationships in which our commitment allows us to share our vulnerable places as well as our joyful places. We need to cry and laugh together. We want to spend many quiet, unhurried hours with each other, finding what pleases and excites us.

COMMUNICATING ABOUT SEX

The true language of sex is primarily non-verbal. Our words and images are poor expressions of the deep feelings within and between us.

Few words in the English language feel appropriate for sex because they convey attitudes and values very unlike how we actually feel. Clinical, 'proper' terms – vagina, penis and intercourse – seem cold, distant, tight; slang terms – cunt, cock, fuck – seem degrading or coarse; euphemisms like 'making love' are vague. We use different words with lovers, children, friends and doctors. Though sex is a natural way of expressing ourselves, we have no natural way of talking about it. Many of us are trying to put together a sexual language with which we are comfortable.

SAYING WHAT WE REALLY WANT

There are certain issues we all face in a sexual situation, whether it's with a date, long-time lover or spouse: How do I feel at the moment? Do I want to be sexually close with this person now? In what ways? What if I don't know – can I say I'm confused? Then can I communicate clearly what I want, what I don't want? Do I feel comfortable saying it in words or letting him/her know some other way? What are the unspoken rules? Is there enough trust and caring between us for this person to listen to my feelings and respect them if I feel differently from him/her? Particularly in any new heterosexual relationship, there is now the additional issue of AIDS. We need to protect ourselves but we may fear hurting our partner's feelings. In reality, both partners in a new relationship are probably relieved if this issue can be brought into the open. See p. 488 for guidelines for safer sex.

Often the question is whether to make love or not. When we want to ask someone to make love with us, we may have to overcome certain inhibitions, for we have been brought up to think that women should not initiate sex. We have to get used to the possibility of being turned down. When we *don't* want to make love, we often face (in men primarily) the assumption that 'women don't really mean it when they say no'. Or someone interprets our not wanting sex as a sign of rejection or 'frigidity'. The more complex truth lies somewhere between the extremes of 'good girls don't initiate sex' and 'liberated women always want it'; often we do, often we don't. Sometimes we love being coaxed into it, sometimes we hate feeling pressured. All we can do is try to be as fully aware as possible of our feelings at the moment, to be honest with ourselves about them, and to practise saying them, with clarity and no apologies.

Communication about our sexual needs is a continuous process. One woman who had plucked up the courage to talk with her man about their sexual relationship said in angry frustration, 'I told him what I liked once, so why doesn't he know now? Did he forget? Doesn't he care?'

Even in the most loving relationships, asking for what we want is hard.

- We are afraid that being honest about what we want will threaten the other.
- Our partner seems defensive and might interpret our suggestion as a criticism or a demand.
- We are embarrassed by the words themselves.
- We feel sex is supposed to come naturally and having to talk about it must mean there's a problem.
- We have been making love with the same person for years (sometimes several decades) and it feels risky to bring up new insights.
- We and our partner aren't communicating well in other areas of our relationship.
- Even with a willing partner, we may as women feel a deep inhibition about asserting our sexuality openly and proudly, which is what we'd be doing if we proclaimed our erotic needs and wishes.
- We don't know what we want at a particular time, or we need to react to something our partner does. The barriers can be inside us, not just between us and our partners.

How do we work on better communication in sex? Making love is one of the special times when we have more than words to use to reach each other. Taking a partner's hand and putting it in a new place, making the sounds that let him/her know we are feeling good, speeding up or slowing down our hip movements, a firm hand on the shoulder meaning 'let's go slow' – there are many ways we have of communicating, if we will use them.

I've liked just saying, 'Watch', and showing.

We were both really excited. My lover began rubbing my clitoris hard and it hurt. It took me a second to work out what to do. I was afraid that if I said something about it, I would spoil the excitement for both of us. Then I realized I could just take my lover's hand and very gently move it up a little higher to my pubic hair.

With all our old stereotypes about who does what in sex, communication doesn't happen overnight – we move gradually away from the old myth that men know all about sex, women just have it done to them, and no one talks about it. However, telling or showing each other what feels good is not complaining or demanding; it's a profound kind of honesty.

EXPLORING LOVE-MAKING

We have many ways of getting and giving pleasure – touching, caressing, looking, teasing, kissing, massaging, licking, sucking, penetrating.

We can spend hours – when we're on holiday or the kids are away on a weekend morning – looking at each other, stroking and cuddling each other, pulling and pushing and feeling our bodies stretch together. If we go past a certain point we'll both know we want to 'make love', but actually we have been making love the whole time.

What we do in sex is a matter of personal preference and ingenuity, who we are with, how much love and understanding we feel, how comfortable we both are with our bodies, how each of us feels that day. At its best, love-making takes its shape as we and our partners move together by mutual (often unspoken) agreement. Sexual equality is as important in bed as it is everywhere else.

TOUCHING AND SENSUALITY

Massages, back rubs, foot rubs, head rubs – these are wonderful at any time. As part of love-making, they can make sex slower and more sensual.

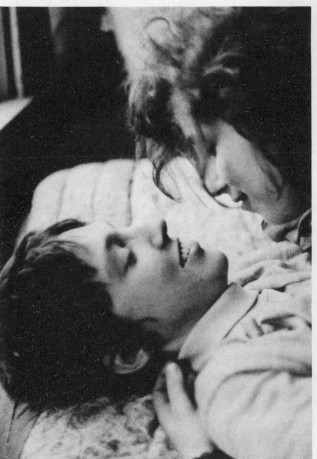

Joy Schneider Kendra

Sometimes it's a thrill to make love fast, whenever and wherever the desire hits. Other times I like to take time to emphasize every little sensual detail. We'll eat something delicious together (not too much or I'll get full and sleepy). We'll put on music, light a candle, take turns rubbing each other with oil or lotion, roll around a lot, caress each other everywhere, let our excitement build up slowly, let orgasm happen if it does. It's like a long sexual dance.

Eric likes me to rub his feet and suck his toes. I think that gives him as much pleasure or more than anything else we do in sex.

Tender touching can be a way of making love.

When a couple has problems in sex, it may turn out that they have been focusing entirely on each other's genitals, and not taking time or learning how to touch and stroke each other lovingly all over. Many men are more focused on genitals than women are, and need to learn the pleasures of touching.

ORAL SEX

We can suck or lick our partner's genitals, which when done to a woman is called *cunnilingus* (slang: going down, eating) and when done to a man is called *fellatio* (slang: going down, blow job). Sometimes oral sex is more intimate than any other kind of love-making. For some of us, it brings orgasm more surely than other ways of making love.

We're really into oral sex, and he's always ready and willing. He'll say, 'Do you want to have an orgasm?' And he'll go down on me. It's terrific.

To enjoy oral sex it helps to like our partner's genitals and feel good about our own. Yet we are often ashamed of our 'private parts'.

For ages I thought my lover was doing me a favour when he did oral sex on me. I couldn't imagine that I tasted good. Finally he convinced me that he loves doing it. Also, I tasted my juices and they're not bad!

At first I was repulsed by the idea of going down on a woman. I thought we smelled bad, that vaginas were nasty. It was a little pungent and intimidating in the beginning (though less so than a penis had been!). I soon learned to lose myself in the wonderful textures, tastes and formations of a woman's genitalia. I realized that lesbian sex is about loving myself, overcoming my hatred of my own body.

One of the pluses of oral sex with men is that we won't get pregnant (though with men or women we may risk a sexually transmitted disease). But like everything in sex, it's good only if we want to be doing it.

If I don't want to have intercourse with a man, I certainly don't want oral sex with him either. I find that far more intimate than intercourse!

My husband likes me to do oral sex on him. Sometimes it's incredibly erotic for me to have his penis moving in my mouth. Since I don't enjoy swallowing his semen, I usually spit it out or let it flow out on the sheets, and that's fine. Sometimes, however, blowing him makes me choke – I don't want his penis filling up my mouth at all. Then we do something else. Or we get in a position where I have more control, like being on top of him with the base of his penis in my hand.

What feels good in oral sex differs from time to time.

I like tongue, lips, moisture, not too much sucking and pulling, and time for exploring – my lover's got to be willing to stay with it for a while.

It can be done rather crummily! I hate it when I feel he's eating me up with his teeth or when the pressure's too hard and it hurts or when he moves around from place to place and doesn't keep the stimulation steady.

For me there's no right or wrong place, just the places I want concentrated on on a particular day. I'm getting better at telling my lover where it feels best.

ANAL STIMULATION

The anus can be stimulated with fingers, tongue, penis* or any slender object. For many of us, it is a highly sexually sensitive area.

I like having something small in my anus during love-making – no pressure or movement, just there.

Having the area around my anus licked during oral sex is a real turn-on. And anal intercourse when I'm in the mood is incredibly sexy. I love the sensations deep inside me, and the thrill of doing something so unusual.

The anus is not as elastic as the vagina, so it is important to go slowly, wait until you're relaxed and use a lubricant – saliva, secretions from the vagina or penis or a water-soluble jelly such as K-Y Jelly. This reduces the risk of damaging the tissue. The seriousness of tissue damage has increased because this leaves us open to transmission of HIV, the virus that can lead to AIDS. See p. 488 for

*Called *sodomy*, often by those who disapprove of it.

guidelines for safer sex. Anal bacteria can also cause serious vaginal infections and cystitis, so don't put anything in your vagina which has been in your anus without washing it first; if a man uses a condom during anal or vaginal intercourse, this will also protect us. If you use your tongue (sometimes called rimming), you may get a stomach infection or a sexually transmitted disease.

Anal sex isn't for everyone.

My husband wants to have anal sex a lot. Once I almost didn't know it was happening. There was lubrication and everything was right and it felt fine. At other times I've really not wanted it and a few times it's been almost painful and I've stopped it. I wish I liked it better because I'd love to give him that pleasure, but I have to be honest – I just don't enjoy it.

In our one great try at anal intercourse I ended up jumping three feet in the air and squealing like a stuck pig. This so terrified him that he completely lost his erection, and we laughed and laughed.

MASTURBATING IN LOVE-MAKING

When my fiancé asked if he could help me masturbate I thought it was kinky at first. Then I showed him how I do it and he showed me how he does. We watch each other to see what feels good. He has trouble sometimes having orgasms inside me, and I know it's a relief to him that he can openly bring himself to orgasm after intercourse.

My lover rubbed her breasts and clitoris while I made love to her yesterday. After I got over feeling a little inadequate (I should be able to do it all!), I found it was like having another pair of hands to make love to her with. It was a turn-on to both of us.

When one person in a relationship wants sex or orgasm more than the other, masturbation is a possibility. Here are some different views.

It's typical for my husband to want to make love at night, but I'm too tired. Then by morning I'm very horny and he wants to get up. I always tease him in the morning, ask whether he jerked off or not. Sometimes he did. Sometimes I'll be going off to sleep and feel the bed shaking.

I've been ill for the past week, and how can you get really turned on when your throat's sore and your nose is running? So I said to my lover, 'I don't have much energy for sex, but if you want to masturbate, please do.'

Masturbation is such a private thing, and I want to keep it for when I'm alone with myself. Also,

doing it with someone else would be the ultimate in showing that I'm a sexual person, and maybe I'm shy about that.

It's a relief to me to know that either of us can give ourselves an orgasm if that's what we want. It helps make coming less the centre of sex for us, and frees both of us from feeling we have to 'do it right' or the other person will be frustrated.

INTERCOURSE

If you have intercourse with a man, think of it as reciprocal – you open up to enclose his penis, you surround him powerfully and he penetrates you. Intercourse can be infinitely slow and gentle, hard and thrusting, or both.

I can so clearly remember moving in and around him and him in me, till it seemed in the whole world there was only us dancing together as we moved together, as we loved together, as we came together. Sometimes at these times I laugh or cry and they are the same strong emotions coming from a deep protected part of me that is freer now for loving him.

When I was trying to get pregnant I found intercourse especially exciting because of the possibility that this might be the time his sperm met my egg.

For intercourse to give you pleasure you must feel aroused, sexually excited, your vagina wet and open. Often it takes women longer – sometimes much longer – than men to become aroused. If you are sexually inexperienced or angry with your partner, or have a partner who practises only the 'in and out' of intercourse and not the love-making which surrounds it, then penetration (especially when your vagina is dry) can be boring, unpleasant, even painful.* Do whatever gives *you* the most pleasure. Sometimes you will feel open and ready for intercourse immediately; more often you will want your partner first to touch, rub, kiss or lick your vulva and clitoris.

Certain positions will feel more exciting to you than others (and may differ each time you make love). The 'man on top' is not a 'naturally' better position at all. You can sit, or lie upon him, or lie side by side. Sit up with your legs over his and his penis in you; or he can enter you from behind and reach around to caress your clitoris. If you want deep penetration and pressure on your cervix, choose positions which make these more possible. We are all different shapes and need to find positions which suit us.

*See The Politics of Sex, p. 255 for a discussion of how our relationships with men are bound up with sexual politics and male power.

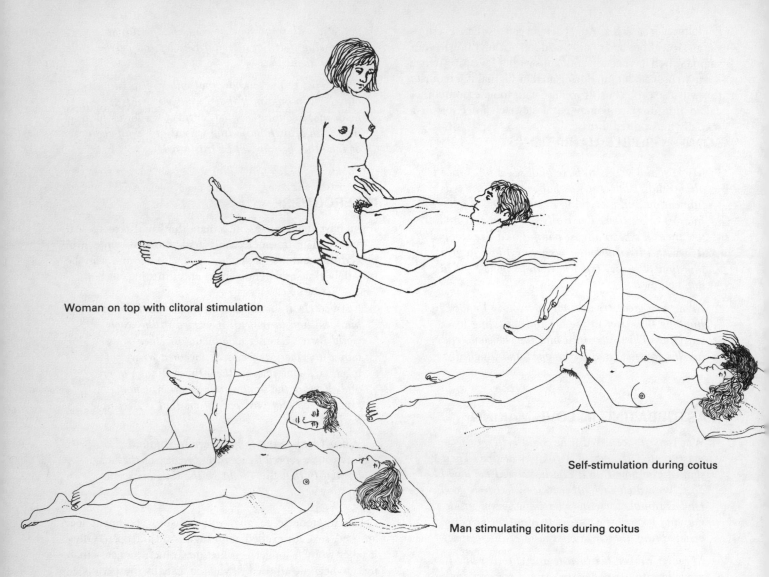

Woman on top with clitoral stimulation

Self-stimulation during coitus

Man stimulating clitoris during coitus

Intercourse is about pleasure and connection for *both* of you, and not necessarily orgasm. Many women don't orgasm during intercourse. Sometimes trying to have an orgasm makes you self-conscious and tightens you up. On the other hand:

Sometimes it's exciting to strive for orgasms – if I don't strive I won't get them, and they feel so good!

If you are not ready for orgasm and your partner is highly aroused when you begin intercourse, he might reach orgasm too soon for you if he moves back and forth inside you and you move your pelvis against his quickly. Both of you can slow your movements until you become more excited yourself. Experiment with holding your bodies still for a time when he enters you, then begin to move together slowly. Moving slowly can help men learn to delay ejaculation, which can make intercourse more pleasurable for both of you.

Pressure of the penis on the cervix can be the key to orgasm for some women, as are clitoral and vulval stimulation.

It is best if you can communicate with words or movements what feels best to you. Yet sometimes talking about it is neither easy nor possible.

He would come almost instantly when we began to make love after marvellous kissing. A little while later we'd make love again, when I'd be more aroused – aching for him, in fact. I never knew how to alter this pattern, never dared talk about it, and later on found out that he had resented 'having' to make love twice.

Over time you and your partner can learn your mutual rhythms of desire and arousal and explore what gives each of you the most pleasure.

AFTER LOVE-MAKING

The hour or so after active love-making can be a special time.

After sex we talk tenderly, laugh deeply, whisper,

cry, sleep like babies in each other's arms. Some of the most important conversations in our relationship have come in those satisfied and intimate moments.

SOME POSSIBLE VARIATIONS

- Changing roles. The one who usually initiates sex can be more receptive, the quieter one more vigorous or noisy. It can take a while to get comfortable with these changes.

I have real difficulty taking the initiative in sex, even though I know my husband would like it. Growing up I was taught that sexually aggressive women are less civilized, and I can't seem to shake off my inhibition. Also, what if I initiate and he says no? What a risk; yet he takes it all the time.

- Making love in different places or positions. (Many of us find, however, that towards the end of love-making one or two positions are best for orgasm.)
- Enjoying sexual fantasies while making love (see p. 238).
- Using sexually explicit materials like books, magazines or photographs, welcoming the images or words that arouse us and free our sexual energy.

There are times when Gwen and I want a little extra turn-on. Maybe we're tired, or preoccupied with work or kids, yet we'd also like to make love. Our own fantasies are usually quite juicy enough, but when they're not, we'll read something sexy together and have a great time.

Unfortunately, most of the erotic material that's available today is based on men's fantasies, not ours. Most of it is pornography, which depicts women's bodies as depersonalized objects and instruments of men's sexual pleasure. The positions usually shown do little for a woman's clitoral stimulation. All this can aggravate the differences between what women and men want in sex.

My husband has read porn magazines since he was fourteen. He gets lots of ideas from them and keeps wanting to try things in sex which don't arouse me and I don't like much. We are both pretty disappointed in our sex life at this point.

It can be important to distinguish between 'erotica' – sexually explicit materials showing sex which doesn't degrade anyone, and 'pornography' – the materials which show someone (usually a woman) being forced or degraded. Women need to create more erotica of our own!*

- Playing games in sex. We can play-act situations and fantasies which excite us, like being kids about to be caught or making love in a public place. We can dress up. We can be our child selves as well as our adult selves, our lusty, vigorous as well as our needy selves.

Sometimes when I'm feeling good I'll create a strip scene for my husband – and for me, since our mirror is strategically placed – and we both get very excited. Now he does it, too, standing in front of the bed, moving his body rhythmically, slowly taking off and throwing down his clothes. I love it. His strength and vulnerability come through at the same time.

In sado-masochistic (S/M) sex play the play-acting is based on fantasy situations of dominance and submission. Partners act out roles like teacher–student, police–citizen, monarch–subject. One will 'enforce' her or his will on the other, often experimenting with activities involving physical pain, until the other gives the signal to stop. S/M is highly controversial among feminists, and has caused debate and even division among lesbians. Women who support S/M point out that between partners who both *fully* want to be doing it, S/M play can increase sexual pleasure and open up hidden issues of power which are present in most human intimacy. Others argue that dominance and pain infliction have no part in 'healthy' sexuality. A major concern is that the many *real* inequalities in our society create a risk that S/M won't be just play, and that one partner will actually *be* dominant, while the other feels forced to acquiesce. S/M can camouflage truly oppressive behaviour.

I was a battered wife. My husband, a professional with a good job, said he was into bondage. I bought into it at first. Towards the end he said that he could relate to me sexually only if he tied me up. At the end he was threatening to kill me. For him, bondage had to do with low self-esteem and wasn't a healthy expression of sexuality.

It's important to say *no* to anything you don't want to do. If you are confused or upset by pressure from a sex partner, discuss the situation with a friend who can help you decide how to respond.

---

*The Dodson and Friday books (see Resources) are erotic for many. For lesbian erotica, see Resources in Chapter 12.

A LIFETIME OF SEX

Over our lifetime we can have many changing feelings about our sexuality.

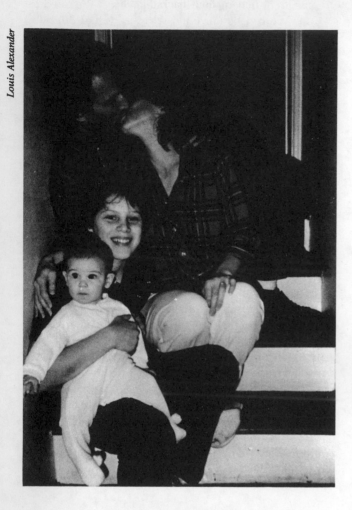

Louis Alexander

Just in the last two years – after fourteen years of marriage – we've been able to talk to each other about sex. We experience a deep kind of uncrazy passion. When you are in love it's crazy passion – you want to swallow each other up and be swallowed. This, in contrast, is a relaxed openness. Anything goes, no hurry, free of guilt. We are more sexually connected than we've ever been in our lives and able just to be with each other.

I have trouble talking about sex right now because there isn't much. I feel closeness and deep connection with my mate, and still I'm disturbed. We used to always count on being able to make love, no matter what else was wrong. And that just isn't true any more. I feel uneasy.

My divorce (at forty-five) has me feeling like a teenager all over again. I get crushes; wonder whether to sleep with someone for the first time; wait passionately for the phone to ring.

I've got so angry at him in fights we've had – little fights, big ones – that I could easier kill him than sleep with him. At first these feelings scared me. Now I know they pass and change and I feel loving again.

We have been married for fifteen years. For several years we were passionate lovers. There was a lot of romance in our lives. Now there is less romance and very deep love and friendship. Sex is no longer the most important thing in our lives. We have sex less frequently and yet our love-making feels good in different ways than in those early years. We feel very warm, intimate and deeply trusting of each other.

I have ebbs and flows within the monthly cycle, and I have bigger cycles that can involve months or years. When I had my two kids, I didn't fuck for two years. I felt completely asexual. I didn't even masturbate. I was lucky because I wasn't living with someone who pushed themselves on me. After this long gap, sex came back into our relationship. And after another period of time, the pattern changed again. I find that if sex goes away, I can rest, put energy into something else, or something happens which makes you suddenly see the person you're with again – what you admire, what you find beautiful. I find that totally the same – in heterosexual or lesbian relationships. There's a kind of phoenix that rises, and sex reappears often in a different guise, but it still reappears. You feel it's died, and all of a sudden it comes back. It can be in a very different form, a different dynamic.

We're forty-eight and fifty, and we're both very private people, but ours is such a success story that somebody ought to hear about it.

I was a virgin when I married and, as such, had quite an undefined sexuality. It quickly became apparent that, while I enjoyed making love, I liked it a great deal less than my husband did. In fact, if he had his way, I am sure he would like to make love at least once a day, now as well as then.

We immediately exploded the myth of the vaginal orgasm and learned to use manual stimulation of the clitoris, which increased my pleasure. But I was terribly afraid of making my own wishes about frequency known; above all I was afraid that, like so many other men, he would 'need' to have his sexual life supplemented by extra-marital sex. I never called it 'rape' when he wore down my resistance over and over again or misused his superior physical strength. I now know that I did sometimes look upon it as rape.

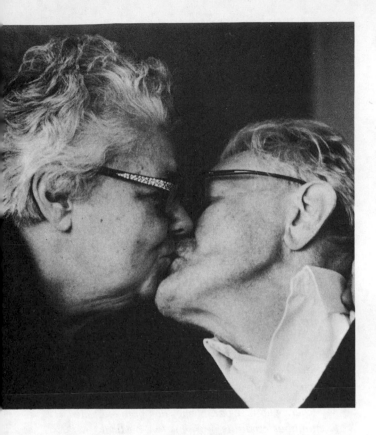

But it doesn't happen any more. When I was forty, for many reasons not related to marriage and sex (and maybe a few that were), I went into a depression. Sexual activity virtually ceased for us. And when I began to come out of the depression about a year later, I continued to call the shots; that is, we made love when I wanted it, and only when I wanted it. My husband had been tender and forbearing all during the worst times, and he continued to be so.

The result is that he waits to make love until I'm ready, and our sex life has never been so good. I think even he has become willing to accept the trade-off: less frequency, more intensity. We try more daring things. But the most interesting development is that I have begun to ask to make love more often. It may have something to do with age – I understand that we women just continue to get better and better – but I think it has more to do with the fact that I was given – no, took – more space for myself. Now I make my wishes known, he respects them and I no longer fear losing him to a more highly sexual woman. Because I'm great in bed, and so is he.

IN BED

Discontinuous we lie
with an old cat asleep
between our backs

where jealous children
used to squirm
wedged in between us.

We grow old, you and I,
to be so equable, lying
back to cat and cat to back.

© ALICE RYERSON

We look forward to a lifetime of ups and downs and growth and change in how we live our sexuality. We will be fascinated to see how our daughters revise this chapter!

SEX AND PHYSICAL DISABILITIES*

Some of the women speaking about sexuality throughout this chapter have a physical disability, either invisible, like epilepsy, or evident, like cerebral palsy, spina bifida or paraplegia. Those of us with physical disabilities are feeling increasingly open and proud about being sexual people. †

Whether we get a physical disability during our life or grow up with it from birth, we too often find other people assuming that we are not sexual at all.

I never get comments from guys. To them I'm an asexual object. It's a side of me that men don't see.

When I went out with my first ever, very good-looking boyfriend, schoolfriends were openly amazed that I had been able to capture such a creature. I was not seen to be a woman, so I did not really see myself as a woman.

*See also the table on Sex and Disability at the end of this chapter, pp. 263–5.
†Please see Chapter 2 for our reasons for speaking as 'we' even though no one in the Collective has a physical disability, and for more on popular stereotypes of women with physical disabilities. Our special thanks to the women of Boston Self-Help for their contribution to this section on sexuality and physical disabilities, and to Michelene Mason for her comments and suggestions for the UK edition.

Those of us with physical disabilities discover early and more painfully something that all women face: that our identity as women and as sexual beings is measured according to our looks and our desirability to men. *

One day the gas man came to read the meter. As he was leaving the flat he asked if I was married. I told him I was, and then a funny look came into his eyes and he asked if I had sex. I was shocked. Then I was angry and said the first thing that came into my head. 'Yes, do you?' He looked embarrassed and hurried away.

Growing up with certain physical disabilities keeps us from getting in touch with many of the dimensions of our sexuality.

Friends have said to me that getting their period for the first time was an important moment in their growing sense of themselves as womanly and sexual. Because my disability required my mother to catheterize me several times a day, she was the one who discovered my period. I understand now why it was so important to me a few years later to learn to change the pads myself.

I spent several months in a body cast when I was eleven and twelve years old, just when my breasts were developing. They kept having to alter the cast around my chest to make room. When my father finally came to take me home from the hospital, he brought a little sunsuit I'd worn months before. There was no way I could get my breasts in there! It was a riot. That was my introduction to puberty!

Yet we may develop some dimensions of our sensuality more than others do.

A nice thing about my disability as a child was that my parents and others held me a lot, touched me all the time when they were helping me dress, kept me on their laps. Touching is still a very sensual thing for me.

Certain disabilities like multiple sclerosis and some spinal cord injuries can be so painful that there are times when we may want sex but can't stand to be touched. For the many times when the medical world can't ease the pain, some of us are turning to non-medical alternatives like visualization or acupuncture (see Chapter 7).

Reclaiming our bodies for our own experiences of sexuality takes time and patience.

In my lesbian illness-support group we have to push past our own censored voices to discover what to do when the vulnerability of the body to pain and to medical manipulation numbs it to the touch of a lover.

I persist in feeling that my body is ugly when I'm naked. Yet my husband clearly loves making love with me. I asked him one day if I made love with a limp. 'Yes,' he said, 'you make love with a rhythm like your walking rhythm. It's nice.'

My lover, who is a paraplegic, has been subjected to enormous amounts of insensitive medical attention all her life. Health-care professionals have handled her body again and again without allowing her control over the process. So obviously it is difficult for her to let go of control over her own body, and to entrust a lover with this control. I need to honour her experience, to know that it is not my fault or my inadequacy as a lover – or hers – that is the reason for sexuality being an issue in our relationship. We have discovered that honest and loving communication, with no blame or criticism, leads us to finding several ways to experience sexual pleasure with each other.

I prefer to relate sexually to women because they are far less judgemental of my 'odd' body and are really far more into sensual expression than men.

I finally lost my virginity at twenty-eight, just before going to college. Even so, it took the guy in question six months of sensitive and gentle persuasion, and then the occasion was for me a joyful and enjoyable one, coupled with a sense of relief.

*It is ironic that with most physical disabilities we are considered asexual, yet if we have a condition which makes us appear unintelligent – mental retardation, emotional or speech disability – we are often thought of as *overly* sexual. For instance, one argument against sex education for mentally retarded or deaf people has been that others didn't want to encourage their 'natural promiscuity'. This reveals an odd warp in our society's assumptions about sexuality.

How to make love is often a challenge, especially with a severe disability. But the 'problems' are often distorted or exaggerated because of the discriminative attitudes and factors we have to face, from others' fears or unrealistic expectations to physical spaces which are poorly designed for our needs. The cultural pressure for sex to be 'spontaneous' is hurtful to those of us who need some accommodation to our disability.

> There is that first moment when the mechanics of your bladder management are revealed. This is the major test. How will he react to a mature woman who wears plastic knickers and pads and requires help when going to the bathroom? Reflection on this count is painful and inhibiting. Time is an important factor, because a considerable amount of physical preparation is required for intercourse. Unexpected disturbances or visitors are impossible to cope with, as I am unable to get up quickly, dress and wash. Even when sexually aroused the spontaneity can soon disappear when your partner has to help empty your bladder and carefully clean and position you . . . My sexual fantasies relate to spontaneous sexual behaviour – sex in a lift, in any room of the house and in numerous positions – on the floor, up against the wall, and so on.[4]

Some advanced sexual planning and open discussion may be necessary, and we need to use our imaginations and be open to whatever makes us feel good. This can be a model for all lovers whether or not they are disabled.

Whether one or both partners are disabled, often we depend on a personal care attendant to help us prepare for sex. Having someone who affirms our sexuality and wants to help us is *crucial*. Then our lover has a choice about how much of the preparation to be involved in, and we can feel more independent in the sexual relationship.

Existing literature and counselling on sexuality and disability is often unsatisfactory for women.* Its terminology, for instance, can undermine our sexuality. If we experience sexual response and orgasm despite a lack of sensation in our pelvic region, for instance, we are said in medical literature to have 'phantom orgasms', as though they're not quite real. The emphasis on 'achievement' of orgasm and on 'performance' and 'sexual adequacy' make us more conscious of what we may not have rather than delighted by what we experience. The literature also focuses on sexual techniques and positions, when sexuality for *all* human beings involves above all affection, touching, communication, caring, sensuality and love.

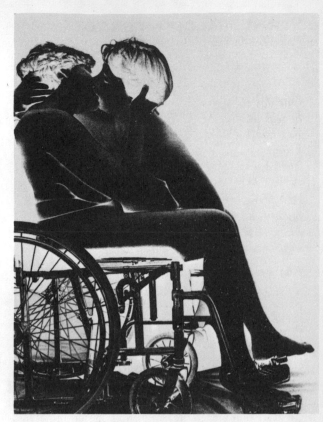

Tee Corinne

We don't do much 'hard-core sex', but find our greatest fulfilment in slow, deep touching and holding. We can't seem to get enough cuddling.

I have no sensation below my waist now, but for some reason my neck, ears and armpits are much more sensitive than they used to be, and stimulation there is really quite exciting to me.

I really like going down on my partner because I can totally control what's going on and I experience so much sensation in my mouth, whereas I can't control my vagina or feel anything there.

I have erratic, vague sensation in my vagina and clitoris. When I have an orgasm, I feel most of the pleasure in my knees – it's a nerve transfer thing, I expect. I'm probably the only woman in the world whose knees come . . .

---

*Most current literature and counselling about sex and physical disability focuses on men, penis-in-vagina intercourse and male concerns about performance and potency. Most books assume that sexual readjustment is easier for a woman, and stress how to be attractive to men rather than how to get sexual satisfaction. They deal almost exclusively with spinal cord injuries, and give little helpful information for women with other disabilities. Those of us who are blind or deaf find even less information. See Resources for a few suggestions.

THE POLITICS OF SEX

It can be difficult, even painful, to be sexual in a sexist, violent society. We have blamed ourselves and been blamed if sex didn't go well. We have accepted cruel labels like 'frigid' or 'cold' or 'dysfunctional' or 'cock-teaser' or 'insatiable'. Yet when we talk with other women, we learn that many others have had the same problems we suffer over in the privacy of our bedrooms.

CONVENTIONAL DEFINITIONS OF LOVE-MAKING

Most people define sex mainly in terms of intercourse, which is why so many heterosexuals are incredulous about what lesbians actually *do* in bed! Yet for women, love-making without intercourse is often what we want. Or at least we'd like more of it.

I feel shy to ask for more foreplay when I know what he's really waiting for is the fucking.

At school we had long periods of petting and I had orgasms all the time. When we 'graduated' to intercourse I stopped having them so easily because we stopped doing all the other things.

I have orgasms easily during intercourse. Sometimes I love his thrusting deep inside me. Sometimes I don't want the penetration, I want something else. But he feels if we haven't had intercourse we haven't actually made love.

Standard (male) definitions call all the touching, licking, sucking and caressing which turns us on 'foreplay' to the big act – intercourse. Most texts even call us 'dysfunctional' or 'frigid' if we don't reach orgasm *during* intercourse. This is not a *female* definition of female sexuality.

In one survey 70 per cent of women did not orgasm during intercourse, while most did during other kinds of sex play or masturbation.[5] Many of us have learned ways of increasing our satisfaction in intercourse. But the more basic answer seems to be to change our definitions of love-making.

Around the time when I learned I could have orgasms through oral sex but not intercourse, I was angry because so much emphasis had been placed on how to achieve them in intercourse. Why did I consume so much energy worrying about that when it seemed you could just have a different concept of what sex is?

It took making love with women for me to see that all the other things – oral sex, having my breasts sucked, rolling around or just lying still and feeling the sensations, touching my lover and turning her on – all these are love-making for me. Now when I make love with men I do it more like making love with a woman – slower, more sensually and tenderly, sometimes without penetration at all.

EMPHASIS ON PERFORMANCE AND GOALS

Sex books focus on techniques and say little about feelings. We worry about being sexy enough, about 'doing it' well enough to please our partners. Orgasms, too, can become a goal: some partners 'work at it' for hours, wanting to please us or to show they are good lovers.

Because my previous relationships with men involved orgasm-centred sex (his orgasm, that is), I have brought to my first woman lover lots of expectations about coming. If one of us doesn't come, I feel we haven't made love 'well'. I think I miss a lot of pleasure that way.

Perhaps it takes someone my age, sixty, who has lived through other times, to point out that this society's glorification of sexual orgasm borders on the excessive. It's almost enough to make a person flaunt her chastity!

The first few years we had a great sex life. We were very attracted to each other and I loved sex with him. I didn't have orgasms and I didn't even know what an orgasm was. Then I learned about orgasms, partly by reading some of the new books and articles and partly by having one while masturbating. It felt so good that I wanted to have it with him. The next two years were awful in bed. We had this goal – my orgasm – and it was like we'd look at our watches and say, 'One, two, three, go', and work at it until we succeeded. Now, finally, we're back on an even keel. Usually I come, sometimes I don't. I let him know which way I'm feeling. We can forget that goal and just do what feels good. But I wish I'd known everything I know now back when our feelings were so intense.

We may judge ourselves by new 'liberated' norms.

I feel vaguely guilty if sex isn't great all the time, as though if I'm a real liberated woman I should have an incredible orgasm every time, instead of accepting that sometimes there will be little ones and sometimes big ones.

With sex coming at us from every direction in the media, we may worry whether we are doing it enough. If we're single, we 'should' be finding more sex partners. If in a relationship, we 'should' be making love a certain number of times per week.

Many couples these days report the 'problem' of lack of interest in sex. This may reflect problems in the relationship or in ways of love-making. But what experts are calling insufficient interest in sex may actually be our own desires measured against today's escalated sexual standards. It may even be a reaction against the general hype about sex in the media, or simple skin hunger – the need to be touched by another human being without sex.

OBJECTIFICATION OF OUR BODIES IN THE MEDIA

We bring negative feelings about our bodies into sex in a particular way. The media's 'ideal' woman often robs us of sexual confidence.

For years I wouldn't make love in a position that exposed my backside to scrutiny, for I had been told it was 'too jiggly'. Needless to say, this prevented me from being sexually assertive and creative and limited my responses.

We have a good sex life with lots of variety, fantasies, games. The fact that my disability prevents me from bending my leg limits us in some positions, but we just try different ones. Yet I don't have orgasms with my husband, only in masturbation. I am still struggling with my body. When I am unclothed I still feel like parts of me are really ugly. I think that when I can finish mourning, cry out my anguish over the disability, then sex will get better for me.

If we like the way we look and feel good about our bodies, we feel better about making love.

One of the difficult things about being large is that more often than not other people are the problem, not me. Many times I have felt that people I know wonder at my friendship with my lover. They wonder how a thin person can make love to a large one. The idea, I suppose, is that large women aren't attractive. Nonsense, of course. I enjoy my body immensely when I make love, either to myself or my boyfriend. I never think about my largeness. I simply am it and positively luxuriate in it. I love my body when I make love. It is beautiful to me and to my boyfriend. For six years we have both exulted in good love-making.

SEX-ROLE STEREOTYPES

Men are 'supposed' to know more about sex, to initiate it, to have a stronger sex drive. Women are 'supposed' to be passive recipients or willing students. Supposedly *they* want sex and *we* want love. Such rigid classifying of people by gender is not only false and silly, it is also damaging.

It makes it difficult for women to take sexual initiatives (even sometimes in lesbian relationships too). As far as heterosexual relationships are concerned, men may *seem* to want sex more often than women do, but it is a fact that men are raised with few ways of expressing their emotions. Sex (i.e. intercourse and/or orgasm) is one of the few permissible ways for men to be close to someone, the only acceptable place for men's tender, loving feelings. It may be

this limitation, rather than an innate, irrepressible 'sex drive', which prompts men to initiate sex so often, and leads to the false notion that women are less sexual than men. The stereotype must also arise from a deep cultural fear of women's sexual passion and power. And it is this fear that has led men as a group to find ways of gaining power for themselves. This affects us in every aspect of our lives and is responsible for much of the violence from men that we are all prey to. It affects our relationships generally, and our sexual relationships with men in particular.

MALE POWER AND SEX

Men as a group have more power in our society than women do. Even if you feel equal to your husband, male lover, friends, colleagues or co-workers, our culture values men more. This supposed 'superiority' (even though your sex partner may not *feel* superior at all) gets played out in sex in the following ways:

- You should make love when he wants to, whether you're in the mood or not.
- You should take care of birth control because condoms interfere with his pleasure.
- You should make yourself attractive for him when he gets home from work (this despite the fact that you have been working, too, inside or outside the home or both).
- You should make sure the kids don't interrupt while you are making love.
- You should have orgasms to show him what a good lover he is.
- If you don't want to make love to orgasm, you should at least relieve him of his sexual tension by oral sex or masturbating him. (It's no more painful for a man to go without orgasm than for a woman.)

I have a physical disability which makes me slow to feel sexual sensations in my genitals. With my husband I am finally going slow enough to get past my terror that I won't feel anything. But for five years I faked orgasms so men would think they were great lovers. I am angry now that I subjected myself to that kind of sexual pretence.

There are so many times I say yes when I don't really want to, just to avoid a long discussion about why not.

When I finally learned to have orgasms and wanted to make love more, my husband seemed to have less of a desire for sex. He wasn't used to my being so turned on and assertive. I think he missed the power he used to have in determining how our love-making would go.

Underlying all my sexual relationships with men was the assumption that my body somehow belonged to him, not me. I thought I owed my partner my sexuality, and should muster it up for him when he wanted or needed it. It was not even as crude and simple as giving over my body to be fucked. I had somehow to give him my ardour as well, let him turn me on. In fairness to the men who were my lovers, these were not superdemanding or overly macho men. Whether or not they thought I owed them my sexuality was irrelevant, because the assumption that I did was deep in the culture and deep in my own sense of myself.

We will have more satisfying sex and begin to know our full sexual potential only when we are in relationships (and eventually in a society) where sexual, racial and class prejudice and dominance are absent.

It is a cruel fact of our lives that many men abuse women, often using sex as a weapon. Rape, an early experience of incest, sexual harassment by a boss or co-worker or teacher, battering in the home by the man we share a bed with: any of these can devastate what sex could be for us. If we don't experience violence directly, the possibility leers at us from pornography, from news stories, films, crude jokes.

Sometimes when I hear about a rape that's happened, I can't make love with my husband, even though I love him and usually enjoy sex. I know he is a gentle person, but for a moment I don't see him, I see all the men who use their penises as weapons to dominate and hurt women.

Making love with Rachel I am sometimes swept over by a feeling of fierce protectiveness. Her body is so precious to me, I want women and non-violent men to become stronger and stronger and to change the things in our world which make sexual violence possible.

All of us as women face the troubling paradox of seeking to open ourselves to the deep vulnerabilities of sexual loving in a society in which we are often *not safe.**

> We must work for a more equal, less violent society in which sex is used not to make money or as an instrument of dominance but in service of love — love of ourselves, love and friendship for others.

---

*For more discussion on relationships with men, and male violence, see Chapters 10, 11 and 13.

APPENDIX

SEXUAL HEALTH CARE

Sexual health is a physical and emotional state of well-being that allows us to enjoy and act on our sexual feelings. We all need to take care to stay sexually healthy. Here is a check-list:

- A *Gynaecological Examination.* (See p. 593).
- *Care of Infections.* (See p. 438). If you get an infection of the vagina or urinary tract, you need to do something about it immediately.
- *Genital Cleansing.* Wash your genital area daily with warm water. Separate the outer lips and pull back the hood of the clitoris to clean away the secretions that collect around the glans. Our body secretions and smells are a natural part of us, and if you are in good health and wash regularly, you smell and taste good. However, some of us like to wash our genitals before love-making. Do what makes you comfortable. Make sure that if you are having sex with a man, he washes his genitals regularly. Since most men don't, you may be wise to insist that he does so before intercourse, and in any case if he has not washed them – or his hands – after working with oily, dusty, or other dirty substances. Lesbians who work with similar substances would be wise to pay similar careful attention to their hands. These measures may well be an important way of protecting women from cervical cancer (see p. 525).
- *Birth Control.* If you do not want to be pregnant and you are having intercourse, you'll need to discuss with the man involved the use of birth control and who will use the selected method. If you cannot discuss it with him or he won't discuss it with you, perhaps the relationship is not ready for sex. Even if you are not having intercourse, if sperm is deposited anywhere near the vagina (even in the mons area), the sperm can reach the vagina on vaginal secretions and up through the cervix to the uterus and fallopian tubes and join with an egg. For more about birth control, see Chapter 15.
- *Prevention Against STDs.* (See Box opposite and Chapter 23).
- *Menstruation.* It's fine to have sex during your menstrual periods if it feels comfortable to you. Some of us have found that orgasm relieves menstrual cramps. A diaphragm usually will hold back menstrual blood.
- *For sex during pregnancy* see Chapter 18.

SEXUAL AROUSAL AND ORGASM

Here are some details left out of the text.

Excitement

The vagina becomes moist (lubricated). (See p. 241.) It begins to expand and balloon and eventually the inner two-thirds double in diameter.

WARNING

While it is possible to transmit STDs between women, the chances of doing so are much greater with heterosexual contact. When embarking on a new relationship we need to consider special precautions to protect ourselves and our partners against sexually transmitted diseases. All STDs have potentially disastrous long-term effects, not only HIV infection (which we discuss on p. 501). We also need to consider precautions in long-term relationships if either partner is involved sexually with anyone else.

We discuss safer sex guidelines on p. 488.

The inner lips swell and deepen in colour.

The clitoris swells, becomes erect and is highly sensitive to touch.

The breasts enlarge and become more sensitive. The nipples become erect.

The uterus enlarges and elevates within the pelvic cavity.

The heart rate increases; breathing becomes heavier and faster.

A flush or rash may appear on the skin.

The muscles begin to tighten, especially in the genital area.

If stimulation continues, the inner two-thirds of the vagina continue to balloon. The outer third narrows by one-third to one-half of its diameter, and is quite sensitive to pressure.

The entire genital area continues to swell, as do the breasts. (You may become increasingly aware of these areas of your body.)

The uterus elevates fully.

We breathe very rapidly; we may pant.

The muscles continue to contract.

With full arousal the clitoris retracts under its hood. Stimulation of the inner lips from manipulation or intercourse moves the hood of the clitoris back and forth over the glans.

Orgasm: the Release of Sexual Tension

For women, if sexual stimulation is interrupted, excitement may decline. This is especially true just before and during orgasm, when we need continuous stimulation. Direct or indirect stimulation of the clitoris (and/or, for some women, pressure on the uterus) leads to orgasm.

During orgasm, muscles around the vagina, uterus and rectum contract (the contractions cause the release of the blood trapped in the pelvic veins). For a half-hour or more after orgasm, if love-making doesn't continue, swelling decreases, the muscles relax and the clitoris, vagina and uterus return to their usual positions.

THE ROLE OF TESTOSTERONE IN SEXUALITY*

Certain hormones play a role in sexual feelings, sexual activity and intensity of orgasm. The most influential is *testosterone*, sometimes called the 'libido hormone' and also, erroneously, the 'male hormone'. Testosterone, like oestrogen, is present in both men and women, though the proportions differ between the sexes. In women it is produced through the operation of both the *adrenals* (two small glands near the kidneys) and the *ovaries*, with the ovaries probably the more important source.

The role of testosterone in sexuality is illustrated in several ways.

1. When one adrenal is removed, women report a dramatic decrease in sexual interest, sensation and frequency of orgasm.

2. When ovaries are removed, many women report a similar loss.[6] Testosterone levels are lower in women after menopause or after ovary removal (oophorectomy) than in healthy young women with ovaries in place, showing that less testosterone is produced as ovarian function slows or stops.

3. When women who have once known libido and lost it receive moderate doses of testosterone, libido increases.[7] Pellet implants of oestrogen and testosterone increase the frequency and intensity of the sexual climax, although pellets of oestrogen alone or placebos have no such effect. †[8]

4. A recent study of sexually active women showed a significant correlation between blood testosterone levels and sexual responsiveness and satisfaction.[9] Knowing the importance of testosterone, ovaries and adrenals can alert us to protecting our sexuality from unnecessary removal of the ovaries or adrenals.

PROBLEMS WITH SEX

At one time or another all of us have problems with sex. Sexual problems in a relationship are relationship problems. Sexual ignorance is the most frequent cause of sexual problems; poor communication patterns, male and female role expectations, a lack of trust or commitment, or unresolved conflicts between us can also lead to sexual difficulties.

How we think and feel about ourselves and sex powerfully affects how our bodies respond. Guilt, shyness, fear, inner conflicts (which we might not even be aware of), ignorance, all can block or inhibit sexual responsiveness. If any of the following is a problem, we owe it to ourselves to explore further. We need not be in total agony to look for help. Sexual problems are common.

*Prepared by Edith Bjornson Sunley.
†The administration of testosterone can have unwanted effects, some of which, such as deepening of the voice, appear to be irreversible. For more information about hormone replacement therapy, see p. 456.

Problems with Orgasm

Many of us experience difficulties reaching orgasm, either by ourselves or with a lover. Shame about exploring and touching ourselves keeps us from learning to bring ourselves to orgasm through masturbation. A variety of problems keeps us from having orgasms with another. Here are some of the reasons why:

- We don't notice or else we misunderstand what's happening in our bodies as we get aroused. We're too busy thinking about abstractions – how to do it right, why it doesn't go well for us, what our lover thinks of us, whether our lover is impatient, whether our lover can last – when we might better be concentrating on sensations, not thoughts.
- We feel ourselves becoming aroused, but we are afraid we won't have an orgasm, and we don't want to get into the hassle of trying, so we just repress sexual response.
- We are afraid of asking too much and seeming too demanding.
- We are afraid of taking an active part and showing our partner what to do.
- We are embarrassed to touch ourselves when having sex with someone else.
- We are afraid that if our lover concentrates on our pleasure we will feel such pressure to come that we won't be able to – and then we don't.
- We are trying to have a simultaneous orgasm, which seldom occurs for most of us. It can be just as pleasurable if we come separately.
- We are in deep conflict about, or angry at, the person we are sleeping with. Unconsciously we withhold orgasm as a way of withholding ourselves.
- We feel guilty about having sex and so cannot let ourselves really enjoy it.
- We rush into sex – swept off our feet just like in films and swept under the rug when it comes to climaxes.

Lack of Interest in Sex: Sexual Aversion (lack of libido)

Often our sexual interest goes in phases, and this is perfectly natural. We may be angry, depressed, too involved in other interests, preoccupied with worries, or too tired (particularly with small children to care for). But sometimes the phase seems to be going on for ever, causing anxiety and tension in a relationship. In this case it is important to find out what is bothering you.

It may simply be that you are past the initial excitement phase and you have not adjusted to this yet. Or you might find that you are both misinterpreting each other's needs. Sexual appetites are as varied as appetites for food.

Sometimes it is hard to accept that sex doesn't always have to be electrifying; it can be gentle, the sensations quite mild. Learn to allow your body to respond to even mild feelings; they will probably build up after a while, and even if they don't you can enjoy the pleasure of physical closeness, as several women report in this chapter.

However, lack of interest may be concealing other profounder problems within a relationship. It could be the result of unresolved conflicts which you may or may not be aware of (see Chapter 8 for discussion on how to deal with these); it might herald the end of an unsatisfactory relationship. Whatever the reason, it is important to be open about how you feel. It may be difficult to remember that your partner is suffering too.

Masters and Johnson developed a technique for re-kindling sexual interest – though no technique will be completely successful if you haven't resolved the deeper problems as well. It is called 'sensate focus'. Each partner must take turns at pleasuring the other without touching genitals or breasts. The passive partner of the moment gives feedback on how it feels. On the second or third days you can move to the genitals but must make no attempt at intercourse and/or orgasm until both partners feel absolutely ready for it.*

Some of us have conflicts about sex which go so deep that we never have any interest in it. We may feel unpleasant sensitivity to touch, or so ticklish we can't relax. If our problems are deep inside our own minds we may need help to unlock and resolve them through some kind of psychotherapy (see p. 128).

Painful Intercourse: Dispareunia

You may experience discomfort, even pain, with intercourse for the following physical rather than emotional reasons:

1. *Local Infection*. Some vaginal infections – candida or trichomoniasis, for example – can be present in a non-acute, visually unnoticeable form. The friction of a penis or finger moving on your vulva or in your vagina might cause the infection to flare up, making you sting and itch (see p. 489). A herpes sore on your external genitals can make friction painful (see p. 496).

2. *Local Irritation*. The vagina might be irritated by spermicide. If so, try a different brand. Some of us react to the rubber in a condom or diaphragm. Vaginal deodorant sprays and scented tampons can irritate the vagina or vulva.

3. *Insufficient Lubrication*. The wall of the vagina responds to sexy feelings by 'sweating', giving off a liquid that wets the vagina and the entrance to it, which makes the entry of the penis easier. Sometimes there isn't enough of this liquid. Some reasons: you may be trying to let the penis in (or the man might be putting/forcing it in) too soon, before there has been enough stimulation to excite you and set the sweating action going; you may be nervous or tense about making love (e.g. it's the first time, or you're worried about getting pregnant); if the man is using a condom you may need to add lubrication. Be sure to give the vagina time to get wet. If you still feel dry you can use saliva, lubricating jelly (e.g. K-Y) or a birth control foam, cream or jelly. (Never use Vaseline to lubricate a condom or diaphragm. It will deteriorate the rubber.) Occasionally, insufficient

---

*See Resources for further reading about techniques like this.

lubrication is caused by a hormone deficiency. After child-birth (particularly if you are breastfeeding or if your stitches hurt) and after menopause are two times when a lack of oestrogen can affect the vaginal walls in such a way that less liquid is produced. Try the lubricants suggested above.

4. *Tightness in the Vaginal Entrance.* The first few times you have intercourse, an unstretched hymen (if you have one) can cause pain. And whenever you are tense and preoccupied the vaginal entrance is not likely to loosen up enough, and getting the penis in might hurt. This can also be a problem after childbirth when the area is tender (see p. 410). Even if you feel relaxed and sexy, timing is important. If you try to get the penis in before you are fully aroused, you might still be too tight, though you are wet enough. So don't rush, and don't let yourself be rushed.

5. *Pain Deep in the Pelvis.* Sometimes the thrust of a finger or penis hurts way inside. This pain can be caused by tears in the ligaments that support the uterus (caused by obstetrical mismanagement during childbirth, a botched-up abortion, rape); infections of the cervix, uterus and tubes (such as pelvic inflammatory disease); endometriosis; cysts or tumours on the ovaries. All these may be treatable, but you need to have them attended to without delay (see Chapter 23).

6. *Clitoral Pain.* The clitoris is exquisitely sensitive, and for most of us direct touching or rubbing of the clitoris (especially the glans, or tip) is painful (many men don't know this until we tell them). Also, genital secretions can collect under the hood, so when washing pull back the hood of the clitoris and clean it gently.

7. *Vaginismus.* This is the term used to describe the involuntary muscle contractions around the vagina which some women experience with penetration. The spasm can be so strong that penetration is impossible. It may be that you are reacting defensively because of a past bad experi-ence such as rape. It could also be that you just do not want penetration or sex.

It is perfectly possible to be sexually responsive and have a very pleasurable sex life without penetration. If pen-etration does not give you pleasure then it has no place (for you) in what is supposed to be a pleasurable experience. There are many ways for you to make love without anything inside your vagina. Your lover can use tongue and hands to make love to you. In a heterosexual relationship you can find ways of enclosing your partner's penis using your hands, between your breasts, under your arm or between your thighs. Finding other ways to make love can increase sexual pleasure for both of you.

If you want your partner to be able to penetrate and you wish you could enjoy it, you may be able to work gradually towards that once you have established a loving and trusting non-penetrative relationship. Take it very gently, using fingers first (yours and then his). Retain the absolute right to say stop and don't make penetration the goal of your relationship. (Read the rest of this chapter; many of the resources listed on p. 266 can also be helpful, and in particular, the section on vaginismus in *The New Sex Therapy* by Helen Singer Kaplan).

Getting Help

If you feel pain during sex, go to a doctor and insist on being examined. Many doctors, if they cannot find an obvious cause, will just dismiss you and say, 'It's all in your head, dear.' Few gynaecologists are equipped to help with sexual problems, and at the very least they should make sure they have carefully checked out the physical ones. We know of one woman who had an exploratory operation in a London hospital; she was sewn up again and told that her problem was depression. On a subsequent examination from another doctor she was diagnosed as having endometriosis (see Chapter 23).

Despite our knowledge about sex, despite the support of friends and partners, sometimes we cannot work through our difficulties. A sex discussion group can help, simply by talking with other women about sex. Women's sexuality workshops, which are now run in many parts of the country, involve a more focused look at sexuality, and often enable women to work on particular problems – e.g. to do with lack of orgasm, so-called 'frigidity', etc. The Redwood Association or a local Women's Therapy Centre (see Organizations) should be able to tell you if there is any possibility of such workshops being run where you live. Counselling can help too. You should be able to find a counsellor through one of the organizations listed in Resources (see also Resources at the end of Chapter 8). Unfortunately, most people seem to believe that psychosex-ual help should only be available to heterosexual couples and are not interested or equipped to offer help to lesbians. Relate (previously called the Marriage Guidance Council), however, try not to discriminate against homosexuals, and lesbians might find there is more chance of getting support-ive help via them than from members of many other organizations. *

Practitioners vary in what they offer. Some concentrate solely on sex itself, often teaching you and your partner certain exercises to do at home. They usually see you together with a partner. Some are prepared to see people who are not in a relationship. Others pay at least as much attention to how you relate to each other generally, since sexual problems may be a symptom of deeper problems – either in relationships or in the individuals concerned. They also vary in quality. Some may hold quite reactionary views about women or about female sexuality; others may be only too willing to help you break free from patriarchal myths that might have been constricting you for years.

If you decide to seek help from a counsellor or sex therapist, read Chapter 8, in particular the section on 'Choosing a Therapist'.

---

*Lesbians may need to concentrate on working with friends, or our partners, or both. See Resources in Chapter 12 for some useful books on lesbian sexuality. Jo Ann Loulan's book, *Lesbian Sex*, is particularly useful.

LEARNING TOGETHER ABOUT SEX

In a group we can discuss factual information, talk out problems, learn to communicate verbally and non-verbally, and learn alternative ways to get what we want sexually. Some women's groups have decided to spend a month or so discussing sex, other women have come together specifically to talk about it. Here are some suggestions for organizing discussion.

At the first meeting draw up a list of topics. Get different members of the group to research on practical aspects and suggest material for other group members to read. Some topics which you might like to discuss are: childhood and adolescent memories of sexuality; your feelings about your body; differences in male and female socialization; masturbation; fantasies; virginity; homophobia; aspects of love-making; relationships with women, with men; sexual problems.

The following 'journey' through one's own sexuality is a stimulating way to begin your discussion. Before your second or third meeting, two of you get together and draw up a list of questions beginning with first memories of sensual pleasure and affection (e.g. 'What kind of touching did you get as a child from your parents?' 'How did you feel?'). You will want to include questions about sexual language, your parents' relationship to each other and to you, sex play with siblings and friends (e.g. playing doctor), your first menstrual period, dating,

petting, intercourse, orgasm, crushes on girlfriends, marriage, sexuality as an adult, and so forth. When you all meet together again, the two of you take the rest of the group on the journey. Ask each woman to find a comfortable spot and close her eyes. The two of you alternate reading your questions very slowly, giving women time to remember. Leave a minute or two between questions. When the questions are finished, leave some more space before joining together to discuss your memories and reactions to them.

Consider activities you think would enrich your talking together. You might keep personal journals throughout the weeks you meet and share from them at a final meeting, make a collage of sex cartoons at the beginning of one week's meeting, see a porno flick or visit a bookshop that sells pornography, make a group list of all the street and slang terms you know for sex, include your lovers for a meeting or two.

When discussing aspects of our lives that we have always kept hidden and private it is important to build up trust in each other. It might help to make it a rule at the start not to discuss anything that happens within the group outside meetings even with other group members. The simple experience of expressing deeply hidden concerns about sex can be enormously liberating in itself.

MALE SEXUALITY

Male Sexual Response

Sexual arousal in men, as in women, leads to vasocongestion (blood-engorged veins) and myotonia (muscle contraction). A woman's first reaction to arousal is vaginal lubrication, and a man's is penile erection. For both sexes the peak of sexual excitement is orgasm, which for a man is defined as ejaculation (when a fluid called semen, which includes sperm, spurts out of the penis). After orgasm a man has a period of a few minutes or even hours (longer as he gets older) when he cannot have another erection.

Male Sexual Problems*

If we are having sex with a man who is having sexual difficulties, it is hard to have the kind of pleasure both partners would like. Further, his difficulties may complicate our own problems – even create some for us.

Men can suffer problems similar to ours, and for many of the same reasons. The common male sexual problems are: *premature ejaculation* – the inability to control the ejaculatory reflex; *impotence* – the inability to maintain, or even be aroused to, an erection; *dispareunia* – pain with intercourse; and *sexual aversion* – lack of interest in sex altogether.

Some sexual problems can be worked through with the help of good books and a caring partner, while others might call for professional help.

*When there are sexual problems in a heterosexual relationship it is often the woman who seeks help first. This may be because culturally it is easier for us to admit to our sexual concerns. It may also be because we too often assume that if sex is a problem, we are the ones in need of help. Sexual problems usually reflect or express relationship problems.

SEX AND PHYSICAL DISABILITIES

PREPARED BY JANNA ZWERNER.

Chronic disease or disability	Effects on our sexuality	Helpful hints and special implications
CEREBRAL PALSY (CP)	Muscle spasticity, rigidity, and/or weakness may make certain sex acts and self-pleasuring difficult to impossible for us. Contractures of our knees and hips may cause us pain under the pressure of a partner, and spasms may increase with arousal. Our genital sensations remain intact but some of us experience a lack of lubrication. Menstruation, fertility and pregnancy are not affected. During delivery, those of us with severe CP might need a C-section.*†	Non-genital love-making, different positions and propping our legs up on pillows may help ease spasms. We can use a vibrator to make love alone or with another person if our arms and hands are involved. A water-soluble lubricant can often help if our vagina lacks lubrication. Inserting spermicidal foam or a diaphragm may be complicated by spasms or poor hand control. Because of an increased risk of clotting, the birth control pill is not advisable for those of us taking anti-convulsants or if our mobility is greatly restricted by severe CP.§
CEREBRAL VASCULAR ACCIDENT (STROKE)	We may have difficulties in sexual positioning and sensitivity because of impaired motor strength, coordination, or paralysis. How much this affects our sexual functions will depend upon the severity of our CVA. Our sex drive may decrease, more commonly when our CVA occurs in the dominant side of the brain (for right-handers usually the left hemisphere with right-side paralysis). Menstruation and fertility are not affected, but there may be complications with pregnancy and delivery.*	If spasms or paralysis persist we can use other love-making positions that do not require strenuous activity. Most persons who were sexually active before CVA remain active; thus one cannot generalize about sex drive and functioning. An understanding friend or partner will often be the best help during the long recovery process. The birth control pill is never good to use, especially if our CVA resulted from diabetes or circulatory disorders.‡§‖
DIABETES	Most of the medical literature is about male sexual functioning and the few reports about women with diabetes show conflicting results. About a third of diabetic women in one study reported that their orgasms gradually got to be rarer and less intense. One possible explanation was that the threshold for orgasm increased because of damage to the nerve fibres in the pelvic region. A lack of vaginal lubrication and recurrent infections may make some love-making unpleasant.*	Some women say that using a vibrator allows them to reach orgasm because the stimulation is more intense. Poorly controlled diabetes may stop menstruation and cause fertility problems. Depending upon how stable our blood glucose levels are, pregnancy may be complicated and should be closely monitored. Birth control pills often aggravate other symptoms of our diabetes and should not be used because of possible cerebrovascular and cardiovascular complications.‡§‖
RENAL FAILURE	In chronic renal insufficiency, menstruation may stop or become extremely irregular. Many women become infertile and rarely carry pregnancies to term. We may have difficulties in becoming sexually excited and as in diabetes, our orgasms may become rarer and less intense. Sometimes we have a decrease in vaginal lubrication and breast tissue mass.*	Maintenance haemodialysis often brings on excessive and sometimes painful menstruations, but may improve our sex drive, though not necessarily sexual functioning. Kidney transplants usually improve both our sex drive and function, and fertility improves dramatically. If our vagina is too dry, a water-soluble lubricant can help. Many of the drugs used to lower hypertension arc likely to dampen our sex drive. The birth control pill is usually not advised.‡

(For footnotes see p. 265.)

Chronic disease or disability	Effects on our sexuality	Helpful hints and special implications
RHEUMATOID ARTHRITIS (RA)	Swollen, painful joints, muscular atrophy and joint contractures may make it difficult for us to masturbate or make love in some positions. Pain, fatigue and drugs may decrease our sex drive, but genital sensations remain intact. Menstruation, fertility and pregnancy are not affected, but birth may be complicated if our hips and spine are involved. However, symptoms may improve during pregnancy due to changes in our immune system.	To avoid pain and pressure on affected joints, we can be creative in sexual positioning. If our symptoms respond to heat, we can plan sex after a compress, or a hot bath with our partner. Choose the best time, when you have the least pain and stiffness, for love-making. Try sex instead of corticosteroids – it is said to stimulate the adrenal glands and so increases output of natural cortisone which alleviates painful symptoms. The birth control pill may not be good for us if we have circulatory problems or greatly restricted mobility. ‡§
SYSTEMIC LUPUS ERYTHEMATOSUS	Many difficulties are the same as in RA (above). However, because different people have quite different symptoms, often connected to other disorders, one cannot generalize. Research on the female sexual effects of lupus is scarce, despite the fact that nine out of ten people with lupus are women. Sometimes we also have sores in and around the mouth and vagina, and a decrease in vaginal lubrication, so we may have pain during vaginal penetration.*	For helpful hints, see above as in RA. Also, we can use a water-soluble lubricant if our vagina is too dry. Choose birth control methods with extreme caution, especially if symptoms or complications other than RA exist. Birth control pills may not be advisable if we have circulatory or kidney problems, or if our mobility is greatly restricted. ‡§
MYOCARDIAL INFARCTION (MI)	For those of us with very serious conditions, chest pain, palpitations and shortness of breath may limit our sexual activities. However, many of us can resume regular love-making once we can climb two flights of stairs at a brisk pace without causing symptoms. (The cardiac responses during step-climbing and love-making are similar, the average being 125 beats per minute.)†	We should consult our doctor to see when and if we can safely begin an exercise regime. We can use love-making positions that require little or no exertion, especially with our arms (for example, on our side or back). Go slow in the beginning to minimize stress and fear of stress, because the majority of sexual problems arise from anxiety and misinformation about this ailment. Birth control pills should not be used. ‡
MULTIPLE SCLEROSIS (MS)	Depending upon the stage and severity of MS, our symptoms will vary and may come and go. Some of us experience difficulty in having an orgasm, decreased genital sensitivity, dryness of the vagina, muscle weakness, pain and bladder and bowel incontinence. There is no change in our menstrual and fertility patterns. Pregnancy and post-pregnancy stress may increase MS symptoms, but the reports about this are conflicting.*†	Because sexual difficulties may come and go with other MS symptoms, it helps to be creative. Drugs for spasms and topical anaesthetics for pain may be helpful. If our balance is not good and we tire easily, we can use love-making positions that require little exertion. A water-soluble lubricant can help with a dry vagina. Some women say that intercourse is painful but having their clitoris stimulated feels good. The birth control pill is not good to use if you have paralysis or restricted mobility, but a recent study showed that it may help symptoms in the early stages of MS.*‡§‖

(For footnotes see p. 265.)

Chronic disease or disability	Effects on our sexuality	Helpful hints and special implications
OSTOMY	Although much more is known about sexual functioning of men with ostomies, it appears that women are better off. Surgery should not impair our genital functioning or fertility and often makes it safe to become pregnant, because a disease process, such as cancer or ulcerative colitis, has been wiped out. However, a few women report pain during intercourse or a lack of vaginal sensations after ileostomy and colostomy surgery.	An ostomy is a 'hidden disability' until our clothes are off; therefore, it may help to find a comfortable way to tell potential partners before sexual relations begin. The opening or appliance may be covered or secured before love-making, both for aesthetic reasons and for support so it does not get in the way. We can use love-making positions where we feel most secure that the bag will not get pulled out. If odours are a problem we can bathe and empty the bag before making love. Consider alternatives and consult a doctor if taking the birth control pill because sometimes it is not absorbed properly. ‡
SPINAL CORD INJURY (SCI)	Our sexual functioning will depend on the location and severity of the injury, and there is great variation even for women with injuries at the same spinal level. Basically, if our injury is above the sacral area there will be reflex sexual responses, and at or below this level (conus medullaris), our reflex responses will be disrupted. SCI may result in paralysis, spasticity, loss of sensation, incontinence, skin ulcers, pain and a dry vagina, sometimes complicating making love with yourself or another. We may continue to have orgasmic sensations or they may be diffused, either in general or to specific body parts, such as our breasts or lips. Our neck, ears and the area above the injury may become more sexually exciting. Arousal, self-pleasuring and love-making may increase spasms and the risk of incontinence. Although we may stop menstruating for several months after the injury, fertility is not permanently disrupted. †	It can help to make love in ways other than vaginal penetration, which may be painful due to increased bladder infections, spasms, vaginal irritation and tearing and autonomic dysreflexia. Routine bowel and bladder programmes can decrease the risk of 'accidents' during sex, and a towel will help if there is any leakage. We can also tape our catheter down or move it out of the way so it does not get pulled out. Spasm medications and a water-soluble vaginal lubricant may be of some assistance. Pregnancy increases the risk of thrombophlebitis and bladder infections, but many women have relatively healthy and painless births. Be on guard for signs of autonomic dysreflexia during labour and delivery, and of uterine prolapse afterwards. Take birth control pills only with extreme caution, if at all, and never if taking antihypertensive medication or if you have circulatory problems. ‡ §‖

*The research literature is severely limited. Information presented here is only meant to be a guide, since it is based on only one or two studies or clinical observations.

†Most of the literature concerning sexuality and this disability is male-oriented, and many studies generalize their findings from men's to women's sexuality. Adequate research on sexual functioning (as opposed to reproductive functioning) has yet to be carried out with women.

‡Many drugs are directly responsible for the negative effects on sexual functioning – often much more so than the disability itself! Examples of such drugs are antihypertensives, phenothiazines, etc. Consult your doctor about alternatives if you think you may have this problem. Be sure to inform your sexual health-care provider about the drugs and dosage you are taking when seeking contraceptive services.

§The diaphragm may not be a good method of birth control if you have poor hand control, recurrent bladder or vaginal infections or very weak pelvic muscles. If the use of your hands is limited ask your partner or attendant to help insert the diaphragm. There are also devices available that can make it easier to insert the coil-spring diaphragm, but some hand control is required.

‖The intra-uterine contraceptive device (IUD) is not good to use for women with a loss of sensation in the pelvic area because of the risk that puncture or pelvic inflammatory disease may go unnoticed. Also, good hand coordination is needed to check the strings every month to make sure the IUD is still in place.

NOTES

1. For many examples of how women masturbate, see Shere Hite, *The Hite Report*. London: Summit/Hamlyn, 1977; Anja Meulenbelt. *For Ourselves*. London: Sheba, 1981; Anne Hooper. *The Body Electric*. London: Allen and Unwin, 1984.

2. Quoted in *Red Herring*, a Scottish lesbian feminist magazine, sadly no longer published. See Resources to Chapter 12 for lesbian magazines currently published in the UK.

3. Quoted in *Spare Rib*, no. 23, May 1974.

4. 'Julie' in Jo Campling (ed.). *Images of Ourselves: Women with Disabilities Talking*. London: Routledge and Kegan Paul, 1981, p. 17.

5. Hite, op. cit., note 1.

6. L. Zussman, S. Zussman, R. Sunley and E. Bjornson. 'Sexual Response and Oophorectomy: Recent Studies and Reconsideration of Psychogenesis', *American Journal of Obstetrics and Gynecology*, vol. 140, no. 7, 1 August 1981, pp. 725–31.

7. U. J. Salman and S. H. Geist. 'Effects of Androgens upon Libido in Women', *Journal of Clinical Endocrinology*, vol. 3, 1943, pp. 253–8; also J. W. W. Studd and M. H. Thom. 'Ovarian Failure and Ageing', *Clinics in Endocrinology and Metabolism*, vol. 10, no. 1, 1981, pp. 89–113.

8. J. W. W. Studd 'The Climacteric Syndrome', in P. A. Van Keep, D. M. Serr and R. B. Greenblatt (eds). *Female and Male Climacteric*. Lancaster: MPT Press, 1979, pp. 23–4.

9. Harold Persky et al. 'The Relation of Plasma Androgen Levels to Sexual Behaviors and Attitudes of Women'. Report to meeting of the American Psychosomatic Society, 25 March 1982 in *Journal of Psychosomatic Medicine*, 1983.

RESOURCES
PUBLICATIONS

For books specifically on lesbian sexuality, see Resources following Chapter 12.

GENERAL

Barbach, L. G. *For Yourself: The Fulfillment of Female Sexuality*. New York: Doubleday/Anchor Books, 1976. Written, though not exclusively, for the 'pre-orgasmic' woman.

Barbach, L. G. and Linda **Levine**. *Shared Intimacies: Women's Sexual Experiences*. New York: Bantam Books, 1980. Includes lengthy, informative and explicit quotes from women in many kinds of sexual relationships.

Bell, Ruth et al. *Changing Bodies, Changing Lives: A Book for Teens on Sex and Relationships*. New York: Random House, 1980. By the authors of *Our Bodies, Ourselves* – American edition only.

Belleveau, Fred and Lin **Richter**. *Understanding Human Sexual Inadequacy*. London: Hodder, 1971. Shortened and more readable version of the second Masters and Johnson study, without all the clinical details.

Brecher, Ruth and Edward **Brecher** (eds). *An Analysis of Human Sexual Response*. London: Panther, 1971. This is a very readable analysis of the first Masters and Johnson study.

Brown, Gabrielle. *The New Celibacy: Why More Men and Women Are Abstaining from Sex and Enjoying it*. New York: McGraw–Hill, 1980.

Comfort, Alex. *The Joy of Sex*. London: Quartet, 1974, and *More Joy of Sex*. London: Quartet, 1977. Both give encouragement and helpful suggestions though some people find the cookbook style offensive.

Corinne, Tee. *Labiaflowers: A Coloring Book*. Tallahassee, FL: Naiad Press. Women's erotica.

Country Women magazine, Sexuality Issue. Box 51, Albion, CA 95410. A fine collection of erotic writing.

Cousins-Mills, Jane. *Make It Happy, Make It Safe – What Sex is All About*. Revised edn. London: Penguin Books, 1988. Written specially for young people.

Coward, Rosalind (ed.). *Women's Sexuality Today*. London: Paladin, 1984.

Cox, Gill and Sheila **Dainow**. *Making the Most of Loving*, London: Sheldon Press, 1988.

Demeter, Kass (formerly Teeters). *Reclaiming Women's Sexual Power*. To be published soon. For this and the book below, write to KAT, Inc., P.O. Box 21, Aptos, CA 95003.

Demeter, Kass. *Women's Sexuality: Myth and Reality*. Palo Alto, CA: UP Press, 1977. To order, see entry above. Excellent short book for women and lovers of women. Direct, perceptive, informative, lovingly written, it emphasizes communication, touch, alternatives to intercourse.

Dodson, Betty. *Liberating Masturbation: A Meditation on Self-Love*. Bodysex Designs, P.O. Box 1933, New York, NY 10001, 1974. ($4.00) A classic celebration of masturbation and how to do it.

Ehrenreich, Barbara et al. *Remaking Love: The Feminisation of Sex*. London: Fontana, 1987.

Freud, Sigmund. *On Sexuality*. London: Penguin, 1977. An outline of Freud's basic ideas on female sexuality. We don't agree with some of his theories, but as his texts are slavishly followed by many people we should know what he said.

Feminist Review. *Sexuality: A Reader*. London: Virago Press, 1987.

Friday, Nancy. *My Secret Garden: Women's Sexual Fantasies*. London: Quartet, 1976. Full of women's sexual fantasies, these two books are a kind of natural erotica for some.

Gilbert, Harriet and Christine **Roche**. *A Woman's History of Sex*. London: Pandora, 1987.

Hite, Shere. *The Hite Report*. London: Summit/Hamlyn, 1977. Highly recommended. More than 3,000 women are surveyed about what they really like and don't like, do and don't do in sex. The results challenge many stereotypes.

Hite, Shere. *The Hite Report on Male Sexuality*. New York: Knopf, 1981.

Hooper, Anne. *The Body Electric*. London: Unwin, 1984. A self-help sex therapy book for (heterosexual) women.

Kaplan, Helen S. *The New Sex Therapy*. Male and female sexual 'dysfunctions' and their treatment, primarily according to Masters and Johnson technique. Pictures are particularly fine.

Kerr, Carmen. *Sex For Women – Who Want to Have Fun and Loving Relationships with Equals*. New York: Grove Press, 1977. Especially helpful in identifying power dynamics in sexual loving between women and men. It includes a sensitive step-by-step programme towards having orgasms with a lover (of either sex).

Kirkpatrick, Martha, (ed). *Women's Sexual Experience: Explorations of the Dark Continent*. New York: Plenum, 1982. Essays by diverse writers on women's sexual responses, teen mothers, American Indian women, Afro-American women, ageism in sexual counselling, woman abuse, incest and more.

Kitzinger, Sheila. *Woman's Experience of Sex*. London: Penguin Books, 1985.

Ladas, Alice Kahn, Beverly **Whipple** and John D. **Perry**. *The G Spot and Other Recent Discoveries About Human Sexuality*. New York: Holt, Rinehart and Winston, 1982. This popular but controversial book has met criticism in much of the scientific community for proclaiming a 'theory' based on skimpy data. Many feminists criticize its authors' reinstatement of the old dichotomy between 'clitoral' and 'vaginal' orgasms, and their apparent (though perhaps unintentional) advocacy of the latter. Other readers are more positive about the book as a useful inquiry into women's varied experiences of orgasms. See text for more on the G-spot.

Masters, William H. and Virginia E. **Johnson**. *Human Sexual Inadequacy*. Boston: Little, Brown, 1970. Major research on the nature and treatment of sexual problems. The major drawback is a medicalized and performance-oriented approach to sex and sexual problems.

Masters, William H. and Virginia E. **Johnson**. *Human Sexual Response*. Boston: Little, Brown, 1966. Masters and Johnson's revolutionary research helped open the way to more helpful understandings of women's orgasms, particularly the central role of the clitoris. Tough reading.

Meulenbelt, Anja. *For Ourselves: Our Bodies and Sexuality – from Women's Point of View*. London: Sheba, 1981. Not just for heterosexual women.

Mitchell, Juliet. *Psychoanalysis and Feminism*. London: Penguin Books, 1974. Hard going, a reassessment of Freud's view of female sexuality.

Nelson, James B. *Embodiment: An Approach to Sexuality and Christian Theology*. Minneapolis: Augsburg, 1978. Nelson's feminist perspective on sex and sexual relationships makes this an unusual and helpful book for women who are thinking through the relationship between sexuality and religion.

Off Our Backs. An American monthly women's news journal. Often runs excellent articles on sexuality, and available from some feminist bookshops.

Open University. Course book on *Sexuality* (Unit 4 of 'The Changing Experience of Women'). O.U. Press, Walton Hall, Milton Keynes MK7 6AA.

Pond, Lily (ed.). *Yellow Silk: Journal of Erotic Arts*. Verygraphics, P.O. Box 6374, Albany, CA 94706. Erotic poems, stories, essays, graphics, for women and men. The motto: 'All persuasions: no brutality'.

Reich, Wilhelm. *The Function of the Orgasm*. London: Panther, 1968.
Reich, Wilhelm. *The Sexual Revolution*. London: Vision Press, 1972. Important work on human sexuality which predates Masters and Johnson.
Reich, Wilhelm. *The Invasion of Compulsory Sex-Morality*. London: Penguin Books, 1975.

Rush, Anne Kent. *Getting Clear: Body Work for Women*. London: Wildwood House, 1974. This is a workbook to help us get in better touch with our bodies and ourselves. Fun to use – highly recommended.

Segal, Lynne. 'Sensual Uncertainty, or Why the Clitoris Is Not Enough' in Sue **Cartledge** and Jo **Ryan** (eds). *Sex and Love*. London: Women's Press, 1983. A thoughtful and valuable article that forms a critique of much recent writing on female sexuality, including Barbach, Hite, Masters and Johnson, and Meulenbelt.

Shanor, Karen. *The Fantasy Files: A Study of the Sexual Fantasies of Contemporary Women*. New York: Dell, 1977. Includes guidance on how to interpret your own fantasies.

Sherfey, Mary Jane. *The Nature and Evolution of Female Sexuality*. New York: Vintage Books, 1972. First printed in 1966, this history-making study explores the nature and origins of female sexuality. Critiquing Freudian notions, Sherfey highlights the role of the clitoris in orgasm and the potential intensity of women's sexual drives and satisfactions. A feminist classic.

Silverstein, Judith. *Sexual Enhancement for Women*. Cambridge, MA: Black and White Publishing, second printing 1982. Techniques and sensitively done explicit illustrations of self-pleasuring, pleasure with a partner, becoming orgasmic during intercourse and more.

Stimpson, Catharine and Ethel **Person** (eds). *Women, Sex and Sexuality*. Chicago: University of Chicago Press, 1980. Important essays from a feminist/academic perspective. All first appeared in *Signs: A Journal of Women in Culture and Society*.

Valins, Linda. *Vaginismus*. Bath: Ashgrove Press, 1988.

Vitale, Sylvia Witts. 'A Herstorical Look at Some Aspects of Black Sexuality' in *Heresies: A Feminist Publication on Art and Politics*, Sex Issue, vol. 3, no. 4, issue 12.

Walker, Alice. *The Color Purple*. London: Women's Press, 1983. A powerful novel which touches on many aspects of a black woman's sexuality.

SEX AND PHYSICAL DISABILITY*

Becker, Elle F. *Female Sexuality Following Spinal Cord Injury*. Bloomington, IL: Cheevar Publishers, 1978. Shows the struggle of a woman with paraplegia or quadriplegia in a world that represses and defines her sexual expression and identity, and how others can help.

Bregman, Sue. *Sexuality and the S.C.I. Woman*. Abbott-Northwestern Hospital Research and Education Department, Office of Continuing Education, 2727 Chicago Avenue, Minneapolis, MN 55407. One of the first booklets of its kind, and very helpful.

Bullard, D. and S. **Knight**, (eds). *Sexuality and Disability: Personal Perspectives*. St Louis: Mosby, 1981. Excellent book giving many different kinds of experiences.

Duffy, Yvonne. . . . *All Things Are Possible*. A. J. Garvin and Associates, P.O. Box 7525, Ann Arbor, MI 48107, 1981. More than seventy-five differently-abled women speak candidly about their lives. Chapters on parental attitudes, masturbation, relationships, sexual intercourse, lesbianism, birth control, childbirth and childrearing contain explicit descriptions and concrete suggestions for overcoming difficulties.

Ferreyra, Susan and Katrine **Hughes**. *Table Manners: Guide to the Pelvic Examination for Disabled Women and Health Care Providers*. Sex Education for Disabled People, 477 Fifteenth Street, Oakland, CA 94612, 1982. Written by two differently-abled women; advocates a cooperative approach.

Intimacy and Disability. Institute for Information Studies, 200 Little Falls Street, Suite 104, Falls Church, VA 22046. 1982. A 'guide for people with disabilities who want to develop and maintain intimate relationships.' Clear and concise, this booklet touches many issues, including ways to avoid sexual assault and exploitation. Has a chart showing sexual and contraceptive implications of fifteen disabilities. The main drawback is its exclusive heterosexual focus.

Kolodny, Robert, William H. **Masters** and Virginia E. **Johnson**. *Textbook of Sexual Medicine*. Boston: Little, Brown, 1979. Although not exactly feminist, the authors' attitudes towards sex and disability are excellent. Highly informative book.

Mimmack, Julie. 'Physical Relationships and the Disabled Woman', *Spare Rib*, no. 86, September 1979.

VIDEOS

Rhymes and Reasons. Concord Films, 1981, 32 mins. People of different backgrounds and ages talk about how they learned about sex. Produced by FPA.

True Romance etc. Concord Films, 1981, 35 mins. Interviews with young people about influences on sexuality, challenging sexual stereotypes.

ORGANIZATIONS

Association of Sexual and Marital Therapists, PO Box 62, Sheffield S10 3TS. Send sae for list of therapists. Some of their members work within the NHS.

British Association for Counselling, 37a Sheep Street, Rugby, Warwickshire CV21 3BX. Tel: 0788-78328/9. Keeps a list of counsellors, including those who are interested in, or specialize in, psychosexual problems. For more about BAC see Chapter 8, p. 131.

Family Planning Clinics sometimes offer psychosexual help, or can put you in touch with someone who can (see Chapter 15).

*Our thanks to Janna Zwerner and Barbara Waxman for assistance in compiling this section.

Institute of Psychosexual Medicine, 11 Chandos Street, Cavendish Square, London W1M 9DE. Tel: 01-580 0631. Members are doctors who may work in family planning or hospital-based psychosexual clinics.

London Bisexual Group, BM BI, London WC1N 3XX. Acts as a national contact.

London Bisexual Women's Group, BM Box LBWG, London WC1N 3XX.

Relate: Marriage Guidance Council. Has trained counsellors, some of whom specialize specifically in sexual problems (see Chapter 8 for further information about Relate).

Women's Sexuality Workshops, Redwood Association, 'Invergarry', Kitlings Lane, Walton on the Hill, Stafford ST17 0LE. Tel: 0785-662823. Some may be helpful for lesbians as well as heterosexual women. Send sae for information.

Women's Therapy Centres. These see individuals (including lesbians) and also often run groups. For list of centres that existed when we went to press, see Chapter 8.

See also *Psychosexual Problems: a Directory of Agencies Offering Therapy, Counselling and Support* by Francis Taylor (ed.). British Association for Counselling, 1983, and Resources listed in Chapter 8.

PART III

CONTROLLING OUR FERTILITY

INTRODUCTION

Controlling our fertility is central to controlling our lives. The chapters in this unit present tools for understanding our fertility and making choices about whether and when to have children. Safe, affordable birth control and abortion, though absolutely crucial, are only part of our full reproductive freedom. All women must be free not only to prevent or end unwanted pregnancy but also to have children if, when and how we choose. This means, for example, that no woman should be forced into abortion or sterilization because she can't afford to bring up a child (as many poor women and black women are today). It means that no woman should become infertile due to dangerous birth control methods or misdiagnosed or untreated pelvic infections.

We believe that women have a right to control our own bodies and that we must organize to secure that right in the face of attacks by the church, state and organized right wing.

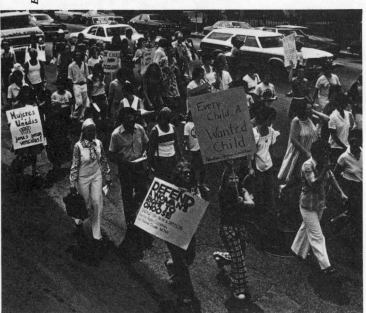

Ellen Shub

RIGHT TO LIFE

A woman is not a pear tree
thrusting her fruit in mindless fecundity
into the world. Even pear trees bear
heavily in one year and rest and grow the next.
An orchard gone wild drops few warm rotting
fruit in the grass but the trees stretch
high and wiry gifting the birds forty
feet up among inch long thorns
broken atavistically from the smooth wood.

A woman is not a basket you place
your buns in to keep them warm. Not a brood
hen you can slip duck eggs under.
Not the purse holding the coins of your
descendants till you spend them in wars.
Not a bank where your genes gather interest
and interesting mutations in the tainted
rain, any more than you are.

You plant corn and you harvest
it to eat or sell. You put the lamb
in the pasture to fatten and haul it in
to butcher for chops. You slice
the mountain in two for a road and gouge
the high plains for coal and the waters
run muddy for miles and years.
Fish die but you do not call them yours
unless you wished to eat them.

Now you legislate mineral rights in a woman.
You lay claim to her pastures for grazing,
fields for growing babies like iceberg
lettuce. You value children so dearly
that none ever go hungry, none weep
with no one to tend them when mothers
work, none lack fresh fruit,
none chew lead or cough to death and your
orphanages are empty. Every noon the best
restaurants serve poor children steaks.

At this moment at nine o'clock a *partera*
is performing a table top abortion on an
unwed mother in Texas who can't get Medicaid*
any longer. In five days she will die
of tetanus and her little daughter will cry
and be taken away. Next door a husband
and wife are sticking pins in the son
they did not want. They will explain
for hours how wicked he is,
how he wants discipline.

We are all born of woman, in the rose
of the womb we suckled our mother's blood
and every baby born has a right to love
like a seedling to sun. Every baby born
unloved, unwanted, is a bill that will come
due in twenty years with interest, an anger
that must find a target, a pain that will

beget pain. A decade downstream a child
screams, a woman falls, a synagogue is torched,
a firing squad is summoned, a button
is pushed and the world burns.

I will choose what enters me, what becomes
flesh of my flesh. Without choice, no politics,
no ethics lives. I am not your cornfield,
not your uranium mine, not your calf
for fattening, not your cow for milking.
You may not use me as your factory.
Priests and legislators do not hold
shares in my womb or my mind.
This is my body. If I give it to you
I want it back. My life
is a non-negotiable demand.

---

*Medicaid is the US state system which enables some poor people access to health care, some of the time.

CHAPTER

15

CONTRACEPTION*

Prepared by
MARGE BERER

INTRODUCTION

In 1843 the first rubber condom was made and in 1882 the diaphragm was invented: important years in the history of contraception. Until quite recently, women and men depended on these methods of contraception and used them successfully, together with abortion, to limit the number of their children.

Birth control is fundamental to our effort to control our bodies and our sexuality, and to have autonomy in our lives. Today we have many more contraceptive methods, yet we still get pregnant when we don't plan to. Worrying about pregnancy can prevent us from enjoying sexual intercourse with men, but we also have to worry about birth control. We may dream of a contraceptive which is perfectly safe, never fails us, is easy to use, is instantly reversible and doesn't interfere with sexuality. But it doesn't exist and never will. We can't be expected to be infallible either: most of us make mistakes and take risks, knowingly and unknowingly, in using birth control.

Contraception is not just about methods and techniques; using it involves our feelings about ourselves, our sexuality and our relationships. Deciding which method to use involves questions about our health, and the amount of risk we are prepared to take. It involves the participation of a man, and his willingness to take responsibility too.

This chapter looks at the differences between women's and men's attitudes to birth control, how to obtain contraceptives and sterilization, where our contraceptive choices come from, and how we make choices for ourselves. Then it looks at each method available in the UK. (See Chapter 3, p. 36 for an explanation of how pregnancy happens.)

WOMEN AND BIRTH CONTROL

It is often assumed that the responsibility for birth control lies with the woman. Women do have a more personal

*References for this chapter are listed at the end, section by section.

interest in preventing unwanted pregnancy than men, because we bear the children and are in large measure responsible for bringing them up. However, this lets men off the hook. It takes two to get pregnant.

Because most contraceptive methods are for use by women, we are the ones who spend time with GPs or in clinics, reading up the different methods, trying to choose one that suits our needs and that we can feel comfortable with. We are the ones who have to remember to take the pills, check the IUD strings, or keep a diaphragm waiting and ready. And we are the ones who put up with any side-effects of the various methods. It's no wonder many men seem freer about sexuality – they are!

These are some of the reasons many women give for not using contraception:

Deep down, I think sex is wrong, so it's hard to admit we're doing it.

Contraception is too premeditated, clinical or messy; sex should be spontaneous; contraception kills the romance.

He'll be angry if I bring it up, and I'm scared of making him angry.

It can't happen to me, I won't get pregnant.

I hate the method I'm using; I hate all the methods; I can't be bothered with it all the time.

It's the wrong time for a baby, but I would love to have someone to care for, and I wonder if I'm fertile.

I don't know who to ask for help, and I'm afraid of having an internal examination.

Worrying about whether the doctor will disapprove and/or tell our parents, added to the newness of the whole procedure, makes young women especially vulnerable.

Facing any of these feelings may be easier when we realize that most women share them. Dealing with them can mean the difference between enjoying sex or not, and at the same time not getting pregnant when we don't want to.

MEN AND BIRTH CONTROL

The attitudes of the men we are involved with can make all the difference. Many men resist talking about or doing anything about birth control, and some don't want us to do anything either.

Being able to talk about birth control with our partners is a first step towards being able to share the decision-making and the responsibility. Men who recognize that unprotected intercourse holds a greater risk for women are less likely to press for it. Making them aware of our cycles, and having to be more careful when we are fertile is another step. Two people prevent pregnancy better than one.

A man can share the responsibility for birth control in many ways. He can get and use condoms, and not just when we remind him to. He can share putting in a diaphragm, cap or sponge. If there's no method available, he can explore with us ways of making love without intercourse (see Chapter 14) or agree to wait till another time. If no (more) children are wanted, he can have a vasectomy.

Clinics that provide contraception are publicizing that they are open for men too, and they have had a big response. Some health authorities, like North Manchester and Brent in London have started sessions especially for men. This is a good beginning but it does require an expansion of services in a period when cuts are the norm. If we want this to become standard practice, we'll have to campaign for it.

BIRTH CONTROL AND SEXUAL FREEDOM

Wider availability of contraception, safe abortion, sterilization and vasectomy have changed many things for women. They have made it possible for us to feel freer about having sexual relationships with men without having to worry so much, at least about unwanted pregnancy. Just because we use birth control doesn't mean we are promiscuous or are available all the time. We need to be assertive about *our* desires, and find the confidence to say what we want and what we don't want. By pressuring us to have sex against our will, men can turn this potential freedom into a new form of oppression. Problems in our sexual relationships, and our view of ourselves as sexual beings, are often reflected in our use of (or failure to use) contraception.

In addition, there are other aspects of having sex that limit our freedom, such as sexually transmitted diseases. The fear of getting HIV, the virus that can cause AIDS, is only the latest in a long line of diseases people have to avoid if they have sex. By itself, contraception is no guarantee of sexual freedom.

Helping Ourselves

Talking to each other, sharing our problems, sharing information about methods, identifying good doctors and clinics – all are ways we can help ourselves and each other.

Availability of contraception depends on good services that meet our needs. As you read this, *be aware that NHS cuts are severely affecting the services described and we shall have to campaign very hard to resist the effects of the Thatcher Government's plans.*

We can campaign against attitudes and laws that restrict our rights, and for facilities that better meet our needs. We can fight for decent housing, jobs and childcare, so that we can choose birth control freely, instead of being forced to use it because we can't afford the kids we want. Whatever we choose to do, we can act together. (See Organizations in Resources.)

WHO CAN GET CONTRACEPTION

By law, anyone who wants contraception can get it. Since 1974 it has been a duty of the NHS to provide contraception free. The law says nothing about age limits.

Young Women

In practice, doctors will encourage young women to talk to their parents about getting contraception. While some doctors may insist that if you want contraception you must tell your parents you are in a sexual relationship, there are many others who are sympathetic if you explain that telling parents would be a mistake. Clinics, especially those for young people, are usually very good about talking this over and helping you reach a decision that is right for you. In 1985, a court case decided that young women under sixteen had a continued right to get confidential advice and help with contraception. Doctors have been told to encourage young women to talk to their parents, but they have no right to require you to. The decision was important, because it meant that no matter what our age, we still have a right to contraception and confidentiality.

WHERE TO GET CONTRACEPTION

Condoms, spermicides and contraceptive sponges can be bought at all chemists. They are usually on display near the till, and you can pick them up and hand them directly to the assistant. Condoms are also available at barbers' shops, in many men's, and some women's, toilets and by mail order. It is becoming increasingly acceptable for women to buy and carry condoms as a result of the public education campaign to prevent transmission of HIV (see p. 501).

You need not pay for contraception. If you go to a family planning clinic or to a GP, contraception is free on the NHS, with one or two exceptions, which are discussed below.

There are more GPs than family planning clinics, and

about 60 per cent of women attend GPs for contraception, as opposed to 40 per cent in clinics. Both types of services are important, and women sometimes consult both.

Going to a Family Planning Clinic

You can find out where your nearest clinic is from your GP, from the phone book (look under 'Family Planning'), from your local Community Health Council, the library, Citizens' Advice Bureau, or from the Family Planning Information Service (FPIS, see p. 308). The FPIS has a list of every clinic in the UK and can direct you to clinics with related services as well.

Only a few clinics are still walk-in, so it is always best to ring first for an appointment. It may take up to two weeks to get your first appointment. These restrictions and delays are due to cuts. Even if you have to wait for an appointment, they can help with supplies of condoms in the meantime.

Clinics tend to be more anonymous than a local doctor's surgery. They have specialist knowledge and experience, and there is a much greater chance of seeing a woman doctor. Clinics increasingly encourage your partner to come with you. They provide the full range of methods, including at least one brand of condom, but not contraceptive sponges. However, some women don't feel comfortable going to clinics because it is obvious to other people why they are there. Nor is it always possible to see the same doctor on each visit, though you can ask for this to be arranged if possible.

Many clinics also offer youth advisory sessions, 'morning-after' contraception, sterilization/vasectomy counselling and operations, cervical smears and breast checks. Some, but not nearly enough, also offer pregnancy testing, abortion advice and referral, sub-fertility advice, psychosexual counselling, menopause counselling and a range of well-woman services. It would make sense if all clinics were to offer this range of services, but many who might have done so cannot because of NHS cuts. However, the stronger local campaigns for improved services are, the more chance that clinics can offer what women want (see Chapter 28).

Going to Your GP

Up to 1974, when the law on contraception changed, many GPs had little or no training in providing contraceptives. Now over 97 per cent of GPs provide contraceptive services. All newly-qualifying doctors get some training for this, but only those who do a specialist course are fully trained. The advantage of going to your GP is that s/he knows your medical history and perhaps knows you. S/he may be easier to talk to than a strange doctor. It may be quicker to get an appointment than at a clinic, and people in the waiting-room will not know why you are there.

The disadvantages are that many GPs still have less training and experience with some methods and are therefore less willing to provide them. Only those with specialist clinic training are likely to offer all methods. You are much more likely to end up with the Pill than any other method.

In 1982, 84 per cent of women who saw GPs for contraception got the Pill, compared with 55 per cent who went to family planning clinics in 1984. *GPs do not provide condoms* (or contraceptive sponges). And GPs do not always provide the kind of follow-up care we can expect from clinics. They are also less likely to encourage your partner to attend with you.

We need to press for GPs to provide condoms and to get full training so that they offer a full service.

Clinics for Young People

There are a number of clinics specifically for young people under twenty-five, such as the Brook Advisory Centres, though their funding is increasingly threatened. These are specially geared to the needs of those starting off in sexual relationships. They can be found in the same way as other family planning clinics (see above and end of this chapter for addresses). Some family planning clinics have separate sessions for under twenty-fives, though fewer than used to.

When we are younger, the question of whether to tell our parents anything about our relationships, and what to tell them, looms large. These clinics can be especially good in helping with those problems. Some also have begun setting up special sessions for young men, which have quickly become popular, proving that young men need information and someone to talk to as much as young women.

Although some people think that providing birth control to teenagers leads to promiscuous behaviour, the fact is that people have sex whether they use birth control or not. The number of unwanted births and shotgun marriages among teenagers, as well as older women, has decreased tremendously in the UK since contraception and safe abortion were made more easily available. This is an improvement in women's lives that we cannot afford to lose.

Domiciliary Family Planning

Domiciliary services were first set up in Birmingham and Glasgow in 1959. By 1975 there were more than 140 units round the country, though all but forty of them had been closed by NHS cuts five years later. More may well have closed since then. With this service a doctor initially and then a nurse visit a woman in her home. Women may refer themselves, their friends may refer them or a health visitor, social worker or doctor may do so.

Some women are thankful for the domiciliary family planning service; others find it intrusive. With these services fast disappearing, the question of how women who use them feel about them is important, particularly whether their needs could be met in the more usual ways.

At the Clinic or GP

If you have not been before, you will be asked your name, address, age, etcetera, and a few questions about your relationship with your partner. You will be weighed and your blood pressure will be taken. This will probably all be done by a nurse. The doctor will ask about your medical history. If you have any illnesses or are taking any type of drug, including cigarette smoking or a prescription drug, it is important to tell the doctor, as this can affect what methods are safe and effective for you. You will then be offered an internal examination (see p. 593), though it can be done on a later visit if you are feeling anxious about it. If this is a first for you, you may feel embarrassed; it can feel like a terrible invasion of privacy, more so if you have never touched that part of your body. If you do a little exploring with a mirror and fingers before you go (see Self-examination, p. 32) you may feel less anxious. Reading the whole of Chapters 3 and 14 may also help.

You may know what birth control method you want. If not, you will want to be told about all the alternatives and their benefits and risks, so that you can discuss your options. You may have to ask a lot of questions to achieve this. If you already know what you want to ask, write it down and take the list with you. You may not be offered every method (particularly by a GP). Ask questions about anything you don't understand.

You should make the final decision about what to use. Then you should be given full instructions on how to use your method of choice. A follow-up appointment will be arranged; the timing will depend on what method you choose.

You may prefer to go with someone else for your first visit – many women do. Don't be afraid to ask if they can stay with you during the examination.

WHERE DO OUR CHOICES COME FROM?

Earlier in this century, as in the nineteenth century, contraception was not an open topic for discussion. It was neither easily available nor legal. Women fought for generations to make it acceptable and legal, and more recently to make it free on the NHS, and we still need to fight to keep FP clinics open, just as we have fought and are still fighting for full abortion rights.

Before the 1950s, rubber companies produced contraceptives. The discovery that progesterone prevents conception, which led to the first birth control pills, was an accident. In the 1950s and 1960s a fear of population growth in Third World countries rapidly took hold among international aid donors (see end of chapter for further reading). A great deal of money was invested in research to find new contraceptive methods, using existing work on female hormones as the basis. Research on intra-uterine devices, crude versions of which had been around in earlier decades and had been removed from use because of health risks, was also initiated. Improvements in sterilization and abortion techniques were also sought.

Many of the methods and techniques now available are a result of this impetus. Drug companies had to be dragged into the contraceptive market at that time because the subject was still not quite polite and they didn't want to be accused of producing 'dirty' products. The aim was the development of reliable, long-term methods, in the hope that their use would lower the birth-rate. Drug companies now make a considerable profit from our use of birth control and have their own interests to protect.

This is how our 'choices' have been influenced in the last few decades. It is no accident that there are many more hormonal methods and IUDs available than there are barrier methods. The vast majority of research money in the last thirty years has been spent on these; population-control ideology favours the development of 'fail-safe' methods.

The perceived need for fail-safe methods of contraception is linked to repressive attitudes about abortion. The belief that prevention of pregnancy is always better than termination, even when an abortion is very early, has led to the acceptance of methods that carry health risks, even though early abortion is a very safe procedure. In countries where abortion is illegal or access to it is very restricted, the risk of death from dangerous abortions seriously alters the risk-benefit ratio when type of contraception is considered. This represents a serious restriction on women's choices. In the UK, where there is access to abortion (though far from ideal), the back-up of early abortion when contraception fails should be an intrinsic part of what women are offered when we seek contraception. Yet because contraceptive failure is not grounds for abortion under the 1967 Abortion Act, this option is rarely discussed. The separation of 'family planning' and abortion services reflects this.

Since it takes decades before we can begin to have any clear idea of the relative risks of methods such as the Pill, IUD and injectables, this makes us subjects in prolonged experiments. The same thing happens with all drugs and drug research, but we do not take contraceptives to prevent or cure illnesses, so how we assess their risks, as opposed to their benefits, is therefore quite different.

We are often given conflicting information and false assurances. The risks of certain methods are sometimes minimized in order to ensure that we don't get scared and stop using them. Some doctors think such information will encourage us to experience side-effects just because we know they might occur, but research shows this is just not the case.*

We need to be aware of all this background, and how it might affect us personally, when we seek birth control. Only then can we begin to make an informed choice from what is on offer. With this knowledge, and as part of an international women's health movement, we can also try to make things better both for ourselves and for the women who come after us.

ABUSES

Our rights in relation to birth control can be abused. Some examples are:

---

*See, for example, S. Berry, 'Patient Package Inserts: Help or Hindrance?', *Contraception Technology Update*, vol. 3, 1982, p. 124.

- We have been told a particular method has no adverse effects, when it has. Or that a particular symptom is not a side-effect of the method, when there is evidence that it is. Or that nothing is wrong, when it is, and we need medical treatment.
- We have been told we have to have an injectable contraceptive with a rubella vaccination, when in fact we could just as easily use – or continue to use – another method in order to avoid pregnancy while the vaccine is active.*
- We have been told the doctor will be fitting an IUD when we have an abortion, or that we will be given an injectable following a second abortion, whether that is our method of choice or not.
- Doctors have not bothered to find an interpreter to explain what they are giving us, when our first language is not English.
- We have been encouraged to accept a method we don't want, or are not yet sure about, because the doctor is convinced that that is what is best for us.

Such abuses can be resisted and challenged. It may help to take someone to the doctor with you. Remember that, if necessary, you can seek contraceptive advice elsewhere. Your community/local health council is there to listen to your complaints and to take action on your behalf. (See Organizations in Resources for other organizations who will help you with this.)

CHOOSING A METHOD

There are seven main questions to consider before choosing a method that is appropriate for you.

1. Are you delaying a first child, spacing your children or not planning to have any (more) children?
2. How would you feel and what would you do if you got pregnant in spite of your method?
3. How motivated are you to use the method and how cooperative will your partner be?
4. Do the advantages of the method outweigh the disadvantages and/or the possible adverse effects and health risks, and which disadvantages are you prepared to put up with in order to have the benefits?
5. How will this method affect your sexual relationship with your partner?
6. Are there medical reasons why you should not use a particular method?
7. How great is the risk of your getting a sexually transmitted disease, including HIV?

Whatever you decide on will involve a compromise, since there is no one perfect method. The method you think you will feel most comfortable with is probably the one you will use most effectively. We choose differently according to the point we are at in our lives – no one method is likely to carry us all the way through our fertile years.

The effectiveness of all methods, apart from the IUD and sterilization, depends on how they are used. With IUDs and sterilization, the skill of the doctor makes a difference. As a result, actual failure rates differ from theoretical failure rates. Actual failure rates include times when women (or men) forget or decide not to use the method as well as times when the method itself fails. So they are higher than the theoretical rate. If a method has a 3 per cent failure rate, it means that of 100 women using the method for one year,

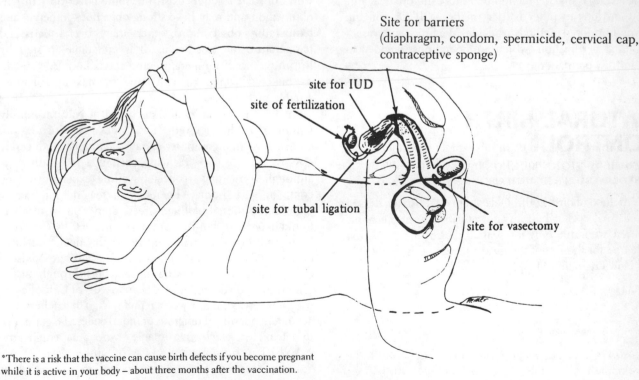

Site for barriers
(diaphragm, condom, spermicide, cervical cap, contraceptive sponge)

site for IUD

site of fertilization

site for tubal ligation

site for vasectomy

Nina Reimer

*There is a risk that the vaccine can cause birth defects if you become pregnant while it is active in your body – about three months after the vaccination.

on average ninety-seven will not become pregnant and three will. Note that, by comparison, a fertile, sexually active woman using no method has a 90 per cent chance of becoming pregnant within a year. We often hear it said these days that no responsible woman need get pregnant accidentally with so much contraceptive choice. Failure rates will never disappear so this is rubbish.

Methods go in and out of favour, particularly for specific groups of women, and recommendations as to who can or should not use them change, according to new information gained from studies and depending on what else is on the market, and also on the attitudes of those providing methods and information. At any point in time, both doctors and individual women favour some methods over others, and not always for scientific reasons. Those of us in the women's health movement can be accused of this too! The more you know about your alternatives, the more real your choice will be, whether what you choose is in favour or not.

The rest of this chapter describes each of the available methods in as much detail as possible. At the end of the chapter, Resources indicate where you can get further information.

We start with Natural Birth Control (fertility awareness)* because learning about this method teaches us best how our bodies work and how to know when we are fertile. This is worth knowing, whether we choose to rely on it for our birth control method or not. It can help us feel confident about choosing a barrier method that doesn't interfere with our bodies' normal functioning. Next we look at condoms, which have been consistently underrated since the advent of the Pill, in spite of their many advantages. Their dual role as contraceptives and protectives against sexually transmitted diseases, including HIV (the virus that can cause AIDS) is making them much more important again. We then look at other barrier methods, IUDs and the various hormonal methods available. We finish with vasectomy and sterilization, which are operations intended to end fertility permanently.

NATURAL BIRTH CONTROL†

Prepared by FIONA McCLOSKY, BRISTOL WOMEN'S HEALTH GROUP

This method of birth control sets out to establish the days of a menstrual cycle when it is not possible to get pregnant. Women are fertile only for a small part of the menstrual cycle and for the rest of the time conception is impossible (see How Pregnancy Happens, p. 36). With this method of

*Not to be confused with 'Rhythm Method' – an outdated and unreliable approach.
†This is the term we prefer to the more commonly used 'Natural Family Planning'.

birth control a woman would have sexual intercourse only on days when she is sure that she will not get pregnant. She could use a barrier method of contraception on the other days (see below), or she could abstain from sex completely or only from sex involving penis/vagina contact (see Chapter 14 for discussion of sexuality and p. 488 for safer sex guidelines).

Culturally and historically, different methods of identifying the phases of the menstrual cycle exist. Evidence from the Bantu people of East Africa and the American Cherokee people suggests that traditional verbal communication between women on this subject has seldom been recorded by anthropologists.

In all fertile menstrual cycles there are noticeable changes in the uterus, vaginal/cervical secretions and temperature. As well as these main indications of fertility there are sometimes other signs such as breast tenderness, spotting, and so-called ovulation pain that can help us understand what is happening. Natural birth control works with, rather than against, our biology, positively using the ordered and precise sequence of events in the menstrual cycle. It does not view controlling our fertility as a purely biological problem that needs to be dealt with by medical intervention; rather the 'problem' is rooted in the social and political construction of heterosexuality and not in female biological inadequacy.

LEARNING ABOUT NATURAL BIRTH CONTROL

If you want to learn how to identify and understand all the bodily changes that take place during the menstrual cycle you will need to contact a teacher who has been trained in cervix, mucus and temperature observations. Several networks of such teachers exist, but some cover only mucus observation and may have strong objections to cervix and temperature observations; others may cover mucus and temperature but not cervix. It is preferable to start by learning mucus, temperature and cervix because you can double-check one sign with another, making it a more reliable method.

In Britain the National Association of Natural Family Planning Teachers (NANFPT) provides a growing network of teachers trained in temperature, mucus and cervix observation (see p. 308). Most teachers work voluntarily, although some may request travelling expenses if they come to your home. There are a few natural family planning clinics, but there are seldom trained teachers found in ordinary family planning clinics or GPs' surgeries. Some centres for alternative medicine provide natural birth control classes at a cost. The Catholic Marriage Advisory Council also has a list of trained teachers throughout the UK. While you do not have to be married – or Catholic – to use their service, many women prefer to go to teachers who act independently of religious or moral codes. To get an up-to-date picture of what is available in your area, contact the NANFPT in Birmingham, or CMAC in London.

Some teachers prefer to teach on an individual or

'couple' basis and others are prepared to take on small groups. Usually it takes about three to six cycles before a woman begins to feel confident to interpret her charts on her own. The number of times you can expect to see your teacher will vary according to how your teacher works and how much support and contact you feel you need. An average example would be three times in the first two cycles and then perhaps once in each subsequent cycle, or until you feel confident.

What is Involved

When you start observing the changes that take place during your cycle you can expect to spend three to five minutes in the morning taking your temperature and about the same in the evening checking your cervix, mucus and noting the changes on a chart. Over a few cycles you will begin to see a pattern emerge which you will eventually be able to interpret at a glance.

Starting from a position of extreme caution during the learning cycles you will quickly observe a clear post-ovulation non-fertile phase of about ten to sixteen days. After six to twelve cycles you will have enough information about your patterns of change at the beginning of the cycle and the onset of fertility to start using some of the early days as non-fertile. The beginning part of the cycle is the most difficult to interpret and the easiest to make mistakes on; much of the teaching time is centred around getting this clear. Women with short cycles will have very few early non-fertile days and may start to become fertile whilst still menstruating. For women with long cycles there may be several days or even weeks between the end of menstruation and the onset of the fertile time of the cycle.

Effectiveness

A completed large-scale study of the combined natural birth control method – involving the monitoring of temperature, mucus and cervix – is not yet available. However, several studies of temperature and mucus only exist and all indicate that motivation and the quality of teaching are crucial factors to the success of the method. Well-taught users who want to prevent further pregnancies have an effectiveness rate comparable to the Pill and IUD. * Women wanting to delay or space a pregnancy, or combine the method with the use of a barrier at the fertile time, have a reduction in effectiveness. If monitoring of the cervix is added to the mucus and temperature method, we can assume that this will increase reliability of natural birth control. That is why in this book we discuss natural birth control in terms of using all three.

Advantages

1. There are no adverse biological effects.
2. Women at any stage of fertility can use it, whether they are breastfeeding, post-Pill or pre-menopausal.

3. Natural birth control can be an empowering experience for women because it validates our biology, depathologizes our fertility and gives us control over our reproductive capacity.
4. It gives us the opportunity to discuss with our partner(s) our feelings about sexual activity and pregnancy, which can bring about a better understanding and closeness. See Sexuality, p. 257 for more discussion on this.

Disadvantages

1. Women who are not in a position to choose when and if to have sexual intercourse are not protected from unwanted pregnancy.
2. Finding a teacher who you get on well with may be a problem.
3. Re-evaluating the 'sexual availability' of women to men can be frightening.
4. For some women, the period around ovulation is the time when they can experience most sexual interest.

BARRIER METHODS

Barrier methods prevent sperm from entering the uterus through the cervix and reaching a mature egg in the fallopian tube. Throughout history men have put things over their penises and women have put things in their vaginas in order to prevent pregnancy. Barrier methods today include condoms, diaphragms, cervical caps, the contraceptive sponge and spermicides. *

CONDOMS (Also called sheaths, Durex, French letters, rubbers, protectives)

Condoms are the most widely-used contraceptive in the world and, made of different substances, have been in use for many centuries. In the nineteenth century they began to be made of rubber and are still today, though they are now much thinner and lighter in weight than they used to be.

Condoms are not only very efficient contraceptives if used properly, they also help to protect against cervical cancer and sexually transmitted diseases (including HIV). Condoms are now being widely promoted for use as protection against HIV (see p. 501) for those who are at risk of transmitting or getting the disease through sex. If condoms are your chosen method of contraception they will serve this dual purpose for you. If you are using another method of contraception and are at risk from HIV, advice commonly given is that you should use condoms as well as your chosen contraceptive method. †

---

*See Rice et al. in References.

*A new, 'female' condom has just been introduced to the market as we go to press. Trials are currently under way at the Margaret Pyke Centre in London (see Organizations).
†You will want to decide whether this makes sense for you, and you may in any case want to take into account the information we discuss in relation to the IUD and the Pill.

Description

A condom is made of thin, strong latex rubber. It is designed to fit over a man's erect penis to prevent semen from getting into a woman's vagina. It consists of a circular cylinder with one closed, teat-shaped or plain end; the other end is open with a thin rim around it. In the UK they come in one size only, packed individually in foil, and are sold in packets of three or more. (In the USA they are produced in more than one size.) It is worth shopping around if you don't like the first brand you try. Men find that some brands feel more comfortable and fit better. Some brands smell more strongly of rubber than others.

Most have lubrication to make it easier for the penis to enter the vagina. Some come with spermicide in the rubber, for extra protection. They can be different colours (though the dye may stain and cause irritation). If you or your partner are allergic to rubber, or to the lubricant used on the condom, anti-allergic condoms are available. There are also condoms made from animal membrane, which are supposed to provide extra sensitivity for the man, but they are much more expensive and may not be as easy to find. They are also not as effective in preventing transmission of STDs, including HIV.

Only those condoms with the British Standards kite-mark (BSI) on the packet have been quality tested for reliability. (*Note*: Those made of animal membrane have not been BSI tested.)

Where to Get Condoms

Men and women can get a limited number of brands of condoms free from family planning clinics, along with spermicides. They are not at present available from GPs. You can also buy them from chemists, barbers and vending machines or by mail order.

Many men say it is embarrassing to buy them the first time (women too). If the chemist asks 'What size?', s/he means how many to the packet.

If this is your chosen method, keep some yourself. Don't rely on your partner alone to have a supply.

How to Use a Condom

Using condoms well takes practice, either alone or together. A family planning clinic will be glad to provide advice if wanted.

The condom should be rolled on to his already erect penis before it comes near your vagina. While rolling it on, the tip should be held between thumb and index finger to prevent an air bubble and to leave space for semen to collect. This prevents it bursting and semen seeping out. Nearly all condoms are lubricated, but additional lubrication can help if your vagina is dry. Use a water-based lubricant, not an oil-based one. A lubricating jelly or a spermicide can be inserted into your vagina, or on to the condom after it is on his penis. Saliva can also be used, but if you or your partner have oral thrush it may be transferred to your vagina this way.*

One of you must hold the rim after he has 'come' and lost his erection. Otherwise the condom might slip off and

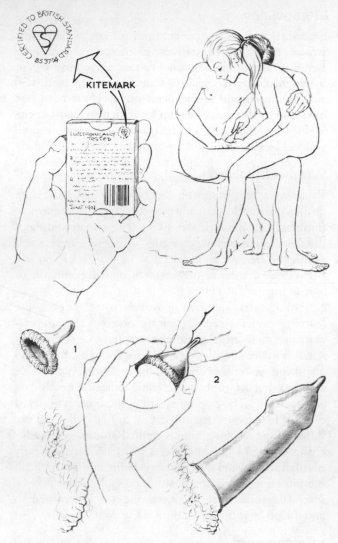

KITEMARK

Helping each other to put on a condom is just one of the ways in which a couple can share fun and the responsibility of birth control.
1 A rolled-up condom with a teat looks like this when it is taken out of its package.
2 Condoms with teats are a lot less likely to burst than those without. One of you has to squeeze the teat as you're putting it on to prevent any air getting trapped in the end of the condom.

semen could get into your vagina. The condom should be removed only after the penis is no longer touching your vaginal lips. It will slide right off.

Condoms can only be used once. Dispose of them in a bin.

Never use condoms after the expiry date on the packet. Store them in a cool place: heat, including body heat if they are kept in a pocket for a long time, makes them deteriorate.

---

*If your vagina is very dry, you may not be ready for intercourse. Sexual stimulation increases vaginal fluids, which makes intercourse easier and more pleasurable.

Effectiveness

Failure rates as low as 2 per cent and as high as 15 per cent are quoted. Effectiveness depends almost entirely on how well you and your partner use them. The commonest reason for failure is not using them properly, particularly not putting one on before penis-vagina contact, or not leaving enough space at the tip for semen so that it bursts during orgasm, or letting it slip off inside your vagina.

If used correctly, condoms are good enough on their own. However, some people like to add a spermicide (see p. 284) for extra reassurance during fertile days.* For almost 100 per cent effectiveness on your fertile days, you can use a diaphragm with condoms. Or you can avoid intercourse and make love in other ways.

Condoms rarely tear or burst unless they are used incorrectly, but it can happen.

In cases where you think semen has got into your vagina by mistake, you can get 'morning-after' pills (within three days) or an IUD (within five days) from your GP or clinic (see Morning-after Birth Control, p. 295). This may not be necessary if it happens during your non-fertile days. Consult your GP/clinic if you aren't sure.

The more your partner and you use condoms, the more comfortable you will feel with them (which means you will use them more effectively), and the easier it becomes to incorporate them into love-making.

Advantages

1. Condoms do not affect or delay fertility in men or women.
2. They are easy to obtain without professional help.
3. With correct use, they have a low failure rate.
4. Except for allergy to rubber (which is relatively rare) or to the lubricant, they cause no adverse effects or long-term risks to health. Indeed, they may protect your health.
5. They provide more protection against sexually transmitted diseases than any other contraceptive. This includes gonorrhoea, chlamydia, trichomonas, thrush, herpes, genital warts and HIV (see p. 488 for safer sex guidelines). They also protect against cervical cancer and should be widely promoted for this reason too.
6. They carry no health risks when used immediately following childbirth.
7. They give a man some direct responsibility for birth control.
8. They may help a man who ejaculates too quickly to keep an erection longer.
9. There's no wet spot in the bed afterwards, and you won't drip for hours.
10. It isn't necessary to use spermicides,† which can be messy.
11. Both of you can participate in using them.
12. You need only use them during intercourse.

---

*See p. 278 for how to work out your fertile days.
†But spermicides do offer some protection against sexually transmitted diseases – see Chapter 23.

Disadvantages

1. The interruption of love-making may be unacceptable to one or both of you, especially if you lack confidence about sex. You can try to get round this by making it part of love play.
2. Some men complain they lose sensation or find it more difficult to get or keep an erection. This can be overcome if you talk about it and alter how you make love too, and it usually disappears when you get used to them.
3. If both of you are not motivated to use them correctly, the chances of using them wrongly or not at all are high.

THE DIAPHRAGM

The diaphragm in its present form – made of rubber – was developed in the nineteenth century. It was very popular until the 1960s, when it was displaced almost overnight by the Pill. Research to improve all barrier methods practically stopped at the same time. Now, because of the risks related to hormonal methods and IUDs, increasing numbers of women are again considering barrier methods, particularly women over twenty-five, though the figures up to 1983 don't show that increasing numbers are using them. The women's health movement is also calling for increased research to improve barrier methods by reducing their disadvantages and making a wider range of choices available.

Description

The diaphragm is a flexible rubber cup-like container, which fits over the cervix and is held in place by a metal spring in the rim. The rim rests against the pubic bone inside your vagina (see diagram) and the cup covers your cervix so that sperm can't get through. You should not be able to feel it once it is in place. There are three types of diaphragm spring: flat, coiled or arcing. Most women are offered the flat-spring type first, and it is the most commonly used. The coiled spring is softer and suggested for

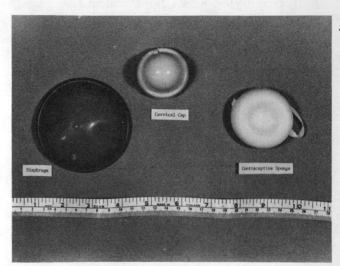

Phyllis Ewen

Diaphragm/cap/sponge

women who get cystitis from, or are made uncomfortable by, pressure on the vaginal walls from the flat type. The arcing type has a very strong spring and is recommended for women with weak vaginal walls, a retroverted uterus or a long cervix.

Women's vaginas differ so diaphragms come in ten different sizes measured by the width, from 55 to 100 cm in multiples of five. If you gain or lose more than 7 lb (3 kg) of weight or have had a baby, miscarriage or abortion since getting a diaphragm, you may need a different size and should be measured for this. If you can feel the diaphragm once it is in place, it is probably the wrong size or the wrong type for you.

It has always been assumed that a diaphragm works only if it is used with spermicide, and that its role is only to hold the spermicide in place. Yet no research has conclusively proved that this is true. A number of clinics are now doing trials which compare the effectiveness of a diaphragm with and without spermicide. Until this has been fully tested, we (have to) assume that spermicide is needed. Unfortunately, it is often the spermicide rather than the diaphragm itself which puts us off using it. We can only wait for the results of these trials to see if our practice can change.

There are obstacles to getting a diaphragm – many doctors do not trust our ability to use them well and many assume we would not be interested and don't even suggest them. In addition, many doctors don't know how to fit them. You may have to insist to get one or try another doctor. Your GP or clinic may not stock all three kinds, but they can be ordered.

Where to Get a Diaphragm

You can get one from a family planning clinic or GP who knows how to fit them. Women who are sure they know their correct size can order and buy one from a chemist. To determine the correct size for you the doctor or nurse measures with two fingers inserted into your vagina. S/he should teach you how to insert and remove it until you feel comfortable with the procedure. You will probably be given a practice diaphragm with spermicide to take home and try every day for a week. The jokes about it flying across the room the first few times are not an exaggeration. It may seem impossible at first, but persevere. It will get easy! You will be asked to come back with the diaphragm in place so they can check again that you have inserted it correctly, that it is the right size, and that the spermicide is acceptable to you. During that week, you should use another method of contraception if you need it.

You should return to the clinic once a year with your diaphragm, or earlier if you have any problems or if it has become damaged.

How to Use a Diaphragm and Spermicide*

1. Make sure the diaphragm is clean and dry.
2. Put a ribbon of spermicide (about a teaspoon to a tablespoonful) inside the cup and around the inside of the rim. Leave a space on either side of the rim for thumb and finger – this makes it less slippery.

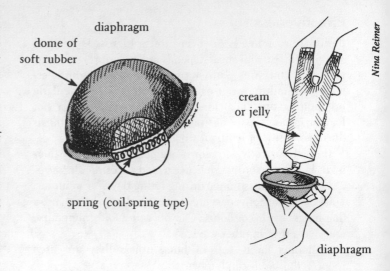

diaphragm
dome of soft rubber
spring (coil-spring type)
cream or jelly
diaphragm

Nina Reimer

3. Holding the rim with thumb and index finger on either side, squeeze the two sides together. With legs apart, either standing with one foot on a chair, squatting, lying down, or sitting on the loo, separate your labia and insert the device into your vagina. Slide it up the vagina in the direction of the small of your back and over the cervix.

4. Check that it is covering your cervix by feeling with your finger. You will need to know what your cervix feels like first (see p. 31). Check also that the rim is sitting on your pubic bone in front. If you squat and bear down (that is, push down with your vaginal muscles as if trying to push the diaphragm out), it should stay in place. If it doesn't try inserting it again. It is also easier to reach your cervix to feel that it's in place if you bear down. The diaphragm can become displaced during (very vigorous) intercourse though not easily if it's in correctly.

5. Spermicide is active for at least three hours. It is recommended that you insert additional spermicide into your vagina, without removing the diaphragm, just before intercourse if more than three hours have passed. Either you or your partner can do this by using a spermicide applicator or inserting a pessary (see p. 284).

6. The diaphragm should be left in place for at least six hours after last intercourse and removed at a convenient time. It is recommended that you do not leave the diaphragm in for more than twenty-four hours, because there is a possible increased risk of toxic shock syndrome, and also because of odour.

7. To remove it, use your index or middle finger. Reach in and hook your finger around the rim and pull downwards. Be careful your fingernail doesn't tear it. If you're having difficulty, try bearing down first.

8. Wash the diaphragm with warm water and mild soap, rinse thoroughly and dry with a clean towel. Do NOT put

*These are the standard instructions given in the UK. They have a wide margin for error and have never been adequately researched mainly because women don't volunteer to be research subjects! You may not need to use so much spermicide. In some countries application on the inside only is recommended.

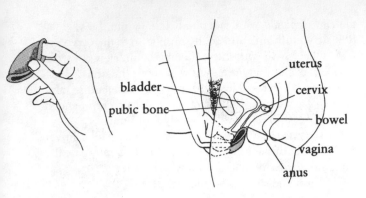 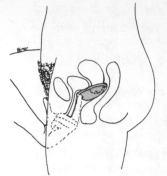 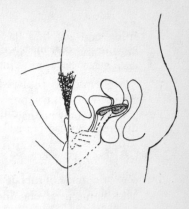

Nina Reimer

talc on the diaphragm before you put it away. This used to be recommended, but it is now thought that talc is associated with some cancers. Store the diaphragm away from heat. Every so often check it for holes by holding it up to the light or filling it with water to see if it leaks, especially around the rim.

Effectiveness

Failure rates between 2 per cent and 15 per cent are quoted. The failure rate depends on whether you are using the right size, and on how well you and your partner use the device. If it's too small, it will be inefficient and is more likely to be displaced. If you do not insert it correctly or before intercourse begins, or do not leave it in long enough after intercourse, or do not use it every time you need protection, you are more likely to get pregnant.

The diaphragm is more complicated to use than a condom, but if the person teaching you is positive about this method and teaches you well, the effectiveness with which you use it will increase and you will probably be more willing to use it.

During your fertile days, for extra protection you can either use extra spermicide or use condoms with the diaphragm. Adding a condom gives almost 100 per cent protection. Or avoid intercourse during your fertile days and make love in other ways.

To make the use of a diaphragm less intrusive in love-making, some women put it in several hours before they expect to need it, and add spermicide to their vagina just before love-making. Others put it in whether they think they will need it or not and treat it like brushing their teeth, as a habit they have every day. This makes sense if you and your partner make love regularly and/or sleep together every night. However, once you are used to using it, there is no reason why you shouldn't keep it by the bed to use when needed. Some women get their partners to put it in, making it a part of love-making.

If the diaphragm becomes displaced during intercourse, and you think you could get pregnant, you can get 'morning-after' pills (for three days) or an IUD (up to five days) after intercourse (see p. 295). This may not be necessary if it happens during your non-fertile days. Check with your GP/clinic if you aren't sure.

Adverse Effects

1. Particular spermicides can cause an allergic reaction

in a small number of women. This can cause itching, vaginal discharge and a lot of discomfort. Try a different spermicide.

2. The diaphragm may cause discomfort or more frequent and/or painful urination. These may be signs of a urinary tract infection or cystitis. Diaphragms are associated with a higher incidence of urinary tract infection. Having a pee before and after sex may prevent this. If not, check with the doctor whether the size is right or try a different type of diaphragm or a cervical cap.

Who Should Not Use a Diaphragm

1. Women with a damaged or unhealthy cervix, with a severely displaced uterus, with cystocele (protrusion of the bladder through the vagina wall), or with fistulas (other openings in the vagina).

2. Women or their partners who are allergic to rubber or all types of spermicide (rare).

Advantages

1. It does not delay or affect fertility.

2. There are few adverse effects and no long-term risks to health.

3. It may in fact protect your health by reducing the risk of getting some sexually transmitted diseases, and may help to prevent cervical cancer, though not as effectively as condoms.

4. It only needs to be used with intercourse, not all the time.

5. If used during your period, the diaphragm can catch the menstrual blood and reduce the messiness, though some now suggest this is not good practice due to possible risk of toxic shock syndrome (see p. 566).

Disadvantages

1. It takes time to learn to use it and feel comfortable with putting it in and removing it.

2. Women who don't like to touch their genitals and vagina will need to overcome this. This isn't difficult and is worth trying to do. (See Chapters 3 and 14.)

3. There may be a loss of spontaneity during love-making if you have to stop to put it in, and this requires motivation from both partners. Try putting it in before you need it (see above) or incorporating it into love-making.

4. Some people find spermicide messy and smelly, and along with semen it can drip for hours. Some people who

enjoy oral sex find the taste and smell of spermicides unpleasant, though some brands are considered better than others.

5. It may be displaced during intercourse if it isn't in correctly or is the wrong size.

6. You may not have the privacy you will want to use it.

CAPS

Caps are made of rubber and are smaller than diaphragms. They come in several different shapes. They fit on to the cervix itself and, unlike diaphragms, they are held in place by suction. As with diaphragms it is recommended to use them with spermicide, despite any clear evidence as to whether or not this makes them more effective. As we go to press, trials are in progress which should provide this information.

Description

There are several types of cap. The most commonly used is called a cervical cap. It is shaped like a thimble and fits very closely over the cervix. There are two variations; one is lighter and made of softer rubber than the other. They come in four sizes.

The vault (or Dumas) cap covers the cervix but does not fit as closely to the cervix, and comes in five sizes. It is mainly used for women whose cervix won't easily hold a cervical cap.

The Vimule cap is a variation of the vault cap and comes in three sizes. It is mainly for women who cannot use the vault cap because their cervix is too long for suction to hold the vault cap in place.

The size of your cervix determines the correct size of cap, but with a limited number of sizes not all women can necessarily get a good fit. Precise fitting is important so that it is not displaced during intercourse or at other times. As with the diaphragm, the size needs to be checked after childbirth, miscarriage or abortion or with weight changes of more than 7 lb (3 kg). As with the diaphragm, you should not be able to feel it once it is in place.

A Comparison of Caps and Diaphragms

Caps can be more difficult to insert and remove than diaphragms at first, especially if you find it difficult to reach your cervix. They may or may not be as effective as the diaphragm; too few studies have been done to say for sure. On the plus side, caps do not cause discomfort, and because they do not put pressure on the bladder they are unlikely to affect urination or cause cystitis. Women with weak vaginal muscles and some types of uterine prolapse will be able to use the cap but not the diaphragm. Women with long vaginas who have trouble reaching their cervix will find it easier to use a diaphragm than a cap.

How to Use Cap and Spermicide

1. Check that the cap has no holes and is clean and dry.
2. Fill about one-third of the cap with spermicide.
3. Sitting, squatting or lying down, compress the top of the cap, separate your labia and slide it into the vagina. Release your thumb and gently push it on to the cervix.

4. Check with your finger that it is completely covering your cervix and that there is no gap above the rim.

5. Leave it in for at least six hours after intercourse, and remove it at a convenient time. It is usually recommended not to leave it in longer than twenty-four hours.

6. To remove, insert your index or middle finger between the rim of the cap and your cervix. Gently ease the cap downwards and withdraw it with two fingers.

7. Wash and store as for diaphragm.

Adverse Effects

1. Rubber and/or spermicides may cause an allergic reaction.

2. Some doctors have noticed that the Vimule cap can cause red marks in the area around the cervix. It is uncertain whether this is significant, and more studies need to be done.

Advantages and Disadvantages

Apart from the comments above, the same as for the diaphragm.

SPERMICIDES

Spermicides are chemicals that block sperm progression and are capable of destroying sperm. The aim with all spermicides is to deposit them as near to your cervix as possible, so that it is covered by the chemical.

Spermicide is meant to be used with diaphragms and caps (see above) but its use is also suggested in other parts of this chapter for extra protection with other methods and as a lubricant with condoms. Spermicide can also be used alone, but this is not recommended except in emergencies because of the high failure rate. However, using a spermicide is still much better than using nothing.

Spermicides containing a high concentration of the chemical nonoxynol-9 have been shown in lab tests to kill HIV, the virus that can lead to AIDS. However, spermicide by itself cannot be assumed to be effective against HIV in practice and therefore it is not recommended alone (or even with a diaphragm or cap) as protection against HIV. You may, however, want to use it for extra reassurance when using condoms as protection against HIV.

Where to Get Spermicide

Your GP or family planning clinic can provide you with spermicide free of charge, though there may be a limit on how much you can have per year. Spermicide can also be bought at chemists.

Description and How to Use Them

Spermicides come in a number of different forms: foam, cream, jelly, pessaries or film. Each packet will have an expiry date stamped on it; after this date the spermicide is no longer effective and should be thrown away. *We must emphasize that it is not recommended to use spermicides alone.*

Foam is the most effective spermicide because it can fill the whole vagina, whereas other types rarely do so. It is a white, aerated cream which has the consistency of shaving cream. It comes in a can with a plunger-type plastic applicator. To use, shake the can well because the spermicide tends to settle in the bottom and because shaking creates bubbles which make it more effective. Put the applicator on the top of the can and follow the directions for filling it. To insert, put the applicator about 3 to 4 inches (8 to 10 cm) into your vagina, aiming it towards the small of your back. Push the plunger, and remove the applicator without pulling out the plunger. Inserting the applicator is similar to inserting a tampon; if you have never done this, practise a few times with the empty applicator. The applicator should be washed with mild soap and warm water after each use, and dried well. This doesn't have to be done immediately after use.

Creams and jellies. Creams are white, while jellies are clear. Jellies can be less irritating than creams, but they can be gooier. Both come in a plastic tube with an applicator.

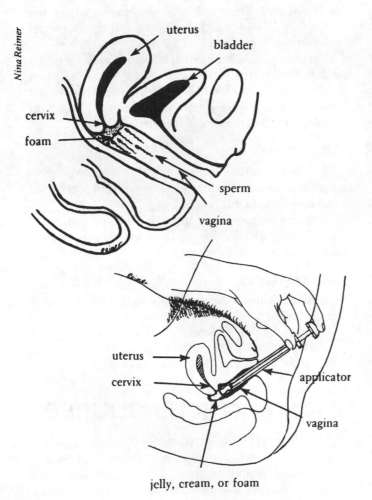

HOW TO INSERT SPERM-KILLING FOAM, CREAM, OR JELLY

uterus
bladder
cervix
foam
sperm
vagina

Nina Reimer

uterus
cervix
applicator
vagina

jelly, cream, or foam

With diaphragm or cap, they can be used directly from the tube. To insert them directly into your vagina, fill the applicator and insert as with foam. Cream or jelly should be inserted a short time before intercourse, to give them time to melt and start working. Clean and dry the applicator as with foam.

Pessaries and film come packed in individual foil packets. Place one in your vagina with middle and index fingers and then push it up towards your cervix with one finger. Once inside your vagina it will melt. A pessary or film should be inserted a short time before intercourse, to give it time to melt and start working.

Effectiveness

Failure rates are reported to be as low as 4 per cent and as high as 25 per cent. Foam can fill the whole vagina, which is why it is the most effective. Other spermicides are not reliable on their own. If you have to use a spermicide by itself, foam is your best choice.

Adverse Effects

Some women may get an allergic reaction – itching, vaginal discharge and discomfort – from one or more types of spermicide. If this happens, try another type and/or brand.

Advantages

1. There are no known adverse effects apart from allergic reactions.
2. They do not affect or delay fertility.
3. Readily available without prescription at chemists if there's no time to go to the GP or clinic.
4. They can provide extra lubrication during intercourse.

Disadvantages

1. Potentially high failure rate if used alone.
2. Messy, smelly and bad-tasting, though some are worse than others.
3. Have to be inserted shortly before intercourse, especially if used alone; or up to three hours before if used with diaphragm or cap.

THE CONTRACEPTIVE SPONGE

This method has only been on the market in Britain since 1985. It was designed as a disposable, over-the-counter alternative to the diaphragm. It is a soft white circular sponge made of polyurethane foam and impregnated with the spermicide nonoxynol-9 (also used in many other spermicides). It comes in one size only. There is a dimple in the middle that fits over the cervix, and there is a loop attached to make removal easier. It acts as a barrier to sperm and the spermicide also kills sperm.

Where to Get a Sponge

The sponge is only available from chemists; it is not available free on the NHS.

How to Use a Sponge

1. Moisten it thoroughly with water and insert high in the vagina. Check that the dimple is over the cervix.

2. Once inside your vagina, the sponge will expand.

3. Leave it in for a minimum of six hours and a maximum of twenty-four hours after intercourse.

4. Intercourse may be repeated as often as desired while it is in place, without extra spermicide.

5. To remove, catch the loop with your finger and gently pull out.

6. You cannot re-use the sponge. Throw it away.

When Not to Use It

Some doctors recommend not using it during menstruation, because the risk of toxic shock syndrome is not yet known.

Effectiveness

A trial at the Margaret Pyke Centre in London and other studies found the sponge to have a failure rate of 7 to 25 per cent. Family planning clinics do not supply them because of this potentially high failure rate and also because of their cost.

Adverse Effects

1. Allergic reaction to the spermicide in some women, that is, itching, vaginal discharge and a lot of discomfort.

2. One woman has recently complained of vaginal numbness, which her doctor confirmed by tasting the sponge with the tip of her tongue, and found it had an anaesthetic effect which lasted several hours.

Advantages

1. You can get them from a chemist without a prescription.

2. No fitting is required.

3. There is no effect on fertility.

4. There is no need to use a separate spermicide.

Disadvantages

1. High failure rate.

2. Sensitivity to the high concentration of spermicide in some women/partners.

3. Some women have found they shred while in place and pieces of sponge keep coming out after it has been removed.

4. They may be displaced or expelled far more easily than a diaphragm.

WITHDRAWAL (COITUS INTERRUPTUS OR PULLING OUT)

Withdrawal is not a method that is recommended by doctors, but estimates are that more people employ it than use the diaphragm or the IUD in the UK and that it is practised by people all over the world.

The method involves the man withdrawing his still erect penis from your vagina just before ejaculation, so that no semen is deposited inside your vagina or on the vaginal lips. Commitment and discipline are needed, and the man must be able to recognize when he is reaching a climax and withdraw quickly before it happens. However, some semen may come out of his penis before he has an orgasm, enough to make you pregnant. Alternatively, he can withdraw well before orgasm and you can use other ways for both of you to come (see Chapter 14). But semen may come out of his penis any time after he has an erection, which makes this method have a potentially high failure rate, particularly around your fertile days.

If you definitely don't want to get pregnant, this method is not for you, though it is a lot better than using nothing. Many people have practised it successfully for years, so doctors don't often hear about them, but many also end up with unwanted pregnancy.

Effectiveness

Failure rates are said to range from 5 per cent to 20 per cent but few studies have been done to confirm this. The more fertile you are, the more likely the method is to fail. Failure mainly occurs if the man doesn't withdraw before he comes or if drops of semen get into your vagina before full ejaculation. If semen gets on your vaginal lips sperm can still swim up your vagina.

For effectiveness, the method is best used in conjunction with fertility awareness techniques. If you then use another method during your fertile days (see Barrier Methods) and 'morning-after' contraception as a back-up if there's an accident, the failure rate will be reduced.

Advantages

1. There is no need to get anything from a doctor or chemist or use anything or talk to anyone about your sex life – it's a very private method.

2. There are no adverse effects or effects on fertility.

3. It's very useful when you have nothing else available and want to have intercourse.

Disadvantages

1. High failure rate, especially with a man who is inexperienced at it.

2. It can limit sexual pleasure if you don't find ways around this. Both of you will be on guard – he to withdraw in time and you hoping that he will manage it.

AVOIDING INTERCOURSE

You don't need to have sexual intercourse to have a sex life. You and your partner can stimulate each other with fingers, hands, mouths and other ways until you both reach orgasm, separately or together. Some women prefer this; all it needs is the confidence to tell your partner.

Sometimes, what we really want is not to have sex at all, which is the most effective form of birth control.

Read Part II, where you will find more discussion about sexuality, ways of making love and asserting our needs.

THE INTRA-UTERINE DEVICE (IUD or coil)

About half a million women in Britain are using IUDs, which is about 8 per cent of women using contraception. They are the third most common method after condoms and the Pill.

IUDs are a very convenient form of contraception. Most women get on fine with them. However, they can cause serious side-effects. The trick to living with an IUD is to know what can go wrong so that you can do something about it before it becomes serious.

Description

An IUD fits inside your uterus. It prevents pregnancy by causing the lining of the uterus to change so that a fertilized egg cannot implant. Copper IUDs also kill sperm. There are threads attached to it which protrude several centimetres into your vagina through your cervix.

There are three types of IUD, though more brands. Only one type is widely used and available in Britain now: this is the copper IUD. It is made of polypropylene or polyethylene (hard rubber-like substances) with thin copper wire wound round part of it. It is smaller than older types of IUD. Some come in two sizes, some in only one. The older copper devices need to be changed every three years and the newer ones every five years because the copper slowly disintegrates.

An inert device called the Lippes Loop is no longer manufactured, but will still be available until supplies run out. It is called 'inert' because it contains no active substances like copper. Many women will still be using it because it does not have to be changed regularly like a copper device, unless there are problems. A second inert device, the Saf-T-Coil is no longer manufactured because it wasn't profitable. A third inert device, the Dalkon Shield, was removed from the market because women experienced too many complications with it. A major international law suit against its manufacturer is being waged in the USA. In late 1987 the court agreed a total amount of compensation but the case is far from over as we go to press. This device caused a high number of cases of septic miscarriage and seventeen known deaths, along with other problems, before it was removed from the market. If you have an IUD in place and don't know what it is, get it checked, particularly if it was fitted in the early 1970s. If it is a Dalkon Shield, have it removed as soon as possible.

The third type of device, which was available in the UK until the end of 1987, is impregnated with progesterone and has to be changed each year. It was rarely offered to women

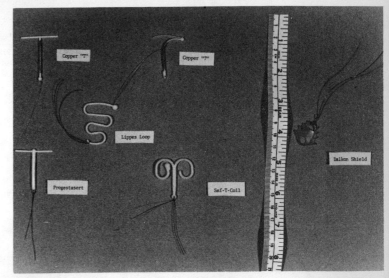

IUDs

Phyllis Ewen

because it is associated with a high incidence of ectopic pregnancy (see p. 439), and offered few advantages over existing IUDs. New ones being researched (but not on the UK market as we go to press) will release progestogen, a synthetic form of progesterone. Both of these continuously release small amounts of hormone in the uterus, which affects the uterine lining and the body in similar ways to the mini-pill.

Where to Get an IUD

IUDs must be inserted and removed by a doctor specially trained in this procedure. The best place to go for this is a family planning clinic where staff will have more practice, and therefore more skill, in inserting IUDs than many GPs. (The skill of the practitioner is important in relation to avoiding any problems that might be caused at insertion.)

Because an IUD can carry infections already present in your vagina or cervix into your uterus, it is important that you have no such infection before the IUD is inserted. If you think you are or have been at risk of acquiring an STD you should go to a sexually transmitted disease (or special) clinic (see p. 489) so that all appropriate tests can be done, especially for chlamydia and gonorrhoea. You would be wise to get an STD check regularly after that, even if you have no symptoms, because an infection can travel up the IUD threads into your uterus. This will minimize the risk of any infection you may get remaining undetected and causing serious damage or possible infertility.

Insertion will normally be done during your period because your cervix is softer, making insertion easier. It should be fitted towards the end of your period as expulsion is less likely than if fitted at the beginning. The doctor will measure the size of your uterus to determine the best size of IUD. To insert it the doctor will put a speculum in your vagina and insert the IUD through a thin tube in your cervix. The IUD is compressed inside the tube and will open into its real shape in your uterus. You can expect this procedure to cause discomfort or hurt, but different women feel different amounts of pain. This depends partly on whether the woman is relaxed and on how skilled the doctor is. Some women feel faint, and nausea is common. You may want to take someone with you to bring you home, just in case. You may get bleeding in the first day or so, and pain or cramps as your body adjusts to the device. These should not continue. If they do, and you feel something is wrong, go back to the doctor. You will probably be told that it will go away, but listen to your body. One of the most common times for infection to start with an IUD is soon after insertion.

You should not be able to feel the IUD once it is in place. Your partner may be able to feel the threads during intercourse but this shouldn't bother him.

You will be told to feel for the threads each month after the end of your period and once or twice in between periods for the first two to three months to make sure it is still in place. You should go for a check-up six to eight weeks after insertion and then once each year.

INSERTION OF A NOVA T IUD

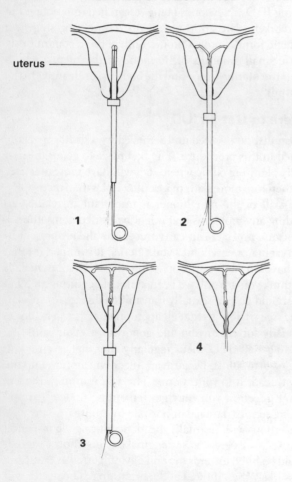

uterus

1
2
4
3

1 Introducer with IUD emerging from end
2 IUD being pushed out and springing into shape
3 IUD fully emerged
4 String protruding into vagina

If you want to stop using the IUD, DO NOT TRY TO REMOVE IT YOURSELF. You could permanently damage yourself and, in fact, risk your life. Go back to the clinic, where it will be removed for you. Removal is done with a speculum in place and the device is gently pulled out by the threads. There may be discomfort, but it doesn't last very long and is usually tolerable. Slight dilatation of your cervix may be needed if it doesn't seem to be coming out easily. If the threads break, the doctor will need to use an instrument to reach into your uterus and pull it out slowly. You will probably need an anaesthetic if there are problems.

Some women, who have wanted the IUD removed, have reported that doctors have refused to do so, belittling their worries that something is wrong, or for other reasons. If this happens to you, contact your local CHC/LHC, FPIS, women's group or WHRRIC in London for advice.

Insertion after Childbirth, Miscarriage or Abortion

You may be offered an IUD at these times. However, expulsion and perforation rates are higher than if there is a delay of two weeks after abortion or miscarriage, or four to six weeks after birth. You may well not be interested in intercourse at this time anyway, so it is better to give your body a rest before getting an IUD.

A number of NHS doctors insert IUDs after abortion as a policy (there is an extra fee in it for them) and they may not discuss this with you much or at all. If you haven't definitely decided that this is the form of contraception you want to use, refuse it. It is unethical for a doctor to make abortion dependent on your accepting a contraceptive. If this happens to you, seek help elsewhere.

Effectiveness

The failure rate is 1–4 per cent per year. Sometimes the IUD just doesn't work, and there is nothing you can do about it. Or it can be expelled from your uterus without you necessarily knowing, which is why it's important to check the strings regularly.

For nearly 100 per cent effectiveness, you can use a condom or spermicide during your fertile days, especially in the first three months when the chance of expulsion is greatest. However, you may want to ask yourself if the risks of the IUD are worth this type of doubling up of methods.

Who Can Use an IUD

It is now mainly recommended for women over 25 who are in relationships in which both partners are monogamous (see 1. below).

Who Should Definitely Not Use an IUD

1. Women who have or have had pelvic inflammatory disease (PID) or infection, or who are at high risk of getting PID (women with more than one sexual partner are at higher risk because they have more than one possible source of infection; women whose partners have more than one sexual partner are also at higher risk for the same

reason). Even if previous infection has cleared up, some studies show the risk of new infection is higher with an IUD. Untreated infection, especially chlamydia, which doesn't always show any symptoms, can lead to infertility.

2. Pregnant women, or women who may be pregnant.

3. Women with undiagnosed abnormal vaginal bleeding.

4. Women with suspected or diagnosed cancer of the cervix or uterus.

5. Women with copper allergy (rare) or Wilson's disease.

6. Women with previous ectopic pregnancy.

7. Women with uterine fibroids, an abnormally shaped uterus or uterine scars from past surgery.

8. Women who already have very heavy menstrual periods.

9. Women having systemic corticosteroid treatment or other immunosuppressive treatment, because this lowers your body's ability to fight infection.*

Who Should Be Cautious about Using an IUD

1. Women with endometriosis or endometrial polyps.

2. Women with valvular heart disease, because of increased risk of infection. If you do use an IUD, you should have antibiotics at insertion and removal to lower the risk.

3. Women with insulin-dependent diabetes. IUDs may have a higher failure rate for you, though studies disagree.

Advantages

1. With an IUD you need do nothing else to prevent pregnancy, except check regularly that you can feel the threads.

2. The device usually needs to be changed only after several years, and you need a medical check only once a year.

3. It doesn't interfere with love-making, so women who get few or no adverse effects find it very convenient.

4. If you do not get any of the complications listed below, an IUD will not affect fertility. You may want to wait several months after removal before getting pregnant to give your uterus a rest, though this is not considered medically necessary.

Disadvantages

The disadvantages of an IUD are the possible adverse effects and long-term health risks.

Complications from an IUD affect only a minority of users but they can be serious and affect you for the rest of your life. *Bleeding, late or missed period, backache, one-sided or other abdominal pain, fever, chills, blood clots, unusual or bad-smelling discharge, pain during intercourse, uterine or pelvic tenderness may be signs of infection, perforation of your uterus by the IUD, a lost IUD, preg-*

*Editors' note: Avoidance of the IUD is also thought to be advisable for women with HIV or AIDS, for similar reasons. See, for example, Judith Bury in References.

nancy, ectopic pregnancy or expulsion of the device.

See your doctor for minor problems lasting more than two cycles but do not delay if it seems serious.

The following are the possible complications that can result from IUD use:

1. *Heavier, more painful periods.* Most women get heavier bleeding during periods, and some get bleeding or spotting between periods, especially just before they are due. Dull ache and cramps may get worse during periods and also happen at other times of the month.

2. *Pelvic infection.* This is caused by gonorrhoea, chlamydia or other bacteria that are sexually transmitted. It is treated with antibiotics, the type depending on the type of infection. The risk of uterine/tubal infection increases with an IUD. Untreated infection can cause not only infertility but chronic inflammation and pain for years, and may even lead to hysterectomy to relieve symptoms and, rarely, even death. If pelvic inflammatory disease is diagnosed (see p. 503), the IUD should be removed and you should use another contraceptive. At least two out of every 100 women per year of use get infection with an IUD – see your doctor immediately if you suspect anything. It may be a good idea to have annual STD checks, or more often, particularly if you or your partner have had intercourse with others. Note that antibiotics taken for other reasons may mask symptoms of infection.

3. *Perforation.* In a very few cases the IUD may perforate your uterus during insertion or afterwards. It is estimated to happen in only one in 1,000 cases, but this may be higher with an inexperienced doctor. It requires immediate treatment. If your uterus is perforated, the IUD may travel into another part of your abdomen, another reason why you can't feel the threads. Again see your doctor immediately. Ultrasound or X-ray will have to be used to find it, and laparoscopy or other surgery will be needed to remove it.

4. *Expulsion.* Your uterus may try to expel an IUD because it is a foreign body, and pain/bleeding may mean it has moved down into your cervix or vagina. This happens to 1–4 per cent of women using it. If you can feel the IUD itself when you feel for the threads, it is coming out. See your doctor immediately. Less often it may come all the way out without you noticing, especially during your period. You may be advised to check tampons or pads for it during the first three months after insertion, which is when half of all expulsions occur. T-shaped devices and the Multiload are said to have lower expulsion rates than others.

5. *Pregnancy.* Pregnancy rates are 1–4 per cent with an IUD and somewhat lower in women over thirty and those who have previously had a child. If you do get pregnant, you will first have to decide whether or not you want to continue the pregnancy. If you decide not to continue, you will need an abortion; the IUD will be removed during it. The pregnancy can go to term with an IUD in place. However, the chance of infection, miscarriage between 12 and 24 weeks, premature labour and delivery, and death of the baby are all increased if the IUD is left in place.

Opinion varies about the degree of risk. Some books give the risk of miscarriage as 25 per cent if the device is removed, compared to 50 per cent if it is left in place. Doctors recommend removing the IUD if you are within the first twelve weeks of pregnancy and the strings are easily visible and offer no resistance during removal. After twelve weeks it may be left in with careful supervision. If the pregnancy continues to term, there is no evidence the baby will be born damaged. Bleeding, fever or leaking amniotic fluid should send you to the doctor. At childbirth, the IUD is normally expelled with the placenta or must be removed by the doctor.

6. *Ectopic pregnancy.* Up to one in twenty of women who do get pregnant with an IUD have a pregnancy that does not implant in their uterus, but in one of their fallopian tubes. THIS IS A LIFE-THREATENING CONDITION. *If you have symptoms of pregnancy accompanied by one-sided or generalized abdominal pain that doesn't stop, a delayed or missed period or a brownish discharge instead of a normal period, go to the casualty or emergency department of your nearest hospital.* For your safety, doctors are advised to treat every pregnancy as ectopic, until proved otherwise. For more information, see p. 439.

7. *Embedding.* The lining of the uterus can begin to grow around the IUD. It will usually still be effective but it can cause more pain at removal, and in difficult cases laparoscopy will be needed to remove it. This is more likely to happen the longer the IUD is in the uterus.

8. *Death.* Five deaths and one near death due to IUD complications were reported between 1973 and 1983 in Britain. All of them could have been avoided if doctors had known what to look for and what to do. Instructions to doctors on IUDs now contain recommendations (as in this section) that, it is hoped, will avoid deaths in future. But this indicates just how seriously you should take any symptoms that something is wrong.

HORMONAL METHODS

In the 1940s it was accidentally discovered that the hormone progesterone affected fertility and soon afterwards that another hormone, oestrogen, prevented ovulation. In the 1950s progestogens, synthetic forms of progesterone, were first produced. These developments revolutionized contraception. Within a few years the first birth control pill had been synthesized and, not long after that, work began on various ways of using hormones to prevent conception. Later, progestogen-only methods were developed when it was thought that only the oestrogen in the Pill was responsible for health risks. Methods now on the market like injectables, implants and vaginal rings were all first thought about in the 1960s as alternative 'delivery systems' for hormonal contraceptives for women. The hormones used are synthetic versions of hormones that women's bodies produce naturally (see Chapter 3). These hormones regulate our menstrual cycle as well as affecting our other body systems. By taking them we are not only preventing pregnancy but changing our entire body chemistry as well.

THE PILL (Oral Contraception or OCs)

In 1960 the first birth control pill was approved in the USA. Although it was not adequately tested, its use spread rapidly all over the world and caused great excitement both in the medical community and among women. It was almost 100 per cent effective in preventing pregnancy and didn't interfere with sexuality. Within a few years millions of women were using it and their numbers steadily rose until the mid-1970s.

Medical literature confirmed that the Pill carried risks as early as 1962. In 1968–9 the first major studies were completed on the risk of thrombosis from the Pill, and this information was widely publicized. From these British studies came guidelines about using OCs containing less than 50 mcg of oestrogen. New information about the Pill is emerging all the time – in fact, the Pill is now the most widely researched drug on the market.

The first Pills contained 150 mcg of oestrogen plus progestogen. This dosage of oestrogen caused serious side-effects, including death, so the amount of oestrogen was steadily reduced until now it is 30 mcg. Fewer women are taking the Pill now than in 1975 but it is still the most widely used method of birth control for women.

The Pill is a powerful drug. Most women get on well with it and don't have serious health problems, but there are health risks which everyone taking it needs to watch out for. There are also women for whom the Pill is dangerous and others who should use it only with caution. As with any drug, signals that something is wrong should be taken seriously.

There are two main types of Pill, the combined Pill and the progestogen-only Pill (POP), described separately below. With both types you take one pill every day for most or all of the month, depending on the brand. There are more than two dozen brands, containing one of two types of oestrogen and one of eight types of progestogen. Newer formulations are coming out regularly.

Where to Get the Pill

The Pill is available on prescription only in the UK, from your family planning clinic or GP. It is important that your medical history is taken, because particular illnesses (or history of illness), or other drugs (including cigarette smoking), will affect whether you should take the Pill. The doctor will go over this with you on your first visit. It is also important that you are monitored regularly (with blood pressure and weight checks and regular cervical smears; see p. 521). You will be offered a cervical smear at the first visit, but can have it at a later visit if preferred. You will be asked to return for a check-up and more supplies three months after the first visit and then every six months thereafter.

THE COMBINED PILL

The combined Pill contains a combination of oestrogen and progestogen. Most women take combined Pills which contain 30 or 35 mcg of oestrogen per pill, while the dosage of progestogen varies from one Pill to another. Pills containing 50 mcg of oestrogen each are used mainly by women who need a stronger dosage, e.g. those on specific drugs that reduce the Pill's efficiency. Higher dosages than that are still available but never prescribed for contraceptive purposes in the UK.

Two newer types of combined Pill are 'biphasic' and 'triphasic' pills. With these the amount of progestogen is varied in two or three phases over one Pill cycle; in some brands, the amount of oestrogen is varied too. The purpose of these is to try and imitate the rise and fall of natural hormones during a menstrual cycle, and to reduce the total dosage of hormones taken each month.

The oestrogen and progestogen in the combined Pill together prevent ovulation by stopping the production of the natural hormones that make an egg mature in the ovary. The progestogen makes cervical mucus thicker and sperm are less able to survive in it (a barrier effect), and prevents the uterine lining from developing so that if an egg happens to be fertilized, it will have difficulty implanting in the uterus. It also affects the motility of the fallopian tubes, which therefore affects the passage of the egg to the womb. The Pill simulates early pregnancy in your body, which is why some of its side-effects are like those of early pregnancy, for example, nausea.

You do not actually get a period on the combined Pill, but you do get what is called 'withdrawal' bleeding in Pill-free days, which is like a period but often lighter and shorter.

There is no way of telling in advance which Pill suits which woman. Some may cause minor side-effects while others don't, so you may have to try several brands in order to find one that suits you.

How to Take the Combined Pill

Combined Pills come in packets which contain twenty-one (or twenty-two) pills. You take one each day, with seven (or six) pill-free days at the end of each packet. With most brands you start your first packet on the first day of your next period, which gives you immediate protection against pregnancy. Some still start on the fifth day of your next period (this used to be the norm); with these, you will need to use another method (condoms or diaphragm or cap) for the first seven days of that first packet until the pills are effective enough to protect you alone.

A few brands of combined Pill are called Everyday (ED) pills because they have seven (or six) 'dummy' pills to take on the days that would otherwise have been pill-free. These are mainly intended for women who are afraid they will not be able to remember when to start their next packet. With ED Pills, you will need additional contraceptive protection with a barrier method for the first fourteen days after you start taking them.

It is important to decide on a time of day to take the pill, and make it into a habit, like brushing your teeth. Common times for many women are just after getting up or just before going to sleep. The combined Pill is effective as long as you take it within twelve hours of your usual time (i.e. within thirty-six hours of your last pill). For example, if you normally take it at midnight every night, and one night you forget, the effectiveness is not reduced as long as you take it before noon the next day. If this happens, you should go back to your regular time with the next pill. (In the example, you would have taken the pill before noon the next day and the next one again that night at midnight.) Sticking to the same time each day avoids a lot of confusion and worry!

Biphasic and triphasic combined Pills have to be taken in a specific order, because of the differing doses in each pill. You will be given directions for this, and all Pill packets have directions enclosed. These written directions can be confusing, so ask if you aren't sure.

If You Miss a Combined Pill

Take it as soon as you remember and take the next one on time, finishing the packet as usual. If you missed the Pill for twelve hours or more, you will need to take extra precautions for seven days because there is a chance that you will ovulate. If the seven-day period runs into your Pill-free week, don't take a break between packets. Start the next Pill packet as soon as you finish the current one. With ED Pills, miss out the 'dummy' pills. You may or may not get breakthrough bleeding, depending on the type of Pill you are using.

If you forget more than one pill, you are not protected during the days you missed and for seven days afterwards, so you will need extra protection.

Effectiveness

If you take the combined Pill correctly, it is said to be almost 100 per cent effective. The actual failure rate ranges from 0.1 to 7 per cent. Many pregnancies are the result of late or forgotten pills. Using extra precautions when this happens should reduce the chances of pregnancy. If you find yourself often forgetting pills, you will need to work out what to do about it or consider another method.

There are other reasons for Pill failure, however. Vomiting within three hours or severe diarrhoea within twelve hours of taking a pill may mean that it is not absorbed into the body, which reduces effectiveness. You should use extra precautions as for forgetting a pill. Interactions with certain drugs can also cause Pill failure. These include: some antibiotics, tranquillizers, anti-inflammatory drugs, anti-convulsants and hypnotics. If you are taking these or other drugs, be sure to tell your doctor. *

Editors' note: While some may recommend an increase in the Pill dosage in these circumstances, this could lead to problems including the possibility of other interactions; see, for example, Orme et al. in References.

How Long to Take the Combined Pill

Young women should not start using the Pill until our menstrual cycle has settled into a regular pattern, as a precaution against effects on future fertility while our reproductive system is still developing.

Studies of long-term effects of the Pill indicate two things. First, any long-term health risks are more likely as the number of years of Pill use increases, particularly after ten or more years. Second, that risks increase with age, as all health risks do, sometimes combined with other factors.

It is currently recommended that women who smoke cigarettes should start thinking about changing to another method at age thirty, and definitely by age thirty-five, because the risk of blood clots, strokes and other blood disorders that affect the heart rises sharply after this point. If a woman has no other risk factors and is healthy, it is increasingly being recommended that low-dose Pills can be used till age forty-five, though we do not yet know the wisdom of this.

Natural fertility declines steadily after age thirty-five, meaning that we can get pregnant less easily than we could at sixteen or twenty-five. Depending on what your relationship is like with your partner, you may find it easier at this age to try other methods which carry fewer or no health risks.

Advantages

1. It is a very reliable and convenient method.

2. Doesn't interfere with love-making and, with the fear of pregnancy reduced, you may feel freer to enjoy sex than you did before.

3. Lighter, absolutely regular periods, no ovulation pain, reduced menstrual symptoms.

4. Women with endometriosis may find that reduced menstrual bleeding on the Pill reduces the severity of attacks of endometriosis.

5. There is evidence that the Combined Pill reduces the risk of the following conditions: anaemia, ovarian cysts* and ovarian cancer, endometrial cancer, benign breast disease (with Pills containing a high dose of progestogen), fibroids, pelvic infection in the uterus and tubes, and possibly thyroid disease. These effects of the Pill are being presented as advantages, but they are not a reason for choosing the Pill as a contraceptive, rather than another method. For example, if you have anaemia, Pill use will perhaps reduce it because of less blood loss, but what you really need is a cure for anaemia. Most of us do not know whether we are at high risk of the other conditions listed, so while it may be reassuring to know that the Pill has these 'advantages' the knowledge shouldn't really affect our decisions.

Disadvantages of the Combined Pill

The disadvantages are the Pill's adverse effects and long-term health risks.

Some of the less serious effects listed below may be

*But see item 15 under 'Disadvantages' concerning biphasic and triphasic pills.

alleviated or disappear with a change of Pill. But if you are worried, see your doctor.

If you get symptoms of major problems, stop the Pill immediately and see your doctor without delay. These include: painful swelling in your legs, pain in chest or stomach, breathlessness or cough with blood-stained phlegm, a bad fainting attack or collapse or focal epilepsy, severe migraine or headaches that disturb your vision, disturbance of speech or eyesight (with or without headaches), numbness or weakness in arms or legs, or jaundice. Bear in mind that having stopped the Pill because of these symptoms, you may get pregnant if you have had intercourse within the previous five days.

1. *Delay in return of fertility.* After stopping the Pill, most women get their first post-Pill period within four to six weeks. About one out of 100 women under thirty experiences greater delays. Women over thirty are more likely to experience longer delays, in some cases up to four years. Most women do get pregnant successfully after going off the Pill. But some, especially those who had irregular cycles before starting the Pill and women over thirty, may have difficulty getting pregnant afterwards. It is of course possible that some women may have had fertility problems anyway, which were masked by the Pill. The Pill has not been shown to cause permanent infertility.

2. *Bleeding problems.* On the 30–35 mcg Pills, some women get breakthrough bleeding or spotting during pill-taking, in addition to the withdrawal bleed at the end of each packet. It happens most commonly in the first two or three months of pill-taking. Keep a record of when it happens and tell the doctor at your next visit. Breakthrough bleeding or spotting can also be caused by forgetting a pill; if it isn't being absorbed properly by your body; if the dosage is too low for you. It could be a sign of cervical or other disease too. See your doctor for advice. If a woman has fibroids, which can cause heavy bleeding, these may occasionally become enlarged when she is on the Pill.

3. *No withdrawal bleeding.* There is a chance you may be pregnant if this happens, so have a pregnancy test that provides immediate results (see p. 309 for where to go). If you are definitely pregnant, and want to continue the pregnancy, stop the Pill immediately. If you are pregnant and don't want to continue the pregnancy, seek abortion advice. If you are not pregnant, start the next packet as usual. Lack of withdrawal bleeding rarely happens with biphasic and triphasic pills.

4. *Headaches.* Headaches, particularly severe ones, may be a serious warning signal, especially if you rarely had them before starting the Pill. They may possibly be associated with increased risk of stroke. Report all headaches to your doctor. See above for severe headaches.

5. *Mood changes.* Some women experience increased irritation, anxiety or depression on the Pill. The progestogen is thought to be responsible for this; it alters body chemistry in such a way that Vitamin B6 levels are decreased. This is more likely if the dose of progestogen is high relative to the oestrogen.

6. *Loss of sexual desire.* This is often linked to depression

WHO SHOULD AVOID THE COMBINED PILL

The Pill can be dangerous if you have any of the following conditions. In some instances, if no other contraceptive method seems possible for you, the doctor may say that you could use the Pill under close medical supervision. However, you will need to weigh up the considerable health risks involved, and are advised to try another method.

- A history of any circulatory disease, including sickle cell anaemia, thrombosis, migraine (crescendo or focal type or you are taking ergotamine tablets), heart disease, arterial disease, clotting problems, bad varicose veins, stroke, high blood pressure. [Women with sickle cell trait can take the Pill.]
- Liver disease or problems, including hepatitis, jaundice, cirrhosis, porphyrias, or tumours.
- Undiagnosed vaginal bleeding.
- Recent hydatidiform mole, a pregnancy in which the fetus never develops but the placenta does.
- Actual or possible pregnancy.
- Cancer of the breast or reproductive organ(s).*
- Herpes gestationis, chorea, otosclerosis or other conditions affected by sex steroids.
- Diabetes.
- Gall-bladder disease.

- Four weeks before or after any major surgery.
- Any condition which means you are confined to bed or are unable to move around on your own, temporarily or chronically.
- Women over age forty and cigarette smokers over age thirty. (Some would say age forty-five and thirty-five respectively.)
- Kidney disease.
- Within four weeks after childbirth or while breastfeeding.
- Severe depression.
- Chronic systemic disease, Crohn's disease.
- DES daughter (see p. 520).
- Varicose veins with phlebitis.
- Epilepsy – attacks may be reduced or increased and a higher dose Pill is needed because of drug interaction with anti-epilepsy medicine.
- Serious overweight, or weight gain of more than 10 lb (4.5 kg) while on the Pill.
- Women taking drugs that reduce Pill effectiveness or increase its potency.
- Women who are HIV positive may also be wise to avoid the Pill because of evidence that it affects the immune system (see Disadvantages, no. 13).†

*See Disadvantages nos. 20 and 21. FPA policy is to favour continued use of the Pill in the event of abnormal cervical smear. You may wish to consider the evidence in favour of coming off it – see Cervical Cell Abnormality and Cervical Smears, p. 521.

†**Editors' note:** While there is no evidence that the Pill affects progression of HIV disease, no relevant research has yet been done. There is evidence that suggests that Pill-users exposed to the virus might be more likely to become HIV positive compared with non-Pill-users (see Judith Bury, *British Journal of Family Planning*, in References). The findings of this research are not clear-cut and further studies are in progress.

---

and with relatively high progestogen content. Your vagina may become drier, which may make intercourse painful. A lubricant should help the dryness.

7. *Weight gain and water retention.* The Pill alters water metabolism, which may lead to water retention, swollen ankles, discomfort with contact lenses or weight gain. Some pills may also cause an increase in appetite, leading to weight gain if you eat more.

8. *Nausea.* This usually goes away after a few weeks. It may be reduced by taking the Pill with food.

9. *Increased breast tenderness.* This usually occurs in the first few months of pill-taking. If it doesn't go away, change your brand of pill or use another method. Enlargement of breasts may also be a sign of pregnancy.

10. *Gum inflammation.* If your gums become inflamed, brush your teeth carefully and see a dentist regularly. Explain to the dentist that the Pill may be at fault and get advice. (This problem also occurs in pregnancy.)

11. *Skin problems.* The Pill is associated with and may make some skin conditions worse, including eczema, hives, rashes and chloasma (pigmentation change like freckles). Consult your doctor. Acne or greasy skin may occur if you use a relatively high progestogenic pill and

have a tendency to these conditions. An oestrogenic pill can sometimes reduce the problems. Skin cancer is increasingly being linked to exposure to sunlight, but there has also been some association with the Pill.

12. *Increased body hair.* This may occur with relatively high progestogenic pills, but only if there is a tendency to this condition anyway.

13. *Infections and inflammations.* Some studies indicate that infections like chicken pox and gastric flu, and inflammations like tenosynovitis and allergic polyarthritis are more common in women taking the Pill. This implies that the Pill may affect the immune system in some way.

14. *Gall-stones.* During the early years of Pill-taking, women who are predisposed to gall-stones may have an increased risk of these on the Pill.

15. *Ovarian cysts.* Biphasic and triphasic Pills may cause the formation of ovarian cysts, which may cause lower abdominal pain. It is not yet clear why these occur, but they may have some connection with the effects of progestogen on ovulation. They tend to disappear if you stop taking these Pills and, until more is known about them, it may be better to find another method or type of Pill. They should not require surgery but may be mistaken

for ectopic pregnancy, which may lead to unnecessary surgery.

16. *Complications following childbirth*. The oestrogen in the combined Pill increases the risk of complications after childbirth (e.g. blood clots). Women are advised not to use it for four weeks after childbirth. The oestrogen in the Pill also reduces the amount and quality of breastmilk, so other contraceptive methods are advised during breastfeeding.

17. *Liver problems*. Jaundice may be a serious sign of a number of liver complications, including hepatitis. If you get it, stop taking the Pill immediately and see your doctor. Liver problems, including benign tumours, are very serious. The risk of benign liver tumours, which are often fatal, is increased by Pill use. There is also some evidence of a link between Pill use and liver cancer, which is nearly always fatal. The incidence of liver tumours and cancer in the UK is low, but in some countries it is much more common and may have serious implications for users of the Pill.

18. *Diabetes*. The Pill affects blood sugar and insulin absorption. However, pregnancy is more hazardous for diabetic women, and the POP is usually advised as an alternative to the combined Pill, though there are also other methods you can use.

19. *Circulatory diseases*. In general, the risk of death due to heart attacks, strokes, blood clots, and other arterial diseases is increased by Pill use and length of Pill use. This increased risk persists even after you stop taking it, if you have taken it for more than five years. Cardiovascular disease is responsible for most Pill-related deaths, which is why after a certain age taking the Pill becomes more dangerous. The Pill can increase the risk of blood clots with sickle cell anaemia. Cigarette smoking greatly adds to the risk of circulatory problems on the Pill. Most women on the Pill get a slight increase in blood pressure, though still within the normal range. About 5 per cent get high blood pressure, however, and this is more likely the longer the Pill is used. It is also more likely if you have a family history of high blood pressure, retain water easily, or are overweight. You should stop using the Pill if your blood pressure becomes high, not least because of the risk of a stroke.

20. *Breast cancer*. There is increasing evidence of a link between the Pill and increased risk of breast cancer, particularly in long-term users.[*] For more discussion, see p. 541.

21. *Cervical cancer*. Studies on this subject in relation to the Pill are far from reassuring. For this reason it is essential that women taking the Pill have regular cervical smears. See p. 525 for a discussion of the evidence.

22. *Interactions with other drugs*. Co-trimoxazole – an antibiotic often given as Septrin – appears to enhance the effects of the Pill, as does Vitamin C. One gram of Vitamin C changes a 'low-dose' Pill into a high-dose one, 'with

resulting toxicological implications', as one review puts it (see Orme et al.). In addition, alcohol levels are increased in women taking the Pill. *Women are rarely told about these effects, although they have been known about for some years.*

THE PROGESTOGEN-ONLY PILL (POP OR MINI-PILL)

The POP is also called the mini-pill because it contains no oestrogen (not because of the dosage). It is mainly suggested for women who want an oral contraceptive but who would be advised not to take oestrogen, e.g. women over forty-five and smokers over thirty-five, breastfeeding women, and women with diabetes or mild hypertension. It works by making cervical mucus thicker (a barrier effect), changing the lining of the uterus so that it is less likely to support a fertilized egg, and altering the motility of the tubes. It sometimes prevents ovulation, in about 40 per cent of cycles. You may or may not get a period or irregular menstrual bleeding or spotting on the POP.

How to Take the POP

POPs are taken one per day every day without a break, starting the first packet on the first day of your next period. It is effective from the first day you take it. Different brands have a different number of pills per packet. You start the next packet the day after you finish the last one.

The POP is most effective about four hours after you have taken each pill. If you usually make love at about the same time of day, it may be recommended to you to take the Pill each day about four hours prior to that (whether or not you make love that day). Your love-making may not be that ordered or it may be totally inconvenient for you to take the Pill at that time of day. If so, find a time of day that is most convenient and take it then.

If You Miss a POP

If you miss a POP more than three hours after your regular time, take it as soon as you can and take the next pill on time, finishing the packet as usual. You will need extra precautions for forty-eight hours afterwards.

If you miss more than one pill, you are not covered on the days you've missed pills and for the next forty-eight hours. You will need to take extra precautions.

Effectiveness

The failure rate of the POP is 1–4 per cent. Most pregnancies are the result of forgetting one or more pills, or not taking them on time, but there are other reasons for pill failure. (See Effectiveness of combined pill re vomiting or diarrhoea, p. 291.) If you are taking anti-rheumatics, anti-epileptics and some sedatives, you will be advised to use extra precautions with the POP, since these drugs may reduce its effectiveness. Antibiotics, however, do not seem to reduce the POP's effectiveness.

---

[*]While some of the evidence is conflicting, this is mainly because even well-conducted studies showing no increased risk have serious drawbacks. See McPherson et al., 1986.

WHO SHOULD AVOID THE POP

The POP may be dangerous for women with:
- any liver problems or disorders;
- any hormone-dependent cancers, e.g. breast or other reproductive organs;
- actual or possible pregnancy;
- menstrual irregularity of uncertain causes;
- previous ectopic pregnancy or any condition that would increase the risk of this, e.g. history of pelvic inflammatory disease or tubal surgery.
- after hydatidiform mole (see p. 293).

'MORNING-AFTER' BIRTH CONTROL

If you have had sex without using contraception, or the sheath broke, or you forgot the Pill (especially at the beginning or end of a packet), or you have been raped, or you are afraid your contraceptive method hasn't worked, there is a good chance you can prevent pregnancy within three to five days afterwards.

There are two methods currently available.

THE PILL

Two Eugynon 50 mcg or Ovran 50 mcg pills taken within three days of intercourse and followed exactly twelve hours later by another two will prevent pregnancy 98–99 per cent of the time. These are available only on prescription. Other brands and doses of pill do not work.

They may cause nausea; to avoid this, eat at the same time as you take them. If you vomit or have severe diarrhoea within three hours of taking them, they may not work. If the clinic has not given you two spares just in case, phone them for further advice.

After you have taken them, your period may arrive at any time, even up to a week later than it was due. You may well ovulate between taking the pills and your next period, because of the change of hormone levels. Take care to use contraception or don't have intercourse! If you don't get a full period, have a pregnancy test.

The 'morning-after' pill is not a good alternative to regular methods of birth control, because if you used it regularly it would make your periods irregular. This means you'd have a greater chance of getting pregnant, as you wouldn't know when you were fertile and when you were due. Also the amount of hormone, if taken regularly, would be high.

If you have epilepsy or are taking antibiotics or antidepressants, this may affect the treatment. Tell the doctor you see, so s/he can advise what to do.

Women who should not use the ordinary birth control pill should check with a doctor whether it is all right to take the 'morning-after' pill. Read the section on the Pill carefully.

THE IUD

An IUD can be inserted in your uterus within five days of unprotected intercourse and will prevent a fertilized egg from implanting. (This method is effective up to ten days after unprotected intercourse, but Department of Health rulings about when birth control becomes abortion make it difficult for clinics to offer the 'morning-after' IUD after five to seven days.)

This method is almost 100 per cent effective as a 'morning-after' method. Only one failure has been reported in the UK so far.

The IUD should be removed during your next period, unless you decide you want to try using it for regular birth control. (See section on IUDs for details, p. 287.)

Women who should not use the IUD for regular birth control should check with a doctor whether it is safe to use it temporarily.

Any woman who is at risk of an STD should be checked for this first, since insertion of the IUD may spread infection to the uterus, where it can cause serious problems (see PID, p. 503). (It is possible that you may not obtain reliable results in time, in which case the IUD would be best avoided.)

Follow-up

You should have a follow-up visit to the doctor four weeks after taking the 'morning-after' pill, or during your next period to have the IUD removed. Although both methods are likely to have prevented pregnancy, you can make sure during this visit and talk about how to avoid a crisis again.

Where to Get 'Morning-after' Birth Control

GPs, young people's and family planning clinics should all offer this service. Ring first for an appointment, making it clear there is a time limit, and to check they offer the service. If not, try to talk them into it, as they ought to be offering it. It may be that no one has asked them before. Or you can go to one of the non-NHS clinics listed at the end of this chapter.

Advantages

1. High rate of effectiveness if taken correctly.
2. Convenient and does not interfere with love-making.
3. No known effect on fertility.
4. Reduced period pains.
5. Appears to avoid many of the adverse effects of the combined pill, and no deaths associated with it have been reported in the UK; however, since fewer women have used the POP, fewer have been studied and we know less about its adverse effects.
6. The POP does not affect production of breastmilk. The POP is often suggested for breastfeeding women who want a hormonal method. Some doctors are reluctant to recommend this, however, because although small-scale studies have been done over a seventeen-year period, no large-scale studies have been done to prove that the small amounts of hormone taken by the baby are harmless.

Disadvantages

1. Affects menstrual cycle. The length of cycles varies widely. Most women get a period every twenty-three to thirty-three days, but about 20 per cent of cycles are less than twenty-three days and 10 per cent of cycles are longer than thirty days. Many women get breakthrough bleeding or spotting between periods. Many women with irregular cycles get no bleeding at all. Most cycles settle down; women whose cycles don't, tend to stop using the method.
2. Difficulty knowing if you are pregnant. In women who get regular menstrual cycles and bleeding on the POP, the Pill is probably not preventing ovulation, which means you have a higher risk of accidental pregnancy. No bleeding at all probably means you are not ovulating, and are therefore better protected, but it may also mean you are pregnant, though this is unlikely if you are taking it correctly.

Adverse Effects

The following adverse effects may be experienced:
1. *Headaches, nausea* and *breast tenderness*.
2. *Weight gain*.
3. *Depression, fatigue* and *loss of interest in sex*.
4. *Lower abdominal pain*. This may be caused by ovarian cysts, which seem to be linked to progestogen-only methods. It is not yet clear why these occur, but they may have some connection with the effects of progestogen on ovulation. Cysts tend to disappear if you stop taking the POP, and until more is known about them, it may be better to find another method. These cysts do not require surgery; they may be mistaken for ectopic pregnancy, however, which could lead to unnecessary surgery.
5. If you do get pregnant on the POP, there is an increased risk of *ectopic pregnancy*, similar to that reported with IUDs. This is a life-threatening condition. See p. 439 for symptoms and what to do.
6. Although some doctors may suggest the POP for women with a history of blood clotting disorders there is evidence that progestogen increases the risk of circulatory

problems such as high blood pressure and stroke (see p. 457).

INJECTABLE HORMONAL CONTRACEPTIVES – LAST-RESORT METHODS

There are two injectable contraceptives currently on the UK market, Depo Provera (DMPA or DP) and Noristerat (NET-OEN). Both are progestogens, though different kinds.

Both of these injectables have been the subject of controversy in a number of countries concerning their safety and how they have been promoted by doctors and family planning programmes. In the UK, women campaigned against the licensing of Depo Provera from the mid 1970s until 1984 when a long-term licence was finally granted.

The Campaign against Depo Provera and later the Coordinating Group on Depo Provera (CGDP) documented evidence which showed abuses of women's right to make an informed choice to use the drug. When a public hearing about licensing the drug was held in 1983, the CGDP challenged biases in the research about the drug and its administration. Partly because of the evidence presented by the CGDP, the panel of experts who presided over the hearing decided to recommend the licensing of DP as a last-resort method only. This was a significant, though only partial, victory for feminists. It was an historic occasion for other reasons too: for the first time consumers' representatives were able to intervene in the drug-licensing procedure, and for the first time part of that procedure was held in public.

Unfortunately, the panel's recommendations for restrictions in the use of DP were given no teeth. No one is responsible for ensuring that the restrictions are being followed, except doctors, some of whom abused the drug to begin with.

Hearings on DP were held in the USA at about the same time as the UK hearings. There, advisers to the US Food and Drug Administration recommended not to grant a licence for DP as a contraceptive. (However, DP is used as a contraceptive in the USA; it is available because it is licensed for other indications.)

Because injectables are so easy to give and not so easy to stop using as other methods, they are open to abuse. Some women are much more likely to be offered or encouraged to use an injectable than others, particularly those of us thought to be unmotivated or irresponsible. Colour, class and level of education have also made a difference. (See section on abuses in the introduction to this chapter for example.) These abuses raise a lot of questions about medical practice generally, and certainly do not apply only to injectables.

DP and NET-OEN have not been licensed as first-choice methods in any developed country, yet are used widely in some Third World countries.

One of the consequences of the controversy over injectables is that women who have chosen them and been satisfied with their use have barely spoken out in the UK. Feminists have been accused of making inaccurate statements about the risks of injectables in order to discourage women from using them, and in some cases this accusation has been justified. At the same time feminists have justifiably accused supporters of injectables of bias and inaccuracies. Because this has left women who need contraception in the middle, it is crucial that information about these, as about all drugs, is as accurate as possible.

UK Licensing Restrictions

Under the restrictions on the licence for Depo Provera in the UK, your doctor should explain the following to you if you are considering an injectable method: Depo Provera is licensed in the UK as a last-resort method only. In other words, it should only be considered when *no* other method is acceptable or possible for you. It is a long-acting method, which may delay return of fertility for an average of eight to twelve months but possibly up to two years after you stop using it. All the benefits and risks should be explained to you, so that you can make an informed decision whether to use it. DP is also approved for one-off use, i.e. one injection, with a rubella vaccination to prevent pregnancy for three months or following vasectomy until your partner's sperm count goes to zero. In practice, it is rarely used with vasectomies because most people will already have a birth control method and will simply continue using it a bit longer. DP has been used often with rubella vaccinations, mostly in women who have just had babies and who are not rubella immune. While it is important not to get pregnant when rubella vaccine is active in your body (because there is a theoretical risk of birth defects), you can use the contraceptive method that you would normally have chosen during this time.

DP is *not* recommended in the UK for women who have just given birth, or had a miscarriage or abortion, or in women who are breastfeeding, at least for the first six weeks. If you are offered DP at this time, refuse it and get advice on other methods, if not in hospital, then from your GP or clinic when you get home.

NET-OEN is approved for one-off use only, i.e. one injection only, with rubella vaccinations or vasectomy, as with DP. It should also not be used following childbirth, miscarriage or abortion. However, you may well be offered NET-OEN for longer-term use. When DP only had a one-off licence, it was also given as a long-term method. This is possible under UK drug licensing, but it means that the doctor takes full responsibility for any consequences.

In fact, these two injectables are the only contraceptives approved under such stringent conditions, and the one-off licence is unique to them.

Description

Both are given as an injection in the buttock or arm muscle. The amount of drug in your body is at its highest point in the first weeks following the injection and gradually decreases. Although the contraceptive effect lasts two months in the case of NET-OEN and three months in the case of DP, the drug can affect your body in a variety of ways for an average of eight to ten months per injection. Both drugs have similar adverse effects.

There have been fewer studies on NET-OEN than DP and until 1985 NET-OEN was available in the UK only for trials. Since NET-OEN is less used, most of the information below is about DP, as indicated. Where 'an injectable' is mentioned, the information applies to both methods.

How to Get DP and NET-OEN

Available from family planning clinics and some GPs. You should be given the injection between the first and fifth day of your period, to ensure you are not pregnant, and not at any other time in your cycle. It takes effect almost immediately. You will be given an appointment for the next injection before you go home.

WHO SHOULD AVOID AN INJECTABLE

- Women who have just had a baby, a miscarriage or an abortion.
- Women who are breastfeeding.
- Women who are pregnant or think they might be.
- Women who might want to try for a baby within two years after stopping the injection.
- Women who suffer from:
  depression
  current liver problems
  diabetes
  weight problems
  arterial disease
  other illnesses that require regular medication, e.g. epilepsy
  undiagnosed vaginal bleeding
  hormone-dependent cancer of the breast/ reproductive organs
  recent trophoblastic disease, e.g. hydatidiform mole (see p. 293)
- Women willing to try or use another birth control method.

Effectiveness

DP is almost 100 per cent effective. The only ways women have got pregnant while using it are: if they were already pregnant before the first injection and didn't know it, or they left much more than three months with DP (or two months with NET-OEN) between injections and got pregnant in between.

NET-OEN is almost as effective as DP, as long as the next injection is on time.

Advantages

1. Lowest failure rate of all methods.
2. You need do nothing else to prevent pregnancy.
3. If your partner has prevented you from using other contraceptive methods, he cannot stop you from using an injection once you have had it. In the short term an injectable may be the solution to prevent pregnancy with such a man. However, any man who, in effect, wants to force you to get pregnant is violating your right to decide not to have a child. The real problem lies with the man, not with you. If you are in this situation, you may want to seek support and help in dealing with him from your doctor or another adviser, or women's group,* who can refer you both, if needed, for counselling elsewhere.

Disadvantages

1. Once you have had an injection, you cannot change your mind about using it. You can decide not to have further injections, but there is no way to remove the drug from your body or stop any adverse effects until they wear off on their own, which can take an average of eight to ten months. (This means it can take less time or more.)
2. If you suffer any adverse effects, you are likely to suffer from more than one of them.
3. Both injectables affect menstrual bleeding in most women who use them, and this is the most common reason why women stop using them. After your last injection, it may take months before your cycle becomes regular again. During this time, it will be difficult for you to know if you are fertile and when, or whether you have become pregnant. This is more common with DP than with NET-OEN.

The majority have either complete loss of periods or irregular spotting or bleeding. Irregular spotting/bleeding may happen only a few days out of every month or every day. You may be told that there is no known danger in not having a period. In fact, no one has ever studied whether it is harmful to our health or not in the long run.

Some women get very heavy and/or prolonged bleeding (that is, heavier and/or longer than normal for them and even every day). The chance of heavy/prolonged bleeding greatly increases if you are given the injectable in the first days or weeks following childbirth.

Heavy/prolonged bleeding can lead to anaemia, blood loss, weakness and exhaustion. You may be unable to work or look after children. The only treatments available if this happens are to give oestrogen, or to give an additional injection of the method, or to have a D & C which requires hospitalization and anaesthesia. None of these treatments will necessarily work or may help only temporarily. For women who have just had a baby, it may be difficult to tell whether the bleeding is caused by the drug or something else. The added risks of any of the treatments after childbirth are totally unjustified.

The CGDP received letters from some women who had bleeding problems after they stopped using DP.* In some cases bleeding was very heavy and lasted up to several months. This had not previously come to light because studies have focused on users, not ex-users of the drug.

4. *Fertility.* If you stop using an injectable in order to get pregnant, it may take up to two years before you are able to conceive. Return of fertility is generally faster with NET-OEN than with DP.

5. *Weight loss or gain.* Either could happen. The majority of women who experience weight changes gain or lose up to 10 lb (4.5 kg). Rarely, weight gains up to 68 lb (31 kg) have been recorded. Some women say their appetite increases, but neither exercise nor diet seems to make a difference, until they stop using the drug. The long-term effects on metabolism that may be linked to weight changes are unknown.

6. *Other possible adverse effects reported by women include:* bloated feeling, headaches, dizziness, sore breasts, back pain, pain in lower abdomen, effect on bowel movement, depression, other mood changes, tiredness/lack of energy, tension, nervousness, loss of sexual desire, red/sore eyes, arm/leg pains, nausea, hair loss/changes, skin changes and acne.

Although these may not all necessarily be related to the drug, but to other factors, many of them are also linked with other methods containing progestogen.

7. *Effects on breastmilk and breastfeeding infants.* Some studies show breastmilk increases while on injectables, others show a decrease. If you produce too much milk, the baby may not get the hind (or last) milk while feeding because s/he is full. (The hind milk is richer in certain nutrients.) A decrease in milk is obviously not a good thing. Both DP and NET-OEN are carried in breastmilk, though not all of it is absorbed by a breastfeeding baby. Studies up to puberty of children are thought by some to be reassuring. However, the UK licence on DP says breastfeeding women should not use it for six weeks after birth. The authors of this book think this caution should apply the whole time you are breastfeeding, and to NET-OEN as well.

8. *Effects on fetus exposed in the womb.* If you are mistakenly given an injectable when you are already pregnant, you should be aware that almost nothing is known about the effects it may have. Progestogens are associated with birth defects, however, so make very sure you are not pregnant before using either injectable.

9. *Arterial disease.* High doses of progestogens increase the risk of arterial disease. As with the Pill, a risk like this could continue long after you stop using the method, and may be important for women who use the drug for a long time. There have been no studies to determine the actual risk.

10. DP appears to reduce a woman's oestrogen levels, in some cases to lower than in women after menopause. As Jill

---

*See also Chapter 10 for help concerning men who violate our lives.

*See CGDP evidence listed in Resources.

Rakusen has pointed out,* in the long term this could increase the risk of serious problems, including thinning and weakening of the bones (osteoporosis) and dryness and thinning of the vaginal walls. We know that such a drastic effect on women's oestrogen levels while young exposes women to a greatly increased risk of serious and premature osteoporosis and other problems associated with the post-menopausal period (see Chapters 22 and 6). Again, no follow-up research has been done on DP's effects in this respect, so we have no way of knowing if this risk is simply theoretical.

11. *Cancer.* One of the main reasons why DP has not got a licence in the USA to date (end 1987) is because the findings about the risk of various cancers are so unclear. Animal studies using very high doses showed both breast and endometrial/endocervical cancers. As far as cancer risks in women are concerned, studies to date are inconclusive and we cannot yet say there is no increased risk. Preliminary results of a recent cross-country study, published in 1984, showed that women who used DP for more than five years had an increased incidence of cervical cancer, compared with women not using it. The final results have not yet been published, and other studies on cancer risks are still in progress.

12. The interaction of injectables with other drugs has barely been studied. This is particularly important if you take other drugs regularly, e.g. for epilepsy.

13. Finally, there is not enough evidence to provide clear assurances concerning any long-term risks of injectables. For further discussion see CGDP report and *Who Needs Depo Provera?* (in Resources).

METHODS NOT YET ON THE MARKET

The vast majority of research on new methods of birth control is on hormonal methods, including implants and vaginal rings, and there are regular trials in different countries to try these out. The trials, as with all drug trials, usually involve small numbers of women in the initial phases and larger numbers as the methods get nearer to being approved on grounds of safety and efficiency. Most of these trials do not make news, though they are reported in specialist journals. More often than not, problems are identified during the four phases of research trials which mean a method is abandoned and does not reach the market at all.† Some of the other methods being worked on include injectables that combine oestrogen and progestogen, vaccines, anti-progesterones, and methods using other hormones such as LHRH (luteinizing hormone-releasing

hormone). Non-surgical sterilization techniques for both women and men are also being worked on. In some cases a method may end up on the market in some Third World countries with or without being licensed there and may never even come to the UK. Combined injectables are a good example. In other cases, it may be approved in a developed country first; implants are an example of this. In other cases, it may be submitted for approval in a great many countries at once, including the UK. This is happening with implants and will probably also happen with vaginal rings.

Little work is being done on barrier methods, partly because less money is available for research and partly because women will not volunteer for clinical trials in large enough numbers to evaluate the methods. The Margaret Pyke Centre in London are doing a lot of work on barrier methods. They did trials of the contraceptive sponge before it came on the market and they are currently testing the effectiveness of diaphragms without spermicides by comparing this with spermicides alone and diaphragms used with spermicides and other new designs for diaphragms and caps.

It is difficult to predict which of the methods currently in trials will end up on the market and which will not. However, two methods which are likely to become available in the next few years are described below. If they are licensed in the UK, you will need to read more about them for up-to-date information.

HORMONAL IMPLANTS

One such implant – Norplant 1 – has been approved for contraceptive use in Finland, Sweden, Ecuador, the Dominican Republic, Indonesia, Thailand, Colombia, Peru, China, Sri Lanka and Venezuela. The manufacturer has applied for a licence in more than forty countries and it has been used in clinical trials in Scotland. Norplant 1 is likely to be available in the UK by the time you read this if the Committee on Safety of Medicines approves it. It was first approved in Finland, where it is manufactured, in 1985.

Norplant 1 consists of six small capsules containing the progestogen levonorgestrel that is also used in some combined pills and POPs. The information below is about Norplant 1. More information is gradually becoming available about other varieties and brands.

The capsules are implanted under the skin in the inside of your upper arm under local anaesthetic through a small incision that heals by itself. They are effective about twenty-four hours after insertion. Removal of the capsules is by a similar process. The capsules gradually release the hormone into the body and can be left in place for up to five years with almost 100 per cent effectiveness in preventing pregnancy. If they are left in for an additional two years they have a failure rate of 3–5 per cent. After that, they continue to release the hormone but rapidly become less and less effective. Studies to date indicate no permanent adverse effect on fertility in women who have participated in trials.

---

*See CGDP evidence listed in Resources.

†As we go to press, setbacks in the development of vaginal rings (adverse effects of one type and withdrawal of the material used to make another type) mean that they will not come on the market as soon as expected, if at all.

Almost all traces of the progestogen appear to leave the body within a week after removal (though this does not mean that any adverse effects on the body will disappear so quickly).

The method works by making the cervical mucus less penetrable by sperm and the lining of the uterus less able to accept a fertilized egg. It suppresses ovulation about 80 per cent of the time in the first year of use and 50 per cent of the time thereafter, but it is not possible to predict whether ovulation will or will not occur in any one cycle. Much more hormone is released in the first six to eighteen months after insertion than afterwards. The amount gradually drops from 80 mg per day initially to 30 mg per day after eighteen months (30 mg is comparable to one progestogen-only pill per day). It then remains relatively steady for about three years after that.

Norplant is not recommended for use in breastfeeding women because effects on infants are not known. Effects of Norplant following childbirth, miscarriage or abortion are also not known because no trials have been conducted to find out. However, experience with Depo Provera suggests that use of a high dose of progestogen at this time may carry a risk of heavy bleeding, so caution is advised.

Norplant will probably be recommended for women who want no further children, as an alternative to sterilization, and to women who do not want to get pregnant for a long period of time. As a long-acting method, its advantages over injectables are that it requires fewer visits to the clinic and can be removed on request.

Adverse Effects

1. *Menstrual bleeding*. Most women experience changes in menstrual bleeding patterns. The majority get frequent or infrequent bleeding or spotting or no periods at all. Some (up to 25 per cent in one small study, but usually fewer in other studies) may have prolonged or heavy bleeding for at least one year. There is no way to predict how your body will react. Irregular patterns in the first year tend to become more regular after that. Variations from month to month are the main reason women have stopped using it.

2. *Headaches*, including very severe headaches, are reported by 4–9 per cent of women in different studies.

3. *Other effects reported include*: dizziness, nausea, depression, loss of appetite, weight gain or loss, nervousness, fatigue/weakness, lower abdominal pain, pain at the implant site or under the arm, acne and other skin problems. These may occur singly or in groups, and may not necessarily be related to the drug.

4. *Minor infections* after insertion and removal have been reported. Pain at insertion has made some women afraid to have them removed, when they might otherwise have wanted to have them out. Removal is more difficult where skin tissue has adhered to one or more capsules.

5. Some women have been found to get *ovarian cysts* while using Norplant, indicated by pain and swelling in the area of the abdomen around the ovaries. There is now some evidence that this also occurs with progestogen-only pills and combined phasic pills. The cysts seem to be temporary but you should seriously consider having the implants removed if cysts are diagnosed. This was done during trials where it occurred. Surgery for the cysts is not necessary, since once the implants are removed the cysts seem to go away. Cysts related to Norplant have been misdiagnosed as ectopic pregnancy (though this is less likely to happen with ultrasound testing), and such a mistake could lead to unnecessary surgery.

6. It is reported from studies that the effects Norplant has on body functions like metabolism, blood sugar levels, glands, etcetera, are present but less than those experienced on the Combined Pill.

7. There were several deaths during a Norplant trial in Latin America, but the cause(s) of death were not stated. This does not inspire confidence in the research.

8. There has been no time for long-term studies on health risks, though the effects of levonorgestrel have been studied in other methods. This will remain true for some considerable time to come.

9. Since progestogen is linked with *congenital abnormalities*, it is very important to ensure that you are not pregnant before starting to use Norplant 1.

10. If the capsules are not removed after the recommended time, they will continue to release small amounts of hormone into your body, even after ten years. No one is sure how long it takes for the capsules to become completely empty. There will be almost no contraceptive cover, however, only possible side-effects. This is a major disadvantage of Norplant, and unique to this method.

STERILIZATION FOR WOMEN AND MEN

Over the past twenty years an increasing number of people, mostly between the ages of twenty-five and forty, have chosen sterilization when they are sure they do not want more (or any) children.

A recent study by Wellings and Mills reported that in 20 per cent of couples in the fertile age range, one partner had been sterilized. The proportion was six female sterilizations to five vasectomies (male sterilization). The majority (75 per cent) had two children or less, and more than one in eight had no children at all.

Sterilization is a permanent step and most of the time it is irreversible. For this reason, the decision to have it must be carefully thought out, not for days or weeks but for months, so that the chances of regretting it are as low as possible. If you are not sure that it is the right step for you, it is best not to go ahead with or agree to sterilization. You can always use another method for a bit longer and decide in your own good time.

If you are in a long-term relationship, you may want to consider which one of you has the operation. Having babies is a woman's job and it is likely that birth control has also been your responsibility. Vasectomy is a safer and simpler operation than female sterilization, and it does not require a stay in hospital. For this reason alone, you and your partner might want to consider whether, at this point, the responsibility should be taken by him.

FEMALE STERILIZATION

Female sterilization prevents pregnancy by closing off a section of each fallopian tube on either side of the womb so that sperm cannot move up to meet an egg and an egg cannot move down to meet sperm.

The first known sterilization was reported in 1834 and was done after a caesarean birth. Since then, the methods of doing the operation have changed and improved many times, so that in most cases it is no longer considered major surgery and has become quite safe. Ways of making it even safer continue to be worked on.*

Sterilization is done in hospital and in almost all cases general anaesthesia is used. There are two stages in the surgery, the first to get access to the tubes and the second to sterilize them. There are a number of possible ways to do this, and these will vary somewhat from one doctor to another.

Access to the Fallopian Tubes

1. *Laparoscopy.* Two cuts are made in the abdomen about 1 cm each in length, one in or below the navel and the other above the pubic hair. A laparoscope (an instrument with mirrors and light) is inserted in the upper cut to give the surgeon a clear view of the tubes, and carbon dioxide is pumped into the abdomen to give better access to and view of the tubes. Instruments for doing the sterilization are then used through the lower cut. (Laparoscopy is also used for other purposes, see p. 596.)

2. *Minilaparotomy.* One cut is made in the abdomen about 3 cm in length above the pubic hair. Instruments are used to bring the tubes, one after the other, closer to the surface in order to sterilize them.

Laparoscopy is much more commonly used in the UK than minilaparotomy. Rarely the operation is done through the vagina, but the chance of complications is higher.

Sterilizing the Tubes

Once the surgeon has gained access to the tubes, the main techniques used to sterilize them are:

1. *Ligation.* This means cutting out a piece of each tube and closing off the two ends. There are more than half a dozen ways of doing this, named after the surgeons who developed them. They vary in terms of how much of the tube is destroyed, how difficult they are to do and how effective they are. The most commonly used is the

---

*There may be medical reasons why your fallopian tubes and/or uterus may need to be removed, which are not related to birth control. Surgery to remove these organs will result in your being unable to get pregnant again, but should never be used for sterilization purposes only, as it is more serious and is unnecessary for birth control. These operations are: salpingectomy (removal of one or both fallopian tubes) and hysterectomy (removal of the entire uterus and possibly the tubes, see p. 597).

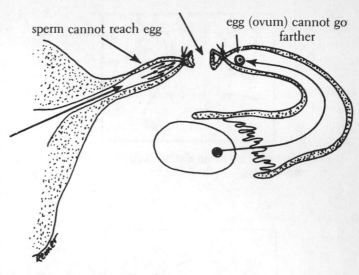

sperm cannot reach egg

egg (ovum) cannot go farther

TRADITIONAL TUBAL LIGATION

1 Ends of tubes are actually folded back into surrounding tissue.

Pomeroy technique, which involves making a loop in the tube and tying it off with an absorbable suture, and then cutting the top of the loop off and closing off the ends. It is considered the simplest and most effective technique, and destroys about 3–4 cm of each tube.

2. *Tubal rings or clips.* These are a more recent development, designed to damage less of the tubes and, it is hoped, to make it more possible to reverse the sterilization later if requested. Only time will tell if this intention will succeed. A rubber-like ring or clip is put round the tube to close it off. The clips damage less than 1 cm of the tube and the rings damage 1–3 cm.

3. *Cauterization.* This involves using electric current or heat to destroy a section of each tube and possibly then cutting out the burnt section afterwards. The potential for damaging other organs, particularly the bowels, is higher with these methods and they are practically out of use.

You will usually be kept in hospital for two or three days after the operation, depending on how much pain and discomfort you feel. No matter which method is used, most women feel some pain and general tiredness for three to five days. Laparoscopy may cause a bloated feeling, discomfort

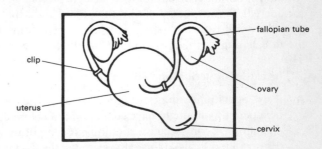

fallopian tube

clip

ovary

uterus

cervix

2a a plastic clip ½–1 in (1–2 cm) long is put on each fallopian tube to prevent eggs moving down towards the uterus and sperm going up them.

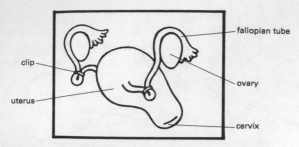

2b Each tube is looped and the loop secured with a silastic ring.

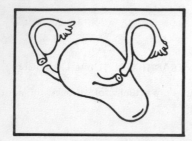

3 Each tube is divided and sealed using cauterization.

and shoulder or chest pain for several days, due to the use of carbon dioxide. Clips and rings cause cramping and lower abdominal pain until the nerve endings near them die: this is worst on the day of operation and usually goes within five days. You will be offered pain-killers for this if you want them.

You should allow several days after you get home before resuming light work, and about a week before returning to full activity. After minilaparotomy heavy lifting should be avoided for about three weeks. Sexual activity can be continued when you feel like it; no contraception is needed.

Effectiveness

Female sterilization is not 100 per cent effective, though many people think it is. According to the FPA Information Service, about one woman in 300 becomes pregnant after sterilization, usually within the first two years after the operation. These numbers are very low, but if you don't know that pregnancy is possible, you may not recognize the symptoms, nor may the possibility of ectopic pregnancy be considered. (Because of the sterilization, the chances that a pregnancy will be ectopic are increased; this condition is life-threatening and requires immediate attention. See p. 439).

The causes of sterilization failure are:

- if the operation is done between ovulation and your next period, you might have conceived just before the operation. A contraceptive should be used right up to the operation to avoid this. However, tell the doctor if you think you might have got pregnant. It appears to be widespread for doctors to do a D & C at the same time

as the sterilization to ensure you are not pregnant. Many may not talk about this with you at all, so it is worth asking about if they don't mention it;

- a clip or ring may not completely close off the tube;
- after ligation, a tube may reconnect on its own in spite of the damage, or an opening may develop in a sealed-off tube that allows egg or sperm through;
- the surgeon may mistakenly do the operation on something other than the tube.

In addition, much depends on the skill of the surgeon and the technique used.

Possible Complications

Any complications are likely to be apparent before you leave hospital, and can be treated quickly. Minor complications occur in about 2–3 per cent of operations and include: injury to surrounding blood vessels, injury to tissues or organs near the tubes, pelvic infection, infection of the incision(s), and urinary tract infection.

Major complications are similar in type to minor complications but require surgery. These occur rarely, only in about two per 1,000 operations. There are also risks from general anaesthesia during and just after the operation, as with all surgery (see p. 596). In the very few cases where women have died during sterilization, anaesthesia was the cause; this should be avoidable.

Longer-term Effects

Up to 15 per cent of women who are sterilized experience heavier menstrual periods or other changes in their periods. There is disagreement over whether sterilization or something else causes this. Some studies show a link with sterilization, others don't. On the one hand, a lot of women will have been using the Pill prior to sterilization; it may be that they would have got heavier periods or irregular cycles after stopping the Pill, regardless of whether they were sterilized or not. On the other hand, some doctors believe that sterilization may injure the blood vessels near the tubes and affect the flow of blood to the ovaries, which could cause hormonal imbalances that lead to menstrual period changes.

In the 1970s a number of doctors identified a 'post-sterilization syndrome' which included shortening of the menstrual cycle with heavier and more prolonged bleeding, more premenstrual tension and painful periods, loss of libido, vaginal dryness (which can make intercourse painful), and tenderness and pain in the area around the uterus. A study in 1978 found that one out of five women having hysterectomies had been sterilized in the previous five years. Sterilization may or may not have led to problems which led to the need for hysterectomy.

Sterilization methods have changed since then, however, and it could be that earlier methods, particularly cautery methods, were responsible for these problems. We will have to await studies of women using newer methods like clips and rings before we will know for sure whether this syndrome will contine to appear. In the meantime, women should be aware that this 'post-sterilization syndrome' might affect them.

VASECTOMY

Male sterilization, or vasectomy, is done by damaging the two vas deferens (tubes) which carry sperm from the testes to the penis. The operation does not stop the production of sperm, which are absorbed into the body instead of entering the semen, nor does it stop the production of semen, which continues to be ejaculated during orgasm. The man will not notice any difference in his ejaculate, because sperm make up only a small part of it, and he will continue to get erections as before.

Vasectomy usually takes less than half an hour. Only local anaesthetic is necessary and it is almost always done on an outpatient basis. A few GPs have been trained to do vasectomies, but the majority are done by doctors in family planning clinics and hospital outpatient clinics.

A small incision is made in the scrotum and a second small incision is made in the internal sheath around the vas. The vas is then made visible and cut or cauterized, and the ends sealed off, as in female sterilization. The sheath and scrotum are then closed, and the same procedure is repeated on the other side. There may be a temporary gap in the skin which requires a daily dressing until healing is complete, which takes one to two weeks.

The man should be accompanied home after the operation if possible. He can expect some scrotal swelling and possible bruising and should wear a support twenty-four hours a day for two weeks. It is preferable to avoid manual work for two or three days, but many men return to work the day after the operation. Sexual activity may be resumed as soon as there is no discomfort, but contraception will still be needed.

The effect of the operation is not immediate, unlike with women, because some sperm will already be in the semen, and will only be washed out by ejaculation. Fertility will decrease with each ejaculation until the sperm count is zero. Two zero sperm counts (when the semen is free from all sperm, dead or alive) are required before a vasectomy is considered successful. It used to be thought that this took three months, but more recent studies have shown that it is not time, but the number of ejaculations, needed for the sperm to disappear from a man's semen. Twenty-four to thirty-six ejaculations are usually enough to reach a zero sperm count, either during love-making or through masturbation. He will be asked to return to the clinic or hospital several times, for a sperm count to be taken. YOU SHOULD CONTINUE TO USE YOUR USUAL METHOD OF CONTRACEPTION UNTIL THE SPERM COUNT IS ZERO.

Effectiveness

Vasectomy fails to prevent pregnancy in about one in 1,000 operations. The causes of failure are similar to those in women. Most failed operations are picked up during semen analysis for a zero sperm count within the first two or three months after the operation. In much rarer cases, perhaps one in several thousand, rejoining of a tube may occur later, after a zero sperm count. In such cases, only a pregnancy is likely to indicate it has happened. Though this is rare, it is still important to know it is possible.

Possible Complications

Vasectomy is one of the safest operations and methods of birth control. Minor complications that may arise are infection or inflammation in the testes within several weeks of the operation. Symptoms include swelling of the testes, pain and tenderness. Antibiotics are used to treat this. While no long-term effects have been confirmed, two recent studies in the USA suggest that there may be a higher incidence of kidney stones and prostate cancer in men who have had vasectomies. With the latter, smoking appeared to increase the risk. Further studies are needed and the FPA believes the findings are as yet inconclusive.

DECIDING WHICH OF YOU HAS THE OPERATION

Men seem to be more anxious about having a vasectomy than women do about being sterilized. Perhaps this is because men are not used to years of dealing with contraception and pregnancy personally, and only face the idea of interference with their bodies when they consider vasectomy. Women may have little patience with this, especially since vasectomy is so relatively safe and simple, but the fact is that most men will not agree to vasectomy without the reassurance of other men who have already been through it. For this reason, many clinics offering vasectomy use only male counsellors who have had the operation. Britain is among the few countries where vasectomy rates are high compared with female sterilizations; the USA and China are two of the others.

The vast majority of men interviewed in a study by Isobel Allen said they decided on vasectomy precisely because it was a less serious operation than female sterilization, not needing a hospital stay, and their wives had done enough in the birth control line. In the same study the majority of wives who had been sterilized said it was because their husbands were unwilling, scared of or against vasectomy, or because the men might want to have more children while they didn't.

There are a number of reasons why a woman or a man may prefer to have the sterilization themselves, rather than let their partner do it. These include not being in a steady relationship, having more than one partner, or for health reasons.

Whatever decision you make, we recommend considering the pros and cons of both options. Using contraception and having babies scare women a lot more and for a lot longer than vasectomy scares men, and if most of the advantages point in the direction of vasectomy, perhaps he should get help in overcoming his fears.

REGRETTING THE OPERATION

At least one out of every hundred people sterilized regrets it later. With the number of people being sterilized increasing, the chances are that there will be more people who may wish they hadn't done it. The main cause of sterilization regret is the desire to have more children some years after the operation. Change of partner following separation or death is the most common reason; a sterilization can make it difficult to get involved with someone who wants children when you can no longer have them. After a separation, if your partner has custody of the children, you may find yourself wanting to start a new family. And there is always the outside possibility that children may die and you will want others.

While sterilization reversal may be possible, in most cases it is not. The decision to be sterilized should be seen as a permanent one, and you should consider whether a major change in your circumstances would make you regret it. Many doctors advise younger people inquiring about sterilization to wait, on the grounds that the younger you are, the more chance there is that you will change your mind later. Many women are not having children in their twenties these days and often decide in their thirties that they would like to. However, no one knows you better than yourself and in the end it is an individual decision. Guidelines can help to prevent sterilization regret, e.g. the decision should never be made at a time of stress, and should be thought over and talked over for at least several months, if not longer. Studies in the USA have shown that people who waited less than a month between first considering the operation and having it were much more likely to regret it later.

Second, if you have any doubts, you should talk to someone about them and think further before you make up your mind. Counselling is always available if you need it, from your GP, family planning and other clinics which offer the operation (see Resources for a list of these).

Third, it would be a good rule of thumb for doctors never to suggest sterilization, but to wait for the person to raise the subject herself. A recent study by Allen, 1985, found that in 19 per cent of cases in one district, a doctor had suggested sterilization to the woman before she had thought about it herself, while this was almost never the case with the men who were sterilized. This does not mean that those women, as opposed to others, will necessarily regret their decision later, or that the others will not. However, as Peter Huntingford says:

> Suggestions made by doctors or others are seldom sensitive to the needs of an individual and carry undue weight, because they are accepted as coming from someone who should know best.

STERILIZATION ABUSE

Abuses of sterilization have been reported internationally, in both developed and Third World countries. Pressure and coercion have been used to get (mainly) women to agree to be sterilized, usually the promise of food or money or access to services or the threat of withholding these. Women have been sterilized without their knowledge, usually after birth or an abortion, and mentally handicapped women have been sterilized 'for their own good' without their informed consent (e.g. see *Women's Global Network on Reproductive Rights Newsletters*, 1985 and 1986).

Abuses have been reported in the UK as well, usually as isolated cases, but no studies have been done to establish how often these occur. Some doctors have made sterilization a condition for doing an abortion, for example. Others have suggested sterilization to women or to their husbands while the women were in labour for childbirth, so that 'they don't have to go through this again'.* In 1980 1–3 per cent of sterilizations were following childbirth and in 1982 about 5 per cent of abortions (mostly on the NHS) were followed by sterilization.** There are regional variations in these figures, which imply that some doctors are doing more sterilizations in these circumstances than others. Again, we do not know if any of these involve abuses. If you had already thought about being sterilized and decided it was convenient to do it in connection with childbirth and abortion, that is one thing. However, if the doctor expects you to make a quick decision about sterilization, this is unethical.

On the other hand, policies or laws forbid sterilization in some countries, and people are forced to pay for it privately or travel to other countries to get the operation. Women from Ireland and Spain travel to Britain for sterilizations as well as safe abortions, for example.

In the UK, many women, particularly those under thirty, with few or no children and/or not in a steady relationship, have been refused sterilization by doctors. Department of Health guidelines suggest that people be at least thirty years old, have at least two children and the consent of their partner, and many doctors refuse to operate outside these guidelines. Their refusal is understandable, both because of their worries about people later asking for reversals and for their own protection under the guidelines, but for the people they turn away it is grossly unfair. In addition, both men and women are being turned away because the NHS budgets in many regions are inadequate to cover all those who want the operation. (See Resources for details of non-NHS clinics doing sterilization and vasectomy.)

STERILIZATION REVERSAL

Studies of both men and women requesting sterilization reversal have indicated that change of partner was the main reason for the request and loss of children was also a factor.

*Information from letters and phone calls to the Women's Health and Reproductive Rights Information Centre, 1983–5.
**OPCS figures quoted in Hansard, 1 August 1984, Part III, vol. 65, no. 205, cols. 367–8.

The first successful reversal of a female sterilization took place in 1934 in the USA. Before 1970 pregnancy rates following reversal were much lower than they are now. New microsurgery techniques for rejoining the tubes have doubled the percentages since then, but they are still not high. Not everyone who requests reversal will be able to have the operation. Availability on the NHS is limited and private treatment expensive. In addition, there may be too much damage to the fallopian tubes or vas deferens or too much scar tissue, or there may be other problems impairing fertility that make it not worth trying. Even if a reversal is attempted and appears to be a technical success, a pregnancy may not result. One large study has shown that if reversal is requested ten or more years after a vasectomy, the chances for a successful reversal are significantly lower.

Reversal in men and women uses similar techniques. Damaged areas of the tubes are removed, along with any scar tissue that has built up. The ends are then joined together with tiny stitches. It is quite a delicate operation, requiring a lot of skill. One of the most common reasons why the operation may fail is that scar tissue builds up again and reblocks the tube(s). There is nothing doctors can do about this except to remove it again, and there are instances of people going back several times for this. However, there is a limit to how often this repeat surgery is advisable.

The success rate of reversal of vasectomy is generally agreed to be higher than with female sterilization. In the USA doctors actually operate on only 30 per cent of those women who request reversal and only two or three of those have a successful pregnancy afterwards. In other words, the operation results in a pregnancy for only 2–3 per cent of those women who have it, and that is with the best surgeons. Success rates with vasectomy reversal have been in the range of 30 to 50 per cent of those having the operation.

In vitro fertilization (IVF) may, in the future, become an alternative to reversal of female sterilization for some women. First, however, the success rate of IVF would have to improve, and the treatment would also have to be much more available on the NHS if this is to become possible for enough women. Some men might in future be able to have their sperm frozen and kept in a sperm bank, before a vasectomy, for inseminations if they want children later. This would only be possible if their sperm can successfully be frozen and if there is a sperm bank available.

However, reversal or other means of bypassing sterilization do not always work, which is why everyone must consider sterilization permanent and irreversible.

SERVICES FOR STERILIZATION IN BRITAIN

Surveys done in England and Wales in 1982 and 1984 showed that 65 per cent of District Health Authorities had no facilities for vasectomy and 88 per cent had none for female sterilization. Services are provided mainly at a regional level, and there are long waiting lists in most regions. (See Chapter 28, on how the NHS is structured.)

For female sterilization, the waiting time in England and Wales can be from three months to a year or more. In Scotland, the waiting time is generally four months or less. For vasectomy, although there is no need for a hospital stay, waiting times still average three to six months in most regions, including Scotland.*

Waiting lists seem to be the longest in regions which budget for a certain number of operations per year and, having completed those, have to wait until the next financial year to continue. Pressure on theatre time, lack of hospital beds and staff, and scarce resources generally are the other main causes of delay.

A reasonable waiting period, perhaps a few months, can be a good thing for those who may change their minds before they have the operation. On the other hand, too long a wait may cause anxiety and involves the chance of unwanted pregnancy before the operation. There are women who have needed an abortion while they or their partner were waiting for a sterilization, so it is important to keep using birth control in the interim.

How to Obtain Sterilization and Vasectomy on the NHS

Both women and men should first consult their GP or family planning clinic. Women will then be referred to a hospital and men will be referred to a trained GP, or doctor in the family planning clinic or a hospital outpatient clinic.

Counselling should be available either from the doctor(s) you see or trained counsellors attached to a clinic or hospital. Some people feel they need quite a lot of counselling while others want little or none. Doctors may or may not be sensitive to people's differing needs.

Isobel Allen found that, for a number of reasons,

medical involvement in vasectomy counselling was considerably less than in [female] sterilization counselling. Men saw fewer doctors less often, and the whole process of consultation with doctors was usually considerably simpler for the men than for the women.

Although female sterilization is medically a more serious operation, Allen rightly raises the question of why this needs to be so, since the outcome is the same – sterilization of one or other partner.

Department of Health regulations recommend that the consent of the partner is obtained, though this is not legally required. In practice, it seems a man's consent for the woman to be sterilized is asked for more often than the other way round. This is a form of sex discrimination; if men are able to take autonomous decisions, women should be able to do so as well. We do not need a partner's consent for abortion, nor should we for sterilization.

METHODS THAT DON'T WORK

You may have been told that douching with water or other special solutions immediately after intercourse will protect you by removing semen from your vagina before sperm enter the uterus. This does not work. The douche may even push the sperm up into your vagina from the pressure of the liquid entering your vagina. In any case, douching is not a good idea (see p. 491).

None of the following works at all: standing up during intercourse, only having intercourse during your period, holding your breath, not allowing his penis to go all the way in, jumping up and down afterwards. Forget them!

And, remember, you don't need to have an orgasm to get pregnant.

REFERENCES USED IN THE TEXT
(listed section by section)

INTRODUCTION

Arnheim, Ann. 'Do We Need a Domiciliary Family Planning Service?', *Health Visitor*, vol. 56, May 1983, pp. 162–3.

Leathard, Audrey. *District Health Authority Family Planning Services in England and Wales*. FPA, 1985.

Margolis, Karen. 'More than Just a Packet of Pills', *Guardian*, 17 November 1980. (On domiciliary family planning.)

Snowden, Robert. *Consumer Choices in Family Planning*. FPA, November 1985.

Wellings, Kaye. 'Trends in Contraceptive Method Usage Since 1970', *British Journal of Family Planning*, vol. 12, 1986, pp. 15–22.

NATURAL BIRTH CONTROL

Rice, Frank et al. 'Effectiveness of the Sympto-thermal Method of Natural Family Planning: an International Study', *International Journal of Fertility*, vol. 26, 1981, pp. 222–30.

BARRIER METHODS

AIDS, vol. 1, no. 1, 1987, pp. 49–52. (Re lower effectiveness of condoms made of animal membrane in preventing transmission of STDs.)

Berer, Marge. *The Diaphragm and Cap: Barrier Methods for Women*. London: Women's Reproductive Rights Information Centre, 1986.

Curtis, Dr Margaret. 'Today Sponge', letter to *British Journal of Family Planning*, vol. 12, 1987, p. 130.

Donovan, Glynis. *The Sheath*. London: Women's Reproductive Rights Information Centre, 1985.

Gregson, Elizabeth. 'Barrier Methods', in Nancy Loudon (ed.), *Handbook of Family Planning*. Edinburgh: Churchill Livingstone, 1985.

Kopp, Zoe. 'Cervical Cap Receives USFDA Approval'. *IPPF Medical Bulletin*, vol. 23, no. 1, February 1989.

Tayob, Yunus et al. 'Female Barrier Methods', *Mims Magazine*, vol. 1, October 1985, pp. 19–25.

Vessey, Martin. *British Journal of Family Planning*, vol. 13, no. 4, January 1988, supplement pp. 41–3. (About the relationship between diaphragms and urinary tract infection.)

IUDS

Berer, Marge. 'The IUCD or Coil'. London: Women's Reproductive Rights Information Centre, 1986.

Bury, Judith. 'HIV-positive Women and Contraception', *British Journal of Family Planning*, vol. 14, 1988, pp. 50–4.

Daling, Janet et al. 'Primary Tubal Infertility in Relation to the Use of an IUD' and Daniel **Cramer** et al. 'Tubal Infertility and the IUD'. *New England Journal of Medicine*, vol. 312, no. 15, 11 April 1985, pp. 937–47; and Correspondence, *ibid*. vol. 313, no. 10, 5 September 1985, pp. 635–7.

Newton, John. 'Intra-uterine Contraceptive Devices', in Nancy Loudon (ed.), *Handbook of Family Planning*. Edinburgh: Churchill Livingstone 1985.

Novak, M. K. et al. 'Long-term Use of Intra-uterine Devices', *IPPF Medical Bulletin*, 22, 1 February 1988.

'Screen for Chlamydia before Fitting the Coil', *Pulse*, 7 July 1981.

Smith, P.A. et al. 'Deaths Associated with IUCDs in the UK between 1973 and 1983', *British Medical Journal*, 19 November 1983, pp. 1537–8.

Snowden, R. and B. **Pearson**. 'Pelvic Infection: a Comparison of the Dalkon Shield and Three Other IUDs', *British Medical Journal*, 26 May 1984, pp. 1570–73.

THE PILL

Bury, Judith. 'Deciding on the Best Pill Can be Difficult', *Pulse*, 5 March 1983.

Bury, Judith. 'HIV-positive Women and Contraception', *British Journal of Family Planning*, Vol. 14, 1988, pp. 50–4.

Caillouette, J. et al. 'Phasic Contraceptive Pills and Functional Ovarian Cysts' *American Journal of Obstetrics and Gynecology*, vol. 156, no. 6, June 1986, pp. 1538–42.

Guillebaud, John. 'Combined Oral Contraceptive Pills', and Nancy **Loudon**, 'Progestogen-only Pills', in Nancy Loudon (ed.), *Handbook of Family Planning*. Edinburgh: Churchill Livingstone, 1985.

Hale, Ralph. 'Currently Available Formulations' and Homer **Ellsworth**, 'Focus on Triphasil', *Journal of Reproductive Medicine*, vol. 31, no. 6, June 1986, Supplement pp. 557–64.

Holck, Susan and K. **Ebeling**. 'Review: Oral Contraceptives and Cancer', *Arch. Geschwulstforch*, vol. 56, no. 2, 1986, pp. 155–67.

McPherson, Klim et al. 'Early Oral Contraceptive Use and Breast Cancer' *Journal of Epidemiology and Community Health*, vol. 40, December 1986, pp. 289–94.

McPherson, Klim. 'On OC Use in Early Life and Breast Cancer Risk', *Family Planning Today*, Third Quarter, 1988.

Orme, M. L. E. et al. 'Drug Interactions with Oral Contraceptive Steroids', *British Journal of Family Planning*, vol. 10, no. 1, April 1984 Supplement, p. 19.

Royal College of General Practitioners. *Oral Contraceptives and Health*. London: Pitman Medical, 1974. (Among other things, the first study to suggest the Pill's effect on the immune system.)

Shearman, Rodney. 'Oral Contraceptive Agents', *Medical Journal of Australia*, vol. 144, 17 February 1986, pp. 201–11.

INJECTABLES

Berer, Marge. *Who Needs Depo Provera?* Community Rights Project, 1984.

Rakusen, Jill, Jean **Robinson**, Marge **Berer** et al. *Submission to the Public Hearing on Depo Provera*. Coordinating Group on Depo Provera (CGDP), 1983. (available from WHRRIC; see Organizations).

WHO Collaborative Study of Neoplasia and Steroid Contraceptives. 'Breast Cancer, Cervical Cancer and Depot Medroxyprogesterone Acetate', *The Lancet*, 24 November 1984, pp. 1207–8.

NORPLANT

Bardin, C. W. and I. **Sivin**. 'Norplant Contraceptive Implants: A New Contraceptive for Women', *IPPF Medical Bulletin*, vol. 19, no. 5, October 1985, pp. 2–4.

Berer, Marge. 'Norplant: the first contraceptive implant'. *Newsletter*, Women's Global Network on Reproductive Rights January–March 1986.
Croxatto et al. *Acta Endocrinologica*, no. 101, 1982, pp. 307–11.
Nilsson C. and P. **Holma**. 'Menstrual Blood Loss with Contraceptive Subdermal Levonorgestrel Implants', *Fertility and Sterility*, vol. 35, no. 3, March 1981.
Sivin, I. et al. 'Three Year Experience with Norplant Subdermal Contraception', *Fertility and Sterility*, vol. 39, no. 6, June 1983, pp. 799–808.
Sivin, I. et al. 'Norplant: Reversible Implant Contraception', *Studies in Family Planning*, vol. 11, no. 7/8, July–August 1980, pp. 227–35.
Studies in Family Planning. June–July 1983. Whole issue, vol. 14, no. 6/7.

MORNING-AFTER BIRTH CONTROL

Berer, Marge and Susannah **Simons**. 'Morning-After Birth Control', Women's Reproductive Rights Information Centre and Pregnancy Advisory Service.

STERILIZATION

Allen, Isobel. *Counselling Services for Sterilisation, Vasectomy and Termination of Pregnancy*. London: Policy Studies Institute, March 1985.
Berer, Marge. *Information Sheet on 'Sterilization and Vasectomy'*. London: Women's Reproductive Rights Information Centre, 1985.
Birth Control Trust. *Sterilisation and the NHS*. London: Birth Control Trust, 1981.
Corson, Stephen et al. (ed.). *Fertility Control*. Boston, MA: Little Brown, 1985. Chapters: 'Female Sterilization' by Carl Levinson and Herbert Peterson, 'Hysteroscopic Sterilization' by Jay Cooper, 'Vasectomy' by Joseph Davis, 'Female Sterilization Reversal' by Stephen Corson, and 'Male Sterilization Reversal' by Stanley Greenburg.
Family Planning Today. 'Prostate Cancer', Second Quarterly Bulletin, 1988.
Geirsson, Reynir et al. 'Prospective Comparison of Postoperative Morbidity after Laparoscopic Sterilisation with Clips and Rings', *British Journal of Family Planning*, vol. 11, no. 2, July 1985, pp. 55–9.
Henry, Alice. 'The Cutting Edge', *Off Our Backs*, December 1980.
Huntingford, Peter. 'Abortion and Sterilization'. Paper presented to the Symposium on Family Planning and Poverty at the Royal College of Physicians, 4 May 1979 (on file at WHRRIC; see Organizations).
Kronmel, R.A. et al. 'Vasectomy and Urolithiasis', *The Lancet*, 2–9 January 1988, pp. 22–3.
'Late Failure of Vasectomy', *The Lancet*, 6 April 1985, pp. 794–5.
Leathard, Audrey. 'Family Planning: Facilities Surveyed', *British Journal of Family Planning*, vol. 11, no. 2, July 1985, pp. 62–3.
Letchworth, A. T. 'Long-term Effects of Female Sterilization', *Update*, 1 February 1987, p. 253.
Savage, Wendy. 'Abortion, Sterilisation and Contraception', *Medicine in Society*, vol. 7, no. 1, 1982, pp. 6–12.
Wellings, Kaye and Angela **Mills**. 'Contraceptive Trends', *British Medical Journal*, vol. 289, 13 October 1984, pp. 939–40.
Women's Global Network on Reproductive Rights (ed.). *Divided in Culture – United in Struggle: Report on the International Tribunal and Meeting on Reproductive Rights, Amsterdam, July 1984*. Amsterdam: 1985 (available from WHRRIC; see Organizations).

RESOURCES
PUBLICATIONS

Allen, Isobel. *Counselling Services for Sterilisation, Vasectomy and Termination of Pregnancy*. London: Policy Studies Institute, March 1985.
Berer, Marge. *Who Needs Depo Provera?* London: Community Rights Project, 1984.
Billings, E. *The Billings Method*. London: Allen Lane, 1981. About natural birth control.
Birth Control Trust. *Men, Sex and Contraception*. London: BCT and FPA, 1984.
Blanco, Ana. *Net-Oen: the Other Injectable*. Oxford: War on Want/ICASC/WRRIC, 1984.

Bury, Judith. *Teenage Pregnancy in Britain*. London: Birth Control Trust, 1984.
Chalker, Rebecca. *The Complete Cervical Cap Guide*. London: Harper and Row, 1987.
Clubb, E. *Fertility – a Comprehensive Guide to Natural Family Planning*. Newton Abbot: David and Charles, 1987.
Davidson, J. and F. *Natural Fertility Awareness*. Saffron Walden: C.W. Daniel, 1986.
Dolto, C. et al. *How to Get Pregnant and How Not To*. London: Sheldon Press, 1985.
Drake, K. and J. *Natural Birth Control*. Wellingborough, Northants: Thorsons, 1984.
Federation of Women's Health Centers. *A New View of Woman's Body*. New York: Simon and Schuster, 1981.
Flynn, Anna and Melissa **Brooks**. *A Manual of Natural Family Planning*. London: Allen and Unwin, 1984.
Goldstein, Marc and Michael **Feldberg**. *The Vasectomy Book: a Complete Guide to Decision-Making*. Wellingborough, Northants: Turnstone Press, 1985.
Gordon, Linda. *Woman's Body, Woman's Right: A Social History of Birth Control in America*. London: Penguin Books, 1977.
Guillebaud, John. *The Pill*. Oxford: Oxford University Press, 1984.
Guillebaud, John. *Your Questions Answered*. London: Pitman, 1985.
Hartmann, Betsy. *Reproductive Rights and Wrongs*. London: Harper and Row, 1987. About population control policies internationally and their effects on contraceptive choice.
Hayman, Suzie. *Sterilisation*. Wellingborough, Northants: Thorsons, forthcoming. On female sterilization and vasectomy.
Homans, Hilary (ed.). *The Sexual Politics of Reproduction*. London: Gower, 1985.
Leathard, Audrey. *The Fight for Family Planning: the Development of Family Planning Services in Britain 1921–74*. London: Macmillan, 1980.
Leathard, Audrey. *Consumer Views and Family Planning Perspectives*. London: FPA, 1987.
Loudon, Nancy (ed.). *Handbook of Family Planning*. Edinburgh: Churchill Livingstone, 1985.
Luker, Kristin. *Taking Chances: Abortion and the Decision Not to Contracept*. University of California Press, 1975.
Mamdani, Mahmood. *The Politics of Population Control: Family, Caste and Class in an Indian Village*. New York: Monthly Review Press, 1972.
Menezes, J. *Natural Family Planning in Pictures*. Catholic Hospital Association in India, 1982. Designed for people who do not read.
Oxford Women's Health Action Group. *Whose Choice? What Women Have to Say About Contraception*. Oxford, 1984 (available from WHRRIC).
Pauncefort, Zandria. *Choices in Contraception*. London: Pan, 1984.
Population Reports. 'Hormonal Contraception: New Long-Acting Methods', Series K, no. 3, March–April 1987. On file at WHRRIC.
Pregnancy Advisory Service. *Post-Coital Contraception: Methods, Services and Prospects – a Symposium*, 1982.
Rakusen, Jill. 'Information or Propaganda?', *Spare Rib*, no. 32, February 1975. By assessing one particular research report (the RCGP study on the Pill), exposes the need to assess all contraceptive research for biased reporting.
Rakusen, Jill et al. *Submission to the Public Hearing on Depo Provera*. Coordinating Group on Depo Provera, 1983 (available from WHRRIC).
Shapiro, Rose. *Contraception: a Practical and Political Guide*. London: Virago Press, 1987.
Snowden, Robert. *The IUD: A Woman's Guide*. London: Unwin, 1986.
Trombley, Stephen. *The Right to Reproduce: a History of Coercive Sterilisation*. London: Weidenfeld and Nicolson, 1988.
Weil, M. et al. *Fertility Awareness*. Emma Goldman Clinic for Women, USA, 1982.
Women's Global Network on Reproductive Rights (ed.). *Divided in Culture – United in Struggle: Report of the International Tribunal and Meeting on Reproductive Rights, Amsterdam, July 1984*. Amsterdam: 1985. (On file at WHRRIC.)
World Health Organization. *Family Fertility Education*. London: BLAT Centre of Health and Medical Education, 1982.

PERIODICALS

Abortion Review (bi-monthly) published by Birth Control Trust.
British Journal of Family Planning (bi-monthly), available from: National Association of Family Planning Doctors (NAFPD), 27 Sussex Place, London NW1 4RG. Tel: 01-724 2441.
Family Planning Today (quarterly) published by Family Planning Information Service.
Medical Bulletin of the International Planned Parenthood Federation.
Newsletter (bi-monthly), the British Pregnancy Advisory Service.
Newsletter (quarterly), the Women's Global Network on Reproductive Rights – international in scope.
Newsletter (quarterly), the Women's Health and Reproductive Rights Information Centre.
Newsprint (bi-monthly), the Brook Advisory Centres.

All of the above publications are in the documentation centres of the Family Planning Association in London and the Women's Health and Reproductive Rights Information Centre, who can also advise on where to obtain copies. These two centres also have extensive documentation, information and leaflets on contraception and many other issues relating to health and reproduction.

EDUCATIONAL MATERIALS

Menstrual Cycle Wallchart: available from Wellwoman Information, 24 St Thomas Street, Redcliffe, Bristol BS1 6JL.
Tape and booklet for 10–16-year-old girls: available from Wellwoman Information, 24 St Thomas Street, Redcliffe, Bristol BS1 6JL.
Books of charts for recording cycles: available from above or NANFPT (see Organizations).
WHRRIC, the FPIS, the Birth Control Trust and the Birth Control Campaign also produce regular information sheets and pamphlets.

ORGANIZATIONS

CLINICS AND COUNSELLING

British Pregnancy Advisory Service, Austy Manor, Wootton Wawen, Solihull, West Midlands B95 6BX. Tel: 05642-3225.
Non-profit-making charitable clinics offering counselling, contraception, abortion, sterilization, vasectomy, sterilization and vasectomy reversal, morning-after contraception, pregnancy testing, and donor insemination. Branches in Basingstoke, Bath, Bedford, Birmingham, Bournemouth, Brighton, Cardiff, Chester, Coventry, Doncaster, Glasgow, Hull, Leamington Spa, Leeds, Liverpool, London, Luton, Manchester, Milton Keynes, Sheffield, Swindon. See Organizations in Resources for Chapter 16, p. 334, for addresses and telephone numbers.
For your nearest 'family planning' clinic, contact:
Catholic Marriage Advisory Council, NFP Service, 1 Blythe Mews, Blythe Road, London W14 0NW.
The Family Planning Association (ask for the Family Planning Information Service), 27–35 Mortimer Street, London W1N 7RJ. Tel: 01-636 7866 (for whole UK), 0222-42766 (for Wales), 0232-225 488 (for Northern Ireland), 041-333 9696 (for Scotland).
Margaret Pyke Centre, 15 Bateman Buildings, Soho Square, London W1V 5TW. Tel: 01-734 9351.
Provide counselling, contraceptive information and methods, pregnancy testing, morning-after contraception, sterilization and vasectomy. Only for men and women living in the area.
National Association of Natural Family Planning Teachers, NFP Centre, Birmingham Maternity Hospital, Queen Elizabeth Medical Centre, Edgbaston, Birmingham B15 2TG. Tel: 021-472 1377 ext. 4219.
Pregnancy Advisory Service, 11–13 Charlotte Street, London W1P 1HD. Tel: 01-637 8962. Non-profit-making charitable clinic offering pregnancy testing, morning-after contraception, abortion, donor insemination, sterilization.

CLINICS AND ADVISORY SERVICES ESPECIALLY FOR YOUNG PEOPLE

Brook Advisory Centres, 153a East Street, London SE17 2SD. Tel: 01-708 1234. For young people up to age 25. Offer free pregnancy testing, advice and counselling, contraception advice and methods, and abortion referrals, and counselling on sexuality generally. Branches in Birmingham, Bristol, Burnley, Coventry, Edinburgh, Liverpool and in London in Islington, Walworth, Shoreditch, Lewisham, Kennington, Brixton, Vauxhall and the West End.
Central Wandsworth Youth Advisory Service, 97 East Hill, London SW18 2QD. Tel: 01-870 5818.
Pregnancy testing, counselling and information on contraception.
London Youth Advisory Centre, 26 Prince of Wales Road, London NW5 3LG. Tel: 01-267 4792. Advice and counselling on contraception. Not a clinic.
New Grapevine, 416 St John Street, London EC1V 4NJ. Tel: 01-278 9157 (helpline: 01-278 9147 Tues. 10.30–2.30 p.m., Wed. 2.30–6.30 p.m.). For anyone under 25. Advice and counselling on all aspects of sexuality, including contraception and abortion. Walk-in sessions, phone counselling, discussion groups. Will accompany you to a clinic. Not a clinic.
Pregnancy Advice Contraception Education (PACE), King George VI Community Centre, Knowsley Road, Bootle, Liverpool L20 5DE. Tel: 051-944 1661.
The U2 Project, The Bakehouse, 6 Church Street, Wolverton, Milton Keynes MK12 5JN. Tel: 0908-220042. Advice and counselling for under 25s on pregnancy and contraception. Clinic once a week. Drop in or by appointment (funded initially till mid-1989).

INFORMATION

Birth Control Trust, 27–35 Mortimer Street, London W1N 7RJ. Tel: 01-580 9360. Publications on birth control laws and services.
Bristol Women's Health Group, c/o Wellwoman Information, 24 St Thomas Street, Redcliffe, Bristol BS1 6JL. Tel: 0272-221925. For information about Natural Birth Control as well as support, teaching and fertility awareness classes. Appropriate for women wanting to plan a pregnancy; with subfertility problems; for getting to know your body; going through the menopause.
Family Planning Information Service see Family Planning Association, under Clinics and Counselling, above. For information about all 'family planning' methods and reproductive health.
Women's Health and Reproductive Rights Information Centre, 52–54 Featherstone Street, London EC1Y 8RT. Tel: 01-251 6332/6580.
Information and advice about all aspects of birth control and women's health. Publications, information sheets, self-help groups, public meetings.

CAMPAIGNS AND SELF-HELP GROUPS

Copper 7 Association, 54 Firgrove Hill, Farnham, Surrey GU9 8LQ. Self-help group for women who think the Copper 7 or Gravigard IUDs may have damaged their health.
Dalkon Shield Association, 24 Patshull Road, London NW5 2JY.
Information and support to women who have used the Dalkon Shield. Co-ordinating legal action in the UK for women damaged by the Shield who are claiming compensation from the US manufacturers.
Women's Reproductive Rights Campaign. Campaign for women's right to decide if and when to have children. Contact 01-490 0042 for information about current activities and local groups nation-wide.

INTERNATIONAL CAMPAIGNS

Women's Global Network on Reproductive Rights, Nieuwe Zijds Voorburgwal 32, 1012 RZ, Amsterdam, The Netherlands. Tel: 010-31-20-20-96-72. Network of women's groups internationally campaigning for women's right to decide if and when to have children.

IF YOU THINK YOU ARE PREGNANT

Rewritten by
ANGELA PHILLIPS

As soon as I missed my period I knew that I was pregnant. I felt differently than I ever had before. There was the going to the toilet, of course. I have always had a very weak bladder, but it was now weaker and more sensitive than ever. My energy seemed to be dwindling.

I sometimes miss my period anyway, or it comes really late. So when it didn't come this time I didn't even notice for a while. Then when I did notice, I thought 'That couldn't happen to me.' So I ignored it a while longer. [These words, from a sixteen-year-old, could also come from a woman nearing menopause.]

The most common sign of pregnancy is a missed menstrual period. Nausea and vomiting, breast tenderness, frequent urination, tiredness, may also be early signs. For some women the vital sign of a missed period doesn't occur immediately. Some of us have as many as three 'periods' after conception and some women bleed regularly throughout pregnancy. 'Periods' during pregnancy are usually different from normal periods, often much lighter and lasting a shorter time, but any bleeding irregularity can be a sign of pregnancy.

If you have just come off the Pill, periods may take a while to return to a normal cycle, and for women who have irregular periods or very long cycles, the start of bleeding may not be a sufficiently dependable sign to rely on. If pregnancy is a possibility and/or you have any of the signs mentioned above, the best thing to do is to get a pregnancy test. If you suspect pregnancy but are not sure, and you don't want to be pregnant, keep using contraception until you have the pregnancy confirmed.

If you are even considering terminating your pregnancy, remember there is a time limit for your decision. *The earlier an abortion is done, the safer it is!* Complication rates for early procedures, while all low, do become higher with each week of pregnancy. The induction procedure (16 to 28 weeks) carries three to four times the risk of earlier abortions, although newer techniques do seem to be safer and

less traumatic for women (see p. 328). Also, as the fetus becomes more developed, abortion becomes more emotionally upsetting both for you and for the medical and counselling staff.

WHERE TO GET A PREGNANCY TEST

Pregnancy tests should be available free from your doctor or a family planning clinic. Some district health authorities have considered withdrawing pregnancy-testing facilities where there are no 'medical reasons' for them. We feel that every woman should have the right to a free test on which she can base decisions about her future health. However, overload at laboratories often means that, even when labs accept their responsibility to women, the delays in getting results can be unacceptably long. If the test results are likely to take more than a few days you will probably be better off paying for a test.

Some women's centres and women's health groups provide tests very cheaply (look on noticeboards and in your local paper), otherwise try a chemist (they advertise in the window), or a pregnancy advisory service (listed under 'Pregnancy testing' in the Yellow Pages or see p. 334). Beware of agencies offering free tests which are only trying to promote something else. Lifeline, for example, offers free testing and counselling but will actually try to persuade you not to have an abortion and will use frightening propaganda to push you into rejecting the option that they disapprove of. You can also buy a 'home kit' (see below).

KINDS OF PREGNANCY TESTS

URINE TESTS

A hormone called human chorionic gonadotrophin(HCG) is secreted into the blood and then the urine by the developing placenta. The most common pregnancy tests are based on a chemical reaction with this hormone. Until recently, most tests could not give an accurate result until about twenty-seven days after conception, when the level of HCG had risen sufficiently to be detectable. Over the last few years newer, more sensitive tests using monoclonal antibodies have been developed which can detect much lower levels of HCG. These tests can be used on the day you expect your period or a few days later. This may seem an advantage but you should remember that a large number of pregnancies are spontaneously aborted in the first couple of weeks. You may prefer to wait a few days to be more certain that a positive test means a viable pregnancy rather than be alarmed, or excited, prematurely.

The new early tests are gradually becoming available through the NHS as well as in home kits, and pregnancy-testing services. No doubt in a few years' time the old tests will have been completely replaced.

Some tests are done on slides and some in test-tubes. Some depend on a fine judgement to detect a change in texture, others have been linked to enzymes which change colour if you are pregnant. Most need to be carried out very carefully if the result is to be accurate.

To collect a good urine sample use a *very clean, dry jar*. Do not use an old medicine container or shampoo bottle, because traces of chemicals or soap can contaminate the sample. Especially if it is early in the pregnancy, take the sample when you first wake up in the morning, because your urine is more concentrated then. A small amount (several tablespoons) is sufficient for the test. Cover the urine and keep it refrigerated. It is best not to use aspirin or marijuana the day before you take the sample, because they can interfere with the test.

Pregnancy test results can be positive, negative or inconclusive. A positive result almost always means pregnancy. A false positive – that is, a positive result when a woman is not actually pregnant – is rare. False positives can be caused by an error in reading the test, drugs (marijuana, methadone, Aldomet, large amounts of aspirin, synthetic hormones like birth control pills, some tranquillizers and other drugs that affect the nervous system), protein or blood in the urine, soap or other substances in the container, hormone changes of menopause* or certain tumours or other rare medical conditions.

A negative test may mean that you are not pregnant, but false negatives are fairly common. Often, it is too early in your pregnancy for the test to measure the small amount of HCG in your urine. Later, the amount of HCG starts to decrease after a couple of months; by four to five months the HCG level may be so low that a test may give a false

negative. Other reasons for false negatives are:
1. the urine became too warm;
2. the urine was not concentrated enough;
3. there was contamination from the jar or from certain medications;
4. it is an unhealthy pregnancy that may miscarry;
5. it is an ectopic pregnancy (pregnancy outside the uterus);
6. there has been a mistake in doing the test.

A health worker can help you evaluate your chances of a false negative and discuss why your period may be late if you are not pregnant. If you suspect that you are pregnant even though a test is negative, have a pelvic examination and/or repeat the urine test. Don't just keep waiting for your period.

In two weeks I had three pregnancy tests; all of them were inconclusive, according to the lab reports I got. By the time I was given a blood test which established my pregnancy as real rather than imagined, I felt angry at the medical establishment for disbelieving me.

HOME PREGNANCY TESTS

Some women prefer a home test because it allows them privacy, convenience and control over the experience. However, it also has drawbacks. If you are extremely

---

A GUIDE TO HOME PREGNANCY TESTS*

The best time to perform the test is five to seven days after a missed period, says Dr Mandy Donaldson, who has checked the reliability of four brands in her laboratory at the Chelsea Hospital for Women. To be sure, women should repeat the test.

Predictor Colour and Discover 2 had the highest rate of failure to spot a pregnancy, but the error rate was acceptably low, at less than 4 per cent.

Clearblue and Discover Colour suggested that the woman was pregnant when she was not in 1 per cent of cases.

Overall, Dr Donaldson concludes that, while Clearblue, Discover Colour, and Eva test Blue 5 are more likely to be correct around the day of the missed period, it is best to wait for five to seven days before testing. Then the Predictor Colour test, which is easier to perform, will give a clear, rapid result.

Clearblue, Discover 2 and Boots own brand provide two tests per kit. 'This is to be recommended,' Dr Donaldson says.

*Andrew Veitch, *Guardian*, 17 September 1987.

---

*Most tests cross-react with luteinizing hormone (LH; see p. 40). For this reason, premature menopause and actual menopause can give false positives. If you are nearing menopause make sure that your age is mentioned in the letter to the lab so that special care is taken with your test. A blood test (serum B HC G estimations) would be more accurate. Also, it is possible, though very rare, that a test at the LH surge at ovulation could give a false positive.

anxious about the result you may find it harder to deal with in isolation. A pregnancy-testing counsellor or sympathetic GP can provide support and advice when you are feeling most vulnerable. The tests are not hard to do but the results may be difficult to interpret and often the instructions are not sufficiently detailed to help. Since most tests are affected by such things as vibration and temperature, the results are not as reliable at home as they would be in the controlled conditions of a laboratory.

BLOOD TESTS (radioimmunoassays, RIAs)

Blood tests are occasionally used because they can detect pregnancy even earlier. In Britain their use is confined to clinical work, for example with fertility investigations.

PILLS

If the doctor suggests pills to see whether they will bring on your period, *do not agree*. This procedure, sometimes called a hormone withdrawal test, is *not* an accurate test for pregnancy, and it is dangerous. The drugs used are synthetic hormones (usually progestogen) which can cause negative effects in a woman who takes them, and birth defects if she is pregnant and decides to have the baby. Though the Department of Health issued warnings against this procedure, some doctors may still use it.

PELVIC EXAMINATION (see p. 593)

To check on the results of a pregnancy test or to find out how far along your pregnancy is, have a pelvic examination at around eight to ten weeks after your last menstrual period (LMP). If you are pregnant:

1. you, or your doctor, will feel that the tip of your cervix (neck of the uterus) has become softened;
2. your cervix may change from a pale pink to a bluish colour because of increased blood circulation (you can see it yourself if you have a speculum and mirror);
3. your uterus feels softer to the person examining you;
4. the size and shape of the uterus change.

Some women just know they are pregnant. Some of us feel we know the *moment* we become pregnant. Perhaps one sign – a missed period, tender breasts – tunes us in to the fact that our bodies feel different.

> With my first child I missed a period and my breasts hurt. With Jesse, I knew the moment I conceived him.

> My period was two weeks late and I was going to get a test but when red wine started tasting like vinegar I knew I was pregnant and didn't bother with the test.

CHECK THE ALTERNATIVES

If your pregnancy was planned and wanted you should organize ante-natal care as soon as possible and start taking extra good care of yourself (see Chapter 18). If you are certain that you do not want this pregnancy turn to Chapter 17. If you are uncertain what to do, you have a little time to consider the alternatives. You can keep the baby, have an abortion, or have the baby adopted. Whichever option you finally decide on it is important that it should be *your* choice, an active decision.

Most of us have found that in coming to a decision, it helps to talk to someone. It may not be someone we know well. Often our closest friends and family find it hard to focus calmly on our needs at this time. It may be easier to talk things out with someone who is not involved first, so that your own feelings are straight and clear. You can call a local women's centre, go to a family planning or Brook Advisory Centre clinic, talk to a teacher, youth worker or welfare officer or possibly your doctor (though many doctors are used to being directive and won't give you the space to make up your own mind). Responsible pregnancy advisory services (see p. 334) provide a counselling service to help you make up your mind.

Once you have made a decision you will need sympathetic support from friends and family to help you see it through. You may or may not want to involve the man concerned.

If we do not share with the man the hassle and pain of the unplanned pregnancy, we allow him to avoid his responsibility or even prevent him from assuming it. We also deprive him of the opportunity to share his feelings and to give support. Of course, some men will not face their involvement, and either leave us or withdraw emotionally. This is when we have to turn to a friend or counsellor for all of our support. It is perhaps hardest when our partner disagrees with what we feel we need to do. His feelings are important, but it's our body, and in this society the parenting will be primarily up to us – so the decision must finally be ours.

HAVING AND REARING A CHILD

Having a child changes your life. Think about how you will feel: consider your job, your relationships, your other children if you have any. If you have a partner, you will have to discuss how a child would alter your relationship. Of course, in practice it may be a lot different to how you imagine it so it may help to talk to other friends who have already had children to find out how they manage. If you are alone, practical considerations may be particularly important. Do you live somewhere suitable for a child? If you share a home, how would the others feel about a child? Would you have to move and could you afford to do so? Will you be able to keep your job and, if not, could you survive on 'income support'? Bringing up a child single-handed may seem daunting but it is worth keeping in mind that many women with partners effectively bring up children alone. We all need help some of the time and we can all help each other.

ABORTION (see p. 314)

For many women abortion is a positive choice. Having an abortion can be much less traumatic physically and emotionally than having an unwanted child. The safest and easiest time to have an abortion is within the first three months (first trimester) of the pregnancy.

This is the first time I really told people because it was such a big thing for me. There are so many women who've had abortions. These women have made these choices, too – so nothing's wrong with me . . . When you are willing to talk about it, it makes another feel she can talk to you.

I was the mother of three little boys. Being a mother and having children has always been very important to me, and this made the decision that much more difficult. Loving children as I do, I also knew that having the baby and then giving it up for adoption would not be an option for me.

My lover was opposed to having the child (as a team) and I didn't want another child without his help, so I decided on abortion. I was not happy with this because I wanted the child and was in love with the father.

I knew that abortions were legal, but that's all. I was afraid to mention it to my doctor. I thought he'd accuse me of being evil. (He didn't.) I also thought I'd be in terrible pain. He explained the procedure the day before. It was very helpful.

I get so bitter hearing people piously stating how those poor babies have a right to live and there are lots of people who want babies and can't have them. A baby isn't just produced and given away and that's that. You're talking about a part of a woman's body. That baby is part of her, and to expect her to give it up after going through a pregnancy is really ridiculous. I know many women could, but many couldn't. I couldn't have. I know that without my abortion I would have gone through nine months of hell, dealing with my boyfriend, my parents, my friends, my job, my financial situation, my health, my whole future and then thinking about the baby, its future, would I keep it or not, how to support it, and so on – one headache after another. At that time in my life, I don't think I could have handled it all. I couldn't even handle it now, and I'm better off now than I was a year ago.

ADOPTION

For some of us, continuing the pregnancy and then giving up the child for adoption seems preferable to abortion, and sometimes the decision is left too long and then adoption may seem to be the only alternative.

Few women these days are pushed into adoptions by social pressure. Those who are tend to come from religious backgrounds with a very strong disapproval of abortion. Since the passing of the Abortion Act the number of babies adopted at birth has plummeted to less than 800 in 1983. Ten times as many children are adopted later on, many after court care proceedings, because their parents are unable to cope. Adoptions at a later stage may also be the result of economic pressure. Parenthood is hard enough for two parents in reasonably good economic circumstances. If you are alone, isolated, living in bed and breakfast accommodation and on income support the pressure can be too much.

Every time I went to the Social Services they pushed me to get him adopted: 'You'll never manage,' they said. 'He'd be better off adopted.' I was just desperate for money. I couldn't cope. I wanted to keep him but I knew I couldn't manage. Afterwards I got drunk. I had never drunk before but I was depressed and had no one to talk to. I thought I was doing the right thing but I bitterly regret it.

Coping with an adoption is hard whatever the circumstances. The baby may no longer be in your care but you will not find it easy to get it out of your mind. You need careful and unbiased counselling before making a final decision. Local authority social service departments and adoption societies employ social workers who will discuss your options with you, but try to talk to other people too. Avoid organizations such as Lifeline. They are set up to stop abortions so they cannot be expected to offer unbiased counselling about adoption.

You will be given some say about the parents your child should go to. You can specify the kind of religious and cultural background you would prefer. Generally, agencies try to match babies to parents of the same race as this is considered beneficial for the child's development. Handicapped babies may be a little more difficult to place but many people are happy to bring up a handicapped child particularly if they have the child as a baby.

Arranging an Adoption

Adoption is a way of transferring parenthood. It is a legally binding arrangement which cannot be reversed. You cannot arrange an adoption yourself unless it is to a close relative and even then courts are very cautious. Even the baby's father has no automatic right to adopt (though if you are married he would have legal guardianship and adoption could not proceed without his permission). All other adoptions must go through an approved adoption agency (see below) and be ratified by the court. The law is very strict in order to protect women and children from financial exploitation.

The arrangements are made by your local social services department (social work department in Scotland), or by a voluntary agency which may have a connection with a particular church.* Although you can start things moving before the birth, nothing legally binding will be done until after the birth and you are free to change your mind at any stage until the adoption is finalized.

After the birth some hospitals allow you to leave the care of the baby to hospital staff, others expect you to care for the child for the first few days. You should find out in advance. The hospital should allow you to make up your own mind, at the time, whether or not you want to care for your baby.

Temporary fostering is arranged in most cases before the baby is placed with the adoptive parents. After six weeks, a 'reporting officer' will visit and ask you to sign an agreement to the adoption. You may be asked to sign a 'freeing order', which gives parental responsibilities to the adoption agency until the adoption is formalized in court, or you may keep your parental rights until the adoption order is granted when the baby has been with its new parents for at least three months. During the first six weeks before signing your consent, you will have the opportunity to change your mind. If you have not signed a freeing order you may also be able to get your baby back at any time until the final adoption. However, once the baby has settled with its new parents you would have to persuade the courts that it was in the baby's interests to be returned to you.

You have no legal right to see your child again once the adoption has gone through. S/he will have a special birth certificate which does not show your name on it. However, when the child reaches eighteen (seventeen in Scotland), s/he has the right to see the original birth certificate and may try to contact you. If you are certain you do not want to be contacted or anxious that you should be, you can write to the Registrar General, Titchfield, Fareham, Hampshire. Your wishes will be kept in strict confidence. According to NORCAP,* the agency which arranges contacts between adoptees and their 'birth mothers', most mothers are delighted to see their children again. Indeed, many mothers dearly wish to make contact themselves. Although NORCAP are not allowed to make contact with adopted children on behalf of mothers, many women contact them, often years after the adoption, in the hopes that their child has been looking for them. In the USA 'birth mothers' have started to meet and talk about what adoption has meant to them. NORCAP can help those women who are still trying to cope with the emotional legacy of adoption through counselling and by putting women in touch with other birth mothers for support.

When I hear people say that adoption is the option women should choose instead of abortion, I get a knot in my stomach and all my memories come back. Adoption may be an option for some people, but it wasn't a good answer for me.

---

*A list of agencies is available from the British Agencies for Adoption and Fostering (BAAF), 11 Southwark Street, London SE1 1RQ.

*NORCAP is at 3 New High Street, Headington, Oxford OX3 7AJ.

ABORTION
(Termination of Pregnancy, TOP)

Rewritten by
ANGELA PHILLIPS

One of our most fundamental rights as women is the right to choose whether, and when, to have children. Only when we have that right can we be free to take a full part in society. While contraception is the first defence against an unwanted pregnancy, no contraception is absolutely effective and those methods that are safest for our health tend to have a higher failure rate. So, for the foreseeable future, abortion will continue to be an intrinsic part of any comprehensive birth control service. We believe that all abortions should be free, voluntary and safe, performed in a supportive atmosphere with sufficient information and counselling.

Around 1 per cent of abortions are carried out to end pregnancies when fetal abnormalities have been detected. Terminating a pregnancy which has been embarked on with pleasure is a very painful experience. It is a choice which women are increasingly expected to consider as technology allows more and more access to the fetus earlier in pregnancy.

We are concerned that women are being expected to make decisions about abortion in a very short time and with very little information about the nature of the potential handicap. We know also that some doctors who are unwilling to grant abortions to women who do not wish to be pregnant have no such hesitation about aborting supposedly 'defective' fetuses. This betrays an attitude which is not only hostile to the rights of women but also to handicapped people. (We discuss these issues in more detail in Chapter 19.)

The circumstances in which we decide to end a pregnancy are enormously varied. The value judgements of others do not have a place in that decision. If we are to be genuinely able to make choices we all need equal access to the resources which would make parenthood, whether of an able-bodied or a handicapped child, a pleasure rather than a burden. We do not all have those resources. In writing this chapter we are acutely aware that, while the decision to have an abortion is never entirely free of conflict, for some of us it is a particularly painful choice. It must nevertheless be *our* choice, made in the knowledge of what is possible in *our* lives, given the responsibility for childcaring that society has placed on *our* shoulders.

We know that some men and women sincerely believe that abortion is wrong. We cannot agree with them that the rights of an unborn fetus should take precedence over those of the woman who is carrying it. While we defend any woman's right not to have an abortion we reject the right of those who oppose abortion to impose their beliefs on others. The Abortion Today section of this chapter explores the tactics of the anti-abortion movement and ways in which we can defend our right to abortion.

ABORTION AND POPULATION CONTROL

There have always been groups and individuals who have supported birth control, not in order to free women, but to control populations. They have turned a tool which we should use in our own interests against groups of people (usually less advantaged groups) whose growth appears threatening to the status quo. Marie Stopes, famed in popular history as an agitator for birth control, in fact believed that it was (at least partly) necessary because 'we have been breeding revolutionaries' or as Harold Cox, another agitator for reform in the 1930s, put it:

> There is a danger that the higher racial or national types may be swamped by the lower types.[1]

While we believe firmly in the right of individual women to choose abortion we utterly reject the use of birth control techniques, on an involuntary or coercive basis, as a way of controlling populations or groups within society. And, while the rhetoric may have changed, we are aware that the population lobby today follows in the footsteps of Harold Cox, quoted above, spreading propaganda in favour of birth control for those people in non-industrialized nations whose rate of population growth is considered threatening to the Western way of life. Aid from industrialized countries for birth control products (some of which have been banned in our own countries) is well organized.

Back home, birth control presents a much cheaper solution to poverty than the provision of decent housing and nurseries which would give women a genuine right to choose. As a result, attitudes towards black and working-class people may also differ from those towards the white, middle classes. There is certainly evidence that certain forms of contraception are more readily prescribed for black women (see p. 276). There is also some evidence that black women are pressured into having abortions. One black woman told the Abortion Rights Tribunal in 1977:

I managed to get an NHS abortion after the usual palavers but I was disturbed by what I learnt subsequently. My GP is more liberal in referring black women because he feels that they 'breed too much'. He does not refer white women for abortions nor does he prescribe the pill for them.[2]

Black and working-class women are also more likely to be expected to accept sterilization at the same time as abortion; a combination which increases the risks of both. The combined procedure is far more common in the NHS than in the private sector.

While it is clear that the need for birth control can be perverted by those who do not care about women's rights, we must also be careful not to be taken in by those men who use opposition to the population lobby as a reason to prevent women from organizing among themselves, and in their own interests, for birth control. A correspondent to *The Communist* in the 1930s expressed a view which can still be heard in some quarters today when he argued against birth control because:

No decently organized society has the right to deny parenthood to a healthy father.[3]

When abortion is freely chosen it is a useful tool for all women. In the words of a black American woman activist:

Many black people on hearing the word 'abortion' immediately think of genocide – the killing of a people. With a racist history and the continuing virulence of racism in the US, there is little question as to why blacks link abortion to genocide. While such precaution is warranted, at the same time many black women are choosing to have abortions. In the struggle to become full participants in the labour force and to overcome tremendously adverse social conditions, the availability and accessibility of adequate and supportive abortion services is essential for black women. A black woman's decision to have an abortion is integrally bound up with her continuing struggle to improve the quality of life for herself as well as her family. It is for these reasons that black women and all women of colour join in the fight to maintain abortions – safe, legal and on demand.

HISTORY OF ABORTION LAWS AND PRACTICE

The anti-abortionists sometimes argue that abortion violates an age-old natural law. But for centuries abortion in the early stages of pregnancy was widely tolerated. In many societies all over the world it has been used as one of the only dependable methods of fertility contol. In Europe and America even the Catholic Church took the conveniently loose view that the fetus became animated by the rational soul, and abortion therefore became a serious crime at forty days after conception for a boy and eighty days for a girl. (Methods of sex determination were not specified.) English and American common law, dating back to the thirteenth century, shows a fairly tolerant acceptance of abortion up until quickening, the moment sometime in the fifth month when the woman first feels the fetus move.

Most of the laws making abortion a crime were not passed until the nineteenth century. In 1869 Pope Pius IX declared that all abortion was murder. In the 1860s, in this country, new legislation outlawed all abortions except those 'necessary to save the life of the woman'.

These mid-nineteenth-century abortion laws did not succeed in curbing our strong natural sexuality. But history has shown that women will seek abortion whether it is legal or not and at considerable risk, and the new laws obliged increasing numbers of women to get abortions illegally. The trauma of illegal abortion is a part of our collective history as women that deeply agonizes and angers us. There was a high rate of complication, infertility and even death among women who desperately tried to abort themselves, or who were forced underground for dangerous illegal operations. There were illegal profits to back-street abortionists, who charged high prices for non-medical procedures done in unsanitary conditions. There was blatant discrimination against poor women, who had to risk back-street abortions while their wealthier sisters could often find and pay a cooperative doctor. And those unable to end their unwanted pregnancies too often found their lives, and those of the children born, twisted by the hardships involved.*

Agitation against these laws started in earnest in 1936 with the formation of the Abortion Law Reform Association. It took ALRA thirty years to get a law through Parliament. Finally, David Steel's Abortion Act was passed

---

*A Swedish study of children of women denied abortion twenty years earlier revealed them to be (as compared to a control group) in poorer health, with histories of more psychiatric care, and with a higher rate of alcohol use.[4]

in 1967. It does not apply to Northern Ireland where women are still forced to use illegal methods or travel to Britain for private treatment. This law does not repeal previous legislation, it only outlines specific cases where to give or procure an abortion would no longer be a crime. They are when:

1. the continuance of the pregnancy would involve risk to the life of the pregnant woman greater than if the pregnancy were terminated;

2. the continuance of the pregnancy would involve risk of injury to the physical or mental health of the pregnant woman greater than if the pregnancy were terminated;

3. the continuance of the pregnancy would involve risk of injury to the physical or mental health of the existing child(ren) of the family of the pregnant woman greater than if the pregnancy were terminated;

4. there is substantial risk that if the child were born it would suffer from such physical or mental abnormalities as to be seriously handicapped.

Under these conditions termination is legal up until 28 weeks (attempts to reduce it are constantly being made). In order to comply with the law, *two* medical practitioners have to certify 'in good faith' that the conditions above have been satisfied. They may take into account present and future environment in making their decision. No terminations may be done after 20 weeks unless resuscitation equipment is available.

This law can be interpreted in many different ways. Some doctors still refuse to perform an abortion unless there is a real risk of death for the mother. Others will do it only if the woman accepts sterilization at the same time. At the other end of the scale there are concerned doctors who believe in the woman's right to decide. These doctors tend to interpret the law very liberally, on the basis that early abortion is always statistically safer than a pregnancy taken to term and will therefore always fall within the terms of the Act.

The partial legalization of abortion has provided a service for thousands of women. But women were not themselves given the right to choose – the decision was left to doctors and hedged about with rules and regulations which have hampered the introduction of safe methods, such as very early aspiration, which could be provided by GPs and family planning clinics. The growing liberalization of medical attitudes has paradoxically endangered even this partial reform. Anti-abortion groups attack the law on the grounds that it is being abused by doctors who interpret it liberally and that it should therefore be restricted.

Our right to abortion will never be assured until we have won the repeal of all legislation which can be used against women or the people who help us to get abortions.

ABORTION TODAY

Extremes in interpreting the Abortion Act, coupled with a cumbersome and expensive bureaucratic procedure and progressive cuts in health-service funding have combined to produce an inefficient, inadequate service across the country. Only about half of all abortions are performed on the health service. Abortion is the only routine medical procedure which is not automatically available to all people irrespective of income and as such is a gross example of sexism in medical care.

There are some areas where the efforts of sympathetic senior staff have ensured that most women can have abortions free, often on an outpatient basis. In many others such as Wales, the west of Scotland and the Midlands, women are forced not only to pay for abortions but also to travel miles for treatment.

The NHS has organized 'agency arrangements' with the charitable abortion clinics (p. 322) in some places and pays for some local women to have abortions. This has not increased the number of abortions done free in these areas. There is no doubt that the existence of abortion charities has done much to help women in need and to lower the price for abortion in the private sector. Nevertheless, they have enabled the health service to duck out of a major obligation to women.

THE ANTI-ABORTION MOVEMENT

The two major organizations are Life and the Society for the Protection of Unborn Children (SPUC). These organizations are strongly supported by the Catholic Church, although they both claim to be non-denominational. The basis of their argument is that the fetus is a person from the moment of conception, and that abortion is therefore murder. On this assumption they would like to deny the right of abortion to all women.

As soon as the abortion law was passed the anti-abortion forces began work. Initially they tried to get amending laws through Parliament. When that failed, they called for a committee to be established to look into the working of the law. When that committee came down firmly in favour of the law as it stands they declared that it was biased. They then started to organize a vast 'grassroots' campaign with highly emotive literature, huge demonstrations and organized letter-writing to Members of Parliament. Their demonstrations included large contingents of nuns, Catholic schoolchildren and church-organized bus loads from all over the country.

On the crest of this wave of support James White, the MP for a largely Catholic marginal constituency in Glasgow, introduced his amendment Bill in February 1975. This time, instead of the previous outright rejections, the Bill passed its second reading (each Bill is read in Parliament three times, with two debates and voted on at each stage), and was referred to a special 'select committee' for further examination.

Since then regular attempts have been made to amend the law or to restrict it by tightening up the regulations covering its operation. In 1985 the anti-abortion organizations tried a new tack: an attempt to provide protection to the fetus via a Bill ostensibly aimed at stopping embryo research. In spite of the campaigns the law remains largely intact but the anti-abortionists have succeeded in blocking any hope of a more liberal law in the immediate future.

Anti-choice organizations are an international pheno-menon. Anti-abortion campaigners in the USA have resorted to violence in attempts to stop abortion. The US National Right-to-Life Committee, which includes most anti-choice groups, claims a membership of 11 million and has a three-million-dollar annual budget. Right-to-lifers also routinely harass staff and patients at abortion clinics. They try to prevent women from entering and disrupt abortions in progress. After struggling with her complex feelings and then deciding to have an abortion, a woman approaching a clinic may be faced with cries of 'murderer'. Since 1977 hundreds of clinics have been bombed, burned and vandalized. Pro-choice supporters have responded with physical defence of clinics and escorts for patients.

THE PRO-CHOICE MOVEMENT

The wave of attacks on the abortion law in Britain stimulated the organization of the first mass movement for the right to choose. The National Abortion Campaign (NAC) was set up almost overnight, taking the feminist demand for a woman's right to choose into political organizations and into the heart of the organized trade-union movement.

The trade-union movement, which had steered clear of such 'controversial' matters since backing the call for birth control clinics in the 1920s, was rocked on its heels by a new wave of women activists determined to take the message of a woman's right to control her fertility into a movement which had previously barely recognized that it had women members.

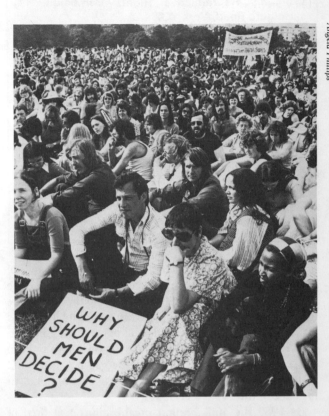

Angela Phillips

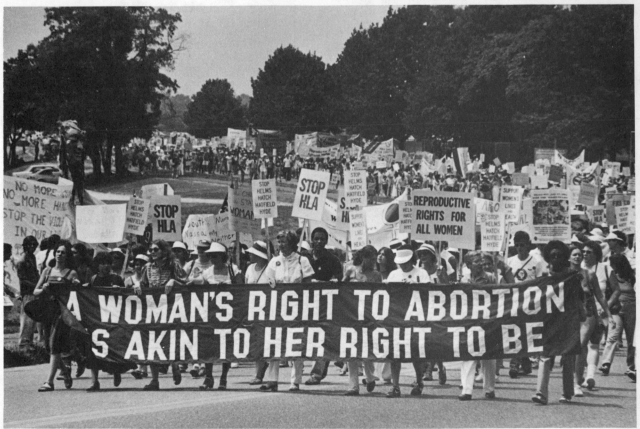

David Beach

PRO-CHOICE ORGANIZATIONS

Women's Reproductive Rights Campaign, 11 Holgate Road, York YO2 4AA.

Abortion Law Reform Association, c/o WHRRIC, 52–54 Featherstone Street, London EC1Y 8RT. Tel: 01–251 6332/6580.

National Abortion Campaign, Wesley House, 4 Wild Court, London WC2B 5AU. Tel: 01-405 4801.

Coordinating Committee in Defence of the 1967 Act (COORD), c/o The Birth Control Trust, 27–35 Mortimer Street, London W1N 7RJ. Tel: 01-580 9360.

Doctors for a Woman's Choice on Abortion, 101 Burbage Road, Dulwich, London SE24 9HD. Tel: 01-274 4901.

While NAC brought together an often stormy alliance of feminists and women from the organized Left to take the issues of sexuality and fertility control on to the streets, the other organizations set about the business of lobbying and applying pressure in the corridors of power. The Abortion Law Reform Association, adopting the 'women's right to choose' campaign slogan, bridged the gap between NAC and the newly formed Coordinating Committee in Defence of the 1967 Act (COORD).

By 1980 the anti-abortion organizations had tired of head-on confrontation and, as the threats receded, the pro-choice organizations adopted a lower profile. Many feminists felt that this was the moment to form a broader movement on fertility control and this eventually led to a split with many women leaving NAC to form what is now called the Women's Reproductive Rights Campaign. Since

Statistics confirm that voluntary legal abortion is improving women's physical and psychological health. According to government statistics, since 1968:

- the infant mortality rate has dropped;
- abortion-associated deaths have dropped to almost nil;
- hospital admissions for incomplete (illegal) abortions have virtually stopped;
- mortality and complication rates of legal abortion have dropped steadily;
- the mortality rate for abortion is now well below that for full-term pregnancy and delivery.

Studies on the psychological effects of legal abortion for an unwanted conception consistently show that women feel more happy than sad, more relieved than depressed, after having a voluntary abortion.[6]

then there has been another failed attempt to amend the law. Nevertheless, with the law as it exists, many hundreds of women are still forced to go through a time-consuming, often humiliating and usually expensive process to obtain services which, as Stella Browne put it in 1935:

> . . . should be available for any woman, without insolent inquisitions, nor ruinous financial charges, nor tangles of red tape. For our bodies are our own.[5]

IMPROVING ABORTION SERVICES

In many areas women's groups have campaigned for outpatient facilities in their local hospitals. Outpatient clinics, properly run, would allow the maximum number of women to get the help they need at an early stage in pregnancy. These clinics would also be cheaper to run than the current facilities, which often necessitate a two-night stay in hospital. However, abortion services should be organized not on the basis of saving money but of giving service. All patients should have the option of talking to a counsellor, and wherever possible that counsellor should be available to stay with them throughout the operation if local anaesthetic is used (see p. 323).

How to Organize

It isn't easy to tackle the monolith of the NHS, but within a NAC or women's group there are a number of things you can do.

1. Contact other local women's groups and local Labour Party women's sections (the Labour Party is officially in favour of the right to choose although a significant minority of Labour MPs disagree and continue to vote for restrictions) to set up a joint campaign.

2. Try to contact members of hospital staff, particularly those who are active in unions, i.e. Confederation of Health Service Employees (COHSE), National Union of Public Employees (NUPE), Medical Practitioners' Union (MPU). If it is a teaching hospital, medical students will be in the National Union of Students. Trade-union members can work through their own unions to establish policy on outpatient clinics, and even when they do not have national policy favouring abortion (some do) they will be invaluable in any local campaign.

3. Write leaflets and hand them out to staff and patients at the local hospital. The organizations listed in the box above can provide information.

4. Organize meetings inside the hospitals with the help of staff, to discuss the issue of abortion with those people who are involved.

5. Contact your local or community health council (see p. 642) and district health authority (or health board) (see p. 644,) and push them to support your campaign. your campaign.

6. Contact the local papers and radio stations with information about your campaign.

HAVING AN ABORTION

FEELINGS ABOUT UNWANTED PREGNANCY

Most of us experience a powerful mixture of feelings when an unwanted pregnancy is confirmed. We may fear that our families will find out and punish us; fear that we won't be able to decide what to do; fear that we'll be all alone in trying to decide; fear the prospect of motherhood. We may also fear abortion even though we know it's legal and safe: Will it hurt? Will it cost more than I can pay? Will I be punished by having some dreadful complication and maybe even be made sterile? Will I feel guilty? Will I later wish I had had the baby?

We feel a lot of anger too. We may feel angry with ourselves or our partners for not being careful enough about birth control. Often, however, we have been using birth control and it has failed:

When I found I was pregnant, I was frightened and angry that my body was out of my control. I was furious that my IUD had failed me, and I felt my sexual parts were alien and my enemy. I felt I was being punished for my femaleness.

Abortion can also be a positive and powerful affirmation of independence:

The fact that I was able, for so many reasons, to choose to have an abortion has made an enormous difference in my life since then. Other decisions that I've made (where to live, to go back to college, to come out as a lesbian, what kinds of work to do) might all have been different if abortion hadn't been available to me in the past. As a woman-identified woman, I feel so strongly that those options should be open to other women. Of course, this means not just abortion but childcare, decent incomes and housing and education, struggling with racism and more. But I know from my own direct experience what is involved, on so many levels, for a woman to decide on an abortion and follow it through. Knowing that afterwards my feelings weren't as simple as I'd expected just makes it clearer for me that no one else has any right to interfere with a woman doing what she needs to do, according to her own wisdom and judgement.

A highly ambivalent experience:

I was extremely anxious and upset. Although a health professional, I panicked. I felt hopeless – depressed, guilty and angry.

Or a relatively straightforward one:

Deciding to have an abortion wasn't a difficult decision or a big deal. From the way everyone I told reacted, though, I started wondering if something was wrong with me for not being upset.

For many of us the decision is more painful because it is based not on personal desire but economic necessity:

I had strong feelings against abortions and knew that I myself could never have one. Pregnancy to me meant that a little soul had chosen to come into my body, and how could I say no to that? But when I found myself pregnant and with two teenage children, a year-old baby and myself and my husband working day and night with barely any time for each other, I knew that I had to have an abortion. It wasn't too hard a thing to do.

But for most of us it is a right worth fighting for:

I have never regretted my abortion. I am just determined that my daughters and my granddaughter can have safe and legal abortion available should they need it. The freedom from unwanted pregnancies that today's woman enjoys is something I wish my mother could have lived to see, as it is something she never dreamed would ever happen. Her struggle to limit her reproduction has left its imprint on me, as we were very close. My father was a tyrant. Birth control was her problem. But it was her wifely duty to satisfy his sexual desires. She used self-induced abortion as a means of limiting her family. She was determined not to have a houseful of cold and hungry kids as her own mother had – eight children and she finally died in childbirth.
My mother suffered a great deal of guilt because of society's attitude about abortion – miscarriage, it was called. She reasoned it a greater sin to bring into the world children to suffer cold and hunger than to abort.

FEELINGS ABOUT ABORTION AFTER ANTE-NATAL TESTING

I felt I didn't have the right to 'play God' but I had other children to think of. I knew a Down's baby would take up time and energy which I simply did not possess.

When I agreed to the amniocentesis I simply had not thought the implications through. It didn't occur to me that the test could be positive. In the event I had thirty-six hours to make a decision. I think I made the right one but I still keep reliving it, trying to justify the abortion to myself.

I don't think I had any feelings then. It was as

HOW PREGNANT ARE YOU?

The length of a pregnancy is usually counted from the first day of the last normal menstrual period (LMP) and not from the day of conception (fertilization). LMP dating is inaccurate and misleading. It can make you think that you are two weeks further along in the pregnancy than you really are. It assumes that every woman not only has a twenty-eight-day cycle but ovulates exactly two weeks after her period began. (Nobody has a regular cycle *all* the time.) The *first trimester* is the first 12 weeks; the *second trimester* is the 13th to the 28th week LMP; 29 weeks LMP and later is the *third trimester*. Abortion is safer, easier and less expensive in the first trimester. It may be difficult to find a clinic that provides second-trimester abortions, and impossible to get a third-trimester abortion unless your life is endangered by your pregnancy.

To date a pregnancy accurately, you must consider whether your last period was normal for you. If it came at an unexpected time or was lighter than usual, conception may have happened before that bleeding.

If you chart your body changes with a fertility awareness method (see p. 37) you will have a written record of ovulation and will be able to recognize pregnancy quite early on. If you do cervical self-examination, you may notice that your cervix has changed colour and become bluish-purple, which happens early in pregnancy.

Signs of pregnancy can help confirm the date of conception (see p. 358).

An experienced doctor can estimate the length of a pregnancy by feeling the size of the uterus during a pelvic examination. This is usually accurate within a two-week range. Ultrasound, another method for determining the length of a pregnancy, also has a two-week margin of error. The doctors signing your 'green form' (see p. 322) make the final decision about how far advanced the pregnancy is and whether to do the abortion. If they refuse, you may be able to find other doctors who will help. Statistically, abortion risks increase as the pregnancy progresses and the uterus becomes larger and softer.

---

though I had died. I went through the next forty-eight hours in a daze. In fact I don't think you could call it a decision to have an abortion. I felt I had been put on a moving belt which didn't stop until about six months later.

I knew only positive results were reported by phone. The image of myself, alone, screaming into a white plastic telephone is indelible.[7]

When ante-natal testing was first introduced, most doctors failed even to consider the emotional aspects. It was assumed that women would be so glad to be relieved of defective fetuses that they would be clamouring for screening and grateful for abortions. Many found it impossible to understand why some women would reject both procedures. Few introduced adequate counselling services and many women have been forced to find their own way through this devastating experience without any help. Research work proving the rather obvious fact that aborting a wanted baby is very different from aborting an unplanned one has resulted in the establishment of a counselling service in some areas before testing and abortion, and then again after the procedure.

Your hospital should provide counselling. If it doesn't, speak to your own GP or health visitor. We should be given unbiased and clear information about the disability which has been identified, the gradations of handicap, the likely outcome and the degree to which the child would need extra help if we decide to continue the pregnancy. Even if we do not wish to discuss the decision it may help a lot to be

DANGEROUS ABORTION METHODS

1. Gin, hot baths, jumping from a height are only likely to dislodge a fetus if you were going to miscarry anyway.

2. Sticking sharp instruments into your uterus may well dislodge the fetus, but it is quite likely to kill you or damage the fetus as well. The same is true of introducing fluids into the uterus.

3. Many pills and potions are sold as abortifacients. The vast majority are either ineffective or extremely poisonous and, even if they do not damage you, there is a chance that they will damage the fetus *without* causing an abortion. Herbs may sound harmless but some are extremely toxic and, if taken without the help of a herbalist, can kill you.

---

able to pour out our feelings. Be sure to find out who you can call to talk to after the abortion as well. Working through grief can help us come to terms with it.

SAFE TECHNIQUES FOR ABORTION

When you are considering an abortion or choosing where to have an abortion, you have a right and a need to know the procedures used at each stage of pregnancy, the risks and possible complications and the cost (if any).

METHODS OF ABORTION

Procedure	Techniques	Weeks LMP
1 Preemptive abortion Endometrial aspiration	suction	4–7
2 RU 486 (mifespristone) (experimental)	'abortion pill'	early
3 Vacuum aspiration	dilatation, suction, sometimes curettage	7–14
4 Dilatation and curettage (D & C)	dilatation, curettage	6–16
5 Dilatation and evacuation (D & E)	dilatation, suction, curettage, use of forceps	12 – upper limit varies from 16 to 24
6 Induction abortion (instillation procedure) (Prostaglandin abortion) (Saline abortion – rarely used)	injection of liquid through the abdomen into amniotic sac; uterine contractions (labour) expel the fetus and placenta	16–24
7 Prostaglandin pessaries (experimental)	drug inserted into the vagina to cause labour and miscarriage	throughout
8 Hysterotomy	uterus is cut open	16–28 or later if woman's life in danger

LMP: last normal menstrual period.
Dilatation: enlarging the cervical opening by stretching it with tapered instruments called dilators, or with laminaria (see p. 328).
Suction: drawing out the contents of the uterus through a narrow tube attached to a gentle vacuum source.
Curettage: scraping the inside of the uterus with a metal loop, called a curette, to loosen and remove tissue.
Forceps: grasping instruments used to remove tissue.
Amniotic sac: sac of fluid surrounding the fetus.
Prostaglandin: hormone-like substance that causes uterine contractions.
Saline: salt water.

In pregnancy, a tiny ball of cells attaches itself to the lining of the uterus about one week after conception. A mass of tissue called the *placenta* develops in the uterine lining to nourish the *embryo*. By the end of the second month, the embryo, now called a *fetus*, is surrounded by a protective fluid-filled sac, the *amniotic sac*. At about 20 weeks the woman begins to feel the fetus move. Sometime between 24 and 28 weeks the fetus reaches the point where it may live outside the mother for at least a short while under intensive hospital care.

In an abortion, the contents of the uterus (embryo or fetus, placenta and built-up lining of the uterus) are removed. Different methods are used, depending on how large the pregnancy tissue has grown, the training of the person performing the abortion, the approaches favoured by the doctor or clinic and the equipment available. The following chart summarizes procedures. They may not all be available in your area, or different names may be used for some of them. Ask for explanations of words and terms that you don't understand.

Aspiration abortion is now the most common technique (see p. 325). Of all the methods it carries the least chance of complications and considerably less risk than pregnancy, labour and delivery. In fact, it is now the safest of all operations, safer than having your tonsils out or circumcisions. It only takes a short time (five to fifteen minutes). This kind of abortion has been the safest and least disruptive for a woman, both physically and emotionally. It can only be done during the first three months of pregnancy.

The new abortion pill RU 486 could possibly supersede surgical abortions in the first three months. It would certainly be less traumatic for women to be able to avoid hospitalization. However, we must await the results of trials before we can feel sure that a drug which acts on the body to provoke an abortion has no significant long-term effects. Given the very low risk attached to early vacuum abortion we would be alarmed by too swift a change to the use of this pill. Women health workers and users will need to monitor the introduction of this method.

HOW TO GET AN ABORTION

It is scandalous that in a country which prides itself on having a fully socialized National Health Service it should be necessary to discuss the facilities of the private sector. However, 50 per cent of women seeking abortions are forced to go outside the NHS. If you are seeking an abortion the first avenue to explore is the local hospital via your GP.

GENERAL PRACTITIONERS

If you have a good, well-informed, caring doctor you are much more likely to get an abortion. Some of us are afraid of discussing abortion with our doctor because we feel that s/he might tell our parents, look down on us, or because we feel too guilty and ashamed to talk to anyone who might have any contact with us in the future. For a number of reasons which we discuss further, it is worth approaching your doctor if it is at all feasible. Remember that most GPs are in favour of the 1967 Abortion Act so there is a reasonable chance that yours is too.

Go to your GP as soon as you suspect you might be pregnant. *If you go within seventy-two hours of a possible conception, you could ask for a 'morning-after' pill (see p. 295). This is not the same as pills prescribed to 'bring on your period'. These pills are ineffective and should not be prescribed.*

Find out at this point how long a pregnancy test would take. Some GPs have testing equipment in their surgeries and can do a urine test while you wait. As this is a cheap and easy process they should all have the equipment, but many don't. There is no reason why you should have to wait more than twenty-four hours for results but some laboratories under pressure of inadequate funding are cutting back on pregnancy testing unless the tests are considered 'medically necessary'. In that case, you would be better to save time and go elsewhere (see p. 309). If you are already convinced that you wouldn't want to go ahead with the pregnancy, say so. His/her reaction will be a good indication of how s/he will treat a request for termination. If you feel quite certain that s/he will not help you, you might as well start another channel of investigation straight away. If s/he seems non-committal or sympathetic go back when your pregnancy is confirmed (see p. 323).

This is what your GP should do:

1. Act as a counsellor, helping you to make up your mind what to do, give you all the information you need and advise on the *medical* aspects of the different possibilities. S/he is not your moral adviser and should not act that way.

2. Sign a 'green form' (H.S.A.1) if s/he considers 'in good faith' that you fall within the terms of the Abortion Act (see p. 316). Many GPs will fob you off by saying that you are 'not eligible' for an NHS abortion and will make no effort to get you one. There is no difference in eligibility between the NHS and the private sector, merely a dif-ference in practice. GPs should make it their business to know which hospitals in the area are sympathetic and which consultants are more likely to do terminations 'on social grounds'. They should be able to send women directly to the right person on the right day. No woman should be sent to a consultant who is known to ill-treat women requesting abortion. However, with the best will in the world no GP is likely to be able to get you an NHS termination if you live in an area where abortions are not done on 'social grounds' at all and many of them are ill-informed about NHS procedure.

3. Your GP should make the appointment for you at the hospital by phone, s/he should not ask you to do it. S/he is, after all, supposed to know the ropes.

4. The hospital will write to you with the date and time of your appointment. That shouldn't be more than a week later. However, waiting lists may be much longer, and some hospitals use their waiting lists as a convenient way of refusing an abortion *before* seeing you. If you will be more than 10 weeks' pregnant by the time you go to a hospital you should consider 'going private'. You can always make an appointment at a pregnancy advisory service for the day after your NHS appointment in case you are refused an abortion. The earlier the abortion is done the better it will be for your health.

If your doctor refuses to help you, or you are unable to get an NHS appointment, or are turned down for an abortion, you will have to try outside the health service. In any case you might like to double-check by phoning WHRRIC or NAC (p. 334) to find out your chances of getting an NHS abortion in your area.

REGULATIONS GOVERNING PRIVATE CLINICS

All private clinics or nursing homes are licensed. No clinic or nursing home may perform terminations after 20 weeks unless they have resuscitation equipment available for the aborted fetus. (This new regulation was aimed at stopping late abortion and many doctors will not now take on women after 18 weeks to give themselves a margin of error.)

All clinics should be inspected regularly and may have their licences removed if they are not up to standard.

Not all clinics are licensed to do day-care abortions and only eight can do abortions after 20 weeks. The big abortion charities, Pregnancy Advisory Service (PAS) in London and British Pregnancy Advisory Service (BPAS) nation-wide, provide both services; PAS tends to be a little cheaper. Both have excellent safety standards. Other private clinics and doctors will provide abortions too. The standards and prices vary.

These clinics also provide a service for some 30,000 women (mainly from Spain and Ireland) who are unable to get abortions in their own countries because of restrictive laws. PAS in London provides a special, multi-lingual service. WHRRIC can provide information about other services.

These organizations employ counsellors to discuss feelings about pregnancy, help you to make a clear decision and to describe the process to you (see 'Counselling', below). BPAS and PAS in London also employ doctors on a sessional basis, who will do the necessary examination and can sign your 'green form' if your GP has not done so. You can go to them direct if you would rather not contact your own doctor, though they do prefer you to have some contact with a GP in your area. You will then be referred to a second doctor who will examine you again and add the second signature to your form. You will then be booked in at a clinic. It usually takes a week to ten days from first contacting the service to leaving the clinic.

Most organizations charge a consultation fee and prices for abortion vary. Sometimes loans can be arranged and in some areas NHS patients are referred to the charities under an agency system in which your operation is paid for by the health service.

Private gynaecologists outside the charities may well charge much higher fees and they are no better qualified. Try not to leave it too late – late abortions are much more difficult to get and to cope with. Many doctors who are otherwise very liberal about abortion referral will refuse to sign the form after a certain time and it is increasingly difficult to get abortions anywhere after 20 weeks.

COUNSELLING

All the good pregnancy advisory services offer counselling to every woman. Some NHS hospitals also employ counsellors (they are usually hospital social workers), but far too many of them offer no discussion other than an initial, and often brief, interview with a doctor.

A counsellor should not force you to discuss things you would rather not mention or push you into taking any kind of action which is not determined by you. She should give any information you require and brief you about the abortion itself.

Questions to ask are:

1. Emergency back-up procedure: serious complications are rare but you should be prepared in case. Both PAS in London and BPAS will give you an emergency number to ring if you are worried but they will encourage you to inform your own doctor so that you can be treated locally if necessary. If you are going to a hospital find out whether you can contact the ward direct in an emergency or whether you have to go through your GP.

2. If you are 12 weeks pregnant or less, most charitable clinics will give you the choice of in- or outpatient procedure provided that you live within two hours of the clinic, have informed your GP and can be collected after the operation. If your local hospital has an outpatient clinic you would automatically be admitted on an outpatient basis at this stage, provided there were no medical problems.

3. If there is a choice between local and general anaesthetic, will you be able to choose which you prefer? (See p. 334.)

4. If you are having NHS treatment will you be in a ward with women with other problems, such as infertility investigations?

5. Can contraception be prescribed by the operating doctors? If so will they provide supplies?

In addition to formal counselling we have found that a lot of support and encouragement can come from the other women who are having abortions with us.

The two rooms where the abortions were done opened on to the porch where the six of us were waiting. One girl from our group, who had said she had never had even a pelvic examination in her life, was just coming out of the abortion room. She had just had her abortion, and she looked OK. That was comforting. A seventeen-year-old girl came in. She was very very scared. I held her hand and comforted her. I hadn't had my abortion yet and was scared too (though I'd had one operation, two children, and a D & C). Something amazing happened when I held her hand. Any fear I'd had disappeared as if it were drawn out of me from all sides. We were all such different women who for varying reasons were having the identical physical thing done to us.

ANAESTHETICS

Local anaesthetic can be used up to 12 weeks with a vacuum suction (or early aspiration) abortion. It does not put you to sleep. You can walk into the operating theatre and lie down on the couch. You will then have an injection in the cervix which numbs it, so that it can be stretched without causing pain. You do feel some pain, similar to period cramps, while the suction is in progress but it doesn't last long (five minutes or so). One advantage is that the doctor is forced to be slower and more careful if you are awake and reacting to what he does. However, if you are very tense and frightened it may be difficult for the doctor to complete the operation properly. The success of local anaesthetic depends on a careful, gentle doctor and the presence of a counsellor or nurse to keep you company and reassure you during the operation. This emotional support is unfortunately not always provided.

General anaesthetic is widely used in this country, too often for the convenience of medical staff who do not want conscious patients so that they can work faster; they are not, therefore, prepared to explain the relative merits of local or general anaesthesia.

The general anaesthetic will probably be light and last only about ten to fifteen minutes, so you wake up with little awareness of what has happened. The disadvantage is that you may feel nauseous, weepy and groggy afterwards; it can affect you for a few days. Comparisons between local and general anaesthesia show that complications such as perforation and haemorrhage are more common with a general and, although the risk of dying from a legal abortion about equals the risk of dying from a shot of penicillin, some women are particularly vulnerable to anaesthetics and a few deaths have been caused directly by their use.[8] (See p. 596 for more on general anaesthetic.)

RISKS AND COMPLICATIONS

As with any medical procedure, there are possible risks and complications. The chance of a complication for a first-trimester abortion is about 5–10 per cent. The later the abortion, the more chance of complications. Signs of a complication will generally appear within a few days after the abortion. Listed below are most possible risks and complications of abortions, their symptoms and treatments; induction abortions carry additional risks (see comparison of risks between induction and D & E abortion, p. 328).

INFECTION

Infection is one of the more common complications. Even though sterile instruments and antiseptic are used, bacteria sometimes travel into the uterus. Signs of an infection are a temperature of 100.5 degrees Fahrenheit or higher, bad cramping and/or vaginal discharge with a foul odour. Treatment consists of antibiotics, usually tetracycline or ampicillin. It is important to have a check-up after finishing the medication to make sure the infection has gone and there is no sign of retained tissue. Left untreated, an infection can cause serious illness, sterility or even death.

RETAINED TISSUE

Since the practitioner can't actually see inside the uterus during the abortion, occasionally s/he leaves some tissue behind. Signs of retained tissue include very heavy bleeding, passage of large blood clots, strong cramps, bleeding for longer than three weeks or signs of pregnancy (for instance, sore breasts, nausea, tiredness) lasting longer than a week. Tissue remaining inside the uterus is likely to become infected. Sometimes the drug syntometrine is given to stimulate the uterus to contract and push out the retained tissue. The other treatment is removing the tissue by an aspiration procedure similar to an aspiration abortion but shorter, or occasionally a D & C.

Doctors should examine the tissue removed during an abortion to ensure that it is complete. This is not always done.

PERFORATION

Perforation of the uterus occurs if an instrument goes through its wall. There is more risk of perforation in a D & E than in a first-trimester abortion. If a woman is awake, she is likely to feel a sharp pain or cramp. If perforation occurs, the medical staff will monitor pulse, blood pressure, cramping and bleeding very closely. The uterus is a very strong muscle and often heals quickly on its own.

However, if there are any indications that a large blood vessel or another organ may have been injured you will need hospitalization and possibly surgery.

HAEMORRHAGE

Uterine haemorrhage (excessive bleeding) during or after an abortion is more likely to occur in second-trimester abortions. Excessive bleeding can sometimes be a sign of retained tissue, perforation or failure of the uterus to contract. Drugs may be given to stimulate contractions of the uterus, or an aspiration procedure may be done to slow down the bleeding.

CERVICAL LACERATION (tear)

There is more chance of the cervix being injured during a second-trimester abortion than an earlier abortion. The practitioner should inform you and record it on your medical record. A small tear heals without treatment. A more serious tear may require stitches, and there may be some bleeding from the tear.

MISSED ABORTION – CONTINUED PREGNANCY

In very rare instances, some tissue is removed and yet the woman remains pregnant. This is more likely early in pregnancy (less than four weeks after conception, 6 weeks LMP). All clinics should inspect the tissue removed from the uterus right after the abortion to be sure that all the pregnancy tissue has been removed. Sometimes one pregnancy is removed but another remains. If this happens, signs of pregnancy are likely to continue. The abortion will have to be repeated in a week or so.

POST-ABORTAL SYNDROME (blood in the uterus)

If the uterus doesn't contract properly or if a blood clot blocks the cervical opening and prevents blood from leaving the uterus, blood collects within it. As blood accumulates, pain, cramping and sometimes nausea increase. Sometimes you can push the clots out by deep massage directly over the uterus (pressing hard with your fingers just above the pubic bone). If this doesn't work, the clots need to be removed by aspirating the uterus.

POSSIBLE EFFECT ON FUTURE PREGNANCIES

When large groups of women are compared statistically, those who have had a legal abortion are no less likely to have a healthy baby in the future than anyone else. Having several abortions does appear to increase the chances of miscarriage and prematurity. However, on an individual level, it is clear that anything which can introduce infection into your uterus (childbirth, miscarriage, STDs) is potentially fertility-threatening. It is therefore particularly important to ensure that you are free of infection before and after an abortion.

MEDICAL PRELIMINARIES

A detailed medical history and pelvic examination (see p. 593) should be taken at the time of referral to the clinic, then some tests (these may be done in the hospital).

The questions will cover: the number of full-term pregnancies you have had and previous abortions or miscarriages or caesarean births; a history of TB, heart disease, asthma, acute kidney disease, bleeding or clotting problems, epilepsy or a recent major operation.

The tests should be: a urine test to check again whether you are pregnant and for your general state of health; a blood test to check for anaemia (if you are anaemic the doctor will have to be very careful about blood loss; if this test is done in advance you may be prescribed a course of iron pills before the operation) and to check for sickle cell anaemia; another blood test determines your Rh factor.

Rh Factor. Everybody's blood is either Rh positive (Rh+) or Rh negative (Rh−). When an Rh− woman carries an Rh+ fetus (which will usually be the case if the father is Rh+), either birth or abortion can cause antibodies to build up in the woman's blood. These antibodies may react against a fetus in a future Rh+ pregnancy. If you have Rh− blood and plan to have children in the future, unless the father of the fetus is Rh− you should be given a shot of blood derivative called Anti D within seventy-two hours after the abortion. Anti D will prevent the antibodies from forming in your blood.

Your *blood pressure* should be taken before, after and during the procedure. A change in blood pressure during the abortion can indicate internal bleeding.

Infection. Few clinics or hospitals will bother to check for vaginal infection unless you ask them to. This is an extremely serious omission as studies show a significantly increased risk of pelvic infection after abortion when there was untreated infection at the time of operation. If tests for infection are not made at your referral visit *we would strongly urge you to visit an STD clinic for diagnosis and treatment of any unsuspected infection before your abortion* (see p. 488). A severe pelvic infection can endanger your future fertility.

PREPARATION FOR THE ABORTION

Take some sanitary towels with you to the clinic as you will probably bleed after the abortion. (You should not use tampons.) You will be asked not to eat for several hours beforehand if the operation is to take place on the day of admission – this is in case you vomit during the operation. It is particularly important if you are having a general anaesthetic because you could choke on the vomit. Most hospitals prefer you to be prepared for a general in case it should be necessary. However, for early outpatient abor-

tions, one doctor reported that 'A woman seems able to cope with the trauma of abortion under local anaesthetic better on a full stomach.'[9]

FIRST TRIMESTER ABORTION PROCEDURES

UP TO SEVEN WEEKS LMP

Early aspiration abortion can be done, theoretically from the time of your first missed period, for up to three weeks afterwards (7 weeks LMP). A syringe attached to a cannula is used to suction (aspirate) the contents of the womb. Since the tube is very narrow this technique does not normally require any dilatation of the cervix.

Most women report some cramping pain during or after

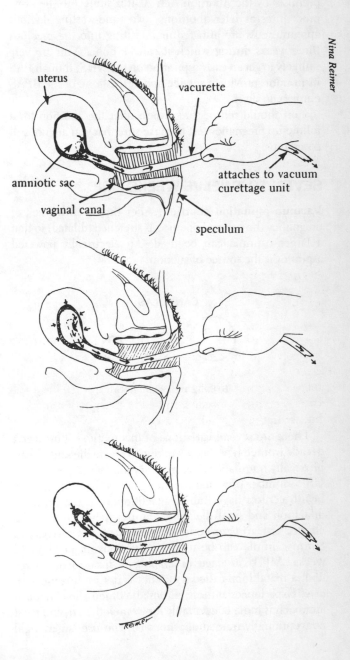

uterus

vacurette

amniotic sac

attaches to vacuum curettage unit

vaginal canal

speculum

Nina Reimer

the procedure. About 34 per cent consider the pain 'severe'. The flexibility of the instruments and the fact that general anaesthetic is not normally used mean that the risk of complications (which is the same as with vacuum aspiration) is much reduced and, because it can be done very soon after pregnancy is suspected, it is probably the least traumatic form of abortion.

One possible complication is that a very early pregnancy can be missed altogether and you remain pregnant. Dr Ros Stephens, who has pioneered the method in Britain, prefers to wait until 6 or 7 weeks LMP because this minimizes the chance of missing the fetus.

It is possible to use this technique before pregnancy is diagnosed (pre-emptive abortion). However, this runs the risk of doing it unnecessarily.

The major drawback in the UK is that the technique, which could easily be available in family planning clinics and health centres, is confined to hospitals and registered premises by the Abortion Act. As it is subject to the same procedures as later abortions, two time-wasting doctor's appointments are also required, eating into the precious three weeks during which it can be done. You are very unlikely to get an early aspiration on the NHS, though PAS in London provide a service and at least one of the BPAS clinics can do it.

You should return three weeks after the abortion for a follow-up pregnancy test to make sure that you are not still pregnant.

SEVEN TO TWELVE WEEKS LMP

Vacuum aspiration abortion. After the seventh week of pregnancy the cervical opening is stretched (dilated) so that a larger cannula can be used. An electrically powered aspirator is the source of suction.

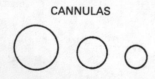

CANNULAS

6, 8, 12 mm diameters

There are several variations of this method. For over a decade women have been working to create the safest, least physically traumatic vacuum aspiration techniques. In the US a number of woman-owned and -controlled feminist health centres have trained practitioners to use minimal dilatation and small flexible cannulas, which reduce the chance of tearing or perforating the uterus or cervix. (An 8 mm cannula can be used for abortions up to 11 to 12 weeks LMP.) Curettage, or scraping the inside of the uterus with a metal loop called a curette, is not routinely necessary. Experiences at these clinics and others show that this approach is more comfortable for women than that of most conventionally trained abortionists, who use larger, rigid

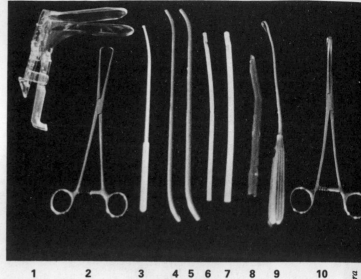

1 Speculum	**6&7**	Flexible plastic cannulas
2 Tenaculum	**8**	Rigid plastic cannula
3 Sound	**9**	Curette
4&5 Dilators	**10**	Forceps

Lynn Vera

plastic or metal cannulas (which require more dilatation) and a curette after the suction.*

Dilatation and curettage (D & C) is a standard gynaecological procedure (see p. 194). Because medical students routinely learn D & C, this used to be the most common method for first-trimester abortions. Now it has been virtually replaced by the quicker, easier and safer aspiration techniques.

RU 486 (mifespristone). Usually used in combination with a prostaglandin. This abortion pill must be taken daily for four days. The side-effects are pain, diarrhoea and vomiting. This drug is still used only in trials. Its potential usefulness to women will be realized only if it can be prescribed by GPs and family planning clinics, which would not be legal under the existing law.

HAVING A VACUUM ASPIRATION ABORTION

The majority of abortions are carried out between 7 and 12 weeks of pregnancy. We want to describe that process step by step. We hope that our outline will give an idea both of what to expect and what to ask for by way of good medical care and emotional support.

In most hospitals and clinics in the NHS, abortion, even at this stage, is an 'inpatient' procedure, often requiring a two-night stay.

For inpatient treatment you will automatically be offered a general anaesthetic unless there are medical problems, or

---

*Doctors are trained to consider new information about medical procedures only if it comes from so-called medical authorities. They are not trained in give and take, or in learning from health workers 'below' them in the medical hierarchy, or from women on whom they do the procedures (patients).

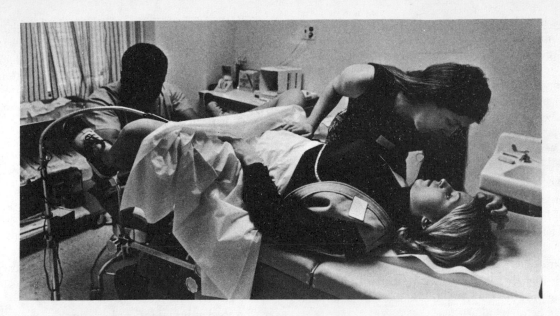

you specifically request a local anaesthetic. Most NHS outpatient clinics and the London PAS clinic give a choice of local or general anaesthetic; BPAS does not provide local anaesthetic.

If you are having an anaesthetic you may be given 'pre-medication' which will make you feel drowsy, or you may be wheeled straight into the operating theatre before getting any medication. In either case, once on the operating couch you will be given an injection which sends you to sleep immediately. The operation is the same for local or general anaesthetic, except that those who have a general will be unaware of what has happened, so we will describe the rest as for a local anaesthetic abortion.

The Procedure

You will lie down on the couch with your feet in stirrups or your legs supported by knee pads. The doctor performs a bi-manual examination (see p. 593). At this point you may be given a tranquillizing injection to help you relax. The vaginal area is thoroughly cleaned with antiseptic solution. It is unnecessary to shave off the pubic hair.

The doctor then inserts a *speculum* (see p. 594) which keeps the walls of the vagina apart and allows a good view of the cervix (the mouth or opening of the uterus). This does not hurt, but it can feel like pressure.

The cervix is then grasped with a *tenaculum*, which feels like a slight pinch. The tenaculum will be held throughout the rest of the procedure to keep the cervix steady.

A local anaesthetic is injected into the cervix. This numbs the cervix. The injection is usually relatively painless.

In most hospitals and clinics you will be given a shot of syntocinon if you are having a general anaesthetic. This drug makes the uterus contract and is thought to prevent bleeding. It also makes the procedure more painful and is not usually used with local anaesthetic.

The cervix is then dilated (opened) slowly with sterile plastic or stainless steel instruments called dilators. They are from six to twelve inches long and vary in diameter from the size of a matchstick to the width of a piece of chalk, and are slightly curved on the ends. The cervix is dilated with the smallest dilator first and then with larger and larger dilators until it is opened wide enough for the tip of the vacurette to enter the uterus.

You may experience what feel like very heavy menstrual cramps while the cervix is being dilated. If the cervix has been dilated before (e.g. during miscarriage, delivery, or previous abortion), the cramping is usually less. Dilatation usually takes less than two minutes.

The aspirator, or suction machine, consists of a vacuum-producing motor connected to two bottles. A hollow tube several feet long is attached to the bottles. A variety of different-sized sterile hollow tips (vacurettes) can fit on the end of this tube. These tips are either stainless steel or disposable plastic and are approximately six inches long. The diameter of the tip used varies with the length of the pregnancy.

This tip is inserted through the open cervix into the uterus. The machine is turned on. The fetal material is removed by gentle pulling on the uterine walls, and is drawn through the tip, through the plastic tube, and into the bottle. The aspiration takes from two to five minutes.

Some doctors will then insert a thin metal instrument called a curette and move it around inside the uterus to check that it is completely empty (see 'Dilatation and Curettage'). Others feel that this extra procedure causes unnecessary extra bleeding, and use tiny forceps to pull out any tissue not taken by the suction.

As the uterus is emptied of fetal material it contracts back to its original size. These muscle contractions may cause quite strong cramps, which generally subside ten to thirty minutes after the procedure is over.

Recovery

You may feel shaky, nauseous and tired. Or you may feel fine. You will lie down (or sit, depending on how you feel) for a half hour to an hour afterwards, in a recovery room where clinic staff can check your blood pressure, temperature, etc. Then in many clinics you will be asked to sit in a lounge or waiting room for a while longer to make sure you are fully recovered, with no excessive bleeding, before you leave.

See p. 324 for Complications and p. 330 for Aftercare.

SECOND TRIMESTER ABORTION PROCEDURES

Dilatation and evacuation (D & E) is a newer method that combines D & C and vacuum aspiration techniques for abortions later than 12 weeks LMP. Because the fetal tissue is larger and the uterus is softer and easier to injure than in the first trimester, a D & E is more complicated and requires a high level of skill on the part of the person performing the abortion. An ultrasound examination may be required beforehand.

The cervix needs to be dilated more than with an earlier abortion so that larger instruments can be put into the uterus to remove the pregnancy.

In the USA *laminaria tent* (a kind of seaweed which expands gradually in moisture) is often put into the cervix the day before to open it gradually. It is very rarely used in the UK because of fear of infection. However, in NHS hospitals, prostaglandin gel may be used to soften the cervix and in post-20-week abortions the cervix may be opened a little on one day and then opened further the next day (two-stage procedure). This is thought to minimize damage to the cervix.

Dilators are used to enlarge the cervical opening. Then the doctor uses forceps, a curette and vacuum suction to loosen and remove the uterine lining, placental and fetal tissue. A drug (syntocinon) may be given to help the uterus contract, slowing down the bleeding that normally occurs.

In an **induction abortion**, the doctor injects (instils) an abortion-causing solution through the abdomen into the amniotic sac which surrounds the fetus or through a tube into the vagina and cervix just outside the amniotic sac. (Before 16 weeks LMP this sac is not large enough to be located accurately, so the procedure cannot be used until this time.) Hours later, contractions cause the cervix to dilate and the fetus and placenta to be expelled. A D & C is often performed after the abortion to remove any remaining tissue. A hospital stay of twelve to forty-eight hours is involved.

The first commonly-used solution was hypertonic saline (salt) solution. In recent years use of prostaglandins has become widespread, as well as combinations of prostaglandins, urea and/or other ingredients. Saline is rarely used in Britain now because it is considered no safer, and is a lot slower, than prostaglandin.

Prostaglandin pessaries placed in the vagina sometimes cause strong uterine contractions resulting in miscarriage. This is the newest, least known abortion method. Nausea, vomiting, diarrhoea, fever and failure to cause abortion are common problems, so the method is not widely used.

In a **hysterotomy** the surgeon removes the fetus and placenta through an incision into the abdomen and uterus, like a small caesarean section. The incidence of serious complications for this kind of major surgery is considerably higher than for other methods of abortion. You may need a hysterotomy when induction methods have been repeatedly unsuccessful or can't be used for medical reasons.

The Advantages of the D & E Procedure

The D & E has several advantages over the induced-miscarriage procedures. Not only is it safer, but it is physically and emotionally easier. D & E is much quicker

EFFECTIVENESS AND COMPLICATIONS OF ABORTIONS PERFORMED AT 13 WEEKS GESTATION BY D & E AND PROSTAGLANDIN F$_2$a[10]

Outcomes	D&E*	PGF$_2$a*	Outcomes	D&E*	PGF$_2$a*
1. Effectiveness			Transfusion	0.19	1.53
Success rate	99.90	92.50	Cervical laceration or		
Induction–abortion time			fistula	1.16	0.64
(hours)	0.50	24.80	Convulsions	0.02	0.32
2. Specific complications†			Uterine perforation	0.32	0.16
Incomplete abortion	0.90	36.10	3. Any complication	5.83	53.26
Haemorrhage	0.71	5.80			

Source: W. Cates, D.A. Grimes, K. Schulz, H.W. Ory and C.W. Tyler. 'World Health Organization Studies of prostaglandins versus saline as abortifacients', *Obstet Gynecol* 52.493, October 1978.

*Data derived from the Joint Program for the Study of Abortion under the auspices of the Centers for Disease Control.

†Complications per 100 procedures.

(ten to forty-five minutes, compared to many hours with an overnight stay in a hospital for induction abortion). You don't have to go through labour and complications are less likely, although more studies are needed. A few doctors are doing the D & E procedures up to 24 weeks LMP with good results, although a limit of 18 to 20 weeks is more common.

The biggest problem with D & E, however, is that it is not widely available and while 60 per cent of 15–16 week abortions are done this way privately, only 12 per cent of NHS abortions are.

There are not yet enough people trained to do D & E procedures, especially in the 18–24 week LMP range because few doctors are willing to accept the personal strain of doing D & Es. Many dislike the idea of removing a second-trimester fetus by performing a D & E, and would rather provide induction abortions. We need more doctors who place greater priority on the fact that *a D & E is both safer and less upsetting for women*, so that many women who have less money are not forced to accept an induction procedure, which involves more pain, more time and more chance of health complications.

HAVING A SECOND TRIMESTER ABORTION BY THE INDUCTION METHOD

Having an abortion from 12 to 28 weeks of pregnancy is a more difficult experience both physically and emotionally than a pre-12-weeks abortion. If you have an induction, as described below, you can go through several hours of discomfort as the uterus contracts to open the cervix and expel the fetus. The complication and mortality rates, though no higher than for full-term pregnancy and delivery, are higher than for earlier abortions.

Emotionally, too, it tends to be a hard experience, even when you are very sure you do not want to have a baby and are feeling great relief at the prospect of being free of pregnancy after long weeks of worry. The pain, the length of time it takes, the similarity of what you go through to what delivery of a baby would have been like; the fact that you have carried the pregnancy for many weeks and probably even felt the fetus move inside you; the fact that a very vocal part of society says what you are doing is 'bad' – all these factors can make late abortion much more upsetting than early abortion.

If you are having an abortion because a fetal abnormality has been diagnosed you will probably feel utterly devastated or numb with shock. Support groups are being established to give women an opportunity to talk through their feelings about abortion in these circumstances (see p. 332).

The very fact that you were not able to have an early abortion may mean that you have had a struggle already. Maybe you had hassles with, or fears about, doctors and hospitals which kept you from getting help until this late; perhaps you ran into opposition or lack of support from someone close to you; perhaps you had felt too confused to make up your mind whether to have an abortion or not;

maybe for many weeks you had pretended to yourself that you were not pregnant because you felt you could not face it. So you come into the experience somewhat emotionally exhausted already. In many cases it will be the medical system itself which has caused the delay.

It is very difficult to find an NHS hospital which will accept you for a late abortion without strong medical grounds or diagnosed fetal abnormality. NHS hospitals tend to be slightly more generous to women who are under age (below sixteen years) or who have a history of severe psychiatric disorder. But many hospitals regularly perform inductions on women who, having been accepted for termination early in pregnancy, have been kept waiting so long that the simpler methods cannot be used.

The quality of care and degree of personal attention vary greatly. Some hospitals insensitively place abortion patients in with women who are having babies. In some NHS hospitals you will be left alone a lot, not told clearly enough what is being done to you, not offered enough pain relief (if you want it). Talk to the doctor and find out exactly what the process will be before you go into the hospital.

The Procedure

There are five phases in an induced abortion: instillation, waiting, contractions, the expulsion of the fetus and placenta, and the recovery period.

Instillation. The process is started when the doctor cleans your abdomen, numbs a small area with a local anaesthetic, then inserts a needle, usually through the abdominal wall a little below the navel (sometimes through a plastic tube into the cervix), and injects the miscarriage-inducing liquid into the uterus. You must let the doctor know immediately if you feel waves of heat, dizziness, backache, extreme dryness.

Waiting. It will take several hours for contractions to begin. You may feel nausea and have diarrhoea. If the waiting period is too long, you may be given an injection of syntocinon to bring on contractions or to speed them up.

Contractions. As contractions begin they will feel at first like mild cramps. At a certain point you may feel a gushing of liquid – this is the bursting of the amniotic sac. After this, and especially for the last few hours before the fetus is expelled, contractions will be stronger and more painful. As a rule the contractions are not as strong as those of full-term labour and delivery, but they can cause you considerable pain. No general anaesthesia is given, but tranquillizers and pain relief should be offered.

Expulsion. After several hours of contractions, the fetus, and then in a few minutes the placenta, will be expelled. The fetus will often show signs of life for a few minutes unless urea is used. It is likely that afterwards the doctor will recommend a D & C (see p. 594) to ensure that the abortion is complete.

Recovery

You will generally stay in the hospital for twenty-four hours or so after the procedure.

AFTER AN ABORTION

AFTERCARE

Women have a variety of physical experiences after an abortion. Most of us feel fine and do not have any problems, but some feel tired or have cramps for several days. Bleeding ranges from none at all to two tó three weeks of light to moderate flow, which may stop and then start again. Signs of pregnancy may last up to a week. Some women experience a variety of changes four to seven days after an abortion because of the drop in hormone levels that happens at this time. Bleeding, cramping, breast soreness and/or feelings of depression may increase or appear if they have not been present.

Here is a list of ways to take care of yourself after an abortion:

1. Try to follow what your body needs – rest for a day or so if you feel tired. (If you can't rest because you have no one to help take care of children or you have to go to work to keep from losing your job, you may recover more slowly.) Avoid heavy lifting or strenuous exercise in the next few days, as it may increase your bleeding. Drinking alcohol may also have this effect. Sometimes ergometrine or syntometrine (drugs that stimulate the uterus to contract) is prescribed on the theory that it may keep bleeding to a minimum and help expel any tissue retained in the uterus.

2. To help prevent infection, don't put anything into your vagina. This will avoid introducing germs that may travel up into your uterus before it has had a chance to heal completely. Don't use tampons, swim, douche or have intercourse for two to three weeks. *

3. Watch for signs of complications. If you have a temperature of 100.5 degrees Fahrenheit or higher, severe cramping or pain, foul-smelling vaginal discharge, vomiting, fainting, excessive bleeding (soaking an entire pad in an hour or less or passing clots) or signs of pregnancy that last longer than a week, report this to the clinic or doctor immediately.

Complications are not likely, but they do happen to some of us. It is not your fault if you have a complication. If a complication is not taken care of as soon as possible, it might turn into a serious situation, so don't ignore possible warning signs. Often a call to the clinic will reassure you that what is happening to you is not a complication after all, but within a range of normal experience.

After the abortion, I had retained tissue. I needed a reaspiration [basically a second abortion] to prevent an infection and remove the remaining

tissue. Although the national rate of complications is very low, I was enraged to be a statistic. I had decided to terminate my pregnancy, but I didn't expect another abortion one week later. I didn't have any choice but to see it through and get my body back to normal.

4. Often the place where you had the abortion is the best source of information and medical advice or care in case of a possible complication. Call them if anything is bothering you, even if you cannot go back there for care. If you need follow-up medical attention, try to consult people who are experienced in treating women who have had legal abortions. Stay away from hospitals, clinics and doctors who believe in forced motherhood and are against abortion. They may try to make you feel that you 'deserve' the complication as 'punishment' for having had an abortion, and they may not be well informed about proper treatment for post-abortion problems.

5. It is important to get a check-up in two to three weeks. * A pelvic examination gives information about the small possibility of retained tissue or infection that may not be causing any symptoms yet. This is often a good time to discuss birth control, which may have been difficult to talk about at the time of the abortion. It can be especially helpful to talk with other women who have had abortions recently. Most of us are reassured by having questions discussed and learning that our experiences have happened to other women, too. If you are one of the few women who has a continuing problem or complication, you need good information and medical help until the problem is over.

6. Your next period will probably start four to eight weeks after your abortion. *You can get pregnant immediately after an abortion, even before your next period, so you need to use reliable contraception if you have intercourse and don't want another pregnancy.* You may say and believe, 'I'll never have intercourse again, so I don't need contraception.' And although there are many wonderful ways of making love without intercourse (see Chapter 14), you may later change your mind. *One thing that you have in common with all women having abortions is that you know you can get pregnant.* If you weren't sure before, you know beyond any doubt that you need to use contraception if you have intercourse again and do not want to become pregnant.

Choosing a contraceptive method is a very individual matter (see Chapter 15). Some clinics will encourage you to use certain methods, especially the Pill, which you can start taking the day of a first-trimester abortion. If you do this, you will be protected after the first cycle of pills, four weeks later. However, the Pill affects your whole body and can cause changes that are similar to signs of pregnancy, which could be confusing right after an abortion. It is not a good idea to have an IUD inserted at the time of an abortion, because of greater risks of infection and perforation. Also

*Some doctors prescribe antibiotics just in case of infection. Studies show that this does reduce the *overall* rate of pelvic infection. However, inappropriate prescribing of antibiotics can cause other problems (see p. 488). It is wise to check for and treat existing infection *before* the operation. You may then prefer to avoid medication unless it is necessary. (Infection may, of course, be introduced during the operation.)

*PAS in London advises four to six weeks because infection, in their experience, can be introduced by early pelvic examinations.

the IUD effects of cramping and bleeding may mask the symptoms of an abortion-related infection. A diaphragm or cervical cap can be fitted or refitted at the post-abortion check-up. You can start a natural birth control class after an abortion or obtain foam and condoms from a chemist without a prescription.

Some NHS doctors insist on sterilization or the insertion of an IUD before granting an abortion. Neither procedure is advisable at the time of an abortion. Insertion of IUDs is better postponed until several weeks later to ensure that there is no infection. Sterilization done at the same time as abortion increases the risk and there is evidence that more women regret the operation when they consent to it at this time.

It is very often black and working-class women who are subjected to this kind of pressure and they are the people least able to refuse pressure and turn to the private sector. Similarly, black, working-class and very young women may be pressurized into accepting an injectable contraceptive at this time. This is certainly not medically advisable, as it may mask abortion complications (see p. 296).

If you are pressurized in this way contact your local Community Health Council or the WHRRIC (see p. 334) for support.

FEELINGS AFTER ENDING AN UNPLANNED PREGNANCY

For most of us the end of an unplanned pregnancy is a tremendous relief. We feel glad to be able to go on with life in the way we need to, and proud that we have made and carried out an important decision. Sometimes the experience of working out the best solution with our lovers, friends or family is a very positive one. We discover strengths and weaknesses which we had not anticipated, both in ourselves and others. It can precipitate discussions which we might otherwise feel unable to start. It is a time for concentrating on our own needs, and for many of us, that may seem a unique experience. At the same time some of us experience a return of some of the same mixed feelings we had in deciding whether to have the abortion. Even the most positive feelings afterwards tend to be mixed with negative ones.

I left the clinic with my friend, feeling two ways about the whole experience: one, that I'd had as good and supportive an abortion experience as a woman could have; and two, I would never put myself in the position of having to go through it again.

Immediately after the abortion there can be a reaction which, like the depressed feelings a woman often has shortly after a full-term delivery, may be related to the lowering in our body of the hormone levels of pregnancy. We may have feelings of inconsolable sadness and periods of crying.

I was so relieved not to be pregnant any more that I didn't think I had any sad feelings at all. Then a few days later, on my way to a friend's house, I saw a young couple walking a new baby and I burst out crying right there on the street.

While society does not allow us a real right to choose by providing material support for those of us who want children, there are bound to be some of us who feel real grief after the abortion. Others of us feel sadness because the experience has brought home for the first time how hard life can be.

There are sometimes also hangover feelings of guilt about what we have done. They are not surprising in a society which has for so long told us that abortion is wrong. Those of us from religious backgrounds may feel particularly guilty. It may be a comfort to realize that thousands of other women whose lives have also been dominated by religion have had to make this same decision in the past. Women have always had to face the contradictions between man-made religious laws and the pragmatic decisions that they have to make for themselves and their families.

Even after the punishment of the operation itself I expected that in some way the odds would be evened in my life for the presumptuous thing I had done. When my favourite aunt got very ill I took it as a sign that I had done something wrong. I felt a nagging fear that I wouldn't ever be able to conceive again.

If we have been able to work through our mixed feelings before we have the abortion by talking to others we are unlikely to feel seriously depressed. In fact severe depression after an abortion is rare (studies in both America and at Kings College Hospital in London have conclusively proved this).

If we do feel depressed, however, this is not a 'punishment' that we have to put up with! The clinic we went to, or any of the referral groups mentioned in this chapter, can refer us to someone to talk with – social worker, counsellor, clergyman. Post-abortion support groups have been set up in some areas to give women the opportunity to air their feelings. Contact the WHRRIC for details (see p. 324). Or maybe what we most need is a chance to share our feelings with friends.

As we move back into our 'real life', the life that was so drastically interrupted by the pregnancy, we can carry a lot of feelings from the experience we've had. Many of us, for instance, feel intense frustration and anger at what we've had to go through. It can take a long time for these feelings to go away.

Even though my husband was very supportive, I felt angry – not so much because he put the sperm in me as because he in no way could understand what I had experienced.

We may feel isolated, even from the people we are close to.

My boyfriend's attitude afterwards was depressingly callous. His idea was: 'Well it's over now, why bother thinking about it.' That's when I started to have to pull away from him emotionally.

Sometimes having an abortion marks the end of a relationship, leaving us with all those mixed high and low feelings of being on our own again, in addition to the feelings from the abortion experience. Sometimes the whole episode strengthens the relationship we are in.

Some of us have negative feelings about sex for a while after the abortion.

For a good month or two I felt like sex was repulsive. We'd start to make love and I'd feel, 'I hope I don't have to pay for this.' Also, we were using a diaphragm for the first time, and I didn't trust it yet. My husband was gentle and tried to help by pulling out to ejaculate outside my vagina. But I never relaxed, and I kept asking him, 'Are you going to come soon?'

Afterwards I felt very much that my boyfriend was potentially my destroyer, or even my enemy, because he had the capacity to impregnate me again. When I used two applicators full of foam while waiting for the Pill to become effective, I used to think that I was arming myself against the act itself. This was not the most pleasant feeling to have just before making love.

On the other hand, some of us had a chance to choose a reliable method of contraception for the first time when we had the abortion, and we feel more relaxed about sex than we ever did. It can be a drag to wait two or three weeks to have intercourse – yet this is a good chance to explore ways of pleasuring each other without intercourse.

Any of the negative or confused feelings we do have after an abortion tend to pass away with time – for some of us quickly, for some of us more slowly. For a few, feelings of depression and loss can come back again in cycles around the time of year when we had the abortion or when the baby would have been born or during some unconnected crisis. This often depends on how good or bad we are feeling about ourselves and our lives at the time.

What's important for us to realize is that positive, negative, ambivalent feelings are all natural after an abortion. We need to accept them all as part of us, give them space in our lives, and not put ourselves down for having them – only then can we make our peace with them. For many of us a crucial part of this process has been the chance to share our feelings with supportive friends.

Fortunately all my conflicts about the abortion were resolved about a year and a half later, when I found the courage to speak of it in a women's group I was in. Because of the calmness and caring the other women shared with me, as well as some of their own experiences with abortion, I came away from that meeting feeling that this thing that had haunted me for so long was finally resolved. I no longer felt bitter about the only choice I could possibly have made in order not to totally wreck my own life and that of others.

FEELINGS AFTER ENDING A WANTED PREGNANCY

Ambivalence, guilt, relief, anger are feelings associated with any abortion. With a pregnancy which was planned and wanted and then ended after ante-natal testing, the predominant feeling will probably be grief. Research into women's feelings after abortion suggests that 'the reaction was akin to that documented after stillbirth or neo-natal death'. Forty-six per cent of the women interviewed were still suffering six months later and some were referred for psychiatric help.[11]

For six months I would wake every night and go downstairs to cry.[12]

Telling the children that I wasn't pregnant any more was the worst part of it and dealing with well-meaning acquaintances wanting to know when it was 'due'.

Making the medical arrangements, going back for counselling, and finally the abortion was the most difficult period of my adult life. I was then 21 weeks pregnant and had been proudly carrying my expanding belly. Telling everyone – friends, family, students, colleagues, neighbours – seemed an endless nightmare. But it allowed us to rely on their love and support during this terrible time. Our community was invaluable, reminding us that our lives were rich and filled with love despite the loss. A few weeks afterwards I talked to another woman who'd gone through 'selective abortion'. She'd returned to work immediately, her terrible abortion experience unspoken. Her isolation only underlined my appreciation of the support I had received.[13]

Talking through your decision and experience with others may help to resolve your own feelings. Your hospital should provide post-abortion support but you may also want to talk to others who have been through the experience. Support groups are being organized. Contact the Disabled Living Adviser, c/o ASBAH, 22 Upper Woburn Place, London WC1H 0EP.

NO RETURN TO BACKSTREET ABORTION

Many younger women do not know what it was like to need an abortion before legalization. Women who could afford to pay skilled doctors or go to another country had the safest and easiest abortions. Most women found it difficult if not impossible to arrange and pay for medical abortions. It is important to keep alive the memory of those days as a reminder of what life could be like again if the 'moral right' achieve their aim of banning legal abortion.

> With one exception the doctors whom I asked for an abortion treated me with contempt, their attitudes ranging from hostile to insulting. One said to me, 'You tramps like to break the rules, but when you get caught you all come crawling for help in the same way.'

The secret world of illegal abortion is frightening and expensive. Many of the laywomen and some of the doctors who performed abortions were both skilled and dedicated. But others cared only about being well rewarded for their trouble. Abortionists often turned women away if they could not pay huge sums, in cash. Some male abortionists insisted on having sexual relations before the abortion.

Abortionists emphasized speed and their own protection. They usually didn't use anaesthesia because it took too long for women to recover, and they wanted women out of the office as quickly as possible. Some were rough and sadistic. Almost no one explained what was happening, discussed contraceptive techniques or took adequate precautions against haemorrhage or infection.

> The abortion took about half an hour and it was excruciating. There was no possibility of anaesthetic. I had to be well enough to leave immediately afterwards. I told him I couldn't walk. He said I must. Illegal abortionists cannot afford to have their clients hanging around.

Typically, the abortionist would forbid the woman to contact him or her again. Often she wouldn't know his or her real name. If a complication occurred, harassment by the law was a frightening possibility. The need for secrecy created isolation for women having abortions and those providing them.

Before the 1967 Act thousands of women each year had illegal abortions. Women came into emergency wards only to die of widespread abdominal infections, victims of botched or insanitary abortions. Many women who recovered from such infections found themselves sterile or chronically and painfully ill. The enormous emotional stress often lasted a long time.

> At about two a.m. I started to haemorrhage. I could hear bells in my ears. I could hardly speak and I couldn't see. I just managed to shout to Mum. Dad went for the doctor, who didn't arrive till morning and then tried to make me tell him who had aborted me. He didn't believe I'd done it myself.

This abortion was in 1966, two years before the law changed. In that year forty-nine women died from backstreet abortions.

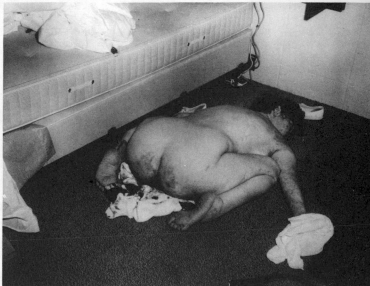

Woman dead on motel room floor. Her death was due to an air embolism suffered during an illegal abortion.

Files of Dr. Milton Halpern, Former Medical Examiner, New York City

NOTES

1. Quoted in Sheila Rowbotham. *A New World for Women: Stella Browne – Socialist Feminist*. London: Pluto Press, 1977.
2. National Abortion Campaign. Report of the Abortion Rights Tribunal, 1977.
3. Quoted in Rowbotham, op. cit., note 1.
4. Hans Forssman and Inga Thuwe. 'One Hundred and Twenty Children Born After Application for Therapeutic Abortion Refused', *Acta Psychiatra Scandinavica*, no. 42, 1966, pp. 71–88. For sections of this study, see Garret Hardin. *Mandatory Motherhood*. Boston: Beacon Press, 1974, pp. 105–33.

5. Quoted in Rowbotham, op. cit., note 1.
6. Wendy Savage et al. 'Abortion Methods and Sequelae', *British Journal of Hospital Medicine*, October 1982.
7. Rayna Rapp. *MS Magazine*, April 1984.
8. Savage et al., op. cit., note 6.
9. 'Doctors for a Woman's Choice on Abortion', *Update*, 15 March 1985.
10. This table appears in Robert A. Hatcher et al., *Contraceptive Technology*. New York: Irvington Publications, 1982, p. 178.
11. Lawrence Lloyd. 'Sequelae and Support after Termination of Pregnancy for Foetal Malformations', *British Medical Journal*, vol. 290, 23 March 1985, p. 907.

12. See A. Phillips. *Your Body, Your Baby, Your Life*. London: Sphere, 1985.

13. Rapp, op. cit., note 7.

RESOURCES
PUBLICATIONS

Bart, Pauline. 'Seizing the Means of Reproduction : an Illegal Feminist Abortion Collective – How and Why it Worked', in H. Roberts (ed.), *Women, Health and Reproduction*. London: Routledge and Kegan Paul, 1981.

British Agencies for Adoption and Fostering. *Single, Pregnant and Thinking about Adoption* (see Organizations).

Clarke, L., et al. *Camden Abortion Study: the Views and Experience of Women Having NHS and Private Treatment*. London: British Pregnancy Advisory Service, 1983.

Francome, C. *Abortion Freedom: A Worldwide Movement*. London: Allen and Unwin, 1984.

Greenwood, Victoria, and Jock **Young**. *Abortion in Demand*. London: Pluto Press, 1976. A history of abortion law reform in Britain.

Kenyon, Edwin. *The Dilemma of Abortion*. London: Faber, 1986.

The Lane Report. Report of the Committee on the Abortion Acts, vols 1–3. London: HMSO.

McDonnell, Kathleen. *Not an Easy Choice*. Ontario: Women's Press, 1984.

Neustatter, Angela, with Gina **Newson**. *Mixed Feelings – the Experience of Abortion*. London: Pluto Press, 1986.

Pipes, Mary. *Understanding Abortion*. London: Women's Press, 1985.

Rowbotham, Sheila. *A New World for Women*. London: Pluto Press, 1977.

Women's Reproductive Rights Campaign (see Organizations). *Abortion Services in London*, and *Mixed Feelings: Ten Women Talk about Their Experiences of Contraception, Pregnancy and Abortion*.

The National Abortion Campaign publishes leaflets and pamphlets on all aspects of abortion including the political fight to establish women's right to abortion. They also have videos and cassette tapes for hire or sale. Send sae for publications list to NAC, Wesley House, 4 Wild Court, London WC2B 5AU.

ORGANIZATIONS

Abortion Law Reform Association (ALRA), see WHRRIC. A campaigning pressure group aiming to defend and extend the 1967 Abortion Act.

British Agencies for Adoption and Fostering (BAAF), 11 Southwark Street, London SE1 1RQ. Tel: 01-407 8800.

Brook Advisory Centres, 233 Tottenham Court Road, London W1P 9AE. Tel: 01-580 2991 and 01-323 1522. For those under twenty-six years old.

Confederation of Health Service Employees (COHSE), The National Officer (women), Glen House, High Street, Banstead, Surrey SM7 2LH. Tel: 07373-53322.

Coordinating Committee in Defence of the 1967 Act, c/o Birth Control Trust, 27–35 Mortimer Street, London W1N 7RJ. Tel: 01-580 9360.

Doctors for a Woman's Choice on Abortion, 101 Burbage Road, Dulwich, London SE24 9HD. Tel: 01-274 4901.

Family Planning Association, 27–35 Mortimer Street, London W1N 7RJ. Tel: 01-636 7866.

London Post Adoption Centre, Interchange Building, 15 Wilkin Street, London NW5 3NG. Tel: 01-284 0555.

MATCH (Mothers Apart from their Children), c/o BM Problems, London WC1N 3XX.

National Abortion Campaign, Wesley House, 4 Wild Court, London WC2B 5AU. Tel: 01-405 4801.

National Union of Public Employees (NUPE), 8 Aberdeen Terrace, London SE3 0QY. Tel: 01-852 2842.

NORCAP, 3 New High Street, Headington, Oxford OX3 7AJ. Arranges contacts between adoptees and birth mothers. Send sae for information

SAFTA (Support after Termination for Fetal Abnormality), c/o the Disabled Living Adviser at the Association for Spina Bifida and Hydrocephalus (ASBAH), 22 Upper Woburn Place, London WC1H 0EP. Tel: 01-388 1382.

Women's Health and Reproductive Rights Information Centre (WHRRIC), 52–54 Featherstone Street, London EC1Y 8RT. Tel: 01-251 6332/6580. Gives advice and has a range of pamphlets and information sheets available; send sae for publications list.

PREGNANCY ADVISORY SERVICES

The following are non-profit-making organizations which can arrange an abortion for you where you will not be harassed or forced to do anything you don't want to do. Beware of an anti-abortion agency called Lifeline. It offers free pregnancy testing and help – but it will never help you to get an abortion.

British Pregnancy Advisory Service (BPAS), Head Office, Austy Manor, Wooton Wawen, Solihull, West Midlands B95 6BX. Tel: 05642-3225. BPAS are a non-profit-making charitable organization and provide a counselling service as well as having their own abortion facilities. They also do pregnancy testing. BPAS operate throughout Britain.

Basingstoke: Church Grange Health Centre, Bramlys Drive, Basingstoke RG21 1UN	0256-59720 0256-782417*
Bath	0225-873321
Bedford	0234-46574
Birmingham: 1st Floor, Guildhall Buildings, Navigation Street, Birmingham B2 4BT	021-643 1461
Bournemouth: 23 Ophir Road, Bournemouth BH8 8LS	0202-28762
Brighton: Wistons Site, Chatsworth Road, Brighton BN1 5DW	0273-509726
Cardiff: Ocean Chambers, Dumfries Place, Cardiff CF1 4BN	0222-372389
Chester: 98a Foregate Street, Chester CH1 1HB	0244-327113
Coventry: Coundon Welfare Clinic, Barker Butts Lane, Coventry CV6 1DU	0203-597344
Doncaster: The Bungalow, 1A Avenue Road, Doncaster DN2 4AH	0302-344893
Glasgow: 2nd Floor, 245 North Street, Glasgow G3 7DL	041-204 1832
Hull: 32 Beverley Road (entrance Norfolk Street), Hull HU3 1YF	0964-626431*
Leamington Spa: Holly Walk Welfare Clinic, 62 Holly Walk, Leamington Spa CV32 4JE	0203-597344 0926-25562*
Leeds: Second Floor, 8 The Headrow, Leeds LS1 6PT	0532-443861
Liverpool: 20 Rodney Street, Liverpool L1 2TQ	051-709 1558
London: 7 Belgrave Road, London SW1V 1QB	01-222 0985
Luton: 3a Upper George Street, Luton LU1 2QY	0582-26287
Manchester: Suite F, Ground Floor, Fourways House, 57 Hilton Street, Manchester M1 2EJ	051-236 7777
Milton Keynes: Eaglestone Health Centre, Standing Way, Milton Keynes MK6 5AZ	0908-663601 0234-46574*
Sheffield: 160 Charles Street, Sheffield S1 2NE	0742-738326 0742-685646*
Swindon: Priory Road Health Clinic, Priory Road, Swindon SN3 2EZ	0793-30366 0793-618865*

Brook Advisory Centres. Offer advice/help and information to all young people (under twenty-six years old) on personal relationships, contraception and pregnancy, including pregnancy testing, abortion referral to

*Telephone answering service.

NHS (where possible and desirable). Most of the services are free, financed by the NHS.

Brook Birmingham. They have four centres. Phone 021-455 0491 or look in phone book.

Brook Bristol, 21 Richmond Hill, Clifton, Bristol BS1 5DQ. 0272-292136

Brook Coventry 0203-412627

Brook Edinburgh, 2 Lower Gilmore Place, Edinburgh. 031-229 5320

Brook London, 233 Tottenham Court Road, London W1P 9AE (Main office). 01-323 1522, 01-580 2991
They have other centres throughout London; ring for details or look in phone book.

London Youth Advisory Centre, 26 Prince of Wales Road, London NW5 3LG. 01-267 4792.

New Grapevine, 416 St John Street, London EC1V 4NJ. 01-278 9147/9157. Offers advice and information to young people under twenty-five years old. Also runs post-abortion groups.

Pregnancy Advisory Service (PAS), 11–13 Charlotte Street, London W1P 1HD. 01-637 8962. A non-profit-making charitable organization. Provides a counselling service as well as having its own abortion facilities. Also does pregnancy testing.

PART IV

CHILDBEARING

INTRODUCTION

Rewritten by
ANGELA PHILLIPS

For healthy, self-confident women, with skilled and caring support, pregnancy, labour and birth are normal and usually uncomplicated processes.

Childbearing brings with it its own strengths: flexibility, determination, patience, humour, endurance and, if we listen to our own bodies, a wealth of self-knowledge. But we have needs too, for:

- enough money and/or community support to take care of ourselves;
- a healthy unpolluted environment;
- nourishing food in adequate amounts to be in as good physical shape as possible and to get sufficient rest;
- a skilled midwife or doctor whom we trust and like, a place of birth which feels comfortable and safe and continuity of care throughout the whole childbearing year;
- confidence in our ability to give birth; people around us who respect us, who have confidence in us and patience with the natural unfolding of our labour; physical and emotional support to help us relax, to sustain and guide us; freedom to adopt the most comfortable labour positions; surgically skilled medical personnel with appropriate equipment reasonably nearby in case of emergency.
- After the baby is born: we need the opportunity to be with her or him whenever we want, and a helping hand during the days and weeks which follow birth.
- Plenty of good food, rest and help in caring for our babies.
- Control over fertility so that we have pregnancies we want and plan for.

We have, in this country, the resources to provide most of these needs. We have enough knowledge of the process of birth (and the means to distribute this information) to ensure that no one need suffer through ignorance and fear; enough money (if it were properly distributed) to ensure that no one need be cold, exhausted or undernourished; medicines and technology to cope with many crises and enough midwives (if they were well organized) to ensure

that every woman could receive care before, during and after birth, from the same small supportive team.*

Sadly, our resources are not being used this way. In twenty-five years, successive governments, bowing to medical pressure, have achieved almost 100 per cent hospitalization. In hospital, pregnancy and birth are regarded as crises which cannot be judged safe until they are over, and the process of pregnancy and labour is divided into unrelated portions with different people assigned to each part. The technology, which has the potential to banish the fear of death which many of our grandmothers faced, is too often used, not to provide back-up to the caring human support which is our first need in labour but to replace it, leaving many women still labouring in fear.

The move to hospital has left both home and hospital birth less safe than it could be. In some areas, adequate emergency back-up for home births is considered uneconomic, while in hospitals some women with perfectly normal labours are exposed to unnecessary interference which actually causes the dangers that the doctors are so eager to prevent. As cuts are made in health service resources the situation becomes worse. In one hospital women are fighting against the over-use of expensive technology and, in another, lack of resources means that women are getting insufficient basic attention.

The over-medicalization of childbirth has led to a situation in which the provision of special-care cots for the treatment of low birthweight and sick babies has become a political priority while women on Income Support are unable to get enough money for food which could perhaps

---

*Most babies in Britain are already delivered by midwives but the service is fragmented and most women find that they are moved from hand to hand like products on a line. If our service were reorganized so that all midwives cared for women throughout pregnancy and birth there would be fewer than one birth for each midwife each week allowing plenty of time for a midwifery team to provide ante- and post-natal care in the community or, if necessary, in hospital – a degree of continuity which has been achieved in some areas with sensitively organized community services.

prevent low birthweight (the major cause of baby deaths).

For many women the greatest tangible drawback of a hospital-based system is the lack of respect it affords us at a time when we feel both very special and very vulnerable. For working-class women, especially black women, hospitals can be particularly hostile. In a small survey of young black mothers, over half complained of overt and covert racial discrimination from hospital staff. Said one of these women:

> I think when you are young and go to hospital to have a baby they should be more helpful, more concerned. This sister said to me, 'You black people have too many babies.' As far as I was concerned, I wasn't 'You black people', I was me. You don't forget something like that. Even now it makes me angry to think about it. I don't see what business she had to say that, she was supposed to be caring for me. *

FIGHTING BACK

In spite of the problems we encounter during our childbearing years there have been some changes since the last edition of this book. Then we looked forward pessimistically to an obstetric service which would have totally obliterated the midwife-based maternity services. In less than ten years the seemingly unstoppable march of technological progress has been forced, by the determination of pregnant women, radical midwives and their allies, at least to pause.

Between 1981 and 1983 two surveys in *Parents* magazine (November 1983) gave some idea of the progress: there was a 75 per cent increase in the number of consultations about pain relief, 50 per cent more babies were now rooming in with their mothers; shaving had dropped by 30 per cent (to 60 per cent) (see p. 340), 28 per cent fewer women were given enemas (down to just over 50 per cent) (see p. 340, and demand feeding was almost universal whereas two years previously nearly half the mothers had been forced to feed four-hourly.

These changes are neither universal (women in the North have not fared so well) nor sufficient, but we women are responsible for them and should take credit. As government reports come out recommending a more sympathetic service and more recognition of the midwives' role, we should take heart from the knowledge that our anger has had some impact. However, we should not be complacent. Promises have been made before, and have not been kept.

It was the action of the pressure groups – the Association for Improvements in the Maternity Services (AIMS), the National Childbirth Trust (NCT), the Maternity Alliance, the Association of Radical Midwives (ARM) – which led the fightback, mainly by preparing pregnant women with the information and confidence to make demands. In hospitals all over the country women, together and individually, have fought their private battles for all of us.

Some changes have been laughably superficial (who needs a picture of Paddington Bear on a labour-room ceiling?) but some changes – introducing birth plans to help women make decisions about the kind of birth we would like; advocate schemes to improve services for ethnic minority women; and continuity of care schemes in the community – have made a real difference to the experience of childbearing for those of us lucky enough to experience them. As we write, chronic under-funding is eroding the midwifery service and the major threat to the maternity services today is lack of staff to run them.

*Jo Larbie. *Black Women and the Maternity Services*, Training in Health and Race, 1985 (available from the National Extension College, 18 Brooklands Avenue, Cambridge CB2 2HN).

PREGNANCY

Rewritten by
ANGELA PHILLIPS

PRE-CONCEPTION CARE

The health of both parents at the time of conception is a crucial factor in determining the health of a baby. As many reports have shown, health and class are very closely related.[1] Poverty, stress, bad housing and working conditions all take their toll on health and this is probably the most important reason why the rate of baby death is so much higher for working-class people than it is for the middle classes.

GETTING PREGNANT

If we have a male partner we may find that getting pregnant is not as easy as we had been led to expect. Single women and lesbians are faced with the practical problem of how to get pregnant. Chapter 21 deals both with problems of infertility and with Alternative Insemination (AI), which is a means of getting pregnant if we have no male partner or if our partner is infertile.

Sperm production can be affected by dangerous working conditions: lead, X-rays, radiation and various chemicals (see p. 151). It is also affected by smoking, excess alcohol and an inadequate diet. Although ova may be less vulnerable before conception, in the early days after conception and before a pregnancy is confirmed, the fetus can be affected, for example, by alcohol and poor diet. On the other hand, a good diet can protect. Studies indicate that a pre-conception diet high in folic acid (found in fresh green vegetables) provides some protection against spina bifida.[*2] See p. 345 for dietary advice.

*Although this hypothesis is not yet proven, and the trial currently in progress may be incapable of proving anything, the existing evidence was considered strong enough to have provoked a recommendation that 'folate should be given to any woman with a history of a child with spina bifida or anencephaly who plans to conceive again'.[3]

Although poverty and bad working conditions are major factors in pre-conception health which can only be improved by collective action (see Chapter 9), there are some small ways in which we can each try to protect our own future children. We can:

- eat as well as our income allows (see p. 345);
- support each other in giving up smoking, drug-taking and moderating drinking;
- get checked and if necessary immunized against rubella (German measles) well in advance of pregnancy (the disease can badly damage a baby if it is contracted within the first three months of pregnancy);
- get a blood test to check for anaemia (improving diet before and, of course, during pregnancy may rule out the need for iron supplements, see p. 345), blood group and, if we are Rh negative (see below), Rh antibodies;
- get checked and treated if there is any chance of carrying a sexually transmitted disease;
- ask to be referred to a specialist well before conception if we suffer from any chronic disease which requires long-term medication or special care;
- seek referral to a genetic counsellor if we suspect that we could pass on a serious inherited disease.

INHERITED DISEASES

There is an enormous range of disabilities which we inherit from our parents and can pass on to our children. Short sight lies at one end of the spectrum and Tay-Sachs disease (which is fatal) lies at the other. Some handicaps vary enormously in severity and it is impossible to find out in advance just how much our own children are likely to be affected. Until recently, pregnancy was a lottery. Everyone hoped that their children would be healthy but no one could know for sure beforehand.

For those who knew that close relatives suffered from disabling diseases the choice lay between having children and risking passing on the disease, or avoiding pregnancy altogether. Now advances in reproductive technology have

WOMEN WITH DISABILITIES

We do not have space here to write about individual conditions and their management. We recommend that women with disabilities make contact with the National Childbirth Trust (NCT) which is in the process of setting up a network for women with disabilities. They have also produced a booklet *The Emotions and Experiences of Some Disabled Mothers*, which is available from them (see Resources).

For women with disabilities the decision to become pregnant will involve extra considerations about present and future health, the practical considerations of childcare and, even more than most other women, the financial implications of parenthood. Many women also have to cope with the negative attitudes of people close to them who may doubt even the existence of sexual feelings, let alone the possibility of pregnancy.

> *My mother thought it was a complete disaster. She feels she will have to be responsible, she sees the baby as just one more person for her to support. Of course I told her that we had considered all the risks. My pregnancy is my responsibility and I have to live with the risks. I was terribly upset by her reaction. I don't think she has any idea how much it hurt.*

Many women with disabilities are under very heavy pressure to accept sterilization and, if they become pregnant, abortion. Negative reactions from health-care personnel at ante-natal clinics are also common:

> *I think people were certainly surprised and found it rather hard to hide and when I turned up for my first ante-natal appointment, I went with a friend who was visiting and they thought it must be her that was pregnant because it didn't cross their minds that it might be me.*

On the other hand, women report the reactions of some specialists and general practitioners who have been enormously supportive.

> *When I first raised the issue of pregnancy with my neurologist he was very excited and encouraging. He has young children of his own and said he felt parenthood was wonderful and that everyone should have the opportunity to experience it.*

Anxieties about pregnancy are something we all have to cope with, particularly in the early weeks. For those of us who have a disability it can be hard to sort out which problems are the normal side-effects of pregnancy and which might signal special problems. It helps to keep in quite close contact with a doctor who knows you and your condition well. Obstetricians may have very little knowledge of your special needs.

> *The doctor seemed to be relying on me for information about my condition, which I found unnerving. I just hope he is doing some reading about it and isn't going to leave it all to me.*

If you belong to a support group for people with your particular disability you may well be able to pick up very useful information about the management of pregnancy and labour from other women. Newsletters, noticeboards or word of mouth may put you in touch. If you do not belong to a group it may be worthwhile finding out now if such a group exists (see Resources).

We all need support after the baby is born. It is so easy to become isolated and overwhelmed. It helps to keep in touch with women who are coping with special problems and who can make suggestions about equipment adaptation and special aids. However, post-natal support groups organized locally are the lifeline for many new mothers. They provide a local reservoir of information about facilities as well as support when our babies are getting us down. In fact, most mothers would benefit from the advice of one mother interviewed by the NCT:

> *I think it is a question of having the confidence that you can cope, also not being afraid to admit to yourself and other people where you find your limitations.*

provided another set of choices. For a wide range of genetic, chromasomal and metabolic disorders, it is now possible to find out with *amniocentesis* (during the sixteenth week of pregnancy), see pp. 370, or *chorion villus sampling* (in the third month), see pp. 371, whether or not a child is affected. Today's decision has moved a stage further: to have an abortion or not.

For those faced with passing on a fatal disability the choice may be easier, even though the process will be

distressing. For others the choice is a great deal harder. Some inherited diseases vary greatly in their severity. In some cases they can be successfully controlled while in others they represent a lifetime of pain and distress. Genetic counselling in advance of pregnancy should provide you with detailed information about the prospects of a baby born with the particular condition you are concerned about. In the case of diseases such as sickle cell anaemia, good information about managing the condition can greatly reduce its severity. It may help also to seek out other people and parents of children with the condition and find out as much as you can before making a decision about screening.

Blood tests can identify carriers of these conditions before pregnancy.

Sickle Cell

One in ten African and Caribbean people carry a sickle cell trait in their blood. When a baby's parents both have sickle cell trait, there is a one in four chance of sickle cell anaemia. If one parent has sickle cell anaemia there is a 50 per cent chance of passing on sickle cell trait and, if both parents have anaemia, it will definitely be passed on. Some people with sickle cell anaemia find that with care for their health they suffer very little, others have frequent 'crises' and suffer a great deal of pain. (You can read more about the disease on p. 558.) If you have anaemia you will need very special care in pregnancy and should be referred to a specialist. (Contact the Sickle Cell Society, p. 592.)

Thalassaemia

Similar to sickle cell but usually more serious, it tends to affect people from the Mediterranean, Middle Eastern countries, India and Pakistan.

Tay-Sachs

This is a disease which affects the nervous system and is fatal after about three to four years. The Tay-Sachs gene is carried by 1 in 27 Jewish people from Eastern Europe and 1 in 300 of the rest of the population. If both parents are carriers, a baby stands a one in four chance of being affected. A few centres in the country can analyse blood to identify carriers (contact the Tay-Sachs Society; see p. 421).

Rh Antibodies (rhesus sensitization)

This can be built up in the blood of a woman whose blood group is Rh negative (Rh−). The antibodies do not affect the mother but can attack the blood of any future Rh positive (Rh+) baby. The antibodies are manufactured in your blood only if Rh+ blood enters your bloodstream. This means that you are unlikely to be affected in your first pregnancy but if you have had an abortion, miscarriage (including ectopic pregnancies), given birth to a Rh+ baby or had a transfusion of Rh+ blood, antibodies may be present. The administration of Anti D, a drug which prevents the build-up of antibodies, has dramatically reduced the incidence of rhesus sensitization.

Injections of Anti D should be given to all Rh− women *whenever bleeding occurs in pregnancy*. If you bleed again you need another dose. If this dose does not happen future pregnancies with Rh+ babies could be threatened. If you already have Rh antibodies ask for a referral to a specialist hospital for advice. There are a few centres which use new techniques for fetal blood sampling and fetal blood transfusions. The decision to embark on a pregnancy when you already have antibodies should be taken after careful consultation and consideration. High technology intervention is extremely stressful and may not work. However, it does provide an option for women who might be otherwise unable to bear children.

> *Before starting another pregnancy I was told I could opt for fetal blood sampling at sixteen weeks. That meant I would know whether or not the baby was Rh− (and would therefore be unaffected by the antibodies). I had already decided that if it was positive I would have an abortion. I just could not face the gruelling blood transfusions a second time, knowing that once again the baby might not survive.*

HIV and AIDS *see p. 558*.

THE PURSUIT OF PERFECTION

Medicine has been pursuing, with ever-increasing intensity, the idea of perfection. This is nowhere more apparent than in the realm of screening for genetic and fetal abnormalities. Indeed, the concept of the perfect fetus is a cornerstone on which current ante-natal care policies are based.[4]

We are all concerned that our children should have the opportunity to grow into healthy and active people. However, we know that every child will be different and that some will be hampered by physical or mental handicaps. Some of these will be brought with them at birth. Others will occur later and many, perhaps unsuspected, difficulties will be inflicted by the process of living in a sexist, racist, warmongering society.

Those of us who will have the major care of children have a particular concern for their health and will do what we can to maximize their opportunities. But we must guard against the expectation that our children will be perfect (none of us is perfect) and we must recognize that our concern for our children's health is also, in part, an expression of our fear that they may be 'different' and therefore 'unacceptable'; fear which may well stem from our own, unconscious, prejudices.

As individuals embarking on pregnancy and parenthood, it is hard to reconcile our justifiable fears for our children's future, our concern about our ability to provide for them, and our political belief in the need to fight the prevailing prejudice in our society against those people who are considered 'different' from ourselves.

It is a dilemma that we all share. We have tried to present information about the burgeoning technology for ante-natal screening, pre-conception care and ante-natal monitoring in a context which will enable all of us to think not only of how these things will affect our emotional and physical state and the health of our children, but also how their very existence and the policy of selective abortion that accompanies them promotes an ideal of perfection which we would be very unwise to promote in our homophobic, racialist society.

Nevertheless, we are aware that mothers still bear the brunt of responsibility for children, whether for a few years in early childhood or for an extended period when a child is severely handicapped. In presenting the dilemmas we believe that we must be able to make our own choices about entering screening programmes and our own decisions based on the results. These are choices which should be supported without moral pressure.

ANTE-NATAL CARE: PREPARATION FOR PREGNANCY, LABOUR AND BIRTH

Ante-natal care is mostly about caring for ourselves. Our ability to care for ourselves is partly dependent on income, working conditions and relationships. Doctors and midwives cannot change an unhealthy pregnancy into a healthy one but regular monitoring and discussion can help pinpoint problems before they start to threaten the baby or ourselves and allow us, in consultation with health-care personnel, to make informed decisions about what action, if any, should be taken.

EATING WELL
Be sure to read Chapter 4.

It is important to eat well during pregnancy. Think of it as eating for yourself (when you are healthy, most likely your baby will be healthy, too). Also think of it as eating for three – you, your baby and the placenta which links you together, through which your baby receives all its nourishment.

By eating well:

- We expand our blood volume to meet the increased demands pregnancy makes on our body. Blood bathes and washes over the placenta where the exchange of oxygen and nutrients takes place.
- We help make sure that our uterus – and all other tissues – grow and increase in elasticity, and that our baby grows to its full potential.
- Adequate birth weight and placental 'sufficiency' increase the likelihood that labour and birth will be uncomplicated. We lower the risk of complications

---

BLACK WOMEN AND PREGNANCY

Statistics in Britain are coded on the basis of class, not race, so it is impossible to know for certain whether black women born in this country suffer from a higher rate of baby deaths than white women. However, we do know that the perinatal mortality rate among mothers born in the 'New Commonwealth' and Pakistan is 15.6 per 1,000 births as opposed to an average rate for British-born mothers of 11.9. The rate is particularly high for mothers born in Pakistan (22 per 1,000 births).

The health of a baby at birth is dependent not only on its mother's health in pregnancy but also on the health of its grandmother during her pregnancy. Given the relative poverty of the non-industrialized nations, a higher perinatal mortality rate is not entirely unexpected. However, evidence in America shows that the differential between black and white rates does not disappear even after several generations. Just as class is the major determinant of perinatal mortality in Britain, in America it is colour. And of course black people in Britain and America are predominantly working class so they share those disadvantages of income, environment and working conditions.

However, those of us who are black have an additional obstacle to health to contend with – racism. Maternity services are 'colour blind' in attitudes, dietary assumptions and language spoken. Routine procedures ignore the needs of black and ethnic minority women. Surveys in Leicester and Bradford show that women of Asian origin are far less likely to get consistent ante-natal care than non-Asian women. They are also less likely to be cared for by GPs with obstetric experience. Few centres carry out routine screening for sickle cell anaemia (which is carried by 10 per cent of African and Caribbean people) or thalassaemia (which is carried by South Asian and Mediterranean people and affects 25 per cent of babies when both partners are carriers). However, routine tests at birth are carried out for the rare condition phenylketonurea which affects white babies. Care of pregnant women with sickle cell anaemia is also uncoordinated and erratic.

On the other hand, those of us who come from India may well suffer unnecessary intervention because our babies are considered to be too small compared with those of most women born in this country. Closer examination of the statistics shows that the average healthy weight for Indian babies is simply lower than British expectations. Black and ethnic minority women suffer the discrimination of having both our real needs and our own knowledge discounted or ignored.

such as infections, anaemia and eclampsia (see p. 361) in ourselves, and prematurity, low birthweight, still-birth, brain damage, and retardation in our baby.

- We contribute to the future health of our child.
- Our body stores the fats and fluids we need for breast-feeding. We will need to continue to eat and drink a lot of healthy foods and fluids after our baby is born.

It is often hard to eat large meals, especially if we are nauseous during early pregnancy or towards the end when the uterus takes up so much room. Most of us find it easier to eat little and often, avoiding long stretches without food which make us feel sick and weak.

Those of us who are on a low income find it harder to eat well, particularly as women often get into the habit of depriving themselves to benefit other family members. It is possible to make some improvements in diet through small changes which may not be expensive. Be sure to claim **free milk and vitamins** if you are on income supplement or a low income.

A Suggested Daily Diet for Pregnancy

To make sure you are getting the best possible value, in the right combination, eat every day:

1. **Vegetables and fruit** (four to five servings). Include some green vegetables and raw fruit every day, and carrots at least three times each week. Be mean with the amount of water you use for cooking, and with the cooking time. Dried fruits make a useful standby for snacks as they are high in minerals and iron.

2. **Meat, fish, dried beans, eggs** (two portions or more if you do not drink milk). If you do not eat meat, make sure you are eating the right combination of foods (see p. 45, Protein Combination).

3. **Cereal and bread** (four to five portions). These are a very important part of most diets, but it is important to eat whole-grain products to ensure that you get the full value. Always ask for *wholemeal* flour and bread (brown bread is not always wholemeal; Asian flours such as Besan are whole products). Look for cereals which state on the box that they are made from *whole wheat*. These include porridge, muesli and some of the more old-fashioned biscuit-type cereals. If you eat rice or pasta buy brown rather than white.

4. **Milk products**. Drink at least a pint of milk a day or the equivalent in yoghurt or cheese (4 oz of cheese is the equivalent of a pint of milk). If you do not drink milk you will need to get extra calcium from green vegetables, nuts and seeds. Since you need plenty of calcium and milk is the major source, you may want to consider calcium sup-plements (consult a dietition or naturopath).

5. **Liquid**. Drink six to eight glasses of fruit juice, water or other liquids. Avoid sugar-loaded fizzy drinks and squash and go easy on coffee and tea (see p. 347).

Some foods do more harm than good. Sweets, biscuits and cakes, fizzy drinks and cheap convenience foods are usually highly refined, short of the many basic ingredients you need for your health, and they crowd out the better food by spoiling your appetite. Wholemeal bread and cheese, pitta and humous, chappati and dal, followed by fresh fruit, can be just as convenient as spaghetti hoops and tinned peaches, and are much better foods.

SPECIAL FOOD NEEDS IN PREGNANCY

Pregnancy increases your need for *calories* and *protein*. If you are still growing yourself, or you are having twins, you must be particularly careful to eat enough. You also need a wide *variety* of food because important nutrients are scat-tered around in different foods. A balanced diet is a better basis for health than vitamin supplementation because by taking too much of one vitamin it is possible to create an imbalance in others. However, you may need some vitamin supplements.

Foods containing Vitamins A and D are thought to be particularly relevant to fetal development and the following are known to be important.

In pregnancy your immune system is depressed so you need to be particularly careful about food hygiene to avoid infection from bacteria such as salmonella and listeria. Any pre-cooked foods should be very well heated before serving, eggs should be hard-boiled. For further advice contact your Health Promotion or Environmental Health department.

Folic Acid

Found in green leafy vegetables, folic acid consists of a group of compounds in the Vitamin B family. It is essential for protein synthesis in early pregnancy and also for the formation of blood and new cells. Your baby needs folic acid to grow. Symptoms of folic acid deficiency are anaemia and fatigue (anaemia may also have other causes). Our bodies don't store folic acid, so if we are anaemic, daily supplements are necessary.

Women who have previously had a baby with a neural tube defect may wish to consider folic acid supplemen-tation (see p. 341). The supplement usually supplied is Pregnavite Forte F for three weeks before and six weeks after conception.

If you have taken birth control pills and are now preg-nant, you may have depleted your supply of Vitamins B_6 and B_{12} and folic acid and may need supplements.

Iron*

Iron is obtained from prune juice, dried fruits, dried beans and peas, lean meat, liver, egg yolk and cooking food in iron pots and pans. It is a main component of haemoglobin (Hb) which, composed of complex molecules of protein and iron, carries oxygen to our baby and our cells. The baby also draws on our iron reserve to store iron in its liver to last for the duration of his/her milk diet after birth. You'll also need a lot of oxygen during labour both for you and the baby, and as a safeguard in case you bleed heavily. Many women are iron-deficient before pregnancy. If you eat a

---

*Some research indicates that zinc is as important in pregnancy as iron. No recommendations have yet been made in Britain.[5]

well-balanced iron-rich diet, your system may contain enough iron and your blood test will show this. A normal pre-pregnancy Hb is 12–24. It will drop in pregnancy but if it goes below Hb 10 it is wise to take supplements. Iron can cause constipation. If so, ask for a different brand.

Calcium

Your need for calcium increases during pregnancy and lactation because you are providing calcium for your baby's bones and teeth. If you do not consume enough calcium it will be taken from your own bones and teeth with serious implications for your health (see p. 469). Avoid eating chocolate with calcium as it prevents proper absorption.

Vitamin D

Calcium absorption is dependent on Vitamin D which we usually obtain through the action of sunshine on our skin. However, it is also added to margarine and occurs naturally in oily fish. Those of us with families from India and Pakistan may need Vitamin D supplements (see p. 44 for a discussion on this) possibly because of the low level of exposure to sunshine in the UK.

Fluids

Fluids aid the circulation of blood and body fluids and the distribution of mineral salts, and stimulate the digestion and assimilation of foods.

THE HEALTH-CARE SYSTEM AND NUTRITION

According to a recent survey, only 58 per cent of women are given advice on diet in pregnancy.[6] In another study of seventy-six London mothers, 95 per cent had lower energy and Vitamin D intakes than recommended by the Department of Health and Social Security.[7] At least half were also low in Vitamin B. (British recommendations are in many cases lower than American recommended levels.)

Even though poor nutrition is thought to be at least partly responsible for a variety of pregnancy problems from subfertility to low birthweight, little attention is given to its place in maternity care. Diet counselling in pregnancy rarely rises above the suggestion that you should eat 'well', drink milk and swallow your iron pills. Diet sheets which are handed out by some hospitals suggest a menu which is well beyond the financial means of many low-income families (who are most at risk).

Obstetric technology is rated so far above the basic right to food that one woman told us:

My doctor suggested taking me into hospital during the strike just to get three meals a day. I was not gaining weight because we didn't have enough money to buy food and the DHSS refused to give us any extra money even though I had already had a threatened miscarriage and my doctor wrote saying I had special dietary needs.

According to the Maternity Alliance, there are 100,000 women in Britain whose poverty puts them at real risk of inadequate nutrition during pregnancy and who are therefore more likely to have low birthweight babies with an attendant higher risk of handicap and stillbirth. If more money was provided for dietary help to pregnant women, we would perhaps not need a campaign to increase the number of intensive-care cots for sick babies.

WEIGHT-GAIN RESTRICTION, SALT-FREE DIETS, DIURETICS AND DIET PILLS

We have passed through many medical fads about restricting weight and diet in pregnancy. Many pregnant women have been told to cut back on calories and salt, and (in the USA) have even been prescribed diet pills (amphetamines) and diuretics (water pills) to reduce water retention and weight.

This was all done in the belief that restrictions of weight and salt intake could cut down the risk of pre-eclampsia (toxaemia), which is described on p. 361. More recent studies show that although increased water retention usually precedes pre-eclampsia, it does not cause it, that women with an inadequate salt intake may be at more risk, and that a degree of water retention is both normal and necessary in pregnancy.

Some doctors, including the American Tom Brewer,[8] believe that pre-eclampsia can be virtually eliminated by eating a high protein diet. His findings are questioned by other researchers but there is certainly evidence to indicate that malnutrition is a contributory factor to pre-eclampsia. Yet another reason why good nutrition should be considered a basic necessity for all pregnant women.

SUBSTANCES AND PROCEDURES TO AVOID

Drugs*

Most of the drugs we take during pregnancy will cross the placenta. Fetuses are extremely susceptible to drugs, especially during the first three months when vital organs are forming. We can classify direct effects of substances on pregnancy and the fetus into three different types: *teratogenic* (can cause birth defects), *toxic* (having a more severe pharmacological effect on the fetus) and *withdrawal* (causing dependence). Although only a handful of drugs have been shown to be teratogenic, few have been adequately researched and there is much we don't know about possible subtle or long-range effects. Therefore, take as few drugs as possible during pregnancy. Sometimes you have to weigh the risks of an illness versus known or unknown risks of the drug in question. For example, if you have a high temperature during the first months of pregnancy, your best course of action may be to take paracetamol to reduce the

---

*Drug research gives us conflicting results because it is difficult to do scientific studies using human beings. Drug dosage can be controlled in animal studies, but as animals metabolize drugs differently from humans, results cannot be directly applied. Also, not all fetuses will be affected by the same dosage.

fever, because prolonged high fever can be teratogenic. If you have a serious condition such as diabetes or hypertension or epilepsy, you may need to take prescribed drugs to control the disorder, since your illness can affect the baby's development. If you are bothered by more common disorders such as headaches, nausea or constipation, diet changes, fresh air or sleep are the safest remedies. If they don't work, consult your doctor before taking *any* medication, prescription or non-prescription. Since the worst drug disasters have been caused by prescribed medicines, it may be best to make sure your doctor has consulted the local drug information centre.

Alcohol

Heavy drinking can harm the baby. Those of us who drink as much as six units a day (see p. 65) should get medical advice. Even two units a day can affect birthweight and increase the risk of miscarriage, and problems are more likely if alcohol is added to a poor diet and cigarette smoking. Alcohol is most damaging in the early months. However, the occasional drink at a party should not cause you anxiety.

Smoking

If we smoke more than fifteen cigarettes a day we run a higher risk of miscarriage or prematurity and our babies are likely to be half a pound lighter than they would be otherwise. The Health Education Council seized on smoking as a risk factor which they could control by trying to change the behaviour of individual women. It is worth keeping in mind that cigarettes *per se* have less effect on babies than the class they are born into. The government could do more for babies by tackling poverty than they can hope to achieve by making individuals feel guilty about smoking. Nevertheless, it is wise to cut down and just as important to encourage close companions to cut down; their smoke also affects the baby. If you cannot stop, try to cut down and eat well.

Mega Vitamins

Taking very large doses of vitamins is not wise in pregnancy. Vitamins are active chemical agents and should only be taken to make up for a definite deficiency.

X-rays

Consider them carefully, and avoid them or delay them until late in pregnancy or after you have given birth. Have the minimum number if you absolutely have to have them. Be aware that the government has withdrawn guidelines protecting women who might be pregnant from X-rays, so it is possible that you will not be asked about this and will have to make sure that technicians know and take special care if X-rays are necessary for you.

Coffee, Tea, Chocolate

All contain caffeine which, in large quantities, could be harmful. Two or three cups a day should present no special risks. Some *herb teas* also contain caffeine and all herb teas should be used in moderation as they have active constituents which, though they have never been researched, could be risky in excess.

For information on *mood-altering drugs* see p. 67 and for *hazards at work* see p. 151.

PHYSICAL ACTIVITY AND EXERCISE

Throughout pregnancy, women do everything from swimming, running or walking briskly to dancing and yoga. Use common sense when exercising. If what you are doing makes you feel good, then continue. If you become too tired or uncomfortable, choose a less strenuous activity. Books on exercises during pregnancy are listed on p. 419. See Chapters 6 and 7 for more information.

YOUR RIGHTS IN PREGNANCY

During the period of Conservative government from 1979, the rights of pregnant women have been gradually eroded. By the time this book comes out most of the income support schemes which used to be a matter of right are now conditional on means-testing or available only through our employer. These changes have been made with little concerted protest (with the exception of the Maternity Alliance) and scant attention from the press. The repercus-

---

PELVIC FLOOR EXERCISES

It is simple to do *pelvic floor exercises* – contracting your pelvic-floor muscles. They help you prepare for childbirth.

A good way to locate these muscles is to spread your legs apart and to start and stop the flow of urine – your ability to do this is one indication of how strong your muscles are. Another method is to try tightening around a man's erect penis during intercourse (this will feel very pleasant to him and can help to enhance your pleasure, too). Or use one or two fingers.

Begin exercising these muscles by contracting hard for a second and then releasing completely. Repeat this ten times in a row to make up one group of exercises (this takes about twenty seconds). In a month's time, try to work up to twenty groups during one day (about seven minutes total). You can do this at any time – while sitting in a car or bus, while talking on the telephone, or even as a wake-up exercise. Some of us have noticed improved muscle tone (and occasionally increased pleasure during sex) in only several weeks. For more detailed instruction on exercises, consult your local childbirth group.

sions, in terms of poverty and ill health, will continue to be felt by women and children well into the future.

Benefits change as governments change; you should check with an up-to-date source to ensure that you claim everything which is yours by right. If you are on a low income or income support, a Citizens' Advice Bureau will help you ensure that you have claimed what you are entitled to.

Free milk and vitamins can be claimed if you are on income support. You will get tokens for seven pints of milk a week during your pregnancy (the same for any children under five). Contact your local benefit office.

Free prescriptions during pregnancy and until a year after the birth (children's prescriptions are also free). Apply on form FW8 (available from your doctor or clinic).

Dental treatment is free for the same period as above and it is sensible to make use of this as your gums need special care in pregnancy.

The **Maternity Grant** of a miserable £25 used to be paid to all pregnant women as of right. It was abolished in April 1987 and replaced by a means-tested grant of £80 available to those of us on income support or family credit. Although this grant is higher than the old one the total amount available to many low-income women is less than it used to be because special single payments worth up to £187 for maternity and baby clothes have been abolished.

Statutory maternity pay can be claimed for eighteen weeks, through your employer, if you have been employed by him/her for at least six months until the fourteenth week before the birth and if you have paid National Insurance for the last eight weeks of this period and stayed at work until the eleventh week before the birth. If you have worked for the same employer for at least two years you can claim an earnings-related benefit for the first six weeks. The money is reimbursed to your employer by the government. If you have any difficulty getting the money, contact your union, the Maternity Alliance (see Resources) or a Citizens' Advice Bureau for help. As this money is taxed, some women may do better on Maternity Allowance, see below.

Maternity Allowance. If you changed employer during your pregnancy, if you are self-employed, or left work early, you can claim Maternity Allowance provided you paid National Insurance for at least twenty-six weeks out of the last fifty-two, up to fourteen weeks before the birth. As Maternity Allowance is not taxable some women may actually be better off leaving work early and claiming the allowance. However, you will need good advice. Contact your trade union or a Citizens' Advice Bureau. Claim forms should be available from a Social Security office or post office.

Job reinstatement after maternity leave is only available by law to women who have worked with their existing employer for two years before the eleventh week before the baby is due. This qualification period (the most stringent in Europe) means that only a minority of women have any job security when they become pregnant. In order to keep your job, you must inform your employer, in writing, not less than twenty-one days before you leave that you are going on maternity leave and intend to return to work. You are then entitled to leave of eleven weeks before and twenty-nine weeks after the birth. You must also let your employer know, in writing, twenty-one days before you intend to return. If your employer writes to you asking you to confirm your intention to return to work, you must respond, in writing, within fourteen days. Failure to comply with this red tape could result in the loss of your job.

Statutory sick pay (SSP) or sickness benefit can be claimed if you are forced to stop work for health reasons in the weeks before the maternity leave period. If you are employed, SSP for the first twenty-eight weeks must be claimed from your employer. Self-employed people can get claim forms from a local Social Security office. *

PUTTING YOURSELF AT EASE DURING PREGNANCY

Childbirth Classes

Pregnancy can be both a frightening and exciting experience. Attending childbirth classes, pregnancy support and ante-natal exercise groups gives us the opportunity to meet other women, learn about pregnancy, minimize fears and make friends whose babies will be companions of our own.

If you live in a city you may have a choice of classes: hospital and clinic parentcraft classes, National Childbirth Trust, Active Birth classes, or classes organized by a local birth centre or community centre. If no groups exist, you can create your own with the assistance of someone (lay or professional) who knows about childbearing and existing groups.

Community-based classes are likely to be smaller, more personal and much richer in content than hospital classes.

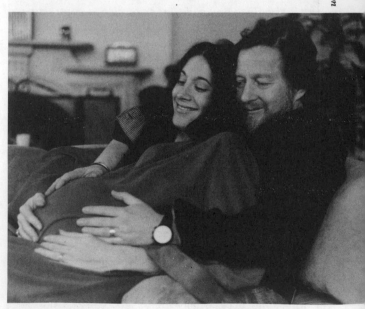

Jim Harrison/Stock Boston

*For more information about maternity rights see *Maternity Rights for Women at Work* from NCCL and the book by Evans and Durwood, *Maternity Rights Handbook* (details in Resources).

The National Childbirth Trust (NCT) has teachers all over the country who organize classes in their homes. As it is a voluntary organization teachers tend to be white and middle class.

It was a shock at first seeing a pink doll come out of a pink pelvis. It didn't seem to have anything to do with my body.

It seemed terribly cosy, like an advertisement for compulsory heterosexual monogamy, but I was very glad I had been. It kept me going through a very long labour.

The NCT has recently started to recognize the unconscious exclusivity of its groups and 'outreach' work is underway in some areas. In Lewisham, for example, seminars for community health workers have been organized and a small group of black women has recently started NCT training. NCT teachers charge fees for a course of classes but they are always prepared to drop the fee if you cannot afford to pay. Book early as classes fill up quickly.

The vogue for active birth classes, with yoga or stretching exercises, has spawned classes which are quite expensive to attend, but you sometimes find active birth teachers funded by the health authority or the WEA (Workers' Education Association) giving classes for a very small fee.

Hospital and clinic classes vary enormously. Many are geared to preparing you to accept hospital procedures.

At our local health centre we did breathing and relaxation. Pain was never mentioned. We were told that labour didn't mean pain, it just meant work. We were also told that 'they never let a woman suffer today; they have a lot of wonderful drugs they can give you if they think your labour needs it' (but not if you think you need it). This brainwashing exercise had a powerful effect on us. We were never given any impression that we had any control over what was to happen to us. This authoritarian behaviour persisted right through to the time I was breastfeeding. It simply produced a frightened and fearful mother. When I was discharged from the hospital, I wondered what on earth I would do with the baby, for I'd never been allowed even to assume I could make a decision before, let alone carry one out.

However, more and more midwives every year are trained by the NCT. Find out if the teachers at your hospital are NCT trained. They are likely to be a lot more open-minded.

Good classes touch on a wide range of concerns – the physiology of labour and birth; visualization of the process (you imagine yourself giving birth); relaxation techniques; the importance of someone (other than hospital staff) to assist you and be your advocate; the practice of supported positions during labour; discussions of fantasies and feelings; risks of routine drugs and interventions, and their occasional benefits; what it's like to breastfeed, to be parents. Mothers, often with partners, visit with their babies to describe their own experiences and answer questions. Films are often shown.

It was the first time I'd ever seen anything be born. Hearing people talk, hearing the sounds, made it real. I see that it's a lot of work; people are working hard to make the birth happen. A person can go through all that and be fine!

Those sounds she made were upsetting. I wanted her to stop. They were so intimate, sexual. I could be making those sounds.

Every class we got to know each other better. During breaks we'd talk about our dreams, problems, questions. After our babies were born we continued to meet every month for two years.

ACTIVE BIRTH

Childbirth preparation is often associated with breathing techniques and instruction on how to relax in specific ways during labour. Critics of this method point out that it fits all too well with the medical way of birth, coexisting with *all* forms of intervention. We are led to believe that we are having 'natural' births when in fact we are lying in bed, horizontal, motionless; our labours accelerated; shaved, hooked to monitors, cut (episiotomy) and sometimes partially drugged. Mentally active – concentrating on breathing, panting away like machines – but physically inactive, we are not 'in control' but controlled by the interventions and by the breathing method itself. In the words of a labour attendant and childbirth preparation teacher:

I've seen women told to 'do your breathing' as they were objecting to painful examinations and procedures.

From a conversation with a midwife:

Teach women how to breathe? Why, we know how to breathe, honey – we've been doing it all our lives!

Rigid breathing techniques are a lot less popular than they were, even with the NCT who pioneered 'natural childbirth' in Britain. The emphasis now is on teaching us to make use of our bodies; to find positions which help to ease pain and speed labour; to move with the physical pattern of labour rather than trying to block it. There are a number of books to read about 'active birth'; the best known is by Janet Balaskas (see Resources).

It helps to involve close partners or friends as much as possible. One father said:

I felt embarrassed at first, sitting on the floor with all those people I didn't know, but it gave me the confidence to feel useful during Sarah's labour.

Many classes go on to form post-natal support groups which can last for years.

To find out what is available locally, inquire at your ante-natal clinic, Community Relations Council (for classes geared specially to women from ethnic minorities), community health council, contact the National Childbirth Trust for a list, look on library noticeboards, and ask friends who have recently had babies.

CHOICES FOR CARE

No matter where you want to have your baby or what your chosen style of care, your first contact with the maternity services will probably be your general practitioner. It is probable that your GP will want to set a hospital booking in motion straight away so it helps to know roughly what you want at this stage, or at least by the time you are twelve weeks pregnant. Your choice of where to have the baby – home or hospital, consultant or GP unit, long or short stay – will also affect the kind of ante-natal care you receive.

Women's experience, now backed up by research,[9] shows that the most effective ante-natal care is provided by a skilled practitioner (midwife and/or doctor) or small group of practitioners who see you regularly throughout pregnancy, providing individual monitoring.

For many women this will mean opting for care organized by a GP often in partnership with local community midwives and, in most cases, shared with care by a hospital clinic. However, some GPs do more than the minimum, some less than that. GP care has been a real problem in some inner-city areas. Ethnic minority women often do particularly badly. At its best, however, it can provide caring, efficient monitoring and support. More districts are now attempting to organize midwives in 'continuity of care' schemes.

Ante-natal care cannot by itself make pregnancy safer. In fact, it often fails in its primary job of detecting possible complications by ignoring the most useful source of information – us. Where ante-natal care could help is in allowing women to express worries. Sharing fears would allow them to be allayed, where appropriate, and provide vital clues to our well-being and the health of our babies. Sadly, lack of proper discussion is something women complain most frequently about.

Hospital-based clinics are rarely organized to provide continuity. Most women's complaints about ante-natal care focus on hospital clinics and they have been criticized in reports over a number of years.

Doctors and consultants talk to the nurses about you

as if you were a prize marrow, lying there on a couch. They should try talking to the patient, not behind her back.[10]

Women are often expected to wait for hours for what has been described as 'a ritual laying-on of hands'. Not surprisingly, some women avoid booking until late in pregnancy or miss appointments. Most of us have better things to do than wait for three hours to have our blood pressure taken.

Women from ethnic minorities make proportionately less use of the ante-natal services which is hardly surprising since the health service is often insensitive to the needs of people who are not male and middle class, and particularly insensitive to those who are not white.

I used to spend ages waiting for a bus, ages waiting to see the doctor. It used to make me cross because when I finally got to see him it was only for about five minutes at most. Sometimes they were afraid to speak to you. I never felt like asking them anything because they used to make out because you're black you're stupid.[11]

After the publication of the Short Report in 1980,[12] some changes have been made (the most significant being that pregnant women now have the right to paid time off work to attend clinics). Some progress is also being made (though with little or no financial help from the NHS) in making services more appropriate and welcoming for ethnic minority women. Nevertheless, long waits, cursory examinations and lack of information are common complaints among all women. If your clinic facilities are inadequate, write and complain either to your community health council, or maternity services liaison committee (these have not been set up in every district as yet). Assertive insistence on your right to decent care can help:

The hospital ante-natal care was so horrendous that being a lesbian was secondary. In the end I wrote a letter of complaint, which got results.

Even if you do not get far with your complaint, it is still worth making it because it will help those who come after you.

Shared care. If you decide to give birth in a hospital consultant unit (see below) you can usually arrange for at least half your ante-natal care to be provided by a GP. In some areas (such as Sighthill in Edinburgh and Hackney in London) most ante-natal care is arranged in the community even if you are having a hospital birth and the consultants visit your clinic rather than dragging you into hospital to see them. In hospital-based GP units, at least two hospital ante-natal visits are usually required but you will otherwise be cared for by your GP and community midwives.

I was rushing to finish a project by the time the baby arrived so every moment was precious. I certainly didn't want to spend any longer than necessary in waiting rooms. My GP was extremely accommodating. I rarely had to wait and visits were friendly as well as useful. I only visited the consultant once in the end because he offered to make the ritual second appointment for the week after the baby was due.

If your own GP is not trained, or prepared, to deal with ante-natal care, you can find another local GP and sign on for the duration of your pregnancy. You will still keep your own GP for all other medical needs. You can find one through the Obstetric List (available at the library) but a far better method is to contact your local National Childbirth Trust organizer or birth centre to get the names of recommended and experienced GPs.

Community care. If you are intending to have your baby at home, or through the domino scheme (see below), your ante-natal care will be centred round the local health centre, your GP's surgery, or in some cases at home.

WHERE TO HAVE THE BABY

This should be your decision and you should have the right to change your mind as your pregnancy progresses.

> Whichever course she chooses, a woman is likely to be better off where she *feels* safest, whether in hospital or at home. Often there is too much emphasis on the 'medical' side and not enough on the woman's own attitudes and feelings. Women should always have the *choice* of the kind of care and medical attention they feel to be most suitable for them. A woman's state of mind is an important factor for happy and straightforward childbirth.[13]

In this section we try to provide as much information as possible to enable a real choice to be made, as well as to show the factors which can affect or limit our choice. Since the scales are so heavily weighted against the possibility of obtaining a home birth, we have devoted a large part of this section to this aspect of the subject. By doing so, we do not intend to imply that women should have a home birth any more than that women should have a hospital birth. We look forward to the time when the right to choose where to have a baby will have become a reality. At present, choice is limited, not only by our own decisions. Government policies for centralizing maternity care have cut down alternatives for women who do not live in cities, and medical attitudes to home birth limit choice by inducing fear (which is not backed up by fact) of the dangers of home births as opposed to hospital births (see below).

None the less, the number of hospital births in Britain has increased from 15 per cent in 1927 to about 99 per cent in 1988. This has been happening gradually and has been due, to some degree at least, to the publication of two particular government reports. The decision to achieve 100 per cent hospital births took place in 1959 with the publication of the Cranbrook Report. The Peel Report, published in 1970, added weight to this decision. The basis of the reports' conclusions was by no means scientific, and social and psychological aspects were not considered. No consumers of the maternity services were represented on the committee, which consisted entirely of doctors. The Department of Health's policy is still based on this 'expert' opinion.

Another reason why hospital births are advocated is an 'economic' one. This is particularly argued where there are new hospitals, which are very expensive to run compared with old ones: unless beds are kept full, the management starts asking questions. In fact, if there *is* a domiciliary service available, and if it is used, as in Holland, the figures show that it is cheaper to have the baby at home. This is not to say that on economic grounds women should have their babies at home. It is simply to point out that there is no economic argument for running down the domiciliary service.

One reason why hospitals are not in themselves particularly safe is because the risk of serious infection is greater in hospital than at home.[14]

THE SAFETY OF HOME BIRTHS

Most of the decisions about phasing out home births have been based on crude and badly interpreted statistics which appeared to show that the baby death-rate for home birth had risen sharply compared to the death-rate in hospitals. Researcher Marjorie Tew was the first person to question the accuracy of those figures. Her work was consistently obstructed and ignored.[15] Since then two studies, one in Cardiff[16] and another carried out by a group of researchers[17] using national figures, have conclusively confirmed her findings that the apparently high death-rate is accounted for by the sharp decline in the numbers of women booking home births compared to those with emergency and unplanned home deliveries.

The perinatal mortality rate for unplanned home deliveries was, not surprisingly, extremely high: 67.5 per 1,000. For those booking home deliveries, the perinatal mortality rate was 4.1 per 1,000 which compares extremely favourably with the national average for that year of 14.7 per 1,000. It is possible that the high death-rate in the unplanned group was increased by the progressive winding down of back-up facilities for home births.

The safety of home births is more than confirmed by a recent study from Holland. The report summarized:

> Among women who had opted for home confinement . . . significantly fewer complications occurred during pregnancy, delivery or puerperium than among those who had their babies in hospital. Morbidity [illness] was also lower among babies born at home. The study suggests that it is a responsible decision for a normal healthy woman given the right kind of ante-natal supervision to have her baby at home with the least risk of complications.[18]

In Holland women are screened early in pregnancy and 10 per cent are referred directly to obstetricians because of 'primary medical indications'. Unless a secondary medical indication crops up during pregnancy the woman may choose where to have the baby. Sadly, in spite of good obstetric back-up and evidence, such as the study quoted above, even in Holland women are bowing to medical prejudice and opting for hospitals. The numbers giving birth at home have declined from 72 per cent in 1960 to 34.7 per cent in 1981.

Some babies will die wherever they are born. Good antenatal screening should ensure that very few vulnerable low-birthweight babies are born outside hospitals and adequate emergency back-up should allow immediate transfer to hospital if labour begins to run into trouble.

As intensive care becomes more centralized, transfer from home to hospital need take no longer than transfer from a local to a regional centre.

Stillbirth may also be easier to cope with at home.

> It was a great comfort to me that I was not lying in the formal atmosphere of the hospital, shut away with soothing words, probably given Valium, not allowed to see the baby. As it was, the fact that she was not going to live dawned on me gradually . . . it was far more bearable than it might have been.[19]

For the mother, the effect of close, personal attention at home may outweigh the accessibility of medical technology. One experienced midwife told us:

> I always preferred home births. I decided they were safer when I dealt with a postpartum haemorrhage at home. The mother was a calm, dignified woman who would never 'make a fuss'. The bleeding came two hours after the birth and was concealed. Having total responsibility for her I acted on my feeling of unease about her colour and weakness. I took her pulse, set up a drip and sent immediately for the flying squad. In a large, busy, post-natal ward, she could easily have died.

Is Home Birth Safe for Me?

Around 90 per cent of pregnancies proceed normally with few or no problems. Most problems can be predicted in advance with good ante-natal care and screening. For women with the following conditions, a home birth is not advisable:

- existing medical conditions such as: heart, circulatory diseases, severe anaemia, kidney disease, epilepsy, diabetes;
- previous problems in labour such as severe postpartum haemorrhage, difficulties leading to a caesarean section (though some women with previous caesars do have home births quite safely), or retained placenta;
- drug or alcohol dependency which may lead to withdrawal symptoms in the baby;

- active herpes virus infection (see p. 499) or any other severe infection;
- known difficulties for the baby such as multiple births, suspected cephalo pelvic disproportion (when the baby is too big to be delivered vaginally), abnormal presentation (when the baby is not coming head first), or Rh sensitization when a blood transfusion may be necessary.

Factors, such as very high blood pressure, pre-eclampsia (see p. 361), premature labour or bleeding in the third trimester, which cannot be predicted at the booking stage would mean a late hospital referral.

Women who are very young (sixteen or under) tend to have more difficult labours and more problems in general so it would be best for them to have their babies in hospital. Otherwise age should not in itself prevent you from having a home birth. The 'ideal' childbearing age, statistically speaking, is between twenty-two and thirty-two, varying from race to race and culture to culture. Pregnant women outside this age range should pay particularly close attention to their health and the preparation for possible complications.

In Britain, the most common reason doctors give for refusing a home birth is 'It's your first baby'. Again, this is not a valid reason for disallowing a home birth. Nor is it necessary for all fifth and subsequent babies to be born in hospital if there are no complications and the previous labour was normal. Age is also a common disqualifier. Some doctors make an upper age limit of thirty-five and a lower one of twenty-two. Risks tend to rise among older or younger women but, obviously, individual factors such as general health can outweigh such statistical generalizations.

Rarely, even in low-risk mothers, problems can occur which are not predictable. These include lack of progress in labour, fetal or maternal distress, abnormal bleeding before, during or after the birth, prolapsed cord (meaning that the cord is being born first). If we are aware of these possible complications they can be spotted quickly and proper action can be taken. This can only happen if there is an adequate emergency service – flying squad – in the area.

> I pee into a bucket and out comes the show which is more red than I expected. This doesn't worry me very much but it was at this time that Kate [the midwife] informed the doctor. The dawn is now coming through the shutters and I'm feeling quite cheerful when he arrives. He and Kate trot out of the room. When they return he tells me he's called an ambulance to take me to Barts because I need hospital cover as I am bleeding. I look at Kate and see that she thinks so too. I am extremely lucky in knowing Kate and the doctor so well that I'm confident that they wouldn't call an ambulance unless I really needed to go to hospital. I feel calm about it. I think I had unconsciously felt that Kate was worried when she saw that I was bleeding. I

can hear Ron asking Kate if she'll come too and help him stop the hospital doing anything unnecessary. [This woman went on to be delivered in hospital by Kate herself with the hospital staff looking on.]

HAVING A BABY AT HOME

Health Authorities have an obligation to see that a midwifery service is available for home births. They must ensure that the provision made is as safe as circumstances permit and that local demand and arrangements to meet it are kept under review.

This is part of the policy statement of the government's Maternity Services Advisory Committee (MSAC). It states the legal position quite clearly. You have an absolute right to give birth at home and the health authority has an absolute obligation to provide you with a midwife.

In spite of the legal position, in many areas you are likely to come up against stiff opposition if you opt for a home birth. You may not be able to find a GP willing to provide medical cover and, although you can legally give birth without a doctor, many midwives will be loath to attend in these circumstances. If they cannot persuade you to change your mind they are quite likely to try and frighten you into it. At the time of writing women in Milton Keynes opting for home births were being visited by the Director of Midwifery Services who made them sign a form (which has no legal standing whatever) taking legal responsibility for their own and their baby's welfare.

A mother who wrote to her local paper complaining that she had been branded as selfish for wanting to give birth at home was threatened with a libel action by her GP unless she wrote a public letter of apology.

You may also be given misleading information about your medical condition. Some women have been persuaded into hospital by reports of 'phantom' high blood pressure or suspected placenta praevia (see p. 387). The former can be double-checked and the latter is most unlikely to be suspected unless there is some bleeding in the last three months of pregnancy (this would be a sound indication for hospital admission) or evidence from an ultrasound scan.

The official attitude endorses this behaviour. The MSAC states that:

> As unforeseen complications can occur in every birth, every mother should be encouraged to have her baby in a maternity unit where emergency facilities are readily available.

As the number of home births declines (it is now down to just over 1 per cent with a slight rise over the last year) GPs and community midwives are getting less practice and are often quite genuinely worried about delivering babies. Fortunately, with the growth in influence of the Associa-

tion of Radical Midwives and various birth pressure groups, younger midwives have joined forces with older midwives (who remember the pre-hospital days), to provide a reasonably responsive service in some areas.

Aside from a competent midwife, the other necessary condition for a safe home birth is the availability of an emergency obstetric unit (flying squad) in your area. Some districts have abolished this vital service even though it is more often needed for unplanned emergencies at home (which will never be phased out) than for planned home births.

What Does It Feel Like to Give Birth at Home?

The birth of my third child was one of the most fantastic experiences my husband and I have ever known. Our son was born at home and it was wonderful . . . We tried to bring the baby into a quiet, gentle atmosphere. In fact the cord was round the baby's neck but the midwife was absolutely marvellous and took it as a matter of course. The baby did not breathe immediately but we stroked him gently and gradually he stirred and took a deep breath. The midwife was cheerful and extremely kind. She gave us both a tremendous feeling of confidence.

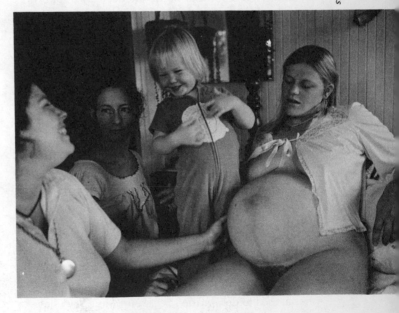

Suzanne Arms

Not every birth planned at home ends up at home but the confidence that you have gained may well spill over into the hospital. A midwife states:

All efforts are made to see birth as a continuum. I tell people who have prepared for home birth, who begin labour at home and then end up at the hospital, 'Who you are never changes: your planning, ideals, values, beliefs, principles never change just because you end up in the hospital, or with a caesarean. You are stronger than you would have been because you've gone through all those decisions and made the choices you did.'

Planning a Home Birth

First find out if your own doctor is willing to take you on. (Do not under any circumstances agree to a hospital booking 'just in case' as this might make it more difficult to get medical cover at home.) If your doctor agrees, you will be asked to sign a form EC 24 which is a contract for care. You will then be contacted at home by a midwife. Unless your district has made some effort to organize midwives into teams you cannot be sure that you will see the same midwife each time or that you will be delivered by someone you know. If your doctor is unwilling or unable to take you on you can find another GP (see p. 629, above) to provide this service.

If you cannot find a willing doctor write to the Director of Midwifery Services or Nursing Officer (community midwifery) c/o the district health authority. Explain that you want to have a home birth, that you cannot get medical cover and that you want to be allocated a midwife. Enclose the name of your doctor too.

You may come under a great deal of pressure to go into hospital. However, once you have weighed up the advice given to you (keeping in mind the stress effects if you fear you will have to deal with a reluctant midwife), it is still your right to give birth at home attended by a midwife.

If you meet a great deal of hostility you can contact local or national support groups for advice. You may, if you can afford it, decide to opt for a private midwife. You can find names through the various pressure groups listed, in particular the Association of Radical Midwives.

I used a natural childbirth method on my first birth in hospital two years ago and had no need of anaesthetics or medical intervention . . . After the delivery and a minimal cuddle my first child was snatched away . . . I want to be free to cuddle my second infant immediately after birth as long as we both want this. When I became pregnant again, to my dismay my GP told me, 'There is no chance of your having the baby at home.' This was the policy of the local practice as it was 13 miles to the nearest hospital. I am now temporarily registered with a sympathetic doctor who will deliver my baby at home; the local midwife has agreed to deliver me . . . so one could say I have won the battle. But should one have to battle for such a basic right?[20]

Preparations for a Home Birth

You will need to make arrangements. The Society to Support Home Confinements (SSHC) provides leaflets concerning what you will need – e.g. nightdresses suitable for breastfeeding, sanitary towels, etc. The midwife will visit you during the third or fourth month and she herself will probably make suggestions as to what you will need and about the arrangement of the furniture. It is often possible to borrow things like bowls and bedpans from either the Red Cross or the local authority. A 'confinement pack' supplied by the health authority will be delivered to you by the midwife ten days before the baby is due. The pack should remain sealed, to be opened by the midwife when labour begins.

HAVING A BABY IN HOSPITAL

Even if we are strong and healthy some of us prefer to give birth in a hospital. We may feel safer there and want to have help after the baby is born. The environment of a hospital can be strange and is often intimidating but the companionship of other women – those giving birth even more than those paid to assist us – can be a great support, particularly with a first baby.

I hated it at first. I felt alone and homesick and scared but, as the ward came to life in the morning, I was drawn into the life of the women around me. They supported me, and in turn I supported those who came in later. The atmosphere was charged with emotion and I think some women found it very hard to take but I felt buoyed up by the common outpouring of love towards our babies and each other.

The baby was unplanned, the labour and delivery prolonged and traumatic, but throughout it all, the help and support I received made the memory joyful.

Sadly, in spite of the potential for providing a loving and supportive environment for women, inhumanity to mothers has been a common by-product of the drive for hospitalization – a fact which is often commented on in reports but with little positive result. In 1959 the Cranbrook Report commented on 'a general complaint that there was in many hospitals too little regard for the personal dignity and emotional condition of women during pregnancy and childbirth'. In 1980 the Short Report returned to the issue but concern focused more on superficial changes (such as providing wallpaper in delivery suites) than the real issues of freedom, choice and dignity. More recently the Maternity Services Advisory Committee has shown a little more concern about these issues. However, we have yet to have evidence that experiences like these are not being repeated:

When I screamed with pain I was told 'pull yourself together, you're not the only person in the ward to have had a baby.'[21]

I've been left feeling sad and disappointed. If I had been allowed to move around more in labour I'm sure I'd have been able to have a normal delivery.[22]

My birth experience was a green cloth over my thighs, and my baby being dropped out by forceps while I was held on to at the shoulders. It was like a chicken being gutted, how can that be enjoyed?[23]

In the 1983 *Parents* magazine birth survey, less than two-thirds of the women had the kind of labours and deliveries they wanted even though 75 per cent of the deliveries were normal. In the 1985 survey there were a few improvements, but there is still a long way to go.

Hospital deliveries can be positive and joyful experiences and in some hospitals a great deal of effort has gone into assembling the staff and creating the sort of atmosphere in which labouring women can feel at home. If you feel that your local hospital is not providing for women's real needs, you could make contact with other women through the local NCT, AIMS, the community health council and add your energy to the long-term job of fighting for change.

Choosing a Hospital

Hospitals vary a lot, even between wards and consultants. In a big city you can usually find out quite a lot about the different hospitals from birth groups and other women, and then choose accordingly. Elsewhere you may have less choice but it is still worth finding out as much as you can so that you are prepared. You can be booked into any hospital of your choice, it may not even be local, though you must take into account the difficulty of travelling a long distance. However, cash limits mean that some hospitals will no longer take women from outside their area and we have yet to find out the effect of the latest reorganization of the health service on choice. If you want to use a GP unit you must be booked in to a local unit by a GP who will take responsibility for you.

Before choosing a hospital it is well worth investigating their different rules and practices and the reasons for them.* The rules are sometimes made for the benefit of mothers, but sometimes they appear to be arbitrary and can be distressing. The following is the experience of one mother at two different hospitals; the first was a teaching hospital in London, the other, a small maternity home in Yorkshire. There is generally still a marked difference in attitude between services in the North and South.

The London hospital was run on flexible and permissive lines – there were no rules that were unreasonable or unnecessary. The Yorkshire home . . . was rule-laden and authoritarian. This structure was reinforced by the whims of some of the nursing staff, who seemed to make up rules and even reverse them to suit themselves. On one occasion I was told to put a pillow under the baby on my lap while breastfeeding, only to be harangued by a sister for 'spoiling hospital equipment'. Patients were not allowed to lie on the bed, except at the official 'rest' periods . . . All baths had to be taken between 7 a.m.

and 8 a.m. and since there was one bath to twelve people and only sufficient water for three baths at a time, the others all had cold baths.[24]

There is no reason why a hospital booking cannot be changed, though it's better to do so early if possible. Here are some questions to ask.

1. *Companions.* The Maternity Services Advisory Committee's advice to hospitals is that companions should be welcomed and encouraged to stay throughout labour. If you want more than one companion it is best to ask in advance and check that they can stay *throughout* the labour if that is what you want.

2. Will you be expected to accept *shaving* and an *enema*? (See p. 340.) Again the MSAC says that such procedures should be carried out only 'if medically advised' or at your request.

3. *Will you be free to move around in labour and find your own position for delivery?* The MSAC upholds your right here 'unless there are overriding medical reasons' against.

4. *Visiting.* Are the hours restricted (you may welcome restricted hours after the birth) and can any other children in your family visit freely?

5. Are *special dietary needs* catered for?

6. Are *interpreters/advocates/linkworkers* available if English is not your first language?

7. *Intervention* rates (current national rates in brackets) vary from one hospital to another. Try to find out the hospital's rates for: induction (25–36 per cent), forceps (13.1 per cent), episiotomy (cutting the perineum during delivery; 55 per cent), and caesareans (10.6 per cent). Low intervention rates may be a sign of a more cautious use of technology, though teaching hospital rates may be inflated by the number of high-risk women being referred to them.

8. *Pain relief.* Will you be encouraged to manage without drugs if you want to? If you would like epidural anaesthesia (see p. 396) is it available?

9. Can you *keep the baby with you?* Most hospitals allow you to spend time with the baby immediately after delivery, though some still insist on keeping babies in communal nurseries at least overnight. You may welcome the rest at night (though you will still need to be woken if you are breastfeeding), but you may find that you are restless without your baby anyway. Research shows that separation can increase the likelihood of depression. Special Care Units should also give maximum opportunity for you to be with your baby (see p. 403).

10. *Feeding rules* are no longer common in hospitals but there may be some old-fashioned units that insist on four-hourly feeding schedules. All the evidence shows that this is the worst way of establishing breastfeeding. It may be wise to let the midwives know in advance that you intend to demand feed.

11. *Going home.* Policies vary about length of stay from six hours to a week. You should have some choice about this. You can always discharge yourself when you feel ready. (See Early Discharge, p. 356.)

*It is also worth checking that stated policies are actually carried out in practice – sometimes they are not. Local NCT teachers are perhaps in the best position to offer advice on this matter, since they have continuous experience of hospitals' practices via their pupils – i.e. other women.

Consultant Units

A consultant is a senior doctor who is in charge of a team of doctors within a consultant unit, or responsible for the pregnancies and labours of the women referred to him or her within a large unit. CUs are usually found in large general hospitals or specialist maternity hospitals. There is at least one in most health districts. Some are also teaching hospitals which means that you can expect to be asked if students can examine you and, perhaps, deliver your baby (you have the right to refuse). These units vary enormously and the treatment you receive will also vary according to the style of the consultant you are booked with. Some of the most progressive places to give birth are run by consultants; others may be autocratic, quirky and insist on procedures as a matter of course which you might prefer to avoid. For example, a consultant in one London teaching hospital is known for insisting that all first-time mothers are given episiotomies (see p. 393); in another, a tremendous row blew up because one consultant encouraged women to give birth in any position they favoured while his senior colleague insisted that all births should take place on beds.

GP Units

GP units may be in a separate building or a section of a hospital consultant's unit. They are run by midwives, and GPs take responsibility for the care of mothers registered with them. In some areas the community midwives who provide ante-natal care also do deliveries (in other areas these functions are separated), but even if they do not, GP care provides reassuring continuity.

GP units only book low-risk women and they therefore have less high-tech equipment and lower intervention rates. In spite of the scope for a more humane service, some GP units are run in an extremely authoritarian manner, but many others provide a much appreciated alternative to consultant units.*

> She [the midwife] had got me into the GP unit and there she stayed with me. It was lovely, just David, me, her and a pupil midwife. I had no medical treatment whatever and all went perfectly. I was given my own room and left in peace with Melanie.[25]

Separate GP units based in the community involve little travelling and are usually less impersonal (though sometimes also less progressive) than the large hospitals. However, they are rapidly being closed down in favour of the bigger centralized facilities. The reasons are partly economic (authorities want to keep hospital beds full even though GP beds are actually cheaper), and partly based on the spurious safety grounds that it is unsafe to give birth without maximum technological back-up.

A Milton Keynes group, fighting to keep two GP units open, produced an excellent document on the comparative safety of GP units.[27] They point out that:

> Analysis of the 1970 PNMR [perinatal mortality rate] shows that if each place [of birth] had had the same proportion of births at each level of risk, the PNMR would still have been four times as great in hospitals as GP units . . . In short, there is an unexplained amount of perinatal mortality *in hospital* which cannot be explained by reference to the mother's level of risk, or to late transfer. It must therefore be associated in some way with factors in hospital care itself. Mothers for whom there is no medical reason to be in hospital may be exposed to *unnecessary risk* by a policy of centralized care.

This group managed to convince its regional health authority of the wisdom of keeping the units open, but the Minister for Health backed the district against it and the units have since been closed.

Early Discharge

If you are having your baby in hospital but want to get out quickly, it is often possible for a six-hour discharge to be arranged. Some hospitals are flexible and allow you to stay as briefly (or as long) as you wish. Health authorities should be encouraged to provide flexibility. Once at home you may find that you can adapt to the baby's routine very easily; breastfeeding is often easier to establish at home when we are relaxed. Often, too, home is much less noisy than hospital and we can sleep better. (But being at home can be a temptation to do too much and get overtired. And visitors may think that, because we are home, we are perfectly fit.) Home helps should be available to all women who need them – and there will be few who don't need a home help after an early discharge. But public expenditure cuts have decimated this service. You are unlikely to get help unless you have a multiple birth.

Increasingly, the promise of an early discharge is used to press mothers into having a hospital rather than a home birth and the new vogue for bed throughput means that few women now are expected to stay longer than forty-eight hours in hospital. If you do not feel that adequate help is available, say so – there is no reason why you should leave early.

If you decide on an early discharge, a midwife will visit you before the baby is born to explain what equipment you'll need. Once you are home, the midwife will call every day for at least ten days after the baby's birth. She is there to look after you and the baby, and is on call twenty-four hours a day, so if you are worried you can contact her.

Domino Schemes

In the domino scheme, a community midwife accompanies you to the local maternity unit, delivers you and returns home with you. This is an excellent way of ensuring continuity of care. However, the Society to Support Home Confinements feels it is hardly desirable to

---

*As we write, a report by the Association of Anaesthetists is threatening the existence of small maternity units. Its evidence has been condemned as biased and self-serving, but it may prove the final straw in the fight against centralization.[26]

move a woman at the height of her labour when this is not necessary: she could remain at home for the birth. Not all areas run domino schemes, one reason being that there are not enough community midwives.

My labour obligingly slowed down for the ten-minute drive to the hospital. Then it went into gear and half an hour later she was born. I was home eight hours later as my son returned from school. I couldn't have asked for a more relaxed birth.

THE PREGNANCY ITSELF

I sit here on the porch as if in a deep sleep, waiting for this unknown child. I keep hearing this far flight of strange birds going on in the mysterious air about me. How can it be explained? . . . Suddenly everything comes alive . . . like an anemone opening itself, disclosing itself, and the very stones themselves break open like bread.[28]

During your pregnancy, several processes are going on at once: you are going through physical changes and emotional changes and your fetus is growing within you. Though your pregnancy will have much in common with other women's, it is yours and unique (and each pregnancy you go through will differ from the others). In talking to women who have been pregnant and who are pregnant, at the same time you are, you will discover that there's no one right way to be pregnant.

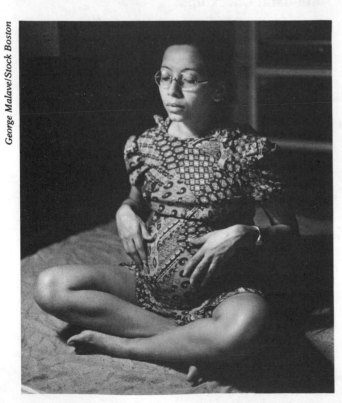

George Malave/Stock Boston

Many changes take place in your body as the fetus develops in you. Some of these changes are just changes but, though we are adapted to bearing children, discomforts can arise. You may feel many changes and discomforts, few or none at all. You'll want to know what they are, why they occur, when they are likely to occur. Eating well and exercising reduce or eliminate many discomforts. Some minor discomforts, if neglected, can lead to major complications. And you should know that in every pregnancy there's a possibility of miscarriage (though the likelihood decreases with the passing months), so that if it happens to you, you won't be totally unprepared.

As for your feelings, they will vary tremendously according to who you are; how you feel about having children; your previous pregnancies and/or abortion experiences, if any; how you feel about your own childhood, your parents or the people who reared you; whether or not you are with a partner – and if you are, how you feel about him or her.

At each stage you may feel conflicts as well as harmonies. Sometimes you'll feel positive, sometimes negative. You'll have doubts and fears. It's important to know that these doubts and fears occur during a 'good' pregnancy, too, for in a very real sense your body has been taken over by a process out of your control. You can come to terms with that takeover actively and consciously by knowing what's happening to your body, by identifying your specific feelings (especially the negative ones, because they are the most difficult to deal with) and also by learning what the fetus looks like as it grows. Its growth is dramatic and exciting. (See p. 359 for more on feelings.)

Our society tends to treat pregnancy as a solitary, clinical experience. Many non-industrialized societies have invested it with religious significance, respect it as an altered physical and psychic state and celebrate it as significant not only for the couple but for the entire community. Making and deepening bonds with people who make you feel special can be an important source of strength.

Expected Date of Confinement (due date)

The length of a normal pregnancy can vary from 240 to 300 days. Each three-month period is called a *trimester*. It's good to know approximately when your due date will be, but don't fix on a particular day. Only 5 per cent of women give birth on their projected due date! If you and your obstetrician disagree seriously about the conception date, this can affect your baby's well-being. For example, if your obstetrician thinks the baby is 'post-mature', s/he may advise induction. If you are right and s/he is wrong, the birth may be premature. If your doctor thinks you are *less* pregnant than you are, you may give birth before anyone is prepared for it.

We have talked with dozens of women whose doctors refused to believe that they knew when their babies were conceived and thus approximately when they were due. Some had problems as a result. Try not to devalue your own knowledge.

The doctors insisted they knew the expected date of

delivery better than I did. They couldn't possibly have done unless of course I had been pregnant for three years. My daughter was induced two weeks before she should have been born. The traumatic birth, on top of her prematurity, was something she could have done without.

Nowadays, obstetricians tend to dismiss their judgement *and* yours, and rely on ultrasound to assess fetal maturity (see p. 368).

THE FIRST TRIMESTER (first 12 weeks)

Physical Changes

You may have none, some or many of the following early signs of pregnancy. If you have had regular periods, you will probably miss a period. However, some women do bleed for the first two or three months even when they are pregnant, but bleeding is usually short and there's scant blood. Also, about seven days or so after conception, the *blastocyst*, the tiny group of cells which becomes the embryo, attaches itself to the uterine wall, and you may have slight vaginal spotting, called implantation bleeding, while new blood vessels are being formed. A pregnancy test can confirm your knowledge (see p. 309).

You may have to urinate more often because of pressure on your bladder from your enlarging uterus and increased hormonal changes; pituitary hormones affect the adrenals, glands which change the water balance in your body, so you retain more body water.

Your breasts will probably swell. They may tingle, throb or hurt. Your milk glands begin to develop. Because of an increased blood supply to your breasts, veins become more prominent. Your nipples and the area around them (areola) may darken and become broader.

You may feel nauseated, mildly or enough to vomit, partly because your system is changing. One theory is that the higher level of oestrogen accumulates even in the cells of the stomach and causes irritation as acids tend to accumulate. The rapid expansion of the uterus may be involved. If you feel nauseated, eat lightly throughout the day rather than taking large meals. Munching crackers or dry toast slowly before you get up in the morning can help a lot. Avoid greasy, spiced food. Don't fast, and at least drink juice. Most of us can manage bread and cereals. Look for wholegrain products, which are high in B vitamins, and eat whenever you feel nauseous. High energy foods seem to relieve nausea for many women.*

Apricot nectar helps some women. Powdered ginger in capsules or as a tea or ginger ale can help too.

You may feel constantly tired.

You may have increased vaginal secretions, either clear and non-irritating or white, yellow, foamy or itchy. The chemical make-up as well as the amount of your vaginal

fluids is changing. If you are very uncomfortable or if such a condition persists, see your doctor.

The joints between your pelvic bones widen and become more movable about the tenth or eleventh week. Occasionally the separating bones come together and pinch the sciatic nerve, which runs from your buttocks down through the back of your legs; this can cause pain.

Your bowel movements may become irregular, in part because the heightened amount of progesterone relaxes smooth muscles; therefore, your bowels may not function as efficiently as they did. Also, if you are resting more often, your decreased activity may cause some constipation. Eat foods high in fibre content and/or add bran to other foods. Eat salads if you can and fresh fruits frequently and drink fruit juices.

During the first ten weeks you'll feel relatively few body changes, though nausea and tiredness can be debilitating.

Early pregnancy surprised me. I was expecting to feel very different and instead was feeling things I'd felt before. It was like premenstrual tension. I was a little nauseous. But it's amazing – once I realized I was pregnant the symptoms were tolerable, because they are not signs of sickness but of a life growing.

I felt at the same time more vulnerable and more powerful than ever.

You can't feel the changes going on inside you. Both the placental systems and the complicated systems of your fetus are developing on a miniature scale. See *A Child Is Born* for wonderful photographs.[29]

Ante-natal Check-ups

Ante-natal checks are primarily intended to screen for insufficient growth in the baby and conditions which could threaten both mother and child. They often lead to over-diagnosis of conditions which are no threat at all. However, a useful baseline of tests does aid diagnosis if problems do occur.

On the first visit a midwife will take a complete medical, reproductive and family history, including menstrual history, previous babies, pregnancies, operations, abortions, illnesses, drugs taken, family illnesses such as heart disease.

You should have a general physical examination for pregnancy, which includes examination of the breasts to see if there are changes in the glands, and a pelvic examination, which shows the position and consistency of the uterus, the condition of the ovaries and fallopian tubes and the consistency and colour of the cervix.

Your weight will be checked and then your blood pressure. The two numbers recording your blood pressure (bp) will be entered on your Cooperation Card.* The lower

---

*See 'Nausea and Vomiting in Early Pregnancy' by Dr Barbara Pickard (leaflet).

*If you have shared care with your GP and the hospital you will be given a Coop Card to take to each appointment. Most important details about your pregnancy will be recorded on it.

number is more important. If it rises by more than 10–15 or goes over 90 it should be rechecked a few hours later and then checked daily – and you may be asked to rest. The anxiety of clinic visits can push your blood pressure up. Relaxation techniques (see p. 107) may help to keep your blood pressure steady. Hospital admission should not be necessary unless there are other symptoms, or it continues to rise (see p. 361). Very high blood pressure can affect the amount of oxygen getting to the baby (it may also herald pre-eclampsia which is dangerous to both mother and baby) so it shouldn't be ignored. However, a moderate rise is no indication for the panic often expressed by doctors.

A blood sample will be taken to check your blood group (and the presence of Rh antibodies, see p. 343), your haemoglobin (to check for anaemia for which you may need iron supplements), rubella immunity,* and for infections such as Hepatitis B** and syphilis. (If you have any reason to suspect any kind of sexually transmitted disease, you would be wise to visit a clinic for specialized tests. See pp. 488–501 for details of the effect of STDs in pregnancy.)

A urine sample will be checked for protein† and glucose. If you have diabetes, or a specific risk factor (large babies, family history of diabetes, or previous stillbirths), checks for glucose are specially important. If the test is positive, another one will be done to check, followed if necessary by a glucose tolerance test and specialist help in following a diabetic diet.

At this first visit you should get an opportunity to discuss the kind of birth you want so it is important to be prepared (see p. 350). If you are having a hospital birth you will be booked in (though you have a right to change later). If you intend to give birth at home make sure you are not booked into a hospital by accident. A midwife should also discuss diet and general health care with you and advise you of your rights to various benefits (see p. 348).

Future visits will be monthly until the 28th week and then fortnightly. Most hospitals perform a routine scan at 16 weeks (see p. 368). During the final month, visits will be weekly. These visits are usually shorter as you will only

---

*If you are not immune to German measles (rubella), try to avoid exposure. When you have it, you may have a rash, tenderness of the lymph nodes in the back of your neck and possibly mild joint pains. If you are exposed in the first trimester of pregnancy and if you get the disease, the fetus may be damaged. At this point you will have to make a decision about whether or not to continue your pregnancy.

**Hepatitis B carriers can pass the disease on to their babies unless they are identified so that the baby can be treated with vaccine and immunoglobulin at birth.

†When you are pregnant you become more susceptible to urinary tract infections because the hormone progesterone relaxes involuntary muscles, and the collecting area in the kidneys and the tube connecting the kidneys to the bladder become larger. Urine tends to stagnate there, aggravating any latent infection. Signs of infection are increased urination, pain and/or a burning sensation. More extreme signs are back pain, chills and fever, bloody urine.

To prevent UTIs, it helps to drink fairly large quantities of fluids throughout pregnancy, especially acidic juices. You add the juice of one whole lemon or lime to a half-gallon of water, keep it cold and drink three to four glasses a day. Also empty your bladder completely and frequently.

In the first trimester of pregnancy your infection should be treated if juices and frequent urination don't work.

---

have a blood pressure and urine test and get your weight checked. Your tummy will be 'palpated' to feel the size and position of the uterus, and later, of the baby. Internal examinations should not be necessary until you go into labour.

During your ante-natal visits you should get the opportunity to discuss matters such as pain relief, breastfeeding and hospital attitudes to active birth as well as getting a clear explanation of how your pregnancy is progressing. However, many women complain that such discussion is inadequate.

> Lack of explanation about procedures, the position of the baby and test results was often put down to shortage of staff but many [of these] reports suggest an unwillingness on the part of the medical staff to regard explanation and reassurance as part of their job. [30]

Most hospitals arrange 'parentcraft' classes where you may have more opportunity for discussion. You may want to send a letter outlining your feelings and preferences to the Director of Nursing (Midwifery) at the hospital. You should ask for the letter to be attached to your notes so that staff, at all stages, are aware of your preferences. Some hospitals provide 'birth plans' for you to fill in (which may be a not-so-subtle way of telling you what the hospital wants you to think). Others resent what they see as pushy behaviour. You will have to judge for yourself whether a letter will actually help, or merely serve to antagonize.

Your Feelings about Yourself and Your Pregnancy: Some Positive Feelings

At the beginning of a first pregnancy, or of any pregnancy, there are many variations in feeling, from delirious joy to deep depression.

You may feel an increased sensuality, a kind of sexual opening out toward the world, heightened perceptions, a feeling of being in love. A lot of new energy. A feeling of being really special, fertile, potent, creative. Expectation. Great excitement. Impatience. Harmony. Peace.

> It gave me a sense that I was actually a woman. I had never felt sexy before. I went through a lot of changes. It was a very sexual thing. I felt very voluptuous.

> It meant I could get pregnant finally after a lot of trying, that I could do something I wanted to do. It meant going into a new stage of life. I felt filled up.

Some Negative Feelings

Shock. I'm losing my individuality. I'm not the same any more; I'm in a new category and I don't want to be. I don't want to be a vessel, a carrier. I won't matter to people now, only my baby will. I can't feel anything for this thing growing in me. I can't feel any love. I'm not interested in sex. I'm scared. I'm tired. I feel sick. I wish I weren't pregnant. I'm not ready. I don't understand motherhood.

Negative feelings are natural. When we deal with them and don't avoid or ignore them, we are better prepared to handle them close to the birth and afterwards. Also, miraculously they usually change a lot from one trimester to the next, most often in a positive direction.

Sometimes it seemed like I got pregnant on a whim – and it was a hell of a responsibility to take on a whim. Sometimes I was overwhelmed by what I'd done. A lot of that came from realizing that I had chosen to have the baby without the support of a man. I was scared up until the third trimester that I wasn't going to make it.

Some of us are too busy to think often about our pregnancies. Others have more leisure. Awareness switches inward at different times.

When I first felt her move, I knew there was life inside me. But I didn't realize I was having a baby until my doctors literally pulled her out of me upside down and she sneezed, and then she lay next to me and I felt her tiny breath on my fingers.

In the last three weeks I started looking at other babies.

At the beginning of pregnancy it's sometimes a relief not to think about it. We may wish we could escape from the inevitability of what is happening to us.

THE SECOND TRIMESTER
(13th to 28th week)

Physical Changes

During the fourth month the fetus begins to take up much more space. Your waist becomes thicker, your clothes no longer fit you, your womb begins to swell below your waist and, around the fourth or fifth month, you can begin to feel light movements ('quickening'). The fetus has been moving for months, but it's only now that you can feel it. Often you will feel it first just before you fall asleep.

You are probably gaining weight now. Eat as well as you can.

Your circulatory system has been changing and your total blood volume increasing, as your bone marrow produces more blood corpuscles and you drink and retain more liquid. Because of the increase in blood production, you may need more iron. Your heart is changing position and increasing slightly in size.

In some women the line from the navel to the pubic region gets darker due to hormonal changes and sometimes pigment in the face becomes darker too, making a kind of mask. The mask goes away after pregnancy. Increased

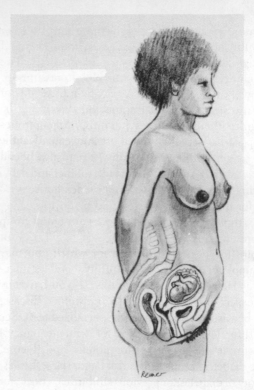

Woman in 16th week of pregnancy

Nina Reimer

colour around your nipples and in the line on your abdomen will not go away, but it may fade.

Some women salivate more. You may sweat more, which is helpful in eliminating waste material from your body. Sometimes you'll get cramps in your legs and feet when you wake up, perhaps because of disturbed circulation. Calcium may relieve these cramps. Just relax – the cramps will go away. Keep your feet elevated and warm, or pull your toes towards your knees.

Your uterus is changing, too. It's growing. Its weight increases twenty times, and the greater part of this weight is gained before the 20th week.

As your abdomen grows larger the skin over it will stretch and lines may appear, pink or reddish streaks in light skin, darker streaks in black skin. Your skin may become very dry; add vegetable oil to your bath and rub your skin with oil.

By mid-pregnancy your breasts, stimulated by hormones, are functionally complete for breastfeeding purposes. After about the 19th week a thin amber yellow or white substance called *colostrum* may come out of your nipples; there's no milk yet. Your breasts are probably larger and heavier than before. If your nipples are inverted (turned in) Woolwich Shells worn under a bra may be recommended to turn them out; there is no evidence that this works and, in any case, your nipples may change by themselves as the pregnancy goes on. If your breasts feel heavy you may be more comfortable in a support bra with wide straps.

Your bowels and your entire digestive system may move more slowly. Indigestion and constipation can occur. You may have heartburn because of too much acid in your stomach. Again, a good diet and regular exercise ease these situations. Eat frequent small meals if possible. Avoid greasy foods and coffee. Drink a lot of fluids and increase bran and fibre. Avoid taking strong, oily laxatives or laxatives containing sodium, such as baking soda or Alka-Seltzer. Some women suggest chewing hazel nuts.

As a result of pressure of pelvic organs, veins in your rectum (haemorrhoidal veins) may become dilated and sometimes painful. To prevent haemorrhoids, practise rectal exercises, which resemble the pelvic floor exercises (see p. 347) except that you contract your rectal muscles instead. When you go to the toilet, prop your feet up on a stool. Eat a lot of fibre. When you have haemorrhoids, lie down with your rectum high and apply ice packs, witch-hazel pads or heat, or take warm baths and apply Vaseline. Vitamin-E oil may help. Eat fewer spices. Continue to exercise. Your doctor or midwife can also prescribe suppositories.

Varicose veins are veins in your legs that have become enlarged and can hurt. Because of pressure, the veins and blood vessels that carry blood from your legs to your heart aren't working as smoothly as before. A tendency to vari-cose veins can be hereditary. Many women find it very helpful to wear support stockings or tights a half-size larger than their ordinary stockings. You can get stockings free on prescription. Get lots of rest, with legs elevated, alternated with walking or mild exercise.

Many women have nosebleeds because of the increased volume of blood and nasal congestion, or perhaps because of increased hormone levels. A little Vaseline in each nostril may stop the bleeding.

Oedema (water retention)

Your feet, ankles, fingers, hands and even your face may swell somewhat. When you are eating well, oedema is normal and no cause for worry, especially during the last half of pregnancy. Pregnancy hormones manufactured by the placenta, principally oestrogens, cause connective tis-sue throughout your body to retain extra fluid, which benefits you and your baby. It serves as a back-up for the expanded blood volume needed to nourish the placenta, protects you from going into shock if you lose blood and assures you an adequate milk flow during early breastfeed-ing. With twins, oedema will increase as will your weight gain. Normal oedema is associated with good infant out-come – higher birthweight and lower infant mortality.[31]

If you are uncomfortable, try to lie down with your feet raised several times a day. Exercise helps squeeze water from the tissue spaces in your blood vessels. Cut down on refined carbohydrates and get more rest.

Pre-eclampsia (toxaemia)

Towards the third trimester of pregnancy, if you develop very high blood pressure, a large amount of protein in your urine with a decrease in the amount of urine, a severe continuous headache or sudden, severe swelling of your face or fingers, you may have pre-eclampsia (sometimes called toxaemia). These conditions can develop in just a few hours, and unless you have them checked immedi-

ately, eclampsia – convulsions and coma – may occur. All serious pre-eclamptic conditions *must* be treated in the hospital; your life and your baby's life are at stake.

If pre-eclampsia is suspected, your doctor should observe your blood pressure on at least two occasions a minimum of six hours apart, and check the amount of albumin (a protein) in the urine.

Raised blood pressure without any other symptoms is unlikely to indicate pre-eclampsia and may be monitored and treated at home. Relaxation techniques (see p. 107) have been shown to be helpful.[32] The incidence of eclampsia has been reduced along with improved living standards and regular blood-pressure monitoring which ensures that the condition is usually caught before it causes harm. A trial is currently going on which should test the effectiveness of taking a low dose of aspirin to prevent eclampsia. We do not know if it will prove useful or whether there are side-effects. If you are asked to join the trial you should be fully informed. Otherwise, it is inadvis-able to take aspirin in pregnancy.

Looking after Yourself

Get as much rest as you possibly can. If you are very busy, try to set aside segments of time for total relaxation, even if it's only fifteen minutes at a time.

Your clothes should be loose and comfortable and shoes should have low heels to avoid straining your back. Many women modify their own jeans by piecing in an elastic stretch panel in the front. Simple unbelted smocks are useful as dresses. Large men's shirts are useful too. Maternity clothes are often expensive; ask your friends for any clothes they may have.

Your Feelings about Yourself

I was excited and delighted. I really got into eating well, caring for myself, getting enough sleep. I liked walking through the streets and seeing people notice my pregnancy.

But many of us watch ourselves growing outward so quickly with mixed emotions.

I don't like being pregnant. I feel like a big toad. I'm a dancer, used to being slim, and I can't believe what I look like from the side. I avoid mirrors.

Your Feelings about Your Baby

Whether you are feeling good, ambivalent or even bad, the first movements you feel your baby make can be beautiful and moving.

I was lying on my stomach and felt . . . something, like someone lightly touching my deep insides. Then I just sat very still and for an alive moment felt the hugeness of having something living growing in me. Then I said, 'No, it's not possible, it's too early yet,' and then I started to cry . . . That one moment was my first body awareness of another living thing inside me.

And after the first movement – in the fourth or fifth month – you may wait days for another sign of quickening. Then the movements will become frequent and familiar. The baby begins to feel real. You can feel from the outside the hard shape of your uterus.

If you are angry or upset by pregnancy, then your baby's movements serve to focus your anger.

Last night its kicking made me dizzy and gave me a terrible feeling of solitude. I wanted to tell it, 'Stop, stop, stop, let me alone.' I want to lie still and whole and all single, catch my breath. But I have no control over this new part of my being, and this lack of control scares me. I feel as if I were rushing downhill at such a great speed that I'd never be able to stop.

Perhaps feeling the baby move for the first time will change you.

Sitting on a rock, trees growing right out of the rock. They cling and flourish on nothing. Images of the growing life inside me, also coming from nothing, getting nutrition from my body the way the tree does from the rock . . . Occasionally I give it warmth, mostly when it moves. The more it moves, the more I like it. I also resent it an awful lot; I feel big, ugly and uncomfortable, and in spite of Len's protestations, I feel alone.

Even during the most positive pregnancies there may be moments, hours and days of depression, anxiety and confusion. These depressions may be connected to all the submerged anxieties you have in relation to your own childhood, doubts that come from our society's ignorance about pregnancy and childbirth, doubts you have about your own identity, economic problems, having too many children already and problems in your relationship with your partner.

It seems that my feelings about my pregnancy, my body, the coming of the baby, were inextricably wound into my feelings, problems, hopes and fears for our relationship . . . It's hard to separate which feelings were a result of my unhappiness about us (a lot of the bad feelings about my body arose because Bob showed very little interest in my enlarged, changing body), which ones were my own negative feelings about having a less functional body (I wanted to keep working and active, but my body was so cumbersome that I was always worn out and tired) and which ones were just moods caused by pregnancy.

We all have general fears, too; there is fear of the unknown, especially if it's a first pregnancy. No matter how much we do know about the physiological changes in our bodies, there's something incomprehensible about the beginnings of life. And by becoming pregnant we open ourselves to changes and complications. We become much more aware of being vulnerable.

I remember feeling overwhelmed by sad things I saw, and was overwhelmed by things that could happen to innocence. I'd wake in the night and think people were going to come in and take things, take the baby from me. I was beginning to be out of control. I was terribly afraid of chance. I've always been afraid of irrationality, of fate.

You may have vivid dreams.

For two nights now my falling asleep has given rise to that old childhood dream-image of falling down a deep, dark, square hole ever diminishing in size.

I'm in a hospital in a room all alone, a cold room. The nurse gives me a shot; I have my baby and I don't feel a thing. I look up and see my baby floating in a beaker, alive. I can't go to her; I'm sad and frustrated.

The baby starts coming out of my belly. I have to hold it in. My skin is transparent.

We fear that our babies will be handicapped. (Around one in fifty of babies in England and Wales are born with malformations of some kind.) Some of us have dreams, fantasies and nightmares about deformity. These are normal and universal.

When I was about six months pregnant and Dick was starting school again, I was home alone, isolated for days at a time. My nightmares and daydreams started around then, really terrible fears of the baby being deformed. All my life I've always been the good girl. I knew I wasn't really good. I knew I had bad thoughts, but I was never allowed to express them. So I thought my baby's deformities would be the living proof of the badness in me.

We fear our own death, the child's death.

In fact, we do have to face the fact that some women miscarry and some babies die. While it's difficult, threatening and sad to think of, we know it happens. Though it's very hard and not usually useful to try to prepare ourselves for death, it helps to know what has happened to some of us, so that if we or our friends experience such tragedy, we can in some way be acquainted with the event. This knowledge is a kind of preparation. It's vitally important to be able to reach out to friends when tragic things happen to them, and to help ease their feelings of isolation. It also helps us to know that we can and need to ask for help if such a thing happens to us.

I went into the hospital for the birth of my first child . . . The child's lungs became infected and he died two days later. I never saw him. When I began to return to myself I found that despite all those times I had told myself that nothing could really happen, I had nothing but an empty belly. I don't know if we should be warned ahead of time to worry needlessly about something that happens to a very few women, but as one of those women, I definitely need to feel some sense of sharing with others in the same position – not to cry over what happened but to work out how to face other people. That's the hardest part – nobody wants to deal with death, especially when your friends are at the childbearing age themselves and can't help being afraid of you for what you stand for. I found that my friends wanted me to pretend nothing had happened – even that there had been no pregnancy. I don't think it was just my particular friends – it's natural to want to avoid those things. And so my fantastic pregnancy, in which a lot of things went on in my head and body that helped me to change and get myself together, had to be buried. Even now, after a year, I can see their pain and fear for me as I start into my eighth month of pregnancy with my second child. I have to be the one who keeps them calm, and I especially must assure everyone that this one will be okay.

We may also feel guilty about having fears. Don't they in some way suggest that as mothers we will be weak and inadequate? The myth is that we can't allow ourselves these depressions because we are supposed to be strong, mature, maternal, accepting, loving all the time.

Our feelings are legitimate. We must feel free to know them, to express them and to be strengthened by them.

Living Alone

If you have no close partner to share your pregnancy there may be times when you feel very much alone.

Most of the time I felt purposeful and businesslike about pregnancy but there were times when I felt very isolated and vulnerable.[33]

If you live in an area where punitive attitudes towards single parenthood still predominate, or if your immediate family are unsupportive, your pregnancy may be a time of great stress. However, in most cities single parenthood is now an accepted variation of family life; though you may still have to contend with medical personnel who insist on calling you 'Mrs' (they will say it's for your sake), or treating you in a patronizing or disapproving way.

There were three of us in a row on the ward, all unmarried. It seemed unlikely to be a coincidence but I didn't know whether we were together for mutual support or because we were regarded as not quite socially acceptable.

Wherever you are, you will find that there are other women around who do not share these negative feelings and will provide support. Friends, particularly those who already have children, can be a wonderful source of tender loving care. Indeed recent unpublished research indicates that single women are less vulnerable to depression at times of crisis than are married women because they are more likely to have built up a network of supportive female relationships.[34] So, accept all offers of help. You will have plenty of time to reciprocate later on with childcare arrangements, and fetching and carrying.

Look also on p. 421 for organizations which provide support to single pregnant women and sign up for antenatal classes locally where you are likely to meet other women to share your pregnancy with you.

Partners' Feelings

If we have partners, their feelings are very important to our experience of pregnancy. They may be men or, for a growing number of lesbians who achieve pregnancy through AI (see p. 432), women. Partners of either sex may feel ambivalent, jealous, afraid of losing you, anxious about your health and your future together. They may well feel excluded from this process which is absorbing so much of your energy. They may also feel impatient and indifferent or just anxious. One woman writing about her partner's decision to have AI wrote:

'Pauline's lover', a weak position, defined by my sexual relationship – what is the relevance of this definition to me or my relationship with a new baby?[35]

A man wrote:

I wasn't ready for the sudden change. I was worried and confused. I had to adjust to a new relationship with you just as you had to adjust to the changes in your body.[36]

If your partner is to be involved during the pregnancy and afterwards, it is important to prepare and learn together, go to classes together and discuss the changes you are going through. A partner who is informed and confident will have a real part to play during the birth and afterwards when your energy will be taken up with the physical acts of birth, establishing feeding and recovery.

Some couples find they are unable to talk easily about the changes and responsibilities that pregnancy implies. Pregnancy and childbirth do put extra demands on a relationship. Some relationships do not survive these changes, others creak under the strain but come out stronger and deeper.*

Dolores Kreiger, Professor of Nursing at New York University, works with childbearing couples using 'Therapeutic Touch' (see p. 87). She has noticed a big change in the way the men begin to relate to the women.

The changes they have undergone – the softness and understanding that they have been able to develop – have been very moving.

Sexual attitudes may be changed too. A male partner may feel close and attracted to you and fascinated by your growing body. Or, for reasons to do with his own attitude and upbringing and particular problems, he may feel repelled, confused and threatened by the changes in your body. His feelings may change from day to day.

Sometimes I thought you were really beautiful and your belly was beautiful, and sometimes you looked like a ridiculous pregnant insect. Your navel bulging out looked strange.

Even our most complex feelings are changeable. Talk can lead to some deep, good questioning about the conventional ideas of beauty we are all brainwashed with.

Living with a Group of People

If you are living with a group of people it is a good idea to think about how you want them to relate to your child. Some communities exist that are themselves large extended families. But many groups are composed of people who will have very different commitments to your child. Often people don't want to have anything much to do with taking care of children. They either don't want to or don't feel ready to. Try to work out just what you are expecting of each person and whether your expectations are realistic. Talk to each person if you can and find out how s/he feels about your coming child. Do it early.

You can't assume that people will automatically help on their own and know you need help. Also, with people who don't have children you have to be explicit and tell them what to do. I don't think it's a good thing to have a lot of people take care of the baby at first, but I was glad that people helped me out. Also find out how they feel about you. Having chosen these people as your new family, you might expect to be cared for and nurtured, and you might find that people won't be able to meet your increased needs.

*Relate (formerly the Marriage Guidance Council; see p. 131) provides counselling which may help you to find a way through these problems.

Making Love during Pregnancy

You will have many different feelings about making love during pregnancy. Your moods and desires will shift.

I wanted to make love more than ever.

I remember feeling very sexy. We were trying all these different positions. I used to feel uptight about sex for its own sake, when I was pregnant I felt a lot freer.

For the first three months I went right off sex. It was even worse the second time when I had bleeding problems. I felt as though I was carrying something very precious inside me and I didn't want anyone to interfere with me. I know it made Dave feel even more remote from the process of pregnancy.

If like many women your pregnancy makes you feel more open and sensuous than before it will be an ideal opportunity for experimenting with new ways of loving. Lovemaking brings you closer to your partner at a time when closeness is needed. As your pregnancy advances you will want to work out new positions for getting close to each other which do not put uncomfortable pressure on your tummy. Many men and women prefer to make love cupped together like spoons with the man behind.

If, on the other hand, nausea and tiredness put you off, don't be dismayed. Your sexual feelings will come back again as your mood changes. Most women feel an increase in sexual interest around the fourth or fifth month. In the meantime there are other ways of showing that you love each other.

There is no evidence that, under normal circumstances, sexual intercourse and orgasm can do anything but good during pregnancy. It is sensible to avoid both if you are bleeding, or experiencing any pain, and you should avoid penetration once your membranes have ruptured as there is then a risk of infection.

If you have oral-genital sex your partner should avoid blowing air into your vagina (in extremely rare cases this has been known to cause air embolism which can kill you). If your partner has been in contact with any sexually transmitted disease, or has open herpes sores, avoid contact until the disease has been treated or it clears.

When your baby is due, love-making may be the best way to encourage labour to start. Nipple stimulation releases oxytocin, the hormone which triggers labour, and the prostaglandin in semen can also start labour. The amounts in both cases are too small to have any effect until you are ready to go into labour.

THE THIRD TRIMESTER
(29th week to term)

Physical Changes

Your uterus is becoming very large. It feels hard when you touch it.

Nina Reimer

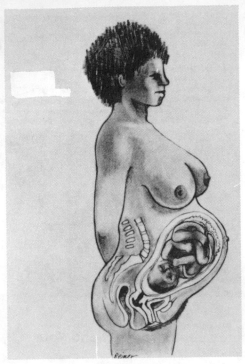

Woman in 40th week of pregnancy

Vaughn Sills

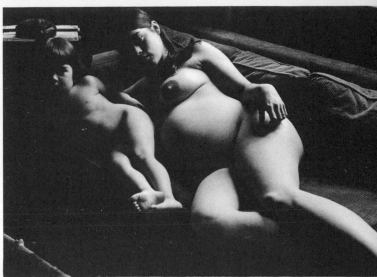

I remember my friends' surprise when they put their hands on my belly to feel it. They expected it to be soft and somehow jellylike and were amazed at its hardness and bulk.

It's a strong muscular container. You can feel and see the movements of your fetus from the outside now, too, as it changes position, turns somersaults, hiccups. Sometimes it puts pressure on your bladder, which makes you feel that you need to urinate even when you don't, and which can hurt a little, or sometimes a lot, for very brief periods. Sometimes towards the end of pregnancy it puts pressure on the nerves at the top of your legs, which can be painful, too.

Your baby will be lying in a particular position, sometimes head down, back to your front, sometimes lying crossways. It moves around often. Your midwife or doctor can help you discover which position the baby is in. By 34 weeks most babies turn head down ready for the birth. You can encourage it to turn (see below).

Sometimes your baby lies still. It's known that babies sleep *in utero*. There should be a regular pattern to movements. If you notice a significant decrease in movements, contact your doctor. See the information on p. 372 (kick charts).

Your uterus will tighten every now and then. These are painless contractions called Braxton-Hicks contractions. They are believed to strengthen uterine muscles, preparing them for eventual labour. Herbalists suggest drinking raspberry-leaf tea towards the end of pregnancy to strengthen uterine muscles. Avoid this herb in the early months.

It becomes increasingly uncomfortable for you to lie on your stomach. You may experience shortness of breath. There's pressure on your lungs from your uterus, and your diaphragm may be moved up as much as an inch. Even so, because your thoracic (chest) cage widens, you breathe in more air when you are pregnant than when you are not.

POSTURES WHICH MAY HELP TO TURN A BREECH BABY

Begin after the 30th week of pregnancy for up to four weeks before birth or until the baby turns.

1. PRACTISE TWICE A DAY FOR TEN MINUTES EACH TIME.

Lie on your back on a hard surface with the pelvis raised by pillows to a level nine to twelve inches above the head. Stomach should be empty. (This posture corrected breech to head-first position of baby for 89 per cent of women in one study.) Lying head down on a collapsed ironing board with one end propped on a couch or chair is sometimes more comfortable than the pillow position.

2. PRACTISE TWICE A DAY FOR TEN MINUTES EACH TIME.

Knee-chest position: on all fours, fold your arms and place head on them, knees about eighteen inches apart, back straight. Bladder should be empty. If you do this posture so that your head is at the edge of your bed, a book can be placed on the floor below and it is possible to read comfortably.

Sometimes when you lie down you may not be able to breathe well for a moment. Prop yourself up with pillows or turn on your side, and the pressure on your diaphragm will be lessened.

The peak load on your heart occurs in about the 30th week (thereafter the load increases only very slowly). After that the heart usually doesn't have to work so hard until delivery.

You are still gaining weight. If you have haemorrhoids or varicose veins, try to avoid standing up for long periods of time, and when you sit or lie down, be sure your feet are raised.

Your stomach is pushed up by your uterus and flattened. Indigestion becomes more common. If you have heartburn, sleep with your head and shoulders raised. Eat small amounts frequently. Don't take mineral oil – it causes you to excrete necessary vitamins.

If you have insomnia or trouble sleeping because the baby's movements make you uncomfortable, take walks and hot baths. Drink warm milk or camomile tea. Avoid sleeping pills. Brisk exercise during the day will help you sleep better.

I think there is a reason for this non-sleeping: there's work getting done. That restlessness needs to happen. Your energy builds up for the coming crisis. I remember pacing around my house at midnight, burning with energy, finally finding the tiny sandals my first child had worn as a toddler. I carefully cleaned and polished them for the new baby. Then I slept fine.

Your navel will probably be pushed out.

Since your body has become heavier, you'll tend to walk differently for balance, often leaning back to counteract a heavier front. This can cause backaches, for which there are exercises.* Your pelvic joints are also much more separated.

At about four to two weeks before birth, and sometimes as early as the seventh month, the baby's head settles into your pelvis. This is called 'engagement' or 'dropping'. (It may not happen after the first pregnancy or if you have a shallow pelvis, which is more common among black women.) It takes pressure off your stomach. Some women do feel much lighter. And if you have been having trouble breathing, pressure is now off your diaphragm. This 'dropping' can cause constipation; your bowels are more obstructed than they were.

As for water retention, a pregnant woman retains on average 5 litres – about 9 pints – of liquid, half of this in the last ten weeks. Swollen ankles are common.

*If you suffer from back problems they may get worse in pregnancy. Try to avoid lifting anything heavy. Osteopathy can help but be sure to use someone who is recommended. A clumsy practitioner can do harm and you are particularly vulnerable now (see p. 98).

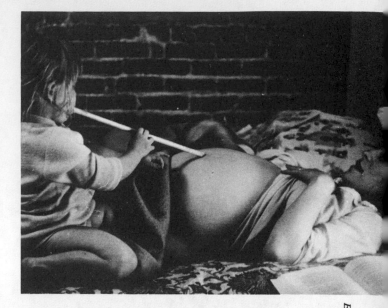

Ed Pincus

Your Feelings about Yourself and Your Pregnancy

I had a feeling of being at the end, of nothing else being terrifically important.

I thought it would never end. I was enormous. I couldn't bend over and wash my feet. And it was incredibly hot.

At the end I started to feel it was too long. Dick took pictures of me during the eighth month. I saw my face as faraway and sad.

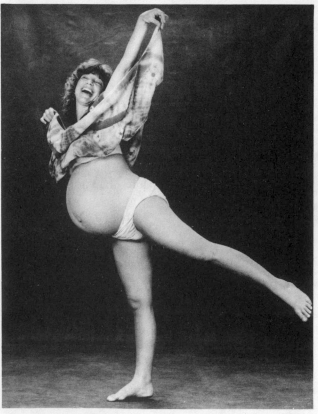

David Alexander

I had insomnia. I couldn't get comfortable. I couldn't sleep, he'd kick so much.

I wonder what it looks like. How fantastic that it only has to travel one-and-a-half feet down to get born.

My kid is dancing under my heart.

The relationship of mother carrying child is the most beautiful and simplest.

I pity a baby who must come out of the womb.

Fairly confidently and calmly awaiting the baby – quite set on a home delivery. Doctor said Thursday I was already dilated two-and-a-half centimetres, so it must be getting close. Getting a bit anxious, listening to every Braxton-Hicks contraction, awaiting with hope – and fear, too – its change into the real thing.

I feel exultant and tired and rich inside. My belly is large, and last night the baby beat around inside it like a wild tempest. I thought the time had come and was panicked and nauseated, then very excited. I woke Ed up. Then at five I fell asleep. Meanwhile I move in slow motion and wait.

TESTING DURING PREGNANCY

New techniques for checking on the health of the fetus during pregnancy have created a whole new set of decisions and dilemmas for women which we discuss on p. 341. While we may have reason to feel grateful for the chance of knowing beforehand whether a fetus is handicapped, and being able to decide whether or not to continue the pregnancy, we also resent tests which could damage the baby, and might bring bad news. Testing allows a very few women to make a choice about bearing a handicapped child, and in some cases can be life-saving, but it also creates extra stress and anxiety for a very much larger number of women. Often we come to believe, in our technological, medicalized culture, that the newly developed pre-natal tests magically 'prevent' disease and birth defects; that by having them we assuage the gods so that we won't be 'punished'; and that we are irresponsible when we decide not to have them. Though tests are appropriate in specific instances for specific women, it is not reasonable for them all to be done routinely for every woman – they may not always be safe for us or our babies and they further medicalize the pregnancy experience. Unfortunately, often their very existence pressures us into having them done. When we decide against them, we have to resist that pressure.

At present 2–3 per cent of babies in Britain are born with congenital handicaps. The rate of major handicap has not changed significantly over the last twenty years except that the number of babies born with neural tube defects (NTDs) is dropping (possibly due in part to screening and abortion of affected babies).

There is no coherent public policy about screening in this country. In some areas, AFP blood tests for spina bifida and ultrasound scans are routine. You may not even be told the implications of the blood test and adequate information about scans is not always provided. Amniocentesis is offered in the majority of hospitals to women over thirty-six, but in others at thirty-nine, though this is likely to change now that blood screening is available for Down's Syndrome (see p. 370). In some areas you may have difficulty resisting routine tests and in others you have to go out of your way to ask for them.

In many hospitals women are expected to decide, in advance of the tests, whether or not to have an abortion if the results show an abnormality; a policy which forces a pregnant woman to cut herself off emotionally from her baby for more than a month just at the time she is likely to start feeling movements. Such a blanket policy also allows no opportunity for discussion about the degree and implications of possible handicaps detected. Testing should be offered, to those who want it, without any precondition.

If your doctor has suggested tests, your decision to have the test or not depends on many personal considerations, such as your family situation, your feelings about medical procedures and risks, your feelings concerning abortion and the way you feel about the possibility of having a child with a disability.

Disabilities differ a lot in their severity. Getting to know children with disabilities and/or their parents can often help you to understand what the situation would mean to you and your partner. Different people feel very differently about this matter, and it is important that you do not feel pressured into a decision you won't be comfortable with.

For the vast majority of women who are tested, the results are negative. However, a negative result on a particular test does not guarantee that the baby does not have some other problems. Many abnormalities cannot yet be tested for. You may want to consider these questions before agreeing to a test.

- Where can I learn more about the conditions being tested for?
- What will I learn from the test? How accurate is it?
- What are the risks to me and my baby if I take the test?
- What are the risks if I don't have the test done?
- How long do I have to wait to learn the results?
- What procedures will be either necessary or available if the test yields positive results? And how far am I prepared to go along with the routines that now exist?

Be sure that you want and need the test in question. Talk it over with your doctor. Ask to talk with a genetic counsellor. Be sure you understand what is happening and why. If you have any doubts, get a second opinion. Try to talk with other women who have had the test.

My son was born fourteen years ago. In the past

three years I had an abortion and a miscarriage. Once again I became pregnant. Though I had planned to have an amniocentesis done that last pregnancy, the miscarriage changed my mind: when the medical centre sent out an informational pamphlet about amniocentesis which said that there was a 1.5 per cent chance of miscarriage or fetal damage, and after Steven and I had done a lot of reading, I realized that if I had to go through another loss I'd be a basket case. So I decided not to have it done.

Then came the enormous pressure: here I was, thirty-eight. My doctor urged me; so did my father, my husband's parents; my sister had had one and so had all my friends, without questioning. I even knew abstractly that I'd rather have a miscarriage than a Down's Syndrome baby.

For three weeks I was a wreck. Then one of my friends asked me, 'What would be the worst thing?' I said, 'The worst thing would be if the baby were healthy and amniocentesis caused a miscarriage.'

That did it: no amniocentesis. I'd really made the decision. We lived with it fine.

And Sarah is wonderful and healthy.

There is no easy answer.

I was thirty-seven, healthy, had had two children and was pregnant again after seventeen years. I just knew I didn't want a needle poking into my womb.

I am planning a home birth and thought long and hard about amniocentesis. You have to use technology selectively. I finally decided to have it done – that if there was something wrong, I owed it to my family to find out. I wanted to have the chance to decide about continuing the pregnancy. After it was over, what a relief! We don't have the results yet, but I'm not at all wondering or worried!

When I became unexpectedly pregnant at forty-three, my doctor told me about amniocentesis, but I told him that because of my religion I wouldn't consider having an abortion no matter what the results of the test. He then suggested I consider having the test just to find the condition of the baby – that probably we would be reassured that it was all right. I talked it over with my husband and he thought this idea made sense. It was very upsetting when we first learned the baby had Down's, but this didn't change our original feelings. Learning the baby's condition early made all the difference. I attended a clinic which helps parents care for children with Down's and talked with many parents. As well as preparing ourselves, my husband and I were able to help our three teenage children know what to expect. We all picked out the baby's name together and the children are waiting for him to come home so they can help take care of him.

It is important to think about why we have these tests, to learn about the procedures, not to feel pressurized and to be comfortable with the decisions we make. Counselling should be offered before any tests are done. The results should be provided promptly to all women. Some centres only give test results when they are positive – a policy which is unjustifiable because it leaves the majority of women in a state of tension and anxiety. Before the tests are done, ensure that you will be informed promptly whatever the results and that you know who to contact if there are delays.

Unfortunately, in the majority of cases, test results will not be known until you are around 20 weeks' pregnant. If you choose an abortion, at this stage it is usually done by induction (see p. 328), which is a painful and emotionally difficult procedure requiring a lot of care and support. (Occasionally a hysterotomy, which is like a caesarean section, will be done but this has the same implication for future childbearing as a caesarean, see p. 394.) A procedure known as chorionic villus sampling (see p. 371) could allow testing in the first twelve weeks of pregnancy but this technique has not yet been evaluated properly.

The emotional reaction of women after an abortion in these circumstances has been described as similar to that after a stillbirth. You must expect to go through feelings of bereavement and you (and your partner) may want to find other people who have been through this experience and can help you come to terms with it.*

ULTRASOUND

Ultrasound uses intermittent high-frequency sound waves to create pictures of the body's inner organs by recording their echoes, much as sonar measures shapes in the water. A technician runs a *transducer* back and forth over your abdomen and a computer translates the resulting echoes into pictures on a video screen so that the fetus's and your inner organs are made visible.

Ultrasound even at its most basic can be used to give a rough idea of where the placenta is lying. This can be useful in late pregnancy if there is an indication that it is covering the cervix (one of the few definite indications for caesarean). Used in early pregnancy, it may wrongly identify placentas as low-lying and cause more anxiety than it allays. It is not very good at dating a pregnancy though it can pinpoint within a fortnight either way if there is no positive evidence to go by. Better accuracy is claimed around 16 weeks. The technique can detect obvious physical abnormalities and modern equipment used by skilled technicians can identify neural tube defects more quickly than other procedures (see p. 369). However, this degree of expertise is rare. In most situations ultrasound is an in-

---

*The Association of Spina Bifida and Hydrocephalus in association with other organizations is setting up support groups for women going through this experience. See Resources for address.

accurate procedure compared with amniocentesis (see p. 370). It is also used to guide other procedures such as amniocentesis and fetoscopy (see p. 371) and is used continuously in electronic fetal monitoring during labour (see p. 392).

When used competently it is a valuable, non-invasive tool which can give immediate, important information when it is required. However, in the hands of inexperienced people it can cause at best anxiety and at worst misdiagnosis. If an abnormality is detected on ultrasound alone, it may be worth asking for a second opinion at another hospital.

I was being scanned after a threatened miscarriage. In the last twenty-four hours my spirits had sunk and then began to climb as the bleeding stopped. The scan was really done to reassure me that the baby was still alive so you can imagine how I felt when two operators failed to find a heartbeat. After what seemed like a century, a third woman appeared and found the little flickering pulse immediately.

No obvious problems associated with ultrasound have appeared as yet; however, it took thirty years for the regular use of X-rays in pregnancy to be questioned on safety grounds. * Genetic effects from ultrasound could take that long to be revealed and, as it is brought in on a routine basis into ante-natal care, the number of babies who are not subjected is dwindling to the point where no proper control group can be found with which to measure the long-term safety of the technique.

Although there is no convincing evidence that ultrasound harms babies, we cannot be convinced that it is totally safe. The Department of Health, following World Health Organization guidelines, has recommended that it should not be used routinely. However, the Royal College of Obstetricians and Gynaecologists dismisses fears and has enthusiastically recommended routine scanning of every pregnancy. As with so many other techniques, the doctors' enthusiasm for looking into wombs has run ahead of any systematic evaluation of the technique. We would question any routine use of it, particularly in very early pregnancy.

ALPHA-FETOPROTEIN TESTS (AFP)

Approximately two in 1,000 infants in the UK are born each year with a neural tube defect (NTD). In this disorder, the developing neural tube, which forms the brain, spinal cord and spinal column, does not close over completely. The defect, which usually leaves an open lesion, can occur anywhere along the neural tube. If the tube remains open at the top, the baby will be born with only a rudimentary brain and open skull. This condition, called *anencephaly*, is always fatal. If the opening is along the backbone, the severity of the defect will depend on several factors: whether the lesion is covered with skin, whether nerve tissue protrudes from the defect, and the size and location of the lesion. This condition is known as *spina bifida* or *meningeomyelocele*. Children with open lesions almost always have severe medical problems and some are mentally handicapped, many have no bladder or bowel control and most have some degree of paralysis. Many do not survive and many require extensive medical and surgical procedures. However, many forms of spina bifida are much less disabling, and people with the condition lead rich, full lives. * Unfortunately, the AFP blood test gives no indication of the severity of the problem, although ultrasound can help with the diagnosis in some cases.

During the last decade, researchers discovered that the amount of alpha-fetoprotein was higher for women who carried an affected fetus. The alpha-fetoprotein test can diagnose about 85 per cent of fetuses with an open lesion. About 10 per cent of fetuses with neural tube defects have lesions covered with skin. They are not detectable and usually less serious.

Although the blood test itself is easy to do, the results are difficult to interpret for the following reasons:

1. The amount of AFP varies during pregnancy. The test must be done at 16 weeks to be accurate. Therefore it is important to know when you became pregnant.

2. The blood test may give 'false positives', due to multiple births, certain rare disorders, an incorrect estimate of fetal age or simply because you have a normally high level of AFP. Doctors may want to monitor your pregnancy more closely if your AFP level is high because these babies do seem to be more vulnerable for reasons which are not yet clear.

Because of the many false positives, further tests are done on women who have a high AFP reading. These include a second blood test, ultrasound to check the fetus's age and look for abnormality and finally, if necessary, amniocentesis. Each step increases the accuracy with which the relatively few cases are diagnosed.

Medical and laypeople have raised objections to routine AFP screening, which subjects numbers of women to several tests when so few will actually have the problem and will have to wait so long for the results. Inadequate counselling, lack of information and the procedures themselves can cause inordinate stress for the women who decide to have repeat testing.

If you decide to have an AFP blood test, remember that a series of tests may be necessary to be sure that a normal baby will not be diagnosed as having a neural tube deficiency. If

*The possibility that X-rays could harm the fetus was first raised in 1926. The 1937 edition of F. J. Browne's *Antenatal and Postnatal Care*, asserts: 'It has been frequently asked whether there is any danger to the life of the child by the passage of X-rays through it; it can be said at once that there is none if the examination is carried out by a competent radiologist or radiographer.' It was not until the late 1950s that research into childhood cancer revealed a link with X-ray and in the early 1970s X-rays were still widely used.[37]

*Contact the Association of Spina Bifida and Hydrocephalus.

you are having amniocentesis anyway, the AFP blood test is unnecessary since the AFP level in the amniotic fluid should be measured routinely.

Researchers do not know what factors can produce neural tube defects, and believe them to be brought on by a combination of genetic and other unknown factors. One study found that supplementary vitamins around the time of conception and for the first month of pregnancy may help prevent the disorder (see p. 341).

BLOOD SCREENING FOR DOWN'S SYNDROME

A blood screening test for Down's Syndrome was about to be introduced as we went to press. This test would be done at the same time, and on the same sample, as the AFP test. It measures the amount of HCG and oestriol in your blood. This information, added to the AFP level and information on your age, can then be fed into a computer and an individual estimate made of your personal risk of carrying a Down's Syndrome baby. On the basis of this risk estimation you can decide whether or not to opt for a follow-up amniocentesis (see below), which will give more accurate information.

Like the AFP test, this means that a large number of younger women who would have gone through pregnancy relatively untroubled by the health of their baby will now have to face the stress of having doubts raised by a positive test. In forty-eight cases out of forty-nine, the follow-up amniocentesis will be negative and the anxiety will have been for nothing.

Older women who are uncertain about amniocentesis may find the blood test a great help in making a decision because it can assess risk more accurately than age alone. The test takes age into account, so the *average* woman of forty will still have a higher assessment of risk than the *average* woman of twenty. However, when other factors are taken into account, your risk may come out equivalent to the average risk for a woman of twenty-five. In this case you may feel happy about opting out of amniocentesis. If, on the other hand, your risk seems higher than normal for your age, it may help you to make a decision in favour of amniocentesis.

However, when considering having the test, women should understand that it is only a screening test. It will pick up only about 60 per cent of pregnancies with a Down's Syndrome baby. That means that the other 40 per cent will be undetected. Older women, who are at highest risk of Down's and other related chromosome abnormalities, may anyway wish to opt for an amniocentesis because it is a diagnostic test that can determine accurately whether a particular fetus is affected.

AMNIOCENTESIS

This procedure can be used to reveal approximately eighty disorders including chromosome abnormalities such as Down's Syndrome (see p. 367) and certain genetic and metabolic disorders. It is also used to follow up AFP tests for the detection of neural tube defects (see p. 369).

Some consultants still use the technique to assess fetal lung maturity late in pregnancy if caesarean section or induction is being considered. It is a hazardous procedure at this stage, though it may be offered when an elective caesarean is necessary and there is doubt about gestational age and the maturity of the baby's lungs. However, not all consultants would be happy about it. According to consultant Peter Huntingford:

The logic of using it has always escaped me. If there is an indication to deliver a baby then it must take its chance. If there is no overriding reason to deliver the baby, then the result [of the test] is dubious support for delivery.

The test has a high level of positive accuracy (it is very rare to get a false positive) but it does not reveal all handicapping conditions or even all of those babies affected by the conditions which are tested for.

The major drawback with amniocentesis is the risk of miscarriage. There has also been some evidence of an increase in respiratory problems though this has recently been largely discounted. The miscarriage risk varies according to the skill of the operator, between 1.5 and about 0.2 per cent.[38] It tends to be higher when a high level of AFP has been diagnosed. Nobody knows why, but a high level of AFP does seem to be associated with vulnerability even in babies who do not have any kind of handicap.

The correct needle size and proper use of ultrasound scanning are important. Doctors at Queen Mother's Hospital, Glasgow, 'regarded the use of real-time ultrasound to provide uninterrupted guidance as mandatory'. Real-time scanning machines allow the doctor to see the placenta and the fetus while doing the amniocentesis. Some older machinery provides only one fixed 'shot' at a time and, of course, the fetus may then move. Ask your doctor to refer you to a hospital which does a large number of these procedures using the correct equipment.

Because of the risks associated with amniocentesis, it is not routinely offered except where the benefits outweigh the risks. With the introduction of blood screening (see above), only those women at highest risk will be offered amniocentesis. Each of us will tend to have our own view of the potential benefits of such a procedure and should be able to make our own, informed, choices accordingly.

If you have Rhesus negative blood you should be given an injection of Anti D when you have amniocentesis.

The procedure: a doctor performs amniocentesis on an outpatient basis using ultrasound to check the location of the fetus and the placenta. (Some use a local anaesthetic to numb the skin, others don't.) The doctor then inserts a long, thin needle through your abdominal wall into the womb and draws off approximately four teaspoons of fluid into a syringe. On rare occasions s/he may have to try a second time to get enough fluid. You may experience pricking or stinging of your skin, cramping when the needle enters the uterus and pressure when the fluid is withdrawn. These reactions are normal and don't mean that anything is amiss, but they should diminish and disappear within a day. If they don't, call your doctor.

While some women find the procedure easy, others find it an unpleasant, upsetting experience. Most women agree that it is wise to rest afterwards for at least a day as you may well feel quite shaky and shocked.

I found the procedure itself absolutely painless but my knees started to shake and I was very glad to get home to bed.

First they showed it on the ultrasound screen and then made a pen mark on my stomach where the needle was to go in. The whole procedure turned out to be completely painless. My doctor talked his way through: 'Now I'm going to do . . . Now you'll feel . . .' It was reassuring. Then he told me to take it easy for a day. After, we spoke to a genetics counsellor and asked a lot of questions. She told us as much as we wanted to know and showed us 'pictures' of imperfect chromosomes which cause birth defects. It was abstract but it hit home. It helped that nothing had gone wrong during the procedure.

No one had prepared me for how important it was to have someone there holding your hand and being supportive. The doctor couldn't get the needle in the right place and kept moving it around for a long time. This really hurt and I was upset and anxious. Finally he took the needle out and tried again. The second time there was no problem but I was quite distraught by that time. The staff and doctors were wonderful but I wish I had talked beforehand to someone who had gone through the experience.

The procedure itself wasn't bad. My husband went with me. I found it kind of creepy thinking of that long needle so I didn't look. It took longer than I thought. Afterwards, however, I had bad cramps and was in great pain. I found it traumatic to hear (from the counsellor) about all the genetic deformities that could not be picked up and why the test might have to be done again. The cramps did go away but I stayed in bed for two days because I had lost a baby a few years before and was afraid of miscarriage. When it became clear that things were all right I felt better.

It takes three to four weeks to culture the amniotic fluid and examine the cells. It is a time which many women find profoundly disturbing.

It seemed a very long time and I had some very disturbing dreams. I think the knowledge that you are flirting with your child's life outrages some very

deeply held sense of protectiveness. The results felt like a reprieve.

CHORIONIC VILLUS SAMPLING (CVS)

This is a new technique, still in the experimental stage which must be done very early in pregnancy, between 8 and 11 weeks. The test carries a higher risk of inducing miscarriage than amniocentesis, but the miscarriage rate is being reduced as operators gain skill. In 1986 world rates were between 6 and 2 per cent, but without any reliable figures on the normal rate of miscarriages at this stage these figures are hard to evaluate. It seems clear that the skill of the operator is important. Miscarriage rates are lower at the centres with most experience.[39]

The procedure is not widely available and, as it does carry a significant risk (both known and possibly unknown), it is offered only when there is a high chance of severe handicap and, in some centres, as part of a randomized controlled trial. We do not know as yet whether there are any long-term risks involved for the baby. If this test is found to be safe it could, in time, take the place of amniocentesis.

The value of this technique is that the results are available within the first three months of pregnancy. This means that if an abortion is decided upon it can be done with less physical and emotional trauma (see p. 321). The material examined from the chorionic villi (where the embryo joins the placenta) contains the same cell material as the baby. It can therefore be examined for chromosome, metabolic and genetic disorders such as sickle cell disease and thalassaemia, sex-linked abnormalities, Down's Syndrome, and Tay-Sachs disease. However, in practice the technique provides problems: it is not always possible to get a good sample for analysis and false positives are possible.

The procedure is usually done vaginally via a very fine tube through the cervix, but in the future doctors may prefer to do it by passing a fine needle through the abdominal wall, similar to amniocentesis. (This cuts down the risk of infection.) A small cell sample is taken for examination.

FETOSCOPY

This is a method of literally looking at the baby in the womb. It is available only in a few specialist centres. A very fine tube carrying a minute lens is inserted through the abdominal wall into the womb. The lens can then be replaced by a needle with which to take samples. The whole operation must be guided by ultrasound scanning. It can allow fast, direct examination of the baby, blood sampling and cell sampling. The needle can also be used for some treatments, for example, to give a transfusion to a baby whose blood is being attacked by Rhesus antibodies (see p. 343), and limited *in utero* surgery.

As has been shown in the USA, this raises the issue of who is the patient – the mother or the fetus? One can envisage a time when women's rights over their own bodies could be sufficiently eroded to allow doctors to operate on the baby without the mother's consent.

The method of testing can only be done after 16–18 weeks and it carries a miscarriage rate of 3–4 per cent, which is higher than the risk in amniocentesis, as well as other possible risks such as infection and damage to other organs. It should not be used unless other tests have indicated that intervention is necessary and you want it.

TESTING BEFORE BIRTH
(ante-partum fetal testing)

Another set of tests exists, originally designed as screening and diagnostic tools for women with health problems (diabetes, heart or kidney disease or excessively high blood pressure) or for women who have had a previous problem, such as stillbirth. These tests are also performed when a woman or her doctor thinks that a baby is overdue – usually after 42 weeks of pregnancy – or that a fetus still in the uterus has stopped growing (IUGR – intra-uterine growth retardation), for the placenta can reach a point where it no longer functions at its peak. The goal of these tests is to discover whether the baby is healthy enough to remain in the uterus. While sometimes successful in reassuring worried women and doctors, and sometimes leading to a truly life-saving caesarean, these tests, like the tests previously discussed, do not *guarantee* a healthy baby. In addition, researchers have not performed enough randomized clinical trials to prove that testing and knowing the results actually do reduce the perinatal death rate. The tests have high false-positive rates and medical people disagree as to which results constitute 'normality' and which mean danger.

The tests can be useful if you are faced with a consultant who is very keen to induce for post-maturity simply on the basis of dates.

Kick Charts

If you do have any of these tests, first do what is simplest. As a start, some women simply check to see if the baby moves at least ten times in twelve hours. Any marked decrease in movements could indicate stress and should be reported to a doctor or midwife who will listen with a stethoscope to the baby's heartbeat after each of several movements to determine whether the heart tones speed up (accelerate) after each movement, an indicator of good health. You can ask for a 'kick chart' to give an easy-to-read record of movements.

Oestriol Determination Series

The placenta provides a high amount of the hormone oestriol towards the end of pregnancy. Oestriol is excreted in the blood and urine, and the level can be determined by tests, the blood test being the most accurate. The oestriol level indirectly indicates whether the placenta is functioning properly or not. You must have several tests; just one isn't enough. A gradual or sudden drop may indicate a problem. Oestriol counts by themselves are never accurate enough to provide the basis for a decision to perform a caesarean section, though they are often used as a reason to induce.

Fetal Heart-rate Monitoring

This test may also be performed, based on the idea that when a healthy baby moves in the uterus, its heart-rate will speed up with each movement. The test takes twenty to forty minutes and is usually performed in a hospital maternity ward or wherever an external fetal monitor is available. The midwife determines fetal heart-rate by hooking you up to the fetal monitor as you lie on your left side or sit up. The baby either moves by itself or when you or your doctor push at it. The test is 'reactive' if fetal heart tones accelerate fifteen beats above baseline (120 to 160 beats a minute) twice or three times within twenty minutes. However, doctors don't all have the same standards as to what a normal response should be, or they may misinterpret their findings. Negative results – a 'non-reactive' baby – don't necessarily mean that the baby is in danger. This test is almost always performed before the contraction stress test.

Blood Flow Studies

Using ultrasound to monitor blood flowing through the placenta and baby's circulation is being done experimentally and may come into more general use.

Contraction Stress Test

Known as the oxytocin challenge test, or OCT, a small amount of syntocinon (synthetic oxytocin) is introduced via an intravenous drip. You lie on your left side or sit up, hooked up to an external fetal monitor. Contractions begin within twenty to forty minutes, and usually much sooner. You should have three moderate contractions within ten minutes, each lasting around forty-five seconds. The monitor records the fetal heart's response to each contraction.

The aim of this test is to determine your baby's condition by seeing how the placenta responds to the stress of a contraction. It is possible to stimulate contractions by the less invasive method of nipple stimulation. Rubbing your nipples releases a small amount of oxytocin which may be enough to stimulate contractions. You could ask to try this method before syntocinon is used but be prepared for some surprise from medical staff.

Once contractions begin the fetal heart tones are checked. The OCT has a high false-positive rate with results sometimes difficult to interpret and different observers giving different readings. Its risks lie in the fact that it is an unnatural intervention. It can lead to artificial induction of an entire labour, to caesareans and to hospital-caused (iatrogenic) prematurity – a baby simply may not be ready to be born.

NOTES

1. See Sir Douglas Black et al. *Inequalities in Health.*

2. K.M. Lawrence et al. 'The Increased Risk of Recurrence of NTDs to Mothers on Poor Diets and the Possible Benefits of Dietary Counselling', *British Medical Journal*, vol. 281, 1980, pp. 1592–3; K.M. Lawrence et al. 'The Role of Improvement in the Maternal Diet and Preconceptual Folic Acid Supplementation in the Prevention of NTDs', in J. Dobbing (ed.), *Prevention of Spina Bifida and Other Neural Defects*. London: Academic Press, 1983, pp. 85–110.

3. M.J.V. Bull. 'Pregnancy', *British Medical Journal*, vol. 284, 1982, p. 1162.

4. Jill Rakusen. 'In Pursuit of the Perfect Baby', WHRRIC Newssheet, 1982.

5. See D. Bryce Smith, letter to *The Lancet*, 7 December 1985.

6. Catherine Boyd and Lea Sellers. *The British Way of Birth*. London: Pan, 1982.

7. W. Doyle et al. 'Dietary Survey in Pregnancy in a Low Socio-economic Group', *Human Nutrition: Applied Nutrition*, no. 36A, 1982, pp. 95–106.

8. Gail Brewer and Tom Brewer. *What Every Pregnant Woman Should Know*. London: Penguin Books, 1977.

9. Sighthill Maternity Team, 'Community Care, the Way Forward', *Scottish Medicine*, April 1982.

10. A woman from Harrogate CHC quoted in Angela Phillips, *Your Body, Your Baby, Your Life*. London: Pandora, 1988.

11. Quoted in Jo Larbie. *Black Women and the Maternity Services*, Training in Health and Race, 1985 (available from the National Extension College, 18 Brookland Avenue, Cambridge CB2 2HN).

12. *Perinatal and Neonatal Mortality*, second report of Social Services Committee (the Short Report). London: HMSO, 1980.

13. See Society to Support Home Confinements, *Maternal Deaths and the Place of Confinement* (critique of DHSS report 1970–72) and *Opting for a Home Confinement*.

14. R.E.O. Williams et al. *Hospital Infection: Causes and Prevention*. London: Lloyd-Luke, 1966.

15. Marjorie Tew, 'The Case Against Hospital Deliveries: the Statistics', in Sheila Kitzinger and John A. Davies (eds), *The Place of Birth*. Oxford: Oxford Medical Publications, 1978.

16. Murphy et al. 'Planned and Unplanned Births at Home: Implications for Changing Ratios', *British Medical Journal*, 12 May 1984.

17. Rona Campbell et al. 'Perinatal Mortality According to Intended Place of Delivery', *British Medical Journal*, 22 September 1984.

18. S.M.I. Damstra-Wijmenga, 'Home Confinement: the Positive Results in Holland', *Journal of Royal College of General Practitioners*, August 1984.

19. Quoted in Kitzinger and Davies, op. cit., note 15.

20. Letter to the *Guardian*, 17 October 1975.

21. Quoted in survey in *Parents* magazine, November 1983.

22. Ibid.

23. Boyd and Sellers, op. cit., note 6.

24. Sue Lees, *New Society*, 25 April 1984.

25. Letter to Society to Support Home Confinements, 1975.

26. Association of Anaesthetists of Great Britain and Ireland. *Anaesthetic Services for Obstetrics – A Plan for the Future*, 1988.

27. Westbury and Bletchley Action Groups. *Maternity Care in Milton Keynes – the Case for an Alternative Proposal*. Submission to the Milton Keynes District Health Authority and District Management Team, February 1983.

28. Meridel Le Sueur. 'Anunciation' in *Ripening*. Old Westbury, NY: Feminist Press, 1982, p. 128.

29. Lennart Nillson. *A Child is Born*. London: Faber & Faber, 1977.

30. Boyd and Sellers, op. cit., note 6.

31. Dr Leon Chesley (author of the section on toxaemia in *Williams Obstetrics*, the most widely used ob/gyn textbook in the USA), quoted in Brewer and Brewer, op. cit., note 8.

32. Betsy C. Little. 'Treatment of Hypertension in Pregnancy by Relaxation and Biofeedback', *The Lancet*, 21 April 1984, pp. 865–7.

33. Quoted in Phillips, op. cit., note 10.

34. Brown and Harris quoted in Heather Hunt, 'Women with Young Children and Mental Health', unpublished paper, 1986.

35. Quoted in 'Self-insemination', Feminist Self-insemination Group.

36. Quoted in Phillips, op. cit., note 10.

37. See Ann Oakley. *The Captured Womb: a History of the Medical Care of Pregnant Women*. Oxford: Basil Blackwell, 1986.

38. Margaret McNay et al. *British Journal of Hospital Medicine*, 31 June 1984.

39. Bruno Brambati. 'Chorionic Villus Sampling – A Safe and Reliable Alternative in Fetal Diagnosis?', *Research in Reproduction*, vol. 19, no. 2, April 1987 (International Planned Parenthood Federation).

CHILDBIRTH

Rewritten by
ANGELA PHILLIPS

CREATING CONFIDENCE

For my first labour I was flat on my back for twenty hours with electronic monitors and drips. It terrified the life out of me. At the end everyone just filed out of the room without a word. I didn't want to go through it again but this time it's been different. I just cannot believe it. Seeing the same people each time, knowing that one of them will be there. It will be so much better with someone who cares about me.

One midwife told us: 'The midwife's best medical aid is the ability to inspire confidence in the woman's ability to give birth.' Sadly, women do not always find themselves giving birth in an atmosphere in which they are inspired by the confidence of those around them. It is an attempt to capture the atmosphere which leads to the kind of stressful battles with the authorities to which no pregnant woman should be subjected.

One woman fought her GP, two consultants and the local midwifery hierarchy until the 34th week of pregnancy in an attempt to get a straightforward midwife delivery for her twins. Her previous experience of a twin delivery with humiliating and unnecessary intervention and separation from her two healthy babies was not an experience she cared to endure again. It was finally an NCT contact who suggested another hospital in another town. She got what she wanted:

Everyone was laughing and joking. People popped in and out and said, 'Ooh, that twin delivery, can I watch?' and that was fine. I also consented to a fetal monitor which I hadn't wanted. It was the kind of atmosphere which made the difference. Nothing I wanted was considered odd. I needed no drugs and none were pushed on me. The babies were both delivered normally by a midwife. When

the paediatrician came to check them I was afraid he was going to take them away. He just said, 'Nobody wants them but you.' I was euphoric.

Few women have this degree of determination when they are pregnant. It is a time when we need to be supported, not opposed. It takes very little to crush the fragile self-confidence that we need in order to approach labour without fear:

I wanted to have my second baby at home. The doctors at my local health centre have decided that at thirty-six I am too old. Their guidelines end at thirty-five. Of course, if I insist, they will deliver me at home, but I don't want to insist. I want them on my side, not against me. I don't know what I am going to do now. I feel lost. Which will be worse: to go into a hospital (which I dread) or deliver at home feeling that if anything goes wrong I will be to blame?

For many women the atmosphere of home creates that confidence. The presence of familiar people and surroundings gives us a sense of control over our own labour which may be harder to achieve in the sterile and alien atmosphere of a hospital where pregnancy is seen as a disease, and rather a common one at that. Nevertheless, it is possible to create that climate of confidence even when hospital staff do not themselves inspire it.

But to feel confident, we must have a clear knowledge of what labour is, what interventions we can expect and how to decide for ourselves whether they are needed. We need also a companion who is clear about our needs and will argue for us when our minds are on the work we are doing in labour. For most of us, birth preparation classes will provide that knowledge. This chapter is not intended as a substitute for birth preparation but as a guide to it.

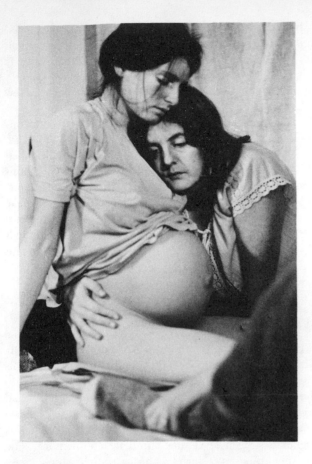

Suzanne Arms

SOME ATTITUDES WHICH CREATE AND SUSTAIN A CLIMATE OF DOUBT

Taking their own bodies as the norm, most doctors see women's bodies as abnormal. Influential obstetricians in this century have come up with some striking descriptions of labour and birth, among them Joseph B. DeLee who in 1920 compared labour to a crushing door and birth to falling on a pitchfork, the handle driving through the perineum:

> In both cases, the cause of the damage, the fall on the pitchfork and the crushing of the door, is pathogenic, that is disease provoking, and anything pathogenic is pathologic and abnormal.[1]

The well-known author of *Birth Without Violence*, Dr Frederick Leboyer, says:

> One day, the baby finds itself a prisoner . . . the prison comes to life . . . begins, like some octopus, to hug and crush . . . stifle . . . assault . . . the prison has gone beserk . . . with its heart bursting, the infant sinks into this hell . . . the mother . . . she is driving the baby out. At the same time she is holding it in, preventing its passage. It is she who is the enemy. She who stands between the child and life. Only one of them can prevail. It is mortal combat . . . not satisfied with crushing, the monster . . . twists it in a refinement of cruelty.[2]

The orthodoxy reflects an anxious view of birth . . . as a treacherous course mined with sudden, unexpected disasters requiring the medical equivalent of a military alert.[3]

These ideas and others less dramatic but equally negative underlie and shape many routine obstetric practices. The practices then reinforce our fears that our bodies won't work correctly and something will go wrong, cause new doubts, disrupt the physiology of labour, distort our experiences or completely prevent them from taking place normally. Attitudes themselves – our own and our doctors' – affect the course of labour – slowing it down, speeding it up – as much as any drug or mechanical intervention.*

Childbearing has always involved a perfectly natural fear of something going wrong, of the unknown, of pain and the risk of death. We can never be completely certain of the outcome wherever and however we have children. Medical attitudes and practices encourage, indeed thrive on, these fears. One mother says:

> It is as if our confidence is a large, bright piece of fabric. When little pinprick holes of fear and doubt appear, the medical mentality makes them larger and larger until the once beautiful cloth is nothing but gaping holes.

Doctors and, increasingly, midwives trained in medical schools and hospitals rarely see a normal spontaneous labour and birth. To many students, childbirth means a woman lying on her back during labour, her bag of waters broken artificially, labour 'accelerated', often hooked up to a fetal monitor, drugged or anaesthetized, given an episiotomy, with a possibility of forceps or perhaps a caesarean section.

As a result, they don't know how to relate to a fully-conscious, unanaesthetized woman. They don't sit through labour from beginning to end to learn how or what a woman feels, to become acquainted with the rhythm of her labour, the positions she chooses and the sounds she makes, to encourage her and simply to do nothing at times – 'mastering the art of inactivity', as one childbirth educator said.

> My first home birth . . . was also the first time I had ever been alone with a woman throughout her whole labor. It took hours. There were . . . no shifts, no system to shield me from how long having a baby really takes. I remember opening my obstetrics book, examining the course of labor charted on the page and feeling reassured, for the hours of labor were no longer than the hours of the curve.[4]

We also may have no one at all with us for periods of

*When we accept medical descriptions of what we should feel, do and take during labour and birth we allow our powers to be diminished and tamed.

time. *Few cultures leave labouring women so alone.* Midwives change shifts and the doctor, appearing briefly, or just at the end of labour, may be someone we have never seen before. When the baby is born, we often have a new set of midwives and doctors.

This terrible care distracts us, causes insecurity and confusion at a time when we should be relaxing, comfortable, concentrating on ourselves and our babies.

Isolation and immobility during labour increase pain, which increases tension and fear, which brings on more pain. In such surroundings, women end up 'needing' pain relief, and obstetricians, anaesthetists, researchers and drug companies hasten to provide it in abundant variety.

Many doctors learn to manipulate us into accepting and submitting to interventions 'for our own good' and 'for the safety of the baby', strongly suggesting that if we don't agree to undergo certain procedures we do not care about the baby. They also learn that unless they use or have close at hand every available tool and instrument, they may be sued at some point in their future career. Drugs and intervention used routinely in the name of safety become instruments of control and debilitation.

After such training it is no wonder that doctors genuinely believe that we cannot and should not give birth without medical intervention and hospital assistance. Sadly, midwives trained in hospitals learn to defer to doctors. They have learned to doubt their own skills and rely on machines rather than hands, eyes and ears. Midwifery skills, such as delivering without episiotomy, are fading as a generation of midwives, with no memory of independent practice, comes out of training. Attempts by radical midwives to halt this drift into obstetric nursing are keeping skills alive and the Association of Radical Midwives and MIDIRS (Midwives' Information and Resource Service) provide the means to inform and support midwives who want genuinely to be practitioners in their own right, working with women.

THE NORMAL PROCESS OF LABOUR*

Your body prepares for labour. During labour, uterine muscles gradually stretch the cervix open for the baby to come out, and the muscles also push the baby down into the vagina so it can be born.

Throughout your pregnancy you have been having contractions regularly – called Braxton-Hicks contractions – as uterine muscles tighten, then loosen, exercising the uterus and preparing it to work efficiently during labour. Towards the end of pregnancy you may feel these contractions pulling and stretching more intensely and frequently; occasionally they are uncomfortable. Your cervix is softening, ripening.

*The vast majority of labours could progress as we describe but interventions, necessary in some cases, alter the pattern for a very large number of women.

Both effacement (thinning and drawing up of the cervix) and dilatation (opening of the cervix) can occur before you *feel* your labour beginning. Some women remain slightly dilated for weeks before labour begins. Others go into labour *before* dilatation starts and have their babies a few hours later!

When you feel contractions stronger than Braxton-Hicks, more like menstrual cramps, you may think you are beginning early labour (and sometimes you are!). Called 'false labour' by the medical profession, these contractions are another form of preliminary labour and play an important role in initial dilatation and effacement. They make your cervix contract and relax rather than contract and pull back. These contractions usually stop after a while, though they can last for hours. When you feel them, get up and walk around, and see if they continue or if the intervals between contractions become longer or shorter.

WHAT CAUSES LABOUR?

We know a lot about labour, but we don't know exactly what sets it off. It may be that when the fetus matures, its own glandular system sends out hormonal messages into the woman's bloodstream, altering maternal hormonal levels. As a result, the woman's pituitary gland secretes the hormone oxytocin, which causes the uterus to contract. A higher oestrogen level may stimulate contractions. The uterine lining may secrete prostaglandins which cause secretion of oxytocin. And the baby's head pressing on cervical nerve endings may help initiate labour. Our emotional state as well as physical position can also affect labour, stopping or slowing it down if we feel afraid and tense, speeding it up when we relax.

SOME FIRST SIGNS OF LABOUR

Some body-signals let you know that you are about to go into labour. Your Braxton-Hicks contractions may become more intense and frequent. You may have diarrhoea for a few days or on the day labour begins, your body's way of emptying itself so that labour is less obstructed. You may feel an extraordinary burst of energy and want to cook, clean, organize – a kind of nesting instinct. You may suddenly want to do nothing.

The Show

As your cervix begins to stretch open, the small mucus plug which seals it comes out, not usually in one piece but as pink mucus, 'bloody show', blood-tinged from broken capillaries in the cervix. Many women never have a 'show'. Others have it all through early and active labour.

Waters Breaking

As your baby's head presses down against the membranes containing amniotic fluid, they may break. (Most often they break when you have been in active labour for a while. Rarely, they remain intact until after the baby is born.)

Your 'waters' may rush out or, more commonly, just trickle out, usually clear and odourless, or milky. Some women think they are wetting their pants. Check colour and smell. If you can't stop it by holding it back, it is probably amniotic fluid. *No matter how much fluid comes out, your body replaces it every few hours. There is no such thing as a 'dry birth'.* After your membranes break, labour will probably begin within a few hours, though some women trickle for a few days or even weeks. Doctors disagree about what should be done after your waters break. Most say that you should come to the hospital to prevent infection. Some of them routinely induce labour after twelve to twenty-four hours if you haven't started on your own. Others tell you to relax, that labour will begin soon.

Even if you are planning to give birth in the hospital, consider staying at home; there's usually *less* chance of your getting an infection at home in your customary environment. *Don't* take baths, put anything into your vagina (no internal pelvic exams) or have sexual intercourse. Stay clean. Drink a lot of fluids. Take your temperature regularly, twice a day or more. After twenty-four hours, another thing you could ask for is a white-blood-cell count to make sure there's no infection. Your midwife or doctor may want to check your baby's heartbeat periodically.

If your waters break *suddenly*, contact the labour ward or your doctor or midwife. You should be checked to ensure that the baby's head fits right into your cervix so that the umbilical cord isn't swept through your cervix (which happens sometimes if the baby is in breech position or presenting 'high'). A cord prolapse could endanger your baby's life. Once you are sure the head is fully engaged you can stay at home or return there until labour starts. Also, if you notice any brown or green staining, let your practitioner know, as it means that meconium (the tarry substance in your baby's bowels) has been squeezed out – common but occasionally an indication of fetal stress or distress.

Contractions (one of the most common signs of labour)

Your uterus will begin to contract regularly and/or strongly after a while. At first it may feel like wind, menstrual cramps, backache, a pulling and stretching in your pubic region. In early labour, contractions may be as regular as clockwork – perhaps ten minutes apart – or they may be irregular, inconsistent, widely spaced. (For some women they remain irregular or widely spaced all during labour.) If you begin labour during the daytime, go about your daily routine, especially if this is your first baby, when labours usually take longer. More often, labour begins at night when you are relaxed. It's a good idea to get some more sleep if you can.

At five a.m. I felt period cramps, was really excited. They weren't particularly painful. I knew something was happening! I waited for other signs.

LESS USUAL PRESENTATIONS

In our description of labour, we have assumed the baby's position in the uterus to be the most common – *left occipito anterior* (LOA). This means that the baby is head down in the uterus, lying on its left side, with the occiput, or back part of the skull, towards the mother's front. It is the most effective way for a baby to slip past the pubic bone and into the birth canal.

Another position is head first but faced the opposite way, with the baby's face towards the mother's front. This is called *posterior presentation*. It can mean a longer labour, since the baby usually turns around during labour in order to be born in the more favourable way, facing the mother's back. With a posterior baby, you may experience labour pains in your back. Feel free to take labour positions most comfortable for you – often on 'all fours'.

Some babies present buttocks down or feet (footling) first. They are in the *breech* position, which can mean a long back-labour. Sometimes you can turn a breech baby around yourself from the 30th week of pregnancy on (see p. 365). They may turn themselves during labour or may not turn at all. A *skilled obstetrician may be able to turn them from the outside (external cephalic version).[5] If your pelvis is big enough and the baby small enough, you'll be able to deliver her/him vaginally. In the UK, breech deliveries are usually done with the mother's feet up in stirrups. Forceps are common. If you can find an obstetrician prepared to deliver this way, *squat: it widens your pelvic outlet significantly!* A danger in breech births is that after the body is delivered the head will be trapped, and the baby will try to breathe and will suffocate. Knowledgeable midwives and obstetricians wrap the baby's emerging body in warm blankets to keep cold air from shocking her/him into taking a breathful of mucus; they also insert a finger into the woman's vagina, clearing a passageway for air. Footling breeches are usually delivered by caesarean (unless they are the second of twins, when the cervix has opened wide enough). These days obstetricians in training rarely learn the necessary skills to perform external cephalic versions or to help deliver breech babies vaginally; they perform caesareans instead which carry more risk to the mother and can have implications for the baby too (see p. 394).

Some babies lie horizontally (*transverse lie*) or present shoulder first, and their heads never engage. They must be born by caesarean.

Had 'bloody show'. Beryl examined me. I was fully effaced and not dilated at all. We thought about what we wanted to do with the day. I baked a birthday cake, we took naps, had a quiet day together. I ate lightly all day, had spaghetti for dinner. We went to sleep; I woke up at eleven-thirty p.m. truly in labour.

Some women know when they are about to go into labour, and some can make it happen.

My body felt different the night before, as if I'd become lighter and the baby had shifted position.

I went into labour with my second child very consciously because I needed to. I don't believe in trying to control a process like labour, but it was wonderful to know I could invite it/allow it to start. My blood pressure had been climbing the last weeks of the pregnancy because of overwork and extreme stress. The midwife said to me firmly, 'Just have the baby,' so I went home to try. I thought about it, we made love, I let go of the reasons why it wasn't a good day, and in two hours my waters broke with mild contractions starting up soon.

I know a midwife who covers the delivery service for only twelve hours a week at a large city hospital. She has delivered four babies for this one woman with whom she has a deep rapport. The woman has managed to time all four labours to fit into the midwife's twelve-hour segments, which shift around from week to week.

EARLY LABOUR

In early labour, walking around, taking long walks, taking long baths or making love if your waters haven't broken, orgasm without intercourse if your waters have broken, showering, hugging, kissing, stroking your nipples or hav-

ing them sucked all can stimulate your contractions and relax you.

When we went for a walk it was fun running into friends: 'What are you doing up? I thought you were in labour.' It was fun changing people's image of a woman in labour.

We went to the cinema because our flat was small, and it was too cold out to take a walk. I don't remember much of the film.

We made love while I was in labour. We went to bed and had a wonderful time. I was happy to be giving – to him and to myself – and not just concentrating on contractions.

When you rest or go to bed, the baby's head no longer presses on your cervix, and contractions may slow down. Alternate moving around with brief naps. Stay rested.

Some women prefer to stay at home until contractions become frequent and strong. *The longer you stay out of the hospital, the less likely you are to have your labour intervened in.* Others prefer to go and settle in before contractions become so strong that walking and riding in a car are uncomfortable. (Afterwards, some wish they had never gone to the hospital, others that they had left home sooner.)

ESTABLISHED LABOUR

When labour really gets going, contractions are strong and rhythmic. You feel them building like a wave, pulling and tightening first in one place, then expanding throughout your uterus, into your back or groin, and then lessening. In between you can rest, sleep, stay still, walk, talk. *Make sure to empty your bladder regularly.* Relaxing deeply *between* contractions gives you energy for each new one. Relaxing deeply *during* them helps reduce pain sensation.

Contractions when most intense felt like a belt around my lower back and abdomen. Most of the feeling was in my lower back. Contractions had a curve: strong at the beginning and then slowing down. You get to know them. What surprised me was that you're in two worlds. You have to concentrate on them when they happen, but when they stop, you're just regular. I've never felt so lucid, so clear, as in between contractions.

Language was really important, and I didn't like the word 'contraction' . . . I found when I was having my babies that if I thought 'contraction' it meant making something tight. It's true the uterine muscles are contracting, but if everything's working right, at the same time the cervix is expanding. It's much more helpful to think of the expansion.[6]

You adapt to labour. The hardest part comes early sometimes. Then you accept that it's really

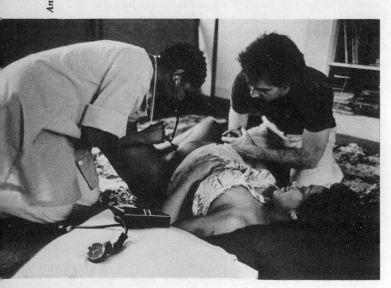

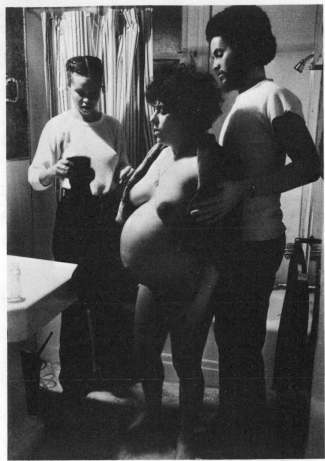

Suzanne Arms

happening, it's a baby, it hurts – no abstractions. Later it can get easier, though contractions may be much *stronger.*

You may feel exhilarated during labour, mellow and peaceful between contractions, especially when your labour is progressing naturally and uninterruptedly. Some researchers now believe that when you are relaxed, your body produces its own substances for pain relief, called *endorphins*, which have a morphine-like effect. (High levels have been found in the placentas of animals and humans after birth.[7]) Tension and fear may inhibit the secretion of endorphins, causing you to secrete adrenalin instead, which tenses you up, slows your labour and makes it more painful. If labour is painful, don't blame yourself. Deep relaxation can be difficult, even in an ideal environment.

There is a lot else going on besides the pain in the belly . . . I saw the colors in the kitchen getting brighter and stronger. I'm not into mystical things, or thinking about auras, but yes, labor is a kind of high if you flow with it, and a room full of loving people does produce energy . . . gives you strength.[8]

Keep changing position if you feel able to (your partner can help). If you can be reasonably upright, or on hands and knees during contractions, you allow gravity to help

you (see box). Over the last ten years, British midwives and birth educators have started to relearn lessons from other cultures and encourage women to get off their backs while giving birth; lessons which may have been learned sooner if they had listened to the women in our midst who have given birth in other ways.

Long before the hospital introduced its birthing room for local active birthers, I talked to a woman having her fourth baby. She had given birth to the first three in India and was outraged when the staff strapped a monitor around her and made her lie down. She knew that you cannot give birth like

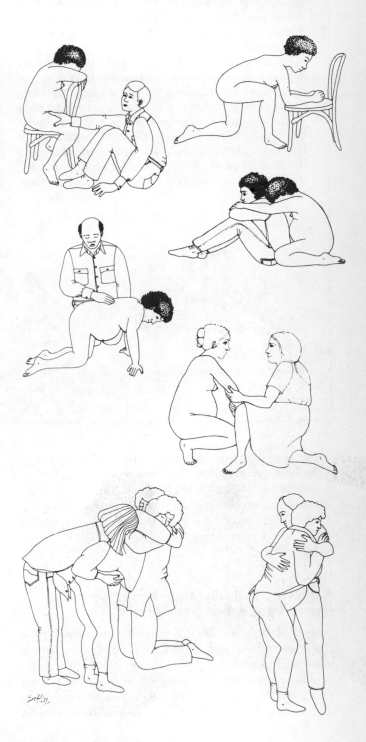

POSITIONS FOR LABOUR AND DELIVERY

According to a *Parents* Magazine survey (November 1983), 50 per cent of British women were unable to move around in labour. Lying flat on your back (in the 'dorsal', 'supine' or 'lithotomy' position) is neither the most efficient nor the most comfortable position, and it is quite possibly the most dangerous one. There is much evidence that the supine position not only produces more pain, but that it also leads to slower labours and more maternal and fetal distress. Fetal distress can be caused by the uterus pressing on the major sources of blood to and from the uterus, thus cutting off the oxygen supply. Furthermore, if we are lying flat, gravity cannot help us push the baby out.

Paediatrician Peter Dunn wrote in 1976 that less efficient uterine contractions when the woman is lying down have been a 'clinically recognized fact for hundreds of years'. He went on to report how a study in Spain compared the effect of the supine position with the standing position, each woman alternating her posture every half hour throughout the first stage of labour. The effectiveness of contractions in dilating the cervix was *doubled* in the standing position and it was also much less uncomfortable and painful.[9]

The best ways of giving birth were well known long ago:

> A vast and important fund of knowledge may be derived from a study of the various positions occupied by women of different peoples in their labours . . . According to their build, to the shape of their pelvis, they stand, squat, kneel, or lie on their belly [see illustrations]; so also they vary their position in various stages of labour according to the position of the child's head in the pelvis.[10]

Modern obstetric practices have invaded most societies but, in a few, traditional methods of giving birth are still used. In Yucatan, for example, a woman may give birth in a hammock:

> The pregnant woman is suspended in space, accessible from all sides; she can be held, supported, touched, rubbed – whatever her needs are at the moment.[11]

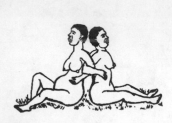

A Madi woman of Central Africa supported by another woman while delivering

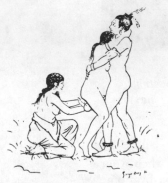

Delivery of an Iroquois Indian

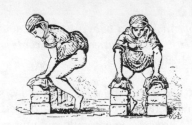

Obstetric positions of the Persians

that and finally found the strength, in spite of the hostility and amazement of those around her, to get the belt off, get off the bed and deliver, squatting, on the floor. At the time her knowledge of the birth process was not valued at all. Now it has been endorsed by white women and incorporated.

Achieving Full Dilatation and Effacement (sometimes called transition)

A range of signs indicates that your uterus is coming to the end of stretching and opening fully. You may have a powerful 'opening up' feeling, contractions may come rapidly or be more intense than before. The more relaxed you are at this time, the better you'll feel. You may need others especially now to help you breathe deeply and focus your energies, to hold you, encourage you.

You may be very vocal during contractions, and doze or be very still in between. Or you may be inward and concentrated throughout. Many women choose one particular position at this time – kneeling, on hands and knees, on their side in bed. This time has been associated with nausea, shaking, trembling of thighs and legs, chills and irritability, though these things can happen at other times, too. Some women are comforted by the incredible intensity, even by their own irritability, because they know it means that they are close to the end of this part of labour.

When you reach full dilatation labour often slows down, with contractions farther apart for a while, as if your body were taking a rest. Or contractions may come so close together they feel like one long one. Or you may scarcely have time to take a breath before your enormous uncontrollable 'pushing' contractions begin.

LABOUR

During each contraction your upper uterine muscles pull the cervical muscles upward ('thinning', 'taking up', effacement) and pull open the muscles around the cervix (dilatation). Effacement is often measured by percentage (50 per cent, 80 per cent effaced) and dilatation in centimetres or fingers (two centimetres equal one finger). When you've dilated ten centimetres, or five fingers, your baby is ready to be born, and then the uterus can push her/him through your vagina and out of your body. A while later your uterus contracts a few more times to expel both placenta and membranes (the transparent bag which contained your baby and the protective amniotic fluid).

Medical tradition divides labour into three stages:
1. the time it takes to become fully effaced and dilated,
2. pushing the baby out,
3. expelling the placenta.

Many doctors and midwives and hospital personnel set strict time limits in which they expect each of these stages to take place. These limits vary from one practitioner and place to another. Some hospitals use a graph of the average process of labour and accelerate if labour deviates from this 'norm'. Most doctors don't like 'second-stage' labour to last more than one or two hours.*

Some midwives say there are only two stages: before the baby is born and afterwards. A practitioner skilled in normal labour knows that each labour has its own rhythm and takes its own time. S/he will not set arbitrary limits for the length of each phase but will decide whether labour needs to be helped along at a certain point. S/he also knows that these medically defined stages refer only to the relation of the baby to the woman's body, and not at all to labour as the woman experiences it. Some first stages can last up to forty hours with a one-hour second stage, or last two hours with a four-hour second stage. Other midwives and childbirth educators refer to the end of the first stage as 'transition'.

All practitioners agree that the placenta must come out within a reasonable time (see p. 386).

*Often this is because if you have received anaesthesia, it has a depressant effect on the baby.

CERVICAL DILATION IN CENTIMETRES
Shown actual size

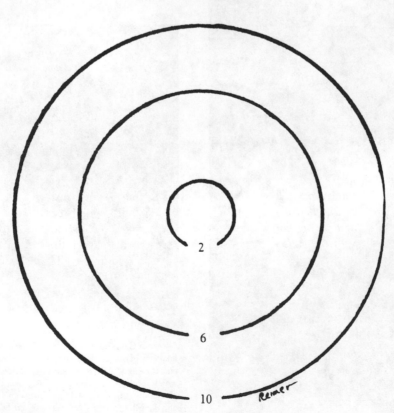

2

6

10

Nina Reimer

The Baby Moves Down through Your Vagina

You may suddenly feel an amazing urge to bear down. Breathe lightly or blow if your attendant says that you are not completely dilated. Many women are disappointed when this phase turns out to be more painful or longer than they expected. Others, who expect the expulsion to be the most painful part, are surprised by how exhilarating and painless it can be to push out a baby. A few women never feel that strong urge to push.

Women are often taught to practise pushing by taking huge, deep breaths, holding them and bearing down as hard as they can. Yet strenuous active pushing doesn't necessarily get the baby out faster.[12] In fact it can lead to the baby's being deprived of oxygen.[13]

Your uterus contracts involuntarily and will push the baby out itself most of the time if not interfered with. *Feel it* pushing and bear down only when you feel the urge. Don't close your throat unless your body wants to. (Breathe deeply or sigh between contractions.) You may want to grunt, moan, howl or simply 'breathe' the baby out.

Today many physicians emphasize having a short second stage (typically two hours or less) without evidence to prove that a longer one hurts the baby.* This phase of labour can, in fact, take a few minutes or five hours, as long as the baby's heartbeat is fine. When you relax between contractions and don't push hard, you don't get as tired as you would if you were pushing. Your perineum has more time to stretch around the baby's head as it moves down during the contraction, then back a little, down during the next, then back again. (Don't be disappointed if the process takes a long time; many women think it only takes a couple of pushes and wonder what is wrong if it takes longer.) Sometimes you will be asked to breathe lightly so as not to be pushing at all as the midwife guards the perineum to ease the baby out. Gentle pushing means fewer or no perineal tears. During contractions, let your belly bulge out; relax your whole body, especially your mouth and jaws. Consciously direct your energy downward, outward.

I was holding back. This thought raced into my mind and out the other side: If I push hard enough, I'm going to become a mother. Ann said, 'Next time you have a contraction, push a little bit; think open; *you'll feel better.' Amazing – I could feel her coming down; it did feel better.*

You can be in any position to let the baby come out, but upright ones often work best. When you are on hands and knees or squatting with knees apart, your pelvis is at its widest. You may feel most comfortable kneeling or on the toilet at first, then go to kneel on the bed or sit, or lie on your side with one leg up on an attendant's shoulder.

Pushing was the strangest and in some ways the nicest sensation I've ever had. I could actually feel the shape of the baby, feel myself sitting on the head as it moved

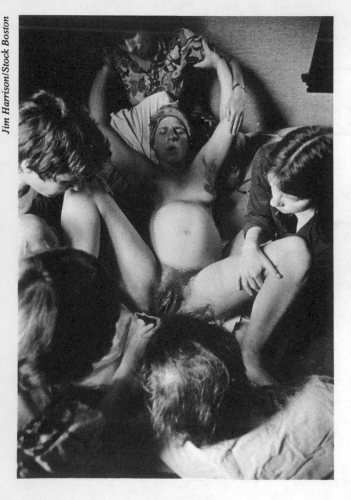

Jim Harrison/Stock Boston

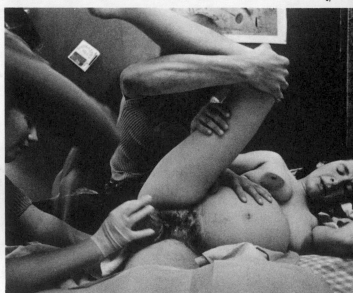

Suzanne Arms

*Roberto Caldeyro-Barcia, a well-known South American ob/gyn, says that fetal lack of oxygen (hypoxia) has been a 'reason' to push the baby out quickly and thus have a short second stage, when in fact it's the sustained pushing which can cause hypoxia in the first place. Physicians often feel hysteria at the idea of the baby 'trapped' in the 'birth canal' and rush to pull it out. Midwives also contribute to the rushed atmosphere by calling doctors in too soon. Since they're all there they say, 'Let's get her delivered', especially when they are very busy.

WHAT YOU CAN DO

Plan ahead to ensure that your companions and medical attendants know what you want. Then you can concentrate on yourself with confidence.

Choose people you feel comfortable with. It is important that the presence of others, their touch, advice and actions give you comfort and strength and make you happy and confident, and that they feel comfortable with you.

> *The pain was like a hurricane shaking me apart. I yelled a lot and walked around and took showers. I remember looking at Paul and thinking, What are you so happy about? This is terrible. Yet I know that the grin on his face sustained me. I needed his touch and his joy, and I needed – very differently – the midwife's words and knowledge and reassurance.*

Choose people who can understand what you want and don't want without having their feelings hurt. Too many and/or the wrong people (sometimes even your partner) can hinder labour by being too solicitous, too anxious, too noisy, too bossy.

Choose comfortable surroundings. When you feel comfortable and safe, with familiar people around you, you are better able to relax. Women give birth at home to be in familiar territory where they are free to be themselves. If you go to the hospital, bring 'home' along with you – favourite clothes, photographs, pictures, beloved objects, a rug or blanket, records or tapes for music.

Breathe deeply. Whether or not you've practised breathing beforehand, deep breathing can help you to relax. Imagine your breath carrying oxygen to every part of your body. Breathe in whatever way is comfortable. Loosen your jaw. Open your mouth and throat. Smile. Laugh. But beware of over-breathing which can make you feel dizzy and numb. It's easy to cure, just cup your hands over your nose and mouth for a couple of breaths.

> *I found my own way of breathing. I knew I had to relax into the tenseness.*

Some women may use the breathing they've practised and become too controlled, too tense. Combine breathing with different positions, with sounds.

> *I was with a woman doing rigid strong labour breathing she had learned in a childbirth class. She was tight, exhausted. I said, 'You don't have to do that.' 'What will I do?' 'Just see what happens.' She began to relax. When she let go trying to keep her control, her energy started to flow. Over the next few hours she started doing little sighs which became moans at the end. On the floor, kneeling, she breathed into her husband's lap and rocked her pelvis. He started to breathe and rock with her.*

Change position and move around. Positions in which your spine is upright, as when you are walking or rocking, can help you relax, alleviate pain and make contractions work more effectively. Being on hands and knees also helps, especially when you have back labour. You can rock back and forth, dance slowly and rhythmically and move in ways you'd never dream you'd move! Many women find sitting on the toilet most comfortable.

Eat and drink. When you drink and eat – light foods at the beginning of labour, tea with honey, ice cubes (avoid acidic juices) as it becomes more intense – you keep up your strength and blood sugar level. You don't become dehydrated and you are better able to handle contractions. Drink, and remember to pee often.

> Birth is a time of great energy: no one would be expected to run a marathon or swim the English channel if she had been deprived of sustenance and was unable to continue to nourish herself from time to time.[15]

Express emotion if you want. Some women don't want or need to make noise, but many find that expressing strong emotions of the moment – anger, exaltation, fear, pain – groaning, grunting, shouting, moaning, laughing, singing, chanting – can loosen them up. During second-stage labour as you breathe or push the baby out you'll probably be making sounds along with the pushing. Low sounds seem to work better than high-pitched ones – more of a *downward* feel to them, say some midwives.

Experiment with water. Baths and showers can relax and soothe us during labour. Some women stay in the shower for hours. (When your waters have broken, avoid baths.) When tub water is shallow, someone can pour warm water over your belly during contractions. (A midwife we know says, 'It's better than syntocinon for getting contractions going!') When the water is deep, your uterus will be lifted up and away from your body, which can reduce the intensity of labour, especially back labour. Lying mostly under water, leaning against supports, you can float slightly and relax deeply.

Ask for physical support, touch, massage and holding. Ask your partner, friend, birth attendant or nurse to help you when you squat, stand or kneel; to lean against you; hold you under your arms; let you hang from his/her shoulders; hold you however you want to be held.

'Drink in' touch and massage. Human contact can make you feel at ease, sustained and loved. Your partner or attendant may know exactly what to do without being asked. Or s/he may not. If the touch doesn't feel right, ask until something feels better.

continues overleaf

This kind of caring enables you to relax and makes pain more bearable.

I asked my two friends to massage deeply and hard, putting a lot of pressure on my lower back muscles to counter all that force. I liked feeling their hands supporting my belly at the same time.

Actively imagine opening up. In South India, birth attendants place a flower near the labouring woman; as its petals unfold, her cervix opens. Opening is a ceremony, a celebration.

Imagine being in a place you love the best, where you are most happy. Imagine you are a flower opening, light exploding. Open your mind to images. Imagine your baby hugged by your uterus, pushing down, ready to be born in its own way, opening you. Say to yourself, 'I feel my baby moving down my pelvis, I feel my muscles letting go; my cervix is stretching, opening, opening MORE – open . . . open . . . OPEN.'

Suggestions for people attending a birth: what they can do. Look at her. Does she look comfortable?

Check her breathing. Is she relaxed? Say, 'Relax'. Use your hands. Run them down her back, over her muscles. Stroke or massage her in a way that helps her relax more. Move slowly, breathe slowly, stay calm. As you touch her, think of what your hands are communicating. Don't expect her to be stoic. Don't expect her to tell you politely what she wants. Sometimes she may not want you to touch her at all. If she tells you to go away, don't take it personally. It's just labour. Don't feel sorry for her. Yes, it hurts, but show your belief in her strength. Or she may say, 'I can't stand this any more.' Tell her she can. She is. Change what's happening. Make it better. Maybe a walk, a shower, a bath, a change of position will make her feel better. Keep her focused on the present. If she is losing her concentration, help her focus. Hold her, sing, chant, laugh, moan, rock with her. Just before the baby is born, at the most intense time, she may need touch, eye contact. Breathe along with her. Hold hot compresses against her perineum; she can relax into the heat. Or let her lean against/on you.*

*Thanks to Becky Sarah.

---

down . . . the thought of moving, especially from a good, comfortable, well-supported seated position, to flat-out on a bed seemed ridiculous. So there I was on my rocking chair, with my feet up on two little kitchen chairs, with Hersch on one side and the doctor on the other . . . it was like moving a grand piano across a room: that hard, but that satisfying.[14]

BIRTH

Your baby's head will be born first, unless the baby is in breech position (see p. 377). You must usually wait for the baby to rotate a quarter-turn in order for the rest of it to be born – shoulders, one at a time, then body. During this time your midwife may ask you to pant and not push as s/he checks to see if the cord is around your baby's neck and perhaps also to suction mucus from its nose and mouth if this is necessary (it should not be done routinely).

Within a few minutes, the baby was coming. I knelt on the bed, leaning forward against Thomas. It was a wonderful position, very solid and stable, yet my hands were free to reach down and feel her head. My older daughter was ready with a blanket to wrap the baby, and I will never forget the feeling of the little body sliding out and into my hands just as the sun came up. It's a great moment – the baby is there, it doesn't hurt any more, both in the same instant. The room was full of light.

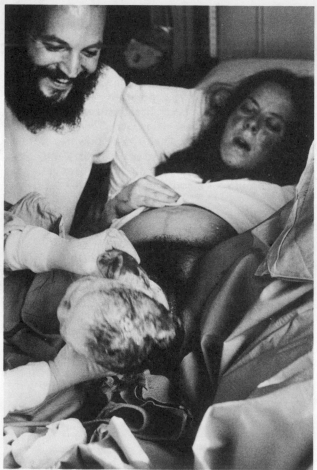

Vaughn Sills

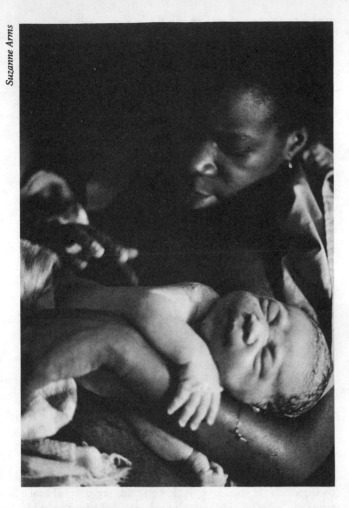

Suzanne Arms

*I was shouting, 'That's enough, that's enough.'
'My haemorrhoids hurt,' I was blubbering. Marya
said, 'Run some water; take a bath.' It felt good to
have all that water sloshing around. Nothing was
happening on the bed; it seemed so much easier in
the water. Everything I needed was there at the
time. I said, 'I feel kind of open!' Then I saw my
son float out. It was great. He was so peaceful and
calm. His eyes were open under the water.*

*I felt godlike – a miracle worker. It was the best
moment of my life. I felt my baby's head, then saw
his face – I got to cut his cord and put him to my
breast. I felt like I did the impossible. I couldn't
believe he was finally out into the light. I felt holy.*

RIGHT AFTER*

If your baby breathes as soon as the head is completely out,
s/he may be born looking pink or brown. Otherwise s/he
will look very still and bluish until breathing becomes
regular and sustained. Black babies are usually very light
coloured at birth. The full colour may not come in for a few

days. Not all newborns cry. Some cry for a moment, then
stop. They may just breathe, blink and look around or
snuffle.

After the birth, hold your baby close. S/he's your own;
you have waited all this time and laboured hard. At home
and in most hospitals you can hold your baby right away. It
can be easier to hold your baby when you are sitting up.
Cover her/him with blankets for warmth and hold her/him
naked against your breasts and belly in order that s/he may
touch your skin, smell you, feel you, hear you, look at you
and your partner. You'll want to caress, touch, talk to her/
him. Enjoy this slow time. If you are exhausted, your
partner can hold the baby against you or close to him/
herself. (In some cultures, babies are always cleaned before
being handed to their mother. If this custom is important to
you, ask the midwives to make a note of it in advance.)

So much has been written about this moment. We want
hospitals to respect how crucial it is for us, our partners and
children to be close to our babies. Most babies have the
capacity to form a strong attachment to another human
being after birth. Yet this process, called 'bonding', cannot
be forced or created just by going through the motions. As
Sheila Kitzinger said in one of her talks, 'Some hospitals act
as if it's a special glue that can be sprayed on and will take in
five minutes. After that they think it's too late.' One mother
fighting separation from her baby was told, 'You're bonded
to her now, so what's the problem?'

And if for some reason the first moments after birth don't
turn out the way you want, you will have many ways of
becoming attached to your baby and her/him to you.
'Bonding' in humans is an ongoing process.

Right after the birth, midwives evaluate your baby's
heart-rate, respiration, muscle tone, colour and reflexes.
Their conclusions are expressed in the one- and five-
minute Apgar score (from one to ten). Most infants score
between seven and ten. Your practitioner will have oxygen
and suctioning equipment at hand in case the baby needs
help with breathing, which is vital since lack of oxygen can
cause brain damage. Gentle suctioning of the nose and
throat is done if needed. It must always be carefully done to
prevent injury to delicate tissues. The baby will be wet-
looking, may be covered with a waxy substance called
vernix and usually is not very bloody. Her/his head may be
oddly shaped temporarily, having been moulded during its
passage through your vagina.

Your baby may or may not suck straight away.* Some
do, and know exactly what to do. (They have been sucking
in utero.) Others aren't quite ready yet or need a little
guidance. Babies born to unsedated and/or unanaesthetized mothers often have strong sucking reflexes. This is

*This section is about births with a happy outcome. Sadly, not every labour
ends this way. See Chapter 21.

*When you have received drugs, your baby may not want to suck or be able to
until the drugs wear off. In some cultures the colostrum is not offered to the
baby at all and feeding is delayed until the milk comes in.

a good time to let your baby suckle even if you don't plan to breastfeed later. Babies need to breastfeed in order to receive important antibodies and nutrients from your colostrum. If the baby doesn't seem to want to suckle right away, offer the breast as often as you can and encourage, but don't force him/her. It will come. If hospital staff object, remember that *you are in charge.* Sucking is important for you, too. It stimulates oxytocin, which makes your uterus contract to expel the placenta and stay contracted afterwards. It also slows down the bleeding.

You are still connected to your baby by the umbilical cord, attached to the placenta inside you. The cord will usually be cut as soon as the baby breathes or cries; some midwives wait five or ten minutes until the cord has stopped pulsating and all the blood has gone out of it into the baby. This enables the baby's circulatory system to get going on its own and provides extra blood supply, including iron. However, in most hospitals the drug syntometrine (see below) is given by injection during the birth. It is not wise to leave the cord pulsating in this case because too much blood may be pushed through it. The cord is clamped in two places and cut between the clamps a few inches from the navel. Sometimes partners cut the cord. In a week or so, the bit of cord left on the baby's navel dries up and falls off.

DELIVERY OF THE PLACENTA

After a short interval the cord lengthens, you may feel a contraction, have a rush of blood and expel the placenta. You may not feel a contraction and be told to push. Contractions usually come sooner when you are sitting up or squatting. It is extremely important to expel the placenta completely, which completes the birth cycle.

Until this happens, blood vessels remain open and women are especially vulnerable to infection and haemorrhage. Once the entire placenta is born, blood vessels close down. The pregnancy cycle reverses itself; your uterus clamps down and begins to shrink. Breastfeeding helps this process. Expulsion of the placenta usually happens within ten minutes to a half-hour or so; sometimes it takes longer. If all else is normal, it's reasonable to wait, watchfully. Usually the placenta comes out by itself, helped along by your baby suckling. In Britain the process is usually speeded up by the use of syntometrine. The midwife then delivers the placenta by pulling very gently on the cord (Controlled Cord Traction). If syntometrine is given, CCT is necessary or the uterus could clamp shut before the placenta is delivered. The aim of this is to prevent postpartum haemorrhage. You may prefer to wait and deliver the placenta without drugs or CCT, knowing that it can be given if heavy bleeding occurs or the delivery is delayed. If you are at home and have problems at this point, you may have to go to the hospital to have the placenta removed.

THE FIRST FEW HOURS AFTER THE BABY IS BORN

MOTHER AND BABY

It is best if your baby stays with you for as long as you want after birth. At home parents and child sleep and wake together, get to know each other, and the baby sucks whenever s/he wants. In over 50 per cent of hospitals mother and baby stay together. (It is important to check this in advance.)

There is no medical reason to separate healthy mothers and babies after birth. It is your right to keep your baby with you. Babies with minor and even major health problems benefit from being close to their parents; they also may need medical observation at the same time. A midwife or doctor will do a complete physical examination of your baby. It is not necessary that they do it right away (unless there is an obvious problem). In the hospital ask to have it done in your presence so that you can see exactly what is happening, and ask any questions you may have.

Babies born in hospitals may receive Vitamin K after birth to prevent a rare (one in 2,000) disorder known as haemorrhagic disease of the newborn (when the blood doesn't have enough clotting factor). In out-of-hospital births, Vitamin K may or may not be given. If it has been a traumatic birth with excessive head-moulding, Vitamin K is necessary. You can give Vitamin K orally to the baby, or by injection. If you have sickle cell trait (see p. 343) make sure your baby has a blood test to check for the trait or sickle cell disease.

WHERE YOU ARE AFTER YOU GIVE BIRTH AFFECTS HOW YOU FEEL

The comfort of being at home cannot be overestimated, being in my own bed afterwards, familiar cracks in the ceiling, my family all around.

After a normal delivery in a hospital, a first-time mother usually stays between two and five days. Expenditure cuts mean that many women are being sent home before they feel ready. Experienced mothers stay between six and forty-eight hours. You can leave earlier (or later) if you want to.

We had planned a home birth, but because of an unexpectedly long labour, wound up delivering in the hospital instead. Our disappointment, however, was tempered by our doctor's promise that if everything went OK, we could return home right after the birth. Megan was born that day at noon, and by five p.m. I was back at home taking a much-needed shower, while Peter and my mother and his parents prepared supper and admired the baby. Then we all sat down to a celebration birthday supper, complete with cake and champagne and Megan in the middle of the table in her basket. By nine p.m. Peter and I were asleep in bed with Megan snuggled between us. The next day, the midwife came, checked me and the baby and answered my barrage of questions. Later in the day, friends came bringing food and baby presents. I remember those days as among the happiest in my life.

You may want to stay in the hospital a few days, especially if you have other children at home or no household help.

I have five kids at home. I look on this as my only holiday this year!

If this is your first baby you may enjoy the support and companionship of a hospital ward. 'I loved it. I could have stayed a fortnight!'

Your hospital may have 'rooming in', where your baby stays with you all the time; it may have 'modified rooming in', where your baby stays with you whenever you want, or just during the day, and then goes back to the central nursery whenever you are tired or at night. (One midwife found that mothers who kept their babies with them were more rested than mothers whose babies stayed in the nursery!) But some hospitals still separate mothers and babies routinely between feeds. You and your baby may find it difficult to adapt to hospital routines. Rigid policies of four-hourly feeds and restricted visiting, while much less common these days, can interfere with the natural process of recovery and with getting to know your baby; they can make feeding more difficult to establish and cause or aggravate depression. Many women simply find hospital exhausting.

I had my first baby in the hospital. For the next four days I hardly slept. My roommate was nice but she liked the TV on all the time. Then there were the nurses who came in every couple of hours to take my temperature or give me a laxative or scold me for feeding 'too long' on one side. During visiting hours and at night, they took the baby to the nursery, and I would fantasize that she was the one I heard crying. I felt tense and depressed most of the time.

There are good reasons for going home as soon as possible. Babies in hospital nurseries are at significant risk of infection.* There's an advantage to immediate hands-on practice in taking care of your baby.

SOME SIGNS OF ABNORMAL LABOUR AND DELIVERY

If complications should arise during labour, your body will usually give you some warnings. It is, of course, of vital importance that you be aware of them and make your midwife aware of them. When you are awake and not drugged, you will have a much clearer sense of what is going on. Also, some complications are set in motion by anaesthesia.

Here are a few signals that should warn you to notify your midwife immediately.

Continuous and Severe Lower Abdominal Pain, Often Accompanied by Uterine Tenderness

This is different from the pain of normal labour contractions, which comes on with increasing intensity and then gradually disappears completely until the next contraction – a pain which comes and goes.

An Abnormal Presentation or Prolapse of Cord, Placenta or Limb

If any of these occurs, an experienced practitioner must decide if a caesarean is required. Prolapsed cord (when the cord falls into the vagina and there is the danger that it might be compressed, thereby cutting off oxygen to the baby) and placenta praevia (placenta first instead of baby first) generally call for a caesarean section.*

Excessive Vaginal Bleeding (ante-partum haemorrhage)

There are a number of reasons for this, such as cervical laceration, placenta abruptio (when the placenta suddenly becomes detached from the uterus) or delivery before the cervix is fully dilated. It is normal, however, to have a bloody mucus discharge just before complete dilatation, especially when the cervix is opening up very quickly.

Abnormally Slow Dilatation of the Cervix

When contractions are severe and the cervix is still not dilating regularly, then the ineffective contractions may be creating undue stress on the fetus, the mother or both. This is a particularly hard condition to diagnose, since pain is subjective and many labours last much longer than others. This is discussed in Caesarean Section (p. 394). Many midwifery techniques can help this type of labour. However, sometimes even then there will be little or no cervical dilatation, possibly because the baby's head is in a posterior position and not bearing down effectively on the cervix.

*Central nurseries used to be considered sanctuaries where babies were kept safe from infections, chilling, mucus problems and over-exhaustion from medicated or operative deliveries. Yet in large nurseries, infants receive intermittent and often impersonal care, a poor substitute for mothering. Some nurseries breed *Staphylococcus aureus*, *Streptococcus* and *Salmonella*, which cause 'nosocomial' infections – infections acquired in hospital. These clearly iatrogenic – hospital-caused – illnesses can be serious, sometimes resulting in infant death.[16]

*Michel Odent, in *Birth Reborn*, discusses the possibility of vaginal birth if only a bit of the placenta covers the cervical opening.

Abnormality in Fetal Heartbeat

This condition is a sign that the baby may be in trouble. Fetal heartbeat should be checked regularly throughout labour.

Any Adverse Change in Condition of Mother or Baby

If the pattern of heartbeat and/or blood pressure changes, if the woman develops a high temperature or if some other difficulty arises, it is essential that an experienced doctor or midwife be present to interpret the signs.

PRETERM LABOUR AND DELIVERY

A preterm baby is one who is born before the 38th week of pregnancy. Low birthweight babies, born with a weight at or below 2,500 grams, are also treated as preterm as they share many of the same developmental problems. Preterm babies who are also 'small for dates' are particularly at risk.

Preterm birth and low birthweight may be caused by infectious diseases, thyroid disturbances, other maternal illnesses such as kidney disease, placental and fetal abnormalities, multiple pregnancy and pregnancies which are very close together. Smoking can also have an effect. However, poverty, and all that goes with it, is still the single most important factor affecting low birthweight. Only 7.1 per cent of the babies born in 1981 weighed less than 2,500 grams, but this group accounted for over 60 per cent of the baby deaths in that year.[17]

Preterm delivery proceeds like normal full-term labour. It may be a little slower owing to weaker contractions or more rapid because the baby is smaller. Some obstetricians prefer to deliver all preterm babies with forceps to 'protect' the head. Others maintain that vaginal delivery unassisted is safer. An episiotomy (see p. 393) *may* be necessary if the baby is distressed and second stage is delayed.

Preterm babies are very susceptible to drugs used in labour. If you are prepared to handle labour without drugs you will do your baby a great service.

Preterm delivery may be by caesarean if investigations show that you or your baby are in danger from, for example, pre-eclampsia (see p. 361), ante-partum haemorrhage (see p. 387) or if investigations show that your baby is not thriving. Tiny babies as small as 24 weeks can occasionally be saved by intensive care. However, we have to understand that it is still rare for a baby at this age to survive and there is a chance of handicap or long-term medical problems. By 29 weeks the vast majority of babies can now be saved though they still need intensive care and are far more vulnerable than full-term babies.

Small or sick babies require immediate intensive care. You may be transferred to a regional centre before the delivery so that facilities are available immediately. If you have delivered in a hospital without an intensive care unit your baby should be transferred by ambulance to a regional centre with intensive care cots. You need your baby and your baby needs you. Your companion should insist on having you transferred with the baby or, if you are not well enough to be moved, make sure that a bed will be prepared for you near the unit as soon as you can be moved (see Neonatal Intensive Care Units in Chapter 20, p. 403).

OBSTETRIC ROUTINES, INTERVENTIONS AND DRUGS

The mechanism of labour is both powerful and delicately balanced. Each part and process has a function in helping the baby be born well. Our attendants must respect the process and not interrupt it, hinder it or speed it up (unless absolutely necessary). Contractions massage the baby to squeeze excess fluid out of its lungs, amniotic fluid equalizes pressure and cushions the baby's head, membranes hold the waters in until the perineum has a chance to stretch slowly. Like any other animal, we need a calm environment for labour to proceed at its own pace, and we tense up when we are afraid, causing labour to slow down. Like elephants and dolphins, we labour best with females like ourselves nearby.

Occasionally things go wrong and we need medical intervention. We are fortunate it is being refined. At the same time we must be aware that most commonplace drugs and hospital procedures have never been scientifically proven beneficial for healthy mothers and infants.[18]

A government-sponsored report from the National Perinatal Epidemiology Unit quietly underlines this fact:

> Regional intervention rates have been compared with regional perinatal mortality rates and no statistical association, either positive or negative, can be seen between them . . . Of course there are occasions when the use of caesarean section, or instrumental delivery, is crucial to the baby's chance of survival. With the increasing use of the procedures, however, it is likely that the numbers of these cases are increasingly swamped by the numbers of instances where the use of intervention may not have been of such critical importance.[19]

Most of the time medical obstetrics interferes with our bodies in outrageous ways, as if male doctors over the course of the past century had sat down and systematically figured out how to interrupt each natural step of the labour process, one by one. When Jean Robinson was chairperson of the Patients' Association, she found that the only people who complained about treatment given against their will were women concerned about their experiences during childbirth – and such complaints were common. Childbirth appears to present medical practitioners with what seems to be a unique opportunity to provide treatment against a woman's wishes. If this occurs, it is legal assault. We do not know with any certainty how common this is, not least because the cost of taking legal action is prohibitive, and also because only the most articulate and courageous among us feel able to make even the most mild complaint. However, we do know that women often have to struggle in order to maintain a modicum of control over the way their birth is handled. If you feel you have been abused during childbirth, you may feel the need to talk to informed and sympathetic people. You can contact the NCT, the AIMS or the Maternity Defence Fund.

It is a credit to our basic health and resilience that, despite such assaults, we and our babies emerge so healthy. It is sad that so many of us expect intervention as the norm and rely on it for safety and pain relief when it is not always safe. It makes no sense for us to accept routine tampering with our bodies, our strengths and the safety of our children. It makes sense to learn as much as we can so that we use medical resources during labour only when we really need them.

DRUGS AND INTERVENTIONS IN HOSPITAL BIRTH

Like a snowball rolling down the hill, as one unphysiological practice is employed . . . another frequently becomes necessary to counteract some of the disadvantages, large or small, inherent in the previous procedure.[20]

Before booking into a hospital you can ask what their

SOME IDEAS FOR COPING WITH HOSPITAL ROUTINES

- Go in with your partner and/or birth companion. It's better to be with someone familiar, never necessary or helpful to be separated. You may want to bring two support people – one to help you physically during labour and one to troubleshoot in case you have problems getting what you want.
- They may bring you a wheelchair. Ignore it if you feel comfortable walking; take advantage of it if you want to. There is no medical reason for you to use it.
- They may give you a hospital gown to wear. You can wear your own clothes if you prefer. You may feel more independent and less like an invalid. Be sure to bring soft, stretchy socks, preferably knee socks, and a shawl or dressing gown as you may get shivery.
- You may be asked to sign a patient consent form, but you do not need to, and may prefer not to, do so.
- A midwife will ask you some questions about your pregnancy and your labour.
- Hospital staff may listen to the fetal heartbeat with a Pinard stethoscope or sonicaid (Doppler) to see if the fetal heart remains steady during and after contractions. Since the sonicaid is a form of ultrasound, you may want to ask for a Pinard stethoscope instead.
- During all these procedures you can stand or sit. You don't need to get into bed or lie down, though you may be urged or expected to. A mother who laboured and gave birth twice lying flat on her back observed:

  I've often thought that the best thing a woman can do for herself when she gets into the hospital is to stay upright, standing, sitting, kneeling, squatting. That way she remains active, in control.

- In some hospitals the midwives may want to do a 'test strip', using the external fetal monitor (see p. 392) to check the course of the baby's heartbeats during a series of contractions. They will ask you to lie still for twenty minutes to an hour. Remember that when you lie down, your contractions change. If you are in early labour they may slow down and even stop altogether. They may become more uncomfortable, making you tense up, which affects their efficacy. You can ask for a human monitor instead!
- You will probably have an internal examination to check dilatation. Usually a midwife will do this. Sometimes a doctor.

  I'd brought tapes and music, was walking and dancing. We'd created a wonderful mood. Then the doctor came in and blew it. He examined me internally, causing more pain than ever in my life.

- You can refuse to participate in teaching programmes. You can always refuse any procedure from anyone. Your partner or companion can advocate for you and protect you.
- Midwives will be your most constant medical attendants. Let them know what you want. Many midwives are encouraging and helpful.
  If you have a bad rapport with one midwife, ask for another. It's not always easy or possible to do so, but it's worth a try.
- If, during any of the procedures mentioned above, you are having a contraction, let the people around you know. They may not be aware of it. Hold up your hand, tell them. Your partner can tell them. They should stop what they are doing and wait. You should not be distracted. Focus on what you want and need. This is your labour and your birth.

rates are for various obstetric interventions. You may not be able to get the information very easily as some hospitals do not keep very detailed records. The Association for Improvements in the Maternity Services (AIMS) is trying to collate as much of this information as possible. You can reinforce your desire to avoid unnecessary intervention by writing to the Senior Nursing Officer (Midwifery) explaining what kind of birth you would like. The response to your letter will give you a good idea of the hospital's attitudes.

'PREPPING' (shaving pubic hair)*

This is totally unnecessary. It is just one part of the male medical ritual of depolluting, purifying women.[21] Prepping desexes us, makes us look like little girls again. Doctors believe that pubic hair contains germs and prepping decreases the risk of infection. In fact, prepping *increases* the risk of infection, when surface skin cells are scraped off and sometimes razors nick skin. As hair grows back, it is itchy and uncomfortable.

Since the last edition of this book many hospitals have dropped the procedure but it is still routine in some hospitals.

ENEMAS

Enemas are still routine in some hospitals but many no longer give them. They are not necessary. Women often have a natural diarrhoea before labour begins or during labour. You can request an enema if you think it will make you feel better or if faeces in your rectum seem to be holding up your labour; often enemas stimulate labour. But if you are in active labour already, it can make your contractions stronger and more uncomfortable, which in turn may make you ask for drugs, thereby setting off the chain of procedures related to their use (it can also encourage haemorrhoids; see p. 361). One 'medical' reason for giving enemas is to prevent contamination of the perineum by faeces. Yet enemas result in watery faeces which may be less 'clean' than natural diarrhoea.

INDUCTION AND THE ACTIVE MANAGEMENT OF LABOUR

Induction refers to labour which is started artificially. Active management refers to the use of artificial acceleration of labour according to a predetermined norm. In the mid-1970s induction was very much in vogue. Since then, after an outcry among women and in the media, the rate of induction has levelled off at around 20 per cent (which is still far higher than necessary). Rates vary a great deal between different consultants. In one AIMS survey (autumn 1984), induction rates in hospitals with a similar

*Two British studies conclude that routine prepping and enemas constitute 'unjustified assaults' on women, and that there is no evidence of benefit.[22]

population varied from 9 to 12 per cent in East London to 25 per cent in Glasgow and 42 per cent in Manchester.

As induction rates have dropped, the rate of acceleration appears to have risen (though no clear figures exist). So the overall number of 'managed labours' is probably no lower than during the mid-1970s peak.

Reasons for Induction or Acceleration

Induction is medically necessary in only 5–10 per cent of cases when, for example, the mother's very high blood pressure is threatening the baby's survival or her own health. Or there is concern that the placenta may be failing to give adequate nourishment (see p. 372 for tests which should be done if induction is contemplated in these circumstances). If there is clear evidence that the baby itself is distressed, an emergency caesarean section is usually necessary. It is in the grey area when the baby's health appears to be compromised but there is as yet no evidence of distress that induction is most often used. In fact, the most frequent reason is simply that the labour has gone two weeks over the expected date of confinement. (See p. 357 for more on dating.)

Acceleration is like induction, but the process is initiated after labour has started. It is intended for use in a labour which is both long *and* distressing to mother and/or baby.

In a study carried out by the National Childbirth Trust, of the minority who were not unhappy about the experience and would choose it again, most had had particularly long and arduous previous labours.[23]

> 'If I ever had a third child,' remarked one woman, 'I would do everything in my power to arrange for an induced birth' . . . One woman was very happy after a seven-hour labour which she said was 'like a holiday' after a previous thirty-six-hour labour, and another after a twelve-hour labour compared with nineteen-and-a-half hours with a severe backache labour . . .

However, long labours are not necessarily distressing and we are concerned about the routine acceleration adopted in some hospitals when labours last longer than predetermined norms.

> They said it would take too long without the drip. Too long for whom? I wondered.

The Procedure

Prostaglandin pessaries are now used in most British hospitals to soften the cervix if an induction is intended. The pessaries are inserted into the vagina. They should never be given orally or intravenously. You should be carefully monitored for a short period after insertion (see below). If you were ready to go into labour the pessaries will probably start you off with no further intervention.

Oestradiol may be used to soften your cervix if placental insufficiency (see p. 372) is suspected. This drug will not trigger contractions and so continuous monitoring is not necessary at this stage.

ARM (Artificial Rupture of Membranes) may be performed if the pessary does not start labour. An ARM may also be used as a first step procedure to initiate labour if your cervix is already slightly open and it may be done after contractions have started to accelerate labour. In fact, an ARM may be performed without your knowledge to 'hurry things up'. You may not want to 'hurry up' and this procedure should not be carried out without your consent.

It is described as like a 'long vaginal examination' and some women find it painful, though, if it is done carefully, it shouldn't be. You will feel the water gush out and will continue 'leaking' throughout labour. Once an ARM is performed, delivery should take place within twenty-four to thirty-six hours because the risk of infection is greater than it would be with a natural rupture of the membranes.

Oxytocin infusion using the drug syntocinon may be used either to induce or accelerate labour. If the waters have not broken, an ARM must be performed (see above). A scalp electrode may be attached to the baby's head for electronic monitoring of the heartbeat. Close monitoring is essential when syntocinon is used because the contractions are more vigorous than in normal labour. The syntocinon is delivered through a drip attached to your arm which is controlled through a pump to ensure an even delivery of the drug. Some machines measure the intensity of contractions (via a catheter in the cervix or a pressure gauge on the abdomen) and dole out syntocinon accordingly. The internal pressure gauge increases the risk of infection and, according to Professor Peter Huntingford, 'can never be justified'.

Side-effects

Most of the information we have about adverse effects of induction/acceleration refers to the use of ARM and syntocinon. It is probable that some of these disadvantages apply also to prostaglandin.

Failure to progress is the chief risk attached to induction. If labour is started before the cervix is ripe (ready to open), it may fail to dilate properly and the baby runs the risk of needing to be delivered by forceps or caesarean. Even Irish obstetrician Professor O'Driscoll, a leading advocate of routine acceleration, believes that 'an embargo on inductions would improve maternity care'.

I was put on a drip which was switched up at frequent intervals to 'get some action here'. After four to five hours I was told that my baby was distressed and I was only two centimetres dilated. I believe this was because I was induced when my cervix wasn't ready.

They were helpful and sympathetic but they could not allay my feeling that the baby's distress and the caesarean section could have been avoided if I'd been left alone.[24]

Failure to progress is not a significant risk with acceleration when it is used in established labour. However,

syntocinon infusion used when waters have broken or after an ARM which has failed to trigger labour, though it may be referred to as an acceleration, is effectively an induction and runs the same risk of failure. The use of prostaglandin pessaries to ripen the cervix cuts down the risk of failure.[25]

Fetal distress can be caused by extra-strong contractions which may reduce the blood supply carrying oxygen to the uterus and exert extra pressure on the baby's head (which is no longer cushioned by amniotic fluid after the ARM). The more accurate control of syntocinon has reduced these risks since the last edition of this book. However, there have been reports of similar risks using prostaglandin when placental insufficiency (see p. 372) is suspected.[26] Close monitoring of induction or acceleration is therefore of vital importance. Some doctors recommend continuous monitoring for the twenty minutes before and forty minutes after the insertion of prostaglandin pessaries.[27]

Immobility. The necessity for constant monitoring means that women are usually expected to lie immobile with monitors attached. This in itself makes the labour appear more oppressive and may slow it down (leading to an increased dose of the syntocinon).

Every time I had a pain I couldn't move because I was fastened both sides by thongs. The drip kept coming undone and bleeding if I put my weight on it.[28]

Special care. More babies subjected to syntocinon-induced contractions end up needing special care. This could be because they were at risk in the first place but figures certainly suggest that it is a direct effect of the procedure.

Jaundice is more common in syntocinon-induced babies.

Pain. Syntocinon and ARM induce sharper, more painful contractions which women find harder to cope with. In the National Childbirth Trust study, thirty-four out of fifty-three women felt that in spite of preparation to cope with induction it was worse than last time and they would try to avoid an induced birth in future.

I approached the birth in a state of happy expectancy and confidence, since the procedure [induction] had been explained to me. However, I received a severe shock. The membranes were ruptured, causing extreme pain and great mental distress. Then the oxytocin drip was set up, and about ten minutes later contractions started, roughly four minutes apart at first. Later they were coming every two minutes and were very painful; at no time could I control the pain and 'ride it'. Injections had no effect, and I was thankful to be given gas-and-air, but the pain was so great and so regular that I could not use it without assistance. Afterwards I had a great deal of pain, and required three weeks to recover, compared with eleven days on the previous occasion. The whole birth was a very distressing experience and one I will not repeat.

Prostaglandin has not been in use for long and we cannot be sure of all its effects, but it appears to be more acceptable to women than syntocinon. In one study comparing them, prostaglandin labour followed more closely the normal curve, with a slower beginning and then faster delivery than with syntocinon (only four women in the prostaglandin group needed additional syntocinon); 72 per cent of the syntocinon group needed epidurals or narcotic pain relief, whereas 42 per cent of the other group managed with Entonox (gas and oxygen). Eighty-six per cent of the prostaglandin group found the experience 'favourable' whereas none of the syntocinon group considered it so. This could be at least partly due to the fact that women using prostaglandin do not have to lie down and do not suffer the restriction of a drip. In this study remote control monitoring was used so there were no restrictive monitor wires either.[29]

Avoiding Induction and Acceleration

Although techniques have been improved since the last edition of this book, they still carry significant risks and should not be used unless there are clear medical reasons. There is no justification for inducing simply on the basis of dates alone, particularly since dates are often difficult to establish; ultrasound scans can vary two weeks in either direction unless a very early scan has established a clear baseline. If you know the date of conception, and your knowledge does not tally with the scan, stick to your knowledge and insist that it is taken into consideration. Other tests should be used to establish the condition of the baby (see p. 372) before induction is performed.

Alternative Methods of Starting Labour

Acupuncture and *homoeopathy* can be effective in triggering labour, though these techniques have not been well evaluated. A simple, and now clinically proven alternative, is nipple stimulation.* You can do it yourself or get your partner to help. It isn't dangerous, doesn't need monitoring and you may even enjoy it.

Prostaglandin is a natural constituent of semen. So making love may be a good method of induction for heterosexual couples. Don't do it after the waters have broken because of the increased risk of infection.

ELECTRONIC FETAL MONITORS

These are machines which electronically record the baby's heart-rate during labour. There are two basic kinds of monitors: external (non-invasive) and internal (invasive). The external monitor is applied by temporarily sticking gummy electrodes on to the labouring woman's abdomen or strapping an ultrasonic transducer on to her belly, to

*A study of self-stimulation of the breasts from 39 weeks reduced the incidence of 'postmaturity' from 17 to 5 per cent.[30]

monitor and record the heart-rate. The electrodes are more accurate. In addition, a strap about two to three inches wide, is placed around the woman's abdomen to hold the tocodynamometer, which records the intensity of the uterine contractions.

Internal fetal monitors are now almost routine in many hospitals. Electrodes connected to wires within a plastic tube are introduced into the woman's vagina and attached directly to the baby's presenting part (usually the scalp) by means of metal clips or screws. (No one has bothered to find out if this causes pain to the baby; if the waters have not already broken an ARM (see above) will be done.) The wires coming out of the vagina are held in place by an elastic strap around the woman's thigh. These electrodes measure the baby's heartbeat. The woman's contractions are measured either by a catheter designed for that purpose, introduced into her uterus through her vagina, or by the external tocodynamometer strap described above. A print-out shows the baby's heartbeat, which is also audible.

While most British hospitals can now monitor electronically, only 40 per cent of them are equipped to do fetal blood sampling. Without the facilities for analysing the acidity of the baby's blood (a sure sign of distress) the evidence of the monitor is only *half* as accurate as it should be. The errors lead to excess diagnosis of distress which then results in unnecessary forceps or caesareans.[31]

Several studies have been done to try and evaluate the effect of electronic monitoring on the perinatal mortality rate and the incidence of brain damage. A large-scale study by Adrian Grant of the National Perinatal Epidemiology Unit[32] showed no difference in perinatal death or disablement (after one year) in babies monitored electronically or intermittently with low-tech midwives' Pinard stethoscopes. There was an increase in neo-natal seizures in the intermittent group but only in labours which had been accelerated. Fetal blood sampling was carried out for both groups to minimize false readings. In this particular study the instrumental delivery and caesarean rate was no different either, but this is probably due to the unusually conservative use of such intervention in this hospital and to the routine blood sampling.

Though the monitor may be useful in some truly high-risk situations and necessary when labour is induced or accelerated or the woman anaesthetized, it entails many discomforts and risks to women and babies.[33]

1. Ultrasound has never been proven safe.

2. Many women say that the straps and the pressure of the transducer are uncomfortable.

3. Ironically, fetal stress picked up by the monitor may be a product of invasive hospital routines/procedures, including the monitor itself.

4. Since women with a monitor cannot move around much, if at all, labour may slow down or stop. (Though some hospitals now use remote-control monitors which allow the heartbeat to be recorded without restricting the mother's movements.)

5. Machines get old and break down. They often interpret normal signs as pathological or indicate normality

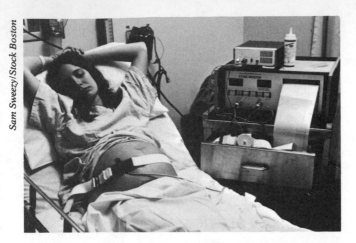

Sam Sweezy/Stock Boston

tears extending to the anus (third-degree lacerations); that they prevent damage to the baby's head; that they keep the pelvic floor from becoming too stretched and guard against uterine prolapse, cystocele and rectocele (when the uterus falls into the vagina, when the bladder or rectum protrude into or through the vaginal walls). Yet there has never been any evidence to prove this.[35]

AN EPISIOTOMY

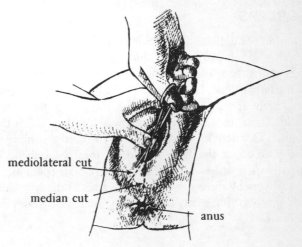

mediolateral cut

median cut

anus

Nina Reimer

when something is really wrong. The machine may lose the baby's heartbeat when s/he moves, or the electrode may slip out of the baby's scalp.

6. Hospital personnel tend to pay *less* attention to women with monitors. Also, partners and attendants may direct their attention and support away from the woman and pay attention mainly to the machine.

7. Hospital personnel may interpret machine data incorrectly. Incomplete understanding of the range and fluctuation in fetal heart-rate during and between contractions has led to unnecessary forceps and, these days, unnecessary caesarean deliveries.

8. Women and babies run a much greater risk of infection with the internal monitor. The baby's scalp may bleed because of the way the screw has been attached. Post-delivery rashes are common where the electrode was attached (85 per cent in one study), and scalp abscess is not uncommon (20 per cent).

9. Monitoring has contributed to the recent rise in caesareans (due to an increased rate of false diagnosis of fetal distress), an added risk for mother and baby.

EPISIOTOMY

Episiotomy is the most frequently performed obstetric operation in the West. It is one of the most intense and dramatic ways in which the territory of women's bodies is appropriated, the only operation performed on the body of a healthy woman without her consent. It represents obstetrical power: babies can't get out unless they are cut out. It prevents women from experiencing birth as a sexual event, and is a form of ritual genital mutilation.[34]

An episiotomy is an incision through skin and muscles in the perineum, the area between the vagina and the anus, to enlarge the opening through which the baby will pass. The procedure is necessary only when forceps are used, when previous damage to the perineum means that a severe tear is likely, and in case of fetal distress, when the baby must come out quickly and the woman's tissues just won't stretch any more.

Doctors believe that episiotomies will prevent perineal

There is no justification for routine episiotomy, yet some consultants insist on its routine use and midwives are, as a result, getting insufficient training in those midwifery techniques which can prevent or minimize tearing. For instance, in most births you will have little if any tearing when you are upright, sitting or squatting to breathe or push your baby out, resting between contractions; when your practitioner helps you to control your pushing, open up and relax while s/he carefully supports your perineum.

If you have an episiotomy you are unlikely to feel it at the time. A local anaesthetic injection is usually given. The stitching of a tear or episiotomy is usually done by a doctor (often a student). A local anaesthetic injection should be given if you have not already had one. Make sure the doctor waits until it has taken effect before starting. The stitches may be itchy and extremely painful for a few days and often several weeks (depending on the number of stitches needed, a superficial tear will heal quicker than a cut). Some women are allergic to stitches, sometimes stitches don't dissolve. Many women report that penetrative sex is painful for many weeks and, for a minority, the discomfort impairs sexual pleasure for many months. In a few cases, when overtight stitching is to blame, the stitch line must be cut and resewn. Given these difficulties it is shocking that perineums are considered suitable practice material for students and that a few doctors deliberately stitch tightly in the belief that they are doing our male partners a favour:

I saw my doctor at the check-up six weeks after my baby was born. Full of male pride, he told me during my pelvic exam, 'I did a beautiful job sewing you up. You're as tight as a virgin; your husband should thank me.'

You can minimize problems by keeping stitches as clean and dry as possible. An old detergent bottle filled with warm water can be used to wash the area after a bowel motion and a hand hairdryer will dry without causing pain. It helps to avoid penetrative sex until your own explorations tell you that your perineum is no longer tender. *

FORCEPS

In a forceps delivery the doctor pulls the baby out with a double-bladed instrument which resembles salad tongs, except that the blades are longer and curved to fit the shape of the baby's head. Each blade is introduced into the vagina separately and placed carefully on the side of the baby's head. Then the two blades are clamped together outside the vagina. Different kinds of forceps will be used according to the position of the baby's head. A local anaesthetic is usually used unless you already have had an epidural.

Delivery by forceps has saved the lives of many infants and mothers, but many unnecessary forceps deliveries are performed.

The incidence of delivery by forceps and vacuum extractor [see below], combined, rarely rises above 5% in countries where mothers actively participate in the birth of their babies.[36]

The rate in Britain is 13.1 per cent. Forceps deliveries can result in damage to the baby. They are also thought to increase the risk of infection in the mother and should not be performed without good reason.

The usual reasons for a forceps delivery are:
1. they speed up second-stage labour if there is severe fetal distress;
2. in case of unusual presentations (see p. 377);
3. if regional anaesthesia doesn't allow the mother to push out her baby;
4. to shorten a very long second-stage labour;
5. extremely high blood pressure or heart disease where straining could be dangerous.

Normal second-stage labour can go on from half-an-hour to three hours and unless there is some indication that the baby is having trouble getting out, there is no medical reason for introducing forceps. Women are designed to be able to give birth to babies. The survival of our species depended on it and still does.

VACUUM EXTRACTION (or the ventouse)

This is occasionally used as an alternative to forceps (in 1 per cent of deliveries). When the cervix is fully dilated and the baby is ready to be delivered, a small metal cup is placed on its head and this is connected to a vacuum which makes it stay on the scalp. Traction then results in the baby being delivered. The baby will have a swelling on its head but this will disappear. Some British doctors never use it: however, recent trials show that the ventouse causes less 'maternal trauma and less blood loss at delivery' and is usually quicker than forceps delivery.[37] It is widely used in Europe and Scandinavia. Women need to be aware that there are just as many studies condemning the ventouse so it is mostly a matter of personal opinion.

CAESAREAN SECTION

Caesarean section appears to be a sometimes useful and needed technique presently utilized in an undocumented, unclarified and uncontrolled manner.[38]

Caesarean sections are life-saving operations when women have certain problems before or during labour – severe pre-eclampsia, transverse lie of the baby, failure of the baby to descend at all, cord prolapse, placenta praevia, baby much too large, active herpes lesions, sudden unexplained fetal distress.

She had been head down for three months before the birth but somehow she turned, put her foot through the amniotic sac, tore off the placenta and the uterus collapsed. My contractions were very painful and came every three minutes. Then I started bleeding. We watched her heart-rate go down on the monitor. The doctor said a caesarean was necessary. They tried a spinal [epidural] three times; it didn't take. My husband was going through hell; he couldn't do anything. Finally I was given general anaesthesia. I came to three hours later. I'd lost a lot of blood.

Afterwards every day I asked the doctors and nurses if there was anything I could have done to make it less traumatic, more normal. I got the facts. There was nothing I could have done. I kept reliving it, asking my husband lots of questions like a child. The hospital people were wonderful.

Not having seen her born really hurts. They gave her to my husband to hold right after. It took me three days to unwrap her and look at her naked and see that she was really all right.

It was so quick and different than we'd planned. So much happens in such a short time; there's no time to process it. I wish there had been some way to prepare for it. It was good that it was done; it saved my life and hers.

Please let women know that in regard to caesareans there is a 'grey area' between the life-or-death emergency situation and the absolutely unnecessary operation. In my case, I had been in extremely painful labour for hours and hours, with

---

*See also Sheila Kitzinger, *Episiotomy: Physical and Emotional Aspects* and *Some Women's Experiences of Episiotomy*, London: National Childbirth Trust, 1981.

back-to-back long-lasting contractions (unexpected because my first labour had been intense, but short and manageable). David held me, massaged me; I walked, stood, squatted, took baths. Now, I'm no martyr, but I think I could have stood it if there had been any progress, but there was very little. Most discouraging, the baby's head wasn't engaged. After nine hours I said to my doctor, 'I need a caesarean.' Not one to jump into a C-section, he didn't want to do it right away. Finally, I had an epidural. When it took effect, I could smile again. We waited a while longer – no progress. When he finally did the caesarean, he was amazed by the size of my baby. She was a giant! I know that some people believe that women can birth just about any size baby vaginally. Perhaps I would have been able to do so, too, if I had done other things and been willing to labour for twenty-four more hours. Maybe not. I wonder whether the intense pain wasn't my body's way of telling me that vaginal birth was impossible this time.

Caesareans must be performed in hospitals with anaesthesia, antibiotics and blood transfusion equipment. The upper part of your pubic hair will be shaved and a catheter (tube) inserted into your urethra to empty your bladder. You will be washed down with an antiseptic solution. You'll have either epidural (when your abdomen is numb but you are awake) or general anaesthesia. With general anaesthesia you should receive as small a dose as possible (epidural doses will be greater than for labour-pain relief). If you are awake for the operation, nurses may place a screen below your shoulders so that you don't see it, though sometimes you can see in a mirror. When your abdomen has become numb or when you are unconscious, the obstetrician makes a small horizontal cut in your abdominal wall, low down near the line of your pubic hair. (Sometimes a vertical cut will be necessary to get the baby out quickly.) The obstetrician then cuts horizontally through the uterine muscle and eases the baby out. If you are awake, ask to see the baby being born. The baby's nose and mouth will be suctioned with a mucus catheter. When s/he is breathing well, you or your partner can hold her/him. The obstetrician then removes the placenta and sews you up, layer by layer. In some hospitals your baby will be automatically admitted into Special Care (see p. 403).

Risks of Caesareans

The risk of maternal death, though generally very low (about 9 per 100,000 births in 1981) is nine times higher for caesareans. Of course, the higher rate must be partly due to the disproportionate number of high-risk pregnancies delivered by caesarean. Nevertheless, since the risk has not declined with the increasing number of caesars, a substantial part of the excess risk must be attributed to the procedure itself. Other common problems are: a post-operative infection rate of around 23 per cent,[39] difficulty in establishing feeding with a drugged baby, problems in coping

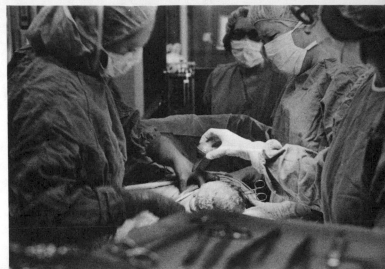

Caesarean birth

Vaughn Sills

with a newborn while recovering from a major operation, possible long-term problems with adjustment as a result of this early experience.[40] For the baby caesarean is also traumatic and babies delivered this way are often slow to start breathing and may be shocked. Problems with feeding may require an early switch to bottles with the attendant risks of allergy and infection (see p. 407).

In spite of these acknowledged drawbacks, the caesarean rate continues to climb from one in every twenty-two deliveries in 1963 to one in nine in 1982. According to a Maternity Alliance report,[41] the rate between hospitals varies dramatically from 5 to 18.9 per cent.

Some doctors defend this rising rate on the grounds that it is directly responsible for the improving perinatal mortality rate. However, a study at the National Maternity Hospital in Dublin showed that between the years of 1965 and 1980, although the caesarean rate at that hospital remained steady (between 4.1 and 4.8 per cent) the perinatal mortality rate fell from 42.1 to 16.8 per 1,000 births. The report concludes that:

> These results do not support the contention that the expansion in Caesarean birth-rates has contributed significantly to reduced perinatal mortality rates in recent years.

When the Maternity Alliance asked obstetricians what they saw as the reason for the rising rates, their comments made instructive reading. Most pointed out that caesars were more commonly done for breech deliveries these days. (Studies on the safety of deliverying breech babies vaginally or by caesarean do not conclusively support either method as safer.) Several obstetricians also pointed to a shortage of doctors trained to handle complicated births and one commented that:

> *Shortage of qualified theatre nursing staff makes us do caesarean sections sooner rather than later in case there is no one to assist at the operations.*

Caesars may also be performed in difficult labours to avoid the possibility of a negligence suit if something goes wrong. One particular legal case was quoted many times in the report as a reason for 'Defensive Obstetrics' (when a doctor was sued for using forceps instead of a caesarean and the baby subsequently suffered brain damage). *

One other major reason for increasing rates is the wider use of electronic fetal monitoring. As one obstetrician commented: 'if fetal distress is diagnosed by heart recordings alone then this will steeply increase the number of caesareans performed – the majority of them unnecessarily.' When a woman has had one caesarean she is very often led to believe that all future deliveries should also be by caesarean. This in itself increases the rate. However, the risk of uterine rupture (which doctors may quote) is extremely small and, provided that there is no good reason for a subsequent caesarean, a vaginal delivery is usually quite safe.

Women who have prepared for a 'natural' birth and end up with a caesar may feel bitterly disappointed and even guilty that they have 'failed' to give birth as they intended.

---

*Pressure can work both ways. Obstetrician Wendy Savage was called before a disciplinary tribunal in 1986 because, in the opinion of her colleagues, she did not perform caesareans readily enough.

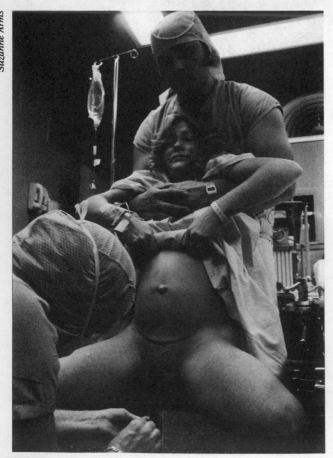

Suzanne Arms

Vaginal birth after caesarean

The knowledge that the operation was necessary plays an important part in coming to terms with the event. Some women have found it helpful to discuss their feelings with others who have gone through similar experiences. Support groups have been set up around the country to provide a place for discussion (see Resources).

PAIN RELIEF IN LABOUR

Labour without pain is not a common experience even with careful preparation. However, preparation, psychological support and a sense of being in control help most women to handle pain successfully.

> Women who feel in control of their own pain are less anxious during pregnancy and experience less pain during the labour itself. Feeling in control of the labour was also linked with suffering less pain during it.[42]

For example, in Holland it is reported that 'skilful psychological management of labour usually precludes the need for obstetrical medication'.[43]

Whereas, in Britain,

> many women who were given a second dose of pethidine or other analgesic when they found it difficult to cope with contractions would have preferred to have been given more emotional support at that point, and obviously felt that the pharmacological pain relief did not really take the place of encouragement, praise and oral guidance.[44]

It is, therefore, not surprising that 95 per cent of British women receive obstetric pain relief compared to 5 per cent of Dutch women.

The need for pain relief is also linked to the use of induction:

> In 1973 in Cardiff, 27.7% of Cardiff mothers asked for an epidural block at a time when the induction rate was 36.8%. By 1980 the induction rate had fallen to 4.3% with an epidural rate of 15.5%.[45]

DRUGS FOR PAIN RELIEF

Almost every drug given to the mother just before or during labour crosses the placenta and reaches the baby. If the baby is premature, smaller than average or in poor health, the effect will be greater. Even a normal baby can suffer temporarily and we mothers can sometimes suffer more from the after-effects of the drugs used in labour than we might have from labour itself. The problem is compounded because along with each drug often come two or three other procedures designed to ensure, as much as possible, the safety of the drug used. Each of these procedures carries its own potential risks and side-effects.

Drugs intended to reduce pain during labour can be grouped under the following headings:

1. Sedatives or tranquillizers: sedatives relieve anxiety and induce a feeling of calmness or drowsiness; tranquillizers simply relieve anxiety.

2. Analgesics: these decrease our sensation of pain; in large doses they will usually cause loss of consciousness.

3. Anaesthetics: these remove the sensation of pain altogether.

Drugs given just before or during labour which dampen down the mother's reactions will have the same effect on the baby. This can last for the first week of life or more, and can thus affect the baby's ability to suckle. Since the baby's sucking reflex soon after birth is important for ensuring a good milk supply, the ability of the mother to produce milk can also be affected by these drugs – and this in turn can affect the mother-child relationship.

Infants whose mothers had received analgesia and anaesthesia during labour and delivery have been shown to have delayed muscular, visual and neural development in the first four weeks of life. This effect wears off quite quickly but as Martin Richards, a Cambridge psychologist who has done some work in this area, says:

> My own guess, and it can only be a guess at present, is that drug effects in themselves are not of vital importance. If both mother and baby are healthy and they live in a supportive social situation the drug effects will be lost among all other chance experiences of life. However, where a baby is already 'at risk' for medical or social reasons, things might be very different and in this situation a drugged baby might become the straw that breaks the camel's back.[46]

What knowledge that is available very strongly suggests that these drugs should not be used routinely during labour, nor should they be used unnecessarily.

1. Sedatives and Tranquillizers

These are commonly given in the first stage of labour 'to take the edge off your contractions'. They may be given to reduce high blood pressure. They may also be mixed with pethidine (see below). They can have depressant effects on some newborn functions.[47] For example, sluggish respiration is common among babies whose mothers receive sedation, and diazepam (Valium) is thought to interfere with a newborn's ability to cope with cold. Diazepam may also cause jaundice in the baby if given around the time of labour. Other tranquillizers used are promazine (Sparine) and promethazine (Phenergan). Sparine may cause labour to slow down or even cease altogether.

Tranquillizers may be helpful in allowing the mother to relax between contractions. However, she may find herself falling asleep until the contraction reaches its peak, and then she may panic and actually experience more pain than she would have without the drug.

2. Analgesics

Narcotics. The most commonly given analgesic is pethidine, a narcotic. (In some hospitals Meptid, a newer drug, is now used.) It is usually given by injection, takes fifteen minutes to take effect, and can last for four hours. In spite of its widespread use, it is not particularly effective and it does have side-effects. One paper by Holdcroft and Morgan[48] shows that three-quarters of the women investigated received no relief from pain at all, though other studies show better results. All narcotics have a depressant effect on fetal respiration, and the newborn's behavioural responsiveness may be significantly decreased by these drugs. Contrary to popular belief, the most dangerous time to give this drug is two to six hours before birth. In the hour before delivery the drugs will still get to the baby but in a form which it can more easily cope with.[49] If you are given too much pethidine, the baby may have to be given another drug – naloxone – to counteract its effects. Pethidine is commonly given in far too high a dose: 150 mg or 200 mg is sometimes routine instead of the 50 mg or 100 mg recommended in midwives' textbooks. Although some women just feel 'high' from the effects of pethidine, others experience nausea, a sense of unreality and loss of control. Some people believe that many unpleasant experiences during labour are in fact caused by the effects of even small doses of pethidine on women not accustomed to hard drugs. If you have been on certain anti-depressants (monoamine oxidase inhibitors), you will need to be watched carefully, since they can increase the effect of pethidine.

If pethidine works for you, and if you are in need of analgesia, it may well be the best drug to use, in spite of its side-effects.

> In the short-term, at least, it may be better to continue to use the well-established drugs like Pethidine, when required, because we at least have some knowledge of their side-effects. Where a mother of a drugged baby is having feeding difficulties it may be very helpful for her to know that the baby's reduced sucking response is the temporary result of the drug and not an indication of her 'mishandling' of the baby.[50]

The following provides a glimpse of the range of experiences women can have with pethidine. It is taken from the NCT's survey 'Some Mothers' Experiences of Induced Labour'. For a more detailed look at women's experiences of pethidine, pain relief and hospitalized childbirth in general, see this pamphlet.

> Those who liked pethidine found that it took the edge off contractions without imperilling their control or that it gave them a chance to sleep and they 'woke refreshed'. Those who disliked pethidine said 'It was a great mistake. It stopped contractions', or slowed down the progress of dilatation, or made remarks such as 'I lost control and understanding'. Women who were left completely free to choose whether or

not they had pethidine and who felt they had good emotional support, were those most likely to find it helpful . . . The very ease with which pethidine can be given – 'It was shot into my thigh as I was lying down with my eyes closed' – contributes to its being used without the woman's consent, and sometimes when she has asked not to be given it.

Inhalation analgesia. This is pain relief that you inhale, usually by means of a face mask. (If you don't like the idea of a face mask, you could try making inquiries in advance about using a disposable mouthpiece instead.) The one most commonly used is gas and oxygen (usually Entonox, which is a mixture of oxygen and nitrous oxide). It appears to be more effective than pethidine though the two are very often used together, producing satisfactory relief for almost half of those who use it. It is particularly effective if used with good teaching and support and could thus be used much more widely than pethidine.

As yet there is no evidence that Entonox has harmful effects on the baby. Like Trilene and Penthrane (see below), Entonox does not greatly depress fetal respiration. Very little nitrous oxide reaches the baby via the placenta and the use of oxygen at the same time – and its benefits to mother and baby – outweighs the possible disadvantages of nitrous oxide.

One overwhelming advantage of inhalation analgesia is that you can administer it yourself. Entonox takes some fifteen seconds to work so you should start breathing the mixture at the beginning of a contraction, tailing off at its height. Most hospitals explain well before labour how to use the machine.

Penthrane takes slightly longer to take effect than Entonox but it gives prolonged relief. Unfortunately, it has a smell which some people find unpleasant. Like Entonox, it helps you to become mentally and physically relaxed but a few women become very drowsy. Unlike nitrous oxide it is absorbed by the mother and does get through to the baby although the effects are minimal with the amount used.

3. Anaesthetics

Regional anaesthesia. The pudendal block anaesthetizes only the vulva, or external female organs. Lignocaine is injected into the vaginal wall and a less painful forceps delivery (see p. 394) is then possible. Even this relatively minor anaesthetic can cause 'a persistent decrease in oxygen saturation in the newborn during the first thirty minutes of postpartum observation'[51] but the effect quickly wears off.

Perineal infiltration is an injection of local anaesthetic given if an episiotomy is considered necessary. It may also be given when the cut or tear is sewn up. It takes two or three minutes to work.

Epidural anaesthesia. This is a local anaesthetic (usually Bupivacaine) which is administered continuously and should numb the body from waist to knees while leaving the labouring woman completely alert. It can be administered at any time during labour but hospitals often prefer to do it fairly early in the first stage.

Epidurals can be useful when a woman has serious respiratory disease as the drug involved reduces the work the lungs have to do. It may make it easier for a diabetic woman, for it reduces the demands on her metabolism. It can slow down precipitate labour and also moderate a premature urge to push as with a footling breech. It is increasingly used in caesarean operations instead of a general anaesthetic. In some large hospitals it is available for anyone who requires it but this is not true of hospitals without the requisite twenty-four-hour cover by experienced anaesthetists. Access to epidurals varies widely.

The drug is administered through a tiny catheter placed in the back. An injection is made in the middle of the woman's back and the catheter, on a needle, moved into her epidural space (not the spinal column), the space between the bone at the base of the spinal cord and the membranes which cover the cord.

When administered properly epidurals should eliminate all pain. (In fact, in some 15 per cent of cases the epidural fails or only partially succeeds.)

Risks of epidurals. The anaesthetic travels rapidly to the baby and studies show lack of responsiveness and other minor effects which persist for up to six weeks.[52] This does not seem significantly to alter the baby's behaviour but it could affect the ability to suck which may in turn have an effect on the relationship between you and your baby.

Maternal complications with epidurals are not automatically notified so we have no real information about the level of complications. Some women report after-effects such as tingling and numbness in their legs and occasionally bad headaches, which may last for days. Epidurals can cause maternal hypotension (low blood pressure)* which reduces blood flow to the fetus. This is usually prevented by lying the woman on her side and setting up a drip which can be used if the blood pressure starts to drop. Transverse arrest (the baby getting stuck sideways) is another possible complication because the anaesthetic can cause the uterine muscles to relax too much.

Serious accidents have occurred during setting and topping up of epidurals which should only be carried out by an experienced anaesthetist. According to AIMS, in spite of the fact that few such accidents have come to light there have been around 300 out-of-court settlements involving epidurals. A survey by the Birthday Trust published in 1988 has drawn attention to the fact that some hospitals have been providing this service without adequate numbers of suitably trained staff – an extremely dangerous practice.

---

*Some effects of hypotension on the mother may be shock-like symptoms, altered pulse rate, nausea and vomiting. Its effects on the fetus are slowed heart-rate, decreased flow of blood through the placenta and insufficient oxygen intake. These effects tend to show up within twenty minutes.

When we choose epidurals we also invite a number of interlocking procedures, most of which increase the risks of the method. These include:

1. An intravenous hydrating solution attached to one arm to treat low blood pressure.

2. Blood pressure gauging. Your blood pressure will probably be checked every fifteen to thirty minutes, since a drop in blood pressure is common and can have serious effects on the fetus as well as on the mother. You will probably have to wear a blood pressure cuff continuously on the other arm.

3. Artificial rupture of the membranes (bag of waters). If your membranes have not already ruptured by themselves your doctor will probably rupture them before you are given an epidural. This is routine, but it is also done to make sure that the baby's head is firmly positioned in the birth outlet and to prepare for the attachment of an internal fetal monitor.

4. Syntocinon may be needed to accelerate a labour which has been stopped or slowed down by the anaesthetic. Ruptured membranes plus syntocinon create very strong uterine contractions which *must* be monitored.

5. A fetal monitor, with all its attendant risks. It is especially important during continuous anaesthesia to check the baby's heart-rate, since fetal distress rises with the length of time the anaesthesia is administered.

6. Much higher (three to four times) incidence of forceps delivery. As the urge for and coordination of pushing are decreased, many babies remain in an occiput, transverse or posterior position. The mother can't push her baby out and ends up 'needing' forceps.

7. A caesarean section. With epidurals there is a higher caesarean rate. Because the monitor is used almost routinely these days and the epidural is usually administered early in labour, it is difficult to separate the influence of the epidural from the monitor in increasing the caesarean rate. 'Failure to progress in labour', the prime indication for caesareans, is often the direct iatrogenic result of a labour slowed down by epidural anaesthesia.

> It was a real pleasure to give birth under these conditions [under an epidural], whereas 'natural childbirth' might have given rise to complications. We enjoyed every bit of it. When our baby was born, I thought I was dreaming, it was so easy . . . Having had such a tireless labour, I recovered very quickly, producing lots of good milk for the baby and was able to enjoy him. The baby became a satisfied and easy-going child. [53]

> I refused to have an epidural, and I was the only one in my ward not to have stitches or a hangover for the next couple of days. [54]

General anaesthesia. According to a consultant anaesthetist at Queen Charlotte's Hospital, general anaesthetics (GAs) should be administered as rarely as possible in pregnancy. A pregnant woman is at particular risk from the effects of anaesthetics (the third commonest cause of maternal death) because it is hard to prevent the stomach contents trickling into the lungs and, as the cardio-vascular system is already under strain, anaesthetics add to the risk. Black women run an even higher risk from GAs partly because changes in skin colour are one of the main signs of trouble an anaesthetist watches for, and they are trained mainly with white patients.

In order to minimize the risk to the mother, the anaesthetic has to be delivered in a dose which will act quickly and wear off quickly. The fine judgement needed (every woman varies in her response to these drugs) means that mistakes occur and there have recently been horrifying cases reported in which women have been insufficiently drugged to mask pain but have been unable to move or speak. Careful monitoring can decrease this risk.

There are a few cases in which a GA is recommended for caesarean; for example, in placenta praevia when heavy bleeding is possible and when a sudden change in the baby's heartbeat means that speed is essential. In virtually all other cases epidural analgesia is a safer option when complete pain relief is medically necessary.

PAIN RELIEF – OTHER POSSIBILITIES*

Homoeopathy (see p. 91)

A good homoeopathic doctor can help prevent or treat all sorts of problems during pregnancy and labour. S/he will prescribe individually-tailored doses of whatever is appropriate for you. One particular remedy – Squaw root – is very useful for pain relief. Taken during pregnancy it may result in much easier labours; it helps expel the placenta and helps postpartum discomfort.

Herbal Remedies (see p. 90)

Raspberry-leaf tea is an old, well-known remedy for the uterus and relieving the pain of labour.

> Somewhat shamefacedly and surreptitiously I have encouraged my expectant mothers, who felt so inclined, to drink the infusion . . . In a good many cases in my own experience, the subsequent labour has been easy and free from muscular spasm. [55]

Raspberry-leaf tea is usually taken during the last few months of pregnancy. It should be avoided in the first sixteen weeks.

Acupuncture (see p. 94)

Acupuncture can be a very effective method of pain relief. While it is not often used in this country, and it would usually have to be arranged privately with an acupuncturist,

---

*For more on these, see books listed in Resources for Chapter 7.

it is becoming more common for NHS hospitals to consider it and, occasionally, to use it. According to one study in the USA, acupuncture not only reduced pain and shortened labour, but 'a majority of patients experienced a sensation of peacefulness and relaxation together with a feeling of warmth'.[56] One British woman recently had acupuncture at hospital for her first baby – her comment: *The whole thing was marvellous*. However, it is important for the acupuncturist to be properly trained in the use of acupuncture in obstetrics.

Hypnosis

For those people who are susceptible to hypnosis, it is possible to achieve a pain-free labour while remaining totally conscious and aware of what is happening.

Transcutaneous Electric Nerve Stimulation

This is being tried in some hospitals. Four pads placed on either side of the spine are linked to a little box which the woman then operates herself. The current is soothing and provides some pain relief, particularly in a backache labour. In Swedish trials women rated it as effective as pethidine and women using it had shorter labour and delivered lively, undrugged babies.

Birth Preparation

Classes teaching techniques for getting in control of labour, providing information on massage, relaxation and birth positions can be more useful than most forms of artificial pain relief. Local classes can be contacted via AIMS, NCT or your local clinic. See page 421.

NOTES

1. Joseph B. DeLee. 'The Prophylactic Forceps Operation', *American Journal of Obstetrics and Gynecology*, no. 1, 1920.
2. Frederick Leboyer. *Birth Without Violence*. London: Fontana, 1983.
3. Stanley Sagov et al. 'The Issue of Safety', in *Home Birth: a Practitioner's Guide to Birth Outside the Hospital*. Rockville, MD: Aspen Systems Corp., 1983, ch. 2.
4. Michelle Harrison. *Woman in Residence*. New York: Penguin Books, 1983.
5. Three small-scale studies on ECV (external cephalic version) have shown that the technique can halve the caesarean rate for breech babies. In 70 per cent of cases babies were turned successfully and stayed head down for delivery. See *The Lancet*, 18 August 1984, p. 385.
6. Ina May Gaskin. 'Practising Midwifery – a Talk by Ina May Gaskin', *Childbirth Alternative Quarterly*, Summer 1981.
7. C.D. Kimball, C. M. Chang, S. M. Huang and J. C. Houck. 'Immunoreactive Endorphin Peptides and Prolactin in Umbilical Vein and Maternal Blood', *American Journal of Obstetrics and Gynecology*, vol. 140, no. 2, 15 May 1981, pp. 157–64; Michel Odent. 'The Evolution of Obstetrics at Pithiviers', *Birth and the Family Journal*, vol. 8, no. 1, Spring 1981, pp. 7–15.
8. Barbara Katz Rothman. *In Labour: Women and Power in the Birthplace*. New York: W. W. Norton, 1982, p. 290.
9. Peter M. Dunn. 'Obstetric Delivery Today – for Better or Worse?', *The Lancet*, April 1976.
10. G.J. Engelmann. *Labour Among Primitive Peoples*. St Louis, 1882.
11. Nancy Fuller and Brigette Jordan. Paper in *The Monthly Extract*, vol. 3, no. 1, 19.
12. Constance Beynon. 'The Normal Second Stage of Labour: a Plea for Reform in its Conduct', *Journal of Obstetrics and Gynaecology of the British Empire*, vol. 64 no. 6, December 1957, pp. 815–20.
13. Roberto Caldeyro-Barcia. 'The Influence of Maternal Bearing-Down Efforts During the Second Stage and Fetal Well-Being', *Birth and the Family Journal*, Spring 1979. (Available as a reprint from *Birth*, Blackwell Scientific Publications, 3 Cambridge Center, Cambridge, MA 02142, USA.)
14. Rothman, op. cit., note 8.
15. Nancy Wainer Cohen. *Birth: A Commentary* (available from the Boston Women's Health Book Collective).
16. See Ruth Lubic. 'The Impact of Technology on Health Care – the Childbearing Center: a Case for Technology's Appropriate Use', *Journal of Nurse-Midwifery*, vol. 24, no. 1, January–February 1979, pp. 6–10.
17. Alison Macfarlane and Miranda Mugford. *Birth Counts*. London: HMSO, 1984.
18. *Obstetrical Practices in the United States, 1978*. Washington DC, 17 April 1978, 95th Congress, 2nd session. US Senate, Committee on Human Resources, Washington, DC: US Government Printing Office.
19. Macfarlane and Mugford, op. cit., note 17.
20. Doris Haire. *The Cultural Warping of Childbirth*. International Childbirth Education Association (available from National Childbirth Trust – see Resources in Chapter 20), p. 32.
21. See Ann Oakley. *Subject Women*. London: Fontana, 1985.
22. M.L. Romney. 'Predelivery Shaving: an Unjustified Assault?' *American Journal of Obstetrics and Gynecology*, vol. 1, 1980, pp. 33–5; M.L. Romney and G. Gordon. 'Is Your Enema Really Necessary?' *British Medical Journal*, no. 282, 18 April 1981, pp. 1269–71.
23. 'Some Mothers' Experiences of Induced Labour', NCT, 1975.
24. From the 'That's Life' survey, *The British Way of Birth*. London: Pan, 1982, p. 97.
25. A.A. Calder et al. *British Journal of Obstetrics and Gynaecology*, no. 84, 1977, pp. 264–8.
26. Van Eyk et al. Letter to *British Medical Journal* cautioning against the use of prostaglandins for ripening, 6 March 1982, p. 742.
27. Beck and Clayton. Letter to *The Lancet* on the hazards of prostaglandin in postmaturity, 17 July 1982, p. 161.
28. *The British Way of Birth*, op. cit., note 24, p. 98.
29. Kennedy et al. *British Journal of Obstetrics and Gynaecology*, September 1982.
30. *American Journal of Obstetrics and Gynecology*, vol. 149, 1984, pp. 628–32.
31. Philip Stein. *British Journal of Obstetrics and Gynaecology*, September 1982.
32. 'Dublin Randomized Controlled Trial of Intrapartum Fetal Heartrate Monitoring', National Perinatal Epidemiology Unit, 1986.
33. 'Antenatal Diagnosis'. Bethesda, MD: National Institutes of Health Consensus Development Conference, NIH Publication no. 79–1973, 1979; A.D. Haverkamp, M. Orleans, S. Langendoerfer et al. 'A Controlled Trial of the Differential Effects of Intrapartum Fetal Monitoring', *American Journal of Obstetrics and Gynecology*, no. 134, 1979, p. 399; A.D. Haverkamp, H.E. Thompson, J.G. McFee et al. 'The Evaluation of Continuous Fetal Heart Rate Monitoring in High-risk Pregnancy', *American Journal of Obstetrics and Gynecology*, no. 125, 1976, p. 310.
34. From Sheila Kitzinger's talk at Boston College, Autumn 1981.
35. Jennifer Sleep. 'West Berkshire Perineal Management Trial', *British Medical Journal*, no. 289, 8 September 1984, pp. 587–90.

36. Doris Haire. *The Cultural Warping of Childbirth*. International Childbirth Education Association, 1984 (available from the NCT).

37. A. Vacca, A. Grant et al. 'Portsmouth Operative Delivery Trial; a Comparison of Vacuum Extraction and Forceps Delivery', *British Journal of Obstetrics and Gynaecology*, no. 90, 1983, pp. 1107–12.

38. Helen Marieskind. 'An Evaluation of Cesarean Section in the United States', Report submitted to the Department of Health, Education and Welfare, June 1979; National Institutes of Health, *Report of the Task Force, Cesarean Childbirth*. NIH Publication no. 82–2067, October 1981, p. 25. Also see Jeanne Guillemin. 'Babies by Cesarean: Who Chooses, Who Controls?' The Hastings Center Report, vol. 11, no. 3, June 1981, pp. 15–18.

39. Alison McFarlane and Miranda Mugford. 'An Epidemic of Caesareans', *Journal of Maternal and Child Health*, February 1986.

40. M.P.M. Richards. 'Caesarean Birth and the Development of Children', *Midwife, Health Visitor and Community Nurse*, September 1983.

41. Catherine Boyd and Colin Francome. *One Birth in Nine: Caesarean Section Trends Since 1978*. London: Maternity Alliance, 1983.

42. J. Scott Palmer. Paper presented to the British Psychological Society's Social Psychology Conference, 1984, reported in *New Society*, 20 September 1984.

43. Haire, op. cit., note 36.

44. 'Some Mothers' Experiences . . .', op. cit., note 23.

45. Rosen and Rees. Letter to *The Lancet*, 13 November 1983.

46. M.P.M. Richards. 'Obstetric Analgesics and the Development of Children', *Midwife, Health Visitor and Community Nurse*, vol. 12, February 1976.

47. Haire, op. cit., note 36.

48. Holdcroft and Morgan. 'An Assessment of the Analgesic Effect in Labour of Pethidine and 5% Nitrous Oxide in Oxygen (Entonox)', *Journal of Obstetrics and Gynaecology of the British Commonwealth*, August 1974 (an early paper to give a 'current' statistic, see p. 481).

49. Sally Inch. *Birthrights*. London: Hutchinson, 1982.

50. Richards, op. cit., note 46.

51. From an article by N. Cooperman et al. 'Oxygen Saturation in the Newborn Infant', quoted in Doris Haire and John Haire, *Implementing Family-centred Maternity Care with a Central Nursery*, 3rd ed. International Childbirth Education Association, 1971, pp. iii–13.

52. Rosenblatt et al. 'The Influence of Maternal Analgesia on Neonatal Behaviour: 11 Epidural Bupivacaine', *British Journal of Obstetrics and Gynaecology*, no. 88, April 1981, pp. 407–13.

53. From a letter to *Peace News*, March 1976.

54. Letter to *Spare Rib*, no. 22, April 1974.

55. Dr Violet Russell in a letter to *The Lancet* in 1941.

56. *World Medicine*, 4 December 1974.

CHAPTER

20

POSTPARTUM

Rewritten by
ANGELA PHILLIPS

BECOMING A MOTHER

The months after having a baby are a mix, a real mix. Some days you love it. Imagine having the chance and time to roll on the bed and drink in the smell of a baby and find the tiny daily changes in a body your body made. Other days you're on a bus with a wet baby and a push-chair that's rolling down the aisle. You look at the neat, childless people in the other seats and you feel messy, clumsy, alone and in the way. I remember Mondays when I could barely shuffle between my part-time job and the sitter's, with the baby wailing in the car seat. Then Wednesday would roll around, she'd wake up laughing with her arms out, we'd sail through the morning and I'd come to work thinking, This isn't easy. But, God, does it matter!

Celebration and change surround the birth of a baby. But the new life isn't just the baby's – it's yours, too. Being a

mother can bring deep pleasure, intimacy and skill.

But in this culture, at this time, motherhood also challenges our well-being. As mothers, many of us assume the role of the 'all-time giver', and bury our own needs for adult company, nurturance, sexuality. Increasing numbers of us are under the chronic stress that comes from balancing the roles of mother, worker and lover. We neglect our own physical and mental health, even those of us who wanted children and who have the protection of enough income, help and closeness with friends or lovers. The strain is even greater for low-income and single mothers and for women who do not fit the motherhood 'ideal' (like lesbian women or women who do not want their babies).

Motherhood can be a time of insight. Birth gives us a new respect for our bodies. Caring for, playing with and cuddling children, we discover new dimensions to loving. Many of us wake up, as never before, to the politics of being women and care-givers. As we move between homes and workplaces, our own lives teach us the changes in housing, health care, wages and work structures that families need. Hours spent caring for others make us more concerned about what sexism, racial prejudice and nuclear weapons mean for the future.

When we move into the first year of motherhood prepared and aware, we can wrestle with the issues and take hold of the possibilities. In this chapter we present the stories, wisdom and strategies of many new mothers: women who had difficult and easy postpartum experiences, women who became mothers alone or with partners, women with male and female partners, first- and many-time mothers, mothers who worked at home and mothers who chose or had to take on or continue outside work.*

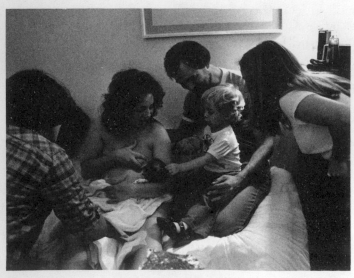

*In this chapter we have focused on the post-birth experience and do not discuss adoptive mothers' or stepmothers' transition to motherhood with older children (see Relationships, p. 199).

Suzanne Arms

THE POSTPARTUM EXPERIENCE

Many women describe three phases of postpartum experience. During the first days after delivery, we deal with the emotional and physical effects of having given birth. Over the next few months we learn what it means to be parents and adjust to life with a baby. Eventually, after daily life becomes more settled (usually in the second half of the postpartum year), we begin to face some of the long-term issues motherhood raises for us.

This doesn't mean, however, that you will experience postpartum in terms of defined phases or that postpartum ends when a year is up. You will probably have some of these feelings at various times and at various levels of intensity for years to come. Postpartum, like birth, is a very individual experience.

THE FIRST PHASE: TRANSITION TO PARENTHOOD

During the first few days postpartum we make the transition from pregnancy to motherhood. This is a time of enormous change; physically our bodies recover from birth and begin to nourish the baby; emotionally we may feel everything from exhilaration to exhaustion, uncertainty and sadness. Our birth experience may also affect how we feel, as may our readiness to become mothers and whether or not we have support from a partner, family and friends.

FEELINGS ABOUT THE BIRTH

If the birth has gone well and the baby is healthy, you may feel incredibly high, tremendously relieved and proud of what you have just accomplished.

Even though I'd had a long and difficult labour, I felt ecstatic after the baby was born. I wanted to leap out of bed and run around the room to celebrate. Then, after a couple of hours, fatigue caught up with me and I began to feel utterly exhausted. Every muscle and bone ached. Still, I didn't mind somehow. It was a good kind of tiredness – the kind that comes when you've been pushed to the limits of your capabilities. Along with the weariness came new, quieter feelings of peace, happiness, tenderness for my baby and a connection to all womankind!

But you may have other feelings, too, especially if the birth did not live up to your expectations, or if you encountered unexpected intervention or complications.

We had planned a birth with no intervention, and I had an emergency caesarean instead. Even though I was relieved that everything was OK and thrilled with my baby, I had the nagging sense that I had failed somehow. Later I got over feeling that it was my fault, but I still felt cheated out of the birth experience we had hoped and planned for. Sometimes I still can't help feeling a little jealous when I hear women talk about their wonderful birth experiences.

In the days following delivery you may think about the birth a lot, want to talk about it in detail and try to resolve your feelings about it. You may relive it over and over, perhaps fantasizing different outcomes for parts you feel ambivalent about. (See p. 413 for more.)

When your baby is ill your feelings of joy at giving birth may be mixed with agonizing fear and even anger.

When she was brought over later that day to me she was lovely. It was then that the floodgates of emotions opened and I couldn't stop crying. Why me, why my child?[1]

Within a few days after birth, whatever the outcome, you may experience the 'baby blues'. They can appear as anything from a fleeting sense of inexplicable sadness to a full-blown depression which temporarily incapacitates you. You may cry unexpectedly, feel worried about your lack of maternal feelings or frightened by the reality of the sudden responsibility thrust upon you. Many of us have vivid dreams and fantasies. For more on 'the blues' and more serious depression see p. 413.

SPECIAL CARE

Some babies are likely to need special care. They may need oxygen-controlled intensive care, possibly with the help of ventilators for breathing and tube (gavage), or intravenous, feeding.

The rate of admission to special care is about 7–10 per cent of all deliveries. In some areas there is an acute shortage of neonatal intensive care cots and sick babies have to be ferried to other hospitals as space allows. On the other hand, a few hospitals admit all small babies and those who have been through long labours or instrumental deliveries into special care units.

These blanket policies are being questioned. Edmund Hey, writing in the *British Medical Journal*,[2] suggests that babies over thirty-five weeks' gestation do not normally need special care unless they have problems other than simply a low weight. In Cambridge, even babies requiring tube feeding are cared for on a ward by their mothers' bedsides, unless there are special problems. After all, mothers automatically provide watchful nursing which a busy unit cannot easily supply.

In countries where few small babies survive due to lack of resources for incubators and a high rate of infection, it has proved possible to improve survival rates by caring for tiny babies at home strapped upright between their mothers' breasts. This position allows for good temperature control, constant stimulation, a ready supply of nourishment and less risk of infection. Survival rates are better in the high technology neonatal units in this country, but close skin contact brings other rewards.

> We have tried this with a number of mothers at the Hammersmith Hospital and have been encouraged by the pleasure of mothers who spend hours holding their tiny babies (naked except for a nappy) between their breasts. Relaxation of the mother and baby (and in some cases the father too) by this close contact seems to be very beneficial in families who have come through a stressful period of neo-natal intensive care.[3]

Even in hospitals without such policies, be assertive about staying with your baby as much as possible – your presence, your voice, your touch and your love will help your baby to thrive. All hospital staff should be aware of your feelings, encourage you to spend time with your baby, welcome your questions and answer them as completely as possible. This does not always happen:

> Nobody at all deemed it necessary either to talk to me or my husband about how I felt or what my child was afflicted with. Racism and prejudice are dirty words, but not dirty enough to be discarded. The only thing that helped me in achieving what I knew my daughter needed was by being assertive, by persisting until I got what she needed or at least a satisfactory reason as to why not.[4]

Very small premature babies will be fed intravenously but if you want eventually to breastfeed it is important to express milk at this stage to stimulate your milk production. The antibodies in colostrum fight the infections to which the baby can succumb. If your baby has not yet learned to suck, you can pump your own milk with an electric or hand breast-pump. Not all babies can be given breast milk.

Advances in neonatal technology mean that some babies as young as twenty-three weeks can be resuscitated at birth and kept in intensive care until they are mature enough to feed and breathe independently. However, the number who survive at this stage is tiny; most die on or soon after delivery.

For parents, the strain of coping with what can be several months of intensive care may be devastating[5] and we do not know what the long-term psychological effects on the baby might be. Follow-up research is under way but it is hard to keep up with the pace of medical change.

Many hospitals now have attached psychologists working with parents and babies and the organization NIPPERS has a network of support groups and can provide much-needed help and advice.

HAVING BABIES WITH DISABILITIES

Between 2 and 3 per cent of babies are born with a disability of some kind. These vary from non-life-threatening disabilities such as cleft palate and mild spina bifida to heart and lung defects which may be fatal. Surgery and other forms of invasive medical intervention may be required at a very early stage and, as parents, we may be called upon to make difficult and distressing decisions at a time when we are already reeling from the emotional shock of the birth.

As with miscarriage and death, discussion about our babies being sick or handicapped is usually taboo during pregnancy, even though many of us experience worrying dreams or fantasies about such a possibility. If the discussion of such fears were common practice during ante-natal classes, it would be much easier to call on our friends, teachers and advisors for support when the fear becomes a reality.

Surveys of parents of Down's Syndrome babies indicate that most are given too little information too late and often the information is provided in an abrupt and unhelpful manner. Nevertheless, the majority of mothers in a survey by Cunningham and Sloper felt that they had got over the shock within a fortnight (90 per cent within a month) and by the fourth month most reported feeling 'at ease with the situation' in spite of 'occasional days of despair'.[6] By this time many mothers may find that the major impediment to accepting their own situation is not their feeling about the baby but the lack of comprehension and support from those around them.

> In all of this, the hardest thing has been my own sense of isolation . . . Often I want to scream 'Why don't you listen to me? Why do you assume I need help to sort out my confusions when I'm trying to get you to consider your own ways of seeing?' I feel people want to talk to me about my problems. I want to say that the problems are theirs, not mine.[7]

The fear of disability which is engendered and nurtured in a society which puts less-abled people into ghettos makes it hard even for us to express our love for our less-abled children or to discuss positively their uniqueness rather than their inabilities.

> I remember my midwife said, it's like a cake, you put in all the ingredients for an ordinary cake but accidentally a little coconut falls in. It's still a nice cake, but it has a little extra. Well, I think that little extra in Melanie is love. She loves everybody and she is happy and smiling from morning to night. She seems to spread happiness around her, my children adore her.[8]

> Having a handicapped child can be an exciting adventure. Somehow his limits also free us from society's expectations. He is free to be and become a person with much more scope than the rest of us.[9]

In spite of the love and sense of uniqueness there are times when we need extra help in caring for our children. For a start we need information about the particular disability. Your GP should refer you to a paediatrician as soon as you feel sufficiently calm about the situation to ask for and cope with the information you need. You should have access to the paediatrician whenever you need more information. On a practical day-to-day basis a support group of parents with similarly affected children may be very helpful. More and more of these groups are springing up. Your local social services department or health visitor should be able to provide addresses of local branches. Your health visitor may be able to help you make contact with other parents in a similar position (in person or by letter) through the contact service in the *Health Visitor's Journal*.

PHYSICAL CHANGES AFTER BIRTH – TAKING CARE OF OURSELVES

For me, physical recovery was no big deal. Because I had an easy birth and no episiotomy, I healed very fast and felt back to normal within a few days. The only thing that bothered me was sore nipples (for the first couple of days) and night sweats, which lasted about a week. Otherwise I felt terrific. Maybe I was just high from the birth, but I seemed to have a lot more energy then than I do now, several months later.

For at least two weeks after the birth I was very uncomfortable. In addition to feeling the episiotomy stitches, my whole pelvic area ached, and it hurt to stand for more than a few minutes. I couldn't sit for a week! Even after I got home, I found I couldn't do anything. I hated the feeling of being helpless. Because I was in so much pain, I was very touchy and found it hard to respond to my husband or to the visitors who came to see me and the baby.

Our bodies undergo enormous changes after birth – a pregnancy in reverse. Your uterus will become firm, contracting often, reducing in size so that by the tenth day after delivery you will no longer be able to feel it above the pubic bone. Breastfeeding your baby speeds up this involution process by releasing the hormones you need to trigger uterine contractions and keep them going. (Sometimes milk not coming in can be a sign of retained placenta.) These post-delivery contractions of the uterus are often strong and may startle you, especially following a second or subsequent child, but they will ease within a few days. Resting with a hot water bottle on your belly will help.

In another dramatic change your blood volume is reduced by 30 per cent during the first two weeks postpartum. Under any other condition this loss would be felt as exhaustion, but many women are exhilarated instead.[10] If you do feel very tired or weak, you may be anaemic. Be sure to eat enough iron-rich foods and/or continue taking iron and vitamin supplements.

As the uterine lining breaks down, it is expelled in a discharge called lochia, similar to a heavy menstrual flow, which usually lasts from two to four weeks after birth. If bleeding is unusually heavy or suddenly resumes after this time, or if the lochia smells bad (a sign of infection), talk with your doctor or midwife. The immediate postpartum period is a time when infection can occur easily. Be on the lookout for signs – excessive bleeding, high temperature – that something might be wrong.

Many women find that after delivery, their pelvic floor and abdominal walls are very slack. Pelvic floor exercises (see p. 347) immediately after birth, followed by gentle abdominal exercises and leg lifts, will help restore your muscle tone.

It may take a while for your bowels to start up and become regular. Drinking a lot of liquids keeps bowel movements soft and helps prevent urinary tract infections as well. Eat high-fibre foods. Sit well back, press a pad folded in half against your perineum, relax and let your body take over. As long as you don't strain, you won't dislodge your recovering organs (a common fear), tear your stitches or aggravate haemorrhoids (varicose veins of the anus) which sometimes appear during pregnancy or the second stage of labour. If you have them, wipe them with toilet paper soaked in water or witch hazel after each bowel movement and take frequent shallow baths (with a strong brew of comfrey tea in one and a half inches of bathwater to promote healing) or the midwife can give you some cream, such as Anusol.

During the first twenty-four hours after delivery, apply ice-packs to the perineum, labia, anus, etc., to reduce swelling, and take warm baths (see above). Some midwives recommend calendula cream or Vitamin E to heal stitches and tears; others prefer keeping the area dry (a hairdryer helps) and exposing it to infra-red light for a few minutes at a time.

As your tissues rid themselves of excess fluids stored during pregnancy, you may drink, urinate and perspire more than usual. The sudden loss of oestrogen can also cause night sweats, which may last for several weeks after birth. (These are similar to night sweats at menopause.) Some women also experience 'hot flushes' during breastfeeding, as their milk lets down.

When you suckle your baby from birth onwards, and according to the baby's demand for food, engorgement (painful swelling of breasts) will probably not occur. If you are not feeding frequently, your breasts may become markedly engorged when your milk first comes in, during the second or third day after delivery. Feeding frequently (to keep the breasts empty); applying heat in the form of hot showers or compresses; and massaging the breasts (to promote circulation and letdown) should relieve engorgement quickly. Some women also recommend ice-packs for pain. Whatever you do, don't stop feeding!

Some hospitals give new mothers injections of

Bromocriptine to suppress their milk supply if they do not intend to breastfeed. Drugs are not necessary. If you do not breastfeed your baby, binding your breasts tightly will ease discomfort when your milk comes in and will inhibit the supply.

After a normal delivery you will probably be out of bed within a few hours. Getting on your feet soon after birth means fewer bladder and bowel problems and a quicker recovery of energy. This doesn't mean, however, that you should resume normal activities right away. Even if you are at home, or return home within forty-eight hours, it is very important to take care of yourself during these early days after birth. Resuming strenuous activity too soon can prolong the healing process and leave you feeling exhausted a week or two later. Even when you are feeling terrific, let other people take care of household chores and any other children you may have. If you are alone at home, ask friends, relatives or neighbours to run errands and bring in meals. You may feel overwhelmed by visitors. Feel free to put up a 'Don't disturb' sign if you are tired.

Our friends set up a great system. Each night for the first week they would bring over a pot of something to eat. But they liked to stay and eat with us. We had to be their hosts! Finally, we asked them just to bring the food and let us eat by ourselves. We were too tired for company.

You may be eligible for a home help. Apply to your local social service department or discuss this with ante-natal clinic staff who may approach the hospital social worker to arrange it. Home-help policies vary. You are unlikely to get one unless you have twins or are ill.

RECOVERY AFTER A CAESAREAN BIRTH

If you had a caesarean birth, you may feel sick and weak for a day or so, as well as very sore around the incision. As you cannot drink or eat, you will have an intravenous feeding tube (drip) and a catheter (to drain the bladder) for twelve to twenty-four hours. Many women find the catheter very uncomfortable; you can ask for it to be removed as soon as possible. Also ask that the drip be placed so that it doesn't interfere with feeding the baby. If you had general anaesthesia during the operation, your lungs will have accumulated fluid which must be coughed up. Raising your knees up to your chest may help you to cough painlessly. Many women also experience wind pains and/or constipation. Eating light, easily digested foods for the first few days will help.

After a caesarean, you should be helped to get on your feet within a day. Walking may be painful, but it helps you to get your digestive system going and avoid blood clots in your legs (thrombosis). Within a few days you can begin exercises which speed healing and restore muscle tone, but you should avoid heavy lifting and strenuous exercise for at least six weeks.

Because you have had major surgery, you will be in the hospital for several days, so it's important that you feel cared for during your hospital stay. Postnatal staff are often rushed and under pressure. They may forget that you have had a major operation and will need extra help, for example, with picking up your baby for feeds. Ask for whatever makes you feel better.

On the second day, I insisted on getting up and taking a shower. Washing my hair was a big step toward recuperation. It made me feel that I was taking charge of my body again. Exercising helped, too – I started stretching my legs and doing ankle rotations immediately.

You can expect to stay in hospital for about six days, or twelve hours after your stitches are removed. You should not be sent home until you feel ready. When you are feeling well enough, and have adequate help at home, ask if you can leave. If you want to leave early, and have enough help at home, your stitches could be removed by a district midwife.

FEEDING YOUR BABY

Most of us working on this book breastfed our babies because we wanted to and were proud that we could provide the best possible nourishment for our children. Even after returning to work, many of us found ways to continue breastfeeding. The importance of breastfeeding is continually stressed by all experts in the field. Doctors and midwives are, theoretically, committed to encouraging it. However, conflicting advice and lack of encouragement often leads to problems in establishing feeding. Sadly, midwives are still very quick to advise a bottle in the crucial early days 'just to settle the baby'. This advice may seem helpful at the time but it is rarely justified and can lead first to supplementary feeds and then to complete bottlefeeding.

On top of this, manufacturers continue to promote formula by sponsoring literature given to new mothers in hospital. Although they are careful to stress the superior quality of breast milk in the text, women who either cannot read or cannot understand English are often led to believe that these heavily-illustrated pamphlets are medically-endorsed encouragement to bottlefeed.*

There are social pressures too. Our society tells us (in subtle and not so subtle ways) that breasts are sex symbols and bodies are sex objects; we may feel embarrassed or uncomfortable about using our breasts to feed our babies. We hear that breastfeeding 'spoils our figures' or ties us down so that we can't resume work or other activities.

*The export of milk formulas to the Third World has caused many baby deaths. Mothers who can ill-afford to buy milk have been persuaded by advertising to switch to bottlefeeding. This is particularly dangerous when adequate sterilization is impossible and water is contaminated.

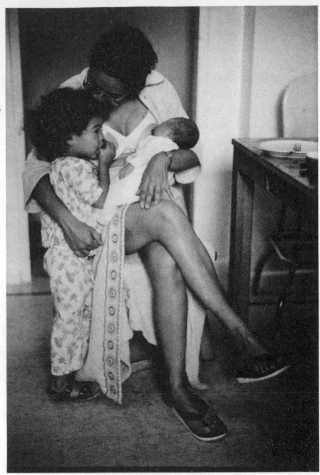

These myths serve to discourage women from making the choice to breastfeed.

Research shows that there are many good reasons to breastfeed and almost no reasons not to. Human milk (unlike cow's milk) is ideally suited to a baby's needs. It provides exactly the right balance of nutrients, which adapt to your baby's changing requirements. Even babies who can tolerate no other food digest breast milk easily. In addition, breastfeeding helps to strengthen the infant's resistance to infection and disease, something no formula can do. Colostrum, the liquid in a new mother's breasts before the milk actually comes in, is especially high in antibodies that protect the tiny newborn against staphylococcus infections, polio virus, Coxsackie B virus, infant diarrhoea and *E. coli* infections, the very germs to which infants are usually most susceptible. Breastfeeding also gives our babies a natural immunity to almost all common childhood diseases for at least six months, and often until we stop breastfeeding completely.*

You can continue breastfeeding for as long as you, and your baby, enjoy it. If you are concerned about allergies it is best not to introduce cow's milk or wheat products in the first six months. But if your baby seems hungry, you may want to supplement breast milk with solid food some time between four and six months.

In general, breastfed babies have fewer problems with infections, allergies, constipation, indigestion, skin disorders and future tooth decay than bottlefed babies. Breastfeeding is even thought to encourage better development of the dental arch.

There are practical advantages, too. Formula must be prepared for each feeding in sterilized bottles. Breast milk is economical and always available at the right temperature, and there are no bottles to carry around! In addition, the milk supply adjusts to the baby's needs; the more the baby suckles, the more milk the breasts produce. As the baby weans, the milk supply tapers off.

From right after birth, breastfeeding helps your body to expel excess fluids and tissue. Because the body burns about 1,000 calories a day to produce breast milk, nursing mothers tend to lose weight gained during pregnancy gradually during the first few months postpartum.

Finally, breastfeeding can be relaxing and sensual, close and satisfying. Some women become sexually aroused and even have orgasms while breastfeeding. This is because oxytocin, the hormone that triggers orgasm (and labour), is also responsible for the letdown of milk when stimulated by the baby's suckling. The breastfeeding mother and her baby have an intimate and interdependent relationship; many women feel extraordinarily close to their babies while nursing.

If you decide to breastfeed your baby, it is a good idea to have access to advice from experienced, successful nursing mothers. The National Childbirth Trust (NCT) and La Leche League provide just this kind of advice, plus literature and support groups. Breastfeeding is a learned skill that takes determination and practice, especially since most of us don't grow up among a lot of women who do it. You can solve most breastfeeding problems with patience and the right kind of support.*

Some women choose to bottlefeed so that others can feed their babies, and because it is easy to tell exactly how much milk the baby is getting. Occasionally women who want to breastfeed have severe difficulties which lead them to switch to partial or complete bottlefeeding at some point. If you decide to bottlefeed for these or other reasons, be assured that you can still have a close relationship with your baby. Whether you feed babies by breast or bottle, they like to be held close and cuddled during feeding. This physical closeness is important to the baby's emotional health, for it satisfies her/his need for touching and sucking, which is especially strong in the early months.

---

*Because of immunities in breast milk, some women delay having their babies inoculated against diseases until they stop breastfeeding. You might discuss this with your practitioner.

*Some common problems include difficulty with letting down milk and maintaining an adequate milk supply when the baby grows quickly. If you do have problems, we recommend consulting nursing mothers or supportive groups (such as NCT) rather than relying on doctors or midwives for advice. Few doctors or midwives are experienced and/or supportive enough of breastfeeding to be really helpful; many actively discourage women from breastfeeding if the slightest problem arises.

BREASTFEEDING UNDER SPECIAL CIRCUMSTANCES

There is no reason why women who have had caesarean births cannot breastfeed their babies, though it may be a little more difficult getting started if the mother is uncomfortable after surgery and/or the baby is sleepy from drugs used during delivery. Since sleepy babies find sucking difficult, some caesarean mothers choose not to take pain-killing drugs after surgery which will pass through their milk to the baby.

Mothers of premature babies can feed their babies.* If your baby is too small and weak to suck, you can express milk to be fed to her/him via a tube until s/he is strong enough. This takes enormous determination so don't blame yourself if you can only manage it for a short time. Even a few days will help your baby. If you are separated from your baby by a prolonged hospitalization, you can usually make arrangements to breastfeed part-time (see below).

With some exceptions, mothers with illnesses requiring medication can and should continue to breastfeed. If you are taking drugs that will pass through your milk to the baby, you and your doctor can often make substitutions, lower the dosage or eliminate the drug. Make it clear to your doctor that you want to continue to breastfeed your baby.

If for some reason you must stop breastfeeding (or choose not to initially), you may be able to reactivate your milk supply later by allowing the baby to suckle frequently. It may take some time for your milk to come in, and the process can be frustrating and difficult. Some determined women have resumed nursing weeks or even months after stopping completely. Occasionally, mothers of adopted children have even managed to breastfeed their babies successfully.

Mothers of twins can breastfeed successfully. The Twins Clubs Association's leaflet *Breastfeeding Twins* may help and Sheila Kitzinger who fed her own twins successfully provides helpful advice in her books (see Resources). The NCT publishes leaflets *Breastfeeding if Your Baby Needs Special Care* and *How to Express and Store Breast Milk*.

SHARING FEEDINGS

If you plan to return to work, want time for yourself or feel it's important for a partner or other members of the family to feed the baby, it is possible to establish a part-time breastfeeding arrangement, especially after the first couple of months. You can express milk (by hand or breast-pump), chill or freeze it (if it is not to be used within a few hours) and leave it for others to give to the baby. Alternatively, you may be able to find another mother who would be willing to breastfeed your baby while you are out.

If you miss feedings on a regular basis, be sure to express milk at the appropriate feeding times to keep up your milk supply. Remember breastfeeding is a matter of supply and demand. We know of airline stewardesses who express milk while they are travelling and breastfeed their babies on the days that they are home.

Some women find that expressing milk is a real inconvenience. Others have trouble expressing enough milk to keep up an adequate supply. As long as you are missing the same feed each day, your breasts will quickly adjust to feeding only at those times. In between you can give your baby formula or, after three or four months, wean her/him on to solids.

BREASTFEEDING AND CONTRACEPTION

When you are totally breastfeeding your baby (i.e. no supplementary formula or solid food), your menstrual periods usually do not return for seven to fifteen months after birth, because the hormones which stimulate milk production also inhibit menstruation. Breastfeeding, however, is *not* a reliable form of contraception after four to five weeks postpartum. It is possible (though rare) to ovulate and conceive before getting a period. Once you have resumed menstruation, you are even more likely to become pregnant.

Combined oral contraceptives are not advised because they may reduce the milk supply. (They also get through to the baby.) You may be offered the 'mini-pill' containing progestogen only. Although this will have little effect on your milk, no long-term studies have been done on its effect on the baby. Likewise, injectable contraceptives containing progestogen, which is also associated with postpartum bleeding, should be avoided. IUDs cannot be inserted for at least six weeks and a diaphragm (cap) cannot be refitted until six weeks. Sheaths and contraceptive foam will provide safe protection until then. See Chapter 15 for more on contraception.

TIPS FOR SUCCESSFUL BREASTFEEDING

In order to establish and maintain a good milk supply, you must take care of yourself. This means eating well (a pregnancy diet should be enough; see p. 345). Be sure to include foods rich in Vitamins B and C, iron and calcium. If you have been taking ante-natal supplements, keep taking them until your doctor advises otherwise. Don't try to lose weight at this time. The ten or so extra pounds you retained after birth will help your body sustain milk production during the first few months. In addition, sudden weight loss can be harmful: if your body is forced to mobilize its fat supplies, your milk may contain higher amounts of some of the potentially hazardous chemicals found in our environment and food supplies.[12]

Remember to drink plenty of fluids whenever you are thirsty. A good rule of thumb is to drink a big glass of juice, milk or water every time you feed. Keep one by your bedside at night, too.

---

*Research shows that the milk of mothers of premature babies contains more protein than that of mothers with full-term babies.[11]

Getting enough rest is *very* important. It is difficult for your body to produce increasing amounts of milk when you are tired and run down. If you feel your milk supplies are inadequate, try to cut down on outside activities and rest whenever possible. Some women also recommend supplemental brewer's yeast (which contains high amounts of B vitamins) or brown ale or stout (which contains yeast). You can also drink teas made from blessed thistle, chamomile, fennel or fenugreek seed thirty minutes before feeding.

Remember, whatever you eat or drink will be passed on to your baby via your milk. For this reason, it is wise to avoid caffeine and drugs* (including over-the-counter remedies). Also, don't take more than a drink or two containing alcohol.

SOME PROBLEMS YOU MAY ENCOUNTER

Sore Nipples

Some women have sore nipples during the first few days of breastfeeding. While hospitals often advise women to feed only five minutes on each breast at four-hour intervals, many women find that nursing more frequently actually works better because the breasts don't become engorged (see below) and the baby sucks less vigorously at the nipple. If your nipples do become sore, exposing them to sunlight and air whenever possible will help, as will sparing applications of calendula cream. Other ointments may contain ingredients that could be toxic to the baby. Check that your baby is latching on well. To feed properly, the underside of your nipple should go well into the baby's mouth (see Resources for books on breastfeeding).

Engorgement

When your milk comes in on the second or third day, your breasts may feel full, heavy and painful to the touch. In some cases, they are so full you may have to express a little milk by hand before the baby can grasp the nipple. Frequent feeding on demand often prevents engorgement, but if it occurs, hot showers or hot compresses made with comfrey applied before nursing will usually remedy the situation within a day or so (some women recommend cold compresses followed by hot just before a feed). By that time, your body will have adjusted its supply to the baby's demand for food.

Sore Breasts

If you have swelling, redness or a painful lump in one area of your breast, you may have a plugged duct, which can be caused by engorgement, infrequent feeding, tight clothing and/or stress and fatigue. Hot compresses, massaging the area and increased feeding will usually ease the discomfort. If the swelling is accompanied by high temperature and a tired, rundown, achy feeling (like flu), you probably have a

*Before taking any drugs, consult your doctor or midwife as to whether they are safe for nursing mothers. Contact the NCT for information about drugs to avoid while breastfeeding.

breast infection (mastitis). In that case, contact your doctor who will probably prescribe an antibiotic,* and make sure to get more rest. It is extremely important to keep emptying your breast. The NCT or your midwife may be able to lend you an electronic breast-pump. Keep feeding your baby. Rarely, a breast infection develops into an abscess that may have to be surgically drained. In most cases, however, early treatment will prevent this.

THE SECOND PHASE: ADJUSTING TO LIFE WITH A BABY

During the first few months after birth we learn what it means to have a baby in our lives. Many women describe early postpartum as a period of fragmentation and disorganization.

During those early weeks I felt as if I was disappearing. I seemed to exist only in terms of other people's needs. Sometimes I wasn't sure where the baby ended and I began. I felt that I had lost my old self and was too tired, physically and emotionally, to find her again. But I was also discovering a new part of myself that I hadn't known about before: unexpectedly intense feelings for my new baby, a resurgence of love for my mother, connection with other women. I went from despair to overwhelming feelings of tenderness, all within the space of an hour.

During this time we have to find ways of coping with the changes this upheaval brings about.

FATIGUE

Of all the stresses associated with postpartum, fatigue is the one mentioned by almost all parents. At some point most of us 'crash' under the pressure of night after night of interrupted sleep – some for only a short while, others for months, especially when there are other children at home and/or little outside help.

For the first week after the birth I was flying. I seemed to have plenty of energy for everything – my new baby, my husband, even the constant stream of visitors who filled the house. Then, one day, it just caught up with me. Suddenly I could hardly get through the day with two or three naps. By nine A.M. I was exhausted. In addition, my perineum, which was nearly healed, suddenly began to ache and feel sore again. My body was

*This may cause thrush in your baby. Be prepared for a nappy rash with little raised spots. It is easily treated with Nystatin cream from your doctor.

clearly sending me a message. When I slowed down and began to take care of myself, I felt better, but I never did recapture that initial high of those days after the birth.

The first six months of my third baby's life are a blur to me. Constantly tired and irritable, I somehow got through each day, but it certainly was no fun for us all. The older children (three and six) suffered from not getting enough attention. Because the baby was breastfeeding six times a day there was almost no time to take the kids out or even get through the daily housekeeping. I still feel spread thin most of the time.

Some physical discomforts also contribute to fatigue. Common ones which last two to three weeks after birth are sweating (especially at night), loss of appetite, thirst (due to loss of fluids and breastfeeding) and constipation. If you continue to lose sleep, you build up a backlog of REM* sleep loss, which can lead to emotional and physical disturbances. Your partner may also suffer the effects of sleep deprivation.

Some women get enough REM sleep even though the baby disrupts their usual sleep pattern. However, if you feel exhausted, getting someone else to take over one feed may allow you a long enough stretch of sleep to refresh you. Keep housework to a minimum and ask for help with it and any other children you may have. If possible, nap whenever the baby naps.

SEXUALITY

Some of us have little or no interest in sex for a while after childbirth. Others resume sexual activity fairly quickly. We each need to set our own pace.

Low sexual interest can result from having your life shaken up, feeling exhausted, having to take care of your new baby, a mate and possibly other children. You may need to be nurtured and cared for, too.

All that first year, our old forms of go-to-it sexuality were just too much. I was too tired and I'd fall asleep in the first five minutes, leaving Jack frustrated, even angry. Other times I'd have the feeding and holding of the baby on my mind and intercourse seemed rough and crude. Also, I think that by the end of a day I had had a lot of skin-to-skin rubbing and touching and didn't feel sexually hungry at all. But Jack hadn't had much at all. The unevenness of it all was driving us nuts. After months and months of snarling, we just had to invent 'middle ways' of being physical with one

another. I think I picked it up from watching each of us with the baby – the nuzzling and the snuggling that goes on with no expectation of orgasm, just affection.

Low sexual interest can have physical causes. If you had an episiotomy or tear in the perineum during birth, the area may be sore for several weeks. Your vagina may feel dry, lacking its normal lubrication because of lowered oestrogen levels (more common in breastfeeding mothers).

If the vaginal area feels OK and the bleeding (lochia) has stopped, there is no medical risk in vaginal penetration when you feel ready.

If it is uncomfortable, an unscented lubricant such as K-Y jelly or a clear vegetable oil may help. Be aware that some breastfeeding mothers also experience painful cramps during and after intercourse.

You can get pregnant again, even if you haven't had a period yet. (For a discussion of contraception, see Breastfeeding and Contraception, p. 408.)

LEARNING HOW TO BE MOTHERS

We may have grown up believing that because we are women, we are supposed to know how to care for a baby. Yet it is really experience that teaches us to be good mothers, including our own experiences babysitting or watching our mothers care for younger brothers or sisters. In the beginning we may be uneasy and afraid to trust our own good sense, especially with a first baby. Talking with other mothers about our feelings and fears can give us the confidence to try different things.

The first month was awful. I loved my baby but felt apprehensive about my ability to satisfy this totally dependent tiny creature. Every time she cried I could feel myself tense up and panic. What should I do? Can I make her stop – can I help her?

After the first month I got the hang of it,

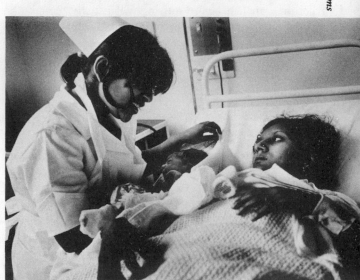

Suzanne Arms

---

*REM (rapid eye movements) are associated with dreaming, which occurs during the deepest phase of sleep and is believed to be necessary for physical and psychological replenishment.

gradually my love for her overcame my panic. I relaxed, stopped thinking so much about my inadequacies and was just myself. It was pretty clear from her responses that I was doing something right.

I didn't know how to change a nappy any more than my husband did. In fact, I may have been more nervous about it, since I was 'supposed' to know how. I learned to do it because I had to learn, and my husband learned, too.

Don't expect to love being a mother all the time. For instance, when your baby sleeps a lot, wakes up for feeding, smiles at you and goes back to sleep again, the baby business is a breeze. But when a baby is colicky (a catchword to describe baby discomfort, fussiness, crankiness) and cries sixteen hours out of twenty-four (that is not an exaggeration; one couple we know just went through forty-eight hours of constant wailing), your physical and mental powers may be stretched to their limits. There is nothing quite so jarring to the nerves as your own baby's cries. Watching the baby writhe in discomfort or pain fills a new parent with feelings of impotence, guilt and understandable anger. No amount of preparation can really equip you to withstand this calmly. But just realize that most babies are colicky for only a few hours each day – often in the late afternoon and evening – and usually outgrow it by around four months.

At around two weeks old she started crying from ten or eleven P.M. until six in the morning. We tried everything – walking, rocking, massage – but nothing seemed to help. Underneath I was sure it was my fault. One night, in desperation, Mark started dancing around the floor with her. I was so tired and they looked so funny that I started to laugh. Mark began to laugh, too, and the baby was so surprised that she stopped crying for a minute. It was enough to break the tension. After that, it seemed to get gradually better. I stopped blaming myself and realized that this was something she just had to go through, and all we could do was be there with her. After a few hard weeks she tapered off.

In many cases, colic is thought to be due to the immature digestive system of the baby.* Sometimes, however, an allergy to a protein in cow's milk is responsible. If you are breastfeeding, you can try to avoid dairy products for a week to see if it helps. Some vegetables (onions, garlic, cabbage, broccoli, cauliflower, brussels sprouts) and occasionally wheat are said to cause wind pains in breastfed babies, although there is no clear evidence of this. It's a good idea to avoid any foods to which you are allergic, as the baby may

also be sensitive to these substances. If you are bottlefeeding, you might try changing the formula.

You can try massaging your colicky baby's tummy, getting in a warm bath with her/him (heat often has a soothing effect) and offering weak solutions of chamomile or spearmint tea. The drug Dicyclomine – Merbentyl – is no longer prescribed for young babies because of dangerous side-effects. Beyond that, the only advice we can offer is to have lots of people around to hold and walk the baby so you can get away for a period each day. If you are alone with your baby this may seem impossibly difficult to arrange. Talk to your health visitor. She may be able to arrange some support for you. If you are afraid you could hurt your baby, put her/him in a cot. Make sure s/he is safe, go into another room and get away from the noise until you feel able to cope again. A lonely baby is better off than a battered one. Try strapping your baby on your back using a large shawl or baby sling. You may find that, as you walk around, the gentle rhythm and closeness calms her down.

Whether your baby is 'easy' or 'colicky', getting along with her/him may take some time and work.

OTHER CHANGES

Living with a new baby means changing our lives in many ways. We discover we are on twenty-four-hour call.

I was used to getting out of the house in five minutes when I wanted to go somewhere. Now it can take me an hour to get organized for even a simple expedition. By the time I've gathered up the nappies, blankets and rattles, fed and changed the baby and put her in the snuggly, sometimes it's almost too late to go. And if I ever want to go out alone, I've learned I need to start phoning babysitters a week in advance.

Many babies are unpredictable in their sleeping and eating habits for the first few weeks. Some breastfed babies continue to feed frequently and wake at night for months. We may be overwhelmed by the constant demands of baby care and find it difficult to get on with the rest of our lives.

I had been told that most babies ate every three or four hours and slept the rest of the time. Not mine! She wanted to feed every two hours and sometimes more often than that. Sometimes she would sleep for an hour, sometimes for fifteen minutes. I loved her, but I also felt consumed by her needs. It was hard to adjust to the fact that I couldn't get anything finished, whether it was an article I was reading or folding the laundry. At the end of the day I would realize I hadn't accomplished anything. Once I accepted the fact that I was not going to function at my old efficient rate (at least for a while) and stopped feeling guilty about what I wasn't getting done, I felt freer to enjoy the time I was spending with my baby.

---

*During the 1950s, colic was usually thought to be caused by maternal hostility to the baby. Some doctors still believe this. If your doctor questions your feelings about motherhood, switch to another topic. What you need is practical help, not psychoanalysis.

Some of us are reluctant or resentful about giving up activities we used to take for granted; for others, it's a holiday if we can stay home for a while. Though it may seem like for ever when you are living it, this phase passes. Within a few months, when the baby is older and on a more predictable schedule, you'll have more flexibility.

ISOLATION

For many of us, life with a new baby means coping with the monotony and isolation of long hours spent alone with an infant. This is particularly true after the first weeks when you do not work outside the home, the excitement of the birth event has worn off, friends and family no longer come around to visit and partners return to work. There may be day after day without adult company.

You can get very nutty from being alone at home. I get so that I invent errands. I go outside just to buy a loaf of bread, just to see people. I notice that the streets are full of people like me, mothers with babies in prams and buggies. I stand behind them in line and see how they try to engage in a bit of conversation because they want someone to talk to, just like me.

It is only in industrialized cultures that women are expected to 'go it alone' with children. In other cultures, postpartum mothers live among mothers, aunts, sisters and cousins and are able to draw on their time, interest and wisdom.[13] Many of us feel more connected with our own mothers after giving birth, but when we are geographically or psychologically separated, we may overlook them as an important source of help and affection.

Nancy Hawley

In fact, research into postpartum depression suggests that one of the most important protections a woman can have is a network of social relationships. For single mothers especi-

ally, family and friends are, as one woman put it, 'better than vitamins, more than money'.

When Alison was still a baby, I was in pretty bad shape. I didn't have to work; I'd dropped out of college. The man I was living with was having a real bout with drinking. It would have been worse if it hadn't been for one of my brothers. He'd come down to the cottage after school in the afternoon. We'd just hang out together. He adored both of my kids. I think he really took the hard parts out of being a mother alone.

When my baby was just a few months old, I joined a playgroup with several other mothers in the area. While the group was formed to get the babies together, its real function was as a support group for the mothers. It was reassuring to hear that someone else's baby was colicky and had been up all night and trade information and suggestions as to what we could do. It was also a help to share some of my ambivalent feelings about motherhood and discover that I wasn't the only one. I came to look on the playgroup as an oasis in what was otherwise a somewhat lonely existence.

If it's important to us, we can and should maintain our friendships with people who don't have children. But it may mean taking the initiative.

Before we had a baby, we used to go to dinner a lot with some friends. For a couple of months after the baby, they went on calling us on the spur of the moment. We couldn't get organized fast enough to find a sitter and go. They stopped calling. I missed them, so I called up and asked them to our house. Of course, the baby cried on and off, and they were put off. I could see what was happening, so I just said, 'This isn't working. How about you call us way in advance, we'll be able to plan, and we can go.'

There are other ways of avoiding isolation. Small babies are *very* portable, especially if you have a baby sling (a frontpack or backpack) or pushchair. As long as they are fed and changed regularly, babies make surprisingly good companions for almost any outing.

After a week, I was going crazy being alone at home with the baby. So I borrowed a baby sling and just took her everyplace with me. I learned how to nurse in public without being obtrusive, and discovered she would sleep anywhere – in the carrier, on the floor of a friend's house, in a shopping cart, even in restaurants and cinemas. Being mobile made me feel less confined and kept me in touch with the world.

NEGATIVE FEELINGS DURING POSTPARTUM

Once the full impact of living with a baby hits us, many internal conflicts, thoughts and fears may surface: I am supposed to be fulfilled because now I am a mother, but I feel ambivalent; I have to go back to work and fear losing touch with my baby; I have to be around all the time just to meet my baby's needs, so I don't have time for my other interests; I've lost my independence; I feel scared and inadequate – I need mothering myself.

All the time I was pregnant, people took care of me. But after the baby was born, she became the focus of everyone's attention, and I was reduced to the role of caretaker. I remember going shopping with the baby in the sling, and people would come up and say, 'What a lovely baby,' and never even look me in the eye. I was proud of my baby, but I felt a non-person myself. I wanted to say, 'I'm the one who cleans up the messes and gets up at night. Pay attention to me, too!'

We may feel angry at ourselves, our partner or our babies when we are particularly exhausted or isolated, or when we are not the perfect, nurturing, endlessly patient mothers we expected to be. Anger does not fit in with our fantasies about motherhood. But acknowledgement is the first step in dealing with our feelings.

I am a psychiatric nurse and therefore was aware of how angry thoughts about a baby postpartum are a normal part of the adjustment process. But I was unprepared for the enormous amount of anger I felt. I was angry about everything, it seemed. First, we had so carefully planned the conception (scientifically) of a baby girl, and I gave birth to a boy; then my sister-in-law, who had given birth six weeks before me, used the name I had reserved for my child for her baby. Then I realized how much my son resembled my father, who thirty years ago had rejected me. I also heavily identified with my oldest child about his displacement as kingpin. When I attempted to share child care with my husband, who worked at home, I found myself at the mercy of two schedules, the baby's and his. It wasn't until six months later that I knew my anger was dissipating. It was a full two years before I felt myself again. During this time I had obsessive fantasies about hurting the baby, how fragile he was, how easily I could drop him, how maybe I would forget him and leave the house, etcetera. I hated myself for such thoughts, but they persisted. It wasn't until I finally accepted the fact that a 'nice woman like me' could have such anger that the fantasies abated. Postpartum for me was learning to deal with more anger than I've ever felt
in my entire life. It felt like one long temper tantrum – unscreamed.

POSTNATAL DEPRESSION

In modern technological societies, almost every mother (as many as 95 per cent)* experiences periods (not just moments) of fear and depression. Almost a third suffer recurring depression. Up to two women out of each thousand experience depression which is deep and disabling enough to require hospitalization. Clearly we need information about postpartum depression in order to act to prevent it, to identify it, to cope with it in ways that will reduce its lasting effects.

Types of Depression

Not all postpartum depression is the same. The range includes:

1. *The 'baby blues'*. A several-day period of feeling weepy, frightened, uncertain or lonely, which typically occurs within a week to ten days after birth. In this type of depression the bleakness and fears do not persist, and can be dispelled with rest, relief from another care-giver, comfort given by a relative, lover or friend. Your interest in living and caring for your baby, your sleep patterns and appetites are undisturbed.

The birth of my baby was wonderful, but the next day I kept having the sense that something was missing, that I'd lost something in the process. Looking at my soft, flat belly, I finally realized what it was: I missed being pregnant. For days afterwards I found myself wanting to feel the baby kick. Even though I had a real, live baby to deal with, I felt hollow inside. It took a while to accept the fact that this baby was the same one I'd carried for so long.

2. *Mild depression*. In this form of depression, bouts of feeling unable, lonely or frightened reappear, and may make it difficult to eat, sleep, make love, work. The feelings may be provoked by a specific incident, such as your baby crying all night or a talk with a childless friend who seems so much more energetic and interesting. Depression may descend when you are run down or under pressure (when you have guests or a job interview). Periods of depression last up to several days or a week. However, rest, time away from the house and child care, or talking with someone who knows what it is like to care for an infant can break through the depression.

The six or eight months after my baby was born were hard. My physical energy started to return

*Estimates of the number of women affected and the seriousness of their depressions vary depending on the orientation of the researchers and the interview techniques they use. These figures are taken from Ann Oakley's *Women Confined* (see Resources).

when he slept through the night and more when he stopped needing a ten P.M. feeding. But my mental and emotional energy seemed to have disappeared for good. It was all I could do to get through a day. I took long naps and cried often. I got jealous about women my husband saw at work. I was out of touch with the me who had been an interesting, active and humorous person. Love him as I did, in some moods I resented my baby for even existing. To most people I pretended to be a 'happy, young mother', but I was quite depressed. I didn't know about postpartum depression, so I blamed what I was feeling on my own failure to be a good mother. I think I also blamed my husband, as though he could have made me feel better. He was worried about his job and resentful that I was too low to give him any comfort. He accused me of having a child and now 'not wanting one'. (He didn't know about postpartum depression either.)

A lot of things contributed to my feeling better. I began admitting to friends how bad I was feeling; I began a cooperative playgroup with four other mothers. Most important, I went to a women's health group and learned that many women are depressed for several months after childbirth. All of a sudden I knew it wasn't my fault. I wasn't a bad person for what I was feeling.

3. *Chronic depression.* If you suffer a serious postpartum depression the bouts of anxiety are frequent and last over weeks, even months. Under these circumstances, activities as basic as cooking, dressing and caring for your child seem impossible. This kind of depression is disabling – women suffering from it cannot get out of bed or out of their homes. The depression is not brought on by specific events but is the lasting result of feeling helpless. If you (or a woman you know) are suffering these feelings, it is very important to seek outside help from someone whom you trust – a family practitioner, your health visitor, a National Childbirth Trust contact, the Association for Post-Natal Illness (see p. 421) or perhaps a healer.

What Causes Postnatal Depression?[14]

There are two sets of theories about postnatal depression: one that it is basically hormonally based and the other that it is a response to a dramatic change in lifestyle. Those who stress the physical aspects of depression see the massive postpartum decrease in circulating oestrogen and progesterone as the trigger.[15] They point out that this hormone swing is similar to that which occurs in other high-stress situations such as combat. On the basis of these theories, postnatal depression is chemically based and can be cured by mood-altering drugs or hormones.[16]

This theory may have some basis to it but it does not explain the particular vulnerability of certain groups of women. Ann Oakley writing in *Medicine in Society* points out that:

In my study, degree of 'technology' used in birth was related to post-natal depression, not simply the blues for the first few days but a disabling, symptomatic depression appearing several weeks later.

The other factors which Oakley associates with depression are: poor housing conditions, little previous contact with children, lack of employment outside the home, lack of shared interests with the baby's father. She points also to the 'depressing effect of divergence between expectation and reality', noting that the vast majority of women questioned found that birth, pain and adjusting to motherhood had been different to what they expected.

Who is Most Likely to Develop Depression?

Those who are most vulnerable are women who for various reasons do not have a network of reliable support close at hand and a supportive, sharing partner; those with memories of loss (especially of parents) or childhood abuse which make them anxious about parenthood; those with a previous history of stress-related illness or who are physically unwell.

Coping with depression

Mothers who have been through it themselves make the following suggestions:

* Find a group for new mothers. These are often organized by the same people who provide ante-natal classes but all new mothers are welcome. Contact the local National Childbirth Trust, look on noticeboards at your health centre or baby clinic, ask your health visitor or community relations council.
* Ask your health visitor or NCT contact if you can talk to a postnatal supporter.
* Talk to a friend, specially someone who has been through it and can give you a 'long view'.
* Go out, with or without the baby, as often as you can. Make an effort to talk to other adults you meet.
* If you are alone at home try to find someone to team up with so that you can do household chores together. If you have a partner, don't take on all the housework just because you are at home more.
* Take care of yourself. Go to postnatal exercise classes, find an exercise class which has a crèche, eat well, make time to do something you enjoy even if it is just reading a book (instead of washing up) while your baby sleeps.

If your mood doesn't change you may need outside help. Signs which indicate you may need help:

* You have lost interest in doing anything on your own behalf.
* You have become dependent on alcohol or drugs.
* You feel suicidal.
* You have abused your child/children.
* You and your partner have serious, constant difficulties coping with the changes brought by parenthood; these

difficulties include long, insulting arguments, physical abuse, affairs that threaten your ability to stay together, desertion.

- As a single person, you find yourself so desperate for affection that you become involved in a series of brief relationships which drain your energy and self-esteem without providing the affection or comfort you hoped for.

If you seek outside help, try to find someone who will look outside as well as within you to find the cause of your depression. Someone who will take your depression seriously and will help you learn to be assertive and constructive about making the changes in your life that may protect you from later depressions (see Psychotherapeutic Help in Chapter 8, p. 127). Ask for recommendations through parent groups, women's centres, doctor or health visitor or a self-help group such as MAMA or the Association for Post-Natal Illness (see Resources).

CELEBRATING THE PLEASURES

I had heard about the negatives – the fatigue, the loneliness, loss of self. But nobody told me about the wonderful parts: holding my baby close to me, seeing her first smile, watching her grow and become more responsive day by day. How can I describe the way I felt when she stroked my breast while nursing, or looked into my eyes or arched her eyebrows like an opera singer? This was the deepest connection I'd felt to anybody. Sometimes the intensity almost frightened me. For the first time I cared about somebody else more than myself, and I would do anything to nurture and protect her.

We are surviving. Just. Why don't they give medals to people who can go without more than two hours' total daily sleep for five weeks? I thought babies ate at six-ten-two-six-ten-two – mine does. He also eats at five-seven-nine-eleven and four-eight-twelve. I am getting rather used to going around with my breasts hanging out. They are either drying from the last feed or getting ready for the next one. But the love – I never knew, never imagined that I would love him like this. This incredible feeling of boundless, endless love – a wish to protect his innocence from ever being hurt or wounded or scratched. And that awful, horrible, mad feeling in the first week that you'll never be able to keep anything so precious and so vulnerable alive.

THE THIRD PHASE: LONG-TERM ISSUES

For many of us there is a special quality to the later postpartum period (usually the period between six and

twelve months after birth). It is often a time when chaos, fatigue and uncertainty ebb away and a tide of confidence and energy washes in. This is partly because our babies begin to sleep through the night, eat solid food, take predictable naps in the morning and afternoon. For many of us it marks the return to paid work and, in spite of the additional strain, the feeling of independence adds to our self-worth. But this return to normal also comes from our own practising, experimenting and learning during that first chaotic half-year.

I was getting together all the stuff I needed to go out – you know, the blanket, the nappies, the toys. I did it very smoothly, thinking all the time about the different buses we had to take. 'This is it,' I said to myself. 'Being a mother is under my skin, in my brain, part of the way I pick things up and put them down.'

No matter how much smoother daily life becomes, parenthood alters practically all of our 'old' ways.

When I think back on it, adding a baby was like sending our relationship through a wringer and planting a garden smack in its middle – both at once.

Throughout the first year, adult caresses or conversations often lose out to a cry from the crib. Our partner becomes less a lover or a companion than 'the other babysitter'. Earlier in this chapter, we talked about practical issues in sexuality and child care which come up during the first months. Some deeper or more complicated issues arise as the people in a couple relationship undergo a gradual shift to parenthood. This is not an easy transition. First, whether we have children at eighteen or thirty-eight, we have to balance being a parent with all the other concerns of our lives, whether it's finishing our education, finding work or caring for our own parents. We discuss further how children affect our relationships in Chapter 11.

THE HEALTH AND WELL-BEING OF MOTHERS

There are plenty of manuals on health care for infants. But almost nowhere is there a discussion of health problems women encounter because they are mothers.

THE STRESS THAT COMES OF BEING A MOTHER

Caring for infants and young children is rewarding but *hard* work. If you have a child between one and three, you are doing something for or with that child about every five minutes, for as long as she or he is awake. Studies of stress have tended to ignore women at home with young children. Howell's studies of child care workers found that *six hours* marked the limit of an adult's patience and endurance when working closely with young children.[17] To avoid being worn down, we have to find ways of providing breaks, even holidays. This is especially true for those of us who are on our own whether by choice, through separation from a partner or because our partners are uninvolved;* it is vital that women at home organize to provide 'breaks' for each other through trading child care hours, playgroups, or sharing the cost of hiring a sitter.

Mothers experience a second type of stress. Everything from myths to current research has made us believe that a woman must always put her family's needs before her own.

> *Getting ready to leave in the morning is a good example. It doesn't only mean me getting breakfast. It means being sure that each of the kids has what they need: the oldest one needs lunch money, the middle one needs boxes for art class, the baby needs eardrops and the right blanket for daycare. But it also means to me that everybody should go away feeling loved and safe and ready. If one of them cries, I get to work feeling sad and like I failed.*

Researchers have repeatedly found that almost twice as many women as men suffer recurrent or serious depression.[18] Until recently this fact has been hard to explain, because men have been thought of as suffering higher levels of stress. Currently, we are coming to see that what men suffer are periods of high stress (e.g., job pressures, illness). What women, and especially mothers, experience is *chronic stress*, the continuing feeling that we must respond to what others ask of us, that we should, but rarely do, meet everyone's needs. All this may help make us vulnerable to depression during the postpartum months and throughout our years as mothers.

> *I have this dream that keeps coming back, since just a couple of months after my second baby was born. In it, I am caught in a wall, so that I am part of what is keeping the room from falling in on itself. In the room there are a lot of people – mostly family – eating and drinking. I want to come out, but they can't or don't hear me. I want to leave the wall, but I am caught and it seems like I am invisible to them.*

For as long as we nominate ourselves as what one mother called the 'universal shock absorber', we are bound to fall short. We have to give some of the responsibility to others,

whether through shared parenthood, community living or asking older children to pitch in.

WHO CARES FOR THE CARE-GIVER?

It usually feels right to be completely absorbed by a newborn baby. Once routines and basic skills are (more or less) in hand, however, it is essential to balance this preoccupation with an interest in caring for ourselves.

> *On a recent outing I started to hand out drinks, apples, raisins, and produce pullovers in and out of various bags. I had thought of my child's needs and his friends'. I had completely forgotten to include any food or drink for myself.*

Research on maternal health is beginning to show that we look after the physical and mental health of our children but skimp on our own well-being. We insist that our children sit down and eat a nutritious meal while we eat leftovers. We send children out to play, to get exercise, sunlight and fresh air, while we stay inside and clean the living room. After the stitches heal, past the six-week post-natal check-up, medical programmes usually ignore maternal health in favour of children's.

We may well spend fifty additional years – or more – in the bodies which gave us the children we so carefully watch

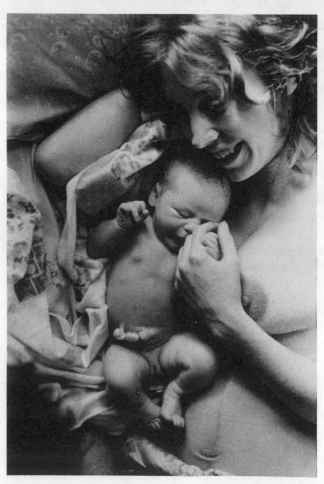

Jim Harrison/Stock Boston

---

*Many married women who are entirely responsible for the daily care of children live lives similar to those of single women, though they may have more money. Women who have distant or uninvolved partners may benefit from talking to single mothers about how they cope.

over. We have to stand back from the ideals of self-sacrifice and monitor our own health just as we do our children's: tooth for tooth, vitamin for vitamin.

THEORIES OF ATTACHMENT:[19] THE COST TO MOTHERS AND CHILDREN

Any time we leave our babies and feel guilty sinking sensations, we are responding to a cultural myth which states that any mother who loves her child should not be parted from her. Bowlby's[20] theories of maternal deprivation have caged women in guilt for thirty years, suggesting that any separation is traumatic for children and that group care is positively damaging. Psychologists have refuted his theories over and over again.[21] They point out:

1. Individual care by one person is the norm in only a minority of cultures. It seems unlikely that practices which are positively damaging to children would be so widespread.

2. Studies indicate that in the right environment children as young as one year old positively benefit from interaction with other children. Attachments to other children work best in small groups which meet consistently. Drop-in groups which do not allow children to become familiar with each other cannot provide a good framework for attachment.

3. In countries where it is the norm for mothers to go out to work there is no evidence of any ill effects on their children, providing the alternative care is of a high quality.

In spite of these findings our government continues to use outdated theories of attachment against the development of publicly-funded day-care.

BEING WORKERS AND MOTHERS

The real personal decisions and compromises involved in going to work while you have a baby at home are enough for any woman. Sometimes the baby is sick, some days she cries when you leave, other times you love her to bits. But the tangle of guilts and shouldn'ts and dangers that have come to surround making that decision has just got to be cut away.

For many of us the prospect of working when we have very young children is complicated both practically and emotionally. We have to find child care and juggle the double demands of home and workplace. We love and miss our children; we are afraid of being replaced in their affections; we want to know that other care-givers will care deeply, too.

These kinds of anxieties and questions are normal signs of caring. However, *the deep doubts and guilt that many of us feel in making and carrying out the decision to work are not a necessary part of being a working mother.* These doubts are our response to being raised as females in a culture which insists that nurturing, and especially child care, is 'women's work'. Of course most mothers do go out

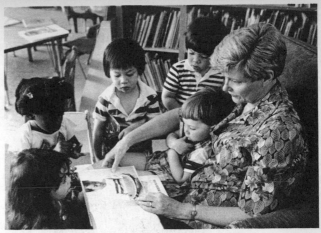

to work. However, in contrast to other industrialized countries, in the UK the majority wait until their children start school. This is probably because our government has presided over the most regressive policy on parenthood and work to be found in virtually any industrialized country. It has cynically manipulated our feelings for our children in order to try to force women out of the labour market while, at the same time, pretending to support equal opportunities.

While moaning about lack of parental responsibility for child care, our government has taken no responsibility whatever for providing the good-quality care that young children need. As a result many of us are forced to choose between affordable child care which we fear is not good enough, and staying home. Some of us are forced into years of dependence on supplementary benefit or on our partners. Most of us lose out in terms of lifetime earnings and career prospects.

Good-quality child care costs money. Without subsidies the majority of those who are employed work back-to-back shifts with partners.[22] Some persistent and energetic parents have fought for and won council funding for small community nurseries or company funding for workplace nurseries. A small number of parents are experimenting with co-ops which combine a voluntary rota and a paid worker. While we resent the pressures that force us into such voluntary solutions, we are glad of the opportunity to be involved with, and to monitor, our children's care. However, we are acutely aware of the fact that voluntary rotas and parent management committees also have a cost in time which many women cannot afford.

Until campaigning for child care comes a little higher up the political agenda, women who could be fighting for political change, taking better care of themselves, earning a living, will continue to be trapped in the day-to-day struggle of coping with the conflicting demands of child care and work.

WORK OPTIONS AND CHILD CARE*

If you are returning to work with a baby it is worth considering the following.

1. Negotiate a return to work on a part-time basis to start with. This will help you to balance demands and ease yourself back into your job. It may even be worth trading

*See p. 347 for maternity rights.

FINDING QUALITY CHILD CARE

What each of us wants from child care varies, but there are some basics:

- Care-givers must be responsive to children, even when children are tired or cranky. They must care enough to notice when children are unhappy, sick or needing new activities. Children are growing human beings and need more than just watching.
- The physical space should not be overcrowded, dirty or chaotic. It should include areas for resting, quiet play, active play.
- The experience should have variety: indoor and outdoor time; rest periods and playtimes. Even small babies need this kind of variety.
- You should be able to find out what goes on during child care hours, should be free to observe and to talk with care-givers about things which concern you and them.
- The environment should be safe: no detergents within reach, no open doors to the street, no stairways without protective gates.

Beyond these basics, choosing child care is a matter of what you feel comfortable with, can find, can afford. But whatever situation you choose, you must trust the care-giver.

As much as you want the child care you choose to be perfect and trouble-free, it is a human arrangement and requires attention, planning, looking after. Remember that the care-giver is a worker who has rights just as you do. S/he deserves reasonable pay, holidays, national insurance and consideration. Get to know the person(s) taking care of your child. Tell her/him what you know about your child. Ask them what they notice. If you have a feeling that something is not right, look into it. Talk to the care-giver(s), observe, ask other parents. If you are still concerned that the care is less than you want, get together with other parents to try to change the situation or find something else if you can. Try not to communicate your doubts to your child. Unless you have no choice, don't go for a stop-gap situation just 'to tide you over'. Multiple changes are hard on children and on parents.

---

the last month of your leave for two months working part time.

2. Investigate the possibility of job-sharing.* This practice is becoming more widespread because it allows you to work short hours and keep your place in the job hierarchy. Most other part-time jobs are routine, low paid and without promotion prospects.

3. Home working is often presented as a useful option for mothers. Be wary. Home workers are usually underpaid, work long, unregulated hours and suffer isolation which cuts them off from fellow workers and prevents any organization to improve their conditions.

4. Even if you have a longer leave, try to organize some kind of child care before your baby reaches six months old. Between six and eight months your child will go through a clingy stage which could make settling in a new environment more difficult.

5. Settle your child in gradually, giving her/him time to feel secure in the new surroundings.

6. If you are returning to a full-time job you may want to organize your child's sleep routine so that she/he is awake later in the evening to give you more time together. This solution is common in the black community where many mothers work full-time and people are far more accepting of children at social events.

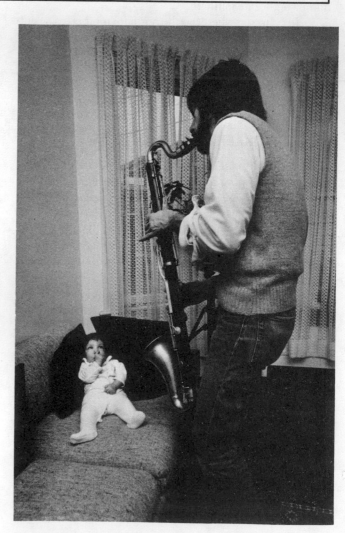

Jerry Berndt/Stock Boston

*Contact the Job Sharing Project, 347a Upper Street, London N1 0PD.

INVENTING A DIFFERENT KIND OF MOTHERHOOD

Having female reproductive organs need not and should not determine how we spend what could be the fullest period of our lives. Women will never be able to participate fully in society until society lifts some of the burden of caring from our shoulders. There are many ways in which the worlds of money and caring could be more equitably combined but so far it has not been in the interests of men or the capitalist system to make these adjustments. It is cheaper to con women into carrying the whole weight – without pay.

NOTES

1. GLC Women's Committee. *Women and Disability*, Bulletin, no. 26, January 1986.

2. E. Hey. 'Special Care Nurseries: Admitting to a Policy', *British Medical Journal*, 19 November 1983, p. 524.

3. A. Whitelaw and K. Sleath. 'Myth of the Marsupial Mother: Home Care of Very Low Birth Weight Babies in Bogota, Colombia', *The Lancet*, 25 May 1985, p. 1206.

4. GLC Women's Committee, op. cit., note 1.

5. Angela Phillips. 'Miracle Babies or Meddling with Nature?', *Parents*, no. 147, June 1988.

6. Cliff Cunningham and Tricia Sloper. 'Parents of Down's Syndrome Babies: Their Early Needs', *Child Care, Health and Development*, no. 3, 1977, pp. 325–47.

7. Jane Elliot. 'Born Different', *Spare Rib*, no. 106, May 1981.

8. Cunningham and Sloper, op. cit., note 6.

9. Elliot, op. cit., note 7.

10. Riva Rubin. 'Puerperal Change', in Nancy A. Lytle (ed.), *Maternal Health Nursing*. Dubuque, IA: William C. Brown, 1967.

11. *Breastfeeding Your Premature Baby*, La Leche Information Sheet no. 13, December 1980 (available from La Leche League – see Organizations in Resources).

12. Gail Brewer. *The Pregnancy After Thirty Workbook*. Emmaus, PA: Rodale Press, 1978.

13. Sheila Kitzinger. *Women as Mothers*. London: Fontana, 1978.

14. For an excellent discussion of challenges to older theories of post-partum depression, see Ann Oakley. *Women Confined*. Oxford: Martin Robertson, 1980.

15. For a discussion of these physical-stress or hormonal theories, see D. A. Hamburg, R. H. Moos and I. D. Yalon. 'Studies of Distress in the Menstrual Cycle and the Postpartum Period', in R. P. Michael (ed.). *Endocrinology and Human Behaviour*. London: Oxford University Press, 1968. See also J. A. Hamilton. *Postpartum Psychiatric Illness*, St Louis: C. V. Mosby, 1962, quoted in H. F. Butts, 'Psychodynamic and Endocrine Factors in Postpartum Psychosis', *Journal of the National Medical Association*, vol. 60, no. 3, May 1968, pp. 224–7; see the chapter on postpartum depression in Maggie Scarf's *Unfinished Business: Pressure Points in the Lives of Women*. New York: Ballantine, 1980.

16. See R. E. Gordon, E. E. Kapostins and K. K. Gordon. 'Factors in Postpartum Emotional Adjustment', *Obstetrics and Gynecology*, vol. 25, no. 2, February 1965, pp. 158–66; and V. Larsen et al. *Attitudes and Stresses Affecting Perinatal Adjustment*, final report, National Institute of Mental Health, USA.

17. M. Howell. *Helping Ourselves: Families and the Human Network*. Boston, MA: Beacon Books, 1975.

18. For more on stress and the effects of stress on women, see George Brown and T. Harris. *Social Origins of Depression. A Study of Psychiatric Disorders in Women*. London: Tavistock, 1978.

19. See Barbara Tizard. *The Care of Young Children: Implications of Recent Research*. London: Thomas Coram Research Institute, 1986.

20. John Bowlby. *Child Care and the Growth of Love*. London: Penguin Books, 1953.

21. Michael Rutter. *Maternal Deprivation Reassessed*. London: Penguin Books, 1972.

22. C. Roberts. *Women and Employment: A Lifetime Perspective*. London: DHSS, 1984.

RESOURCES
PUBLICATIONS

Anderson, Mary. *Pregnancy after Thirty*. London: Faber & Faber, 1984.

Arditti, Rita, R. **Klein** and S. **Minden** (eds). *Test Tube Women*. London: Pandora Press, 1984.

Asquith, Ros. *Baby*. London: Macdonald, 1988. A cartoon book to cheer up the early months of parenthood.

Association of Radical Midwives. *The Vision: Proposals for the Future of the Maternity Services*. London: ARM, 1986.

Badinter, Elizabeth. *The Myth of Motherhood*. London: Souvenir Press, 1982.

Balaskas, Janet. *Active Birth*. London: Unwin Paperbacks, 1984.

Balaskas, Janet and Arthur **Balaskas**. *New Life*. London: Sidgwick and Jackson, 1979.

Bampfyle, Heather. *Countdown to a Healthy Baby*. London: Collins, 1984. A guide to nutrition during pregnancy.

Beech, Beverly Ann and Ros **Claxton**. *Health Rights Handbook for Maternity Care*. Local government and Health Rights Project, 1983.

Beels, Christine. *The Childbirth Book*. London: Granada, 1978.

Borg, S. and J. **Lasker**. *When Pregnancy Fails*. London: Routledge and Kegan Paul, 1982.

Boston, Sarah. *Will My Son: the Life and Death of a Mongol Child*. London: Pluto Press, 1981.

Boston Women's Health Book Collective, *Ourselves and Our Children*. A book by and for parents. British ed. Michele Cohen and Tina Reid, London: Penguin, 1981.

Boyd, Catherine and Lea **Sellers**. *The British Way of Birth*. London: Pan, 1982.

Breen, Dana. *The Birth of a First Child – Towards an Understanding of Femininity*. London: Tavistock, 1975.

Brewer, G. and T. **Brewer**. *What Every Pregnant Woman Should Know*. London: Penguin Books, 1977. A book about diet and drugs in pregnancy.

Chard, Tim and Martin **Richards**. *Benefits and Hazards of the New Obstetrics*. London: SIM Publications with Heinemann, 1977. Very sound introduction to many of the controversies and, though written for a medical audience, has many chapters which are not too difficult to read.

Comport, Maggie. *Towards Happy Motherhood. Understanding Post-natal Depression*. London: Corgi, 1987.

Dale, Barbara and Joanna **Roebert**. *Exercises for Childbirth*. London: Century, 1985.

Dalton, Katharina. *Depression after Childbirth*. Oxford: OUP, 1985. She sees postnatal depression as a hormone problem and proposes hormone treatment for it.

Donnison, Jean. *Midwives and Medical Men*. London: Heinemann, 1977. A history of inter-professional rivalries and women's rights.

Elbourne, Diana. *Is the Baby All Right? – Current Trends in British Perinatal Health*. London: Junction Books, 1981.

Evans, R. and I. **Durwood**. *Maternity Rights Handbook*. London: Penguin Books, 1984.

Flint, Caroline. *Sensitive Midwifery*. London: Heinemann, 1986. A must for radical midwives and a great help to birth partners.

Gaskin, Ina May. *Spiritual Midwifery*. Granby, Mass.: Bergin and Garvey, 1982 (available from Compendium Books, 234 High Street, London NW1).

Grey, Pat. *Crying Babies*. London: Wisebuy, 1987. A complete guide for distraught parents.

Hughes, Mayall, Moss, Perry, Petrie, Pinkerton. *Nurseries Now.* London: Penguin Books, 1980.

Inch, Sally. *Birth Rights: a Parent's Guide to Modern Childbirth.* London: Hutchinson, 1982.

Kane, R. *The Cervical Stitch.* London: Miscarriages Association, 1986. Women's experiences of pregnancy with a 'stitch' to prevent miscarriage.

Kitzinger, Sheila. *Birth at Home.* Oxford: OUP, 1979.

Kitzinger, Sheila. *Birth Over Thirty.* London: Sheldon Press, 1982.

Kitzinger, Sheila. *The Crying Baby,* London: Viking, 1989.

Kitzinger, Sheila. *The Experience of Breastfeeding.* London: Penguin Books, 1970.

Kitzinger, Sheila. *The Experience of Childbirth.* London: Penguin Books, 1970.

Kitzinger, Sheila. *The Midwife Challenge.* London: Pandora Press, 1988.

Kitzinger, Sheila. *The New Good Birth Guide.* London: Fontana, 1979. Based on women's experiences of different hospitals throughout the country.

Kitzinger, Sheila. *Pregnancy and Childbirth.* London: Penguin Books, 1986.

Kitzinger, Sheila and John A. **Davis** (eds). *The Place of Birth.* Oxford: Oxford Medical Publications, 1978.

The Know Your Midwife Report, 1987. Report of the continuity of care trial at St George's Hospital in South London. Available from 49 Peckarmans Wood, Sydenham Hill, London SE26 6RZ (£8.50).

Larbie, Jo. *Black Women and the Maternity Services.* Cambridge: National Extension College, 1985.

Leboyer, Frederick. *Birth Without Violence.* London: Fontana: 1983.

Leigh, Gillian. *All About Twins.* London: Routledge and Kegan Paul, 1983.

Loader, Ann (ed.). *Pregnancy and Parenthood.* Oxford: Oxford University Press, 1985.

Lux Flanagan, Geraldine. *The First Nine Months of Life.* London: Heinemann Medical Books, 1963. Beautiful photographs of various stages of fetal development.

Madders, Jane. *Stress and Relaxation.* London: Martin Dunitz, 1979.

Maternity Alliance. The Maternity Alliance is a voluntary organization campaigning for the rights of mothers, fathers and babies, and publishes the following leaflets and reports:

Maternity Action, their bulletin, includes news, features and comments on all aspects of maternity.

Money for Mothers and Babies – Know Your Rights, no. 1: guide to cash benefits for expectant mothers and parents of new babies.

Single Payments for Baby Goods – Know Your Rights, no. 2: a claim form and guide to claiming single payments for maternity needs.

Getting Fit for Pregnancy – Know Your Facts, no. 1: a guide to preconception health.

Pregnant at Work: a checklist for employers, personnel officers and trades union representatives.

Healthier Babies, Happier Mothers. Report of the inaugural conference of the Maternity Alliance, November 1980.

Is Poverty Affecting the Health of Babies in Tyneside? Report of a conference on the effects of poverty on the health and welfare of mothers and babies, held in Newcastle in March 1982.

It All Depends Where You Live. Survey on ante-natal screening for congenital abnormalities.

Maternity Care – Progress and Problems. Report of a series of four seminars on current issues of concern in maternity.

Maternity Alliance Annual Report 1983–84.

One Birth in Nine – Caesarean Section Trends Since 1978. Survey on recent trends in caesarean section rates in England and Wales.

A Bibliography on Health before Pregnancy.

At Work and Pregnant in the West Midlands. Report of a conference held jointly with Central Birmingham Community Health Council in May 1983.

Rights of Working Parents. A charter for improved health and employment rights for all employees with responsibility for children.

Multi-Racial Initiatives in Maternity Care. A directory of projects for Black and Ethnic Minority Women, 1985.

Born Unequal. Perspectives on pregnancy and childbearing in unemployed families, 1985.

Maternity Rights at Work. London: NCCL, 1987. (National Council for Civil Liberties, 21 Tabard Street, London SE1 4LA.)

Maternity Services Advisory Committee to the Secretaries of State for Social Services and for Wales:

Maternity Care in Action
Part I Ante Natal Care (1982)
Part II Care During Childbirth (1984)
Part III Care of the Mother and Baby (1985)
DHSS

McKenna, Polden and **Williams.** *You – After Childbirth.* Edinburgh: Churchill Livingstone, 1980.

Messenger, Maire. *The Breastfeeding Book.* London: Century, 1982.

Monaco, Marianne and Vicki **Junor**. *The Home Birth Handbook.* London: Souvenir Press, 1984.

National Childbirth Trust (see Organizations for address).

Pregnancy and Parenthood
Emotions and Experiences of Some Disabled Mothers
Mothers Writing about Postnatal Depression
Mothers Writing About the Death of a Baby
Nursing Beyond One (breastfeeding toddlers)
Growing Up With Good Food
Some Mothers' Experiences of Induced Labour (by Sheila Kitzinger)
Thinking about Breastfeeding
How to Express and Store Breast Milk
Introducing Solids
Breastfeeding – a Good Start
Breastfeeding – Avoiding Some of the Problems
Breastfeeding – Returning to Work

New, Caroline and Miriam **David**. *For the Children's Sake. Making Childcare More Than Women's Business.* London: Penguin Books, 1985.

Noble, Elizabeth. *Essential Exercises for the Childbearing Year.* London: John Murray, 1980.

Oakley, Ann. *From Here to Maternity – Becoming a Mother.* London: Penguin Books, 1981.

Oakley, Ann. *Women Confined: Towards a Sociology of Childbirth.* Oxford: Martin Robertson, 1980.

Oakley, Ann. *The Captured Womb.* Oxford: Basil Blackwell, 1984. A very jaundiced history of the medical care of pregnant women – excellent.

Oakley, Ann, Ann **McPherson** and Helen **Roberts**. *Miscarriage.* London: Fontana, 1985.

Odent, Michel. *Birth Reborn.* London: Souvenir Press, 1984.

Phillips, Angela. *Your Body, Your Baby, Your Life.* London: Sphere, 1985.

Phillips, Angela. *Who Cares for Europe's Children?* EEC, 1988. Short report of the EEC child care network.

Phillips, **Angela**. *Until They Are Five, A Parents' Guide.* London: Pandora Press, 1989.

Pickarel, B. *Be Fit and Healthy Before You Start a Baby.* Leeds: University of Leeds Press, 1984.

Polden, M. and B. **Whiteford**. *Postnatal Exercises: a Six-month Fitness Programme for Mother and Baby.* London: Century, 1984.

Price, Anne and Nancy **Bamford**. *The Breastfeeding Guide for the Working Mother.* London: Century, 1984.

Price, Jane. *Motherhood: What It Does to Your Mind.* London: Pandora Press, 1988.

Rakusen, Jill and N. **Davidson**. *Out of Our Hands: What Technology Does to Pregnancy.* London: Pan, 1982.

Rich, Adrienne. *Of Woman Born: Motherhood.* London: Virago Press, 1977. Discusses the meaning of motherhood in present-day patriarchal society.

Rothman, Barbara Katz. *The Tentative Pregnancy: Prenatal Diagnosis and the Future of Motherhood.* London: Pandora Press, 1988.

ROW (Rights Of Women) Lesbian Custody Group. *Lesbian Mothers' Legal Handbook.* London: Women's Press, 1986.

Royal College of Midwives. *Successful Breastfeeding.* London: RCM, 1988. Good, if rather prescriptive, advice for midwives and mothers.

Saffron, Lisa. *Getting Pregnant Our Own Way.* London: Women's Health Information Centre, 1986. A guide to alternative insemination.

Savage, Wendy. *A Savage Enquiry.* London: Virago Press, 1986.

Savage, Wendy and Fran **Reader**. *Coping with Caesarean and Other Difficult Births*. Edinburgh: Macdonald, 1983.

Scott, Hilda. *Sweden's Right to be Human*. London: Allison and Busby, 1982.

Stanway, Andrew and Penny **Stanway**. *Breast is Best*. London: Pan, 1983.

Wellburn, Vivienne. *Post-natal Depression*. London: Fontana, 1980.

Whiteford and Polden. *Postnatal Exercises*. London: Century, 1984.

Working Mother's Association. *The Working Mothers' Manual* (available from WMA, see Organizations).

Zentner, Carola. *Twins: the Parents' Survival Guide*. Edinburgh: Macdonald, 1985.

ORGANIZATIONS

Active Birth Movement, 55 Dartmouth Park Road, London NW5 1SL. Tel: 01-267 3006. Runs conferences and classes in 'active birth'.

Association for Improvements in the Maternity Services (AIMS), 163 Liverpool Road, London N1 0RF. Tel: 01-278 5628.

Association for Post-Natal Illness, 7 Gowan Avenue, Fulham, London SW6. Tel: 01-731 4867.

Association of Breastfeeding Mothers, 10 Herschell Road, London SE23 1E6. Tel: 01-778 4769.

Association of Radical Midwives (ARM), c/o Ishbel Kargar SRN, SCM 62 Greetby Hill, Ormskirk, Lancashire L39 2DT. Tel: 0695-72776 (up to 9.30 p.m.). Campaigns for shift to community-based groups of midwives caring for women and babies throughout pregnancy, childbirth and puerperium. Regional groups, national meetings and conferences; quarterly magazine.

Baby Milk Action Coalition, 34 Blinco Grove, Cambridge CB1 4TS. Tel: 0223-210094. Involved in international action to halt the commercial promotion of bottlefeeding and to encourage good and appropriate infant nutrition.

Caesarian Support Network, 2 Hurst Park Drive, Huyton, Liverpool 36 (for local group contacts).

Cervical Stitch Network, 15 Matcham Road, London E11 3LE. Publications, local contacts, support and information, for women who have had a 'stitch' to prevent miscarriage. Send sae.

Child Poverty Action Group, 1-5 Bath Street, London EC1V 9PY. Tel: 01-253 3406.

Children's Legal Centre, 20 Compton Terrace, London N1 2UN. Tel: 01-359 6251.

Compassionate Friends, 5 Lower Clifton Hall, Clifton, Bristol. Tel: 0272-292778. Counselling and support for bereaved parents.

Cry-sis, BM Cry-sis, London WC1N 3XX. S el: 01-404 5011 or (Scotland) 041 638 8602. For desperate parents of crying babies.

Disabled Parents Contact Register, c/o National Childbirth Trust (see below).

Foresight (The Association for the Promotion of Preconceptual Care), The Old Vicarage, Church Lane, Witley, Surrey GU8 5PN. Tel: 042879-4500, 9.30 a.m. to 7.30 p.m.

Gingerbread, 35 Wellington Street, London WC2E 7BN. Tel: 01-240 0953. Organization for one-parent families.

In Touch, 10 Norman Road, Sale, Cheshire M33 3DF. Tel: 061-962 4441. For parents of children with disabilities.

Independent Midwives' Association, 65 Mount Nod Road, Streatham, London SW16 2LP.

La Leche League, BM 3424, London WC1N 3XX.

MAMA, 5 Westbury Gardens, Luton, Bedfordshire. Tel: 0582-422253. Local Groups for new mothers.

Maternity Alliance, 15 Britannia Street, London WC1X 9JP. Tel: 01-837 1265.

Maternity Defence Fund, 33 Castle Close, Henley-in-Arden, West Midlands B95 5LR.

MIDIRS (Midwives' Information and Resource Service), Westminster Hospital, Dean Ryle Street, London SW1P 2AP. Tel: 01-834 3240.

Miscarriage Association, PO Box 24, Ossett, West Yorkshire WF5 9X6. Tel: 0924-264579.

National Childbirth Trust, Alexandra House, Oldham Terrace, Acton, London W3. Tel: 01-992 8677.

National Childcare Campaign Daycare Trust, Wesley House, 4 Wild Court, London WC2B 5AU. Tel: 01-405 5671/8.

National Childminding Association, 8 Masons Hill, Bromley BR2 9EY. Tel: 01-464 6164.

National Contact Register for Parents with Disabilities/Parents with Disabilities Group, National Childbirth Trust, c/o J. O'Farrell, 6 Forest Road, Crowthorne, Berkshire RG11 7EH. Tel: 0344-773366.

National Council for One Parent Families, 255 Kentish Town Road, London NW5 2LX.

New Ways to Work, 347a Upper Street, London N1 0PD. Tel: 01-226 4026. Mainly campaigns for job-sharing.

NIPPERS (National Information for Parents of Prematures; Education, Resources and Support), c/o Caroline Kerr-Smith, 49 Allison Road, Acton, London W3. Tel: 01-992 9310.

Pre-eclamptic Toxaemia Society (PETS), c/o Sharon Copping, Eaton Lodge, 8 Southend Road, Hockley, Essex SS5 4QQ. Tel: 0702-205088.

ROW (Rights of Women) Lesbian Custody Group, 52-54 Featherstone Street, London EC1Y 8RT. Tel: 01-251 6576/7.

SATFA, 29-30 Wolburn Square, London W1. Tel: 01-439 6124. Support after termination for fetal abnormality.

Society to Support Home Confinements, c/o Margaret Whyte, Lydgate, Lydgate Lane, Wolsingham, County Durham DL13 3HA. Tel: 0388-528044.

Stillbirth and Neonatal Death Society (SANDS), 28 Portland Place, London W1N 4DE. Tel: 01-436 5881.

Tay-Sachs Society, c/o Alan Harris, 17 Sydney Road, Barkingside, Ilford, Essex.

The Twins Clubs Association, c/o Mrs D. Hoeseason, Pooh Corner, 54 Broad Lane, Hampton, Middlesex.

Twins and Multiple Births Association, 41 Fortuna Way, Aylesbury Park, Grimsby, South Humberside DN37 9SJ. Tel: 0472-883182.

Working Mother's Association, 77 Holloway Road, London N7 8JZ. Tel: 01-228 3757.

Workplace Nurseries Campaign, 77 Holloway Road, London N7 8JZ. Tel: 01-200 0281.

CHAPTER

21

INFERTILITY AND PREGNANCY LOSS

Rewritten by
JILL RAKUSEN

INFERTILITY

Infertility is a life crisis. It is usually unexpected; often we don't know how to cope with the feelings raised by the experience of discovering we are infertile. There is an initial reaction of shock and denial.

I, like every other woman in this society, always believed that I would have children without any problems – as many as I wished, and when I decided it was the right time. Unfortunately, after four years of trial and error, tests, operations, etcetera, my husband and I are realizing that life does not always happen the way we plan it. I have found it quite hard dealing not only with our infertility problem but also with the reactions of people around me.

I'm sick of people telling me to 'relax', 'stop thinking about it', 'adopt and you'll get pregnant', and all the other wonderful clichés that, although said to be comforting, ring of insensitivity. Friends and family can never possibly know the pain that I feel inside, the anger and resentment I feel every time I see a woman walking down the street with a big belly. How could they understand? How could anyone capable of having children understand?

Often you find yourself putting off making decisions, or changes, because 'six months from now you will be pregnant'.

I stopped teaching five years ago to become pregnant. When that did not happen, everyone wanted to know what I could possibly be doing at home all day if I didn't have kids. Neither a mother nor a career woman, I stayed in limbo because I kept thinking, Maybe it will happen this month! I was drifting, and it is hard to believe so much time has gone by with just this single purpose in mind.

When women you know have children, it may be hard for you to relate to them. Feelings of envy, jealousy and 'why them and not me?' are common. Because holidays are so child-centred, they can become stressful, lonely and depressing times for you. You may feel isolated from friends or your partner.

My husband is disappointed with our failure to conceive, but he could easily accept a child-free life. He says he understands my feelings and sympathizes, but doesn't care to hear any more about the subject. His view is 'Play the cards dealt you' – you go on about your business no matter what. His disappointment is mitigated by involvement in a job he likes and other alternatives. I have not found a satisfactory alternative.

Infertility is not only a problem for childless women. Difficulty in conceiving a second or subsequent baby is not uncommon.

I didn't feel I had the same right to grieve as a woman who had no children. Yet the loss seemed particularly intense because I knew what it was that I was losing. I was being denied the pleasure of holding my own baby in my arms again. I could feel what it felt like but I couldn't have it. All I had learned about mothering would be wasted. For fifteen months my life seemed to have been suspended while I waited to fill the hole inside me.

Anger is a common feeling, but it is hard to know where and towards whom to direct it. We tend to look for a reason for our infertility. We may feel that something we did in the past caused our present inability to conceive. Some people irrationally think that masturbation, unusual sex practices, etc., have caused this form of 'punishment'. They do not cause infertility, but our minds can trick us into believing it and make us feel terribly guilty. Or we may feel that we are to blame because we had an abortion. As we discuss in the abortion chapter, while abortion *can* result in infertility, this is very rare, unless the abortion was badly performed or wasn't carefully followed up.

Depression, sadness and despair are common.

I grew up surrounded by the idea that if you were willing to work or study hard and always did your best, nothing was beyond your grasp. Generally I have found this to be true. The theory fell apart when I began to deal with my infertility problems. Not only did I become very depressed, but without the help of a friend of mine who shares the same problem I seriously doubt whether my marriage would have remained intact.

It is only through a great deal of pain and anguish that I have begun to accept the idea that I may never have children. After the initial shock wore off, my husband and I became closer than ever.

I wish that more doctors dealing with infertility would address themselves to the feelings of their patients instead of leaving them floundering, looking for their own resources.

I'm tired, I'm tired of an empty, longing, aching heart that yearns to hold a little baby of my own. Oh, I've tried everything. I've tried praying, relaxing, furthering my education, working hard at my career, social clubs, church work, service work, slimnastics, cross-stitch – you name it, I've tried it. And I still cannot get rid of that aching, yearning, longing emptiness that can only be known by barren women.

Infertility is defined by most doctors as the inability to conceive after a year or more of sexual intercourse without contraception. The category includes women who conceive but can't maintain a pregnancy long enough for the fetus to become viable (able to live outside the mother). You have the right to seek help or advice whenever you begin to feel concerned about your failure to become pregnant. Infertility may be a temporary or permanent state, depending on your problem and on the available treatments. Many people are surprised to learn that infertility is not unusual. Commonly quoted figures are that between *15 and 20 per cent* of couples are infertile, although there are no reliable data on the subject (see Pfeffer and Quick in Resources).

CAUSES OF INFERTILITY

Fertility involves complex physiological events, some of which are poorly understood.

Male infertility may be connected with:

1. Problems of *production and maturation of sperm*, e.g. because of previous infection, such as mumps; undescended testicles; environmental factors (including chemicals in the workplace and drugs – both prescription and otherwise).[*] Extremely intensive exercise – e.g. marathon running – has been found to lower sperm count too; infertility has been recorded in some male Olympic marathon runners according to Professor Rose Frisch of Harvard Medical School. The effect is reversed when exercise is reduced.

2. Problems with *sperm movement* ('*motility*') – but little is known about what causes this.

3. *Blocked tubes* through which the sperm travel, possibly caused by untreated infections. (Vasectomy involves blocking these tubes deliberately.) Varicoceles (swelling of the veins from the testis) may also affect some men's fertility.[1]

4. *Inability to deposit sperm sufficiently near the cervix*, because of disability, impotence, premature ejaculation or malformation of the penis (e.g. when the opening is either on the top or underside of the penis instead of the tip).

5. *Poor nutrition and poor general health.* See Diet p. 425.

6. It is possible that *psychosomatic causes* may also play a part (see p. 425).

Female infertility may be connected with:

1. *Hormone problems*: failure to ovulate regularly or irregular menstrual periods may be due to a problem in the ovaries, pituitary, hypothalamus, thyroid or adrenal glands, or to the normal ageing process – as we approach menopause (see p. 454), we ovulate less frequently.[*] Women often develop amenorrhoea (absence of periods) following use of the Pill or Depo Provera (DP). While there is as yet no clear evidence that Pill-use can result in permanent infertility, it can certainly cause infertility for many, many months and for several years in women who are in their thirties and have never had a baby. Prolonged Pill-use seems to increase this risk in older women. Women who have irregular periods or who are older when they begin menstruating also seem to be more prone to this 'post-Pill syndrome'.[2] We do not know enough about DP to be specific about its effect on fertility. Sometimes fertilization does occur but low progesterone levels may mean that implantation does not occur, or the pregnancy is lost in the first twelve weeks.

2. *Scarring on tubes or ovaries* from endometriosis (see p. 485) or untreated infection due to STD (see p. 503), gynaecological procedures such as a D&C or abortion, or

---

[*]See Chapter 9, p. 151 for certain environmental factors; for information about drugs known to affect the male reproductive system, see *Out of Our Hands* by Jill Rakusen and Nick Davidson.

[*]Schwartz et al. found that older women tend to take a little longer to get pregnant than younger women.[3] Although they did not establish what proportion, if any, of women over thirty-five failed to get pregnant at all, this study has been widely referred to as indicating that women should get pregnant in their twenties or face infertility. This is not only groundless on the basis of the evidence cited, it also fails to take into account the negative effects of having a child early – see for example Daniels and Weingarten, who found that, without exception, couples who had their first child in their early twenties later wished they had delayed parenthood until they had developed as individuals and as a partnership.[4]

the use of an IUD (see p. 287). Even infection following childbirth can cause infertility.

3. *Abdominal surgery*: it is possible that some medical emergencies in childhood, in particular a perforated appendix, could be responsible for subsequent infertility, particularly if the emergency was not treated with this in mind. But there is more evidence that poorly conducted abdominal surgery (e.g. that is rough or unnecessarily damaging) is a cause. Dr Robert Winston, whose research has highlighted this problem, has found that a considerable proportion of infertility cases he sees are iatrogenic (i.e. caused by medical treatment). See *Out of Our Hands* for further discussion.

4. A *badly done abortion*, or as a result of an *untreated infection* after abortion (see Chapter 17). Abortion is widely believed to be a cause of infertility; while this was indeed the case when abortion was illegal, the risk of infertility with a legal abortion, particularly early abortion, is minimal, and with late abortion the risk is mainly due to cervical damage if the doctor is not careful.

5. *Structural problems in the uterus*, due to congenital problems or exposure to certain drugs such as DES and other hormones while being carried in their mothers' womb, can cause infertility in some women (by preventing conception or affecting the ability of the uterus to sustain a pregnancy).

6. *Other factors*, such as genetic abnormalities, fibroids, extreme weight loss or weight gain, excessive exercise (see Chapter 6), poor nutrition, stress and chemicals at work or in the environment at large may affect a woman's fertility (see Chapter 9). So, too, may subconscious feelings of fear or anger (see p. 425).

A couple may have a combination of problems which results in infertility. For example:

1. Sperm being unable to penetrate the cervical mucus; this problem tends to be defined solely as the woman's problem – the woman having 'hostile mucus' (which may be due to an infection like chlamydia or T mycoplasma – the treatment of which can often result in pregnancy). However, as Hull et al. conclude: 'The usual terms "cervical infertility" and "mucus hostility" are . . . inappropriate', except in unusual circumstances. They found that 'defective sperm function' is a frequent hidden cause of so-called hostile mucus.[5]

2. They may not know when the woman is fertile, how often to have intercourse during this time or what to do to make pregnancy more likely (see Self-help below).

It is thought that the causes of infertility are roughly equally divided between male factors, female factors and joint factors. However, in around 10 per cent of cases, it is not always possible as yet to diagnose the cause of infertility; when the cause is not understood (which may sometimes be because of inappropriate sequencing of tests) it is referred to as 'idiopathic infertility'. We must press for more research about the causes and prevention of infertility, and for recognition and application of future and existing know-ledge. In particular, the effect of 'environmental' factors on both sexes' fertility, including stress, drugs, chemicals present in the working or home environment, or in the environment at large, is largely unknown, but all are thought to be relevant, at least to some extent (see *Out of Our Hands*). We do know about certain drugs (e.g. people of both sexes who as fetuses were exposed to DES in the womb have an increased risk of fertility problems) and this can teach us lessons about other drugs and chemicals, many of which are used with little thought about long-term effects. Effects on fertility, for example, can take more than one generation to show up, but they'll only show up at all if they are looked for, and to do that accurate records must be kept and the will to look at them must exist.

SELF-HELP

Learning about Our Fertility

This can help a lot. Masters and Johnson stated that one out of five couples who attended their infertility clinic over a twenty-four-year period conceived within three months with no treatment other than use of this basic information: if your menstrual cycle is regular, whether it be long or short, you will probably ovulate fourteen days (give or take twenty-four hours either way) before the beginning of your next period. In other words, you should try to become pregnant on the thirteenth, fourteenth and fifteenth days before your next period. During these three days, spacing your love-making is important (see Fertility Awareness, p. 37). A man's sperm production decreases if he makes love too often, so you should have intercourse no more than once every thirty or thirty-six hours to keep active sperm in your genital tract during that period of time. Infertility clinics suggest a four- or five-day 'abstention' period in order to get a high sperm count.

Use no artificial lubricant when having intercourse and never douche afterwards. If lubrication is necessary, saliva is the safest choice. Your partner's penis should remain inside you until it has gone limp. Approximately 60 to 70 per cent of the sperm are contained in the first part of the ejaculate. Since it usually takes about twenty minutes for sperm to reach the uterus and fallopian tubes, it is a good idea to lie on your back with your knees elevated for about thirty minutes.[*] If your uterus is not tilted back, your chances of conception may be increased by having intercourse with your partner above and facing you, and a folded pillow under your hips to raise them.

You can also get a good indication of whether or when you are ovulating by using a basal temperature chart, and monitoring the type and amount of your cervical mucus (see Fertility Awareness, p. 37 for how to do this). You can then time intercourse to coincide with your fertile time.

Planned sex can really affect your sexual life. You have to plan intercourse around your menstrual cycle; it becomes

---

[*]Some women recommend douching with baking soda thirty minutes before intercourse to change the consistency of cervical mucus and make it less viscous, so that sperm encounter less resistance.

less an act of loving and pleasure and more a medically necessary response. Recording the times of your intercourse on a temperature chart may make you feel that nothing is private or sacred in your life any more!

> I started with the temperature charts. This was quite taxing for me, and mentally depressing. I felt very regulated and calculating, both with my own body and in my relationship with my husband. I need not say what it did to our natural sexual impulses. But a child at all cost – this was how we felt. My husband woke me every morning at six A.M. so that I could take my temperature. Afterwards he charted it. I needed his involvement.

Learning about Ourselves

There is some evidence that subconscious feelings – e.g. fear, at some level, of having a child – may be responsible for infertility. Dr Paul Entwistle has had considerable success in enabling such feelings to surface and be resolved through hypnosis – with ensuing pregnancies[6] – and it is possible that therapy, self-therapy or co-counselling (see Chapter 8) may be helpful in this area, as well as hypnosis.

Learning Relaxation and Similar Techniques

The link between stress and infertility in women with no 'structural' reasons for their infertility may sometimes be due to increased prolactin secretion. Although little research has been done on this, there is evidence to suggest that reducing prolactin levels by reducing stress alone may indeed help such women get pregnant, or doing this in combination with hormone drugs where appropriate (see p. 428).* Of course, the whole process of trying to get pregnant can be extremely stressful. Anything you and your partner can do at this time to find ways of experiencing inner peace and calm on a regular basis is likely to be helpful generally; it will help you cope with the pain and turmoil, and may even increase your chances of getting pregnant. *Self-healing techniques* such as visualization may also help. See Chapter 7 for further information.

Diet

Poor diet contributes to your stress too. There is also evidence that women who live on refined foods appear to secrete smaller quantities of the hormone responsible for ovulation than women who have a diet rich in unrefined cereals and fresh vegetables.[8] Indeed, a naturopathic approach has reportedly been successful. This approach assumes, for example, that the vaginal secretions can be affected by diet, and if the secretions are too acid, sperm can be destroyed. To ensure alkaline secretions, we need to eat a lot of vegetables (preferably raw) and fruit. Alkaline pessaries or solutions can also be used. If you have a constant, heavy discharge (leucorrhoea), diet can also deal with this. Kelso's *Women's Ailments* (see Resources, p.

441) recommends a specific diet along the lines suggested above, as well as other naturopathic ideas.

Women who are underweight may also find that weight gain increases their chances of conceiving.[9] In addition, it has been suggested that deficiency in 'essential fatty acids' can lead to infertility, especially in men. As their name suggests, these fatty acids are essential nutrients. For information about them, see Chapter 4. Some researchers also recommend that men with infertility problems increase their intake of zinc, Vitamin C and Vitamin E, as reported by the Boston Women's Health Book Collective. There is certainly evidence of male cases of subfertility responding to zinc supplementation.[10] At the very least, men, like women, should pay careful attention to their diet.

'Social' Drugs

If we take 'social' drugs, we can try cutting down on these, or eliminating them altogether. Drinks containing *caffeine* are associated with decreased fertility. *Alcohol* and *tobacco* are potentially harmful to sperm production, as is heavy use of *cannabis*, which also seems to be associated with irregular ovulation in women. Smoking in women decreases fertility – the greater number of cigarettes smoked, the greater appears to be the risk.[11] (Ex-smokers do not appear to be unduly at risk from infertility problems.) Heavy alcohol consumption may also impair fertility in women, although the evidence is mixed. (For more about drugs, see Chapter 5.)

SEEKING MEDICAL HELP

Ideally, ask your GP to refer you to a clinic which specializes in infertility and where the same doctor sees both you and your partner. Many family planning clinics run infertility sessions; you can refer yourself to these. You usually have to wait for an appointment at a fertility clinic – but it should not be more than three months. Clinics do not always offer help to all women; sometimes, for example, they will only see married women. If you feel obliged to go outside the NHS, bear in mind that private treatment does not mean better treatment, but it may mean getting help more quickly. The charitable, non-profit-making organization BPAS (see p. 442) is a good bet for single or lesbian women, and in general provides a model service, which the NHS would do well to emulate. For more on where to go for help, see Pfeffer and Woollett, and Pfeffer and Quick, listed in Resources.

Since, overall, the causes of infertility are equally distributed between women and men, it is obvious that in any couple the man and the woman should be diagnosed and treated together. If the man has the problem, then tests and treatment involving the woman alone have no value. A man, because of his anatomy, is easier to diagnose: semen analysis is one of the logical tests to perform first.

Everyone seeking help for infertility needs support – from partners (if we have them), close friends, family or an infertility support group. The experience of infertility can be very isolating. If at all possible, take someone with you to your appointments.

*In an as yet unpublished paper, Mona and Rory O'Moore of Dublin studied thirteen infertile couples who were taught autogenic training – a form of relaxation. It reduced prolactin levels and 'anxiety scores', and three of the women got pregnant.[7]

DIAGNOSIS

British clinics vary a lot in the type and quality of diagnostic tests they do. In some clinics the man is not even examined. This is an unacceptable way to investigate infertility. Make sure that both of you are examined and that full medical histories are taken.*

Though a sequence of diagnostic studies will vary with both doctors and individuals, it should include the following:

1. A *general physical examination and medical history of both man and woman.*

2. A *pelvic examination of the woman.* Your reproductive tract, breasts and general development will be checked for hormone balance. Tell your doctor about your menstrual history, its onset and pattern; about any previous pregnancies, STD episodes or abdominal operations; about your birth control history; about your sexual relations (e.g. frequency of sexual intercourse); about where you live and what contact you and your partner have (had) with chemicals, and about drugs either of you are taking.

3. A *basal temperature chart.* You may be instructed in the use of a special thermometer and chart, and taught how to record your temperature to see if and when you are ovulating (see Self-help above).

4. *Semen analysis.* Your partner ejaculates a sample of semen into a clean container. It must be kept at body temperature and examined as soon as possible under a microscope to determine the sperm count and motility. A count over 20 million sperm per cc is considered in the normal range; below 10 million per cc is considered poor. Yet doctors disagree about how to assess fertile sperm and men with low sperm counts *can* impregnate. If the sperm count is zero the man will be examined for blockage in his tube.

Ask to repeat the semen analysis at least one more time: the test is notoriously unreliable, not least because of ignorance in some clinics, and a man's sperm can fluctuate in count and motility for many reasons, including stress.[12] If the semen analysis continues to be worrying, your partner should pursue his own diagnosis and self-help strategy (see above) before you have further tests.†

Any diagnosis of infertility can make things difficult for both man and woman.

My husband's sperm count was very low; we were both crushed. I don't think my husband believed it was actually happening. In fact, he often talked in the third person, not truly accepting the results. I didn't know what to say. I couldn't say the typical 'Oh, it's all right' because we both knew it really wasn't all right. For some reason, I found I could handle a problem with myself but found it very difficult to handle my reaction to his problem. I was even more concerned that he couldn't handle his problem.

5. *Blood levels of the hormones* oestrogen, progesterone and prolactin as well as urine tests to determine your hormone levels and whether ovulation has occurred. Hormone tests are also done following treatment with certain drugs (see p. 428).

6. *STD tests,* particularly for chlamydia, which can cause infertility in both men and women. Make sure you both are tested for this (you may have to go to an STD clinic, see p. 488).

If all male factors are normal, you may have:

7. *Post-coital test (Sims-Hühner test).* Just before you expect to ovulate you have intercourse and visit the clinic within several hours without washing or douching. The doctor takes a small amount of mucus from your vagina and cervix to study whether, and how many, sperm have survived in the cervical mucus.

We were supposed to make love at seven o'clock in the morning and then I had to run to my doctor's for the post-coital test. Who feels like making love at seven in the morning during a busy week anyway?

I had to make two appointments for the post-coital because the first time he couldn't do it. They were very nice about it and said it happens all the time.[13]

Thankfully, this test is now becoming less common with the advent of a similar test – a *sperm/mucus cross-hostility test* – which can be done in a laboratory without one having to provide a sample following intercourse.

8. *Hysterosalpingogram* (HSG), which allows for direct visualization of the tubes and provides a permanent record that can be used for comparison if future X-rays are needed. Doctors usually perform this procedure in the first part of the cycle, before ovulation, to prevent possible X-ray exposure of a fertilized egg if conception has occurred.* It involves injecting a dye into the vagina and uterus which should pass up through the uterus to the tubes and out into the abdominal cavity. If it doesn't, it means that the tube is blocked, and that an egg is probably unable to pass through it. A series of X-rays are taken during this process. The dye then passes out into the surrounding cavity and your body reabsorbs it. This test can be painful, and it's a good idea to be prepared for this. Take someone who can take you home; learn some relaxation techniques to help you through it. It's also worth discussing pain relief with the

---

*See 'The Trouble with Infertility Testing' in Rakusen and Davidson, *Out of Our Hands.*

†It may be possible for the man's blood to be tested for anti-sperm antibodies, although this is a new area of research; antibodies can be suppressed by large doses of corticosteroids.

*But since all X-rays in the region of the ovary are potentially harmful to unfertilized eggs too, you may want to bear this in mind before considering this test.

doctor beforehand (it can be done under a general anaesthetic).

9. *Tubal insufflation (Rubin test)*. This is much less common than the HSG test. Carbon dioxide gas is blown under carefully monitored pressure into your uterus through the cervix. Normally it will escape out of the tubes into the surrounding cavity, causing shoulder pain when you sit up. (It is eventually absorbed into your body.) If the results are abnormal, it may be repeated or confirmed by X-ray studies. The Rubin test can indicate blockages but can't tell where they are located and can lead to pelvic infection.

10. *Laparoscopy* (a hospital procedure) which allows direct visualization of the exterior tubes, ovaries, exterior of the uterus and the surrounding cavities (see p. 596) and can yield a great deal of information, such as whether you have small pieces of endometriosis at critical sites; treatment for this may lead to pregnancy. Sometimes a dye is pumped into the uterus during laparoscopy, to see if it can pass through the tubes and out into the pelvic cavity (see HSG above).

Feelings about Going for Tests

Clinics tend to be very pressured and you may rarely see the same doctor twice. Some tests can be painful, and they can also leave us feeling undignified and emotionally exhausted and depressed. It takes a lot of strength to go through some or all of the above tests. A good, supportive doctor makes a difference; try to change your GP if yours isn't. Relatives may not be too helpful either:

My parents and parents-in-law want grandchildren and make me feel a failure because I'm not producing them. My husband wants children very badly and sometimes reminds me that other women could provide him with them. I always feel guilty about my jealousy whenever any of my friends becomes pregnant.

Jane and Ann had very similar experiences and feelings, and derived much support from each other when they discovered that they were not alone.

Jane: *Just decided we'd like kids and thought we ought to go ahead straight away, as I was twenty-eight. As the months went by, the worry and tension mounted. I was worried anyway as I'd always taken lots of risks and nothing had ever happened, and I'd had gonorrhoea and knew this could cause infertility. The doctor wouldn't help, as I wasn't married and he said my fellow would leave me, and if I had a baby it would grow up homosexual! The FPA told me I'd got to try for at least two years before they'd begin investigating although I was worried about my age. I kept getting ill with other things, and eventually saw a partner of my doctor who was sympathetic and could see the worry was affecting my health and who referred me to the infertility clinic.*

The tests were terrible and long drawn out – well over a year. Never once were the emotional problems referred to. Each new test was a major trauma.

Ann: *My tests went on for the best part of two years. My overwhelming feeling was hoping something would be found – I couldn't even be treated if there was nothing wrong.*

For both Jane and Ann, sex became very difficult.

Ann: *This was one of the worst aspects, so dominated by the idea of reproduction it ceased to be an expression of anything for each other and became much more mechanical.*

Jane: *Quarrels assume enormous proportions when they mean you don't make love on the crucial day, or terrible bitterness is caused when your partner just doesn't feel like it on the crucial day.*

Ann: *The other side of it is quite as bad – if you don't feel sexy on the 'right' day – it becomes dominant enough to turn you off anyway. That causes huge problems with any other relationships too. I didn't know which came first: the totally unexpected feeling of jealousy or the idea that someone other than I might conceive by my husband. It totally squashed any ideas or practice we'd had of not being exclusive – I couldn't face using contraceptives (emotionally) at that time and couldn't do to him what I couldn't face and get pregnant by someone else. And the aftermath – it must have been nearly two years after the last tests before I felt really relaxed and spontaneous about sex again, which used to be good before it had to be functional.*

Not all people feel the pain of living through this period with equal intensity. With luck we can call on help from our partners, and can find support from close friends, family or an infertility support group.* But we need to be prepared for investigations and/or treatment to go on for many years. Here, a woman GP who has herself had to come to terms with being infertile speaks:

It is easy to let the tests and procedures take over your life, and to lose your other interests. This is a pity even if you eventually succeed in having a child; if you don't, it can be a disaster. So while you are undergoing tests and treatment, it's a good idea to make a conscious effort to develop other

---

*The National Association for the Childless sees as one of its main functions the support of people going through tests and treatment for infertility. The WHRRIC can also put you in touch with support groups. For addresses see p. 442.

sides of yourself – perhaps your career, perhaps a hobby, or a network of friendships. If you end up with a child, you'll have more to offer as a parent; if you don't, your life won't feel as empty.

TREATMENT

In this section we focus solely on 'orthodox' treatment. We cannot discuss 'alternative' approaches in any depth because so little research has been done in this area. This does not mean, of course, that any alternative practitioner's claims of success are necessarily bogus, but it is impossible to assess effectiveness without adequate research. Nevertheless, most 'alternative' systems and techniques, if practised well, aim to improve our general health and well-being – which can, theoretically at least, have spin-offs for our infertility and in any case are potentially worthwhile in their own terms.

I knew I couldn't cope with batteries of tests and medication. I felt the need to harmonize my body and allopathic treatment would do the opposite. I don't know whether it was the acupuncture that restored my fertility or whether the feeling of well-being simply made me feel relaxed enough to conceive. Maybe it was just a matter of time. But the treatment certainly made me feel better.

Most 'alternative' systems also have something to offer us in relation to stress (see Chapter 7).

Turning to orthodox medicine, we also have to report that no controlled studies have been done which would clearly establish its value with regard to infertility either.*

In general, male problems have so far responded poorly to medical treatment with drugs, though surgery is sometimes successful. Insemination with your partner's sperm is sometimes used if his sperm count is low, in the hope that with careful placement of sperm, the chances of conception will be increased. This procedure is called AIH (Artificial Insemination by Husband). A method of separating out fertile sperm from others and inserting them directly into the uterus or using them for 'in vitro fertilization' (see p. 429) is currently being tested; it is too early to know how successful it is. If infection is causing a decrease in sperm motility, it may be corrected by antibiotics. Otherwise, AI (Alternative Insemination) is the only hopeful solution for male infertility (see AI, p. 432).

For women, treatment of hormone disorders currently offers the highest degree of success, although the advent of microsurgery means that many more surgical problems can be tackled compared with in the past.

Drugs

The main drugs to induce ovulation are clomiphene citrate (clomid), HCG (human chorionic gonadotrophin – a hormone extracted from the human placenta), and HMG (human menopausal gonadotrophin – extracted from the urine of menopausal women, who have very high levels of the hormones LH and FSH that induce ovulation); HMG is also called menotrophin, and its trade name is Pergonal.

Clomiphene citrate was introduced in the 1960s and is commonly used. It appears to act directly upon the hypothalamus in the brain and causes it to produce more LH and FSH. About 80 per cent of women will ovulate with the help of this drug, and about 50 per cent will become pregnant, with a slightly higher risk of multiple pregnancies.*

Potential side-effects of clomiphene include visual disturbances, abdominal discomfort, a throbbing feeling in the ovaries at the time of ovulation, hot flushes, nausea, breast tenderness, depression, weight gain, skin rashes and hair loss. Clomiphene can over-stimulate the ovaries (which can damage them): for this and other reasons, the British National Formulary recommends that 'It should only be administered under specialist supervision in carefully selected patients.' You should have a check-up at the end of each cycle to check that the ovary is not being over-stimulated, but this is rarely done; you may wish to ask for it and also to make sure that it is an appropriate treatment in your case (Pfeffer and Quick discuss the inappropriate use of this drug – see Resources).

HCG may be combined with clomiphene. It acts like LH on the ovary and helps the egg ripen and release. Side-effects include headache, tiredness and mood changes.

HMG is used to induce ovulation. It is a very potent hormone and should only be prescribed when other hormone treatment has failed. It requires particularly careful monitoring to avoid over-stimulation of the ovaries, possible rupture, and multiple pregnancies. This means that you might have to travel some way to specialist centres. It involves frequent injections and often daily visits to a laboratory for blood and urine checks. This can play havoc with your life, and employers are not always understanding.† Some doctors use ultrasound to monitor the development of the ovarian follicle(s).**

Bromocriptine (trade name Parlodel), introduced in the 1970s, is used if levels of the hormone prolactin in the blood are high (this occurs in a small minority of infertile

---

*Publicity has centred on 'fertility drugs' because they sometimes cause multiple births. If clomiphene is used carefully and the woman is properly monitored, it only increases the incidence of twins – at most. Pergonal has a higher risk (up to a quarter of pregnancies result in more than one fetus, usually twins).

†Following pressure from infertile women, one trade union has managed to negotiate an agreement for infertility leave on a par with maternity leave.

**The effect of ultrasound on the ovary is virtually unknown. There is, however, evidence to suggest that the use of ultrasound on ovaries around the time of ovulation reduces fertility somewhat. With regard to other possible effects, we are unlikely to know about them until the second generation.[15]

---

*Most infertility clinics appear to have a conception rate of 50–60 per cent. However, this is not necessarily due to treatment. One recent study found that over 60 per cent of infertile couples' pregnancies were completely unrelated to treatment.[14]

women). It appears that high prolactin levels can disturb normal ovulatory patterns. Side-effects of bromocriptine may involve nausea, dizziness, headache, constipation or drowsiness.

The newest development involves *LHRH*, the hormone that enables LH to be released (LHRH stands for LH-releasing hormone). Until recently, use of LHRH was ineffective; then it was discovered that the key was to administer the hormone in short, tiny bursts – mimicking the way the body itself releases the hormone. Several studies have now shown this treatment to be extremely effective for women with certain types of amenorrhoea (in one study, out of twenty-eight women whose ovaries had not responded to clomiphene, all ovulated, and all conceived, nineteen of them within three months).[16] In addition, the incidence of multiple pregnancies was low. Now that a convenient, portable pump has been designed, pulsatile LHRH administration appears far safer, simpler and, above all, more effective for suitable women, than gonadotrophins. Moreover, as *Out of Our Hands* concludes:

> Because this treatment so closely mimics the natural bodily process, in theory it is less likely than most to have powerful side-effects.

Problems in the luteal phase of the menstrual cycle may be treated with clomiphene, HCG, and/or natural progesterone.

Progesterone is given either as vaginal pessaries or as injections. Side-effects include weight gain, gastro-intestinal disturbances, breast discomfort and acne. Synthetic forms of progesterone (progestogens) are not advised as they can be harmful to fetal development.

Cervical mucus problems, depending on their cause, are treated with hormones or a form of steroid (not a common treatment; effects are fluid retention and masking of other infections). Special douches can help if the mucus is overly acid. Diet may help too (see p. 425).

Deciding on what treatment to go for, and for how long can be difficult.

> Only you can decide where to draw the line . . . Properly administered and monitored drug treatment for female infertility can be extremely successful. However, as with all medical technology, some doctors are better at using it than others. If you are thinking about drug therapy you should be aware of the potential complications and side-effects and be prepared to stop if these get too serious. Drug treatment is something of a balancing act in which you need to weigh the desire to have a baby against the possible costs.[17]

Apart from the costs to you, you may also need to consider the possible costs to the baby. As with all drugs taken during pregnancy and around conception, there is the theoretical possibility of causing damage to the fetus.

With regard to embryos resulting from drug-induced ovulation, it is possible that many may have limited potential for continued development at all.[18] In addition, there have been reports which suggest that clomiphene *might* be associated with fetal abnormalities.[19]

Surgery

Surgical techniques can often correct structural problems of the uterus. It is also possible that *dilating the cervix* may improve the chances of conception; this was discovered as a by-product of IVF (see below).

The development of *microsurgery* (involving the use of very fine instruments, guided by a microscope) has made it possible to try and repair blocked or damaged reproductive organs. Successful pregnancies following microsurgery are quite high at the Hammersmith Hospital in London (over 50 per cent for certain types of problem).* However, they have pioneered and developed the techniques at the Hammersmith and success rates are unlikely to be as high where staff have less experience; nor is microsurgery generally available, because doctors have been slow to pursue it. Instead it appears that they much prefer IVF, partly because to do microsurgery well you need to be extremely skilled.

Gamete Intrafallopian Transfer (GIFT) is basically a surgical technique that has been developed recently, where eggs and sperm are placed in a fallopian tube together, under laparoscopy (see p. 596). Obviously it is impossible if both tubes are blocked, but it has already been used with egg donation (see p. 430), for example, where women have had a premature menopause or had their ovaries removed. Birth rates with GIFT have been quoted as one in four in a *Lancet* leader,[20] but no reference is given for this figure.

Laser surgery, for example to clear the follopian tubes, could also be a possibility in the future – the first baby conceived following laser treatment was born in Glasgow in September 1988.

In Vitro Fertilization (IVF)

IVF involves a variety of procedures, so we are devoting quite a lot of space to explaining what is involved. By doing this, we do not mean to imply that IVF is a viable option for many women; indeed, there may be a case for pressing for the availability of more microsurgery than more IVF programmes.

In vitro is Latin for 'in glass'. At its simplest, *in vitro fertilization* involves extracting a ripe egg from the ovary, fertilizing it with sperm in a glass dish (not a test tube, as the media would have it) and replacing it in the womb. At the time of writing, it usually involves the following.

- Hormonal treatment with *gonadotrophins* (see HCG and HMG above) to get several eggs to mature so that more than one embryo may be implanted at the same

---

*The success rate depends on the extent of the damage. It can be as low as 10 per cent. Possible adverse effects of surgery also need to be considered: from anaesthetics (see p. 596), reformation of scar tissue or post-operative infections.

time which increases the chances of a successful pregnancy – see below)

- *Ultrasound* examinations (see p. 368) and hormone level checks, in order to ascertain when ovulation is about to take place (the eggs have to be collected just before they would normally be released). Ultrasound is also being developed to enable collection of eggs on an outpatient basis via the vagina – as opposed to on an inpatient basis involving laparoscopy (see footnote on p. 428 about possible effects of this).
- Removal of ripened egg(s) from the follicle in the ovary by means of *laparoscopy* (see p. 596); (the extraction procedure is not dissimilar to the procedure involved in *amniocentesis* (see p. 370).
- Placement of egg(s) in a sterilized dish containing nutrient solution, to which semen is added; the dish is then placed in an incubator so that fertilized eggs can start to grow.
- Several embryos (technically still conceptuses at this stage) are transferred to the womb in the hope that one of them will attach itself and continue growing. (This can possibly lead to multiple pregnancy.) The transferral process involves a similar procedure to inserting an *IUD* (see p. 287). Other embryos (if any) may be frozen and stored if subsequent IVF attempts are required. The first child from such frozen beginnings was born in 1984.

As with the initial stages of most technological innovations – from X-rays onwards – doctors have argued that the risks are negligible. They have been proved wrong many times, including in relation to X-rays, the administration of certain hormones in pregnancy, and numerous other procedures. It is difficult to ascertain what effects if any there might be from IVF and all the procedures involved. Many of the procedures (such as hormone administration) have themselves been used as infertility treatments for far longer than IVF, and we know little about their effects either. Doctors argue that if an egg or embryo is damaged during IVF, it simply won't develop. But we don't know whether that's true until thousands of babies conceived in this way have had a chance to grow up, and possibly reproduce themselves. As far as freezing of embryos is concerned, even less is known about the risks.* However, set against any possible risks to the fetus are (1) the fact that the timing of embryo insertion can be chosen so that it is most favourable for implantation (the administration of hormones can throw off the cycle), and (2) the lessened risks to the woman, who in the long run won't have to have a series of operations each time IVF is attempted.

IVF is usually considered only for a woman whose ovaries and uterus appear to function normally, but whose fallopian tubes can't function, although it seems to be particularly unsuccessful for women with endometriosis.[21]

It could, however, be used for a lot more women, including those with 'unexplained' infertility;[22] there have also been reports of some IVF successes where male infertility was the problem, for example because of inability of sperm to survive in the cervical mucus.[23]

You don't necessarily have to be married, but a male partner is required, and we know of no cases where lesbians have had access to IVF using donor sperm.

IVF is being practised (with emphasis on the word 'practise') in relatively few clinics, and it has a low rate of success. We can be forgiven for assuming the success rate is good because of the media hype, and also because the doctors involved tend to restrict their programmes to healthy women, usually under thirty-five, and carefully avoid talking about the numbers of *births*, restricting themselves to the number of pregnancies – which sounds more impressive.[24]

Usually it takes several attempts before implantation is achieved, let alone before it proceeds to a live birth, if at all, and the chances are lower for some women than others (so far, the success rate declines with increasing age). While many of us are prepared to come back if it is unsuccessful, clinics may limit the number of times a woman can try.

While IVF is arguably high-tech, it is certainly high cost at present, * and is mainly an option only for the well-off. It also causes tremendous upheaval, with daily, and sometimes more frequent, visits to hospital for tests.

IVF, though as yet possible only for a few, and successful for even fewer, opens up two more possibilities: *egg donation* which enables IVF to be performed using another woman's egg (the first such baby was born in Australia in 1984); *embryo donation*, likewise, is a possibility, where neither partner can produce *gametes* for the production of an embryo, or where to produce such an embryo would be genetically risky. (The use of a surrogate mother – see p. 436 – to carry an embryo conceived by another has been condemned by the Royal College of Obstetrics and Gynaecology Ethics Committee.)

These techniques mean that more than one man and woman can contribute to the many stages involved in creating a fertilized egg, carrying it in pregnancy and raising the resulting child. This brings up many social, emotional and legal questions. It is likely that pressure from religious, medical and political sources will aim to put tight controls on how this technology is allowed to be used.

INFERTILITY TREATMENTS: THE DILEMMAS THEY RAISE

The development of IVF, egg transfer, etcetera and future possibilities (see p. 613) has led to public concern and stimulated debate about the development of reproductive technology in general. As far as women are concerned, they

---

*The same applies to frozen eggs – if and when egg freezing is found to be successful (which may well be by the time you read this).

*However, as a leader article in the *British Medical Journal* (28 July 1984) suggests, eventually, IVF could be a cheaper way of treating infertility than current methods. Along the same lines, *The Lancet* (5 December 1981) suggested that IVF might eventually be possible on a day-care, outpatient basis.

herald the need to question afresh what the implications are when doctors – and possibly the state itself – intervene regarding decisions we can make about our own bodies (in the same way that both intervene now with regard to our right to choose abortion). While many of the Warnock Committee's recommendations are helpful,[25] they barely consider women's rights: for example, the committee felt the need to 'discourage' widows from using husbands' frozen sperm, and concluded that 'as a general rule', children should be born into two-parent families, with both father and mother. The report thus lends support to many current practices which are, by the time you read this, likely to be enshrined in law.

Yet despite the media hype about 'test-tube babies', the resources available for infertility treatment have been consistently very low, resulting in scandalously long waiting lists, and poorly coordinated research and treatment. Infertility is a low priority issue, and will remain so unless we make our voices heard – through organizations such as WHRRIC and the National Association for the Childless. It is particularly important now, with medical interest in the newer technologies, that progress is clearly in the interests of women. There is much glory to be gained by the predominantly male medical élite which is jumping on the 'test-tube baby' bandwagon, and this search for glory (which may well be connected to a more unconscious search for the ability to give birth) can all too easily obscure the issues as women might see them.

Medical approaches to infertility, as currently practised, represent yet another example of how doctors are developing high technology 'solutions' to the exclusion of:

1. improving their all-round services and developing an understanding of preventive strategies which could serve many more of us. For example, they could emphasize and promote the importance of good gynaecological practices, less damaging forms of contraception, and sheer good nutrition. Indeed, it is possible that many of us who end up wanting infertility treatment would not need it if we had known about possible causes and preventive measures and if our doctors had been more careful;

2. considering the effects of their treatments when they are unsuccessful – which is the case for many women, and the vast majority of us when it comes to such procedures as IVF;

3. considering the overall effect of their activities in support of the ideology of motherhood. Perhaps we would feel less obliged to put ourselves through semi-permanent emotional turmoil and what are often extremely invasive and at times degrading medical manipulations if a woman's worth in our society were no longer measured in terms of her fertility.

Approaches to infertility treatment can represent a technological fix for something that has at least in part been socially created.* Sometimes the treatment works . . . or

*This belies the question of how often we are told about the chances of success of any particular treatment.

we manage to have a child anyway. All the torment and treatment then seem worthwhile. But the very existence of sophisticated treatments, however slim their chances of success, can simply increase the pressure on us to try everything – with all the attendant pain and uncertainty that this process entails. It can make it all the more difficult to accept what may well have to be a fact of life for us.

> I used to cling to every story I heard about people having babies against innumerable odds, as I wanted so much to believe there was hope. It made adjusting to the whole problem so much harder.[26]

We also may suffer from the attitudes of other people, perhaps friends or family, if they see technology as the answer to our (and perhaps their) problems.

> *I feel trapped in other people's belief systems. It's like I'm not allowed to give up hope. But until I do I can't begin to really live again.*

And as a psychotherapist says:

> *It's very problematic helping people come to terms with infertility if a baby is something they might be able to have, however remote the chances are, if, say, they undergo IVF.*

Coping with living – as with dying – is painful. Technology can help. Sometimes. But if we look to it as the answer to our pain, we court disaster. It can create a prison for us, particularly if that technology fails us. Yet through our pain we can discover parts of ourselves, of others, of life, that enrich us beyond our wildest dreams. Maggie Jones ends her book *Trying to Have a Baby?* with the following quote.

> I remember walking up the hill – it was a bright day in early summer – after having the final results of the tests and thinking, that's it, I shall never have children. The thought gave me a lot of pain, but as soon as I had thought it, I had the sensation of a huge weight being lifted off my shoulders. I no longer had to go on thinking, if, when, somehow, if only . . . it was all suddenly settled. I walked past the children's playground on the corner of the street and two small boys were playing on the swings. I stood and watched them for a while, and again, I was no longer thinking, if only, perhaps one day, and feeling that familiar stab of jealousy; instead I was standing in the warm sunlight and listening to their high, clear voices with something approaching joy. Suddenly I felt completely washed clean, and at peace – and freer than I had ever felt in my whole life.[27]

We must try to ensure that any available medical help recognizes the problems that that very help creates for us. We need to ensure a more sophisticated understanding by the medical profession of the repercussions of infertility, and guard against their using their power (yet again) both to protect themselves from their own pain at being of such limited help and/or to exercise powerful control over us. We must guard against doctors playing god – not just in terms of wanting to produce babies themselves (consciously or unconsciously) but also in terms of deciding who 'deserves' their treatment. Doctors' 'power-tripping' over women is linked to all reproductive issues, not just infertility. The difference is that, with infertility, it can be harder to see what's happening because of the intensity and complexity of the emotional pain.

COPING WITH INFERTILITY

It is difficult and painful to acknowledge that our infertility is permanent. Particularly when there are no clear-cut medical reasons for infertility, it can be difficult to know when to stop the investigations and treatments, and to put away the thermometer. Feelings of hopefulness may give way to depression. We now have to begin to examine our lives. We may feel grief for the loss of a part of womanhood or manhood, for the parts of us that don't work or have been cut out of us. If we deny or repress this feeling of grief, we prolong the process of its resolution.* Somewhere inside we are dealing with the experience. We have the choice of living it as consciously and directly as we can or suppressing these very natural but painful emotions. The pain of infertility is never completely resolved but is accepted as a familiar ache which may recur, unpredictably, throughout life. Grieving often takes a long time.** The support of friends, family and other people who have experienced infertility can be helpful.

Last year I had a hysterectomy at the age of twenty-nine. Needless to say, I was crushed with grief. I never had the chance to have a baby and then all hope was snatched away. In my case it had to be done – fibroid tumours had practically destroyed my uterus (there were twenty-one, to be exact). I was very bitter for a while, but now I am healing. That is not to say I don't hurt sometimes; I think a pain this deep will always come back from time to time.

After learning of my untreatable infertility five years ago, I experienced the usual shock and denial. Unfortunately, I pushed down all other stages and feelings by submerging myself in work. Eventually we adopted a son and all seemed right with the world. I thought I had everything together, as I rarely thought of my infertility and was very active.

Then, for no obvious apparent reason, my infertility again became a prominent concern, and all the feelings I had submerged five years ago resurfaced. After four unstable months I ended up in severe, crippling depression.

Only with the help of counselling have I been able to begin to work through the feelings and to come out of my depressed state.

I share this only in the hope of helping someone else not to fall into the trap of thinking they have worked through to resolution their infertility, when in reality they have only dealt with the problem on an intellectual level. The pain of the past four months has been as intense as when I first learned of the diagnosis of infertility. I feel that somehow I failed myself because five years ago I was too frightened of the pain to face it. The truth is, it has to be faced sooner or later, and hopefully all the way to resolution.

It was relieving to meet and talk openly with other couples experiencing infertility. Each of us had our own specific difficulties but our feelings and reactions were quite similar. After the initial nervousness that accompanied our first two meetings, I began to feel much more accepting and able to deal with the previous two and a half years that had given us two pregnancies and two miscarriages. My almost constant obsession with pregnancy was lifted. I began to feel in touch with myself and somewhat alive again.

ALTERNATIVE INSEMINATION (AI)*

This can be used by single or lesbian women who do not wish to have intercourse in order to become pregnant, and also by fertile women whose partners are infertile.

AI is a technically simple procedure that can be done in a clinic or at home. A fertile donor male masturbates into a container (clean, preferably boiled and then cooled). The sperm may be frozen and put in a sperm bank, or it may be used fresh – in which case it should be kept at body temperature and inserted into the woman's vagina as near to the cervix as possible; as sperm die fast, insertion should take place as soon as possible after thawing or masturbation, within two hours at the outside. AI should take place around ovulation, so you need to establish this in advance (see Fertility Awareness, p. 37).

A clean, needleless syringe is usually used to insert the semen but women doing self-insemination on their own have used anything from eye droppers to turkey basters. The woman lies flat on her back with her rear raised on a

---

*Since we often need to repress our feelings in order to cope with infertility tests and treatments, it is particularly important to allow ourselves to feel them at some point.
**Some people immediately block this feeling of grief by planning to adopt. The adoption is more likely to be happy and successful if you can 'work out' the grief.

*This is the term being increasingly used by feminists for what is described in medical circles as Artificial Insemination by Donor (AID).

pillow. Ideally she should stay like that for half-an-hour so that as little semen as possible leaks out of her vagina. AI may be repeated on successive days if frozen semen is used; or alternate days with fresh semen from one donor. On average, women who become pregnant from AI do so after trying for three to five cycles; at BPAS 40 to 50 per cent of couples achieve pregnancy within a year. If you aren't pregnant after having tried for six to eight months, you may want to explore the reasons at the clinic or hospital.

Getting AI can be much more problematic than the technique itself. Currently it is not widely available on the NHS, and there are long waiting lists; those clinics that do provide a service often restrict it to couples where the man's sperm production is very poor – as opposed to just averagely poor. They often decide who should receive AI on the basis of whether they consider you to be a suitable parent. And as a *Lancet* article on AI in 1982 concludes:

> Some practitioners provide AID services for single women, for lesbian couples, and for people with psychosexual difficulties – when there is clear evidence that children brought up in such circumstances can be seriously disadvantaged.[28]

It is worrying that such prejudiced and ill-informed attitudes can masquerade as scientific truth. (See chapters on relationships.) This attitude is reflected in the Warnock Report (though in a more circumspect manner), which in addition recommends that the provision of AI without a licence for the purpose should be an offence. While this recommendation, if enacted, should ensure a well-run service (something that is not necessarily the case at the moment), it does not augur well for those of us deemed 'unacceptable' either because of our colour, class, disability or sexual orientation, whose only recourse would be *self*-insemination.*

Until we are able to improve the NHS service, many women therefore consider seeking AI privately. Some clinics have been known to charge scandalously exorbitant sums (upwards of £1,000 per course of insemination). Others, like the charity BPAS (see Resources) are non-profit-making (BPAS currently charges a maximum of £40 for two inseminations per month; there are additional costs, e.g. for counselling and initial examination). If all AI clinics were regulated, they would at the very least be obliged to offer a suitable service – ensuring first the anonymity of both donor and recipient (which can forestall possible emotional and even legal complications) and secondly that all donors are properly screened for possible health problems, particularly HIV, the virus that leads to

AIDS (see p. 501). *Because of the risk of contracting HIV or other sexually transmitted infections from donors, it is important that all donors are adequately screened. High-risk men are advised not to donate sperm.* Current Department of Health recommendations are that, to allow for a valid test for HIV, all semen should be frozen and stored for three months. (Conception rates with frozen semen are slightly lower than with fresh, but this may be connected with busy clinics not defrosting semen carefully enough.)

All clinics should have access to sperm banks. This means you don't need a donor on call to produce semen when you ovulate; finally, although insemination often takes place in a clinical setting, some clinics send you home with special portable containers for the semen, so that you can do it in less stressful surroundings with a partner.[29]

A big problem with AI is the shortage of men willing to be donors, particularly men who are from minority groups. If male readers and partners of women readers would consider becoming sperm donors, there might not be such a problem.

Deciding on whether to try for AI, and the process of trying, can both be very stressful.

> *I've never felt so isolated in my life. Despite comparatively few hassles and BPAS being very encouraging, I was going through it as a single woman. There was no one else as interested or as committed to this baby as I was. In the end, I just couldn't cope any more with watching to see if I'd got pregnant, getting false symptoms, not being able to concentrate on anything else. I was aware of every movement in my body. Then there were the emotional demands of going to the clinic each time. It all got too much and I decided I couldn't take any more after nine months of trying.*

> *I never expected it not to work. But after three to four attempts, I began to worry. I started remembering all the women I knew who needed more than a year to get pregnant to try to make myself feel better.*

Some women have said that AI made them feel they were committing adultery or being promiscuous. (The Roman Catholic and Orthodox Jewish religions consider AI adultery.) As you think about your situation, as well as about alternatives (including structuring your life without a child), you may find it helpful to talk with others who have used AI, and to read about other women's experiences. Listed in Resources are publications and organizations that may be helpful. There may also be an infertility support group in your area that could help.

If you decide to try for AI, it is important to consider what you will tell close friends and family and – most importantly – what you will tell your child. Many parents in the past have kept AI a secret, but it is gradually being recognized

---

*For more about self-insemination, see Resources or contact WHRRIC. Since AI is such a simple procedure, as many doctors acknowledge, attempts to restrict its use illustrate perhaps even more clearly than the abortion issue the extent to which it is deemed that women's right to control our own bodies should not exist. However, at present at least, self-insemination remains legal.

that secretiveness can create problems for AI children, just as it creates problems for adoptees.*

> *Our daughter is really extraordinary – enormous energy, very strong-willed and totally different-looking from either of us. I am reminded constantly that her father was a stranger.*

> My husband and I had more than our share of doubts right up until the moment of our daughter's birth. When we saw our baby girl, all our doubts disappeared.[30]

Francie Hornstein, discussing AI for lesbians, wrote in 1984:

> My decision to conceive a child by donor insemination was a long time coming. It was nearly seven years between the time I first considered the possibility and when I began trying to get pregnant. The one recurring reservation in what had become a passionate desire to have children was my fear of how the children would cope with being from a different kind of family. I knew I would be sorry if I never had children; sorry not only for giving up a part of life I really wanted, but for not making a decision I believed was right. I felt I was as worthy of having children as any other person. To not have children simply because I was a lesbian would have been giving up on a goal that was very dear to me.[31]

Two lesbian partners, who plan to raise children together, told us about the bond it created between them for the one to help the other with her insemination. We need to assert the right of all women to AI. And as Francie Hornstein says:

> We need to establish and protect the rights of partners of lesbians who may not be biological parents of the child, but who may be parents in every other sense of the word.[32]

ADOPTION

> *After we had stopped trying to have a baby, I baulked at the idea of adopting a child – bearing one, having the mixture of us had seemed important as well as living and changing with a child. I felt I had to really believe I would never produce children before I could even consider*

adopting because if I had the slightest 'perhaps' in my head, I couldn't know I would totally accept an adopted child. That took a long time. But it gradually became clear that living through growing up with a child was far more important to me than producing one.

> *My sister-in-law hasn't been able to have children. It's been very frustrating for her. But, although it's still very rare in our Asian society, she's adopted two children. It's made her very happy.*

While adoption may be an alternative to consider for many of us,* it is becoming increasingly difficult to adopt a *baby* unless s/he has a form of mental and/or physical disability.** Although it is impossible to be precise about waiting times, a wait of at least two years is not uncommon. For children with 'special needs' (i.e. any child over five or any child with a handicap), the waiting periods may be much shorter.

Organizations such as Parent to Parent Information on Adoption and Family Care (see p. 442) have originated the idea of holding group discussions for prospective adopters. It can be very helpful to talk over thoughts and feelings in an atmosphere free from the pressures of an interview with a social worker or with an adoption agency, where we are likely to feel under a great deal of pressure to appear 'perfect'.

> *Getting together with other would-be adopters of special needs children was very important and helpful to me. Socially I didn't know anybody who had adopted a special needs child, and it made me feel very sane and good about what I was doing. One of the best things about the adoption group was sharing experiences of loss people had experienced (infertility, miscarriages and children dying), and being able to acknowledge my own grief in losing potential children of my own was very important in the process of preparing to adopt a child. Somebody else's child isn't second best, neither is a special needs child less 'good' than a 'normal' child. It is about the resources you have to give and being able to fulfil your own needs in that giving that is important, and since most people who apply to adopt have experience of loss around children, it seems to me that help to grieve is an essential part of preparation for adoption.*

---

*The National Association for the Childless has received letters from a group of grown AI children, angry at the secretiveness about their origins. To put AI in perspective, however, a by-product of some research on blood is the discovery that in one English town, at least 30 per cent of husbands could not possibly be the fathers of their children.

*Though bear in mind that adoption agencies have a 'ceiling' age limit on prospective adoptive parents (between thirty-five and forty years).
**This is partly because of the Abortion Act, and partly because societal attitudes have made it easier for women to bring up children as single parents, though as yet it is still very much harder to contemplate bringing up a child with a disability on your own.

THE PROCESS OF ADOPTION

If you try to adopt, the process *can* be long, difficult and painful, so be prepared. You may have to try a large number of agencies, particularly if you are trying to adopt an able-bodied baby. Some agencies close their lists if they know they will never be able to find enough children for prospective adopters. Most are choosy – though their criteria will vary. You will have to give up any infertility treatment.

Adopting a 'special needs' child can in theory be a lot easier. Parents for Children, an organization concerned solely with placing special needs children with adoptive parents, has opened its doors to less conventional would-be parents, and many other agencies have followed suit. As Parents for Children says, special children need special parents. Often people with unusual relationships, lifestyles or life experiences are more successful at parenting children with multiple problems.

To adopt a child, you will need to approach either your local authority (in which case, write to the Director of Social Services) or a registered voluntary adoption agency. It is illegal to adopt through any other third party, unless you are a relative of the child or you are 'acting in pursuance of an order of the High Court' (Children Act, section 28). You have to go through an approval process which might take a few months. It involves being allocated to a social worker with whom you will have several interviews. If you are in a couple, you are seen together and separately. You will also have another interview with a different social worker. Police records are looked into and you also need to go to your GP for a medical; your GP will be required to furnish a report to the social worker about your medical history.

I think I was lucky. My GP discussed with me what should go in his report. I had had a period of depression some years before and he was aware that the way he presented this information might make a difference to whether I was approved of or not.

Then your 'case' goes to an 'adoption panel', which may include professionals as well as adopting parents. The panel is the approving body, although in practice most seem to go almost entirely on the social worker's report. Social workers, therefore, have a lot of power (though they are at times overridden). If you don't feel you're getting on with your social worker, you can ask for another one. You can also check whether the particular adoption agency concerned has an appeals system in case your application fails. If it doesn't, all you can do is try another agency.*

*You can also try to adopt from abroad, though the issue of removing children from their culture and roots is very controversial. The least potentially exploitative approach is through a government agency. BAFA and Parent to Parent have lists of bona fide agencies abroad. Beware unscrupulous ones that kidnap children from Third World countries: in 1988 a conference of the International Bar Association was told by Margaret Bennett, a London solicitor, that approximately 16,000 newborn babies were likely to have been abducted from their mothers' bedsides each year in Brazil alone.

The adoption process raises many negative feelings, often surprisingly similar to the ones experienced during the first stages of coping with infertility. Feelings of powerlessness, anger and frustration are common, especially during the time of the approval process when the social worker is evaluating and 'testing' you on your potential as a parent. Families and friends may not be as supportive as you would like, and you may go through periods of anxiety and desperation.

My husband and I found out we might become prospective parents in April. That gave us about seven to eight weeks to think about this. I had many things going through my mind. So many things could happen in the interim. The natural mother could still change her mind. I wondered what the child would be like. The baby's looks, personality, health – everything is unknown . . .

I thought a lot about bonding. I wondered what I'd feel like when someone put an infant in my arms saying, 'Congratulations! You are a mother. This is your child.' Who is this stranger? How am I supposed to love someone I do not even know? How am I supposed to feel? I believe these are healthy feelings, but still it is frightening to think about . . .

I believe couples facing adoption go through the same feelings that biological parents go through – the fears, insecurities, the great change of lifestyle. The only problem is that you do not have nine months to work your feelings through. It is like being told you are eight months pregnant.

I have found most other people trying to adopt, feel desperate to have a child. I had all sorts of feelings of divine intervention stopping me from having my own.

It is quite normal to feel desperate in a society that tells you that having your own child is the only way you can have that particularly special relationship of responsibility with a child growing up. Also your dependence on the approval process can bring up all the previous powerless feelings of depending on fate as to whether you will ever be able to have a child or not. However, the process may in fact be very helpful. A single woman speaks:

My experience of the 'assessment' process was very positive. I was lucky in having a social worker who obviously had a lot of respect for me right from the start and so I felt safe to express all sorts of feelings. It gave me a chance to explore all the feelings and questions of why I wanted a child, what was it about a child that I wanted and I found I did really want to be with a young person growing up and discovering the world and I would be quite happy to do that with a child with a physical handicap. Five months after this process was begun, I was approved as a potential adopter, and have since adopted a child with 'special needs'.

Once you have been through this process, you are likely to experience all sorts of feelings resulting from your decision being officially approved. You are one step nearer the possibility of having a child. You will feel a mixture of excitement, anxiety, vulnerability and joy at the prospect of a child being placed in your home. But be prepared that things may still not be easy, and whether they are or not, you will still need the support of family and/or friends.

Usually there are several people who are informed about a child awaiting adoption. All of those are likely to want to be considered, and will therefore go through the process of mentally and emotionally adjusting their lives in anticipation. When the prospective parent(s) have been chosen, this can be emotionally devastating for the others. And this process may be repeated several times.

Adoption poses a number of problems which prospective adoptive parents need to think about in advance. In particular, when adopted children start to grow up they may have very powerful feelings about being adopted which they do not always express. The Children Act of 1975 also gives adopted people the right to see a copy of their birth certificate when they reach eighteen.

It is important to recognize the suffering of 'birth mothers' – as they are now called – who have had to give up their children for adoption. To do this is not an easy option, nor is it a decision that is possible to forget. Increasingly, birth mothers are beginning to speak about not being able to have contact with the children they have given up. Many birth mothers can never begin to heal from the 'surrender' experience until they have been reunited with their children.

The few studies concerning the adoption process which have been done demonstrate that the feelings and experiences of all those involved in the adoption process are often neglected. We need to challenge the assumptions and practices of social workers who label certain feelings and lifestyles 'abnormal' and distort the experiences and needs of adoptees, birth mothers and adoptive parents alike.

FOSTERING

Fostering is a way of providing a home for a child who cannot be with its own parents – although they are still the parents. Usually, but not always, the aim is to enable the child to return to the original family at some stage. Fostering can be short- or long-term, or 'fostering with a view to adoption'. Many people have successfully adopted after taking this latter fostering option, but securing the adoption can be a long and painful process, and there is always the chance that it won't go through.

The process of becoming a foster parent is easier than for adoption because it does not require the approval of the courts and is solely at the discretion of the local authority. This means that people with 'unconventional' lifestyles, including single women, are more likely to be able to foster.

However, fostering itself is by no means easy. Forming ties with a child can be very difficult if you don't know when s/he's going to be taken away, and children's responses to the situation are understandably confused.

ADOPTION AND FOSTERING FOR LESBIANS AND SINGLE WOMEN

The law now states that a single person or a married couple may adopt (an unmarried heterosexual couple cannot adopt as a couple). At least one local authority – Hackney in London – has changed its policies so that lesbians may adopt or foster children, and a few other authorities, such as Camden in London, are considering similar moves. Single women, including lesbians, have been fostering children for years. The only change in recent years is that this is now being acknowledged more publicly. We do not know how recent changes in attitude towards homosexuality, condoned and promoted by the present Thatcher Government, may affect lesbian parents of all kinds – either now or in the future.

SURROGATE MOTHERHOOD

Practised in its simplest way, this involves one woman – the surrogate – bearing a child that another woman raises as her own. Where a woman in a heterosexual relationship is infertile or unable to give birth herself, the possibility may appeal to use her partner's sperm to inseminate a surrogate, either through intercourse or AI.

Surrogate motherhood raises a host of social, legal and financial questions. Much discussion followed media coverage of the first known surrogate birth in the UK, with the result that it is now illegal to advertise for, or offer, surrogacy, and for all third-party intervention on a commercial basis. However, surrogacy arrangements on a non-profit-making basis are still legal according to the 1985 Surrogacy Arrangements Act. Nevertheless, it is another question whether such contracts would be enforceable by a court of law.

The Department of Health has recommended to all local authorities that any child of a surrogacy arrangement should be made a Ward of Court if there is any indication that the child might be at risk, thus endorsing what happened in the 'Baby Cotton' case, where the child was kept 'in care' (but actually deprived of parental care) for the first ten days of its life. Although it is still legal to make a non-commercial surrogacy arrangement, the courts may well intervene where the people concerned were in dispute (e.g. if the surrogate decided she wished to keep the baby). At the time of writing, the possibility of further legislation is being considered which could confirm the unenforce-ability of all surrogacy contracts. Meanwhile, an additional and unforeseen legal issue has emerged following the enactment of the Family Law Reform Act 1987, whose effect is that if a *married* woman plans to become a surrogate mother by means of *artificial insemination*, and *with her husband's consent, her husband* will become the legal father of the child.* (In Scotland, where the Act does not apply, the child would be regarded as illegitimate.)

It is possible that a form of surrogacy involving IVF *might* be enforceable, whereby the fertilized egg of another woman is implanted in the womb of a surrogate – a curious commentary on how the intervention of doctors via tech-nology appears more acceptable even than loving and non-commercial arrangements between people.** The first such recorded gestures are documented in the Old Testa-ment of the Bible: Hagar bore Abraham's child, so that he and his 'barren' wife Sarah could have one; Rachel and Jacob brought up a child whose surrogate mother was Bilhah (though in this latter case Bilhah may or may not have been willing – to have intercourse *or* a baby). Sur-rogacy is indeed a traditional practice among families in many parts of the world, particularly between relatives, including parts of the UK.[33] The legal status of all such children, however, is illegitimate.

There has been a recent outcry against surrogacy. It has to an extent been echoed by some feminist opinion – although the outcry has been dominated by precisely the sorts of people who seek to curtail women making decisions about our own bodies in other spheres. Aside from the legal issues, there are immense social, political and psychologi-cal issues surrounding surrogate motherhood, and femin-ists have only begun to get to grips with them. For the debate so far, see Rita Arditti et al, *Test Tube Women* and the WHRRIC newsletter (see Resources).

MISCARRIAGE (NATURAL ABORTION)†

It is a surprising statistic that in women who know they are

pregnant, about one in six pregnancies ends in miscarriage. About 75 per cent of these occur before twelve weeks. Miscarriage, then, is a fairly common event. We need to be at least minimally prepared to know how it feels and what to expect. Miscarriage is both a physical event for a woman and a serious emotional crisis which may be shared or experienced in very different ways.

When I found out I was pregnant, I danced around the house. My pregnancy was an easy one. . . . My body was slowly and pleasantly changing. Because it was a conscious and well-thought-out decision to have a child, I felt free to revel in my pregnancy and motherhood. It was a special time. I mention all of this because having a miscarriage has to do with the loss of something so deeply ingrained for so long that it is partially by understanding the depth of the joy that one can understand the depth of the loss.

The medical term for miscarriage before twenty-six weeks is *spontaneous abortion*. You may experience a *threatened abortion* beforehand, with cramps and bleeding or staining. Often bed rest is advised (though there is very little evidence that it makes any difference, apart from calming you down), and your doctor may order specific blood tests to check your hormone levels. In *inevitable abortion*, bleeding becomes heavy, cramps increase and the cervix may begin to dilate. The fetus, amniotic sac and placenta, along with a lot of blood, may be expelled completely intact. You'll probably know when this is happening. If you are not in hospital, you must do the difficult task of collecting fetus and afterbirth, putting them in a clean container and taking them to your doctor or hospital so that they can be examined. Some doctors do not consider doing an examination, or only if you've had several miscarriages. Since an examination may yield important information as to why you miscarried, you may want to press for this. Ask that specialized as well as routine tests be done, such as cultures for infection and genetic examination of tissues. If tests show you have lost a 'blighted pregnancy' (where egg and sperm together have failed to divide correctly) then you can try to be more at ease, knowing that this has been a random event and that the chances of it happening again are small. If a study of the fetal tissue shows genetic abnormalities or suggests that you had an illness or infection, you can work with your doctor on how to proceed. If the fetal tissue is normal, you may learn that your hormone levels were insufficient or that a weak cervix was the problem. Both of these conditions may be treatable.

An *incomplete abortion* means that only part of the 'products of conception' has been passed. Part remains within, and bleeding will continue. Usually a doctor will do a dilatation and curettage (D & C) to clean out your uterus so that it will heal. A *complete abortion* means that everything in your uterus has been expelled. You will continue to bleed, but less and less. If you think you are

---

*If she becomes pregnant under different circumstances – e.g. by intercourse – then the Act does not apply.

**At the time of writing, WHRRIC has been contacted by several women interested in acting as surrogates out of love for friends or relatives unable to have babies themselves.

†A miscarriage is often referred to as an abortion – thus confusingly, and sometimes distressingly, implying that the miscarriage was deliberately in-duced. We prefer the term miscarriage, but we do have to use the technical term on occasions.

bleeding too long, consult your doctor. (Perhaps a D & C may be necessary after all.)

During a miscarriage, you may not believe what is happening. Feelings of helplessness may develop as cramping and bleeding increase. Many women fear that they may bleed to death. Having to go to hospital may intensify your anxiety and fear.

We went home from the hospital dazed and tired. I was weak and enormously sad. I don't know that I've ever experienced such deep emotional pain. The loss was so great and so complete in the way that only death is. For the first few days I couldn't talk to anyone, but at the same time it was painful to be alone. I would just cry and cry without stopping. One of the clearest reminders that I was no longer pregnant were all the speedy changes my body went through. Within two days my breasts, which had grown quite swollen, were back to their normal size. My stomach, which had grown hard, was now soft again. My body was no longer preparing for the birth of a child. It was simple and blatant. Tiredness was replaced with weakness. And then there was the bleeding. My body would not let me forget. I knew things would improve once we could make love again and would be even better when we were full of hope. But it seemed so far away.

You may also experience a *missed abortion*. In this case, a fetus dies in the uterus but is not expelled. It can remain within for several months. Signs are lack of menstrual periods coupled with cessation of signs of pregnancy; sometimes there is spotting. If it is not eventually expelled spontaneously, the fetus must be removed with a D & C or induced labour – a procedure which will be very hard to accept emotionally.

Some possible causes for miscarriage are structural problems of the uterus, infection, weak cervical muscles, hormonal imbalances, environmental and industrial toxins. According to Dr Ian Murray-Lyon of Charing Cross Hospital, drinking alcohol during pregnancy (more than ten units a week) has been shown to increase the risk of miscarriage. Genetic error is associated with a high number of early miscarriages, and blood incompatibility between a mother who is Rh negative and the fetus who is Rh positive can also lead to miscarriage. If you are Rh negative, it is very important to ensure that the drug Anti D is given if you bleed at all during pregnancy to prevent this reaction and safeguard future pregnancies. Some doctors recommend Anti D daily throughout the period of bleeding (see Chapter 18, p. 343).

Try to learn why you had a miscarriage. Some of the diagnostic procedures outlined above for infertility will be useful here. Ask to see the pathology report, and ask that all terminology be explained fully. If you are not satisfied with the explanation, ask if there are other tests that can be done.

It is your right to learn as much as possible about your miscarriage.

One miscarriage does not mean you are infertile. There is a 70 per cent chance that you will have a successful pregnancy even after two miscarriages. However, if you have two or more in a row you may want to begin investigating. Try to find a doctor who specializes, or is interested, in the problem (the Miscarriage Association may be able to help). Plan with your doctor to check out each detail of your next pregnancy as it progresses, including possible reasons for any spotting or cramps, definite ways to deal with contingencies, tests to be made as they become necessary and so forth. You will need encouragement in this project from your partner (if you have one), family, friends and/or a support group, possibly one geared to childbearing problems.

The time following a miscarriage is difficult. Physically, your body may still feel pregnant for a while, your breasts full and tender, your stomach enlarged. You may continue spotting for several weeks. If you have increased flow or odd- or foul-smelling discharge or a high temperature, contact your doctor, as you may have an infection which should be treated immediately. It is usually safe to have sexual intercourse after four to six weeks when your cervix is closed and there is less risk of infection.

You will almost always feel grief and anger. You will need family and/or friends.

Most people didn't know how to give me support, and perhaps I didn't really know how to ask for it. People were more comfortable talking about the physical and not the emotional side of miscarriage. I needed to talk about both. It was also difficult for my husband, because people could at least ask how my body was doing. Unfortunately, he would sometimes be completely bypassed when someone called to talk with us, despite the fact that he, too, was in deep emotional pain.

Feelings of grief are often complicated by guilt. This can cause tension between partners. You may wonder if either of you did something 'wrong' (too much activity, too much sex, but neither is known to cause miscarriage, so blame is inappropriate). Dispelling the tension will take a while, longer for some than for others. It is best if you acknowledge and talk out your feelings. The effects of the miscarriage can last for months. On the date when the baby would have been born, there is usually a resurgence of grief.

If you experience more than one miscarriage, you will need compassion and understanding of the losses you have experienced, and of how very precious these pregnancies were to you. Unfortunately, doctors who can offer this are rare. Your helplessness and hopelessness may increase if you begin or return to treatments for your infertility and start working on becoming pregnant again.

For further help and support, see Resources.

FEELINGS WHEN THE BABY DIES

The death of your baby – either at birth or soon afterwards – is utterly devastating. As well as the emotional pain is the physical pain – a constant reminder of the loss. In fact, your body knows nothing about the baby's death; your breasts are filled with milk, never to be used. You will require help and care on every level at this time: physical, emotional, practical and spiritual.

If the baby's death takes place before delivery, maximum pain relief and delivery in the quickest and least hazardous way are desirable. You should have the chance to decide if and when you want to go into labour spontaneously. Your partner if you have one should be present as long as either of you wish. Once the baby is delivered, many women find it helpful to spend time with it, touching and holding it.

That was all I saw of him; the soles of his feet when he was born and then the top of his head. They brought him to me all wrapped up, even his face was covered. I didn't know if I could unwrap him or not. If I'd known he was only going to live two hours, I'd have unwrapped him and held him next to me all that time. They tell me he had arms and legs, but I don't really know because I didn't see.

I was gently coaxed into holding him, and my initial revulsion disappeared. Time passed all too quickly and allowing him to be taken away to the mortuary was the hardest thing I had to do.

Many hospitals now provide photographs, which can be a godsend later.

The photographs and slides have been a great source of comfort to us, and to our parents.

You should be put in a room away from the nursery and hospital personnel should be told that you have lost your baby. Above all, you and your family must be allowed your grief, in privacy if you need and want it.

You might need to withdraw at first and not confront the reality which may be too much to bear. There might be a period of numbness. If you ask for help in grieving, we hope it will be intelligently and humanely extended. Platitudes such as, 'You'll have another baby before you know it', or, 'Think of your wonderful children at home', have no place. The death of this particular child is being experienced – no other actual or potential children have any relevance to the situation. Perhaps the best help others can offer is sympathetic listening and close physical comforting. And we can often need a lot of listening to, even for months afterwards.

I developed an irresistible urge to describe our ordeal in minute detail to anyone who would listen and have since discovered that this is a common reaction.

Since the last edition of this book, hospitals have begun to improve in terms of their ability to respond to the death of a baby. But maternity units are geared to producing life, and unless staff are given help to cope with their own feelings about the death of a baby, they can be of little help to us. They may have a strong tendency to prescribe routine sedatives, yet such drugs can interfere with our ability to grieve – and grieving at this time is as necessary as breathing.

While procedures for registering stillbirths have been made easier, there are more improvements we can press for: more sensitivity during the time we have to make decisions about burial, and more care to ensure for example that we are not put near mothers and/or their babies.

It is important to understand if possible why the baby died. Most likely whatever happened was totally beyond anyone's control, but if you suspect negligence, you should seek legal advice quickly so that the facts can be analysed. AIMS could probably help you with this (see p. 442).

It can take a long time to get over the death of a child. Feelings of guilt or shame are not uncommon. Be prepared for this and, if possible, make contact with people who will understand the problems you are facing. Compassionate Friends (see p. 442) is a national network of people who have lost a child. It is a non-religious society. By contacting them we can give and/or receive much-needed help. The society acts as a twenty-four-hour service for bereaved parents, however long ago the death occurred, as well as a pressure group to urge research into children's diseases.

Nobody wants to deal with death, especially when your friends are at the childbearing age themselves and can't help being afraid of you for what you stand for. I found that my friends wanted me to pretend nothing had happened. I don't think it was just my particular friends – it's natural to want to avoid those things. And so my fantastic pregnancy, in which a lot of things went on in my head and body that helped me to change and get myself together, had to be buried. Even now, after a year, I can see their pain and fear for me as I start into my eighth month of pregnancy with my second child. I have to be the one who keeps them calm, and I especially must assure everyone that this one will be OK.

ECTOPIC (MISPLACED) PREGNANCY

Whether we intend to get pregnant or not, it is always possible to develop an ectopic pregnancy. *Such a pregnancy is dangerous. There is a danger of severe blood loss, shock, and even death unless appropriate medical attention is given (see below).* If your blood group is Rhesus negative, you will need injections of Anti D, as for miscarriage (see p. 343).

Fertilization of the egg by the sperm almost always occurs in the fallopian tube. If the function of the tube is impaired in any way, for example by pelvic inflammatory disease, then it is possible that the fertilized egg might attach itself to part of the tube instead of proceeding on into the uterus. This results in an ectopic pregnancy; more rarely an ectopic pregnancy can begin to grow in the abdominal cavity, the ovary or the cervix.

Between 5 and 10 per cent of women who have had previous tubal surgery may experience ectopic pregnancy, but it can happen to any woman. Ectopic pregnancies are on the rise because of the increased incidence of PID and use of IUDs, which can result in scar formation on the tubes or inflammation of the uterine lining, which then 'resists' implantation of the fertilized egg. *If you're of childbearing age, have had intercourse and feel constant abdominal pains you don't understand, it's possible you have an ectopic pregnancy.*

Because all the hormonal changes are similar to those of a normal early pregnancy, you can have all the early signs of pregnancy, such as fatigue, nausea, missed period and breast tenderness. As the pregnancy progresses, causing pressure in the tube, symptoms such as stabbing pain, cramps or a dull ache may become severe. In addition, you may or may not have menstrual-type bleeding. To diagnose an ectopic pregnancy, an ultrasound is needed, and/or a beta blood test can be done to pick up levels of HCG in the blood. If levels are low, an ectopic pregnancy should be suspected.

If an ectopic pregnancy is misdiagnosed and the tube ruptures, you will need emergency treatment in a hospital. If you have severe pain, it may be better to go straight to a casualty department than wait to go through your GP. You may need an emergency operation.

It should be stressed that an ectopic pregnancy can be very hard to diagnose. You may need to be persistent.

I kept on going to my GP with various symptoms and was told it's an early miscarriage, all in my mind, etc. This went on for a month, until I was admitted to hospital with severe pain, and even then was only operated on four days later!

Ectopic pregnancy is sometimes misdiagnosed as an early spontaneous abortion. It is essential that any tissue passed from the uterus be checked for developing fetal tissue.

If the doctor detects an ectopic pregnancy early enough, s/he may be able to remove the pregnancy and save the tube. In some cases it is necessary to remove the whole tube and/or the adjacent ovary. Careful surgical technique is important; the less bleeding and consequent adhesions and scar tissue, the better the chance for a normal pregnancy later. In any case, if you have already had a tubal pregnancy, there is a higher risk of having another.

The outlook for future pregnancies is somewhat changed by this experience: you may feel depressed and frightened by the possibility that this could happen again. In addition, if the pregnancy was wanted, you are likely to feel all the feelings that result from a miscarriage. In a future pregnancy it may be worth asking for a very early scan.

POSTSCRIPT

We hope that this chapter provides help and support for women who have experienced infertility or pregnancy loss. Yet while medical approaches may develop and change, we can never assume that they can solve all our problems. This is an uncomfortable fact of life that we are not helped to face by medical professionals who so often fail to disabuse us of the myths that they themselves have created. In fact, the medical profession can neither cure life's problems, nor can it cure many medical ones. By stimulating awareness on this point, we can contribute to creating a more hopeful approach to infertility and pregnancy loss, to life and death. If we tackle this issue alongside the fundamental issue of women's role in society, then women in the future will be better equipped to face infertility and pregnancy loss, and other devastating events in our lives, unclouded by the belief that only medicine can heal the pain with which we have been confronted.

NOTES

1. H.G.W. Baker et al. 'Testicular Vein Ligation and Fertility in Men with Varicoles', *British Medical Journal*, 14 December 1985, p. 1678.

2. M.P. Vessey et al. 'Return of Fertility after Discontinuation of Oral Contraceptives: Influence of Age and Parity', *British Journal of Family Planning*, vol. 11, 1986, p. 120.

3. D. Schwartz et al. *New England Journal of Medicine*, no. 306, 1982, pp. 404–6.

4. P. Daniels and K. Weingarten. *Sooner or Later: the Timing of Parenthood in Adult Lives.* New York: W. W. Norton, 1982.

5. M.G. Hull et al. *The Lancet*, 4 August 1984, p. 245.

6. Francesca Turner. 'Give Me the Moonlight', *Guardian*, 14 June 1986.

7. M. and R. O'Moore. 'Investigations and Treatments in the Manifes-

tation of Stress in Infertile Couples'. Paper presented to a conference in Beijing, 1985.

8. See Jill Rakusen and Nick Davidson. *Out of Our Hands.* London: Pan, 1982.

9. J.L. Treasure et al. *The Lancet*, 21 and 28 December 1985, p. 1379.

10. J. Piesse. *International Clinical Nutrition Review*, vol. 3, no. 2, 1983, pp. 4–6.

11. G. Howe et al. 'Effects of Age, Cigarette Smoking and Other Factors on Fertility Findings in a Large Prospective Study', *British Medical Journal*, 8 June 1985, p. 1697.

12. See, for example, J.P.P. Tyler et al. 'How Representative are Semen Samples?' *The Lancet*, 22 January 1983, p. 191.

13. Naomi Pfeffer and Anne Woollett. *The Experience of Infertility*, London: Virago Press, 1983, p. 103.

14. J.A. Collins et al. 'Treatment-dependent Pregnancy among Infertile

Couples', *New England Journal of Medicine*, 17 November 1983, p. 1201.

15. A. Demoulin. 'Is Diagnostic Ultrasound Safe During Periovulatory Period?' *Research in Reproduction*, vol. 17, no. 2, April 1985.

16. P. Mason et al. 'Induction of Ovulation with Pulsatile Luteinising Hormone Releasing Hormone', *British Medical Journal*, 21 January 1984, p. 181.

17. Rakusen and Davidson, op. cit., note 8.

18. Craft et al. *The Lancet*, 31 March 1984, p. 732.

19. See Rakusen and Davidson, op. cit., note 8, p. 108; W.D.A. Ford and K. E. T. Little. *The Lancet*, 14 November 1981, p. 1107; I. Melamed et al. *New England Journal of Medicine*, 23 September 1982, p. 820 (this last report tentatively implicated Pergonal as well).

20. 'Clinical Status of IVF, GIFT, and Related Techniques', *The Lancet*, 24 October 1987, p. 945.

21. See e.g. R.T. O'Shea et al., 'Endometriosis and Fertilisation', *The Lancet*, 28 September 1985, p. 723.

22. M.G.R. Hull et al. 'Human In-vitro Fertilisation, In-vivo Sperm Penetration of Cervical Mucus, and Unexplained Infertility', *The Lancet*, 4 August 1984, p. 245.

23. J.L. Yovich et al. 'Treatment of Male Infertility by In-vitro Fertilisation', *The Lancet*, 21 July 1984, p. 169: J. Cohen et al. 'Application of In-vitro Fertilisation in Cases of a Poor Post-coital Test', *The Lancet*, 8 September 1984, p. 583.

24. For example, R.G. Edwards and P.C. Steptoe. 'Current Status of In-vitro Fertilisation and Implantation of Human Embryos', *The Lancet*, 3 December 1983, p. 1265; and C. Wood et al. 'Clinical Implications of Developments of In-vitro Fertilisation', *British Medical Journal*, 13 October 1984, p. 978. In an unusual reference to actual birth-rates, a *Lancet* leader, op. cit., note 20, suggests that at best, birth-rates of only one in five or six per treatment cycle can be expected. Since no reference is given for these figures, even these should probably be treated with scepticism. And in a recent editorial in *Fertility and Sterility* authors were actually asked to 'be honest with one another'! (M.R. Soules. 'The In Vitro Fertilization Pregnancy Rate: Let's Be Honest with One Another', *Fertility and Sterility*, vol. 43, 1985, p. 511.)

25. Report of the Committee of Inquiry into Human Fertilisation and Embryology (the Warnock Report), Cmnd 9314. London: HMSO, 1984.

26. From Maggie Jones. *Trying to Have a Baby? Overcoming Infertility and Child Loss*. London: Sheldon Press, 1984.

27. Ibid.

28. 'Whither Human Donor Insemination in Britain?' *The Lancet*, 6 March 1982.

29. E.A. McLaughlin et al. 'Use of Home Insemination in Programmes of Artificial Insemination with Donor Semen', *British Medical Journal*, 15 October 1983, p. 1110.

30. From Barbara E. Menning. 'Donor Insemination: the Psychosocial Issues', *Contemporary Ob/Gyn*, October 1981.

31. Francie Hornstein. 'Children by Donor Insemination: a New Choice for Lesbians', in Rita Arditti et al. (eds), *Test Tube Women: What Future Motherhood?* London: Pandora Press, 1984.

32. Ibid.

33. As a Royal Society of Medicine meeting was told recently, 'It happens every day in Rochdale.'

RESOURCES
PUBLICATIONS

GENERAL

Arditti, Rita et al. (eds). *Test Tube Women: What Future Motherhood?* London: Pandora Press, 1984. An international collection of feminist writings, mostly very critical of technological development.

Dowrick, Stephanie and Sybil **Grundberg** (eds). *Why Children?* London: Women's Press, 1980. Invaluable collection of writings by eighteen women, each talking about her feelings/decisions/non-decisions.

Holmes, Helen B. et al. (eds). *The Custom-Made Child? – Women-Centered Perspectives*. Clifton, NJ: Humana Press, 1981. Part of a two-volume collection that came out of a meeting in which community workers, doctors, scientists, ethicists and government planners – most of

them women and feminists – spent several days discussing women's reproductive health issues.

Houghton, Diane and Peter. *Coping with Childlessness*. London: Unwin, 1984. By the funders of NAC (see Organizations, below). Includes chapters on 'Assisting the healing process' and 'Being childless in later life'.

Jones, Maggie. *Trying to Have a Baby? – Overcoming Infertility and Child Loss*. London: Sheldon Press, 1984.

Overall, Christine. *Ethics and Human Reproduction: A Feminist Analysis*. London: Allen & Unwin, 1987.

Piercy, Marge. *Woman on the Edge of Time*. A feminist novel that envisions a world where reproductive technology exists for the benefit of women. London: Women's Press, 1979.

Rich, Adrienne. *Of Woman Born*. London: Virago Press, 1977. A moving and inspiring book that recognizes patriarchal control of our reproductive capacity *and* of our attitudes to it.

Stanworth, Michelle (ed.). *Reproductive Technologies – Gender, Motherhood and Medicine*. Oxford: Polity Press, 1988. A collection of feminist writings taking a different view from Arditti et al.

INFERTILITY (see also GENERAL, above)

First Report of the Voluntary Licensing Authority for Human In Vitro Fertilisation and Embryology. London: MRC, 1986.

Harrison, R.F. et al. 'Stress in Infertile Couples', in R. F. Harrison et al. (eds), *Fertility and Sterility*. Lancaster: MTP Press, 1984.

Hull, M.G.R. et al. 'Population Study of Causes, Treatment and Outcome of Infertility', *British Medical Journal*, 14 December 1985, p. 1693.

Kelso, Isa Anderson. *Women's Ailments*. Wellingborough, Northants: Thorsons, 1973.

Pfeffer, Naomi and Anne **Woollett**. *The Experience of Infertility*. London: Virago Press, 1983. A very thoughtful and helpful guide; a must.

Pfeffer, Naomi and Allison **Quick**. *Infertility Services – A Desperate Case*. London: Greater London Association of Community Health Councils, 1988.

Rakusen, Jill and Nick **Davidson**. *Out of Our Hands: What Technology Does to Pregnancy*. London: Pan, 1982. Contains chapters on infertility testing and treatments, plus information on the effects of drugs.

Winston, Robert. *Infertility: A Sympathetic Approach*. London: Martin Dunitz, 1986. Useful on the subject of surgery among other things.

ALTERNATIVE INSEMINATION

Berer, Marge. *Donor Insemination*, available from WHRRIC.

'Case Conference, "Lesbian Couples: Should Help Extend to AID?" ', *Journal of Medical Ethics*, vol. 4, 1978, pp. 91–5.

Feminist Self Insemination Group. *Self Insemination* (1980): no longer in print, but on file at WHRRIC and Feminist Library.

Hornstein, Francie. 'Children by Donor Insemination: a New Choice for Lesbians', in Arditti, *Test Tube Women* – see General, above.

Klein, Renata Duelli. 'Doing it Ourselves: Self Insemination', in Arditti, *Test Tube Women* – see General, above.

Saffron, Lisa. *Getting Pregnant Our Own Way – a Guide to Alternative Insemination*, 1986 (available from WHRRIC).

Snowden, Robert and G.D. **Mitchell**. *The Artificial Family – a Consideration of Artificial Insemination by Donor*. London: Allen and Unwin, 1981. Considers social and legal issues prior to any changes in the current law. Attempts to be liberal. See also *The Experience of Infertility* and *Out of Our Hands* in General, above, both of which contain sections on AID.

FOSTERING AND ADOPTION

Adopting a Child, 1984–5 (booklet available from BAAF, see Organizations).

Argent, Hedi. *Find me a Family – the Story of Parents for Children*. London: Souvenir Press, 1984. A must for people considering adopting 'special needs' children.

Rowe, Jane. *Fostering in the Eighties*. London: BAAF, 1983.

Rowe, Jane. *Yours by Choice*. London: Routledge and Kegan Paul, 1982. A guide to the adoption process.

MISCARRIAGE AND STILLBIRTH

Borg, Susan and Judith **Lasker**. *When Pregnancy Fails: Families Coping with Miscarriage, Stillbirth and Infant Death.* London: Routledge and Kegan Paul, 1982. A sensitive and helpful book, though American, for anyone who has been through the tragedy of their child's death.

Leroy, Margaret. *Miscarriage.* London: Optima, 1987. Based on the experiences of the Miscarriage Association.

National Childbirth Trust. *Miscarriage* (leaflet available from the NCT, see Organizations).

Oakley, Ann, Ann **McPherson** and Helen **Roberts**. *Miscarriage.* London, Fontana, 1983. A helpful book that looks at causes and treatment and women's experiences.

Standish, Liz. 'The Loss of a Baby', *The Lancet*, 13 March 1982, p. 611.

ORGANIZATIONS

GENERAL

Association for Improvements in the Maternity Services (AIMS), 40 Kingswood Avenue, London NW6 6LS

British Organization of Non-parents (BON), BM Box 5866, London WC1N 3XX. Support group for those who believe that being child-free should be a seriously respected option in society.

British Pregnancy Advisory Service, head office: Austy Manor, Wootton Wawen, Solihull, West Midlands B95 6BX. Tel: 05642-3225. Has branches in many parts of the country – see Resources in Chapter 16 or your local phone book. A charity that can help with AI, infertility testing, etc.

Child, 367 Wandsworth Road, London SW8 2JJ. Tel: 01-486 4289. Supports infertile people through support groups, telephone counselling, etc.

National Association for the Childless, Birmingham Settlement, 318 Summer Lane, Birmingham B19 3RL. A self-help organization, registered as a charity, offering advice, information and support to people experiencing infertility. Tends to be orientated towards heterosexual couples, but has about 100 contacts throughout Britain, and many support groups. Produces factsheets and an invaluable newsletter, all of which are free to members. Also holds seminars, e.g. on inter-country adoption. NAC also aims to improve NHS infertility treatment.

Single and Infertile, 293 Meadgate Avenue, Chelmsford, Essex. For both single men and women who are infertile.

Women's Health and Reproductive Rights Information Centre (WHRRIC), 52–5 Featherstone Street, London EC1Y 8RT. Tel: 01-251 6580/6332. Provides information about self-help groups generally and infertility support groups in particular, as well as general information, including about AI.

ALTERNATIVE INSEMINATION

BPAS (British Pregnancy Advisory Service) provides AID (AI) in many parts of the country and does not limit their service to heterosexuals or to couples. Also offers counselling and other services, such as sperm testing and sperm storage facilities. See General Organizations above for address, and for other organizations which can advise on availability of AID.

FOSTERING AND ADOPTION

British Agencies for Adoption and Fostering (BAAF), 11 Southwark Street, London SE1 1RQ. Tel: 01-407 8800; Scottish Centre: 23 Castle Street, Edinburgh EH2 3DM. Tel: 031-225 9285. Has useful leaflets for prospective adopters, adoptees, stepchildren and on issues such as 'a child from the past'. Very helpful on adoption altogether.

Contact-a-Family, 16 Strutton Ground, London SW1 2HP. Tel: 01-222 2695. Contact Line 01-222 2211. Links parents of children with special needs. Runs local groups: national telephone link-up service, Contact Line.

Family Care, 21 Castle Street, Edinburgh EH2 3DM. Tel: 031-225 6441. Information and counselling service on all aspects of adoption and on childlessness; also provides social work service for single-parent families and a befriending scheme.

Jewish Association for Fostering, Adoption and Infertility (JAFA), headquarters: PO Box 20, Prestwich, Manchester M25 5BY. Tel: 061-773 3148/776-3199. Provides support, advice and assistance, and has branches nation-wide.

Lesbian and Gay Fostering and Adoption Network, c/o London Friend, 86 Caledonian Road, London N1. Tel: 01-837 3337.

National Foster-Care Association, Francis House, Francis Street, London SW1P IDE. Tel: 01-828 6266. Exists to encourage high standards of foster care and increased opportunities of a foster home for children 'in care'.

NORCAP (National Organization for the Reunion of Children and Parents), 3 New High Street, Headington, Oxford OX3 7AJ. Helps adult adopted people who are trying to get in touch with their birth parents, and parents who have given up their children for adoption, as well as adopters. Send sae for information.

Parents for Children, 222 Camden High Street, London NW1 8QR. Tel: 01-485 7256/7548. Specializes in especially difficult to place children and also 'unusual' parents and families. (see Hedi Argent's book above).

Parent to Parent Information on Adoption Services, c/o Lower Boddington, Daventry, Northamptonshire NN11 6YB. Tel: 0327-60295. A self-help support and information service for prospective and existing adoptive families.

MISCARRIAGE AND STILLBIRTH

The Compassionate Friends, 6 Denmark Street, Bristol BS1 5DQ. Tel: 0272-292778. Helps bereaved parents.

Foundation for the Study of Infant Deaths, 15 Belgrave Square, London SW1 8PS. Tel: 01-235 1721.

Miscarriage Association, PO Box 24, Ossett, West Yorkshire WF5 9XG. Tel: 0924-264579.

National Childbirth Trust, Alexandra House, Oldham Terrace, London W3. Tel: 01-221 3833. Can also put women in touch with others who have experienced miscarriage and who hold regular meetings.

The Stillbirth and Neonatal Death Society (SANDS), 28 Portland Place, Argyle House, London W1N 4DE. Tel: 01-436 5881. Helps bereaved parents.

Twins and Multiple Births Association (TAMBRA), Secretary: 41 Fortuna Way, Aylesbury Park, Grimsby, South Humberside, DN37 9SJ. Tel: 0472-883182. Support networks for people who have experienced death of one or more babies.

PART V

WOMEN GROWING OLDER

WOMEN GROWING OLDER

Rewritten by
FIONA POLAND AND JILL RAKUSEN

I am so busy being old that I dread interruptions. This sense of vigour and spaciousness may cease, and I must enjoy it while it is here.

A long life makes me feel nearer truth . . . I want to tell people approaching and perhaps fearing age that it is a time of discovery . . . If at the end of your life you have only yourself, it is much. [A woman aged eighty-two][1]

Several groups of women took part in discussions which led to the original US chapter covering the period in a woman's life from the forties to the eighties and beyond. A Menopause Collective, an older women's group (ages fifty-two to seventy-eight) and a midlife group (ages thirty-nine to fifty-six) met to talk about their lives, identifying important resources and issues, gaining perspectives on their own lives and those of their parents and contributing to the writing and editing. For this UK version many different women in groups and individually have contributed their ideas.

Women experience so many changes – physical, social, economic and emotional – during these decades that we can't do justice to them in a single chapter. Yet, older women's concerns are so often overlooked, even in feminist books, that it is important to begin.

In our older years we may feel entitled to do what pleases and satisfies us, to slow down, to let go the strain of former obligations, to express our thoughts and feelings more strongly than ever before.

Old age, because of its time perspective, can be a period of emotional and sensory awareness and enjoyment. I savour life more often. When I draw an iris, I see that iris more vividly than I did when my physical sight was better. When I read a book now, I read it more slowly. Several books I have reread, one I have just finished reading the third time.

Elemental things of life have assumed greater importance. I spend more time looking at sunsets.

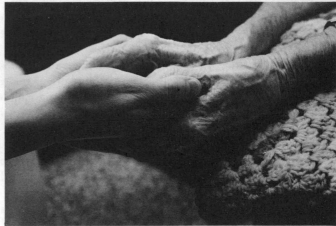

Bonnie Burt

I am more aware of the importance to myself and others of touching (both physical and emotional), of communication, of tenderness.

Space and time for quiet reflection is more available for me now. In a strange way, impossible to put into words, I am experiencing a unity beyond space and time.

Sometimes I feel guilty to be happy when there are so many things wrong in the world and I'm not doing something about making joy possible for others. Yet the universe is going to have to get along without me sometime and so I don't have to change everything. Many of my companions are interested in a better, more compassionate world; I don't have to rush to do it all. [A woman aged seventy-eight]

. . . I know myself better and have more time to pursue my own interests. I enjoy less tempestuous relationships with children and grandchildren. I enjoy a personal growth not possible in my busier years. [A woman aged seventy-three]

Some of us, however, miss these possible pleasures due

to illness or to the loss of certain capacities, or to the combined effects of poverty, sexism, racism and/or ageism, which we discuss first. Later on in this chapter we discuss various aspects of medical care in later life.

THE CONTEXT IN WHICH WE GROW OLDER

AGE AND AGEISM

Most of us want to live a long life but our white, male-dominated culture devalues ageing and being old, especially where women are concerned. While people are often separated by age and generation, women's experience, labour and capacity to adapt are relied on throughout their lives, by people of all ages. There is no retirement age for women's work as 'carers', yet this work, while being taken for granted, is consistently devalued economically. As our bodies change we can sometimes be made to feel that we are losing our only valued asset.

Ageism is the systematic discrimination against persons because of their age. It permeates our thinking in many subtle and unconscious ways so that the discrimination against older people which goes on in all of our social institutions seems to be 'just the way things are' – until we name and confront it.

Ageism has several sources. First, our society tries to deny the reality of infirmity and death, and to avoid acknowledging our interdependence and our own fears. This massive denial discourages us from planning for our later years and feeds the myth that 'old age' – a period covering perhaps a quarter of our lives – is synonymous with ill health. The majority of us will consider ourselves healthy and lead independent lives and will actually only be 'ill' for a very short time before we die.

Second, we devalue all those who are not seen as 'economically productive' – the old, the young and their care-givers. Some older people are pushed aside before we are ready to retire from paid or other work because it is assumed that, once past a certain age, we can make no significant contribution.

Ageing deepens class and gender differences. Wealthy people are often able to maintain their economic positions. Low-income people inevitably grow poorer if they become ill and can no longer get paid work. As women we spend less time in paid work because of our care work, and what jobs we have are worse paid and carry lower pensions if any. This greatly affects our ability to pay for what we need to maintain our home lives as older women. Racism, too, adds to the impact of being an older woman, affecting income and therefore resources in later life and often hindering access to services and benefits for older people.

Third, isolation of older people and dismissal of their skills and wisdom tend to be more acute in times of rapid social and technological change, when we may forget that we can still learn much about living in a difficult world from those who have a greater reservoir of experience of doing so. (Nevertheless, many of us from a range of cultures may feel a sense of pride in the knowledge of becoming a member of the community whose age and experience *are* respected.)

Even as we ourselves age, we may discriminate against older people.

I had always said, 'Oh, I want to be with people of all ages, or with young people,' but in fact I was avoiding being with people my own age – which would mean admitting I'm an old person – and missing out on a lot because of it!

I signed up for a weekend of hiking through a group for older people, and that changed my mind. Everyone was so alert. We were all in sports clothes and we didn't worry about keeping every hair in place. We're not Amazons by any means, just people interested in vigorous outdoor activity. [A woman in her seventies]

Some older women have taken action against stereotyped media images which foster ageism. The Gray Panthers (in the US) and pensioners' action groups here conduct 'media watches' and many individuals are keeping alert.

Every time I see a positive image of an older woman on TV, I write a complimentary letter to the sponsor of the programme. And when I see something offensive, I let them know that, too.

There have been successes, such as the television programmes 'Open Space' and 'Years Ahead'.

Ageism, not age itself, is what limits older people. The fact that I can do things at seventy that when I was sixty would have been frowned upon as inappropriate for an older woman shows how absurd ageism is, and how much difference changing social attitudes can make. Every time we speak out we change attitudes. Affirming ourselves is now in the air. That makes a lot more things possible.

THE FEMINIZATION OF AGEING

The majority of older people are women. Women live, on average, six years longer than men. Today more people are living longer than ever before.*

---

*In 1983 all over sixty-five represented 15 per cent of the total population whereas in 1901 they were 5 per cent.

RATIO OF WOMEN TO MEN IN TWO AGE GROUPS
(1986 figures)

Age	Percentage in UK Population	
	Women	Men
45–64	51	49
65 and over	61	39

Source: *Social Trends*, no. 18. London: HMSO, 1988.

Until the age of forty-five, numbers of men and women are approximately equal, then the gap starts to widen. Women over sixty-five are the fastest-growing segment of the UK population. Between 1901 and 1970 the number of women over sixty-five increased twice as fast as the number of men over sixty-five.

EXPECTANCY OF LIFE IN UK

	Women	Men
1931	62	58
1981	76	70

Source: *Social Trends*, no. 17. London: HMSO, 1987.

The problematic issues of age – chronic illness, poverty, care-giving, needing care, surviving one's relatives and closest friends – are therefore predominantly women's problems, and affect us throughout our lives. Yet researchers and policy-makers have mainly been men who overlook older women's special concerns. Because we are statistically and politically 'invisible' *as women*, our needs are not addressed.

A positive side of our growing numbers is our potentially greater clout politically. People over sixty-five now make up more than 15 per cent of the UK population. The government and the press are paying more attention to us – although often public discussion focuses on 'the problem of how we will care for all of them'. Yet the queues for treatment which would make daily life easier, such as hip-replacement operations, grow ever longer. Extra hospital beds for the elderly are provided without extra nursing and rehabilitative staff in some places.[2] In others hospital places are cut back without provision for adequate community care.[3] This drastically affects the quality of life of elderly people (mostly women) and their hard-pressed carers (usually women).[4]

We need to take advantage of our greater presence to create, demand and fight for policies that respond to mid-life and older women's needs. Age Concern, the Older Feminist Network and the Older Lesbian Network are national organizations which voice older women's concerns.

With partners or without, our friendships with women matter, for it is other women of all ages who will most likely sustain us when we are older. Large numbers of women outlive their husbands, often by a decade or two and a significant number even outlive their eldest sons.

I had never particularly liked women. When I was younger I remember thinking that men were 'it'; they knew what was what and they did things. I've rethought that a few times, especially after my experiences with death, divorce, major problems with children. We all have to deal with loss because we women are the ones who care for men when they are ill, and they are the ones who go first. It's given me a tremendous compassion for other women. [A woman in her sixties]

I was brought up to believe that the people in my biological family were the most important people in my world. I'm still very attached to immediate family members but I have consciously extended my family to include my 'sisters' in the women's community. [A woman in her fifties]

My loneliest times were during my marriage. I came out as a lesbian and my life with women has been a revelation. But so many women I meet don't understand my problems as a single parent and are younger than me. Coming to an older women's meeting has made me realize that I want to meet more women my own age. [A woman in her forties]

AGEISM AND SEXISM – THE DOUBLE-EDGED SWORD

The ageism we face is reinforced by sexism. Why are women seemingly considered old and 'past it' at an earlier age than men?

It was hard for me to tell the man I have been going out with how old I am. When I told him, I felt terrible as if I were telling him I had some socially disgraceful disease. You can't imagine! [She is sixty-two, her friend is sixty.]

Yet women have greater vitality. In terms of life expectancy, it can be argued that women are 'younger' than men of the same age, and our work continues past 'retirement age'.

This double standard for ageing leads us to define older men as 'craggy', women as 'wrinkled'; a man's grey hair is 'distinguished', a woman's shows she is 'over the hill'; maturity makes a man sexually attractive, a woman, grandmotherly.

Our culture sees the sexuality of midlife and older women as a source of humour – grotesque, threatening and inappropriate. Such prejudice arises in part from falsely equating sexuality with reproductive capacity and is perpetuated by the male-dominated media.

When we made love for the first time, I wept for shame at my marred and sagging body, certain that she would have found me repulsive . . . As our relationship develops, though, I'm beginning to feel easier . . . I can see that ageism isn't only to do with how we feel about others, it's to do with how we feel about ourselves, too . . . Nowadays my weeping is for pity for all of us who have for so long been trapped in the prison of men's dictates about what is valuable and desirable in women . . . Now I may look older, since I no longer wear cosmetics or constraining clothes, but I feel as young as I feel, and that's as young as time, as young as a ninety-year-old, as young as the infant I still am. [Jenny, aged fifty-four][5]

AGEISM AND RACISM

Information about help for older people is often not made available to older members of ethnic minority communities. And services often do not reflect our variety of different needs. Assumptions are made about such communities 'looking after their own' – which is simply to shift the burden of responsibility, denying such older people access to treatment and care which is everyone's right. The Standing Conference of Ethnic Minority Senior Citizens is one organization that is beginning to have an impact on racist attitudes and services. See p. 479 for details about them and other resources.

POVERTY

After a lifetime of being either unpaid or underpaid, it is no accident that older women are considerably poorer than older men.*

The poverty rate for women over sixty-five is more than double that for men over sixty-five. Forty-two per cent of those on low incomes *at* or *below* supplementary benefit level (as it used to be called) are people over sixty-five. Because of our life expectancy, most of these are likely to be women. More of the elderly are likely to be living in bad housing conditions, without basic amenities – like a bath and indoor lavatory – than the general population.[6]

The causes of women's poverty are political:

- Women often have to withdraw from the waged workforce because of caring responsibilities, either full-time or part-time. If and when we return to the workforce later in life, we often must take jobs with very low wages or, indeed, find ourselves 'unemployable' for lack of 'recent' experience. Low wages, the low rates of bene-

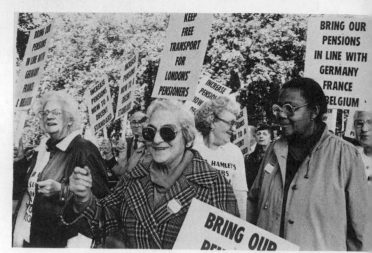

Pensioner's Day of Action, 1984

Joanne O'Brien

fits and the non-availability of social care are problems of the whole society and the political decisions which shape it, not simply accidental happenings in our individual lives.*

- Sex discrimination means women earn less and receive less income from superannuation and employers' pensions.
- Men are more likely to be supported and cared for. When women need care, we are more dependent on benefits which are constantly under threat of cuts.
- Many benefits for which a woman may apply are assessed on the basis of marital status and assume that our financial needs are met through a sexual relationship with someone we live with. Benefits are then reduced accordingly without any notion of how money is controlled and shared out in different household arrangements. However, even on a single person's state benefit or pension women cannot afford a decent standard of living. This is no way to guarantee in later years that we can afford a lifestyle which does not cut us off from everyday life and contact.
- Many occupational pensions for women limit benefits for our dependants more than is done for men. For instance, widows' pensions may be provided but not widowers'. However, there are several which do treat men and women more equally. Lesbians may wish to choose schemes which include provision for a partner. Better schemes refer to 'members' not 'partners'.

ECONOMIC PLANNING

Many of us have begun to realize how important it is to take ourselves seriously and do economic planning which lays

---

*Recent studies of poverty in the 1970s and 1980s find that the new poor are the unemployed, elderly and increasingly 'one-parent families' – mostly young women.

*In 1983, male adult manual workers averaged gross weekly earnings of £140. Adult women averaged £87. Forty-nine per cent of men received overtime pay compared with 19 per cent of women. Between 1979 and 1984 the number of men unemployed more than doubled. The number of unemployed women trebled.

the groundwork for having choices in our later years. Sometimes the death or departure of a partner means having to learn about managing money for the first time.

Because we are all growing older, we all have a stake in supporting older women's demands and concerns. We have to ensure at workplaces and through unions and other organizations that our work is upgraded, that we apply for better-paid jobs and use tribunals to break down the barriers between 'women's jobs' and 'men's jobs'. Many social changes that would help older women to participate more fully in the workplace are similar to those needed by younger women with children: care-giving services for children and sick family members, more appropriate health care, flexibility in homes and jobs.

Working a nine-to-five job is not the only way of being 'productive'. We know that whether we work for pay, bring up children or grandchildren, care for a sick family member or work in the community as volunteers, our work is real yet undervalued. The fight to ensure that our ability to maintain ourselves in later life is not tied to a partner or dependent only on our history of waged work is a vital feminist issue. The present feminist community of younger women has not sufficiently acknowledged its roots in the work done by our mothers in birth control, education, housing and welfare. There is a danger of not acknowledging the resources and needs we all share with women whose lives made our past.

It is the ultimate irony and triumph of patriarchy that the women's movement has built itself on a shame of mothers instead of a glory of them.[7]

THE MIDDLE YEARS

EXPLORATION, GROWTH AND EXPANSION

The midlife years between forty-five and sixty-five can be experienced as less to do with how much time is passing than to do with particular life events that are often linked with 'being that age'. The possibility of becoming pregnant retreats, children become older and maturity can bring more confidence in skills, relationships and sexuality. This can often be a time when we have a surge of new energy, take stock of our lives and look for ways to use our time and abilities in new and different ways.

One day after twenty-odd years of marriage and three children I asked myself, 'Who am I? What am I doing? Where am I going?' The only answer I could come up with was 'I am a wife and mother.' That was only part of me – not all of me. When I was younger I used to have fairly clear edges, but over the years being the mother and wife with unmatched fervour made those edges fuzzy.

I loved my work as a nurse. I'd never married or had children. I always denied that I experienced sexism until, when I was thirty-eight, a new male nurse was promoted above me. That left me fuming. I used my life savings to return to study and then medical school. I've never been sorry.

I just want more! More time free of kids to focus on my work; more time to myself; more passion in my marriage or from somewhere else! [A woman in her forties]

This surge of energy may come with release from two decades of child-rearing. Even while we miss our children, we can use the time freed to refocus – to acquire new skills, refine old ones, spend more time with people, get a job, work harder at our present job, enjoy time to reflect. It can feel, as one woman puts it, like 'getting myself back'.

I returned to college for several reasons – a response to a suddenly very empty house (three sons leaving at once) and a major change (just moving to the country from a large city) to increase my knowledge of social work and to finish a degree begun thirty years earlier. I wanted to prepare for what I dimly perceived might be the beginning of a new chapter – and what turned out to be a whole new edition!

The unexpected results were that I rediscovered my own intelligence and found skills I had been unaware of. I met up with younger women and forged relationships that have continued long since. I encouraged several contemporaries to jump in and try it! In my field work, I came in contact with various local decision-makers, and immediately found the door wide open for getting involved with community issues. As my professional focus and confidence deepen, I learn valuable lessons from those older people who are not only my clients but my teachers.

We may experience a change in our perspective – a heightened awareness of the passage of time and of the value of the time we have left.

Now is the time to do the things I've always wanted to do. I'm no longer thinking in terms of 'someday', but 'soon'. [A woman aged fifty]

It was a shock when a friend of ours, a middle-aged man, died suddenly. It got me thinking that I don't know how many years Dan and I have left together. I've been working hard with some gains. This is still very important to me, but I no longer want it to absorb my whole life. Now that we're in our forties, I want to spend time together and have fun.

When I was fifty I was the oldest person in my community and quite conscious of being older. I thought (this seems ridiculous now that I am seventy-six) that I certainly had to plan ahead because I wouldn't have much time left. In the next five or ten years I wanted to travel a lot before I died.

Enjoy now as much as you can because there is almost never a tomorrow the exact way you would like to have it. [A woman aged eighty-five]

LOSSES DURING THE MIDDLE YEARS

In addition to growth and expansion, the middle years can bring a number of changes which, experienced in quick succession, can feel like 'a crescendo of losses'. Statistically, many of the important losses women face cluster in the forty-five to fifty-five year period. We may mourn them, often without knowing how to express our feelings or to whom.

Some losses undermine our image of ourselves as young, healthy, even immortal, such as when diseases attack the wholeness of our bodies. The risk of breast cancer increases considerably as we reach our fifties (see p. 545) as does the chance of our having a hysterectomy (the latter further increases in our sixties). We all lose our fertility at menopause (see p. 453). If we have children, they often leave home at about the time our fertility ends.

Other important relationships may end or change. Our partners may die (the average age of widowhood is fifty-six). Or they may move on to younger women. Our parents may become ill or die. We have to care for them or for our partners and we may have to give up or postpone long-awaited changes or adventures. All these situations can leave us with less money or no pension and cause considerable stress.

However, in other respects, hysterectomy and menopause, children leaving and changes in partnerships can be tremendously 'freeing', encouraging us to reassess ourselves, our time and value. Although it is women who live longer and can, therefore, be assumed to suffer more of life's losses we also often seem to have more resilience. The highest rate of suicides is among men over seventy-five. The rate of suicide among women over seventy-five is less than half that of men.

Changes in Body Image

The surface signs of ageing mean that we have to develop a new body image. We are taught that much of our value is in our youthful looks (see Chapter 2) and we may experience such changes as a painful loss.

When I walk down the street with my daughter now, I notice that when male heads turn in our direction they are looking at her. My pride in her blossoming young womanhood is bittersweet, because I miss getting that attention myself.

Employers may unfairly dismiss us as incompetent or useless if we don't present a youthful ('contemporary')

image and deny us opportunities if we 'look our age' or have 'let ourselves go' by refusing to diet or dye our hair. In our social groups and relationships, youthful appearance may be overvalued.

A few months ago I let my white hair re-emerge after some years of dyeing it. I thought it was more authentic. The man I am seeing now is about my age (sixty-two). He said that because he doesn't have white hair he would like me to continue colouring my hair. After thinking it over, I decided that I prefer it coloured too.

Most lesbians' culture is youth-orientated, and I feel better with my hair brown rather than grey. People don't look at me as though I'm old. [A woman aged fifty-two]

Some of us feel more confident when we can delay the outward signs of ageing by using make-up and hair colouring.* A growing number of us believe that our years of experience entitle us to wear our greying hair, wrinkles or extra pounds with pride – as mature women. Becoming older can give us the chance to experiment with changing our image – different styles, colours and ways of presenting ourselves.

I look in the mirror and am always a little surprised that, with my greying hair and some new wrinkles, I don't feel what I'm 'supposed' to be feeling. If I were not constantly bombarded from reading, media and society in general with reminders that now that I'm fifty-three I'm supposed to be in crisis, withdrawing, feeling depressed, isolated, incapable or ashamed, these ideas wouldn't occur to me. I am simply building on what was before, seeking out new opportunities. I am, as always, energetic and involved.

GRANDMOTHER ROCKING

Last night I dreamed of an old lover.
I had not seen him in forty years.
When I awoke I saw him on the street,
his hair was white,
his back stooped.
How could I say hello?
He would have puzzled all day
about who the young girl was
who smiled at him.
So I let him go on his way.

© EVE MERRIAM

---

*Research indicates that cosmetics, especially some commercial hair dyes, contain cancer-producing chemicals.

When Our Children Grow Up and Leave*

At this time, many of us feel the satisfaction of a job well done or at least over.** Yet we may feel sadness at losing a daily relationship with our child(ren), some of whom may have become close friends or confidants.

When child-rearing has been our main work and we haven't planned what to do next, we may be at a loose end. Identity crises have less to do with the 'empty nest' (no other purpose in life) and more to do with the question, 'What am I going to do with myself now?'

As we continue to develop our own skills and interests, we can acknowledge missing our children, yet be glad of the extra time for our other pursuits, which may take us outside the home and into new and different activities. †

The 'Dependency Squeeze' of the Middle Years

When children are older, we may be ready to focus on what *we* want, only to find that new family demands from both older and younger generations may actually increase.

As a single parent with young children and ageing parents having health problems, I am pulled between two sets of needs. The pressures are most intense on Sundays when I 'should' visit my parents. (They get home help and meals-on-wheels on weekdays but not weekends.) At the same time, since I work every day and go to night school twice a week, I want to do something healthy and 'outdoors' with my children. When Monday morning dawns I haven't had a day to sleep late, scan the Sunday papers, bake bread or meet with a friend – and when I try to take one I end up feeling guilty all the next week.

A further complication is that our partners may resent attention being given to ageing parents just when children have left – yet many also expect women to care for in-laws. Brothers usually expect their sisters to care for elderly parents, and unmarried sisters (this often means lesbians) particularly experience this pressure.

Because of the economic situation, some adult children continue living with us or they may come back home to live. We can easily end up feeling used and abused.

I still do all the washing and shopping for my sons in their twenties. They don't really pay much towards the household running costs, but you feel like you're just running a boarding house.

*Child-rearing is such a major part of so many women's lives that we cannot possibly do it justice here. For a whole chapter on parents' feelings when their children leave home, see *Ourselves and Our Children: a Book by and for Parents* (see Resources in Chapter 20).

**In Lillian Rubin's study of middle-aged women, at least a quarter of the women expressed relief when the last child left home.[8]

†Laurie Shields, an American woman, has written a book called *Displaced Homemakers: Organizing for a New Life* (see Resources).

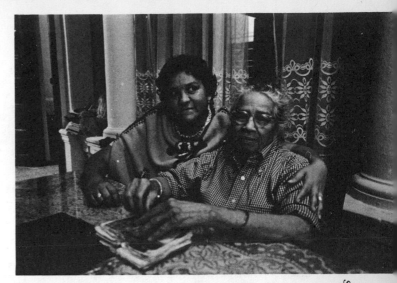

Sarah Putnam

Other mothers, feeling newly independent, are better able to create new kinds of relationships.

After my children were grown up and wanted to return home, I made it clear they were welcome only as equal adults bearing their share of the responsibilities of the home, not in a mother–child role.

We may have a respite between child-rearing and the care-giving demands of the middle and later years.

One of the main reasons I'm going on a longer holiday now is that I feel I have this golden moment when Deborah doesn't have a baby she needs help with and my parents are still well.

Often we may feel we don't have many choices. Yet even as we attempt to meet many demands on our time and energy, we are entitled to make some time for ourselves and it is important and necessary that we do.

Loss of People We Love

As we watch our parents and relatives age, we begin to prepare ourselves for their deaths.

Two of my favourite uncles died a few years ago. Now my favourite aunt at seventy has cancer of the pancreas and a third uncle has just had his second heart attack. I wept and wept about these real and threatened deaths of people who are like stalwart, familiar trees in the landscape of my childhood. I shouted, 'No, I can't stand this; not my favourite aunt!' I know that it's inevitable. I dread my mother's phone calls now because every time she announces another illness, another death. Such present and imminent loss makes me value everyone I love, and life itself.

My mother now suffers both from a chronic and a progressive disease in an advanced state and from some of the debilitating effects of being in poor health and approaching eighty. She seems to be gradually fading away, her hair becoming whiter, her skin paler.

In my own life at the same time I have been going through a difficult transition – the end of a fifteen-year marriage – and experiencing some physical changes of midlife. For a while I equated them with my potential decay and imminent death, as a parallel to my mother's decline. My periods had become prolonged and heavy, I was anaemic, looking pale (like my mother), and my hair was greying. I chipped a tooth twice in one month and began to worry about whether this meant my bones were becoming fragile. The bleeding got worse; I wore sanitary pads for weeks because tampons were insufficient; it felt like an incontinence pad, which is what my mother has to wear. My gynaecologist recommended a hysterectomy. I felt totally sexless, listless and lifeless. Now I see that some of these changes were transitory health problems which I got help for, and others simply the normal changes of middle age, with depression and stress exaggerating my feelings and fears.

Some of my relatives had criticized the decision to place my mother in a home. Part of my identification with her decline came from guilt that I could go on and live and even enjoy my life when my mother was in such poor health.

One night during that time I dreamed of my own death. Instead of fear, I felt peace and completion. My work on earth had been accomplished. My only sadness was regret at not being able to attend my daughter's wedding. I transformed myself into a beautiful rainbow – nature's chuppah [a Jewish wedding canopy] – and protected the festivities from bad weather. I could feel that my daughter recognized the rainbow as my gift to her.

When I awoke I was at peace with saying goodbye to my mother when the time came. I knew she would no more want to take me with her, frightening as it is to die alone, than I would want my daughter's life to end with my death.

Most women will experience the death of their partners. Only a third of women over sixty-five and one-eighth of those over eighty-five will still have husbands and many more will have lost 'unofficial' partners, male and female, whom they had been loving or living with. A widowed woman lives, on average, eighteen years after the death of a spouse. Chances of remarriage are low and decrease with age because three out of four elderly men are married compared with only one out of three elderly women.*

The stress of partner loss or widowhood is enormous, one of the most difficult life situations we live through. Grief is compounded when we:

* have found our main identity in being a wife or through our partner;
* are isolated and lonely after the initial mourning period;
* find that most of our friends are in couples;
* have to seek new friends as a formerly married person;
* have not been able to discuss the loss fully because the relationship was not a marriage or it was a lesbian partnership;
* have to face a reduced income;
* are unused to handling finances and are faced with having to do so for the first time when still numb with the shock of loss.

The full impact of loss may come months or even a year later. Counsellors claim that grief can take anything up to five years before we are able to enjoy life fully again and still be 'normal'. Be wary of doctors who try to medicate away our normal grieving or label it pathological if it takes 'too long'. There is no right time or right way to grieve.

We need people to ring us, visit, bring food, invite us to do things and leave us alone when that's what we want. Yet some may pull back, especially after the initial formalized mourning period or be embarrassed or frightened by our grieving or our needs. Many women have found special support and understanding from other women who have lost partners (see Resources). Ultimately we can build new lives.

When my husband died five years after our divorce, I experienced, with the utter finality of his death, the absolute end of our relationship. Suddenly the years of separation were obliterated and I mourned deeply the loss of my husband, the father of my children, and the ending of the whole life we had shared.

My lover died of breast cancer at sixty-two. Although we had lived together for nearly thirty years I was not able to talk openly about the depth of loss I experienced. I decided to move to a city where I would be close to a number of friends from earlier years who had known us both. I found that by building a new life near them and as I had to look after a cousin in bad health for two years I was able to feel that my life had more meaning. Involvement in the lives of my women friends was very important to me at this time, especially as many of them were experiencing similar events themselves and we were able to support each other.

My husband died after a seven-year period when his health had been deteriorating and I had looked after him. My mother died within six weeks of his

---

*The majority of men who have lost their wives remarry. Those who remain single have higher death and illness rates. It is thought that women adjust better to widowhood despite the stresses because of our greater ability to make and keep friends.

death. So, in addition to losing a husband and a mother, I lost a part of myself, my role as a helping, caring person.

I went out to my mother's house and stayed there for six weeks. I did a lot of different things, but I spent a lot of time writing about what I had left now that I no longer had that identity: who am I?

And what I had left was that I was a woman and I was growing older, and that was the beginning of both my feminism and my understanding of the concept of ageing. That became a new identity for me.

A lot of us women are not brought up to believe that we can make something of what we are. I had been my parents' child and my husband's wife and my children's mother. Now I had the opportunity to be a person in my own right.

Coping with a Series of Losses

This process is one of the most difficult tasks of middle and later life.

A psychiatrist gave me Valium when I was in my forties. I took it regularly or fairly frequently for about five to ten years. Now I think that tranquillizers suppressed or sent underground the pains of that period (divorce, death of mother, betrayal by a lover). These pains still surface with agonizing strength. Maybe if I had fully faced them and 'digested' them at the time they happened, this would not be the case.

When devastating losses occur in a cluster, we feel stunned and very much alone. We shouldn't expect too much of ourselves at this time. One of the best things we can do for ourselves is accept our feelings as normal and not try to carry the load without help. Watch out for doctors who offer drugs to suppress legitimate feelings of despair, anger, guilt, emptiness, fear, anxiety, confusion. Remember, there is no right time or right way to grieve. Each of us has her own unique rhythm. Talking with women who have 'been there' often helps, as does reminiscing, writing or keeping a diary. It is often now possible to find workshops designed to help us come to terms with despair or anger. Many bereavement counselling projects and self-help groups now exist which provide support – sometimes related to particular illnesses or as part of the activity of women's organizations or community groups. (See Resources at the end of Chapters 8 and 10, as well as p. 479.)

It takes enormous energy to rebuild your life. Don't exhaust yourself trying to take care of the emotional needs of others. Take special care of yourself. You will probably need more rest than usual. Go slowly – give yourself time to heal, to regain your trust in the world and in your own capacities.

MENOPAUSE*

PREVAILING SOCIAL VIEWS

Stereotypical thinking about menopausal women includes many myths (many created and perpetuated by doctors and psychiatrists).

The first thing that comes to my mind about menopause is FALLACIES: menopause is blamed for every mood change and unexplained feeling, the way menstruation is with younger women; also discrimination and derision – 'she must be going through the change'.

Helene Deutsch, a disciple of Freud, referred to menopause as women's 'partial death'. Mastering psychological reaction to menopause was, she said, 'one of the most difficult tasks of a woman's life'.[9] It would be more accurate to say that our most difficult task is mastering reaction to the cultural stereotype of menopausal women, a process which is complicated and made even more difficult by the fact that we cannot help internalizing that image to some degree.

The 'raging hormones' myth describes menopausal women as so incapacitated by hormone fluctuations that we are incapable of rational thought and behaviour, and should certainly not hold any kind of responsible position.† A more recent myth, part of the 'superwoman' mystique, suggests that the usefully busy woman will hardly notice menopause at all. Neither extreme is accurate or helpful to women.

Particularly damaging is the myth linking menopause and depression. In the first half of this century, doctors and families hospitalized thousands of women for a 'disorder' called 'involutional melancholia', a 'mental disease' which supposedly occurred during or just after menopause. Though contemporary studies fail to demonstrate that depression among midlife women is associated with menopause, the fear of going crazy at menopause is still part of our culture. Yet involutional melancholia is not a disease but a myth.**

Even when a menopausal woman feels comfortable with herself, her family and others around her may resent her independence, mood swings or irritability, perhaps even fear these as signs of her growing older. They may even urge drugs, surgery or psychotherapy on her rather than being willing to live with her through the changes.

Misogyny taints much of the medical literature. A well-known gynaecologist/writer has referred to menopause as 'a

---

*See Stages in the Reproductive Cycle p. 34.
†Nineteenth-century doctors taught (and practised on) the belief that the uterus was a source of disease and hysteria, especially once reproduction was over. Male doctors used myths about menopause to keep women out of medicine by casting doubt on their emotional stability.
**Involutional melancholia has been dropped from the current edition of the *Diagnostic and Statistical Manual of Mental Disorders*.[10]

living decay',[11] and another has said that menopausal women are a 'caricature of their younger selves at their emotional worst'.[12] In his best-selling book, Dr David Reuben continues that the menopausal woman is 'not really a man but no longer a functional woman', and after menopause will 'just be marking time until she follows her glands into oblivion'.[13] After helping to create the above stereotypes, some doctors reinforce them by treating menopause as a deficiency disease to be managed with hormone replacement 'therapies', tranquillizers or surgery. In our efforts to counter such myths, we may unwittingly suggest that we can sail through menopause without even noticing its physical discomforts and emotional changes, not to mention the social realities facing midlife women. If we overlook the changes of menopause, we run the risk of trivializing our experience. Menopause is an important physical and emotional life transition, and we are different after we have gone through it. We can be strengthened and empowered by acknowledging the reality of our experiences and giving one another support during this transition.

DEFINITIONS OF MENOPAUSE

Definitions of menopause vary in medical literature, with little consensus on when it begins and ends and disagreement about its definitive signs. Since the term menopause literally means the cessation of menstruation, the term *climacteric* is more appropriate as a definition of the period during which menstruation ceases and the body gradually adjusts. This period of adjustment usually starts well before menstruation stops and continues for some time afterwards. Going through menopause is experiencing the whole period which begins when we first have menstrual irregularities (if we have them – see below) until menstruation finally stops completely and our bodies adjust to the hormonal changes, in particular to lower levels of oestrogen production.

We may each have our own definition of menopause.

I think of menopause as the psychological and emotional shifting of gears we experience when our hormone production changes, preparing us for a new stage of life.

Menopause is a slow turning in life. Your insides are changing but you remain the same person. Some people battle with this period as if trying to stop it. Some accept it and go through it more easily.

It's the end of periods and birth control. What a relief!

In the past twenty years, research into menopause has at last increased, partly because of the increased visibility of midlife women. Unfortunately, drug companies have performed or influenced most of the research.[14] Women-initiated research might choose more relevant issues based on our own experiences, and our conclusions might be more holistically- and preventively- rather than drug-orientated.

PHYSICAL CHANGES

Although medical and popular literature often discuss numerous menopause 'symptoms', only three signs can be directly attributed to changes in oestrogen production:

1. changes in menstrual cycle;
2. hot flushes and sweats ('vasomotor instability');
3. vaginal changes (decrease of moisture and elasticity in the vagina, sometimes called 'atrophy').

Yet changes in oestrogen production do not necessarily lead to 'symptoms', and since stress has been shown to influence oestrogen levels – or lack of them – in both pre-menopausal and post-menopausal women,[15] it is clear that hormone balance can be helped or hindered by our lifestyle and socio-economic situation.

Menstrual Changes

For most women the first signs of approaching menopause are changes in the menstrual cycle. Some of us menstruate more frequently than before, others skip periods or find that they are more widely spaced. We may have shorter periods with lighter bleeding or longer and/or heavier bleeding, sometimes with clots and 'flooding'.

I'd just got off a train and noticed I was flooding (though bolstered by a tampon and two pads). I rushed along the platform to the loos. Blood flowed down my stockings and into my shoes. More dripped onto the carpet. Both loos were occupied, of course. I waited, breathing deeply and resisting the very strong urge to kick in both doors.

Because very heavy or extended bleeding is such a frightening, disruptive and debilitating symptom, we can easily be pressured into taking drastic action, such as unnecessary surgery. (See hysterectomy p. 597.) While it is true that heavy and irregular bleeding is a possible sign of cancer, this is true only in a small minority of cases.* It is a possibility, so do check it out by asking for an endometrial biopsy or a D & C (see p. 596 and p. 594). Some women choose hysterectomy simply because of the disruption that the flooding causes in work and social life. However, we can learn to cope by talking with other women who have this problem and by discovering new ways to decrease the flow, such as non-medical approaches and alternative healing methods. If you want to consider these techniques, you should know that the most serious health risk you face, once cancer has been ruled out, is that of becoming

---

*Only 6 per cent of women develop uterine or ovarian cancer during the menopausal years, forty-five to fifty-four. The risk of cancer increases as we *pass* menopause, climbing to 14 per cent for ages sixty to sixty-four, the years of highest risk.[16] The risk may be increased if we have taken HRT, however, particularly in the form of oestrogen alone (see p. 456).

anaemic. Have your haemoglobin checked regularly and take iron if yours is low.*

Premenstrual symptoms may intensify or change, too, or begin to be noticeable for the first time.

The worst discomfort for me has been a great increase in premenstrual tension, extreme nervousness, breast soreness, headaches and insomnia for a week to ten days before my period.

One woman in five has no changes in her menstrual cycle at all until menstruation suddenly stops.[17]

It is hard to tell exactly when menstruation stops for good; periods may stop for several months, then start up again, and such fluctuations can last for a year or longer. Pregnancy is still possible during this time. The current rule of thumb is that there is a risk of pregnancy for women under fifty until they have been period-free for twenty-four months, and for women over fifty until they have been period-free for twelve months.

Hot Flushes

The sign most commonly associated with menopause is hot flushes. Some women describe it as a sensation of heat in the face or moving through or across the upper half of the body. Sweating may follow, and sometimes you may experience a feeling like suffocation. Chills frequently precede or follow. Hot flushes vary in intensity, duration and frequency. They can be aggravated by stress and diet. Some women get hot flushes when their bodies become overheated – during a heat wave, for example – when they eat highly spiced food or drink coffee or alcohol.

During hot flushes, blood vessels dilate and constrict irregularly and unpredictably. No one knows exactly why this occurs. When ovarian oestrogen production declines, the pituitary gland (located in the head) sends signals for the production of more oestrogen. One theory is that hot flushes may be the body's attempt to respond.

Hot flushes may begin when menstruation is still regular or just beginning to fluctuate and continue after your periods end. Some women never experience them, while others have them off and on as late as their eighties. Many women are not bothered by their hot flushes. Some flushes are so mild that at first the woman experiencing them may think the room is too hot, there are too many blankets on the bed or the weather has changed. Some of us, however, are incapacitated by them. The sweating that follows can be so profuse that we need a complete change of clothes or bedclothes. Some women wake up five or six times a night or more, so that sleep may be seriously disturbed.

Some of us are embarrassed by hot flushes and particularly by their unpredictability, an embarrassment due in large part to the negative status of the ageing woman as well as to the taboos, still prevalent, about 'noticing' menstruation and menopause. Though you may feel hot or sweaty,

most onlookers fail to notice what is usually a very slight change in colouring. Check your face in the mirror the next time you have a flush and you'll probably be reassured. Many of us find hot flushes less burdensome after we discuss them (and menopause in general) with other women. Some women carry folding fans to cool themselves, making themselves more comfortable and at the same time showing others that menopause is a perfectly normal occurrence.

Vaginal Changes

Changed oestrogen levels may produce changes in the vagina (see p. 460).

Ovarian Function

When our ovaries no longer produce enough hormones to trigger the release of eggs or to build up menstrual blood and tissues on the inside wall of the uterus, both ovulation and menstruation eventually stop. *Contrary to popular and medical myth, these changes in ovarian function do not mean that our bodies or our ovaries stop producing oestrogen.* Long before the ovaries slow down, alternative sources of oestrogen production are functioning in the fatty tissues of the body and in the adrenal glands, and the ovaries themselves usually continue to secrete small amounts of oestrogen for ten years or longer after periods cease.

Adrenal Glands

Throughout life our adrenal glands help us cope with stress and maintain our resistance to disease.* As oestrogen from our ovaries begins to decline (beginning about age twenty-five), our adrenal glands gradually take over until they become our major source of oestrogen after menopause. This is accomplished by converting a secretion called *androstenadione* into *oestrone* (a non-ovarian type of oestrogen) in body fat. Exercising speeds this conversion process, and having a little fat on our bones makes it easier. While all living is stressful, we can make the adrenals' job easier by eating a healthy diet (including enough Vitamins C and B) and getting adequate exercise and rest. Also, you may want to try relaxation practices and other ways of minimizing the effects of stress (see Chapter 7). At this time in our lives comfortable habits, such as drinking coffee and alcohol and eating sweets, may actually become additional stresses on the adrenals, especially since the protection once provided by ovarian oestrogen to heart, bones and skin and other organs must now come from the adrenals.

Other Changes**

Some women cry more easily, feel irritable, depressed or anxious at times, are less patient or feel disorganized. Some

---

*You should not take iron unless a test shows you are anaemic; you may take too much.

*The adrenal glands are situated just above the kidney (see illustration on p. 507). Many researchers believe that resistance to cancer is related to adrenal function.

**For more about symptoms that might occur during the menopausal period, and their possible causes – and how to deal with them – see Jill Rakusen, *Menopause: a Guide for Women of All Ages* and Judi Fairlie et al., *Menopause: a Time for Positive Change* (see Resources for details).

of these emotional changes may be related to hormonal fluctuations. They may, however, also be a response to a culture which devalues older women or to the traumatic events which so often occur in midlife.

I definitely feel emotionally different. I am more assertive, my tolerance of people is lower, I get hurt and at times am confused about my feelings.

In what used to be a two-handkerchief film, I may have to use four.

Minor physical changes also occur during these years, more or less at the same time as menopause. Our hair may turn grey, we may grow more facial hair, need reading glasses, gain weight. It is difficult to distinguish between signs of menopause and signs of ageing; menopause itself is a sign of the ageing of the female reproductive system. It is a common myth that all changes in midlife women are caused by menopause, with the implication that a woman's reproductive cycle is the major factor in her life and that once it stops, she is a changed person. In fact, men as well as women go through many of the changes, proof that they are not caused primarily by 'oestrogen deficiency'. And research has shown that unemployment and poverty in general can be more closely associated with many psychological and bodily symptoms than a woman's menopausal status as such.[18]

I welcomed the end of my menstrual periods because for years I had experienced premenstrual tension and heavy bleeding. The hot flushes were not a bad trade-off if I could be free of periods at last. I have not had a period for four years; I feel healthier than ever, have an active and joyful sex life with no 'dry vagina' problems, and do a lot of physical activities. This is definitely the best period of my life. [A woman aged fifty-one]

MEDICAL APPROACHES TO PROBLEMS DURING MENOPAUSE

We must stress that it is only a minority of women who experience problems that require medical treatment. Those of us who do need help can often find what we need from the self-help and alternative approaches discussed on p. 458. If we go to our doctors, we may find them less than helpful.

My doctor told me anyone not able to cope with the menopause was just neurotic.

My doctor will only give me pain-killers and Valium, and I still get the most awful headaches, flushes and night-sweats. Intercourse is now so painful my husband does not dare to come near me.

Women's Health Care (now called Women's Health Concern), an agency concerned with providing informa-tion about hormone replacement therapy (see below), alone received 8,000 inquiries in 1975 from women who were unable to obtain either proper advice or treatment for their symptoms. While over ten years later many more GPs are willing to provide appropriate help for menopause symptoms, and many more gynaecologists are running 'menopause clinics', this is a double-edged change; for it is leading to the medicalization of menopause – something that has already occurred in the USA – whereby doctors are increasingly seeing menopause as a disease, with attendant medical 'solutions'.

While the medical approach 'protects' us from the normal discomforts and changes of outlook which accompany menopause and other transitions of the ageing process, it can lead us to believe that these changes are so painful or dangerous that we cannot get through them without drugs and/or surgery; that non-medical alternatives are ineffective, or that we are incapable of finding our own ways of coping. The danger is that doctors will not only do to menopausal women what they do to women in child-birth – intervene in advance to prevent us from really *living* the experience of change – but also that they will hinder us from finding real solutions to our problems at this time, *very* few of which can be solved by doctors.*

HORMONE REPLACEMENT THERAPY (HRT)

This involves taking oestrogen and/or progestogen (pro-gestogen alone is more rare) in the form of pills, injections, implants or skin patches. HRT is now in considerable vogue as a treatment for problems both during and after menopause. However, it is not *the* answer to menopausal symptoms, nor is it protection against old age. Some people believe that HRT should be every woman's right, that HRT given during and after menopause will liberate us for ever. But it does have risks, both known and unknown (see below).

What Can HRT Do?

Most cases of hot flushes and vaginal dryness – both of which can result from lowered levels of oestrogen in the body – are relieved by HRT. It is sometimes used to treat other problems – such as insomnia, irritability, nervous-ness, depression, nausea and constipation. Though it may help these conditions, in some cases a placebo effect may be operating (i.e. a 'dummy pill' would be equally effective). In fact, placebos can be effective in relieving hot flushes as well.[19]

HRT is now also being widely promoted as a way of preventing osteoporosis,** a bone problem that affects a

---

*For more on living through, and coping with, change at this time, see Jill Rakusen, *Menopause: a Guide for Women of All Ages* in Resources.
**The promotion of HRT as *the* means of preventing osteoporosis can be seen as an attempt by gynaecologists on the one hand to maintain control over treatment of menopause, and drug companies on the other to maintain their profitable interests in hormone replacement therapy, both of which suffered a serious setback when HRT's connection with cancer was raised in the 1970s.[20]

large minority of women some years after menopause and which is connected with lowered oestrogen levels. We discuss this on p. 469.

Side-effects and Risks

Despite the burgeoning of research since the last UK edition of this book, the relative long-term risks and benefits of HRT are still not clear. This is partly because it has not been used for long enough, partly because so much research has prompted more questions than it has answered, and partly because, following the endometrial cancer scare in the mid-1970s, the recommended HRT regimen for most women has been changed (to include a progestogen as well as oestrogen – see below), so that research prior to this change sheds little light on the form of HRT currently being promoted.

1. *Cancer.* The most emotive scare has centred around cancer. Several studies have pointed clearly to an increased risk of endometrial cancer with HRT involving oestrogen alone. Dosage and length of use appeared to increase the risk. Since then, evidence has been produced which strongly suggests that the addition of a progestogen minimizes or obliterates risk. However, it is possible that the addition of progestogen might increase the risk of other serious progestogen-associated problems, which could more than cancel out the 'benefits' of reducing the risk of endometrial cancer.* These problems, particularly heart disease and stroke, are linked with progestogen and are discussed below. With regard to breast cancer, some studies appear to suggest a protective effect (with progestogen added), while others – and the more well-conducted ones – suggest an increased risk in some groups of women on HRT, particularly long-term users.**

2. *Circulatory problems.* Some people are now claiming that oestrogen replacement therapy protects against heart disease, and even strokes.[22] However, much research is contradictory and the issue is still unresolved, particularly since progestogen is now often added (see below). Those studies suggesting that oestrogen replacement therapy protects against circulatory disease are not all well designed, nor are they in agreement with other studies, such as the Framingham study, which suggested significantly increased risk of stroke and heart disease and circulatory disease in general.[23] Although the authors of this latter study emphasize the need for caution when interpreting its findings, and it has recently been reanalysed to produce reassuring findings,[24] it should be remembered that the vast

majority of women in this study and in most others were on oestrogen alone – without the possibly further increased risk arising from progestogen use.

3. *Fibroids.* These tend to get worse on HRT.

4. *'Minor' effects.* Women can experience a variety of effects similar to those experienced by women taking the Pill, particularly if they take progestogen as well as oestrogen. These can include: nausea, breast tenderness, headaches, mood changes such as depression, dizziness and bloatedness.

5. Finally, taking hormones can create *vitamin imbalances*,[25] and HRT can interfere with, cover up, distort and delay the body's natural adjustment to decreased oestrogen levels, a transition which most women can pass through without major difficulty.

When and How to Use HRT

Usually, HRT is appropriate only for hot flushes and vaginal dryness, and sometimes as a preventive measure to protect the bones (see p. 470). Given the risks, known and unknown, you may decide to take HRT only if you have tried the self-help and alternative approaches discussed on p. 458. If you decide to take it, try and find a doctor who knows what s/he is doing. Bear in mind that most GPs have not studied endocrinology (study of glands which secrete hormones), so if at all possible it might be best to ask your GP to refer you to a menopause clinic. Women's Health Concern (see p. 480) has an up-to-date list of clinics. Some clinics allow women to approach them direct.

Listed below are various safeguards which are considered to be good medical practice when HRT is prescribed.

- Women should be screened beforehand, including blood pressure, pelvic examination, urine and thyroid tests, and checked regularly during treatment. Apart from anything else, the dosages may need changing.

- The lowest effective dose should be used, and only for as long as it is essential. (If the drug is tapered off gradually, this is thought to minimize the risk of symptoms such as hot flushes returning.)

- Women who have not had a hysterectomy should probably be prescribed a progestogen as well as an oestrogen, on the basis that this seems to protect against endometrial cancer. However, the addition of progestogen may lead to life-threatening or disabling circulatory problems – and more of them than the numbers of endometrial cancers it 'prevents'. For this reason, some people are wary about giving progestogen at all.[26] Unfortunately, it is not known exactly what dose of progestogen causes least risk (if any) and most benefit. As far as endometrial cancer is concerned, progestogen given for twelve to thirteen days each month is now thought to protect against this disease. Each time you stop taking the progestogen pills, you are highly likely to experience a 'withdrawal bleed' from your uterus: this is quite normal. The addition of progestogen does sometimes mean that HRT is less effective.

- Women should be monitored carefully and any

---

*As discussed, for example, at a Symposium held at the Royal Zoological Society, 8 June 1984, entitled Steroids, Safety and Sex in the Over-forties.
**Brian MacMahon, a leading American cancer epidemiologist, calculates that long-term use of menopausal oestrogens (seven to ten years) increases the risk of breast cancer *two times* over what it is for women who do not take them (personal communication). This means that *approximately one in six women who take oestrogens at menopause may develop breast cancer.* Even British epidemiologists – usually more cautious than their American counterparts – are beginning to express concern about data suggesting a relationship between HRT and breast cancer, particularly in long-term users (the risk seems to begin to increase after HRT use for thirty months).[21]

unexpected bleeding investigated. This is normally done with an *endometrial biopsy*, or *endometrial aspiration* or *lavage* can be done instead (see p. 596). In women who are taking HRT for a long time, endometrial biopsy or a similar investigation may be advisable once in a while, to make sure that HRT is not causing changes in the endometrium which could develop into cancer. However, some doctors consider this is no longer necessary if progestogen is prescribed as well.

● If oestrogen cream is prescribed (usually for vaginal dryness), it should not be used every day. After an initial two-week course of applications, it will then only be necessary to apply the cream say twice a week thereafter. The effects of the cream last around one to two weeks, and it works by being absorbed by the body (in a roughly similar way to HRT in pill or implant form) – NOT as a lubricant.*

Who Should Not Use HRT?

It is not usually considered advisable for women with a history of *breast cancer* or recurrent *breast cysts*, *endometrial*, *vaginal* or *ovarian cancer*, diseases of the *liver*, *kidney* or *pancreas*, certain types of *heart disease*, *stroke*, *thrombo-embolism*, *high blood pressure*, *diabetes*, *fibroids*, *migraine*, *endometriosis* or *gall-bladder disease*. Nor is it considered wise if you are *very overweight* or *smoke* heavily. However, exceptions may be made in some of these cases, although HRT should be prescribed under very careful supervision in these circumstances. As Trevor Powles writes concerning breast cancer: 'it is potentially dangerous to alter the endocrine status of any woman who has had, or is at high risk of developing, breast cancer, and this should be done only under expert supervision.'[27]

Women who are expecting to have an operation, particularly if it is a major operation, are often advised to come off HRT for at least six weeks beforehand to reduce the risk of blood clotting.

For some women who cannot use oestrogen, progestogen-only HRT *may* be suitable. It has been known to help in some cases, particularly with regard to hot flushes, but not with vaginal problems. It may sometimes succeed in controlling excessively heavy or prolonged bleeding. Progestogen can cause a variety of effects, such as breast tenderness, depression, water retention and vaginal dryness. It can make premenstrual tension worse. Little is yet known about the use of progestogen-alone HRT during menopause. (See, however, Safeguards, p. 296 and Depo Provera, p. 296.)

Some doctors believe that HRT can, or even should, be given for the rest of a woman's life; most believe that it

should be given for the shortest possible time and that treatment should be stopped periodically to see if it is still needed. Whatever doctors feel, *we* should be able to make the decision about HRT from the facts available and from our own feelings about the kind of lives we want to lead. It seems to us that women should be on HRT for the shortest possible time. We believe that women should have the right to be fully informed of the facts – or lack of them – and should be free to choose if, when and how to use HRT. One problem we face is sifting out the grains of truth from propaganda, 'pro-woman views' from profit-making motives, anti-HRT views from anti-woman or pro-woman views. As with all areas of health care, we will not have a choice unless:

1. we have access to reliable information;
2. the medical expertise and clinics are available;
3. we have the power to make decisions about how we wish to be treated.

ALTERNATIVE AND SELF-HELP APPROACHES

Bear in mind that stress adversely affects oestrogen levels, so anything you can do to reduce stress in your life may help.

Poor diet stresses our bodies and minds, so eating well is essential. In addition to a good diet, many midlife women find vitamins and minerals helpful. Vitamin C, Vitamin D and calcium are essential for bone formation. Vitamin A deficiency has been associated with heavy menstrual bleeding, as have low calcium and/or iron levels; supplements in moderate doses may help.* Magnesium can help relaxation. Some women find that Vitamin E reduces leg cramps, and others note that it modifies or reduces hot flushes. (Avoid Vitamin E in large doses if you have high blood pressure, diabetes or certain heart conditions.)** Some women find that Vitamin B complex reduces oedema, and others that it helps joint pains and eases stress. (See also Eating Well, p. 463.)

Some women use herbal teas to reduce or control heavy menstrual bleeding and to reduce the discomfort of hot flushes and headaches. Since instructions vary or are not specific about which herbs to use, how strong these teas should be and how much you should drink, consult a herbalist or holistic practitioner who knows about herbs. If you want to try these yourself, consult several books. Pay particular attention to any cautions (see Herbs in Chapter 7).

Relaxation techniques, such as meditation, giving and getting massages, and yoga, can reduce stress and depression. Sex, including masturbation, can be relaxing and also helps prevent insomnia and vaginal dryness. (See also Vaginal Changes, p. 460 for further discussion.) Many women find these approaches, as well as acupuncture,

---

*Don't apply it to aid lubrication during sex. Apart from anything else, your partner may absorb more than you, and unwanted breast development has been observed in males who had absorbed oestrogen cream through intercourse. It can also, of course, be absorbed via the mouth, and to a certain extent at least through the skin on the fingers – in the same way that the skin absorbs oestrogen from face creams that contain the substance.

*Vitamin A in high doses can be toxic. Try increasing foods containing carotene, with low-dose Vitamin A (no more than 10,000 IUs daily) first.
**Water-soluble Vitamin E, taken in moderate doses, is unlikely to affect blood pressure.

helpful for head and neck aches, tension and lower back pain and especially for menstrual problems like heavy bleeding. In addition, some homoeopaths report great success with treating 'menopause problems', particularly hot flushes. (See Chapter 7 for more information about these approaches.)

Finally, and most importantly, daily moderate exercise is essential for good health throughout menopause. See Chapter 6, for strategies on how to start exercising even if you've been mostly sedentary for years. *In fact, exercise can produce in midlife many (if not all) of the things that the oestrogen literature of the early seventies claimed would follow oestrogen intake, including (for some women) reduction of hot flushes!*

During my holiday I hiked eight to ten miles a day in good, fresh country air. I cannot recall a single hot flush during that time, although I had them both before and after the trip. Perhaps I was tired enough to sleep without being aware of the flushes, but I don't think that was the case – I never felt healthier.

A few years ago when I was going through change of life I started having joint aches and swelling of hands in the morning. I increased the amount of exercise and took some mineral supplements and Vitamin E, and the condition disappeared within a few weeks.

While these are all useful hints, they are not magic, and many may not be enough by themselves. An equally important part of any non-medical approach is to avoid or cut down your consumption of certain substances which tend to aggravate menopausal signs: e.g. alcohol, caffeine, sugar, chocolate, white-flour products, as well as many prescription drugs: tranquillizers, sleeping pills, anti-depressants.

Support Groups

Women have always relied on one another for information and understanding. The networks of support groups that have begun to proliferate in recent years can be an especially important source of strength for midlife women. In these groups we get emotional support, increased understanding of our particular experience of menopause, and 'body' information. Best of all, we reduce the sense of isolation so many of us have known as we recognize the social, economic and political context of our common condition.

I had never been in any kind of support group before. I thought it would be a discussion group and everyone would be an expert except me, and I'd be embarrassed because I wasn't an expert on anything. But that's not the way this group worked. There's a lot of mutual help; people really listen to each other and laugh a lot. Now I don't

worry about menopause or growing older the way I used to.

Validated by the new knowledge that I had the same powerful physical and emotional experiences as all women, I was proud to have gone through menopause and some difficult life changes at the same time – for instance, creating a new life for myself after my divorce. I love my friends and know they have gone through similar challenges.

For more detailed information and suggestions about self-help and alternative approaches (ranging from vitamin supplements to how to set up a menopause group) see books by Judi Fairlie et al., Jill Rakusen, and Rosetta Reitz, listed in Resources. See also Chapter 7 for healing ideas in general.

MATURE WOMEN AND SEXUALITY

Sexuality continues throughout a woman's life. Some women first become fully aware of their sexuality in their middle years, and have unexpectedly powerful sexual feelings.

I have a new surge of interest in sex. But at the same time society is saying, 'You are not attractive as a woman; act your age; be dignified,' which means to me, Be dead sexually. It's a terrible trap for a middle-aged woman. I say, acknowledge and enjoy your sexuality! Get rid of the stereotypes! Change the image of women to include middle-aged looks and sexuality! [A woman in her fifties]

If you are sexually involved with men, keep using contraception until you haven't had a period for one year if you are over fifty, two years if you are under fifty. While the chances of pregnancy at this time are relatively low, erratic bleeding patterns may mean it is a long time before you realize you are pregnant.

Many older women who would like to be sexually active with men lack the opportunity, especially since with each year of age there are fewer men in their age range, while many men prefer younger partners who they suppose are more sexually active. Even with a partner, we may not be as sexually active as we might like if our partners lose interest in sex.

Our society admires older men who have relationships with women much younger than themselves but makes older women with younger partners the butt of jokes and derision. Yet some of us have younger partners.

It's hard to read the younger-man older-woman thing. We have to send out signals if a sexual relationship is what we want. I've had a problem if the man is the same age as my son, although after thinking about it I've decided it's OK for me. What really bothers me is my vanity – exposing a middle-aged body to a beautiful younger man.

The joy of making love with a young man who is so full of energy and straightforward is wonderful.

Some midlife or older women are for the first time considering or having sexual relationships with women:

When I was younger I used to go out with boys and then married in my twenties because that's what you did. But I always stayed in touch with a number of the woman friends I grew up with and there were two I felt especially close to. I was so upset when one of them moved to America ten years ago. I couldn't settle in my marriage. I thought it was my job or the houses we lived in. We were always moving and doing each house up more elaborately than the last. Eventually I realized I couldn't live with him even though he was a lovely man. I got a job back in the town I'd grown up in and lived by myself. It was only after a number of years, when I was in my late forties, that my other special friend and I felt able to acknowledge that we loved each other and wanted to live together. [A woman in her fifties]

Others of us have been lesbian for many years. (See Older Lesbians, p. 219.)

Many of us would rather not have sex at all, or prefer to limit our sexual expression to masturbation and fantasy rather than changing our sexual orientation or a lifetime pattern of being involved in one special relationship.

I frankly don't need it, and I don't miss it at all. I had a very, very full sex life – and I was mad about my husband which is a nice way to be. When he died it was a real shock, but that's twenty-five years now. I've gone about with a few men since, but nobody that I really wanted to stay with. You have to have a certain desire towards a person and I haven't discovered another person that I had that desire for in twenty-five years now. I'm used to my life the way it is now, and I don't think that my life is incomplete. [A woman aged seventy-three]

Many single older women miss not just sex but touching, gentleness, closeness and the excitement of romance.

Some of you say you have husbands at home that won't go anywhere. I have buried three husbands, and I wish I had one to sit at home with me now. [A woman in her sixties]

It's the intimacy that I miss more than the actual sex act. Shared jokes – you know. I'm finding this with a number of women as well as with men, but the whole romantic aspect of my life seems to have gone by. I miss that. [A woman in her seventies]

SEX AND AGEING: PHYSIOLOGICAL CHANGES

We are physically able to enjoy sex more. With sexual experience we develop a large, complex venous system in the pelvic area which enhances our capacity for sexual tension and improves orgasmic intensity, frequency and pleasure.*

Older women who seek any form of sexual expression, whether pleasuring ourselves or making love with others, face changes too.

Vaginal Changes

Changed oestrogen levels may produce changes in the vagina. Thinning of the vaginal walls, loss of elasticity, flattening out of ridges, foreshortening or narrowing of the vagina and especially dryness or itching may make intercourse less comfortable or even painful. These conditions may lead to irritation and increased susceptibility to infection (see Vaginal Infections, p. 485). It is not clear whether these vaginal changes are caused by the changed oestrogen levels of menopause or simply by ageing. Since there have not been many studies of this condition, no one knows how many women are troubled by it. Doctors, with their gift for naming, call it 'vaginal atrophy' and describe it in medical texts as occurring five or more years after menstruation ceases. Yet many women experience vaginal changes earlier, and others at age sixty or later. In addition, little is known about how long such a condition lasts, how troublesome it may be or how easily it can be corrected.

Many 'experts' recommend 'regular intercourse' to maintain easy vaginal lubrication.

I asked a woman gynaecologist with an excellent reputation, 'Does it have to be intercourse? What about widows, or divorced women, or lesbians, or women whose husbands aren't too interested in sex or are ill?' And I couldn't get a straight answer from her, even though I kept trying.

In fact, we can maintain and improve our ability to lubricate through *any* type of arousing sexual activity. There is nothing unhealthy about losing interest in genital sexual activity; we are not sex machines obligated to keep our bodies perpetually in condition for potential partners. There is also no evidence that vaginal dryness is irreversible.

---

*Sexual activity and pregnancy also contribute to the complexity of the pelvic venous system – see Mary Jane Sherfey, *The Nature and Evolution of Female Sexuality*.

I had a problem with dryness when I started having sexual intercourse again after a few years. In a month or two, my vagina began to get wet faster. [A woman in her sixties]

You may take longer to become amply lubricated. Sometimes lubrication does not take place at all: saliva, K-Y jelly or a vegetable oil can reduce dryness. Itching can be relieved by applying bancha tea or Vitamin E oil on the pubic and vaginal area.

The slower arousal time of older women and men has compensations.

When Geoff used to lose his erection I would think that I had failed as a woman because I couldn't keep him aroused. But now I see that it can mean more time to play around and a chance to start again so that love-making lasts longer. [A woman in her forties]

Sexual activity, masturbation and pelvic floor exercises (see p. 347) all help maintain vaginal muscle tone and intensity of climaxes. Testosterone is also sometimes given – often together with oestrogen replacement therapy – to increase sexual interest (see p. 259 and p. 456).

Drugs and Disease

Some drugs may affect sexual function or interest. For example, medication for high blood pressure can prevent erections, as can too much alcohol. The depressive effect of alcohol becomes more pronounced as people get older. Diabetes can make erections difficult for a man; its effect on the sexuality of women is not well understood. L-dopa, prescribed for Parkinson's disease, may increase sexual interest. Ask your GP about the effects on sexual interest, arousal or functioning of any drug prescribed for you or your partner.

Changing Attitudes and Communication

The physiological changes of ageing invite both men and women to break through old patterns, assumptions, misunderstandings and miscommunication. Men may misinterpret their slowness to arousal as a sign that their sexual capacities are eroding, and often seek out other (younger) women. Women may fear that our ageing bodies' changing appearance has diminished our partner's arousal, or interpret our own lack of lubrication as loss of attraction to our partner. It is important for both partners in a relationship, whether heterosexual or lesbian, to realize that changes are normal and to talk together to find out what is pleasurable. Such communication may be difficult at first and requires practice. You may want to get some help. (See Part II – Relationships and Sexuality.)

If we act on the knowledge that there are alternatives to intercourse and that we can, for example, initiate sex, this may mean shedding years of training. We can take courage to do what pleases us and our partner, even if it seems unusual or strange. It is quite likely that if we like it, other people do, too. A greater capacity for empathy and loving, developed through the years of living, can make sex better. A seventy-year-old woman, recalling a love affair at fifty says:

My immense pleasure and response were for him an incredible high, and that made me feel so marvellous. It was not just the physical part but our delight in each other that was so enormously exciting. It was a circular or spiral effect, because I had not realized that another person could enjoy my passion. Before this, I had experienced my passion and my partner would experience his passion. But this was different. And of course it's very much that way in a lesbian love affair, that delight in the other woman's total experience, the total emotional response. Danny took great pride in that just as a woman does with another woman. He thought it was marvellous that I would have several climaxes. After he died, I was in a state of shock for over a year. The mutuality we shared was rare with a man. My subsequent love affairs have all been with women.

Some people continue to be sexually active in their seventies, eighties and even nineties.

I am seventy-four years old and have been married for fifty-two years. We are fortunate to have good mental as well as physical health. This is not entirely a matter of luck. We have worked at it. Our good times have been more numerous than our bad times. The medical profession has only recently discovered the healing power of laughter. In our fifty-two years together we have had a lot of laughs. A sense of humour is as important as food, especially within marriage. For us the sharing that comes with having a warm and loving sex life over so many years deepens our joy in one another.

AGEING AND PREVENTIVE HEALTH CARE – SPECIAL ISSUES

Ageing brings physical changes, most of which have little to do with sickness. We cannot simply equate getting old with getting ill.

At sixty I am more vigorous and healthy than I was twenty years ago. My eighty-five-year-old mother shows me that by the eighties certain things in your body do start to give way, but even though she gets around less easily, she's certainly what I'd call healthy.

In our fifties and beyond, debilitating disease could well

be the result of a lifetime of exposure to occupational health hazards and low income. One American study of 1,100 persons over fifty found that a main factor influencing health was occupation, past or present.

> Those persons who have, or had, low-income occupations (and the disadvantages that go along with a lifetime of low income) were in poor health much more frequently than those with middle income or high-income jobs.[28]

Yet, while disease and chronic ill health are among the realities of the older years for many of us, they are not the only reality. Social factors can disable us more than is necessary: isolation from family or friends; care-giving for relatives and family without outside help; poor medical care; lack of stimulating activity, both mental and physical; and a sense of uselessness.

Poverty, too, is a special health issue for older women. Money worries due to being on a small, limited income and the fears of cutbacks to social security, for example, add greatly to the unhealthy stresses of daily living. Inadequate income also makes it harder to take care of ourselves in simple but crucial daily ways.

It is difficult, for instance, to get enough exercise if we don't feel safe on the streets or have little access to indoor exercise facilities. A worsening economic situation and drastic cuts in public expenditure make it more difficult each month for thousands of older women to get adequate calories, let alone vitamins and special diets. Some are homeless or without adequate heat.

Without a major turnaround in social priorities and policies, the health of great numbers of older women will clearly worsen over the next few years, with more emergency hospitalization for anaemia, dehydration and hypothermia and collapse and deaths from all causes.*

Here we will address special issues** for all older women as we seek to keep as healthy as possible.

Throughout our lives we can take active steps to maintain good health and lessen the impact of illnesses or chronic conditions when we are older. We can rethink the ways in which we take care of ourselves and acquire new habits which will serve us well for the rest of our lives. We can stop smoking, exercise more, eat as well as possible, reduce our dependence on sugar, caffeine, tannin in tea, alcohol, tranquillizers and sleeping pills. We can involve ourselves in activities which stretch our minds too. Currently there is growing evidence that many of the changes of

ageing, even those once thought biologically inevitable, are preventable and even reversible with changes like these.[29]

The point is not simply to live longer but to have the highest possible quality of life as long as we live.

> *By reading many books and articles on women, mental health, nutrition and exercise I began to see that my life could and should change. The changes did not come easily. My husband resisted. After all, I was rocking the boat in which we had become quite comfortable. I took up Tae Kwon Do [Eastern self-defence]. To my amazement, after a few months of kicking and hitting an imaginary opponent, my chronic insomnia and stiff neck disappeared. Gone also were the painful attacks of gastritis. I began feeling more energetic. Encouraged, I decided to put into practice some of the nutritional advice which I'd been reading. I stopped eating white sugar in any form. No more of my favourite cream-filled doughnuts. No more processed food, including white bread, noodles and spaghetti: in came more fresh vegetables and grains. Out went sleeping pills, aspirin and other medication: in came vitamins. It was not an overnight sensation. After all, I was trying to undo the damage done over forty-odd years. That was more than five years ago. Today, all the ailments I mentioned earlier are completely gone. No more of that headachy feeling from constipation – I count my blessings every day for being freed from this debilitating condition from which I suffered for so long. No more pains in my legs from varicose veins (some of my friends had surgery for this). No more stiff neck from internalized stress and tension. If you never suffered from chronic insomnia, you don't know the joy of being able to sleep all night, every night. All these things which I thought I would have to live with the rest of my life are gone.*

EXERCISE

Exercise becomes increasingly important. Women begin to lose bone mass at around age thirty-five leading to the possibility of severe osteoporosis (see p. 469), yet this may be largely due to inactivity. Weight-bearing exercise such as running is more likely to increase bone density compared with swimming. The exercise doesn't need to be very long and hard to do your bones good, but it's best if it's vigorous and non-repetitive.[30] Free dancing is an ideal form of exercise to protect the bones . . . and it's fun too.

Many of the benefits of exercise for older women are already evident. Exercise can also lower blood pressure and may reduce atherosclerosis, risks of heart attack and stroke, arthritis and emphysema. It is central in finding and keeping a comfortable weight. It can help keep chests clear when we have a cold or other virus infection, preventing the secondary infections that prolong the effects of a cold, leading to sinus trouble, bronchitis or pneumonia. It helps

---

*Low income means cutting down on heating. Many older women stay in bed for long hours for warmth; less exercise means more chance of chest infection among other things. Food intake is often insufficient to keep up body heat. State allowances for heating are far too low in colder weather. Older women are frequently less able to move about easily.

**Several of the more serious health problems which affect midlife and older women appear elsewhere in this book because they affect younger women, too: e.g. hypertension, cancer, heart disease. The troubling but not life-threatening problems – visual impairments, hearing loss, difficulties in walking – along with osteoporosis, which mainly affects women over sixty, are discussed on pp. 464–71.

us sleep, improves bowel functioning, often relieves depression and generally makes most people feel better.

My grandmother in her early nineties noticed that when she moved around more, her memory improved.

There seems now to be clinical evidence that after exercise blood rushes to the skin, bringing with it extra nutrients, and the skin's temperature rises as well. The collagen content then increases and skin actually thickens and becomes more elastic and less wrinkled. Delightfully, it is never too late to start exercising, and there are forms of exercise which fit almost any kind of physical limitation. A few tips: start slowly; watch less TV or exercise when you watch; better yet, exercise with a friend for company and support; try dancing (yes, even on your own!), walking, yoga or swimming; take an exercise class to help you break sedentary habits. See Chapter 6 for other ideas.

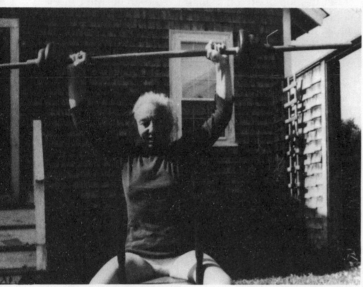

Deborah Wald

EATING WELL

While the same basic principles of healthy eating apply throughout life, nutritional requirements change somewhat with age. You need fewer calories (unless you are working or exercising hard), but the same nutrients and more of certain ones. See Chapter 4 for all but the following few items of special interest to older women, and for sources of nutrients listed below.

Protein

Since we don't absorb as much protein as we age, try to make protein foods a higher proportion of what you eat. However, be sure to balance with a sufficient amount of complex carbohydrates (whole grains, etc.; see p. 49).

Calcium, Magnesium and Phosphorus – A Balance of Nutrients

Calcium is an essential nutrient, as it prevents the bone loss that can lead to osteoporosis.[31] Unfortunately, women over thirty-five absorb calcium less easily, so we must make a special effort to get more exercise (this is indispensable to helping our bodies absorb calcium), eat a calcium-rich diet, learn about the other nutrients that aid or inhibit calcium absorption and get the right balance of such nutrients.*

- Phosphorus intake should equal but not exceed calcium. If phosphorus is too high, the parathyroid glands are stimulated to draw calcium from the bones. Most of us who eat meat and drink cola drinks probably have overly high phosphorus levels which inhibit calcium absorption. If you avoid milk because of its fat, replace it with skimmed or part skimmed milk or milk products. If your body can't tolerate dairy products (lactose intolerance) refer to Chapter 4, for non-dairy sources of calcium. Lactose intolerance may increase with age.
- Magnesium intake should be half of calcium intake. If our magnesium level drops lower, calcium will be lost. There is some evidence that the older we are, the more magnesium we need (around 450 to 500 milligrams daily), especially when we are under stress.[32] Magnesium can help muscles and nerves relax – and is safer than tranquillizers.

Vitamin D

When our skin is exposed to the sun, our bodies produce Vitamin D. This vitamin helps the body to absorb calcium properly. The more skin you expose, and the longer you expose it, the more Vitamin D your skin makes. In Britain, because of our climate, we tend to rely on the Vitamin D stored in the body from exposure to sun during the summer. Perhaps not surprisingly, elderly and housebound people are at risk from Vitamin D deficiency, as is anyone who cannot expose their bodies: not everyone has a private garden, or a park nearby, and some of us in any case have religious or social reasons for not exposing our bodies, including fear of racial and sexual harassment.

While being in sunlight is the best way to get enough Vitamin D, you can also get quite significant amounts from other sources (for example, canned fish such as pilchards, tuna and salmon, and eggs). People who eat margarine often get enough without knowing it, because manufacturers are required by the government to add the vitamin to their products. The government does not so far impose similar requirements on manufacturers of other foods, but some manufacturers add Vitamin D anyway. If you don't eat margarine, therefore, and you don't get much sun, it

---

*Calcium supplements can help us be sure we are getting the recommended 1,500 or so milligrams we need after menopause, but we need to balance this with about 750 or so milligrams of magnesium. Dolomite has often been recommended as containing the proper amounts of calcium and magnesium, but recently there have been reports of harmful trace minerals, such as arsenic and lead, found in dolomite, so until this controversy is resolved it is better to buy calcium and magnesium supplements separately in a two to one ratio.

See Notelovitz and Ware, *Stand Tall!* – a good guide to how to ensure adequate calcium and other mineral levels to prevent osteoporosis. See also *What Everyone Needs to Know about Osteoporosis*, free from the National Osteoporosis Society (see Organizations in Resources).

may be worth checking the labels of some of the products you eat: some breakfast cereals, yohgurts, drinks such as Ovaltine, and even some milk have Vitamin D added. Otherwise, try to discuss the idea of a Vitamin D supplement with your doctor or someone at your nearest well woman clinic (if there is one in your area). Like calcium supplements, they can be bought or prescribed, but while too little Vitamin D can cause serious problems, so can too much! The normal amount required is no more than 10 micrograms a day. A teaspoon of cod liver oil a day should provide enough if you are housebound.

Note: You can't get too much Vitamin D from the sun or from your diet.

Potassium

Plentiful in fresh fruits and vegetables, potassium becomes especially useful to women at midlife because it helps:

1. heart action, which may be less effective during the oestrogen transition;

2. the elimination of fluid build-up, which continues cyclically for many post-menopausal women because of other sources of oestrogen;

3. to balance sodium, which we may now have in greater quantities than we need;

4. to lower blood pressure (along with a low-sodium diet). Coffee, tea, alcohol and too much sodium deplete potassium.

Fibre

The fibre in vegetables, fruit, whole grains and bran helps with constipation, which is extremely common in people who are elderly, especially if they are on drugs or not very mobile. Although constipation is usually treated as trivial, it can make us feel very uncomfortable and unwell. If you are *already* constipated, don't add bran, as this will make it worse.

Fats

Ageing makes us less able to resist the damaging effects of all fats. See Chapter 4 for which fats to eat and how to cut back.

Some of the hints here and in Chapter 4 become less easy to follow in our older years, especially when we can't easily get out to shop or are on a small fixed income and cannot afford to buy fresh foods. If we have dentures or problems with teeth or gums, small changes in diet may be all we can manage – but even cutting down on junk foods can help a lot. If you put off cooking because you are preparing meals just for yourself, try designating one day per week as

WEIGHT AND WEIGHT GAIN AT MIDLIFE AND LATER

As older women we are probably more preoccupied with food, eating and dieting than any other group in society, with the possible exception of teenage girls. One out of two of us puts on weight at midlife because our metabolism is slowing down and we no longer need as many calories to sustain us. Often, too, we are more sedentary than before. If we continue the same food intake and get no more exercise (or even less) than before, we will tend to gain weight. In fact, women on the average gain almost ten pounds between thirty-five and forty-five and two more between forty-five and fifty-five. *There is good evidence that this weight has an important function*: the conversion of androgens into oestrogen in our body fat is one of the three sources of oestrogen after menopause. Some fat, therefore, is crucial: women who are very thin have a higher rate of osteoporosis. It is also true that above a certain level, too many pounds can contribute to ill health – diabetes and high blood pressure in particular. There is controversy today, however, over what constitutes 'too many pounds' (see Chapter 4). It may be that the ideal weights have been set too low.

Consider the several factors below in assessing your weight. If all these factors and their total combination are within the normal range and you feel well, your weight is probably fine.

1. Are you getting a reasonable amount of regular exercise?

2. Are you eating well?

3. Is your weight stable or changing slowly? Sudden weight gain or loss is dangerous at any age and more so as we grow older. If you plan to lose weight, do it slowly, as a result of long-term permanent changes in eating and exercise patterns.

4. Is your blood pressure within normal range? After menopause, blood pressure tends to rise with increases in weight.

5. Is your blood sugar well within the normal range? As your weight increases, the likelihood of getting adult diabetes increases, and the disease often signals itself by slight rises in blood sugar.

6. How is your lung power and control? The lungs have been overlooked until recently as an indicator of general health. The simple, risk-free pulmonary function test is a good indicator and predictor of long-term health and longevity (for women better than for men). It is sometimes done as part of a general check-up; it measures lung power and control as you exhale. Yoga is a good way to build lung capacity.

7. Do you have signs of arthritis or osteoporosis? Either one can indicate that you need to change your diet and exercise patterns. Women who are overweight are more prone to osteoarthritis, while women who are underweight are at higher risk for osteoporosis.

cooking day. Prepare several dishes, including a main dish and a soup you like, and then eat them on alternate days.

Since we absorb nutrients less well as we age and require fewer calories altogether, we may need supplements. (See the discussion of menopause on pp. 455–9.) However, try to get as much of the nutrients you need from your food. See p. 51 for the advantages and risks of supplements. Though the particular balance needed by women over thirty-five sounds complicated, resources like *Laurel's Kitchen* (see Resources section of Chapter 4) can help you work out whether you are eating well or what to change.

GETTING MEDICAL CARE IN LATER LIFE

Because of a combination of ageism and sexism, which is compounded by racism for those of us who are black, many of us suffer from poor medical care in later life.

MISDIAGNOSIS AND FAILURE TO TREAT REVERSIBLE CONDITIONS

Especially when we are past sixty, doctors often blame any physical and emotional problems on 'ageing' rather than looking for treatable disorders. They may be very quick to label emotional or mental confusion as 'senility' (see p. 469), when these may be signs of poor nutrition, treatable physical problems, grief or responses to inappropriate drug treatment. Time after time, they may offer us psychotropic ('mind-bending') drugs such as tranquillizers (see Chapter 5), instead of looking for what's really wrong. As a nurse puts it:

> When a man complains of dizziness he gets a check-up; an older woman gets Valium.

We ourselves may play into this pessimism about whether we can actually get better.

> I was afraid when I broke my wrist that it would take ages if ever to heal, and so I hesitated to do a more 'aggressive' type of therapy for it. Now it's much better, and I'm going to begin that therapy. My fear and a stereotype of being old held me back.

INAPPROPRIATE PRESCRIPTION OF DRUGS

The scandalous inappropriate prescription of drugs to elderly people has been highlighted in recent years. Yet many doctors still do not seem to realize that people over sixty are more sensitive to drugs and drug interactions, and that they should prescribe lower doses if they should prescribe any at all.[33] Many older people are still on far too many drugs at a time, for various chronic conditions. Sometimes they are prescribed by different doctors,

sometimes by the same doctor. In both cases they have neglected to take the crucial step of checking out what drugs we are already taking before prescribing others.

If we are at all concerned about drugs being prescribed for us, we can ask to be referred to a doctor who specializes in caring for older people (a geriatrician – assuming, that is, that the geriatrician is not already doing the prescribing). Geriatricians are often much better informed than many others about the sorts of drug regimes that are suitable for us as we get older, and many of them play an important role in reducing inappropriate drug regimes that have been prescribed by other doctors. They should also be experienced in identifying when our symptoms may be the side-effects of any drugs we have been given. For instance, some drugs can cause depression (for which we may be offered more drugs – which may then interact with the first ones) or mental confusion; symptoms often stop when we stop taking the drugs.*

Research has shown that GPs tend to have a very partial idea of all the drugs we are taking.[34] It's therefore a good idea to bring a list to your medical appointments. One woman we know asked her doctor to review all her prescriptions. He cut down the dosage of most of them and cut out a few completely. Pharmacists may also be able to advise on medications and answer any queries we may have.

Many women are literally 'tranquillized' into quiet and compliance. If you believe that you or a relative or friend is being prescribed drugs inappropriately or excessively, do all you can to change the situation.

> I went to visit a ninety-four-year-old friend who lives in a nursing home. She was recently diagnosed as having various ailments which require anywhere from three to ten pills a day. She was never told what the pills were or what they were for. When the nurse came to her room to give her the pills, my friend looked her squarely in the eye and said, 'The doctor only knows my body and how it works for a short time. I know it for ninety-four years, and nothing is going in it until I know what it is.'

SPECIALIST CARE TEAMS

To get good care it may be best, if we don't have a helpful GP or health visitor, to ask to be referred to a specialist care team – often based in a geriatric unit. These units have multi-disciplinary teams that, although headed by a consultant geriatrician, do include a range of other health workers, including occupational therapists, physiotherapists, dieticians, speech therapists, as well as nurses and social workers. They should also have good contacts with all those providing help for elderly people in the com-

---

*Drugs which are especially problematic as we get older include tranquillizers, alcohol, methyldopa, digitalis, beta-blocking agents, all barbiturates, and mefenamic acid. Some non-prescription drugs, such as aspirin, can also interact dangerously with prescription drugs.

munity. The whole emphasis of a geriatric unit is on helping us stay as healthy as possible for as long as possible, and to retain our independence.

Staff involved in geriatric units, and other specialist community care teams (such as Well Pensioner clinics) that exist in some localities, can be less likely to share our culture's negative attitudes towards old people, compared with other professionals. Nevertheless, it is wise to be prepared for ageism, sexism and racism, and to gain support to challenge insulting and oppressive behaviour – which does nothing for the quality of our care and can endanger our health.

We can only hope that, increasingly, those who specialize in the care of elderly people will become as sensitive to sexism and racism as some of them are becoming to ageism.

BECOMING ACTIVE PARTICIPANTS IN OUR OWN HEALTH CARE

Making changes means, for many of us, turning around decades of a certain kind of dependency on doctors. It may involve changing their stereotype of us, asking more questions, going in with a friend for support and advocacy, learning all we can about our health problems and making informed decisions, seeking second opinions more assertively, checking the negative effects of any drugs they prescribe, and looking for non-medical alternatives. Doctors who are taken aback when younger women use these tactics may be even more surprised, and even hostile, when their long-time patients ('their girls') begin to change. It takes courage to break old patterns, especially when you are feeling sick or frightened. Probably the most helpful thing you can do is to join or create a self-help or self-health group of women your age – even two or three people – to talk openly about your body changes and go to appointments together to help each other get the best care you can. You can provide support for each other when undergoing treatments which may be painful or scary.

The system itself must change too, especially in research and medical training. Proud of the years we have lived and the contributions we have made to society, we must insist on health and medical care which enable us to live our lives as fully as possible.

PHYSICAL IMPAIRMENTS AND CHRONIC CONDITIONS

While recent research has shown that mental capacity stays the same, or may increase with age (only the speed of reaction time decreases), the majority of women over sixty-five have some chronic health problem or condition which may limit activity over a period of time. We should never automatically assume that *any* of these are the inevitable result of ageing; instead we must investigate what we can do. Be suspicious of any practitioner who dismisses most complaints with 'What do you expect at your age?' Many problems are as treatable now as they are at any age.

When we do have to give up a degree of independence or a cherished activity because we can't see, hear or move around as well as before, we may need time to get used to our limits and find alternative ways to manage.

If we are used to driving a car, for example, no longer being able to do so (during day or night) may force us to give up cherished activities and even social relationships.

I loved my job and would have been happy to work for several years more, but it was getting more and more difficult commuting back and forth because my vision was so impaired. Driving back home in the dusk was scary. I felt as though I had my nose right up against the windscreen.

Organized around the nuclear family and individualized transport, this society magnifies the isolation of older women, so many of whom live alone. To live in more interdependent ways – sharing a house, organizing pooled transport – might be better for us. We must work for more and improved public transport, and communities in which it is safe to walk around.

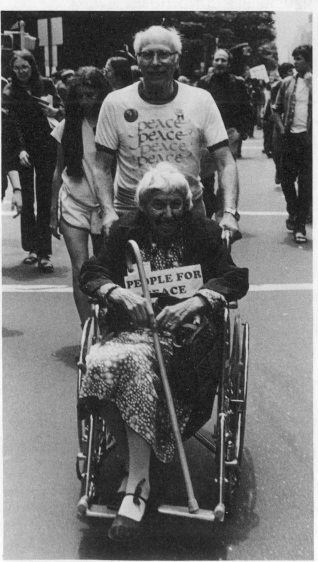

Julie Harper

Eyes

Our eyes have less elasticity by midlife. If you are long-sighted, you probably will need stronger glasses, or perhaps glasses for the first time. Some shortsighted people can give up glasses, except for driving or other distance viewing; others may require bifocals. We may have trouble adjusting to them or feel embarrassed about wearing them.

If you experience sudden flashing light and black spots, get medical attention at once. These could be symptoms of a detached retina – an emergency. In our seventies and eighties or even earlier, cataracts (cloudy lenses) may develop. While there isn't much evidence yet that these specific conditions can be prevented and not much is known about cause, eye repair is one of the few areas where medicine's heroics really pay off, restoring sight or improving it. Until cataracts are 'ready' for surgery, however, the impaired vision can be limiting and discouraging. The main problem with cataracts is long waiting lists for surgery – one of the effects of underfunding of the NHS. It may also be due partly to the fact that ophthalmologists (who specialize in eye diseases) tend to have large private practices.

Glaucoma is a chronic eye disease, usually appearing at midlife or later, in which the pressure of fluid inside the eye becomes too great. This excess pressure can damage the optic nerve and cause blindness if untreated. Although glaucoma may be symptomless, early symptoms include seeing 'halos' around objects. Very acute glaucoma may involve a painful red eye – in which case treatment should be sought immediately. Because it affects women more than men and rarely causes early pain or symptoms, be sure you are tested regularly for glaucoma after age forty-five, or possibly earlier if there is a family history of the condition.*

If detected early, some mild glaucoma can be treated effectively with drops taken regularly. More severe glaucoma requires surgical treatment with regular follow-up, since there are no permanent cures.

Feet

If you've always been active, you probably take your feet for granted. If you begin to notice aches and pain, not just when walking but when you rest as well, this may be part of skeletal or bone changes (e.g. see Osteoporosis, p. 469). But it is more likely to mean that you simply need more regular exercise to avoid stiffness. Some people swear they notice the effects of sugar and caffeine on their bones, especially their hands and feet.

Foot problems you already have may get worse as you age, especially if you have put on weight. Well-designed shoes with a firm, supportive arch may prevent fatigue as well as bunions** and other foot problems.

Most of us notice an increase in corns, calluses and other dry, scaly, hard skin on toes, heels and soles. Toenails often become much thicker, harder and sometimes yellower. This may be a sign of a fungus, so check with your doctor. Soaking your feet regularly, an old-fashioned custom, is vastly preferable to harsh chemicals or carving off dead skin with a razor blade. After a long soak, try a pumice stone to work off the excess skin.

Caring for our feet, especially cutting our own toenails, may gradually become a near-impossible chore, especially if we cannot bend as well as we used to and must ask others to help us. It can be frustrating to need others for such simple acts. Chiropodists – who deal with feet – play a big part in foot care of elderly people. Unfortunately, chiropody services are severely underfunded and many people are not getting the service they need. Contact your Community Health Council if you experience problems getting chiropody treatment. Some chiropodists use homoeopathic remedies very effectively. See Resources Chapter 7.

You can do foot exercises with a friend or by yourself: rise on your toes, walk on them; flex heels and ankles, pick up a pencil with your toes, etc.

Before going to sleep at night, give each foot a slight massage. It will warm your feet and help you to get to sleep more quickly, and the stretch may help you to maintain enough flexibility to care for your own feet. Find a 'foot partner' and massage each other's feet.

Hearing

For those of us who are not, or have never been, deaf, hearing is a function we take for granted. However, as we get older we may suddenly notice that we are missing what is being said or must ask people to repeat more often than feels comfortable.

Every once in a while I miss out on parts of a conversation or don't understand what I am hearing. When this happens, I discover to my later discomfort that, occasionally, I act as if I did hear – bright smile, nod of agreement. When this happens I feel so separate from people that I'm with.

Being hard of hearing is an invisible handicap. No one knows unless you tell them. You have a right to ask people to speak in a manner that enables you to understand.

One of the most important things a hard-of-hearing person can do for herself, I have discovered, is to be very assertive. Tell each person you talk with to speak louder or more clearly, and force yourself to keep reminding that person if she forgets.

---

*Recent research from Moorfields Eye Hospital suggests that people of Afro-Caribbean origin are at risk from developing glaucoma in their *20s and 30s*, and it is argued that they should be eligible for free eye tests from this age.

**Bunions are extremely painful, sudden misalignments of the cartilage under the tendon of the big toe. They can be caused by inadequate exercise and poor shoes, or sometimes from the stress of sudden exercise, like running, without adequate preparation. Surgical treatment is not always successful.

DEALING WITH HEARING LOSS

'Why a lip-reading class?' my friends ask. The reason is a gradually increasing hearing loss I have had for several years. Unless I'm in a room with good acoustics and with people who speak clearly, I have trouble following the conversation.

In the meantime, here I am in the lip-reading class, learning a lot about how to face up to hearing difficulties. The mutual support of the group is reassuring.

While there's no magic cure, hearing aids, signing and lip-reading can help. Lip-reading is hard work. Many sounds can't be seen, so we are learning to be aware of other body clues and are improving our visual skills in general.

TIPS FOR TALKING WITH A PERSON WITH A HEARING DIFFICULTY

- Don't talk from another room or from behind her.
- Reduce background noise. Turn off radio or TV if possible.
- See that the light falls on your face, so she can use visual clues.
- Get her attention before speaking.
- Face her directly, and on the same level if possible.

- Keep your hands away from your face. Avoid speaking while you are smoking or eating.
- Don't shout. Speak naturally but slowly and distinctly – and continue that way without dropping your voice.
- She may not hear or understand something you say. If so, try saying it in a different way rather than repeating.
- Recognize that she will hear less well if tired or ill.
- Be patient. Even hints of irritation or impatience hurt.
- Be an attentive listener. It's probably easier for her to talk than to listen.

Hearing aids can be obtained on the NHS, at audiology clinics, to which you can be referred by your GP. There are many different types of hearing aid and not all of them are available on the NHS. If you decide to consider buying one, e.g. at a hearing aid shop, remember that these are commercial enterprises and some of them have been known to mislead older people. The Fair Hearing Campaign (see p. 479) is trying to improve NHS facilities, including the long waits for hearing aids many people encounter. Contact them for further details.

Common as it is, hearing loss is not an inevitable accompaniment of ageing, though it does seem to run in some families. The enormous increase in the volume and range of noise accompanying industrialization has contributed significantly to hearing loss in the present generation of over-sixty-fives, especially among factory workers and urban dwellers.

It is crucial to obtain an accurate diagnosis of the cause of hearing loss, because treatment varies depending on whether one has nerve or conduction deafness. Conduction deafness, unlike nerve deafness, can often be corrected with surgery.

Urinary Tract Infections and Urinary Incontinence

As we age, the environment in the vagina and urethra becomes less acid; therefore more of us are vulnerable to urinary tract or bladder infections. Cutting back on white flour, sugar and caffeine products; drinking more clear fluids and unsweetened fresh citrus fruit juices; and adding Vitamin C and magnesium sources may help (see the discussion on cystitis, p. 507).

Starting around the time of menopause, some women begin to notice a slight loss of urine as they cough, sneeze, laugh or exert themselves during strenuous activity. The tissues around the urethra begin to thin out just as the vagina does, in response to reduced oestrogen, sometimes

making bladder control more difficult. Women who already have a history of this problem may find it getting worse. Pelvic floor exercises (p. 347) and sit-ups or leg lifts to strengthen the abdominal muscles may help control this problem.

A very common form of urinary incontinence as we get older is 'bladder instability'. This is when we get the urge to empty our bladder, but before we make it to the lavatory, and with no warning at all, the flow starts – not just a slight dribble, but all of it. The first time this happens it is very worrying, as well as acutely embarrassing. 'Bladder retraining', which is very simple to learn, can often stop the problem from recurring. This involves initially 'peeing by the clock' – i.e. making sure you go every hour for, say, a week, and gradually extending the time, over a period of about four weeks. Gradually the bladder becomes 'retrained', and the problem disappears. If it doesn't or if you want help, seek advice – e.g. from your district nurse (see p. 629), who is usually very knowledgeable about incontinence. District nurses can provide free incontinence pads, and social services can provide help with laundering in certain circumstances.

Memory Loss and Confusion

It is frightening to become aware that simple everyday tasks have become a problem, or to notice a decline in your capacity for sound judgement. If you observe either an increasing confusion or loss of memory in yourself, a friend or family member, don't assume 'That's it! It's all downhill from here.'

What does it mean to have memory lapses? We may simply be slowing down, our memory declining just as vision or hearing do, so that we will have to work a little harder at remembering and give ourselves more time. As we get older we have more memories, so retrieving a particular memory may be more difficult.[35] When we are depressed and haven't had a chance to express grief or other emotions, preoccupation with these feelings can interfere with memory.

As one who copes with considerable memory loss at age sixty-eight, my major aid is list-making. Knowing that I may well forget an idea or 'to-do', I write it down immediately. As a result, I am far better organized than at any earlier time of my life and accomplish more.

Though we experience memory lapses at other times, for example some women do in pregnancy, we worry about them more when we are older. It isn't helpful when younger persons say that they also forget things because it trivializes the fear older women experience.

We can exercise memory or prevent memory loss through 'mindfulness', paying attention to everyday tasks, making small (and large) decisions for ourselves.

If severe memory loss and confusion are prolonged, this is called *dementia* (sometimes, pejoratively, called 'senility'). There may be reversible causes, such as drug toxicity (from over-medication or drug-interactions), alcohol, depression, chronic infection, Vitamin B12 deficiency, anaemia, and hormone disorders (particularly of the thyroid – which is commonly under-diagnosed). It is possible that nutritional deficiency could be a major and as yet poorly recognized cause. For example, cases of dementia due to folic acid deficiency have been reported, as has confusion associated with thiamine deficiency; very low intakes of Vitamin C, riboflavin, pyridoxine and thiamine have been noted among people with dementia.[36] It is important that a prompt and thorough assessment is made (this may well involve a specialist's opinion), to avoid inappropriate labelling of 'irreversible' dementia.

Unfortunately, the majority of people with dementia have an irreversible cause, either due to hardening of the arteries or senile dementia of the Alzheimer type (sometimes called 'Alzheimer's disease'). This is a chronic deterioration of the brain and the cause is unknown. It may be related to a virus or environmental toxins.

Sudden confused states may be due to drug toxicity, dehydration, hypothermia (severely reduced body temperature), a small stroke, a traumatic event or accident, a series of losses or an abrupt relocation, and many other causes. Advice should be sought promptly. If the underlying causes are treated, the chances are that we can return to normal.

Depression

Please do not listen to doctors or others who imply that being depressed is typical of ageing, because it need not be. If we lose our appetite, don't feel sexual, sleep too much or can't sleep and can't enjoy anything, if such symptoms continue for over a month and if talking to friends doesn't help much, we may need professional help. A specialist care team (to which you can ask to be referred by your GP – see p. 465) may well be able to help practically with any social or emotional problems we are having, as well as our physical ones.* See also Chapter 8, for different ways of helping ourselves and being helped.

While drugs can sometimes help, they should be taken with extreme caution because as we get older we experience more and greater effects from psychoactive drugs, and some drugs may even cause or deepen depressions.

OSTEOPOROSIS

Normally a woman's bone mass peaks at age thirty-five, after which she tends to lose about 1 per cent of bone mass every year (10 per cent per decade). At sixty-five the loss declines to 3 or 4 per cent every ten years.[37] In osteoporosis, which may start in earlier years but usually does not show up until much later, bones become thin and brittle as the amount of bone mass decreases more severely, and they become liable to fracture – particularly the spine, hip, and wrist. This is a serious health problem for a large minority of elderly women: spinal fractures can result in as much as five inches' loss of height; fractures can be very painful, and only a minority of women regain their previous mobility. Osteoporosis seems to be increasing, possibly because of the poor diet that many pensioners are forced to live on, and because of socially-induced immobility. If present trends continue, by the year 2016, 24 per cent of women will fracture their hip before the age of eighty-five, compared with the present level of 12 per cent. While 10 to 20 per cent of women with a fractured hip die following their falls, these deaths may be more connected with poor nutritional intake rather than to the fall or the osteoporosis as such.[38]

Contributing Factors

In fact, lack of important nutrients is probably a significant factor in the majority of cases of osteoporosis; and in particular inadequate calcium intake – by women of *all* ages (see Calcium, p. 463).

I was born in Islington in North London in 1925. Like so many others at that time, my father was often unemployed and we were a big family, so there wasn't much money for food and clothes. I remember my older brother wearing mother's shoes

---

*In some areas there are doctors specializing in the mental health of elderly people. They are called psychogeriatricians.

to school, as she couldn't afford to repair his. I think now that the poor diet I had then possibly paved the way for the osteoporosis I developed later. [Lillian Lolley, speaking to the National Osteoporosis Society]

Lack of exercise is also highly relevant:[39] apart from anything else, it makes it much more difficult for the body to absorb calcium. Lack of exercise may also be a major cause of 'postural instability' – whereby keeping one's balance becomes difficult – and posture instability leading to falls is not unlikely to lead to fractures in elderly people, whether osteoporosis is present or not.[40] The over-prescription of mood-altering drugs to elderly women may also contribute to the high incidence of falls and resulting fractures.

Yet it is widely believed by the medical profession, and particularly by gynaecologists, that oestrogen lack is the cause of osteoporosis. And since, after menopause, oestrogen levels are reduced, menopause itself is being seen as the cause – and osteoporosis as an oestrogen deficiency disease.* Yet it is possible that low oestrogen levels are relevant simply because they make it harder for the body to adapt to a low calcium diet[41] – and remember, many, if not most of us, have been eating far too little calcium for years. Some long-term medications, such as cortisone for arthritis, or anti-convulsants, also contribute to osteoporosis. The profile of a woman most at risk for osteoporosis includes the following characteristics: white or possibly of oriental background, aged sixty and over, small-boned, slender and sedentary. Usually she has exercised very little and taken in insufficient calcium during her growing years (for example, because of excessive dieting). Often she also smokes and drinks alcohol excessively.

Symptoms

During its early stages, osteoporosis produces no symptoms, or only mild ones such as backaches or back-muscle spasms. An older woman may be unaware she has osteoporosis until she fractures her spine, hip or wrist in a simple fall. Repeated fractures are common once the process starts. A possible sign in post-menopausal women is pain in the upper or lower spine lasting for several days and then stopping, which may be caused by disintegrated vertebrae which collapse spontaneously. In a more advanced form, these 'compression fractures' in the upper spine cause a condition commonly called 'dowager's hump'; the resulting shortened chest area may make digesting food more difficult.

Diagnosis

The National Osteoporosis Society has found that many women are misdiagnosed or not diagnosed for years. When a woman's spine is crumbling, they report that it is not uncommon for her to be told 'It's just your age, dear', and to be offered no information or treatment at all. Largely because of the work of the Society, this situation seems to be improving.

Although routine X-rays may show signs of osteoporosis, they also show reduced bone mass caused by other conditions, so they do not make a definitive diagnosis of osteoporosis possible. If either you or your GP suspects early osteoporosis it might be possible to get a referral to a metabolic bone disease unit, whose diagnostic methods are likely to be more sophisticated.

Treatment

If a serious fracture has occurred, women tend to do better if operated on by a consultant and if the waiting time in casualty is less than an hour. A recent report by the Royal College of Physicians (1988) catalogues a long list of problems that need to be tackled in the NHS if emergency and follow-up treatment are to be improved. It makes many useful suggestions for improving orthopaedic care, around which women's groups and CHCs could campaign.

Predictably, most doctors emphasize treatment of existing osteoporosis, usually once a dramatic fracture occurs, and neglect early prevention (apart from promoting HRT). They may even prescribe, after the fact, the very activities that might have prevented the condition from developing in the first place – replacement calcium, Vitamin C and D supplements, weight-bearing exercises such as walking, special back-exercise regimens and physical therapy (physiotherapists have a very important part to play in the treatment of osteoporosis). However, most are likely to want to prescribe hormone replacement therapy, possibly with sodium fluoride.

Hormone Replacement Therapy and Sodium Fluoride

In recent years the emphasis of medical research and practice has shifted to prevention of osteoporosis through medical intervention with HRT* and/or sodium fluoride. These approaches are still somewhat controversial.

The administration of HRT during, or soon after, menopause is increasingly being recommended as a way of preventing severe osteoporosis in later life. At the same time the role of diet (see p. 463) and exercise (see p. 462) is often overlooked. While there is considerable evidence of the beneficial effect of HRT on bone when given within six years of menopause, it is not clear exactly in what circumstances and in what way it has most benefit and least risk. For example, some research suggests that rapid bone loss following premature menopause can be prevented by the

---

*Having 'created' the disease, they then recommend a solution – which is, of course, hormone replacement therapy, in the form of oestrogen (see below). There are significant political reasons for this development: HRT is big business; drug companies are major influencers of the type of research conducted; and medical careers can be built relatively easily in such a climate. For an interesting exploration of how osteoporosis became inextricably linked with HRT, see Kaufert and McKinlay in Resources.

*That is, HRT involving oestrogen – although some research is being conducted on the possibility of progestogen alone also preventing bone loss.

use of HRT, though possibly only if it is continued on a permanent basis – for there is evidence that the positive effect ceases, and that the rate of bone loss may even increase if the HRT is withdrawn.[42] HRT can also be useful once severe osteoporosis has set in. For more discussion on HRT, see p. 456.

Sodium fluoride in measured doses[43] seems to increase bone mass in post-menopausal osteoporosis so that there is less chance of fracture. However, the quality of the new fluoride-induced bone cells is questionable, and the other effects of fluoride can be debilitating – inflamed joints, recurrent vomiting, anaemia in 40 per cent of women in one study,[44] gastric and joint pain and ankle oedema in another.[45] It is normally used only in specialized centres.

For free information on learning to cope with osteoporosis, contact the National Osteoporosis Society (see p. 479).

COPING WITH AND OVERCOMING IMPAIRMENTS AND CHRONIC CONDITIONS – SOME EXAMPLES

Four years ago, at age eighty-one, I got diabetes. It has impaired my living condition, but it doesn't get me down. In fact, I have always had the feeling that the more we have to fight and overcome, the stronger we are. Obstacles are here to be overcome. That's part of life, and it gives us a good feeling that we are not just little ants, we are fighters.

It's not only the physical impairment which has to worry you and the doctor. It is also your state of mind. The healthy mind creates the healthy body, and the healthy body creates the healthy mind. Sometimes a frail body can draw its strength from a courageous mind.

I coped with some of my feelings of loss about my diminished hearing by developing a new interest in foreign movies. I was missing a lot at the theatre* and in American movies, but when I go to a foreign movie I can read the subtitles so I don't miss a thing – and I'm expanding my horizons! [A seventy-eight-year-old woman]

For a number of years I have been living with Paget's disease in my right hip.** The doctor gave me the feeling that there were a limited number of steps 'programmed' for that hip and that I should give up many of the activities I enjoyed.

Fortunately others, professionals and lay friends, suggested I continue more or less as I was, testing

limits and letting discomfort be the determining factor in what I did. When camping, I found I could take some of the easier hikes and avoid the strenuous ones. I had difficulty climbing stairs at a railway station, so I found I could navigate them by putting both feet on a step before I went to another. If I had pain when I got up after sitting engrossed with a book, I consoled myself with the awareness that this, too, would pass as I limbered up. I accepted these limits to my flexibility and found I could live within them. Then, several weeks ago, I found that I didn't have to accept them as completely. It all began with borrowing a bicycle and relearning how to ride one. It took some getting used to, but I found out how to take advantage of my strong left hip and soon was braving traffic and riding, once more, with confidence. I experienced a new freedom, a new sense of my body's resources.

Then I learned from a hiking book that all my life I had been walking incorrectly. Soon I began changing, using a more productive method. I began to feel more grounded and, at the same time, freer. [A woman in her seventies]

CARE-GIVING AND ALTERNATIVE LIVING ARRANGEMENTS

CARE-GIVING – A GAP IN OUR DELIVERY OF HEALTH AND MEDICAL SERVICES*

Approximately 1.5 million handicapped people are living in their own homes in Britain. In most cases, where they need help with bathing, dressing or feeding, this is provided by members of their household: 1.25 million carers are carrying out this role. Most of these are elderly people.

It is the fate of thousands of women (and some men), upon whom the care system depends, to care for the aged, the chronically ill and the disabled. They are the hidden workers without whom the health and social services would collapse. Only 5 per cent of people over sixty-five and 19 per cent of all those over eighty-five are in residential establishments. Of these 90 per cent are women.**

Women are approximately ten times more likely than men to care for an ageing spouse or parent or spouse's parent. When men do this caring they are less likely than women to do the more physically demanding personal tasks. We often marry men who are older than we are; we maintain our health and live longer than they do; everyday household tasks are mostly done by women. When care-

---

*Signing is a way to make cultural events accessible to people with hearing loss. If you are planning a cultural event, be sure to find someone who will sign. Alternatively, choose a venue with a loop system for use by people with hearing aids.
**This involves softening and bowing of the bones which though thicker and enlarged become structurally weak.

*See also Chapter 27.
**Forty-five per cent of women over sixty-five and 60 per cent of women over eighty live alone in private houses.[46]

giving is work we want to do, respected by our family and community, it can be rewarding. Too often, however, others simply expect it of us.

We planned for my husband – I was going to be the person who sustained him until his death. We never worked out who would care for me. It's an unseen social service that women do; if the wife dies first, he finds another woman.

Often the carers of older women are other older women.[47]

Traditionally, women have cared for family members in their own homes, with 5 per cent of elderly people, *both* in Victorian times and the present day, being cared for by the State. In modern times, this 5 per cent means higher *numbers* of older people. The type of care offered outside the home has changed from workhouses to sheltered and residential homes, both local-authority-run and private. None the less, such care work is still, also, done by women, paid at the lowest wage levels.

A variety of services has been developed to help people remain in their homes, from Meals on Wheels and Home Helps to a variety of social and medical day-care services. There is a growing awareness that people prefer to remain in their own homes and often remain in better health there than they do in an institution. Unfortunately, though such services are not only desirable but cost-effective, they are not uniformly available and receive meagre government backing. Thus, family-provided care most often still means woman-provided care, in isolation, without the security of job-retraining or an occupational pension.

For three years I was confined caring for a sick husband twenty-four hours a day. Then my doctor said I had to send him to a home because of my high blood pressure.

We rushed my husband to the hospital with a stroke, and it was a medical miracle. Now I'm not so sure it was a blessing. He is not always rational and cannot be left alone. Naturally, I had to give up my job. Financially, we are in a bad way but disaster will strike when he dies. I am fifty-seven and will be on income support. I can't see any way out.

It cannot be taken for granted that we necessarily like or want to be cared for in later years by family members whom we ourselves have looked after.[48] Moving in with our families can often lead to strain and conflict over where we fit into the household. Much informal care is often provided by friends visiting – but where we need personal care, we often prefer to have this provided without a sense of personal imposition on friends or family. If we need this kind of personal care, we may be able to claim 'Attendance Allowance' to pay for it – whether someone else lives with us or not.

Professional care-givers are becoming aware of the importance of not pushing people to accept what they do not want – such as residential care – and of ensuring people have control over the care they receive. Because of what we have come to expect in our relationships with our family and friends, it may be more difficult to feel in control *and* accept more than a certain proportion of care from them. With our families, we may have been used to doing the giving and with our friends we may have been used to at least returning what they have given us.

For a growing number of us, care-giving conflicts with our jobs. (Nearly half of all married women, and even more single women, aged forty to fifty-nine are in the labour force at a given time.) Women, including married women, should be able to claim an invalid care allowance if they cannot work *and* care for a family member. Clearly we need services which would make continued employment possible, such as day-centres and domiciliary care workers. Short term care-relief – even for a weekend – can help relieve the pressure on a woman doing other work as well as that of care-giving. There are now a number of organizations pioneering support groups for care-givers, such as Crossroads Care Attendant Schemes and the Carers' National Association (see Resources). It is also becoming recognized that the needs of carers cannot be ignored by statutory services and that they, too, need support and resources.

RESIDENTIAL ACCOMMODATION AND NURSING HOMES

We ourselves, or our relatives, may need to go into residential accommodation or nursing homes when we come to need more help or nursing care. Care in such establishments is often poor, putting economics ahead of quality care, paying workers low salaries and skimping on residents' needs. Often, in the interests of 'efficiency', the routines are set up to serve only the neediest residents, depriving the more able of a chance to use their full capacities. Having other people or pets to care for may sustain attentiveness and memory. Physical and mental abilities deteriorate when we have neither mental stimulation nor chances to exercise and carry out simple tasks on our own.

The pattern of cutbacks over recent years has meant on the one hand that private homes have begun to turn people

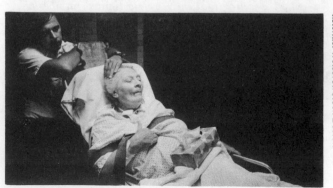

Michael Weisbrot/Stock Boston

away who are wholly dependent on the State, because they are not given enough money to cover their costs, and on the other hand residents in State homes have been admitted only when suffering from advanced physical and mental disability, putting further strain on the staff and resources. We are critical of many aspects of residential care – its impersonal nature, medicalization of everyday life and lack of privacy and choices for residents. We must work for more realistic funding and for improvements that give residents more control and real care. Recent studies indicate that few residents are meaningfully involved in the choice to go into homes in the first place.[49] Some recent innovations include regular visits from schoolchildren and young people, and raised garden plots for persons in wheelchairs; and there is a move to give greater privacy with single bedrooms and different places to meet, talk or pursue activities. A lot more needs to be done and we need the support of our younger sisters in developing and achieving what we want.

Where we are offered a choice of homes for ourselves or relatives it is worth comparing them to find the answers to the following:

- Are there single rooms for privacy?
- Is there a range of activities and what are they?
- What personal possessions (including items of furniture) can be brought?
- Is it possible to keep pets?
- Can residents make snacks or drinks themselves?
- How often does a doctor visit?
- What kinds of opportunities are there for seeing people and going to places outside the home?

Housing and Care Arrangements

As we grow older, health, housing and economic needs are less easily separable into neat compartments. Those of us who live with chronic conditions know that we need concerned persons nearby to help us with everyday tasks that have become difficult. This can contribute more to our well-being and ability to live in the community than GP visits or medical interventions.

Despite vast differences in our well-being, living conditions and income levels, most of us want to be self-sufficient as long as possible. As we have discussed above, a variety of services can help us, as individuals or couples, to stay in our own homes even when we need occasional nursing services or help with everyday tasks. However, while home care – whether in the form of bath aides, home helps or visits by chiropodists or occupational therapists – can be highly cost-effective, it is not consistently available and is continually threatened with cuts. Medical help can also be provided at day hospitals, physiotherapy and outpatient clinics, and transport to and from clinics should be available.

NHS aids provided include: commodes, bed-rests and incontinence pads. People on low incomes can claim exemption from prescription and dental charges, and opticians' fees in certain circumstances.

Personal alarm systems can give confidence to older people with potentially life-threatening conditions who live alone. Various schemes are being explored to make continued living in one's own home a reality:

1. Local authorities and housing associations run specially built or adapted sheltered housing with wardens on site in case of emergency.

2. Expanding 'home equity conversion' – where some insurance companies provide annuities to people who fully own a home which has appreciated in value, but do not have the cash to pay living expenses or upkeep. These are then provided by the company in return for various types of share in the home.

3. Converting part of a home to a flat for additional income and closer neighbours. Some organizations, such as Abbeyfields, will take over a large house, convert it into flats and give one to the owner.

At some point, for many of us, living alone is no longer feasible. We may experience physical changes, reduced energy or fewer resources; we may have problems that require having others nearby; we may be lonely. Yet we probably will not need twenty-four-hour care or medical services on a daily basis. Recent government benefit policies have encouraged institutionalization by subsidizing places in privately-run 'homes' for those living on income support state benefit. If a 'home' has fewer than four residents, it does not need to be registered or inspected by social services. This is currently under review.

There is a growing movement for alternatives, particularly in housing. Cooperatives, inter-generational living with relatives or friends, turning part of a house into an annexed flat, or small group homes are all new patterns of living together. Total privacy is not possible in such schemes but they may give more control, dignity, companionship and security.

We are impressed by the variety and innovativeness of support services for elderly people and their care-givers in other countries.

- The Scandinavian countries provide service buses to bring cleaning and laundry, hairdressing supplies, books and hot food to those who wish to remain in their homes. Home-makers and personal care attendants are provided for those who need them. An alternative is the service house, where all such services are available on the premises to those who live there, and sheltered housing schemes which also provide nursing facilities. The State pays family care-givers.
- In New Zealand low-interest loans, services and subsidies are available to families who wish to care for elderly relatives at home.
- In The Netherlands elderly people's blocks of flats are situated near parks and activity centres, with their own shopping arcades so it is easy for them to do their own shopping and handily situated for people who want to visit as part of their everyday activities.

Many of these services or equally creative ones are available or potentially available to older people in this country. However, our community care policies rely on a patchwork of innovations in health and social services departments and voluntary groups, and on the exploitation of unpaid and badly paid women's caring activities. Both these activities and the framework of health care needed to back them up are constantly threatened by cutbacks.

As a nation we have not deliberately decided (as have the Scandinavian countries) to make the older years a good time of life, free from financial worry and deprivation. As an ever greater percentage of the community enters the older years, we must work through organizations, perhaps some of those listed on p. 479, to press for such a national commitment.

SURVIVAL SKILLS

Most of the older women we spoke with in preparing this section enjoy reasonably good health and adequate economic situations. Though this is not the case for large numbers of women, these experiences highlight the potential for the older years; a potential (the birthright of every person) denied to so many of us because of inadequate food, housing, care, transport and the constant worry about how to pay for all of these.

Many women are still going strong at seventy or seventy-five and beyond. We want to end this chapter with their voices as they tell of the 'survival skills' which help them stay active, creative, involved and feeling good about themselves and their lives.

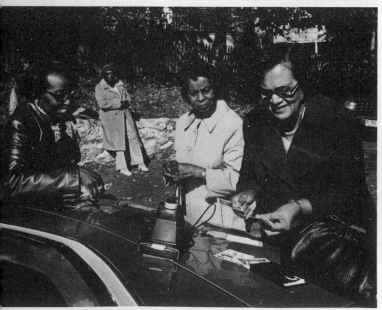

Photography class at Freedom House, Roxbury, MA.

When I was a girl we always seemed to see older women as having to wear clothes we wouldn't want to and as not able to do things or go to places outside the home that we thought were

interesting. As I grew older I noticed some of my friends seemed to just tie themselves to become what they thought was suitable for 'this time of life'. But some of them didn't, and I find as the years pass it has become more, not less, important to me to do things that matter to me and where I feel I count – whether that is meetings or holidays with friends or voluntary work. I feel that we older women are often seen as helpless, or that we don't really count, so some of the work I now do is with other older people to change that, to decide what services we want and to be heard. I always seem to be meeting new people and it's often when I'm talking with people who have lived for many years that I realize what unexpected turns people's lives can take. I'm always being surprised and intrigued.

It is important to challenge the stereotypes of older people as rigid, unable to form new relationships or to experience change and growth. Professionals, researchers and practitioners have contributed to the stereotyping of older people by perpetuating the 'disengagement theory' – the idea that we gradually withdraw from life by divesting ourselves of important roles and commitments as an appropriate adjustment to ageing and approaching death. It would be more appropriate to say that 'disengagement' is forced on many older people by ageism and impoverishment. We have learned from the many lively, vital, older women we spoke with that it is possible to live fully for as long as we live.

There's a discrepancy between my image of an older person in her seventies and the way I feel. In fact, there's no connection. My concept of a grandmother was of someone who didn't do much. But I became a grandmother at forty-seven. I started a vigorous exercise programme at forty-three and am still running every day at seventy-six and love it.

The seventies have been the best decade of my life. From what I have seen with my friends, it is either the best or the worst. My creative work as an artist is what keeps me alive; my friends keep me happy and contented. If I had to give up people, I would never have another happy day, but I would stay alive if I could work. [A woman aged seventy-seven]

It is not so different to be over eighty, except that accidents and illness can make a change. If I had not broken my hip I would probably still be very active today, but I wouldn't have the insight I have. Being confined gives me more time to reflect.

I know I have developed in the last ten years, even at my age. I have become more optimistic. A lot of young people seem to be drawn to me. I don't know if I give more now than I used to, or have more composure and insight. That sounds funny, but it is a fact.

I had to concentrate on getting well, and this makes you rather self-centred. Sometimes I catch myself thinking, I am too busy with my body, what about exercising my mind? That's why I think that mixing with different kinds of people, young and old, is very important. The segregation of the aged is absolutely ridiculous, cruel, unproductive and costly. [A woman aged eighty-five]

STAYING IN TOUCH WITH OUR INNER SELVES

Staying in touch with ourselves helps us to reach out to others, cope with the hard things in our lives and keep on growing. There are many ways we can do this – keeping a diary, reading a book, exercising, meditating, walking in the park, a long hot shower or bath, camping. For some of us, being connected with a spiritual community helps too.

Each week a group of us meet and talk about a spiritual topic in relation to things that are in the news or are happening in our lives. We are talking about things that matter to us, and I find that it helps me feel that ideals like human caring and sharing, which are so much of what we do as women, do matter, there is a wider purpose in my life and that I do have all kinds of things in

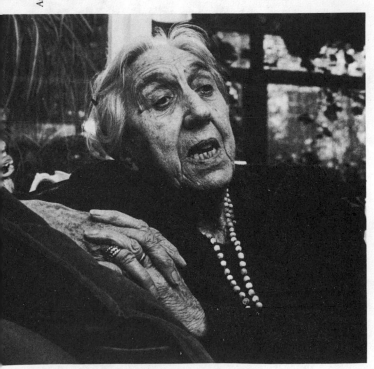

Angela Phillips

Gwen Coleman, suffragette.

common with others. There is a different kind of closeness to what you have with your family – in some ways I feel I'm able to be more open and honest with people in that group. Because I feel there that I'm part of something more important than me, I can also feel that I'm helping to give rise to things that may continue to make things better when my own life has ended.

SUPPORT GROUPS FOR OLDER WOMEN

Friendship is valuable not merely for happiness and mental well-being but for physical health and survival as well. Since ageing in this country too often means increasing isolation, the middle and older years are a good time consciously to build a support and friendship network if you don't already have one. A US study found that, regardless of age, persons with strong social bonds (friends, lovers, marriage, group and organizational links) had a mortality rate 2.5 per cent lower than those who were relatively isolated. The other important finding was that friendship and support from *any* of these sources contributed to survival. It is never too late to build relationships, to exchange different kinds of support.

Although growing older is made to seem such a depressing stage of one's life, I've found it to be exactly the opposite. Now I'm through the menopause I'm in better health than I've ever been, I've never been busier, though I'm only doing the things I really want to do. I feel more assured, confident, comfortable and powerful every day. [A woman aged fifty-nine]

Old age isn't calm
fires burn in bodies of old women
Flutes sing in their ears and they
fall in love now and then
Old women dream of dancing in
moonlight and being held
Old women want you to hug them
and to feel your warmth
I will not speak to you in
platitudes – words of wisdom
'be like me'

I do not have a rocking chair I
have no pattern for younger women
I don't have a richer outlook on
life (life is always confusing)
Except there is joy in the struggle
And in leaping from change to change
But let the struggle be your own
Resist compromise – don't take
anything lying down

© SONIA SAXON

NOTES

1. Florida Scott-Maxwell. *The Measure of My Days*. New York: Knopf, 1968.

2. For example, see T. Collins. 'Demographic Changes and Resources for the Elderly', *British Medical Journal*, vol. 290, no. 6476, 1985, p. 1284.

3. K. Andrews. 'Demographic Changes and Resources for the Elderly', *British Medical Journal*, vol. 290, no. 6474, 1985, pp. 1023–4.

4. See J. Finch and D. Groves (eds). A *Labour of Love: Women, Work and Caring*. London: Routledge and Kegan Paul, 1983. And review by J. Gray of *From the Cradle to the Grave* in *British Medical Journal*, vol. 291, 17 August 1985.

5. Jenny in *Spare Rib*, no. 154, May 1985.

6. *Britain's Elderly Population*, Census Guide no. 1, OPCS.

7. Pauline Long. *Spare Rib*, no. 82, May 1979, p. 17.

8. Lillian Rubin. *Women of a Certain Age: the Midlife Search for Self*. New York: Harper and Row, 1979.

9. Helene Deutsch. *The Psychology of Women: a Psychoanalytic Interpretation*. New York: Harper and Row, 1979.

10. See Myrna Weissman 'The Myth of Involutional Melancholia', *Journal of the American Medical Association*, vol. 242, no. 8, August 1979, pp. 24–31.

11. Robert Wilson. *Feminine Forever*. New York: M. Evans, 1966.

12. See David Reuben. *Everything You Always Wanted to Know about Sex*. New York: David McKay, 1969.

13. Ibid.

14. Rosetta Reitz. *Menopause: a Positive Approach*. London: Unwin, 1982; Barbara Seaman and Gideon Seaman. *Women and the Crisis in Sex Hormones*. New York: Bantam, 1977; *Consumer Reports* (USA), November 1976, p. 642.

15. See, e.g., Susan Ballinger. 'A Comparison of Possible Effects of Acute and Chronic Stress on Post-Menopausal Urinary Oestrogen Levels', *Maturitas*, 3, pt 2, 1981, p. 107.

16. *Surveillance, epidemiology and end results, incidence and mortality data, 1973–7*, US Department of Health and Human Services, Public Health Service, National Institutes of Health Publication no. 81–2330.

17. Vidal S. Clay. 'Menopause', in Patricia Cooper (ed.), *Women's Health and Medical Guide*. Des Moines, IA: Meredith Corp., 1981.

18. Myra Hunter et al. 'Relationships between Psychological Symptoms, Somatic Complaints and Menopausal Status', *Maturitas*, vol. 8, 1986, pp. 217–28.

19. See, e.g., Jean Coope. *British Medical Journal*, 18 October 1975.

20. For further discussion, see K. MacPherson. 'Menopause as Disease: the Social Construction of a Metaphor', *Advances in Nursing Science*, vol. 3, pt 2, 1981, pp. 95–113; P. Kaufert and S. McKinley. 'Estrogen-replacement Therapy, the Production of Medical Knowledge and the Emergence of Policy', in V. Oleson and E. Lewin (eds), *Women, Health and Healing*. London: Tavistock, 1985.

21. See e.g., M. Vessey and G. Bungay. 'Benefits and Risks of Hormone Therapy in the Menopause', in A. Smith (ed.), *Recent Advances in Community Medicine*, no. 2. Edinburgh: Churchill Livingstone, 1982; K. Hunt et al. 'Long-term surveillance of mortality and cancer incidence in women receiving hormone replacement therapy', *British Journal of Obstetrics and Gynaecology*, July 1987, p. 620; and L. A. Brinton et al. 'Menopausal oestrogens and breast cancer risk: an expanded case control study', *British Journal of Cancer*, vol. 54, 1986, p. 825.

22. See, e.g. Robert Beaglehole. 'Oestrogens and Cardiovascular Disease', *British Medical Journal*, 3 September 1988, p. 572; and Anna Paganini-Hill et al. 'Postmenopausal Oestrogen Treatment and Stroke: a Prospective Study', *British Medical Journal*, 20–7 August 1988, p. 519. Colditz et al. in the *New England Journal of Medicine*, 30 April 1987, p. 1105, provide some tentative evidence to suggest that HRT protects against the increased risk of heart disease in women who have had both ovaries removed before menopause.

23. P. W. F. Wilson et al. 'Postmenopausal Oestrogen Use, Cigarette Smoking, and Cardiovascular Morbidity in Women Over 50' ('The Framingham Study'), *New England Journal of Medicine*, 24 October 1985, p. 1038.

24. E. D. Eaker et al. 'Differential Risk for Coronary Heart Disease Among Women in the Framingham Study', Workshop on Coronary Heart Disease in Women, Bethesda, Maryland, 26–8 January 1986.

25. See, e.g., Seaman and Seaman, op. cit., note 14.

26. See, e.g., C. Kay. 'The Role of Progestogens in Peri-menopausal and Post-menopausal Hormone Replacement Therapy', *Postgraduate Medical Journal*, vol. 54, supplement 2, 1978, p. 99.

27. Trevor J. Powles. 'Treatment of Menopausal Symptoms in Breast Cancer Patients', *The Lancet*, 6 August 1988, p. 344.

28. Robert C. Atchley. 'Later Adulthood in Oxford Township', summary of one-year data. Scripps Gerontology Foundation, Miami University, 1975.

29. See, e.g., S. V. Saxon and M. H. Etlen. *Physical Age and Ageing: a Guide for the Helping Professions*. New York: Tiresias Press, 1978.

30. See, e.g., Roger Smith. 'Exercise and Osteoporosis', *British Medical Journal*, 20 April 1985, p. 1163; L. E. Langon and C. T. Rubin. 'Regulation of Bone Mass in Response to Physical Activity', in A. St John Dixon et al. *Osteoporosis, a Multi-disciplinary Problem*. London: Academic Press and Royal Society of Medicine, 1983; 'Osteoporosis and Activity', leader article in *The Lancet*, 18 June 1983, p. 1365; E. Smith et al. 'Physical Activity and Calcium Modalities for Bone Mineral Increase in Aged Women', *Medicine and Science in Sports and Exercise*, vol. 13, no. 1, 1981, p. 60. R. Chow et al. 'Effect of Two Randomized Exercise Programmes on Bone Mass of Healthy Post-menopausal Women', *British Medical Journal*, 5 December 1987, p. 1441.

31. See, e.g. A. M. Parfitt. 'Dietary Risk Factors for Age-related Bone Loss and Fractures', *The Lancet*, 19 November 1983, p. 1181; and A. St John Dixon. 'Non-hormonal Treatment of Osteoporosis', *British Medical Journal*, 26 March 1983, p. 999.

32. Warren E. C. Wacker. *Magnesium and Man*. Cambridge, MA: Harvard University Press, 1980.

33. See, e.g., Margo Gosney and Raymond Tallis. 'Prescription of Contraindicated and Interacting Drugs in Elderly Patients Admitted to Hospital', *The Lancet*, 8 September 1984, p. 564.

34. Charles Claoué and A. R. Elkington. 'Informing Hospitals of Patients' Drug Regimes', *British Medical Journal*, 11 January 1986, p. 101.

35. Alice Lake. *Our Own Years: What Women Over 35 Should Know about Themselves*. New York: Random House, 1979, pp. 215–16.

36. For more information see David M. Shaw et al. 'Senile Dementia and Nutrition', *British Medical Journal*, 10 March 1984, p. 792.

37. Donald G. Whedon. 'Osteoporosis', editorial in *New England Journal of Medicine*, vol. 305, no. 7, 13 August 1981, pp. 397–9.

38. M. D. Bastow et al. 'Undernutrition, Hypothermia and Injury in Elderly Women with Fractured Femur: an Injury Response to Altered Metabolism', *The Lancet*, 22 January 1983, pp. 143–6.

39. See note 30.

40. J. M. Aitken. 'Relevance of Osteoporosis in Women with Fracture of Femoral Neck', *British Medical Journal*, 25 February 1984, p. 597.

41. See, e.g., C. Nagant De Deuxchaisnes. 'Involutional Osteoporosis',

in Dixon et al., op. cit., note 30; D. H. Marshall et al., *Clinical Endocrinology*, vol. 7, 1977, p. 159.

42. For example, this is what Robert Lindsay et al. found in a study published in 1980 ('Prevention of Spinal Osteoporosis in Oophorectomised Women', *The Lancet*, 29 November 1980, p. 1151). See also C. C. Johnston et al. 'Oestrogen and Calcium in the Management of Osteoporosis', in Dixon et al. op. cit., note 30. After Lindsay et al.'s study was published, Christiansen et al. produced another one ('Bone Mass in Menopausal Women after Withdrawal of Oestrogen/Gestagen Replacement Therapy', *The Lancet*, 28 February 1981, p. 459) which appeared to contradict this, suggesting that the effects of HRT on bone may be permanent. Lindsay et al., commenting on this in a letter to *The Lancet* (28 March 1981, p. 729), point out that Christiansen et al. gave women calcium supplements throughout the study, which may account for the apparent benefits after HRT was stopped.

43. B. Lawrence Riggs et al. 'Effect of the Fluoride/Calcium Regimen on Vertebral Occurrence in Postmenopausal Osteoporosis', *New England Journal of Medicine*, vol. 306, no. 8, 25 February 1982, pp. 446–50.

44. Ibid.

45. Joseph Lane. 'Postmenopausal Osteoporosis: the Orthopedic Approach', *The Female Patient*, vol. 6, November 1981, pp. 43–51.

46. Central Statistical Office. *Social Trends*, 1985; *Monthly Digest of Statistics*. London: HMSO, March 1984.

47. National Council for Carers and Their Elderly Dependants. *Granny Caring for Granny*. Available from Carers' National Association (see Organizations).

48. See C. Wenger. *The Supportive Network: Coping with Old Age*. London: Allen and Unwin, 1984.

49. For example, G. Nesbit. Dept of Sociology, Manchester University, 1986.

RESOURCES
PUBLICATIONS

GENERAL*

Age Concern. *Your Rights*. Covers all pensions and benefits, updated annually (available from Age Concern – see Organizations).

Age Well Campaign Unit *Age Well Ideas Pack*. (available from Age Concern – see Organizations).

Allen, I. *Short Stay Residential Care for the Elderly* (available from Policy Studies Institute, 100 Park Village East, London NW1), 1985.

Asso Doreen. 'The Ending of the Reproductive Cycle' in *The Real Menstrual Cycle*. Chichester: John Wiley, 1983.

Attendance Allowance – going for a review (available from The Disability Alliance – see Organizations), 1984.

de Beauvoir, Simone. *Old Age*. London: Deutsch, and Weidenfeld and Nicolson, 1972.

Black and Asian Old People in Britain (available from Age Concern – see Organizations), 1984.

*Blair, Pat. *Know Your Medicines* (available from Age Concern – see Organizations), 1985.

Bloomfield, J. *Devoted, Dedicated and Dog-tired*. A report on informal care for the elderly in Coventry, prepared for Coventry Social Services Department, 1986.

Booth, T. *Home Truths: Old People's Homes and the Outcome of Care*. London: Gower, 1986.

Bytheway, W. D. *Street Care*. ARVAC Occasional Paper no. 5, Wivenhoe, 1983. Details elderly women looking after other elderly people in a neighbourly way in four streets in a Welsh town.

Carers and Services: a Comparison of Men and Women Caring for Elderly People (available free from the Equal Opportunities Commission – see Organizations).

Caring for the Elderly and Handicapped: Community Care Policies and Women's Lives (available from the Equal Opportunities Commission – see Organizations), 1982.

Caring for Someone with Dementia. Broadcasting Support Services for Channel Four, 1983.

Caring from Day to Day (available from MIND – see Organizations), 1980.

Choosing How to Live (available from MIND – see Organizations), 1979.

Claim Your Rights – A guide to benefits for ethnic elderly citizens (available from Pensioners' Link – see Older Women's Project in Organizations) in Turkish, Greek, Chinese, English and five Asian languages.

Cloke, C. *Caring for the Carers 1983: a Directory of Initiatives* (available from Age Concern – see Organizations).

*Cloke, C. *Getting On: a Guide to Positive Ageing*. The College of Health Guide to Homes for Elderly People. London: College of Health, 1984.

Consumers' Association (Which?). *Approaching Retirement*. London: Consumers' Association, 1984.

Copper, Baba. *Over the Hill – Reflections on Ageism between Women*. Freedom, California: Crossing Press, 1988.

Elder, G. *The Alienated: Growing Old Today*. London: Writers and Readers, 1977.

Equal Opportunities Commission. *Equal Opportunities in Post-School Education* (available free from EOC – see Organizations).

Equal Opportunities Commission. *Model of Equality*. A report prepared to show how equal treatment could be achieved between men and women in occupational pension schemes (available free from EOC – see Organizations).

Ethnic Minority Senior Citizens: the Question of Policy (available from SCEMSC – see Organizations), 1986.

Every Solution Creates a Problem (available from Counsel and Care for the Elderly, 131 Middlesex Street, London E1 7JF). Documents effects of social security cuts, forcing elderly people to stay in hospital when they don't want to.

Fennel, G. and M. **Sidell**. *Good Practice Guide. Day Centres for the Elderly*. Norwich: University of East Anglia, Centre for East Anglian Studies, 1982.

Finch, J. and D. **Groves** (eds). *A Labour of Love: Women, Work and Caring*. London: Routledge and Kegan Paul, 1983.

Finch, J. and R. **Sinclair**. *Sixty Years On. Women Talk About Old Age*. London: Women's Press, 1987.

Fitzgerald, K. 'Sex and the Over Seventies', *New Society*, 7 June 1985.

*Franks, H. (ed.). *What Every Woman Should Know About Retirement*, 1987 (available from Age Concern – see Organizations).

Fresh Start: a Guide to Training Opportunities (available from Equal Opportunities Commission – see Organizations).

Godlove, C., L. **Richard** and G. **Rodwell**. *Time for Action: an Observa-*

*Items marked with an asterisk are primarily designed to be of practical value.

tion Study of Elderly People in Four Different Care Environments. Sheffield University: Joint Unit for Social Services Research, 1981. Details the demeaning effects of day-to-day interaction in residential homes.

*Grimshaw, C. 'Keeping out of Hospital', *Openmind*, no. 8, April–May 1984 (available from MIND).

Harman, Harriet and Age Concern. *A Guide to Choosing an Old People's Home.* London: 1989. Available *free* from Community Education Department, Thames Television, 306 Euston Road, London NW1 3BB.

Harrison, J. 'Women and Ageing: Experience and Implication', *Ageing and Society*, vol. 3, no. 2, 1981, pp. 209–35.

Hemer, June and Ann Stanyer. *Survival Guide for Widows.* London: Age Concern, 1986.

Hemmings, Susan (ed.). *A Wealth of Experience.* London: Pandora Press, 1985. Eighteen older women write about their lives.

Home Life: a Code of Practice for Residential Care. Centre for Policy on Ageing (available from Bailey Brothers and Swinfren, Warner House, Folkestone, Kent CT19 6PH), 1984.

Housing for Ethnic Elders. Age Concern/Help the Aged Housing Trust (available from Age Concern – see Organizations).

Jerrome, D. 'The Significance of Friendship for Women in Later Life', *Ageing and Society*, vol. a, no. 2, 1981, pp. 175–97.

King's Fund Centre. *Promoting Better Health among Elderly People.* London: King's Fund, 1988.

Kohner, N. *Caring at Home.* National Extension College Cambridge.

Living in Homes: a Consumer View of Old People's Homes, 1988 (available from British Association for Services to the Elderly – see Organizations).

*Lodge, B. *Coping with Caring. A Guide to Identifying and Supporting an Elderly Person with Dementia.* 1981.

*Mace, N. L. and P. V. Rabins. *The 36 Hour Day.* Sevenoaks: Hodder, 1985. A family guide to caring for persons with Alzheimer's disease.

Mandelstam, D. *Incontinence and Its Management.* Beckenham: Croom Helm, 1986.

McGoldrick, A. *Equal Treatment in Occupational Pension Schemes* (free from Equal Opportunities Commission – see Organizations), 1985.

Midwinter, E. *Ten Million People.* London: Centre for Policy on Ageing, 1983.

Midwinter, E. *The Wage of Retirement. The Case for a New Pensions Policy.* London: Centre for Policy on Ageing, 1985 (available from Bailey Brothers and Swinfren, Warner House, Folkestone, Kent CT19 6PH).

*Mitchell, L. *Healthy Living Over 55. The Getting On Guide.* London: Central Independent Television/John Murray, 1984.

*Montgomery, E. *Retaining Bladder Control.* Bristol: John Wright, 1983.

Moore, P. with C. P. Conn. *Disguised.* Milton Keynes: Word (UK) Ltd, 1986. Fascinating story of what happened to a young woman who dressed and made up as an eighty-year-old over three years in America. The experience of ageism.

*Muir Gray, J. A. and H. McKenzie. *Take Care of Your Elderly Relative.* Beaconsfield: Allen and Unwin, 1980.

Muir Gray, J. A. and H. McKenzie. *Caring for Older People.* London: Penguin Books, 1986.

Murray-Sykes, K., N. North and B. McKay. 'Who Cares about the Carers? The Effect on Family and Friends of Admitting an Elderly Person to Hospital', *Radical Community Medicine*, no. 18, Summer 1984.

National Consumer Council. *Residential Care for Elderly People: a Consumer View.* London: NCC, 1989.

Newton, E. *This Bed My Centre.* London: Virago Press, 1980. Graphic first-hand account by an eighty-year-old woman of her years in a series of nursing homes where she experienced her individuality and independence being submerged and imprisoned.

Norman, A. *Triple Jeopardy: Growing Old in a Second Homeland.* London: Centre for Policy on Ageing, 1985 (available from Bailey Brothers and Swinfren, Warner House, Folkestone, Kent CT19 6PH).

Palmore, E. B. et al. *Retirement: Causes and Consequences.* New York: Springer, 1985.

*Pates, A. and M. Good. *Second Chances Yearbook. An Annual Guide to Adult Education for Women of All Ages.* Cambridge: She Magazine/Great Ouse Press, 1987.

*Perkin, J. *It's Never Too Late. A Practical Guide to Continuing Education for Women of All Ages.* London: Impact Books, 1984.

Radical Community Medicine. 'The Elderly: Who Cares?', *Radical Community Medicine*, no. 18, Summer 1984.

*Rathfelder, M. *How to Claim State Benefits: a Guide to Your Rights.* Plymouth: Northcote House, 1988.

Rayner, G. 'Appropriate Care for the Elderly: Lessons from the American Health Consumer Movement', *Radical Community Medicine*, no. 18, Summer 1984.

Rossi, A. 'Life-span Theories and Women's Lives', *Signs: Journal of Women in Culture and Society*, vol. 6, no. 1, 1980, pp. 4–32.

Russell, C. *The Ageing Experience.* London: Allen and Unwin, 1981. Research in Australia about the effects of career and lifestyle on elderly women's experience of old age.

Scott Hilda. *Working Your Way to the Bottom: the Feminisation of Poverty.* London: Pandora Press, 1982.

Self and Society. 'Ageing', *Self and Society*, vol. 16, no. 1, January–February 1988.

Sherfey, M. J. *The Nature and Evolution of Female Sexuality.* New York: Random House, 1976.

Shields, L. *Displaced Homemakers: Organizing for a New Life.* New York: McGraw Hill, 1981.

Spier, Peter and Barbara Spier. *The State Pension Explained – a Guide for Women.* Greater London Association for Pre-Retirement (Babcock Power, 165 Great Dover Street, London SE1 4YB), 1985.

*Stoppard, Miriam. *50 Plus Lifeguide.* London: Dorling Kindersley, 1983.

Townsend, P. *Poverty in the United Kingdom.* London: Penguin Books, 1979.

Twomey, Mary. 'A Feminist Perspective of District Nursing', in Christine Webb (ed.), *Feminist Practice in Women's Health Care.* Chichester: John Wiley, 1986.

*van Zwanenburg, F. and J. Corder. *Fit for Life: a Help Yourself Guide to Good Health in Old Age* (available from Help the Aged – see Organizations).

Wenger, C. *The Supportive Network: Coping with Old Age.* London: Allen and Unwin, 1984.

Wheeler, R. *Don't Move: We've Got You Covered. A Study of the Anchor House Trust Staying Put Scheme.* London: Institute of Housing, 1985.

Who Cares about Relatives? About support groups for relatives of elderly people who are mentally ill (available from MIND – see Organizations).

Who Cares for the Carers? Opportunities for those Caring for the Elderly and Handicapped (available free from the Equal Opportunities Commission – see Organizations).

Your Pension. Regularly updated, guide to social security benefits for retired people.

MENOPAUSE AND OSTEOPOROSIS

Cooper, W. *No Change: a Biological Revolution for Women* (2nd rev. ed.). London: Arrow, 1983.

Fairhurst, E. and R. Lightup. 'Being Menopausal: Women and Medical Treatment'. Paper presented at the annual conference of Medical Sociology Group of BSA, Warwick, September 1980.

Fairlie, J. et al. *Menopause: a Time for Positive Change.* London: Javelin Books, 1988.

Kaufert, P. and S. **McKinlay**. 'Estrogen-replacement Therapy: the Production of Medical Knowledge and the Emergence of Policy', in V. Oleson and E. Lewin (eds), *Women, Health and Healing.* London: Tavistock, 1985.

MacPherson, K. 'Menopause as Disease: the Social Construction of a Metaphor', *Advances in Nursing Science,* vol. 3, pt 2, 1981, pp. 95–113.

National Osteoporosis Society. *What Everyone Needs to Know about Osteoporosis* (pamphlet). Bath, 1987.

Notelovitz, Maurice and Marsha **Ware**. *Stand Tall!.* A guide to how to ensure adequate calcium and other mineral levels to prevent osteoporosis (details available from WHRRIC – see p. 334).

Rakusen, Jill. *Menopause: a Guide for Women of All Ages.* Cambridge: National Extension College/Health Education Authority, 1989.

Royal College of Physicians. *Report of a Working Party on Fractured Neck of Femur.* London; 1988. Highlights many inadequacies in the provisions of treatment for hip fractures but fails to deal adequately with the question of prevention of osteoporosis, concentrating on HRT to the exclusion of diet and exercise prior to menopause.

Vessey, M. and G. **Bungay**. 'Benefits and Risks of Hormone Therapy in the Menopause', in A. Smith (ed.), *Recent Advances in Community Medicine,* no. 2. Edinburgh: Churchill Livingstone, 1982.

Women's Health Information Centre. *Factsheet about Self-help Approaches to Menopause* and *Broadsheet about Socio-political Aspects of Menopause* (available from WHRRIC – see p. 638).

FICTION

Arnold, June. *Sister Gin.* London: Women's Press, 1979.

Arrowsmith, Pat. *The Prisoner.* London: Journeyman, 1982.

Ba, Miriama. *So Long a Letter.* London: Virago Press, 1982.

Kuzwayo, Ellen. *Call Me Woman.* London: Women's Press, 1985.

MacDonald, Barbara and Cynthia **Rich**. *Look Me in the Eye: Old Women, Aging and Ageism.* London: Women's Press, 1985. A collection of essays.

Marshall, Paule. *Praise Song for the Widow.* London: Virago Press, 1983.

McNeill, Janet. *The Maiden Dinosaur.* Dublin: Arlen House, 1984.

Moos, Lotte. *Time to be Bold* (poems). London: Centerprise, 1981.

Oosthuizen, Ann. *Loneliness and Other Lovers.* London: Sheba, 1981.

Sarton, May. *As We Are Now.* London: Women's Press, 1983; and *A Reckoning.* London: Women's Press, 1984.

Sarton, May. *At Seventy.* London: Norton, 1988.

Wolff, Charlotte. *An Older Love.* London, Virago Press, 1976.

MAGAZINES

Grey Power, official journal of British Pensioners and Trade Unions Action Association (see Organizations).

Spare Rib (see p. 637) has increasingly taken on the issue of ageism, and many back issues – e.g. on ageing and changing no. 154, May 1985 – are worth looking at.

ORGANIZATIONS

AFFOR (All Faiths for One Race), 173 Lozells Road, Birmingham B19 1RN. Tel: 021–523 8076. A multi-racial community resource agency.

Age Concern, Bernard Sunley House, 60 Pitcairn Road, Mitcham, Surrey CR4 3LL. Tel: 01–640 5431. Also 4th Floor, 1 Cathedral Road, Cardiff CF1 9SD. Tel: 0222–371821. Scottish Old People's Welfare Council, 33 Castle Street, Edinburgh EH2 3DN. Tel: 031–225 5000. Northern Ireland Old People's Welfare Council, 6 Lower Crescent, Belfast BT7 1NR. Tel: 0232–245729.

Alzheimer's Disease Society (ADS), 158/160 Balham High Road, London SW12 9BN. Tel: 01–675 6557.

Association to Aid the Sexual and Personal Relationships of People with a Disability (SPOD), 286 Camden Road, London N7 0BJ. Tel: 01–607 8851/2. Also **SPOD** Ireland, PO Box 1000, Dublin 4.

Association of Crossroads Care Attendant Schemes Ltd, 10 Regent Place, Rugby, Warwickshire CV21 2PN. Tel: 0788–73653.

British Association for Service to the Elderly (BASE), 119 Hassell Street, Newcastle-under-Lyme, Staffordshire ST5 1AX. Tel: 0782–661033. A charity furthering better care for the elderly.

British Pensioners and Trade Unions Action Association, Norman Dodds House, 315 Bexley Road, Erith, Kent DA8 3EZ. Tel: 0322–335465.

Carers' National Association, 21–23 New Road, Chatham, Kent ME4 4QJ. Tel: 0634–813981. And 29 Chilworth Mews, London W2 3RG. Tel: 01–724 7776.

Disability Alliance, 25 Denmark Street, London WC2 8NJ. Tel: 01–240 0806. Advice on social security benefits for people with disabilities. Publishes *Disability Rights Handbook* annually.

Elderly Accommodation Counsel Ltd, Eardley House, 182–4 Campden Hill Road, Kensington, London W8 7TT. Tel: 01–243 8545.

The Elderly Pedestrians' Road Safety Project, The Health Education Unit, Department of Education, The University, Southampton SO9 5NH. Tel: 0703–559122.

Equal Opportunities Commission, Overseas House, Quay Street, Manchester M3 3HN. Tel: 061–833 9244.

Fair Hearing Campaign, c/o Royal National Institute for the Deaf. 105 Gower Street, London WC1E 6AH. Tel: 01–387 8033.

Forum for the Rights of Elderly People to Education, c/o Diane Norton, Bernard Sunley House, 60 Pitcairn Road, Mitcham, Surrey CR4 3LL. Tel: 01–640 5431.

Help the Aged, 16–18 St James's Walk, London EC1R 0BE. Tel: 01–253 0253/8000.

National Association for Mental Health (MIND), 22 Harley Street, London W1N 2ED. Tel: 01–637 0741. For Wales Information Office, Wales MIND, N.A.M.H., 23 St Mary Street, Cardiff CF1 2AA. Tel: 0222–395123/4/5. Scottish and Northern Ireland Associations see separate listing.

National Association for Widows, 54–7 Allison Street, Birmingham B5 5TH. Tel: 021–643 8348.

National Federation of Retirement Pensions Associations, 14 St Peter Street, Blackburn, Lancashire BB2 2HD. Tel: 0254–52606.

National Organization for Widows, Widowers and their Children (CRUSE), 126 Sheen Road, Richmond, Surrey TW9 1UR. Tel: 01–940 4818.

National Osteoporosis Society, Barton Meade House, PO Box 10, Radstock, Bath BA3 3YB. Send sae for information.

Northern Ireland Association for Mental Health, 84 University Street, Belfast BT7 1HE. Tel: 0232–28474.

Older Feminist Network, c/o Wesley House, 4 Wild Court, London WC4B 5AU.

Older Lesbian Network, c/o 274 Upper Street, London N1 2UA.

Older Women's Project, Pensioners' Link, 17 Balfe Street, London N1 9EB.

Prisioners' Voice, 4 St. Peter Street, Blackburn, Lancs BB2 2HD. Tel: 0254–52606.

Scottish Association for Mental Health, Atlantic House, 38 Gardener's Crescent, Edinburgh. Tel: 031–229 9687.

Standing Conference of Ethnic Minority Senior Citizens (SCEMSC), 5–5a Westminster Bridge Road, London SE1 7XW. Tel: 01–928 0095.

Support for the Elderly Mentally Infirm (SEMI), c/o University Settlement, 43 Ducie Road, Barton Hill, Bristol BS5 0AX. Tel: 0272–559219. Local Bristol and Avon-based charity; developed from a relatives' support group.

University of the Third Age (U3A), 6 Parkside Gardens, London SW19 5EY. 'Mutual aid' learning groups. Constructive activities for older adults; educational, leisure and creative. Send sae for information and details of over 100 local groups.

Wireless for the Bedridden. 81B Corbetts Tey Road, Upminster, Essex RM14 2AJ. Tel: 04022–50051. Will supply radios and TVs free to the housebound or those on supplementary benefit over sixty.

Women's Health Concern (WHC) PO Box 1629, London W8 6AU. Tel: 01–602 6669. Promotes hormone replacement therapy.

'Years Ahead', PO Box 4000, London W3 6XJ – a topical magazine programme for older people transmitted by Channel Four that publishes some excellent literature, e.g. 'OutrAGEous' which campaigns against ageism, 'Money Matters', 'Caring for Someone with Dementia'. Send sae for copies and full list.

PART VI

SOME COMMON AND UNCOMMON MEDICAL AND HEALTH PROBLEMS

INTRODUCTION

While Part VI is almost a book in itself, we've still had to limit it to looking at those health problems which affect large numbers of women or for which it is difficult to get reliable information elsewhere. Please be aware that information is constantly changing, and make use of the resources listed at the end of each chapter.

We suggest self-help and non-medical alternatives when possible. Please see Chapter 7 for essential information about alternative therapies and in particular for guidelines on choosing alternative practitioners. Please also see Chapter 27 for a discussion of our medical system and suggestions for choosing and using medical care.

First, here is a symptom guide which might help you find your way round the chapter.

SYMPTOM GUIDE*

PAIN AND DISCOMFORT

Pain on intercourse. Pelvic inflammatory disease (PID) (p. 503); endometriosis (p. 515); ovarian cysts (p. 519).

Discomfort on intercourse. Thrush (vaginal irritation) (p. 490); herpes (p. 496); cystitis (p. 507); trichomoniasis (p. 491) or any vaginal infection; insufficient lubrication (p. 260); thinning of vaginal skin (p. 466).

Abdominal pain. Ovarian cysts (p. 519); endometriosis (p. 515); cystitis (p. 507); PID (p. 503); advanced gonorrhoea (p. 492) or chlamydia (p. 493); period pains (p. 510); IUD (p. 287); ectopic pregnancy (p. 439); fibroids (p. 513).

Back pain. PID (p. 503); period pains (p. 510); IUD (p. 287); fibroids (p. 513).

Pain when urinating. Cystitis (p. 507); herpes (p. 496); gonorrhoea or chlamydia (if in the urethra) (p. 493) or PID (p. 503).

Painful swelling of vulva. Infected Bartholin's glands (p. 490).

Painful sores. Herpes (p. 496).

Progressively increasing pain. Endometriosis (p. 515); PID (p. 503).

*See also A Self-help Checklist (p. 21).

Itching in and around vagina. Thrush (p. 490); crabs (p. 502); trichomoniasis (p. 491); anaerobic or bacterial vaginosis (p. 499); vaginitis and vulvitis (p. 489).

DISCHARGE

Thick, white, yeasty. Thrush (p. 490).

White, yellow, bloody or greyish with bad smell after intercourse. Vaginitis (p. 489) or cervicitis (p. 521); anaerobic vaginosis (p. 491).

Yellowish-green, thin, foamy, foul-smelling (fishy). Trichomoniasis (p. 491).

Thin, transparent. Ovulation (p. 35), cervical erosion (p. 521) or early gonorrhoea (p. 491); chlamydia (p. 493).

LUMPS, BUMPS AND BLISTERS

Hard raised skin on genitals. Genital warts (p. 500).

Painless open blister or sore. Primary syphilis (p. 495).

continues overleaf

Painful blisters or sores. Herpes (p. 496); infected Bartholin's gland (p.490).

Abdominal lumps. Ovarian cysts (p. 519); endometriosis (p. 515); ovarian cancer (p. 519).

Uterine lumps. Fibroids (p. 513).

Breast lumps. Breast problems, see Chapter 24.

BLEEDING PROBLEMS

Unusually heavy periods, bleeding between periods or spotting is most likely to be caused by pregnancy or menopause; however, all irregular bleeding should be checked. It could be:

Bleeding without other symptoms. Anaemia (p. 557); polyps or fibroids (benign uterine growths, p. 513); uterine cancer (mainly in older women) (p. 519); mini Pill (p. 294), injectable contraceptives (p. 296); and other conditions which we haven't been able to go into. Sometimes there is no apparent reason for bleeding problems although hormone abnormalities and stress could be the cause.

Bleeding and Pain. PID (p. 503); endometritis Bartholin's gland (p. 490). (p. 439); endometriosis (p. 515).

GYNAECOLOGICAL AND URINARY PROBLEMS

Rewritten by
ANGELA PHILLIPS
(*unless otherwise indicated*)

All women secrete moisture and mucus from the membranes that line the vagina. This discharge is transparent or slightly milky and may be somewhat slippery. When dry, it may be yellowish. When a woman is sexually aroused or ovulating this secretion increases. It normally causes no irritation or inflammation of the vagina or vulva.

Many bacteria grow in the vagina of a normal, healthy woman. Some of them help to keep the vagina somewhat acid and keep yeast, fungi and other harmful organisms from multiplying out of all proportion. In large amounts, the waste products secreted by these harmful organisms may irritate the vaginal walls and cause infections to develop. At such times we may experience an abnormal discharge, mild or severe itching and burning of the vulva, chafing of the thighs, and occasionally frequent urination.

Some of the reasons we get vaginal infections are: a general lowered resistance (from lack of sleep, bad diet, another infection in our body, and similar factors);

PREVENTION OF GENITAL INFECTIONS*

1. Wash your vulva and anus regularly. Pat your vulva dry after bathing and try to keep it dry. Also, don't use other people's towels or flannels. Avoid irritating sprays and soaps (use special non-soap cleansers for skin very sensitive to plain soap) and other chemical bath products. Avoid talcum powder.**

2. Wear clean cotton underpants. Avoid nylon underwear and tights since they retain moisture and heat, which help harmful bacteria to grow faster.

3. Avoid trousers that are tight in the crotch and thighs.

4. Always wipe your anus from front to back (so that bacteria from the anus won't get into the vagina or urethra).

5. Make sure your sexual partners are clean. It is a good practice for partners to wash their hands and for a man to wash his penis before making love. Using a condom can provide added protection, and is particularly important with a new partner.

6. Use a sterile, water-soluble jelly if lubrication is needed during intercourse (something like K-Y jelly, for example, *not* Vaseline). Also, recent studies show that birth control jellies slow down the growth of trichomonads and possibly thrush. Using these jellies for lubrication and/or general prevention is a good idea, especially with a new partner you may not know very well.

7. Avoid sexual intercourse that is painful or abrasive to your vagina.

8. Cut down on coffee, alcohol, sugar and refined carbohydrates (diets high in sugars can radically change the normal pH of the vagina).

9. Applying unpasteurized plain yoghurt (those containing lactobacilli) in the vagina replenishes good bacteria normally found in the vagina, which are often destroyed when we take antibiotics, and helps to prevent infections and cure mild symptoms.

10. Take care of yourself. Not eating well or resting enough makes you more susceptible to infection.

*For prevention of STDs (sexually transmitted diseases) see p. 488.
**Talcum powder has been linked to ovarian cancer, see p. 519.

pregnancy; taking birth control pills, other hormones, or antibiotics; diabetes or a pre-diabetic condition; cuts, abrasions and other irritations in the vagina (from childbirth, from intercourse without enough lubrication, or from using an instrument in the vagina medically or for masturbation); or too much douching.

Chemicals such as bath preparations, 'feminine hygiene sprays' and deodorized tampons or pads can irritate and inflame the delicate vaginal skin. They are unnecessary and often harmful. Vaginal deodorants should be avoided and other chemicals used with caution. Women past menopause are particularly susceptible to these irritants.

SEXUALLY TRANSMITTED DISEASES (STDs)*

STD is a term used to describe any disease acquired primarily through sexual contact. The organisms that cause these diseases (except for crabs and scabies) generally enter the body through the mucous membranes – the warm, moist surfaces of the vagina, urethra, anus and mouth. You can catch an STD through intimate contact with someone who already has the infection, especially during oral, anal

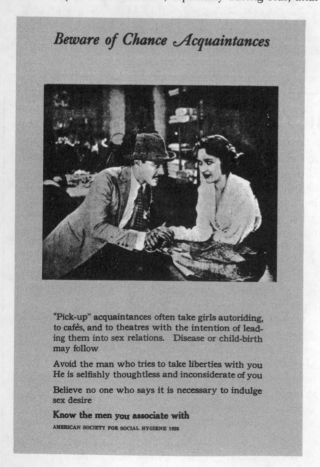

Beware of Chance Acquaintances

"Pick-up" acquaintances often take girls autoriding, to cafés, and to theatres with the intention of leading them into sex relations. Disease or child-birth may follow

Avoid the man who tries to take liberties with you He is selfishly thoughtless and inconsiderate of you

Believe no one who says it is necessary to indulge sex desire

Know the men you associate with

AMERICAN SOCIETY FOR SOCIAL HYGIENE 1926

*The term venereal disease (VD) is no longer much used, partly because it doesn't cover all the infections which can be transmitted sexually, partly because of the moralistic overtones. It is still used on some public noticeboards and in telephone books.

or genital sex. When your partner has more than one STD you can become infected with all you are exposed to; gonorrhoea and chlamydia are often transmitted together.

The stories about how you can get STDs from toilet seats, doorknobs or other objects are not true except under certain rare conditions. (See individual descriptions for more information.) Nor can you catch STDs from heavy lifting, straining or being dirty. Animals don't transmit STDs to humans. Organisms which cause most STDs live best in a warm, moist environment like the linings of the genitals or throat. Outside the body they usually die in less than a minute.

Statistically, if you are young (between sixteen and twenty-four), are sexually active with more than one partner and live in an urban setting you are at highest risk for STD. Your chances of getting an individual infection will also depend on your access to information and screening. Basically, however, if you are heterosexual and have sexual contact with a man who has an STD your chances of catching the infection are high. For example, after just one exposure to gonorrhoea you have a 40 to 50 per cent chance of catching the disease.

If you are lesbian, you are much less likely to get an STD because most STDs are not easily spread between women. It is possible to transmit herpes during oral-genital sex or through skin contact between an open sore and broken skin. It is also theoretically possible, though almost unheard of, to transmit gonorrhoea to the throat during oral sex, or syphilis through skin contact. If you have sex with both men and women, your chances of getting STDs are the same as for heterosexuals. At present, your risk of getting HIV (which can lead to AIDS, see p. 501) is low unless you or your partner are, or have been, involved in high-risk activities (see p. 502). But if we do not all take responsibility for prevention, HIV is capable of spreading at frightening speed.

MORAL ATTITUDES

While there is no doubt about the serious threat of AIDS, there is also a danger that public concern will be manipulated by the right-wing moral minority and any anti-AIDS campaign will become a crusade against sexuality and in favour of repressive sexual standards for all of us. We do not believe that the answer to the spread of this frightening disease is a retreat back to the hypocrisy of 'Victorian Values'. The Victorian pretence of sexual morality coupled with heterosexual monogamy did not stop the spread of syphilis – a disease which in its day was just as frightening and as incurable as AIDS and a great deal easier to contract.

It has taken the more open society of the 1970s and 1980s, compiled with efficient diagnosis and a cure, to bring this killer disease under control. Only in this open atmosphere will it be possible to spread the information about prevention that is necessary to halt the spread of AIDS. Indeed, one of the most hopeful pieces of news to come out of the international AIDS conference in Febru-

BIRTH CONTROL AND STDs

While the Pill does not seem to promote gonorrhoea, one recent study suggests that women using the Pill may be more susceptible to chlamydial infections.[1]

The IUD, on the other hand, does help spread gonorrhoea and chlamydia into the fallopian tubes, possibly by dislodging the protective mucus plug that covers the opening of the cervix and acting as a wick for bacteria. The IUD also irritates the uterus, sometimes causing small ulcerations which can make the uterus more vulnerable to STD infection.

Barrier methods of contraception (condoms or diaphragms with spermicide) provide some protection against STD. For the Pill and IUD in relation to HIV infection, see pp. 293 and 289.

cancer too. What is now needed is the cash to make such voluntary screening programmes a reality.

CHANGES WE CAN MAKE OURSELVES

Many of us still believe that 'nice girls' don't get STDs. When we do, we are labelled 'promiscuous' if we are single, or 'unfaithful' if we are in a monogamous relationship. When news of an infection is the first thing that one partner hears of another relationship the effect can be devastating.

I've been so upset these last few days. My husband told me he'd slept with someone else and might have VD. I didn't know what to do. How could I speak to my doctor and expose myself? If I asked any of my friends what to do, they would be mortified. I saw an ad yesterday for a VD clinic, and after a lot of hesitation I phoned. It was a relief to get information without anyone knowing who I was.

Nevertheless, when fear of damaging a relationship prevents partners from confiding in one another about the disease and the need for treatment, the effect can be far worse. With several STDs there may be no early symptoms in women. An untreated infection can lodge in the fallopian tubes causing chronic infection and even infertility before we are aware that we have been infected. Infection with HIV may ultimately be fatal.

There is increasing awareness among sexually active people of the need for vigilance to protect against STDs of all kinds. One of the biggest categories among the groups of people now visiting STD clinics are those who are discharged without treatment. Clearly, the habit of getting regular check-ups is catching on. Nevertheless, in spite of changing attitudes, the incidence of STDs is growing overall.

STDs can be prevented if we each take responsibility for our own health and that of our partners. In the end, prevention is by far the best solution because:

- there are some diseases which cannot, as yet, be cured;
- the large doses of antibiotics needed to kill infections do our general health no good;
- many of us experience no symptoms and may be, unwittingly, passing diseases on to others;
- serious complications can occur even when there have been no early symptoms to warn us of the presence of disease;
- acting responsibly (see below) and seeking help/advice promptly can break the cycle of disease.

The steps necessary to prevent vaginal infections are described on p. 485. To prevent sexually transmitted infections, special precautions are needed. If none of us ever had sex with another person without first being certain that we were free from infection, the incidence of STD would drop dramatically. We cannot, of course, be certain that new

ary 1988 was that no single new case of HIV had been reported in the gay community of San Francisco for a year.

CHANGES WE CAN PUSH FOR NOW

Some medical professionals maintain that the only way to control STDs is to develop a vaccine. Nevertheless, we can, and should, attempt to contain these diseases now. The rise in incidence of gonorrhoea has already been halted due mainly to increased public awareness, contact tracing, and efficient diagnostic services in clinics. Syphilis has been so well controlled that the old scourge of congenital syphilis has virtually disappeared and the disease is rarely seen in its advanced stages. The same success is possible with the newer diseases through accessible diagnosis and treatment where possible, but, above all, through education for prevention. We can support or initiate campaigns for more complete sex and health education, without moral overtones. When our society accepts sexuality it will be more likely to encourage STD prevention.

At the same time we must campaign for more resources to be devoted to curbing the most common infectious diseases of our young adult population. New diagnostic tests using monoclonal antibodies should soon provide the means for diagnosing a wide range of infections and viruses quickly and efficiently. At present neither the clinics nor the public health laboratories have the funds to establish a diagnostic service which can do any more than check those at the highest risk of contracting a disease.

Voluntary screening for infections such as chlamydia (p. 492) and papilloma virus (p. 500) should be automatically offered along with routine cervical smears (see p. 521). In this way we could cut dramatically the incidence of pelvic inflammatory disease (p. 503) and probably cervical

Safer Sex Guidelines

In order to guard against the HIV virus it is necessary to avoid absorbing your partner's body fluids into your own bloodstream (and vice versa). If you follow guidelines for avoiding HIV infection you will also be protected against other STDs.

Semen and blood both carry a high concentration of HIV in an infected person. Saliva and urine are not thought to be significant risks. Any practices which carry the risk of causing abrasions should be avoided. Vaginal intercourse without sufficient lubrication can damage skin, providing access to the virus. With anal intercourse the skin can be even more easily damaged, particularly if insufficient lubrication is used. Cuts on fingers can provide entry points if they come in contact with infected blood or semen. Mouth ulcers or gum infections may also be a problem in oral sex. As more is understood about the transmission of HIV, guidelines are continually being amended. Check for up-to-date information with organizations listed in Resources (see p. 534). At present the following suggestions are considered to minimize the risks:

1. A sheath is effective against most STDs provided the man puts it on his penis before it touches your genital area. Sheaths should be used for both vaginal and anal sex.

2. Vaginal spermicides[4] (contraceptive foams, jellies and creams), particularly those containing nonoxynol 9 (e.g. Delfen and Ortho) provide some protection against infection (including HIV) even when used alone, but provide a higher degree of protection when used with a sheath.

3. Waterproof plasters can be used to cover any sores or scratches.

4. A contraceptive diaphragm used with spermicide provides some protection against infections of the cervix, and against cervical cancer.

5. If a male partner does not use a sheath it is important that he washes his genitals before sex and after any anal sex (particularly if you go on to vaginal sex). This will not guard against the more serious infections but will help to protect against cervical cancer and some vaginal infections.

6. We do not recommend 'morning-after' antibiotics taken just before or after intercourse. A low dose may mask an existing infection and encourage the growth of resistant strains of bacteria. It also increases the risk of our becoming allergic to a particular antibiotic which then is no longer useful for fighting future infections.

---

partners will follow this code and the spectre of AIDS can leave us with few certainties (see p. 501). However, we can at least follow it ourselves and try to develop ways of being open with each other about the dangers of STDs and the need for caution.

It's one thing to talk about being responsible and another to imagine murmuring into someone's ear at a time of passion, 'Would you mind slipping on this condom or using this cream just in case . . . ?' Yet it seems awkward to bring it up earlier when you are not sure you are going to want to make love. I use a birth control cream the first time and then bring up the subject afterwards for us to consider together.

For those of us who have more than one partner, or who have sex with someone who has more than one partner, it is hard to be certain that infection is not being passed along the chain. It is particularly important for us to be vigilant about changes in our own and our partners' bodies: unusual discharges, bumps, itchiness, redness, swelling or an odd smell. Regular check-ups at a GU clinic should be part of normal health care. The following guidelines are effective against STDs. Though nothing is 100 per cent effective,[2] all reduce the risk.*

*Edward Brecher has compiled a summary of methods tested plus an extensive bibliography on prevention.[3]

DIAGNOSIS AND TREATMENT OF VAGINAL AND SEXUALLY TRANSMITTED INFECTIONS

Once any infection is established it is important to get it checked and treated. *All infections of the genital or urinary tracts are best treated at a specialist genito-urinary clinic.* Not only is the treatment completely free, with no prescription charges, but these clinics, which were set up to deal with sexually transmitted diseases, have developed expertise in helping women manage chronic vaginal and urinary infections which are not sexually transmitted and their diagnostic facilities are far superior to those provided by GPs and gynaecologists. Family planning clinics and other doctors may well spot an infection but they are rarely properly equipped to diagnose and may, as a result, prescribe wrongly.

Many of us feel embarrassed to make use of these clinics. Staff sometimes make the situation worse by acting as though they were guardians of public morality. But attitudes are changing. Some clinic workers have made a constructive connection with sexuality and provide a supportive atmosphere in which we are encouraged to ask questions and participate actively in both diagnosis and future prevention.

You can find out where your local GU clinic is by:

1. Checking behind the doors of a public lavatory (clinic times may be out of date).
2. Looking in the phone book under VD.
3. Asking in a health centre or citizens' advice bureau.
4. Asking (or telephoning) any hospital and asking for the 'special clinic'.
5. Asking your GP.

You do not have to be referred by anyone so you can choose the clinic you prefer even if it is not in your immediate area. Some clinics operate rigid appointment systems, others are more flexible.

WHAT HAPPENS AT THE CLINIC?

When you arrive at the clinic you will be given a card with your name and clinic number for future appointments; you then see a doctor who takes down a detailed case history. This entails asking questions which may seem rather embarrassing but give some guidance to diagnosis. For example: do you have a regular sexual partner? Do you ever have anal or oral sex? Next you go into a consulting room with a couch. You will be asked to undress from the waist down and lie on the couch. The following tests should be done.

- Vaginal, cervical and if necessary anal and urethral swabs which will be examined on a slide and cultured (bacteria are encouraged to multiply so that they can be seen more easily) and examined microscopically.
- A blood test.
- A urine test.
- A cervical smear.
- A bimanual pelvic examination (which they sometimes forget!), see p. 593.
- You may have to ask for a chlamydia test (see p. 493); they are not given routinely.

You will then be asked to wait for the initial test result. Even if this test is negative, cultures must be done for greater accuracy. This takes at least forty-eight hours and it is *imperative* that you return to the clinic within the next few days for your results, as it may take weeks to trace you if infection is found. Test results may not be given over the phone.

When you are given your results you will not necessarily be told what you have by name. 'Don't worry, just a little bug' is the sort of information sometimes supplied. This withholding of information should be strongly opposed. If you are not given a clear diagnosis just go through the possible list by name and get them to say yes or no. (One reason for withholding information may be that your partner has asked for it to be confidential.)

It is important to know exactly what you have and exactly what you are being treated with. Some clinics will prescribe medicine if you are a confirmed contact with infection even if test results are not positive. You may welcome this, as some infections are hard to diagnose and highly infectious. However, you do not have to accept medication and may prefer to wait for a definite diagnosis. This may mean coming back to the clinic several times if you are fairly certain that you have picked something up.

Any medication will be prescribed and given to you immediately, *without prescription charges*. Make sure you finish the whole course, or the infection may recur, and don't have sex until you are clear. If you have syphilis or gonorrhoea you will be asked to see a social worker or 'contact tracer'. There you will be given slips with the address of the clinic to pass on to possible contacts so that they can come in for tests. This is very important; if you have passed the disease on it may have spread to others, all of whom will need treatment. If you feel unable to talk to contacts yourself you can ask the contact tracer to do it for you. Your name need never be mentioned. It may seem hard to do but the health of others may depend on it. Even if you haven't got either of these infections you should bring your partner in for tests. This is important. Your partner may be carrying a symptomless infection which he or she could pass back to you or on to someone else. Although most infections are less likely to travel between women they can do, particularly syphilis and the less fragile organisms like thrush and trichomonas. Women partners should be informed if you have a confirmed STD.

Individual infections are described below.

VAGINITIS AND VULVITIS

This involves any itching, stinging, unusual-smelling or unusually copious discharge. It should be investigated (particularly if you are sexually active). The infection may be either a sexually transmitted infection or an overgrowth of bacteria/yeast, which may also be triggered by sexual intercourse. * In either case you and your partner will need treatment (see the rest of this chapter). If you have recently had an abortion, given birth or had a gynaecological operation or procedure, apparently minor symptoms may be caused by infection introduced into your womb at the time. These could be serious and require investigation and, if necessary, antibiotic treatment.

If you are not sexually active, or specific STD tests have proved negative, consider whether you are using any kind of chemical irritant (bath preparation, deodorant, scented soap, talcum powder) which may be causing the inflammation. This is particularly likely in post-menopausal women or pre-pubescent girls.

A tampon, contraceptive cap, sponge or other foreign body can cause a bacterial infection. It will usually disappear when the cause is removed, though some women who

---

*There is now also evidence that it can result from a man being allergic to a woman's vaginal secretions and producing antibodies against them, which are then transmitted during intercourse.[5] Condom use can end recurring cycles of this type of vaginitis. We do not yet know how, if at all, the man's allergy can be treated, but alternative approaches (see Chapter 7) may help.

are prone to vaginal infections may find that the overgrowth of bacteria caused by the object does not stabilize. In this case some form of treatment is required.

Self-help

Avoid all chemicals, wash only in warm water and pat dry very carefully. A shallow bath with a cupful of salt added can be very soothing, or you may like to try adding herbs such as comfrey to the bath water. Wear clothing which allows as much air as possible to circulate. Cold compresses of yoghurt or calamine lotion may sooth an itching vulva. Avoid intercourse until the condition improves and then use some form of lubricant such as K-Y jelly to avoid chafing.

Orthodox Treatment

If you cannot relieve the itching a doctor or clinic may prescribe a low-dose cortisone cream or other soothing lotion. Post-menopausal women may be given an oestrogen cream. These treatments may help but should not be continued on a long-term basis (see Chapter 22, p. 458).

ANAEROBIC VAGINOSIS (OR BACTERIAL VAGINOSIS)

This is a new term for the vaginal infection which used to be called *non-specific vaginitis*. This common condition is characterized by a watery, fishy-smelling vaginal discharge which is often worse after intercourse.

Anaerobic bacteria are so called because they can survive without contact with oxygen. These bacteria are often found along with bacteria called *Gardnerella vaginalis* and *Mycoplasma hominis*.[6] Although the infection usually produces nothing more than an unpleasant odour, it has been linked with prematurity and postpartum complications so it is worth ensuring that you are clear of infection before embarking on a pregnancy.

Self-help

Approaches recommended for thrush may change the vaginal pH and clear the infection.

Orthodox Treatment

There is a very high recurrence rate for vaginosis. Dr Anona Blackwell of St Thomas' Hospital, London, has done extensive research on anaerobic vaginosis and her chosen treatment is metronidazole (Flagyl).* If taken by both partners the recurrence rate drops. An alternative treatment would be amoxycillin. Flagyl can be taken in suppository form which cuts out the nausea often associated with it (do not drink alcohol with Flagyl).

INFECTIONS OF THE BARTHOLIN'S GLANDS

The Bartholin's glands lie on either side of the entrance to the vagina. They produce secretions which lubricate the entrance. Occasionally the glands become blocked, causing a swelling. If the swelling is painless it is a cyst. If it is painful it is an abscess. An abscess may well form behind a gland which is blocked by a cyst so it is worth treating it.

Orthodox Treatment

If there is an abscess a swab should be taken to identify the cause of infection. Then the relevant antibiotics will be prescribed. Unfortunately, the condition does not respond well to antibiotics alone. It is usually necessary to rest and to take pain-killers at the same time and quite often surgical draining is necessary. If a cyst forms it may be possible to remove it surgically. In some cases the whole gland is removed. The nature of this condition makes it particularly worthwhile to try alternative approaches first.

Self-help and Alternative Approaches

Apply a hot compress for twenty minutes (either Fuller's Earth or Epsom salts on a hot flannel held in place with a hot water bottle). This treatment should be carried out for three days, leaving a two-day gap before repeating it (if you need to). With an abscess you will need to treat the infection too. Apply hot and cold packs to the vulva (or use a shower) to improve the blood flow, go on a raw food diet and try garlic pearles (a natural antibiotic). This treatment can make you feel worse initially before it starts to work (see chapter 7).

YEAST INFECTIONS (ALSO CALLED *CANDIDA ALBICANS* OR THRUSH)

Candida albicans, a yeast fungus, normally grows in harmless quantities in your rectum and vagina. When your system is out of balance, yeast-like organisms may grow profusely and cause itching, usually accompanied by a thick, white discharge which may look like cottage cheese and smell like baking bread. If a woman has a yeast infection when she gives birth, the baby will get yeast in its throat or digestive tract. This is treated orally with nystatin drops or gentian violet.

Candida grows best in a mildly acidic environment. The pH in the vagina is normally more acidic (4.0 to 5.0), except when we take birth control pills or some antibiotics, are pregnant, have diabetes and when we menstruate (when the pH rises to between 5.8 and 6.8, because blood is alkaline). Obviously, we often find ourselves with a vaginal pH favourable to thrush, so preventive measures are especially important.

Orthodox Treatment

Once thrush sets in, treatment usually consists of some form of pessaries which are only available on prescription.*

---

*See footnote on Flagyl, p. 491.

*'One-shot' medication does not seem to be as effective as longer courses.

Cream may be prescribed for partners to avoid reinfection. If the infection is really severe, oral nystatin may be prescribed, but it shouldn't be used in pregnancy and should only be used if it is really necessary because it kills off fungi of all kinds throughout the body. It also occasionally makes you feel nauseated.

Another method which is effective, but less popular these days because it is messy, is gentian violet. It should be painted over the cervix, vagina and vulva. Some people react against it but for the others it is a very effective treatment and a sanitary pad worn during treatment will stop your clothes turning purple. It is important to use an *aqueous* solution, not alcohol, which will burn.

One of the problems with using medications to cure thrush is that all the good bacteria are destroyed with the bad and unless the good ones grow back first we can become reinfected. A change in diet with a reduction in refined foods, combined with a preventive routine, makes more sense, and for those of us on the contraceptive pill it might be worth coming off it until the thrush is cleared. (Use an alternative form of contraception.)

Self-help

Some of us have had success with the following remedies: yoghurt douche* (daily); goldenseal douche (simmer one teaspoon per pint and then dilute 1:1); garlic suppositories (peel but don't nick a clove of garlic, then wrap in gauze before inserting); yellow dock douche (two or three times weekly); vinegar douche (one tablespoon to a pint of warm water); vinegar in the bath; Acijel (from chemists); acidophilus capsules (from some health food stores). Unless otherwise specified, all should be used daily for a week or so at the first sign of an attack, and two or three times a week for three months as a long-term preventive. Also you can acidify your system by drinking 500 milligrams of Vitamin C daily.

> *For a long time I found myself getting a new dose of thrush every month. I would feel the itching start, get a course of Canestan, then two or three weeks later it started all over again, usually just towards the end of a period. Then I bought a douche and used it, first daily, then every second day, with a warm solution of vinegar (about a tablespoon to a pint) from halfway through my period for a fortnight. I didn't have another*

> *recurrence until I got pregnant and had to stop using the douche.*

If you have persistent thrush, you may find that altering your diet will be beneficial. See Leon Chaitow's book *Candida Albicans: Could Yeast Be Your Problem?* for more information about what you can do (see Resources).

TRICHOMONIASIS

Trichomonas vaginalis, or trich, is a one-celled parasite that can be found in both men and women. Many women have trich organisms in their vaginas, though often they are without symptoms. Usually women with trich have a thin, foamy vaginal discharge that is yellowish-green or grey in colour and has a foul odour. If another infection is present along with trichomoniasis, the discharge may be thicker and whiter. Trich is usually diagnosed by examining vaginal discharge under a microscope. It can also cause a urinary infection. It is most often contracted through intercourse but can occasionally be passed on by moist objects such as towels, bathing suits, underwear and flannels. Sometimes emotional stress can cause symptoms to flare up or recur.

Orthodox Treatment

The usual treatment for trich is oral doses of metronidazole (Flagyl) or nimorazole (Naxogin). Anyone taking metronidazole should avoid alcohol, as the combination can make the effects of both worse.**

In some cases, you can treat trich successfully with sulpha creams (low efficacy), Betadine (an iodine-based preparation which should not be used in pregnancy) or self-help remedies (see below). Unless you detect the infection early, however (and often even when you do), these treatments are not as effective as Flagyl.

Self-help

1. Vinegar douches. Trich grows best in an alkaline environment so acidic douches may eliminate a trich infection if applied early enough (see under thrush).

2. Goldenseal douche (see under thrush).

3. Chickweed douche: boil one quart of water, add three tablespoons of chickweed. Cover, let sit five to ten minutes, strain. Douche daily for a week.

4. Garlic inserted every twelve hours (see under thrush).

GONORRHOEA

Gonorrhoea is caused by the gonococcus, a bacterium which works its way gradually along the warm, moist

---

*It is not always easy to get a douche in the UK. You may have to buy a 'vaginal cleansing kit' at a chemist and discard the chemicals which come with it. There is no need for douching except as part of a treatment or prevention programme. Be careful when douching. Too much pressure can force air or fluid into the uterus and abdominal cavity. Use lukewarm water, never have the bag more than two feet above your hips and never squeeze a bulb-type bag hard. Wait until the air is out of the tubing and the solution is running through before putting the nozzle into your vagina. Never douche if you are pregnant. If you experience vaginal pain and/or fever after douching, contact a doctor or go to a hospital the same day. Alternatives to douching include inserting tampons soaked in the solutions, getting your partner or friend to put the solution into your vagina while you lie in the bath, using a speculum to open your vagina, and shallow baths.

**In the last edition we cautioned women to avoid this drug because of association with gene disorders and cancer in animal studies. There has as yet been no evidence of similar problems in humans. While we feel that it is best to be cautious about all drugs particularly in pregnancy and during lactation, there seems to be no special reason to single out this one. No antibiotics should be taken without good cause, particularly for prolonged periods.

passageways of the genital and urinary organs and affects the cervix, urethra, anus and throat. You can transmit this disease to another person through genital, genital-oral and genital-rectal sex. You can get a gonorrhoea infection in your eye when you touch it with a hand that is moist with infected discharge. A mother can pass it to her baby during birth. Occasionally children can contract gonorrhoea by using towels contaminated with fresh discharge or bathing with an infected person. More frequently, children with gonorrhoea are found to have been sexually abused.

The disease is more likely to persist and spread in women than in men. Untreated gonorrhoea can lead to serious and painful infection of the pelvic area called pelvic inflammatory disease (PID), see p. 503. Seventeen per cent of the women known to have gonorrhoea develop PID; of these, 15 to 40 per cent become sterile after just one episode.

A less common complication is proctitis, inflammation of the rectum. If the eyes become infected by gonococcal discharge (gonococcal conjunctivitis), blindness can result. Disseminated gonococcal infection, rare but serious, occurs when bacteria travel through the bloodstream, causing infection of the heart valves or arthritic meningitis. Gonorrhoea can be treated at any stage to prevent further damage, but damage already done usually cannot be repaired.

Remember, it is important to use preventive measures, since a woman often does not have early symptoms. By the time pain prompts her to see a doctor, the infection has usually spread considerably.

Symptoms

Women often have gonorrhoea without any symptoms; as many as 40 to 60 per cent don't notice symptoms because of their mildness, or confuse them with other conditions.

Symptoms usually appear anywhere from two days to three weeks after exposure. The cervix is the most common site of infection. In cervical gonorrhoea, a discharge develops which is caused by an irritant released by the gonococci when they die. If you examine yourself with a speculum you may see a thick discharge, redness and small bumps on the cervix. You may at first attribute symptoms to other routine gynaecological problems or to the use of birth control methods like the Pill. The urethra may also become infected, possibly causing painful urination and burning. As the infection spreads, it can affect the Skene's (on each side of the urinary opening) and Bartholin's glands. Vaginal discharge and anal intercourse can infect the rectum. Symptoms include anal irritation, discharge and painful bowel movements. If the disease spreads to the uterus and fallopian tubes, you may have pain on one or both sides of your lower abdomen, vomiting, fever and/or irregular menstrual periods. The more severe the infection, the more severe the pain and other symptoms are likely to be. These symptoms may indicate PID.

Gonorrhoea can also be spread from a man's penis to a woman's throat (pharyngeal gonorrhoea). You may have no symptoms, or your throat may be sore or your glands swollen.

One to 3 per cent of women with gonorrhoea develop disseminated gonococcal infection (DGI). Symptoms of DGI include a rash, chills, fever, pain in the joints and tendons of wrists and fingers.

A man will usually have a thick gelatinous discharge from his penis and feel pain or burning when he urinates. Some men have no symptoms. If you have had sex with a man who has a discharge from his penis, get him to go for a test right away to identify the infection so that you both will get the correct treatment. It is easier to identify the organ-

Christine Bordante

GONORRHOEA

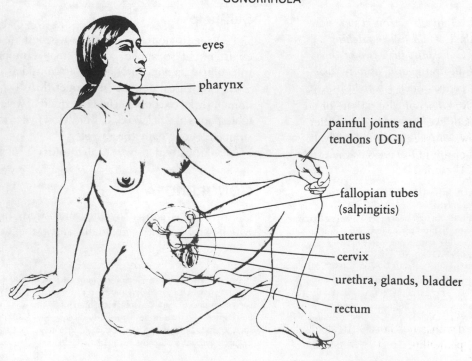

eyes

pharynx

painful joints and tendons (DGI)

fallopian tubes (salpingitis)

uterus

cervix

urethra, glands, bladder

rectum

ism in a man and his infection may be the only clue that you are also infected.

Testing and Diagnosis

It is important to be tested before taking medication, because a test done while treatment is being given is not accurate.

Don't douche right before a test, because you can wash away the accessible bacteria, giving a false negative test result. The gram stain and the culture are two standard tests for gonorrhoea in current use. The widely used gram stain is very accurate for symptomatic men but only 50 per cent accurate for women and asymptomatic men. In this test a smear of the discharge is placed on a slide, stained with a dye and examined for gonorrhoea bacteria under a microscope. If your regular male partner's test is positive, you may want to be treated at the same time regardless of the test results.

The culture test (more reliable, but it takes longer) will be done routinely at a GU clinic. It involves taking a swab of the discharge, rolling it on to a special culture plate and incubating it under special laboratory conditions for sixteen to forty-eight hours to let the gonorrhoea bacteria multiply. The culture test is pretty accurate if it is performed in a specialist clinic with onsite laboratory. Swabs taken by a GP are much less accurate, primarily because it is difficult to maintain specimens in good condition during transport to the lab. Test accuracy also depends greatly on which sites are chosen for testing. If you have the most commonly affected sites (cervix and anal canal) cultured, there is about a 90 per cent chance of finding any existing infection. (Many women with gonorrhoea also have trichomoniasis and/or chlamydia.) The swab from the cervix is the best single test, about 88 to 93 per cent accurate. About 50 per cent of women with infected cervices also have infection in the anal canal. If you have had a hysterectomy, ask for a urethral culture, too. If you have had oral-genital sex, ask for a gonococcal throat culture.

If the initial test is negative but you have definitely been exposed to gonorrhoea, you may want to be treated anyway while waiting for the results of the culture to come back.

If you have any doubts as to how accurate the results of your test were, try to have someone else do one or come back again within a week or two, the sooner the better.

There are several new, quicker, tests currently being developed. At present they are not as good as the existing culture test done at all GU clinics.

Treatment

Many doctors prescribe medication before the culture test is back or diagnosis is certain for three reasons: tests are not always accurate; the doctor is not sure you will come back; and the sooner the gonorrhoea is treated, the easier it is to cure. Ask about medication for your partner.

One argument in favour of waiting for test results is that you should not take antibiotics unnecessarily. Also, chlamydia, often confused with gonorrhoea, is treated with tetracycline rather than penicillin, so it is important to know which infection you have. If you are not sure which you have been exposed to and don't want to wait for the results of the culture, ask to be treated with tetracycline, in addition to penicillin. If you decide to wait for the culture test results, you must consider whether or not it will be easy for you to return for possible later tests and treatment.

An IUD may make cure more difficult since it helps spread infection and increases the chances of getting PID. Have your IUD removed before treatment.

High-dosage injections of penicillin or (more often) high oral doses of ampicillin are the usual treatments for gonorrhoea. Injected penicillin can also cure syphilis still in the incubation stage. You may also receive oral probenecid,* a drug which slows down the urinary excretion of antibiotics and allows them to remain in the bloodstream in high enough concentrations to do the job.

Over the past twenty-five years, gonorrhoea has required increasing doses of penicillin to cure, and new strains of gonorrhoea have emerged which are resistant to the drug. In this case, the gonococcal organism produces an enzyme (penicillinase) that destroys penicillin, making the drug useless for treatment. Tetracycline is also ineffective. If a culture indicates penicillin resistance, another medication, such as spectinomycin, will be prescribed.

Test for Cure

Every woman treated for gonorrhoea should have *two* negative culture tests, including a rectal culture, a week or two apart before considering herself cured. If cultures remain positive, get retreatment with another antibiotic, such as spectinomycin, and a culture for penicillin-resistant gonorrhoea. Pockets of infection in reproductive organs may be difficult to cure. If your partner has gonorrhoea, you can become reinfected very soon after a cure, so it's crucial that he or she be tested and treated as well.

Gonorrhoea and Pregnancy

It may be wise to get tested for gonorrhoea during pregnancy. A pregnant woman with untreated gonorrhoea can infect her baby as it passes through her birth canal. In the past, many babies went blind due to gonococcal conjunctivitis. Antibiotic drops will cure any infection. Pregnant women should avoid tetracycline.

CHLAMYDIA TRACHOMATIS

In the last edition of this book chlamydia was classified simply as a 'non-specific infection' and dismissed as 'usually relatively trivial in women'. We now know that this silent infection is a major cause of pelvic inflammatory disease (see p. 503). It may also cause infection of the urethra and cervix (and if you practise anal sex, an inflammation of the rectum). In rare cases (more frequently affecting men) chlamydia may cause Reiters syndrome, a form of arthritis.

*Those of us of African and Mediterranean ancestry may be sensitive to probenecid.

Symptoms

Ten to twenty days after exposure you may experience cystitis-like symptoms (see p. 507), a thin vaginal discharge and/or lower abdominal pain occasionally with fever. You may experience no symptoms at all until the infection has advanced into the tubes causing scarring and possibly infertility (see PID, p. 503).

Most men will have a burning feeling when peeing and a discharge from the penis about one to three weeks after exposure. The symptoms are similar to gonorrhoea (indeed the disease often accompanies gonorrhoea) but the incubation period is longer and the stinging milder. About 10 per cent of men experience no symptoms even though they are carriers.

Testing and Diagnosis

Chlamydia is the most common form of sexually transmitted disease. Unfortunately, the seriousness of chlamydia has taken a long time to come home to doctors and healthcare planners. Women referred to a gynaecology department for pelvic pain may not have the infection diagnosed, may not be asked to bring their partners in for investigation, and may be wrongly treated and constantly reinfected.

After my first bout of PID I had no more trouble for two years. Then we stopped using contraception to try to get pregnant. Within weeks the infection was back. It wasn't until a non-medical person pointed out that the infection seemed to be associated with giving up the sheath that it occurred to us to get my partner tested. Sure enough, he had chlamydia. He must have had it for five years. Unfortunately by that time my infection was too advanced to yield to ordinary treatment.

The correct diagnosis of chlamydia is impossible without specialized laboratory equipment, including a microscope capable of the magnification necessary to see these extremely small organisms. Blood tests can be used but swabs taken from the cervix (urethra in men) and then cultured produce more accurate results.

At the time of writing these special facilities were not available in some areas of the country and even some large teaching hospitals failed to provide them. When cash limits are tight, the (mostly male, middle-aged and middle-class) people who allocate funding see what they consider 'self-inflicted disease' as having a very low priority.

If you or your partner suspect that you may have contracted chlamydia (remember that it is often classified as non-specific urethritis – NSU – in men) you should telephone your local clinics and ask whether they have facilities for diagnosis. If you have no clinic in your area that can provide this service and your partner has definite symptoms you may want to consider treatment just in case. Remember that *even if gonorrhoea is diagnosed in one or both of you, this does not rule out the presence of chlamydia.* Since the treatment for chlamydia is different, you may cure one disease and keep the other.

Treatment

Tetracycline (or erythromycin if you are pregnant) for a fortnight is the standard treatment for chlamydia. Penicillin is not effective. One specialist who has no facilities for diagnosing chlamydia in one of the clinics he attends automatically prescribes this treatment as well as penicillin when gonorrhoea is diagnosed because the diseases so often come together. Regular sexual partners, or contacts, should take the treatment whether or not they have symptoms. If possible, get a check-up culture one to four weeks after treatment. Heterosexual couples should use condoms until the infection clears. If either of you seems to be getting recurrent attacks you should be checked again to exclude the possibility of another infection.

Chlamydia and Pregnancy

In one American study 8 to 10 per cent of pregnant women were found to have chlamydia.[7] If the infection is untreated it may be transmitted to the baby causing eye infections which are hard to treat, or pneumonia. Chlamydia has also been linked to miscarriage, ectopic pregnancy, premature delivery and postpartum infections. If you have an abortion any infection can be carried into your womb causing post-abortion complications. Given the prevalence of this disease it makes sense to get a check-up at a laboratory with appropriate facilities early in pregnancy (or before).

UREAPLASMA

If your partner has a urinary infection you may also become infected by *Ureaplasma urealyticum* (also called *T-*

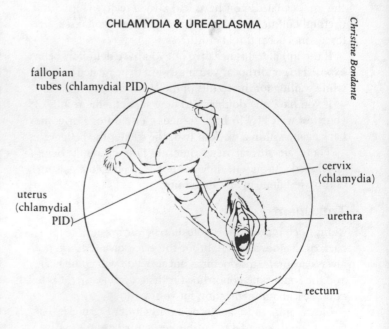

CHLAMYDIA & UREAPLASMA

Christine Bondante

fallopian tubes (chlamydial PID)

cervix (chlamydia)

uterus (chlamydial PID)

urethra

rectum

Chlamydia can also be transmitted to the eyes via the hands.

mycoplasma), transmitted separately from or together with chlamydia. It has been found in the genital tracts of many apparently healthy people who have no symptoms of infection. While ureaplasma causes up to one-quarter of the cases of non-specific urinary infection in men,* it is not generally thought to cause cervicitis or PID in women, though this has been disputed. However, some researchers believe it can cause other genital tract infections and pregnancy complications (see below).[8]** If you are undergoing investigations for infertility make sure you are screened for this organism.

Symptoms

Women may not have symptoms, but for both men and women they are similar to chlamydia (above).

Treatment

The same treatment as for chlamydia, though about 10 per cent will be resistant to tetracycline. A follow-up check four weeks later is recommended.

SYPHILIS

Syphilis is no longer a common infection in Britain. Extensive screening and a simple cure have brought this ancient killer under control. Syphilis is caused by a small spiral-shaped bacterium called a spirochete. You can get syphilis through contact with someone who is in an infectious (primary or secondary and possibly the beginning of the latent) stage via open sores or rashes containing bacteria which can penetrate the mucous membranes of the genitals, mouth and anus as well as broken skin on other parts of the body.

Symptoms

Once the bacteria have entered the body, the disease goes through four stages.

1. *Primary.* The first sign is usually a painless sore called a chancre (pronounced 'shanker') which may look like a pimple, a blister or an open sore, and shows up from nine to ninety days after the bacteria enter the body. The sore usually appears on the genitals at or near the place where the bacteria entered the body. However, it may appear on the fingertips, lips, breast, anus or mouth. Sometimes the chancre never develops or is hidden inside the vagina or folds of the labia, giving no evidence of the disease. Only about 10 per cent of women who get these chancres notice them. If you examine yourself regularly with a speculum (see p. 32), you are more likely to see one if it develops. At the primary stage, the chancre is very infectious. The preventive methods outlined on p. 488 work only if the chemical or physical barrier covers the infectious sore.

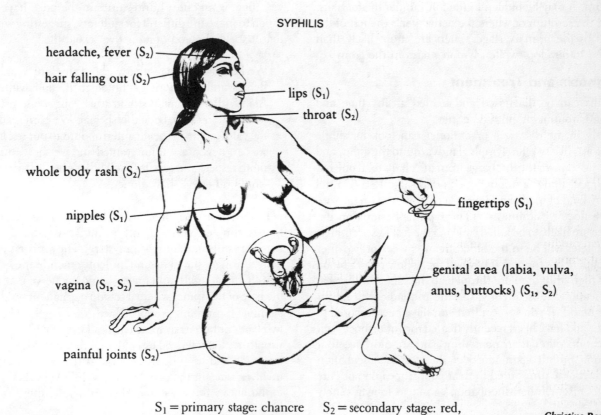

SYPHILIS

headache, fever (S₂)
hair falling out (S₂)
lips (S₁)
throat (S₂)
whole body rash (S₂)
fingertips (S₁)
nipples (S₁)
vagina (S₁, S₂)
genital area (labia, vulva, anus, buttocks) (S₁, S₂)
painful joints (S₂)

S_1 = primary stage: chancre sore area; rash S_2 = secondary stage: red,

Christine Bondante

*Fifty per cent are caused by chlamydia, and the other 25 per cent by unidentified organisms.
**Mycoplasma hominis* (see p. 490) may, on the other hand, cause PID.

With or without treatment, the sore will disappear, usually in one to five weeks, but the bacteria, still in the body, increase and spread.

2. *Secondary*. The next stage occurs anywhere from a week to six months later. By this time the bacteria have spread all through the body. This stage usually lasts weeks or months, but symptoms can come and go for several years. They may include a rash (over the entire body or just on the palms of the hands and soles of the feet); a sore in the mouth; swollen, painful joints or aching bones; a sore throat; a mild fever or headache (all flu symptoms). You may lose some hair or discover a raised area around the genitals and anus.

3. *Latent*. During this stage, which may last ten to twenty years, there are no outward signs. However, the bacteria may be invading the inner organs, including the heart and brain. The disease is not infectious after the first few years of the latent stage.

4. *Late*. In this stage, which is now extremely rare, the serious effects of the latent stage appear. Depending on which organs the bacteria have attacked, a person may develop serious heart disease, crippling, blindness and/or mental incapacity. With our present ability to diagnose and treat syphilis, no one should reach this stage.

Men's symptoms are similar to women's. The most common place for the chancre to appear is on the penis and scrotum. It may be hidden in the folds under the foreskin, under the scrotum or where the penis meets the rest of the body. In the primary stages, men are more likely than women to develop swollen lymph nodes in the groin.

Diagnosis and Treatment

Syphilis can be diagnosed and treated at any time and testing is routine at any GU clinic.

Early in the disease a practitioner can look for subtle symptoms like swollen lymph glands around the groin, and examine some of the discharge from the chancre, if one has developed, under a microscope (a dark-field test). Do not put any kind of medication, cream or ointment on the sore until a doctor examines it. (The syphilis bacteria on the surface are likely to be killed, making the test less accurate.) Spirochetes will be in the bloodstream a week or two after the chancre has formed. They will then show up in a blood test, which from then on, through all the stages, will reveal the infection. Subsequently, specific antibodies will appear in the blood. If you suspect that you have been exposed to syphilis and have been recently treated for gonorrhoea with medication other than penicillin, you should have four tests one month apart to cover the possible incubation period. (Some drugs used to treat gonorrhoea do not cure syphilis.) Remember, incubation can be as long as ninety days.

Penicillin by injection or a substitute such as tetracycline pills for those allergic to penicillin is the treatment for syphilis. Since people sometimes have relapses or mistakes are made, it is important to have at least two follow-up blood tests to be sure the treatment is complete. You should not have sexual intercourse for one month after receiving treatment. The first three stages of syphilis can be completely cured with no permanent damage, and even in late syphilis the destructive effects can be stopped from going any further.

Syphilis and Pregnancy

A pregnant woman with syphilis can pass the bacteria on to her fetus, especially during the first few years of the disease. The bacteria attack the fetus just as they do an adult, and the child may be born dead or with important tissues deformed or diseased. But if the mother gets her syphilis treated before the sixteenth week of pregnancy, the fetus will probably not be affected. (Even after the fetus has got syphilis, penicillin will stop the disease, although it cannot repair damage already done.) A blood test for syphilis is routine during ante-natal care. It should be repeated if there is any reason to think you have been exposed later in pregnancy.*

HERPES

Between 30 and 60 per cent of adults have herpes antibodies in their blood. Only a minority go on to suffer from recurrent attacks of the disease. Although it can be very unpleasant for the 10 per cent of acute sufferers, the disease is not life-threatening and it can be controlled although, as yet, there is no cure. Lurid stories in the press have done much to make life difficult for sufferers, suggesting wrongly that it spells the end of an active sexual life.

> We both felt strongly that without my four years of herpes and my honest attitude to it, and without Alan's utter acceptance and trust, our relationship just wouldn't have been this special. We even realize the value of the herpeatic interruptions to our sex life; we can never take it for granted and we show much more respect and care for each other's bodies than we would otherwise have done.[9]

Herpes (from the Greek word 'to creep') is caused by the herpes simplex virus, a tiny primitive organism whose nature is still more or less a mystery. The virus enters the body through the skin and mucous membranes of the mouth and genitals, and travels along the nerve endings to the base of the spine, where it sets up permanent residence, feeding off nutrients produced by the body cells. There are two types of herpes simplex viruses (HSV). Type I (HSV I) usually is characterized by cold sores or fever blisters on the lips, face and mouth, while Type II (HSV II) most often involves sores in the genital area. While HSV I is usually found above the waist and HSV II below, there is some

---

*Women who have lived in tropical countries may get a false positive test due to an earlier infection of 'Yaws'. This infection is not sexually transmitted and is not dangerous to the fetus.

GENITAL HERPES

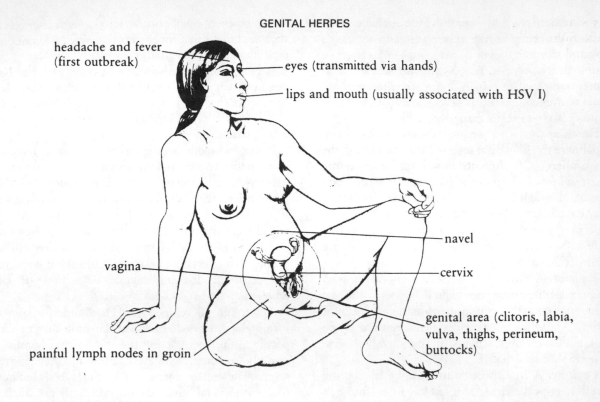

headache and fever
(first outbreak)

eyes (transmitted via hands)

lips and mouth (usually associated with HSV I)

navel

vagina

cervix

genital area (clitoris, labia,
vulva, thighs, perineum,
buttocks)

painful lymph nodes in groin

Christine Bondante

crossover, primarily due to the increase in oral-genital sex. Here we are concerned with genital herpes.

You can get herpes during vaginal, anal or oral sex with someone who has an active infection. You can spread it from mouth to genitals (or eyes) via the fingers. So it is important to wash your hands carefully after touching your genital area. This is particularly important if you wear contact lenses.

The virus can be transmitted from the time the sores crust over and probably for another day or two. Although the virus is sometimes shed in between attacks, there is no evidence that it can be passed on then and there is no reason to avoid sex when you are free of sores.

Symptoms

Symptoms usually occur two to twenty days after a primary exposure, although some people may not have symptoms or may not be aware of them until much later. An outbreak of herpes usually begins with a tingling or itching sensation of the skin in the genital area. This is called the 'prodromal' period and may occur several hours to several days before the sores erupt, or it may not occur at all. You may also experience burning sensations, pains in your legs, buttocks or genitals and/or a feeling of pressure in the area. Sores then appear, starting as one or more red bumps and changing to watery blisters within a day or two. Blisters are most likely to occur on the labia majora and minora, clitoris, vaginal opening, perineum and occasionally on the vaginal wall, buttocks, thighs, anus and navel. Women can also have sores on their cervix, which usually cause no discernible symptoms. Ninety per cent of women have sores on both vagina and cervix during a first infection. Within a few days, the blisters rupture, leaving shallow

ulcers which may ooze, weep or bleed. Usually after three or four days a scab forms and the sores heal themselves without treatment.

While the sores are active, you may find it painful to urinate, and you may have a dull ache or a sharp burning pain in your entire genital area. Sometimes the pain radiates into the legs. You may have an urge to urinate frequently and/or a vaginal discharge. You may also have vulvitis (a painful inflammation of the vulva). During the first outbreak, you may experience fever, headache and swelling of the lymph nodes in the groin. The initial outbreak is usually the most painful and takes the longest time to heal (two to six weeks).

Men may experience pain in the testicles during the prodromal period, followed by sores which usually appear on the head and shaft of the penis but can also appear on the scrotum, perineum, buttocks, anus and thighs. Men can also have sores without knowing it, usually because they are hidden inside the urethra. There may also be a watery discharge from the urethra.

Recurrences

Only about 10 per cent of sufferers experience frequent attacks after the first one. Many more (about 50 per cent) will get occasional attacks within three to twelve months of the first one. Recurrent episodes are usually milder, last from three days to two weeks and usually do not involve the cervix. They often seem to be triggered by stress, illness, menstruation or pregnancy. Most people find that the number of yearly recurrences decreases with time. Because recurrent herpes is associated with lowered resistance, some people believe the infection can lead to secondary infections such as trichomoniasis, bladder infections, venereal warts, yeast infections and vaginitis. Poor diet and drugs that weaken the immune system (such as caffeine, speed, birth control pills and diet pills) may also make you more susceptible to recurrences. People who are deficient in B vitamins or who are unusually tense seem to get more frequent recurrences. Recent studies show that HSV II is much more likely to recur than HSV I.[10]

Testing and Diagnosis

You should visit a GU clinic to confirm that you have the disease. It can usually be diagnosed by sight when the sores are present, although herpes is occasionally confused with other genital problems. Several laboratory tests confirm the diagnosis or indicate the presence of herpes even when no sores are active. This is particularly important if you are pregnant (see below).

The Tzanck test. This test is similar to a cervical smear. A scraping is taken from the edge of an active sore, smeared on a slide sprayed with a cell fixative and sent to a lab for evaluation. A fairly accurate method of diagnosis, it can be used for both men and women. It cannot differentiate between HSV I and HSV II.

Viral culture. A viral tissue culture can be taken using living cells to grow the virus. This test has an advantage in that it can distinguish between HSV I and HSV II. The test is more accurate than the smear and should be done when the sores *first* appear.

Other tests. You can get a blood test to measure the level of herpes antibodies in the blood. (Once you have been exposed to the virus, your body manufactures antibodies to fight off the infection.) For this test, two ampoules of blood are drawn, one during the initial attack and the second two to four weeks later. If you have herpes, the second sample will show a much higher antibody level. (It takes about two weeks to build antibodies.) This test is only effective when performed during the initial attack of herpes. Later, the test results are difficult to interpret.

A *monoclonal antibody* test is being investigated now to determine how accurate it is. It still cannot detect latent cases.

Orthodox Treatment

At present there is no known cure for herpes although more than thirty experimental treatments have been tested and found ineffective. Nevertheless, it is now possible to control very frequent, severe recurrences medically in most cases using the drug Acyclovir (Zovirax). A vaccine is also being tested which appears to boost immunity.

Acyclovir, taken in the correct dose, on a daily basis,* appears to prevent recurrences. Research at the Middlesex Hospital in London has discovered that 200 milligrams of the drug taken four times a day then reduced gradually after three to four months prevents recurrences for most sufferers.[12] However, doctors do not tend to prescribe it unless attacks are very frequent (monthly) because no one yet

knows whether there will be long-term side-effects with such sustained use. For the same reason, it is not usually prescribed for longer than one year.

Recurrences after one year's treatment tend to be less frequent than prior to treatment, though some people find themselves 'back to square one'. Some sufferers find that even a brief respite is enough to help them come to terms with the disease.

It is a very expensive drug and doctors may be reluctant to prescribe it. The Herpes Association has heard of doctors who would only supply a private prescription and of some clinics which will only allow treatment within clinic trials. If you have difficulty getting free supplies from your local GU clinic, contact the Herpes Association (see Resources).

The drug causes inflammation of the liver in some people. The effect disappears when treatment stops but it is not recommended for anyone with liver or kidney problems.

A *vaccine*, developed by Dr Gordon Skinner in Birmingham, seems to be effective in protecting unaffected people against contracting the disease and boosting the immune response of sufferers so that recurrences are less severe. The vaccine doesn't work for everybody but in early trials with several hundred volunteers only two unaffected people went on to contract the disease.

The vaccine has yet to be fully tested with double blind trials; however, the American FDA has given the go-ahead for US trials and UK trials are expected to follow.

Ether or *chloroform* may be prescribed for direct application to stop the stinging and pain.

Self-help and Alternative Approaches

With the growth of self-help discussion groups, many sufferers have found that recurrences can be managed and, once they become less frightening, they very often tail off of their own accord. The Herpes Association feels that any therapies which are aimed at stress control can be useful (see Chapter 7). It may also help to read Get Well Diets on p. 52.

When sores first appear, take warm shallow baths with baking powder three to five times a day. In between, keep sores clean and dry. A hair dryer helps to dry sores. Sores heal faster when exposed to air, so wear cotton underpants or none at all. If it hurts to urinate, do it in the shower or bath or spray water over genitals while urinating (using any plastic squeeze bottle). When sores break, apply drying agents such as hydrogen peroxide, which is available in chemists'. For pain relief, take aspirin.

Many women have found the following very helpful for herpes.* They may or may not work for you. Because some of the products mentioned below must be purchased at a health food store, they may be expensive. We suggest that you pick one or two. Remember, all are most effective when combined with good nutrition and rest. (If you are

---

*Acyclovir in cream form has not been proven to be useful.[11]

*Information adapted from *Herpes*, Santa Cruz Women's Health Center; *Her Pease*, Women's Health Services, Santa Fe, NM; and *Herpes, Something Can Be Done About It*, by N. Sampsidis.

pregnant, don't take medicinal teas or high doses of Vitamin C without consulting your doctor.*)

1. Echinacea is a blood-purifying plant. Capsules made from it are available at health food stores. Take two capsules every three hours, make a tincture and apply (one teaspoon every two hours for three to four days) or make a soothing tea (four cups a day).

2. Take 2,000 milligrams of Vitamin C or two capsules of kelp followed by sarsaparilla tea (four to five cups during the day).

3. Chlorophyll (in powder form) and wheatgrass are good anti-viral herbs. Drink them with warm water. Also, eating blue-green algae (3,000 milligrams daily) may be helpful.

4. Lysine is an amino acid that many women find very effective in suppressing early symptoms. If you stop using it, symptoms may reappear. Take 750 to 1,000 milligrams a day until sores have disappeared. Thereafter take 500 milligrams a day. Lysine seems to work by counteracting the effects of argenine (a substance found in foods such as nuts – especially peanuts – chocolate and cola) which is thought to stimulate herpes. During any herpes episode it may help to avoid argenine-rich foods.

5. Zinc: take 5 to 60 milligrams daily.

6. Acupuncture administered at the first signs of an attack sometimes prevents recurrences. Fingertip stimulation of acupressure points in the feet may also prevent outbreaks (three thumbs forward of the ankle bulge, along the line between the ankle bulge and little toe). See Resources in Chapter 7 for more about acupressure.

For Symptomatic Relief

1. Make compresses out of tea made with cloves, use Indian tea bags soaked in water (tannic acid is an anaesthetic) or take shallow baths with uva-ursi (also known as kinnikinnick or bearberry).

2. Some people believe that keeping the sores moist makes them feel better but they may also last longer. Suggested salves include: peppermint or clove oil, Vitamin E oil, A and D ointment, baking powder, cornflour or witch hazel.

3. Make poultices using pulverized calcium tablets, powdered slippery elm, goldenseal, myrrh, comfrey root or cold milk. Make a paste using any of these and apply to the sores. After applying, keep the paste moistened with warm water.

4. Aloe vera gel soothes and helps to dry out sores and promote healing.

Herpes and Pregnancy

Studies show that women with a primary attack of herpes have an increased risk of miscarriage and premature delivery. When a mother has active sores at the time of delivery, herpes can be transmitted to the baby during the

birth, causing brain damage, blindness and death in 60 to 70 per cent of cases. The risk is much higher when mothers have a primary outbreak at the time of delivery; when they have open sores, their babies have a 50 per cent chance of contracting herpes during a vaginal birth. For a mother with recurrent sores, the risk goes down to about 4 per cent because she has passed antibodies on to the baby through the amniotic fluid and the baby's blood.[13]

Pregnant women who don't have herpes should avoid unprotected sex with partners who have herpes particularly during the last six weeks. If you are pregnant and have recurrent herpes, a viral culture should be tested regularly from thirty-two weeks of pregnancy to delivery. If you have prodromal symptoms or active sores at the expected time of delivery, you will usually have a caesarean section, although women who have negative cultures within three days of birth can deliver vaginally. After birth, take care not to infect the infant. After about three weeks, babies usually do not develop serious infections.

Herpes and Cancer

Studies have linked genital herpes with a greater risk of contracting cervical cancer. However, more recent studies have settled on papilloma virus (warts) as the virus most likely to be associated with cervical cancer. It is probable that the apparently higher risk for those with herpes is simply an indicator that these people are more likely to have been infected with papilloma as well (see Cervix, p. 530).

Prevention

The development of Skinner's herpes vaccine may provide protection in the future. For the moment our risk of contracting herpes can be cut down by following the suggestions on p. 488 and avoiding genital contact with anyone who has open herpes sores. Since the virus can be spread by skin contact from one part of the body to another it is equally important to avoid oral sex with anyone who has mouth sores. If you do touch a sore, wash your hands carefully. None of this means that you should avoid sex with a herpes sufferer. The chances of contracting the disease in between outbreaks is absolutely minute.

Protecting Others (If You Have Herpes)

1. If you have active sores, you might try to keep towels separate and wear cotton underpants in bed at night, since herpes may be transmitted through shared towels or linen.

2. Do not donate blood during an initial outbreak.

3. Some people recommend avoiding swimming baths, 'hot tubs' (also called jacuzzis) and saunas during an initial outbreak.

Living with Herpes

Accepting herpes as a permanent part of your life may be difficult. You may feel shocked when you discover you have herpes, and then frantically search for a cure. You may feel isolated, lonely and angry, especially towards the person who gave you the infection. You may become anxious about staying in long-term relationships or having

---

*If you are on the Pill, be cautious about taking Vitamin C as well – see p. 294.

children. Not everybody experiences herpes in these ways, nor do these responses necessarily last for ever.

After the first big episode of herpes, I felt distant from my body. When we began love-making again, I had a hard time having orgasms or trusting the rhythm of my responses. I shed some tears over that. I felt my body had been invaded. My body feels riddled with it; I'm somehow contaminated. And there is always that lingering anxiety: is my baby OK? It's unjust that the birth of my child may be affected.

If you are in a close relationship with someone who doesn't have herpes, it can affect you both in subtle ways.

Sometimes it bullies both of us. When my lover feels she has to protect me from stress because I'm about to get herpes, she doesn't always ask for attention, time or comfort when she needs them.

How much herpes affects your relationships can depend a lot on how much you trust each other and how comfortable you feel about sharing your concerns.

My lover really trusts me when I say the episode has passed and it's OK to have oral sex. She doesn't second-guess me and say, 'Let's wait a few days so I won't get it.' What a blessing.

The way we experience herpes may have a lot to do with our attitude about disease. For example, people who see herpes as a symptom of stress, illness or other problems rather than as a medical disaster seem to have a much easier time finding their own ways of coping with it.

Herpes is an inconvenience and a pain, but it's something you learn to live with. I think of it as an imbalance. Since I know it's related to stress, I keep myself in as good physical condition as possible and try not to get too upset about it.

The one good thing I can say about herpes is that it keeps me honest in taking care of myself. When I feel my vulva start to tingle and ache, it's immediately a reminder to me to slow down. I take long, hot baths. I try to think relaxing, releasing thoughts and send healing, calming energy to that area. Sometimes I meditate.

Humour is the best way of coping with herpes. There is so much serious, scary stuff about it. You've got to recognize that it's just one of the bad tricks people have to live with.

Herpes may be easier to cope with if you feel comfortable enough to talk about it openly. Some people manage to talk themselves out of recurrences.

What turns out to be really useful is when my family and I talk about the viruses. We say things like, 'They don't want to come down now. It's much cosier up by the spinal cord where they are. The weather is pretty bad out here and everyone's too busy to pay them much attention.' I think what it probably does is calm me and ease whatever is bothering me. Who knows? Maybe they hear! All I know is that sometimes after I get the warning aches we sit at dinner having those discussions about how my little herpes viruses should stay where they are, and they don't come!

The Herpes Association runs a telephone counselling and advice centre and can give you the name of your local group contact. See Resources for the address.

GENITAL WARTS AND HUMAN PAPILLOMA VIRUS INFECTIONS

Genital warts are caused by the human papilloma virus, or HPV, similar to the type which causes common skin warts. The same virus causes invisible warts or flat lesions on the cervix. HPV usually spreads during sexual intercourse with an infected partner. While HPV-caused infections have not been associated with serious complications in the past, studies now show that women with HPV-caused lesions on the cervix have an increased risk for developing cervical cancer. According to a report in *The Lancet*:

There were no differences in sexual behaviour within the study group between women with cervical disease and those without. Moreover there was no cervical disease in the control women, who were as sexually active as the study group and 40 per cent of whom had other venereal diseases. *This suggests that the presence of penile HPV infection in the partner rather than the woman's sexual behaviour places her at high risk of cervical neoplasia.*[14]

Unfortunately, these invisible cervical lesions are not easily detected by either the health-care practitioner or the woman with the infection. For more information about the relationship between warts and cervical cancer, and how to minimize the risk, see p. 530.

Symptoms

Symptoms of genital warts usually appear from three weeks to three months after exposure. The visible genital warts look like ordinary warts, starting as small, painless, hard spots which usually appear on the bottom of the vaginal opening. Warts also occur on the vaginal lips, inside the vagina, on the cervix or around the anus, where they can be mistaken for haemorrhoids. Warmth and moisture encourage the growth of warts, which often develop a cauliflower-like appearance as they grow larger. Cervical lesions, though more prevalent than the visible warts, cannot be seen by the naked eye and have no symptoms.

GENITAL WARTS

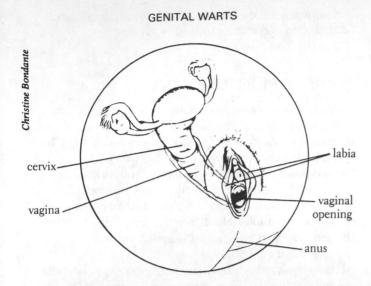

Christine Bondante

cervix

vagina

labia

vaginal opening

anus

In men, warts usually occur towards the tip of the penis, sometimes under the foreskin and occasionally on the shaft of the penis or scrotum. Using a condom can help prevent the spread of warts.

Diagnosis and Treatment

Diagnosis of warts is usually made by direct eye examination. An abnormal cervical smear may indicate the presence of cervical lesions, but a colposcopy (see p. 000) is usually necessary to confirm this. Occasionally you will need a biopsy to check for unusual cell growth, especially if there are ulcerations (open sores) or a discharge, but these are rare.

There are several treatments for warts; all of them should be carried out by a skilled doctor:

1. Laser treatment is now the treatment of choice for cervical lesions because it causes less damage to other tissue than other methods.

2. Clinics often prescribe podophyllin solution (some say ointment is better). It should be very carefully applied to the warts and washed off two to four hours later to avoid chemical burns. The surrounding skin should be protected with petroleum jelly (e.g. Vaseline). Sometimes several treatments are necessary, and they are not always successful.

3. Trichloracetic acid (TCA) is currently used by some doctors but appears to be better than podophyllin in several respects. It is usually equally effective and yet causes fewer problems than podophyllin. The strength of TCA is more easily controlled; it works on first contact with the skin and then stops in about five minutes, reducing the danger of scarring. It does not seem to provoke severe reactions as podophyllin occasionally does. Some doctors use TCA during pregnancy, although no studies have been done to verify its safety at that time.

4. Cryotherapy (dry ice treatment) or acid can freeze or burn off small warts. This hurts briefly and sometimes causes scarring. You may want a local anaesthetic.

5. Surgery or electrocoagulation (using an electric current to destroy tissue) becomes necessary for very large warts

which fail to respond to other treatments. This procedure requires an anaesthetic. If you have a cardiac pacemaker, the electric current may disturb it, so be sure to tell your doctor.

No matter what treatment you get it is important to remove all warts, even those inside the vagina and on the cervix. This may keep the virus from spreading. Sexual partners also should be treated, and it is advisable for men to use condoms.

Genital Warts and Pregnancy

Warts tend to grow larger during pregnancy, possibly because of the increased blood supply to the genitalia. If the warts are located on the vaginal wall and become very large or numerous, the vagina may become less elastic, making delivery difficult. Do *not* use podophyllin to remove warts, as it is absorbed by the skin and is associated with birth defects or fetal death.

HUMAN IMMUNODEFICIENCY VIRUS (HIV) (which can lead to Acquired Immune Deficiency Syndrome: AIDS – see p. 558)

By VICKY WHELAN, CO-ORDINATOR OF MANCHESTER AIDSLINE

HIV is the virus that can lead to AIDS. On p. 558 we discuss how the virus and the syndrome can affect us. Here we discuss how it can be transmitted and what the implications are.

Because HIV is present in body fluids such as semen and blood it makes it more than a sexually transmitted disease (STD), but the response has been to label it a disease of sexuality. In Europe, America and Australia the first group of people to become infected were gay men but there are underlying trends which are now showing an increase among other people whose lifestyle has higher risks of coming into contact with HIV particularly (but not only) among drug users who share needles and syringes and their sexual partners. In Africa HIV infection has always shown itself in men and women equally. The lack of health-care resources to sterilize or replace equipment and unscreened blood in hospitals have helped to spread the virus among the general population.

HIV is difficult to transmit outside certain well-defined activities: it is infectious but *not* contagious. It is not transmitted by droplets in the air, toilet seats, cups, cutlery, money, swimming baths, etcetera. Because it is present in semen it is inevitable that lists of risky sexual activity have been produced. However, these lists have been labelled as 'belonging' to at-risk groups and therefore imply that having sex with people from these groups is always and everywhere risky. This gives a false sense of security particularly to heterosexuals and identifies AIDS as a major crisis which 'belongs' to another group and not to them.

Public discussion about the advantages of gentle sex within open and caring relationships (see Communicating about Sex, p. 246), the use of barrier methods (the condom and spermicidal creams), person-centred counselling and care of those infected would do more to halt the spread of HIV than hysterical press reports and stigmatizing health education campaigns.

An understanding of how the virus is transmitted sexually can give us the information to assess our risk and the confidence to discuss taking the necessary precautions with our sexual partners.

There is a large amount of virus present in the semen of an infected man. In vaginal intercourse semen can be absorbed into vaginal or cervical ulcers, or through tiny tears caused by friction. HIV can also be absorbed through the mucous membrane of the vagina without any tears or ulcers being present. The man using a condom lubricated with a spermicidal cream such as nonoxynol 9 creates a barrier against transmission of the virus via this route.

In anal intercourse there is a risk of tears in the anal wall which would allow direct entry for infected sperm. If the woman is infected tears in her anal wall would expose abrasions on the man's penis to her blood. Damaged piles also pose a high risk of infected blood contact.

Oral sex (penis in mouth or mouth contact with a woman's genitals) would have risk if there were mouth ulcers or sores or bleeding gums. The inside of the mouth is also a mucous membrane like the vagina and this could be a possible route for infected sperm or vaginal secretions to enter. An infected woman's menstrual flow entering mouth ulcers can be a higher risk. Swallowed semen does not seem to be a risk but having stomach ulcers can be a possible route of transmission for infected sperm to enter the bloodstream.

HIV infection and AIDS pose many challenges for women: as sexual beings, mothers and carers. As women we have the unique opportunity to look behind the cold facts at the feelings and emotions this issue brings to us by looking at our sexuality and what we find erotic, how we educate our children and how we set boundaries for ourselves in our caring and giving roles as women. For more discussion, see Part II: Relationships and Sexuality.

AIDS groups and helplines can be contacted right across the UK. The National AIDS Helpline can put you in touch with a local group (see Resources).

HEPATITIS B

Like HIV, Hepatitis B is usually transmitted through blood and semen. However, it is very much more contagious, as it can also be transferred through saliva.

Though most sufferers do survive, there is no effective treatment for the disease, which can last for months, sometimes causing irreversible liver damage. Silent carriers (as well as obvious sufferers) can pass on the disease to others and, during pregnancy, to their babies. Medical personnel are at risk through routine contact. However, a vaccine has been developed which, given immediately after birth, can dramatically reduce the risk to babies and could protect high-risk groups and halt the spread of the disease.

Unfortunately, it is expensive and the government has so far refused to organize a vaccination campaign.

CRABS OR PUBIC LICE

Phthirus pubis is a roundish, crab-like body louse that lives in pubic hair and occasionally in the hair of the chest, armpits, eyelashes and eyebrows. You can 'catch' them by intimate physical contact with someone who has them. As they are passed on from person to person you are unlikely to pick them up from towels or clothes. They are bloodsuckers and can carry such diseases as typhus. The main symptom of crabs is an intolerable itching in the genital or other affected area; they are easily diagnosed because they are visible without a microscope.

Though it may be difficult, try not to scratch. Scratching can transfer lice to uninfected parts of the body. Excessive scratching around the urinary opening can even lead to urinary tract infections.

Orthodox Treatment

Derbac liquid (rather than shampoo) is the preferred treatment as it is less toxic than either lorrexane or quellada which we mentioned in the last edition of this book. These preparations both contain gamma benzene hexachloride which penetrates the skin and is stored in body fat. This is particularly dangerous for pregnant or breastfeeding mothers or small children. Derbac is based on malathion, which, although it is also toxic, is less likely to penetrate the skin and is more quickly dispersed. Do not use any of these drugs in or around your eyes. If you have crabs in your eyebrows use an ophthalmic petroleum jelly.

Alternatively, you can try a very hot sauna, a treatment routinely used in Scandinavia. Either way, it's important that all intimate contacts, including lovers, family members and friends, be treated as well.

Crabs die within twenty-five hours of separation from the human body though the eggs live up to six days. So it may be sensible to wash bedclothes etcetera, although re-contagion is most unlikely if close contacts are also treated.

The itch may persist for some time after treatment, especially if your skin is very irritated from scratching. Soothing skin preparations, such as aloe vera, can ease the symptoms and help your skin to heal faster.

The first time I got crabs I felt embarrassed and humiliated. I'd gone to visit my boyfriend at college and when I came home I began to itch. I couldn't believe that he would give me something like that – especially since I'd mistakenly associated crabs with people who didn't wash enough. I didn't know what to do so I just ignored them as long as possible. When the itching became really intolerable I went to a clinic. Once I learned how crabs are transmitted and that they are both very common and easy to cure, I felt a lot better. The next time I went to visit my boyfriend I took a bottle of Derbac with me. Turns out he hadn't known what to do either!

Self-help

Use essence of lavender oil (from a chemist or health food shop), mix it with a vegetable oil and rub it into the pubic area. Be careful to avoid vulval tissue. As recommended in Billie Potts's *Witches Heal: Lesbian Herbal Self-sufficiency* (see Resources). We know from personal experience that it works like magic with nits (head lice) – better than any of the manufactured toxic chemicals. Crabs are basically the same organism, and orthodox medicine uses the same chemicals to get rid of them.

SCABIES

Scabies are tiny parasitic mites that burrow under the superficial layers of the skin, depositing eggs and faeces and causing intense irritation. Symptoms usually include intense itching (often worse at night) and red, raised bumps or ridges on the skin, which may be found on the hands (especially between the fingers), on or under the breasts, or around the waist or wrists, genitals or buttocks. Scratching the area can break the skin, causing secondary bacterial infections.

According to a report in 1942 by Kenneth Mellanby, 'clothing and bedding play a negligible part if any in the transmission of scabies'. It is usually passed on through close skin contact. If you've never had scabies, it may take a month or more for the skin reaction to develop. During this time you can pass it to someone else without knowing you have it. Once you've had scabies, however, your skin will react much more quickly, often within a day after reinfestation.

Diagnosing scabies can be tricky because it is easily confused with eczema, allergies and other skin conditions. Sometimes physicians will prescribe medication for scabies before they know what you really have. Because these medications can cause allergic reactions, do not apply them until you have a definite diagnosis (made by examining a small scraping of the irritated area under a microscope).

Treatment

The most effective treatment is quellada but, as mentioned above, it should not be used if you are pregnant or breastfeeding, or on small children. Eurax is an alternative treatment for pregnant women but it needs three or four applications. It is no longer marketed for scabies but is still available, without prescription. You could try a sulphur treatment which is considered less toxic although it can cause dermatitis and it smells like rotten eggs. (The recommended mixture is 6 per cent sulphur, 3 per cent balsam of Peru and the rest petroleum jelly.)

You must treat your whole body because the rash does not necessarily appear at the site of infestation, and make sure anyone else with whom you have had intimate contact is treated too. You may want also to wash bedclothes in very hot water to avoid the risk (however small) of reinfestation.

Even after treatment, you may continue to itch for several days or weeks. This doesn't mean you still have scabies; more likely your skin is still hypersensitive and needs some time for the irritation to die down. A soothing lotion (containing calamine or aloe vera) will ease the symptoms. If the itching is really intolerable, an antihistamine may help.

PELVIC INFLAMMATORY DISEASE (PID)

Prepared by THE PID SUPPORT GROUP

Pelvic inflammatory disease is a general term for a group of related infections that affect the fallopian tubes (salpingitis), ovaries (oophoritis), both tubes and ovaries (salpingo-oophoritis) and/or uterus (endometritis). The term PID does not indicate which of the pelvic organs is primarily

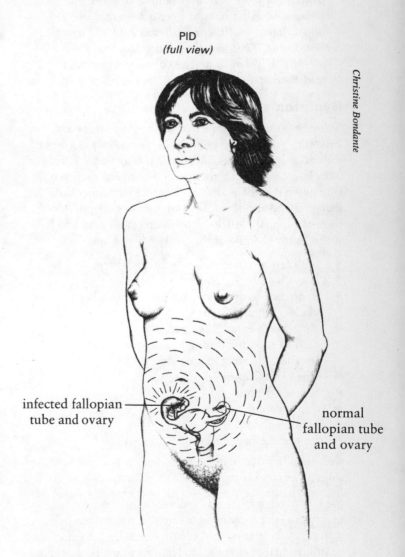

PID
(full view)

Christine Bondante

infected fallopian tube and ovary

normal fallopian tube and ovary

PID can cause a sharp pain at the most infected site and/or can cause pain throughout all or part of the abdomen.

affected, but it is most common for the infection to localize in the tubes. The numbers of women suffering are climbing steadily every year.[15]

Not all women will experience it in the same way – symptoms vary, as do the causes, duration and effect of the infection. Essentially there are four classifications of PID. *Acute* PID means a severe infection often indicated by considerable abdominal pain and a high temperature. A lower level of infection is referred to as *sub-acute* – perhaps with less dramatic pain and no temperature. Sub-acute and acute PID can become acute or *chronic* without proper treatment. With chronic PID a low-grade infection may rumble on in the pelvic organs for years and never seem to clear up. Other sufferers get *recurrent* PID, where flare-ups of infection are interspersed with periods of good health.

I kept going back to my doctor with this abdominal pain and dragging backache. He kept saying nothing was wrong, but eventually prescribed antibiotics in case I had an infected fallopian tube. He didn't take any tests or anything. My periods got more and more painful and sex was impossible. After months I got a hospital appointment and they said it was PID. I'd never heard of it. That was three years ago, and I still get attacks. They've never told me what causes it, and they won't seem to admit they can't cure it.

Symptoms

Symptoms may be so mild that you hardly notice them. For instance, you may be aware of an occasional or constant dull ache in the lower abdomen. It may occur during or after intercourse or increase with movement such as walking. Often it is felt on only one side. On the other hand the pain may be strong enough for you to collapse into the nearest hospital casualty department. You may also have some, most or none of these other symptoms:

- high temperature and/or feeling 'shivery';
- lower back or leg pain;
- frequency of urination, burning or inability to empty bladder when urinating;
- abnormal vaginal discharge;
- pain or bleeding during or after intercourse;
- irregular bleeding or spotting;
- nausea and dizziness;
- fatigue, depression;
- more painful periods;
- swollen abdomen;
- general feeling of illness;
- weight loss or gain.

Causes

PID can be caused by a number of different micro-organisms which make their way past the natural defence system of the vagina and uterus to establish themselves, usually in a fallopian tube, and multiply rapidly. The cause is often a mystery – but in many cases the beginnings of infection can be traced to use of an IUD, abortion, childbirth, miscarriage, or gynaecological procedures involving dilatation of the cervix.

Some experts in genito-urinary medicine say most PID is sexually transmitted, but although STD-linked PID is certainly a growing problem, some women's health groups do not find this emphasis accurate or useful. IUDs are, for example, a major culprit in introducing infection into the uterus. Often women with IUD-related PID are told that their infection is the result of sexually transmitted disease, even though research shows that IUD users run at least double the risk of PID-induced infertility.[16]

Several different micro-organisms can cause PID including the sexually transmitted bacteria that cause gonorrhoea (see p. 492); chlamydia (see p. 493); and other bacteria, including some normally found in the vagina or in the gut.

Effects

PID is a serious disease. If untreated, it can lead to peritonitis, a life-threatening condition. If not treated properly, or treated too late, it can cause chronic pain from lingering infection or adhesions – scar tissue binding the internal organs together. Repeated bouts of infection can permanently damage fallopian tubes, sometimes leading to ectopic pregnancy (see p. 439) or infertility. The disease can drag on for years,[17] flaring up sporadically and draining vitality. With chronic PID, life is a permanent battle against pain and fatigue. The psychological and emotional costs can be devastating. Sex becomes very difficult and relationships can founder.

I seem to be tired all the time. I lost my job because I'd taken so much time off. My boyfriend tries to understand but it's very hard for him when sex obviously causes me so much pain. I keep shouting at my little boy because I'm tired and irritable, and I'm sure my friends think I'm a real drag, moaning all the time. What can I do?

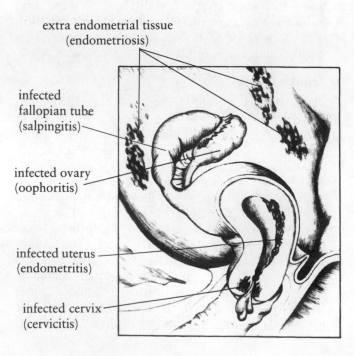

extra endometrial tissue
(endometriosis)

infected
fallopian tube
(salpingitis)

infected ovary
(oophoritis)

infected uterus
(endometritis)

infected cervix
(cervicitis)

It is impossible to measure the incidence of PID in Britain, because figures are kept only of hospital admissions which, at 12,000 per year, represents just the tip of the iceberg. Pelvic infections seem to be increasing as women's sexual activity increases. Yet despite the scale of the disease and its potentially disastrous consequences, PID is largely hidden from view. Most women will never have heard of PID before they fall victim to it, and they soon discover that most GPs are pretty vague about it too.

Diagnosis

The key to treating a first attack of PID is early and accurate diagnosis and identification of the infecting organism, so that you get the correct antibiotic straight away. Diagnosis is difficult because PID symptoms are similar to those of other conditions; for example, endometriosis (see p. 515), pelvic pain syndrome and spastic colon. The best place for correct diagnosis is a genito-urinary clinic (see p. 489). Genito-urinary clinics take infections more seriously and will automatically take swabs. They will also have a wider range of tests available and you will probably get quicker and more accurate results. Many GPs and gynaecologists either misdiagnose or dismiss symptoms; or they may correctly diagnose but fail to appreciate PID's seriousness. They may take swabs from the cervix and vagina, as they should, and then the laboratory may not test for all possible infecting organisms. Tests for chlamydia in particular are expensive, difficult and not even available in all GU clinics (see p. 493). A negative test result leads some doctors to conclude that infection is not present – even though organisms affecting the tubes and uterus often do not show up in a cervical culture.

So, you may not be treated, you may not get the right antibiotics, or you may not get them before the infection becomes established in pockets in the tubes where the poor blood supply cannot bring the antibiotics to bear.

If you think you may have PID don't delay in getting to a doctor. Your sex partner(s) should also be checked in case they are harbouring PID-causing bacteria, perhaps without symptoms. This is important because otherwise you may get reinfected. You may need more than one kind or course of antibiotic to get rid of the infection. Some women's PID is caused by more than one organism. You should expect: an internal bimanual examination (see p. 593) (pain and swelling indicate possible PID); a speculum examination (which may show pus coming out of the cervix); a high vaginal swab taken from the cervix for culture in the lab (some doctors take the swab from too low down and so minimize the chances of a result). This must be done *straight away* at the start of an attack before the bacteria travel up through the uterus and tubes where they can't be detected.

Orthodox Treatment

If PID is diagnosed, a broad spectrum *antibiotic* should be prescribed without delay. Once the results of the culture are known you may have to transfer to a different antibiotic, i.e. one effective against the particular infecting organism.

The good news is that pelvic infections treated early enough with the correct antibiotic stand a very good chance of being cleared up, never to recur. Commonly prescribed antibiotics are tetracyclines, erythromycin and metronidazole (Flagyl). The latter is usually prescribed as a matter of course because it is particularly effective against the pockets of anaerobic bacteria which often invade during PID. This drug may cause nausea and should never be combined with alcohol. See p. 491 for a discussion of Flagyl. Ampicillin is not active against chlamydia, which is a major cause of PID.

Antibiotics, given orally or intravenously, don't always cure chronic PID even if you get the right one, possibly because of reinfection by an untreated partner, or due to a pelvic abscess, septic thrombophlebitis or an incorrect diagnosis. Some women experience repeated bouts of infection and end up taking quantities of different antibiotics over several years. Many such women have given up taking these drugs and have found other ways of coping with PID attacks (see below). Some feel antibiotics make matters worse, and bring additional problems with side-effects, e.g. depression, nausea, diarrhoea, thrush (see p. 490). Certainly, if you have taken many courses to no effect, you might ask whether it is worth taking yet more.

After two and a half years on and off antibiotics, with three hospitalizations and two operations, coming off the antibiotics was the turning point for me. It got worse to start with but I had support from alternative practitioners. I've only taken antibiotics once in the past three years. I'm 90 per cent better than before.

According to the US Centers for Disease Control, *hospitalization* should be strongly considered when

1. the diagnosis is uncertain;
2. surgical emergencies such as appendicitis and ectopic pregnancy must be excluded;
3. a pelvic abscess is suspected;
4. severe illness precludes outpatient management;
5. the woman is pregnant;
6. the woman is unable to follow or tolerate an outpatient regimen;
7. the woman has failed to respond to outpatient therapy;
8. clinic follow-up after forty-eight to seventy-two hours following the start of antibiotic treatment cannot be arranged.

Many experts recommend that *all* women with PID be hospitalized for treatment.[18] You are more likely to be hospitalized for an acute attack or for fertility testing. But, increasingly, chronic cases are also being hospitalized.

In the hospital you can get intravenous (IV) antibiotics which may provide a sufficient concentration of medication in your body to fight the infection.

Whether you are hospitalized or not you must *rest*. This is essential. Don't feel guilty about lying around. It is better to take off a few days from your work/family early on than to risk becoming a chronically ill person later. Some doctors underestimate the need to rest but the PID support group believe it to be of crucial importance in combating this illness. Complete bed rest helps keep the infection from spreading and allows your body time to heal. Continue to rest until you feel completely better. Try to get friends to cook for you – good nutrition is very important. Avoid penetrative intercourse – it can spread the infection. If you feel up to it, orgasm produced other ways may be beneficial because it increases the blood flow. Hot water bottles may ease the pain, and heat applied to the pelvic area may help fight infection by increasing the blood flow.

If you can't get a diagnosis, or if antibiotics don't get rid of your symptoms, you could ask to be referred to hospital for a *laparoscopy* (see p. 596). Laparoscopy is sometimes inconclusive, and can stir up the infection if it is active when the operation is performed. However, it may show whether PID is causing the symptoms and may induce doctors to take you more seriously. Ask whether samples can be taken from the tubes during the operation, so that infecting organisms can be identified in the laboratory. Sometimes doctors seem to neglect this perfect opportunity for taking cultures which may pinpoint the causative organism.

Unfortunately, if you get chronic or recurrent PID there's not much that doctors can offer beyond *surgery* to remove diseased tissue. Before resorting to surgery, it is worth investigating whether the symptoms are being caused by infection (some doctors suggest that stress-related conditions like irritable bowel syndrome can develop, which may explain why pain sometimes persists even after surgery).

Sometimes having one tube removed will clear up the infection. Sometimes surgical separation of adhesions will ease the pain. Some women have more than one 'partial' operation, losing one or both tubes and perhaps an ovary. (Removing both ovaries is a drastic step, as it brings on premature menopause.) Some desperate women resort to complete hysterectomy, and even this in some cases does not wipe out symptoms completely, although it usually does at least reduce the discomfort experienced. Some women who have had PID for years say that partial surgery is worth the risk – you might be perfectly well after, say, an infected tube is removed. Doctors are usually reluctant to destroy fertility, particularly in childless women. But some women wish they had gone for more drastic surgery initially and so avoided repeated operations.

> *After many years with PID you get beyond the stage of wanting to be fertile. You just want to be well.*

You might be offered *pelvic diathermy* or heat treatment – this sometimes helps, but most doctors seem to agree with many PID sufferers that it makes things worse.

Women with PID may occasionally be offered *pre-sacral neurectomy*, the removal of the pre-sacral nerve which carries the 'pain messages' from the pelvis to the brain. British doctors are sceptical of its effectiveness although some reports suggest that it is 75 per cent successful in the elimination of pain.[19] It is a very drastic and complex operation and there can be side-effects, usually temporary, involving loss of control of the bowel and bladder. Its effects on sexual sensations are not known.

Coping with PID

Encounters with doctors often increase our distress and depression. Many GPs and gynaecologists don't take PID seriously, tell you there's nothing wrong with you, or say you'll just have to live with it. It is common for sceptical junior hospital doctors to prescribe tranquillizers, or for patronizing senior gynaecologists to promise miracles through surgery. Many a demoralized woman has dragged herself out of a clinic, almost beginning to share the doctor's conviction that she is imagining her pain. Other women experience aggressive questions about their sex lives. On top of this, you may be made to feel guilty, as if it's your fault that you can't manage to get better.

> *The pains have been variously diagnosed as being due to constipation, a grumbling appendix, a backwards tilting womb, an infection, a spastic colon, fibroids, ovarian cyst and something that would be cured by either going on the Pill or having a baby. They finally decided it was PID and took out one of my fallopian tubes. Four years later I still get the pains and feel ill. Last week the gynaecologist suggested I see a psychiatrist.*

This medical attitude is reflected in one of the standard postgraduate gynaecology textbooks which tells future consultants that 'management of the chronic pelvic woman represents one of the most trying and all too often unrewarding problems for the gynaecologist . . .' and 'patients with this condition are the cross that every gynaecologist has to bear'. This is what we are up against. Also, despite a fair amount of research into STD-related PID, chronic PID receives little attention.

Prevention and Self-help

For first attacks try to insist on correct treatment, as described above. For recurrent or chronic PID, many women have found ways of 'coping' with repeated symptoms. These include plenty of rest, no vaginal penetration, good food, vitamin and mineral supplements, avoiding stress as much as possible, cutting out cigarettes, alcohol and coffee. Very often acupuncture and homoeopathic remedies help control pain and heal the body. Some women get relief through herbal and other alternative medicines. (See Chapter 7 for a discussion of alternative healing including yoga which some women find helpful, and Chapter 4 for Get Well Diets.) For many chronic sufferers sunshine works like magic – lying on a hot beach for a few days is not always possible, but it often does the trick.

Sometimes you can prevent repeated PID attacks by avoiding the things that seem to cause flare-ups – e.g.

PID SUPPORT GROUP

The PID Support Group was formed in 1982 by two chronic sufferers who decided to establish a support network to cut through some of the isolation and anxiety felt by individuals who have this illness.

> We wanted to intercede in the process whereby women who are ill become further undermined by doubting doctors and confused boyfriends/husbands and begin to question their own value or even their own sanity. You would not believe the number of letters we get which begin – 'Am I going mad?'

The group also tries to keep up with research in the PID area and reports on it in its newsletters; it aims to put people in various parts of the country in touch with sister sufferers in their locality; to question and pressurize the medical profession; and generally to bring the issue more to the fore of public and medical consciousness.

Most of the group's work is now carried on by the Women's Health and Reproductive Rights Information Centre; see Resources for address.

---

inadequate sleep, poor diet, stress, over-exertion. If you have never had PID you can reduce your chances of getting it. Here are some precautions.

1. Watch out for signs of infection after abortions, IUD insertion, gynaecological operations, miscarriages and childbirth.

2. Prevent sexually transmitted diseases by following suggestions on p. 488. Get regular checks for STDs if you or your partner have sex with anyone else.

3. Remember that women who use IUDs have a dramatically increased chance of getting PID. Barrier methods of contraception provide some protection.

4. To prevent bacteria getting into the vagina from the rectum always wipe from front to back; never follow anal intercourse with vaginal intercourse.

5. Treat all vaginal infections promptly (see p. 488).

6. Do what you can to stay generally healthy (see Part I) – poor diet and physical and mental stress weaken the body's natural defences to disease.

> *After six years I've learned to live with it. I've abandoned late-night parties, I try to eat wholesome food, and I wouldn't dream of casual sex. It may not sound like fun, but it's better than illness and pain. If I do get an attack, I take to my bed with a hot water bottle, vitamin pills and fruit juice. I'm lucky my employer understands and that I don't have kids – some women are a lot worse off. I'm very angry that the medical world is not interested in women like us.*

URINARY TRACT INFECTIONS (UTIs)

Urinary tract infections are so common that most of us get at least one at some point in our lives. They are usually caused by bacteria, such as Escherichia coli (*E. coli*), which travel from the colon to the urethra and bladder (and

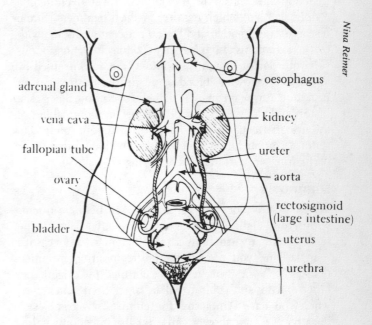

occasionally to the kidneys). Trichomoniasis and chlamydia can also cause UTIs; low resistance, poor diet, stress and damage to the urethra from childbirth, surgery, catheterization, etc., can predispose you to getting them. Often a sudden increase in sexual activity triggers symptoms ('honeymoon cystitis'). Pregnant women are especially susceptible (pressure of the growing fetus keeps some urine in the bladder and ureters, allowing bacteria to grow), as are post-menopausal women (because of hormonal changes). Very occasionally, UTI is caused by an anatomical abnormality or a prolapsed (fallen) urethra or bladder, most common in older women or women who have had many children.

Cystitis (inflammation or infection of the bladder) is by far the most common UTI in women. While the symptoms can be frightening, cystitis in itself is not usually serious. If you suddenly have to urinate every few minutes and it burns like crazy even though almost nothing comes out, you probably have cystitis. There may also be blood in the urine (haematuria) and pus in the urine (pyuria). You may have pain just above your pubic bone, and sometimes there is a peculiar, heavy urine odour when you first urinate in the morning.

It is also possible to get mild temporary symptoms (such as urinary frequency) without actually having an infection, simply because of drinking too much coffee or tea (which are diuretics), premenstrual syndrome, food allergies, anxiety or irritation to the area from bubble baths, soaps or douches or even cold weather. As long as you are in good health and not pregnant, you can usually treat mild symptoms yourself for forty-eight hours before consulting a doctor.* Cystitis often disappears without treatment. If it persists for more than forty-eight hours, recurs frequently or is ever accompanied by chills, fever, vomiting or pain in the kidneys, consult a doctor. These symptoms suggest that infection has spread to the kidneys (pyelonephritis), a serious problem which requires medical treatment. Some researchers estimate that 30 to 50 per cent of women with cystitis symptoms also have 'silent' kidney infections. Consult your doctor if cystitis symptoms are accompanied by any of the following: blood or pus in the urine, pain on urination during pregnancy, diabetes or chronic illnesses, a history of kidney infection or diseases or abnormalities of the urinary tract. Untreated chronic infections can lead to serious complications, such as high blood pressure or premature births (if they occur during pregnancy).

Diagnosis

When cystitis does not respond to self-help treatments within forty-eight hours or recurs frequently, have a urine test. An ordinary urinalysis is not sufficient to test for cystitis – make sure you provide a midstream urine specimen (MSU).** Your urine will be examined for evidence of blood and pus and a culture will be taken. Sometimes, even when you have symptoms, the culture may come back negative (i.e. not show a cause for the infection). False-negative cultures may be due to mishandling or overly dilute urine; you may also get a false negative if your cystitis is caused by something other than bacterial infection (some bladders are easily irritated). On the other hand, a negative culture accompanied by white cells in the urine (called 'acute urethral syndrome') may indicate a chlamydial infection (see p. 493). Sometimes women have bacteria in their urine (bacteriuria) without symptoms. If bacteriuria shows up during a routine urine test, you should be treated to prevent kidney infection and other complications.

A sensitivity test, which shows what kind of antibiotics to use, is usually not necessary unless you have had many infections or severe symptoms indicating pyelonephritis. Women who have had pyelonephritis repeatedly may be tested for abnormalities of the urinary tract. The usual test is an IVP (intravenous pyelogram) in which a dye injected

into the bloodstream collects in the kidneys, showing any blockages or obstructions on an X-ray.

Orthodox Treatments

For symptoms which are severe or indicate a kidney infection, medications are usually started immediately. For milder infections, many practitioners prefer to wait for culture results before prescribing a drug.

Most urinary tract infections respond rapidly to a variety of antibiotics such as ampicillin, nitrofurantoin, tetracycline or sulphonamides (Gantrisin). (Women who may be G6PD-deficient should not take sulphonamides; see p. 558.) The medication may be given in a single large dose or may be spread out over ten to fourteen days. If symptoms persist for more than two days after you start taking drugs, see your practitioner again.

Antibiotics often cause diarrhoea and vaginal yeast infections. Eating plain yoghurt or taking acidophilus in capsule, liquid or granule form helps to prevent this diarrhoea by replacing the normal bacteria in your intestines killed by the drugs. See p. 485 for information on preventing and relieving vaginal infections.

Have a follow-up urine examination when you finish taking the drugs (a culture if you have repeated UTIs) to be certain the organism is gone. If attacks recur the self-help preventive regime explained above and by Angela Kilmartin (p. 533) may well bring the problem under control. Try this before agreeing to any operations. If preventive action does not help, you may wish to discuss more drastic procedures with your doctor. However, none of them is guaranteed to succeed.

Sometimes chronic cystitis will involve the Skene's glands (at the opening of the urethra). In such cases you may think you are cured, then the glands are squeezed (as in intercourse, for example) and release some pus, which starts the cystitis symptoms all over again. Sometimes the Skene's glands are removed (meatotomy) to solve this problem, though specialists disagree about the need for this operation. Recovery takes about a month.

Your doctor may recommend other surgical procedures, such as stretching the urethral opening and/or making a slit in the urethra to help drainage (internal urethrotomy). Ask for documentation of their effectiveness. Surgery is often recommended to correct a prolapsed bladder or urethra, which can be connected with chronic urinary tract infections. Pelvic floor exercises (see p. 347) can avoid the need for this surgery and help prevent future infections.

Treating an Attack*

Many attacks of cystitis can be nipped in the bud by prompt self-help action. Wherever you are, night or day, if you feel an attack threatening try to follow this routine.

1. Take a small urine sample in case you need further medical attention.
2. Drink a glass of cold water immediately.

---

*See the box on p. 509, and *Cystitis: A Complete Self-help Guide*, by Angela Kilmartin (listed in Resources).

**Wash the area carefully, urinate a little, then collect the rest of your urine in a sterile jar.

*Adapted from Angela Kilmartin's *Understanding Cystitis*.

PREVENTING URINARY TRACT INFECTIONS

1. Drink a glass of water every two to three hours to keep up a continuous stream of urine.

2. Urinate frequently; never try to hold on when your bladder feels full; always urinate before *and after* sex.

3. Keep the bacteria in your bowels away from your urethra by wiping from front to back. Keep an empty 'squeezy' bottle and pour a stream of plain warm water over your perineum after a bowel motion.

4. During sex, avoid anything that puts pressure on your urethra, such as prolonged clitoral stimulation or rear entry intercourse. Make sure that you are well lubricated and, if necessary, use a water-soluble lubricant. Anything which irritates the vagina can put pressure on the urethra next door. Make sure that your hands and genitals and those of your partner are clean and avoid activity which could drag bacteria from your anus into your vagina.

5. A very low dose of antibiotics (sulpha, ampicillin, etc.) taken as a preventive measure immediately after sex can break the cycle of reinfection. (This is less harmful to your system than prolonged courses of antibiotics.)

6. Some methods of birth control contribute to or aggravate attacks. Some women find that diaphragms press against the urethra and that certain brands of spermicide cause irritation. A different size or different rim may help and alternative brands of spermicide may not give trouble. Dry condoms may also put pressure on the urethra, while lubricants and dyes may cause irritation.

7. Sanitary protection can be an aggravating factor: tampons can put pressure on the urethra and are best avoided. Pads should be changed frequently (and the vulva washed twice a day).

8. Tight jeans, bicycling or horse riding can all cause trauma to the urethra. Avoid the jeans and ensure that you drink enough to urinate frequently while engaging in sports which put pressure on this area.

9. Caffeine, alcohol and spices may all irritate the bladder and are best avoided as far as possible. Occasional alcohol drunk in association with plenty of non-alcoholic liquid may be all right.

10. Diets high in refined carbohydrates and sugar can also predispose you to infections.

11. Some women drink Vitamin C (500 milligrams four times a day) to acidify their system and prevent bacterial growth in the urine. (However, if you are on the Pill, see p. 294.) Others prefer to make their urine alkaline by taking a teaspoonful of bicarbonate of soda (in water or lemon squash) in the evening.

12. Herbal remedies including teas of uva-ursi, horsetail or shavegrass, cornsilk, cleavers, comfrey, lemon balm or goldenseal have been used (see Herbalism, p. 90).

13. Vitamin B6 and magnesium-calcium supplements are said to be helpful to women who have had their urethras dilated frequently.

14. Keep yourself as healthy as possible and get enough rest (see Get Well Diets, p. 52, and all of Part I).

---

3. Drink a quarter of a glass of orange squash mixed with one teaspoon of bicarbonate of soda every hour for three hours (this should be omitted if you have a heart condition). Drink another half pint of bland liquid every twenty minutes.

4. Take a mild pain-killer.

5. If you are at home fill two hot water bottles. Well wrapped, you can place one between your legs and the other in the small of your back while you continue the routine.

6. Pass urine frequently and wash the perineum each time. Dab yourself dry gently.

UTERUS AND OVARIES

MENSTRUAL PROBLEMS

Menstruation is a normal, healthy occurrence for many years of a woman's life. Yet many women, in very different cultures, experience menstrual problems which range from mild discomfort to acute pain. For those of us who have these problems either occasionally or regularly, it is important to recognize that they exist and to deal with them – arranging schedules so we can get more rest if we need it at that time, planning critical meetings for a time when we are not premenstrual, and so on.

Menstrual problems may well not be inevitable. We simply do not know enough about the interactions of our physical and emotional health and of our external environment (physical and social) and our internal environment (including cyclically changing body chemicals and heredity) to know why some have problems and others don't. We also don't know enough to understand why certain remedies work for some and not for others.

Standard medical views have not been helpful for women. In the past, doctors have attributed cramps and other problems to a variety of physical and psychological causes. Medical remedies sometimes still include general pain-killers (when other medication works better), hormones (sometimes in the form of birth control pills), tranquillizers, a 'pat on the head', a hysterectomy or a recommendation to see a psychiatrist. Many doctors do not respect our self-knowledge. Researchers are finally working to understand the reasons for menstrual problems, but there is still much more to learn.

Women's menstrual problems started to receive more serious attention after 1969 when Dr Katharina Dalton wrote a popular book theorizing about their causes. It was the first book which took women's complaints seriously, a big step forward. However, she still describes women stereotypically as not particularly competent, out of control and ruled by hormonal fluctuations. Unfortunately, many people (including feminists) accepted her book before reading it critically.

Dalton divided women's menstrual problems into two sharply defined categories: *spasmodic*, which roughly corresponds to dysmenorrhoea (see below), and *congestive*, which includes bloating, irritability, depression and various aches. Further research has revealed that many women don't fit neatly into one or the other of the categories.[20] Though women *do* report different types of cramping and specific constellations of symptoms, their experiences vary widely.

Premenstrual Syndrome (PMS)

Despite many shortcomings in her work, Dalton has helpfully identified and popularized PMS, the recurrence of particular symptoms around the menstrual period. PMS symptoms usually include irritability, depression and bloating but actually can include anything. They most commonly start when a woman is in her twenties or early thirties.[21] The latest medical trend for treating PMS is natural progesterone, sometimes used for years. However, the theoretical basis of this treatment is unproven. There have been few controlled studies to test whether progesterone actually works better than a placebo or another remedy. Some studies show that placebos or other treatments dramatically eliminate symptoms for some women.[22] Effects of long-term progesterone use are not known; the few animal studies done indicate problems. Many women find more relief from dietary changes and dietary supplements. Evening primrose oil (an essential fatty acid, see p. 46) and Vitamin B6 (pyridoxine) have both proved useful in trials.[23] As they can be obtained without prescription we describe treatment under Self-help (below). Evening primrose oil is unfortunately expensive and it is not obtainable on NHS prescription. However, improving our intake of essential fatty acids (see p. 46) may help. For more information, see *The PMT Solution* by Anne Nazaro et al. (listed in Resources).

Dysmenorrhoea (Painful Periods)

You can do something about dysmenorrhoea, the sometimes incapacitating cramping during your period. A particular constellation of symptoms, including cramping and often nausea and diarrhoea, may be caused by an excess of a certain type of prostaglandin found in the uterus and perhaps 'leaking' into the intestines. (Prostaglandins are substances found throughout the body, one of which causes contractions of the uterine and intestinal muscles.) With too much prostaglandin, the usually painless rhythmic contractions of the uterus during menstruation become longer and tighter at the tightening phase, keeping oxygen from the muscles. It is this lack of oxygen which we perceive as pain. But we don't know why some women have more prostaglandins in their uterus than others. Since the uterus is a muscle, relaxation exercises help, as do massage and sometimes biofeedback techniques. Anticipation often worsens the pain by making us tense up. Anti-prostaglandins, such as aspirin or mefanemic acid, help some women. In severe cases, you must take the drug before cramping begins; still, it may only lessen the pain. Some women find some of these drugs easier to tolerate than others. The most frequent complaint is upset stomach, which is often avoided by taking the drug with milk or other food. A few women have found that one drug ceases to be effective, and they must try another.[24] Anti-prostaglandins also reduce the amount of flow and shorten the period. We don't yet know how safe these drugs are for long-term, intermittent use, although they seem *relatively* safe so far.

Today, as doctors are beginning to find some physical basis for menstrual distresses, they are prescribing drugs that treat the particular problems. We must understand that the doctors, diagnosing on the basis of symptoms, are *only treating symptoms* and do not know the underlying causes.

Endometriosis and PID also cause menstrual problems, especially cramping, so persistent and, particularly, increasing pain must be properly investigated. Both these conditions are potentially fertility-threatening and can cause severe, long-term problems. They should be identified and treated (see pp. 515 and 503).

Amenorrhoea

Another menstrual problem is amenorrhoea (absence of menstrual periods). Primary amenorrhoea is the condition of never having had a period by the time menstruation usually starts; secondary amenorrhoea is the cessation of menstruation after at least one period. Some causes are pregnancy; menopause; breastfeeding; too little body fat; dieting; starvation; heavy athletic training, especially during early adolescence; previous use of birth control pills; use of some drugs; a congenital defect of the genital tract; hormone imbalance; cysts or tumours; disease; chromosomal abnormalities; stress or emotional factors. Medical textbooks and practitioners pay considerably more attention to amenorrhoea than to PMS or painful periods, although these are far more common.

Weight loss of 10 to 15 per cent below a healthy minimum can stop your periods; a return to *your* minimum weight will correct this. If you've taken the birth control pill, try supplements of B6, folic acid and Vitamin E, and decrease the amount of protein you eat. Severe anaemia can stop menstruation temporarily. For menopausal symptoms, see Chapter 22.

Self-help for All Menstrual Problems

Women have been sharing menstrual remedies for centuries. Some of us have gained new respect for our own knowledge after trying traditional remedies and exploring new ones. Listed here are only those most frequently reported to work. Try one or more of the following suggestions and, *since each woman is unique and has different reactions, pay attention to how the remedy you choose affects you.*

Food. Make sure the food you eat is varied, sufficient and balanced. You can be malnourished and not be underweight. Pay attention to the positive and negative effects of what you eat. Many women find it helps to eat *more* whole grains and whole flours, beans, vegetables, fruits and brewer's yeast and *less* or *no* salt, sugar, alcohol and caffeine (in coffee, tea, chocolate and soft drinks). Some of us avoid salt, white flour and caffeine for at least the week before our periods and find that it helps. (See Chapter 4.) Also, you may need to eat small, frequent meals or snacks rather than two or three bigger meals because your blood sugar level may drop in the day or two before your period, making you feel extra irritable. This is why dieting at this time makes you feel so much worse.

Food rich in linolenic acid (see Chapter 4, p. 46), such as safflower and sunflower oil, may be helpful as LA is a precursor of gammalinolenic acid (GLA), the active ingredient in evening primrose oil. Use pure oil, not margarine.

Sleep. Get the right amount for *you.* Your rhythms may change during your cycle. Allow time for extra sleep if you need it.

Exercise. See Chapter 6 and Maddux's *Menstruation* or Erna Wright's *Periods without Pain* (listed in Resources) for specific menstrual exercises. Some yoga exercises, especially the cobra position, are particularly helpful. Experiment with different positions to find out what helps you, even if it only works temporarily. The Alexander Technique (see p. 104) may also help.

Self-help for Specific Menstrual Problems

Cramps and backache. Herbal remedies: bancha-leaf and tamari (soy sauce), Lady's Mantle, catnip and mint teas (all anti-spasmodic); for water retention and pain: raspberry leaf, marjoram and thyme teas. These are all available at health food or herbal shops.

Some women take calcium and magnesium supplements in a two-to-one ratio for several days before the flow or all through the cycle. Start with 250 milligrams of calcium and half that of magnesium. (Take the tablets separately. Dolomite, calcium containing magnesium, may be contaminated with lead or arsenic. Taking these supplements for a long time in large doses may cause problems.) Some find evening primrose oil works. Heat on your stomach or lower back may help. Orgasm, with or without a partner, may work. Some women use non-prescription drugs such as aspirin, alcohol or marijuana. We encourage moderation in the use of all drugs. All kinds of massage may work. See Menstrual Massage for Two People in the box overleaf and look for others specifically

for menstrual problems in yoga, shiatsu, acupressure and polarity therapy books.

I used to take aspirin but it stopped working. I then tried Melissa – a homoeopathic remedy but that stopped working too. Now I use Solpadeine, which usually kills the pain fast. I've also found that reflexology [see p. 113] occasionally works, so does acupressure.

Depression, moodiness and bloating. Those of us who get depressed premenstrually find, when we think about it, that we are concerned with problems that have usually been there all the time. We just can't handle them as well during our premenstrual period. It is important to remember the problems that bother you, even if it means writing them down, so that when you are feeling better you don't forget to try to work towards solving them.

A week before my period comes I go through a few days of feeling more helpless, stuck or down about things in my life that have been there all along. Sometimes I appreciate being more in touch with the underside of my feelings. Other times it really gets to me. The voices inside my head which are overly critical of what I do get much more insistent when I'm premenstrual. Recently I've identified them more quickly. I'll start to get down on myself for not being a good enough mother, friend, worker, daughter, and so forth, and I'll say, 'Those are your critical voices – go easy on yourself!' It helps.

You might plan to get support for yourself for the times when you feel worst. Ask close friends to drop in, involve the rest of the family more in running the household or get a babysitter for the children. You might start a self-help group by advertising in the paper. If fatigue is a problem, try to schedule time for extra sleeping or for energizing exercise. PMS depression may well be related to diet. (See Chapter 4, Food.)

Many women find Vitamin B6 a great help. Start with 50 milligrams a day and try up to 200 milligrams a day for two weeks up to your period. Use with a general B-complex for better absorption. A lot of B6 is found in whole grains, yeast, peanuts, fresh fish and meats, especially liver. Try to decrease sodium by eating less salt and increase potassium. (See Chapter 4.) Some women use diuretics (plain water, water-reducing teas, foods – consult a book on using herbs – or drugs). Use them with caution; most diuretics except water deplete the body of potassium. Capsules of evening primrose oil often help. Start with one a day. Some doctors recommend up to four capsules a day (half in the morning, half in the evening). Take it throughout the cycle except during your period.

Tiredness or paleness. Check your iron level for anaemia.

Heavy periods and/or irregular bleeding. Try eating foods or take supplements with Vitamin C *and* bioflavinoids (also

MENSTRUAL MASSAGE FOR TWO PEOPLE

Pond/Giles

WOMAN WITH CRAMPS

A. Lie flat on your stomach, with or without clothes. Place a blanket or pad under you for extra comfort.

B. Have your arms straight out or slightly bent at the elbows. Point your toes inward if possible.

C. Tell the other person what feels good and what doesn't. It should feel good.

PERSON GIVING THE MASSAGE

A. Basic movement:
   1. Remove your shoes (or kneel and use the heel of your hand).
   2. Check to see if the woman is comfortable. You might gently shake her feet or legs to help her relax and to establish physical contact.
   3. Stand, placing your outer leg next to the head and *above* the shoulder of the woman on the floor.
   4. Put the *heel* of your inner foot against the edge of the top ridge of her pelvis, on the same side where you are standing (see diagram).
   5. 'Hook' your heel as much under the bone as you can. If you are not sure where the pelvic ridge is, feel for it first with your fingers. It may be higher up on her back than you think.
   6. Keep both of your legs slightly bent.
   7. Gently push away from you, towards her feet, at regular intervals of once or twice a second.
      a. When doing this, rock with your whole body by bending *only* at the *knee* and *ankle* of the leg you are standing on.
      b. Move forward and back. Avoid a circular motion.
      c. When you are pushing firmly enough the whole body of the woman getting the massage will rock, too.
      d. Try not to push towards the floor with your inner foot. Keep your toes pointing upwards to prevent this.

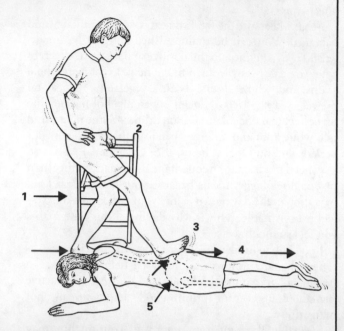

1 Keeping weight on outer leg, rock forward and back
2 For better balance put both hands on hips or one on a chair
3 Toes in the air
4 Direction of push
5 Top ridge of pelvis

      e. Keep your heel in contact with her pelvic bone so the woman getting the massage won't feel bruised.
   8. Increase the frequency and length of the push as long as the woman with the cramps says it is comfortable. You will probably need to work more vigorously than you first imagined.

B. When you feel comfortable with the basic movement:
   1. Move your heel from side to side to different spots along the ridge of her pelvis on the side you are standing next to. Avoid her spine.
   2. Stand on your other leg and repeat A and B-1.
   3. Change sides as often as you want. Continue with the massage until the woman's cramps diminish or go away.

called Vitamin P). Most foods with Vitamin C also contain bioflavinoids. If this problem starts after stopping the Pill,* try Vitamin A. Be cautious; excessive Vitamin A is toxic.

Homoeopathy or acupuncture can be very useful for period problems (see Chapter 7).

ABNORMAL UTERINE BLEEDING

This may involve unusually light or very heavy periods, bleeding or spotting between periods, or cycles that vary widely in length. Abnormal bleeding is frequently due to hormonal changes and is most common in teenagers just beginning to menstruate or women approaching menopause. Many women in their thirties experience light spotting at the time of ovulation, due to the sudden drop in oestrogen. Doctors use a particular term, 'dysfunctional uterine bleeding', to describe abnormal bleeding with or without ovulation. Women who don't ovulate regularly may have late periods and very heavy bleeding due to a build-up of oestrogen. Other possible causes of prolonged, heavy or irregular bleeding include the IUD, birth control pills, pelvic inflammatory disease, ectopic pregnancy, polyps, fibroids, endometriosis and cervical or uterine cancer. (See the sections on each of these conditions.)

In post-menopausal women, abnormal bleeding may be caused by HRT (see p. 456), vaginitis, overgrowth of the endometrial tissues (endometrial hyperplasia), or cancer.

Sometimes, even after extensive testing, no clear-cut reason for bleeding is found.

Self-help and Alternative Approaches

If you are premenopausal, you may be able to stabilize your menstrual flow by reducing stress and improving your consumption of foods high in Vitamins A, E and C, as well as bioflavinoids (in the pith of citrus fruits), zinc, copper and iodine. Supplements of these substances can also help. Consult a holistic nutritionist, if available, to advise you on dosage. Cutting down on animal fat and adding fibre helps to restore normal hormonal balance by lowering cholesterol (which is converted to oestrogen in your body). Acupuncture and other alternative therapies (see Chapter 7) may also help to restore hormonal balance. If you are bleeding heavily, increase your iron intake to prevent anaemia (see p. 345).

Orthodox Treatment

If you are premenopausal and having light, irregular bleeding, your doctor may suggest waiting a month or two to see if your system rights itself. (Sometimes stress can contribute to hormonal imbalances.) If abnormal bleeding persists, however, and diagnostic tests indicate a hormonal disturbance and/or anovulatory cycles, most practitioners recommend hormone treatments (usually combination birth

control pills or intermittent Provera) to help restore normal menstrual cycles. If you want to avoid taking hormones and the bleeding isn't too heavy, you may want to continue self-help measures while observing the amount of bleeding carefully. If you do choose hormone therapy, find a doctor who has skill and experience in it, as mistakes in dosage, duration or oestrogen/progesterone balance can lead to an unnecessary D & C or even a hysterectomy. If you are ovulating and the bleeding is related to the post-ovulation phase of your cycle (see the discussion of menstruation in Chapter 3, p. 35) or if you are anovulatory and wish to become pregnant, you may consider taking Clomid, a powerful fertility drug that stimulates ovulation. Clomid is associated with certain risks, such as the formation of multiple ovarian cysts (see Chapter 21).

UTERINE FIBROIDS (LIEOMYOMAS, MYOMAS)

Fibroids are solid, usually slow-growing and benign tumours* that appear on the outside, inside or within the wall of the uterus, often changing the size and shape of it. About 20 per cent of all women will develop fibroids by the time they are thirty-five, and they are more likely to affect black women. Although they are of unknown cause, these growths seem to be related to oestrogen production: if you are pregnant, fibroids are apt to grow more quickly; this can also happen with HRT containing oestrogen (see p. 457) or with the combined pill (see p. 292).

Fibroids may be discovered during a routine pelvic examination. If they have grown no further when you have a second examination six months later, a yearly check-up will be sufficient.

Small fibroids are usually symptom-free. However, very large or numerous fibroids may cause pain or excessive menstrual flow. (They usually do not cause other forms of abnormal bleeding, so if you have fibroids and experience bleeding between periods or other forms of abnormal bleeding, be sure to be carefully checked for other causes.) Depending on their size and location, fibroids can also

FIBROIDS *(benign growths)*

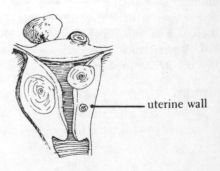

uterine wall

Karen Norberg

---

*See also Chapter 15. Irregular bleeding may come after sterilization and heavy bleeding with IUD use. Psychotropic drugs, either prescribed, such as Valium and Librium, or 'street' drugs, can cause menstrual irregularities. Amphetamines and probably over-the-counter diet aids can increase menstrual flow and cramping.

*The word 'tumour' is very scary to most of us. It is part of an older language of illness that was used by many of our grandparents, both patients and doctors, to disguise the mention of cancer. Actually, tumours are growths of cells which serve no purpose. Over 90 per cent of all tumours are benign and harmless.

cause abdominal or back pain and urinary problems. Large fibroids can make it difficult to conceive or to sustain a full-term pregnancy.

Self-help and Alternative Approaches

If you are taking oestrogen, you may be able to reduce large fibroids by stopping this. Yoga (see p. 109) may ease feelings of heaviness and pressure. If your fibroids cause heavy bleeding, see the nutritional advice given in Abnormal Uterine Bleeding, above. Visualization and other self-healing techniques or alternative approaches (Chapter 7) may be helpful in dealing with fibroids.

Orthodox Treatment

In many cases no treatment is necessary, but if you have excessive bleeding, pain, urinary difficulties or problems with pregnancy, you may want to have the fibroids removed. *Very* occasionally this can be done during a D&C, but usually a myomectomy (which removes fibroids and leaves the uterus intact) is necessary.* This is major surgery with a higher complication rate than hysterectomy. Myomectomy may cause internal scarring, which can lead to painful intercourse, backaches and abnormal uterine bleeding. If you are pregnant, myomectomy can cause miscarriage. In approximately 10 per cent of cases, the fibroids will return.

Many doctors recommend hysterectomy as a treatment for fibroids in women who are past childbearing age or who do not want more children. This surgery may be unnecessary, particularly for women nearing menopause, when the natural decline in oestrogen levels usually shrinks fibroids.

POLYPS

Polyps are usually benign protrusions that grow from a mucous membrane. In women they may appear inside the uterus (endometrial polyps) or along the canal of the cervix, where they grow out of the glands lining the canal. Endometrial polyps are more common. A polyp appears long and tube-like, but is small, easily noticeable by the redness at the tip.

If you have had suspicious bleeding or menstrual flow that seems irregular, it may be caused by polyps. Aside from an abnormal menstrual cycle, bleeding at other times – between periods or right after intercourse – may indicate that there is a growth inside the uterus. This should be checked. A gynaecologist very often will discover a polyp during a pelvic examination.

Treatment

Polyps do not necessarily require treatment. When cervical polyps are small and there is little or no contact bleeding

you can usually just keep track of them with regular self-examination. You may want to have them removed if your symptoms change or the polyp begins to grow. They can often be removed in an outpatient clinic, usually under local anaesthesia. The doctor usually twists the polyp off and seals the base with an electric cautery needle. If your polyp is very large or if you have multiple polyps, you may have to go to the hospital for removal.

If endometrial polyps are troublesome, they can be removed by means of a D&C.

Sometimes polyps recur. While they are almost never malignant, they may occasionally appear similar to cancer, in which case a biopsy of the polyp (in the case of cervical polyps) or a D&C (in the case of endometrial polyps) may be necessary in order to ensure they are not malignant.

PELVIC RELAXATION AND UTERINE PROLAPSE

Pelvic relaxation is a condition in which the muscles of the pelvic floor become slack and no longer adequately support the pelvic organs. In severe cases, the ligaments and tissues which hold the uterus in place may also weaken enough to allow the uterus to 'fall' or 'prolapse' into the vagina. Women sometimes experience pelvic relaxation and/or uterine prolapse after one or more very difficult births, but the tendency can also be inherited. Uterine prolapse is often accompanied by a falling of the bladder (cystocele) and rectum (rectocele) as well.

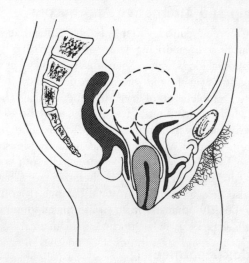

Christine Bondante

Often the first sign of pelvic relaxation is a tendency to leak urine when you cough or sneeze or laugh suddenly ('stress incontinence'). If your uterus has fallen into your vagina you may have a dull, heavy sensation in your vagina or feel as if something is 'falling out'. These symptoms are usually worse after standing for long periods.

Prevention and Self-help

The best way to prevent pelvic relaxation and uterine prolapse is to do regular pelvic floor exercises and leg lifts which strengthen the muscles of the pelvic floor and lower abdomen (see Chapter 19). One way of determining

---

*A new technique, called 'hysteroscopic resection', in which the fibroid is shaved off, is reportedly safer and has fewer complications than myomectomy. It is experimental, however, and should be done only by an experienced specialist.

whether your pelvic muscles are in good shape is to try starting and stopping the flow of urine when you go to the toilet. If you can't stop the flow, you need to do more exercises. Some practitioners recommend doing up to a hundred a day, especially during pregnancy when the pelvic muscles are under particular stress.

> *After my pregnancy I found I was wetting myself each time I sneezed. I did fifty pelvic floor exercises a day and after two weeks felt better. I still get the dragging feeling just before a period but I feel sure I could get rid of it if I kept the exercises up for a few months.*

You may also strengthen a slightly prolapsed uterus by relaxing in the knee-chest position (kneeling with your chest on the floor and your bottom in the air) several times a day. Some women find that certain yoga positions, such as the shoulder and head stands, relieve discomfort from a prolapsed uterus.

Special incontinence pads are available; see p. 468 for further discussion of incontinence.

Orthodox Treatment

Medical intervention is usually not necessary for pelvic relaxation or even mild uterine prolapse. If the prolapse is severe enough to cause discomfort, you can have a pessary inserted (a rubber device which fits around the cervix and helps to prop up the uterus). The disadvantages include difficulty in obtaining a proper fit, possible irritation or infection, and the need to remove and clean the pessary frequently. A surgical procedure called a 'suspension operation' can lift and reattach a descended uterus, and often a fallen bladder or rectum as well. Many doctors recommend hysterectomy for prolapsed uterus but it is frequently unnecessary and should be done only as a last resort.

ENDOMETRIOSIS

Rewritten by THE ENDOMETRIOSIS SOCIETY

Endometriosis is a condition in which some of the tissue lining the uterus (*endometrium*) is also found growing in other parts of the body. This 'normal tissue in an abnormal place' may be referred to as growths, nodules or lesions. They are *not* cancerous. Endometriosis growths are usually found in the pelvic area – on the ovaries, outside the uterus, between the uterus and bowel ('Pouch of Douglas'), on the ligaments supporting the uterus and fallopian tubes. Occasionally they are found on the bladder, intestines or in unexpected places such as the arm, lungs or head. If they are found inside the muscle of the uterus wall, then the condition is known as *adenomyosis*.

Endometriosis growths respond to the monthly variation in the body's hormones in a similar way to the lining of the uterus. Each menstrual cycle, they grow and then bleed slightly during a period. Unlike the menstrual flow, blood from endometriosis cannot escape. Pain and inflammation may occur as the body tries to heal these areas. Over time, the build-up of scar tissue can lead to adhesions, when nearby organs become stuck together (e.g. ovary to uterus, uterus to bowel). 'Chocolate' (blood-filled) cysts can form if there is regular bleeding at sites on the ovaries.

Endometriosis can be an extremely painful disease for some women and yet others do not even realize they have it until it is found during surgery for some other reason. The following symptoms were most commonly reported in an Endometriosis Society survey of almost 800 women definitely diagnosed as having endometriosis:

- *painful periods* (94 per cent);
- painful ovulation (77 per cent);
- swollen abdomen (77 per cent);
- premenstrual tension (67 per cent);
- depression, tiredness, lethargy (63 per cent);
- *frequent/constant pelvic pain* (57 per cent);
- *painful sexual intercourse (dyspareunia)* (55 per cent);
- *painful bowel movements or urination* (48 per cent);
- regular back pain (42 per cent);
- *infertility* (41 per cent);
- insomnia due to pain (32 per cent).

Doctors and medical textbooks recognize only the symptoms shown in italics above as being connected to endometriosis. Some (e.g. insomnia due to pain) may not be directly related to the disease and others are common among women anyway (e.g. PMS); but all the symptoms we have listed are experienced by significant numbers of women who have endometriosis.

Exact symptoms vary, depending to some extent on where the endometriosis is rather than how much there is. For example, patches between the uterus and bowel may cause painful bowel movements which are worse during a period. A tender growth on one of the uterine ligaments can get bumped deep inside during sexual intercourse – very painful and definitely not much fun! The fact that symptoms often come and go with the menstrual cycle, although the disorder is slowly getting worse, means that many women do not realize they have got a physical problem which needs attention:

> *I just kept putting it [pain] down to other things, i.e. PMS, problems with relationships, pressures of bringing up two young children.*

Even if women do see their GP they may need to make several visits before the symptoms are taken seriously:

> *One of the problems is doctors' attitudes towards women complaining of this sort of [sexual] pain – they always seem to think 'She is neurotic, therefore she says she is in pain.' They never think, 'She is anxious because she is in pain!'*

Just to add to the confusion, the common symptoms may be caused by other gynaecological problems (e.g. pelvic inflammatory disease).

Since endometriosis is usually inside the abdomen but outside the uterus, it cannot be seen by looking through the vagina. It is diagnosed by a *laparoscopy* (see p. 596). The laparoscope has vastly improved diagnosis since women can now be checked for endometriosis (or other pelvic conditions) without major surgery. However, it is not a perfect method. Endometriosis usually looks like small bruises or blood blisters but they aren't always visible on the surface or may be hidden among the organs. Some doctors recommend that a laparoscopy should be done just before or during menstruation when the patches are thicker and may be easier to see. However, recent research[25] shows that endometriosis lesions can be microscopic, so future diagnostic techniques using the scanning electron microscope may be more reliable.

No one really knows what causes endometriosis. There are several theories, which are difficult to test. The most popular theory suggests that endometriosis growths form when menstrual blood and tissue from the lining of the uterus flow backwards up the fallopian tubes into the pelvic cavity during period spasms. This process is called retrograde menstruation. However, research suggests that this is quite common in women, most of whom will not develop endometriosis. The theory does not explain why menstrual tissue should implant and grow in some women and not others. Nor does it explain how endometriosis can occur in the lungs and other distant places. Another theory suggests that endometriosis is carried through the lymphatic system. Since growths sometimes appear in scar tissue from previous pelvic surgery, it has been suggested that surgery itself may spread any existing endometriosis. Yet another theory proposes that endometriosis develops from misplaced remnants of pre-natal tissue. Hormonal, immunological or genetic factors may also contribute to the disease's development. For example, in one study, 7 per cent of women with endometriosis had a relative with the disease.[26] Much more basic research is needed to improve the understanding of endometriosis.

The question of who develops endometriosis seems to involve more than its fair share of medical myths. These can be particularly destructive if they contribute to delays in diagnosis and treatment since endometriosis is thought to be a progressive disease with the risk that further damage will occur in each menstrual cycle.

Endometriosis was first described as a separate condition in 1922. Many of the women in early studies were in their thirties and forties and so it was assumed that endometriosis usually occurred in these age groups.[27] Doctors are now acknowledging that this belief reflected the pattern of *diagnosis* rather than the prevalence of the disease. Since the advent of laparoscopy, endometriosis is increasingly reported in young women and teenagers. Similarly, it is now becoming evident that endometriosis is not rare in black women as was once thought.[28] These misconceptions have contributed to the myth that endometriosis is a 'career woman's disease' frequently suffered by egocentric, upwardly striving, white, educated, middle-class women who have deliberately delayed having children. This might

well be true in the sense that these women tend to have the financial resources, knowledge and feeling of entitlement which makes it more likely that they will be diagnosed. This does not mean other women don't have endometriosis! A pattern of late first pregnancies may have a lot more to do with symptoms of painful sexual intercourse and impaired fertility than choice of career.

Orthodox Treatment

Choosing the right treatment depends on several things including a woman's age, location of the endometriosis and its severity, her desire to have children, past experiences with hormones, and family history. Unfortunately, there is no magic, guaranteed cure except the natural menopause, which may be a long wait! The main options are discussed below.

1. *Pregnancy.* There are still doctors who recommend 'getting pregnant as soon as possible'. This is not always a desirable or practical proposition, either for personal reasons or because 40 per cent of endometriosis sufferers experience infertility. As one woman put it:

> *The doctor said the answer was to get married and have a baby. I felt so ill I burst into tears – which seemed to confirm her diagnosis!*

However, pregnancy can relieve the symptoms, which may not return for years after the birth, although they *can* reappear almost immediately. For women who wish to have children, it may be best to go ahead and try before having any other treatment. Breastfeeding is recommended to prolong the time without periods for as long as possible. If conception proves difficult, then one of the common drug treatments for endometriosis, infertility regimes and/or alternative approaches may improve the chances of conceiving.

2. *Hormone treatments.* These are based on the observation that pregnancy and the natural menopause help women with endometriosis. These are both times when women don't have periods. The patches of endometriosis also stop bleeding and if there are no periods for long enough, they seem to wither away. Hormone treatments have therefore been designed to trick the body into stopping the menstrual cycle. This can be done in several different ways.

The drug most commonly used is danazol (17-α-ethinyl testosterone), also known as Danol. It is usually taken for six to nine months in doses of 200 to 800 milligrams daily. During this time it tricks the body into a fake or 'pseudo'-menopause. Unfortunately, it has a reputation for strong side-effects. Some of these can be like the real menopause (hot flushes, dry vagina) while others (increased hair, acne, voice changes) may occur because the drug is very similar to the male hormone testosterone. Further reported difficulties include water retention, oily skin, decreased breast size and joint pains, but by far the most common problem is weight gain. Perhaps not surprisingly, women also mention depression and irritability which may be directly related to the hormone changes produced by the drug or the result of having to cope with unpleasant side-effects over a drawn-out period of time.

Most side-effects are temporary but singers should be aware of the possibility of a permanent deepening of the voice. The Endometriosis Society has also been collating reports which suggest that danazol can exacerbate a previous history of joint problems.

Danazol usually arouses strong feelings in discussions among endometriosis sufferers. Some women have no problems and wouldn't be without it. Most women report some side-effects, while a few cannot tolerate it at all. The decision to continue treatment can be difficult and depends on how bad the side-effects are, balanced by relief from endometriosis symptoms or the hope of conceiving. Some doctors are now working with each woman to find the lowest dose that is still effective, especially since medical research shows that very high doses (e.g. 800 mg/day) are not always necessary.[29] Alternatively, there are several other drugs that can be tried.

Primolut N (norethisterone) and Duphaston (dydrogesterone) treat endometriosis by tricking the body into a fake or 'pseudo'-pregnancy. They are both related to the natural hormone progesterone, which reaches high levels during a real pregnancy. Again these drugs are usually taken for six to nine months in an attempt to stop menstruation. Their side-effects are usually less severe, although weight gain is still a common problem and breast tenderness may be particularly noticeable on dydrogesterone. Occasionally the Pill (taken continuously) is used as treatment but women often get breakthrough bleeding after a month or two because the hormone doses aren't high enough.

Although women can be given years of relief, the current drug treatments are not very effective. For example, in one study more than a third of the sample reported a recurrence after taking danazol.[30] The stress of trying to remember tablets every day for six to nine months, while coping with unwanted side-effects, is not helped by this uncertainty. The anger and disappointment is even worse if we are kept under the illusion that drug treatments guarantee a cure.

Several new drugs are now being tested in clinical trials. Gestrinone is a steroid related to current hormone treatments, but it appears to have far fewer side-effects. A completely new family of drugs called LHRH agonists may be more promising. These drugs (e.g. Buserelin, Nafarelin, Zoladex, 'D-Trp-6-LHRH') are simple protein molecules which block the pituitary's release of luteinizing hormone (LH) which in turn controls the ovary and menstrual cycle. So far, they have not been much more effective at preventing a recurrence of endometriosis than danazol,[31] but their side-effects are limited to menopausal symptoms such as hot flushes and vaginal dryness.

3. *Surgery.* Traditional surgery to treat endometriosis includes a wide range of procedures from 'conservative' (e.g. scraping, cutting away or cauterizing the growths or removing cysts) to 'radical' (hysterectomy – removal of the uterus – with or without the ovaries). Reports at the first International Symposium on Endometriosis (1986) advocated the meticulous use of microsurgery techniques to reduce the risk of adhesions. Advances in laser surgery, though not yet widely available, offer a lot of promise since chocolate cysts and fairly large areas of endometriosis or adhesions can be cauterized through a laparoscope. However, surgery will always be limited to treating visible endometriosis only; since endometriosis cannot always be seen by the naked eye, hormone treatments may also be necessary.

Hysterectomy is a controversial treatment for endometriosis and is frequently performed without a woman's full knowledge or understanding of its special implications for endometriosis sufferers. Many women have believed that in the absence of their uterus, endometriosis would be cured. However, since many endometriosis growths are found elsewhere, it is perfectly possible for them to remain after a hysterectomy. If a woman still has her ovaries after the operation, they will continue to produce oestrogen. This hormone can reactivate any remaining endometriosis, which will go through a monthly cycle of growing and bleeding even though she will no longer have periods. This won't happen in every case and women have gained relief from a hysterectomy, but this major operation should not be regarded as an automatic answer to endometriosis. It isn't!

The real solution to this dilemma may appear to be to remove the ovaries as well. Unfortunately, removing the ovaries will lead to an immediate menopause as oestrogen levels rapidly fall. If a woman is near her natural menopause this may not be important to her, although it has to be said that this will shortly provide its own cure without the need for such drastic surgery. If removal of the ovaries is advised, oestrogen replacement therapy may also be suggested to prevent menopausal changes. However, any endometriosis sufferer taking oestrogen runs the risk of reactivating the disease.* Again, this will not happen in every case, but too many women have faced this catch-22 without adequate discussion or support. In general, removal of the ovaries should be regarded as a last resort when other treatment options have been explored. Please see p. 456 for more discussion on oestrogen replacement therapy, and other approaches to 'menopause' problems.

Alternative Approaches

Many women have turned to alternative therapies such as homoeopathy, herbal and nutritional remedies. The Endometriosis Society is collecting reports of these methods and there are some very positive results:

I am aged thirty-seven and have been trying unsuccessfully for a baby for some time. I have had endometriosis for at least the past six years. I'm in

---

*It is possible that hormone replacement therapy involving progestogen alone may prove to be less risky from this point of view (see HRT, p. 456).

no doubt that the homoeopathic treatment over the past year led to my present state of pregnancy. *

B vitamins (B-complex taken with 100mg B6 [pyridoxine] daily) have been very popular for counteracting the frequent feelings of tiredness, lethargy and depression:

I've felt so much better since taking Vitamin B6. The terrible depression and listlessness I've had, especially since taking hormones, has lifted.

The B vitamins are thought to help oestrogen metabolism and B6 is well known for helping to relieve PMS symptoms. Evening primrose oil can alleviate PMS and it appears to reduce side-effects from drug treatment:

Side-effects from hormones e.g. muscle spasms and crippling pains, vanished completely with Efamol evening primrose oil but returned during the week's trial break I took.

I find almost immediate relief from Efamol – it does not relieve all symptoms but it helps tremendously.

This supplement has an effect on pain-producing prostaglandins and inflammation.[32] Another natural pain-controller that some women have found useful is the amino acid DLPA (D-L phenylalanine):

I have been pleased and amazed at how much the pain was relieved. I had almost begun to forget just how bad the pain was until I stopped taking DLPA.

Selenium ACE (a trace element with added Vitamins A, C and E) has also proved invaluable to many endometriosis sufferers. Apparently selenium and Vitamin E give protection to the body not unlike an anti-inflammatory effect. Selenium is also known to strengthen the immune system, which may be an important factor in fighting endometriosis. Vitamin E often improves adhesions.

I started taking Selenium ACE (two tablets daily) two years ago – after the first six months all my inflammatory pain, which had plagued me for years, had gone and I felt my general health to be better than I ever remember.

Other important supplements for general health are zinc and calcium. Taking calcium and magnesium in the proportion 200–800mg daily from roughly one week before menstruation until the end can reduce cramping and keep the muscles relaxed.

*Please see Chapter 21 for more on alternative approaches to infertility treatment.

Women may need to experiment to find the most useful remedies or the right combination. The potential benefits of a complete change of diet are also becoming evident. Chronic yeast (*candida albicans*) infections can occur in women, especially after antibiotics or with the Pill. In some cases, they may be responsible for weakening the immune system and further ill health. Some authors are now suggesting a possible link between endometriosis and yeast infections.[33] An anti-candida diet has been known to completely relieve endometriosis symptoms and improve general health. (See *Candida Albicans* by L. Chaitow, listed in Resources.)

Self-help

Endometriosis may not be fatal but it can mean suffering from long-term pain, the build-up of adhesions and risk of infertility, not to mention the possible effects on a woman's self-confidence, sexual and other relationships, her ability to carry on paid/home work or her role as a mother. Coping with endometriosis in everyday life is not helped by the sense of isolation women often feel:

I thought that there was only me that suffered from this, as no one had ever heard of it before. When someone asks me what is wrong when I don't look well and I try to explain, they look at me as though to say I'm silly.

These feelings are common in spite of the fact that endometriosis has been quoted as the second most

---

The Endometriosis Society was launched as a registered charity in 1982 after an article by Jill Rakusen in *Good Housekeeping* prompted over 1,000 women to write to the self-help group in London. It is now a national organization with three major goals: supporting women with endometriosis, educating the medical community and general public about the disease and its effects, and funding, participating in and conducting research.

The Society now has a network of over 100 groups throughout the country. Information sheets and a newsletter are available as well as telephone/pen pal schemes. Workshops are held several times a year to explore particular aspects of endometriosis and its treatment. Several hundred case histories of orthodox and alternative treatments are being analysed. On the basis of good reports from members, the Society has negotiated bulk discounts on various alternative medicines.

See p. 533 for the Society's address.

When I told the specialist I had joined the Society he was very amused and said, 'Good grief, there will be an In-growing Toenail Society next!'

common gynaecological disorder after fibroids[34] and has been estimated to affect between 1 and 5 million women in this country.

The Endometriosis Society (see box) offers many different ways in which women with endometriosis can get in touch, find out more and start to participate more actively in their own health care. Many women have been relieved to discover they are not alone and have welcomed the opportunity to share their experiences with other sufferers who know what it *feels* like. This is often an important step towards self-help and being more positive about life.

For more about alternative and self-help approaches to healing, see Chapter 7. See also Get Well Diets, p. 52.

CANCER OF THE UTERUS

Prepared by JILL RAKUSEN

Cancer of the lining of the uterus (endometrial cancer) is the most common pelvic cancer, affecting fourteen out of every 10,000 women yearly. Most women who develop this cancer are past menopause and in their fifties; 10 per cent are still menstruating. If you are overweight, if you have diabetes, high blood pressure or a hormone imbalance which combines high oestrogen levels with infrequent ovulation, or if you take synthetic oestrogen without additional progestogen, your risk of developing uterine cancer is increased (see Menopause, p. 453).

Bleeding after menopause is the most common symptom of uterine cancer. For women who are still menstruating, increased menstrual flow and bleeding between periods may be the only symptoms. Cervical smears are unreliable in detecting uterine cancer. If you are premenopausal, your doctor may suggest a D & C as the first step because it not only screens for cancer but frequently relieves abnormal bleeding from a variety of less serious causes. If you are post-menopausal, you will probably have an aspiration or endometrial biopsy (see p. 596), and if the biopsy is not conclusive, your doctor may suggest a D & C. Before agreeing to a D & C, however, make sure that you have both considered the risks and discussed alternatives for diagnosis and treatment of abnormal bleeding (see p. 513).

Prevention and Self-help

Since endometrial cancer appears to be influenced by factors such as obesity, hypertension and diabetes, controlling these conditions with self-help methods may prevent this type of cancer from developing or spreading.

Treatment

Orthodox treatment for uterine cancer includes surgery, radiotherapy and chemotherapy. There is wide disagreement about which is best. Hysterectomy is the most common treatment, sometimes with follow-up radiotherapy after surgery if the tumour was large, if spread to lymph nodes was suspected or if the cellular changes were more excessive than usual. If you should have a return of the cancer after one of the above treatments, progestogen may help slow its spread.

When uterine cancer is found early, the success rate of conventional treatments is very high.

Please see Cancer, p. 567 for a fuller discussion of treatments (including complementary and alternative approaches) and what you can do to help yourself.

OVARIAN CYSTS

Ovarian cysts are relatively common and often don't cause any symptoms or discomfort. A cyst usually develops when a follicle has grown large – as one or more do every month during ovulation – but has failed to rupture and release an egg. Most of these cysts fill with fluid; others become solid, usually benign tumours. Cysts may be accompanied by symptoms such as a disturbance in the normal menstrual cycle, an unfamiliar pain or discomfort in your lower abdomen at any point during the cycle, pain during sex and unexplained abdominal swelling. Found by a routine bimanual pelvic examination, cysts usually disappear by themselves, though some types may have to be removed.

To determine whether a cyst requires treatment, wait a cycle or two for it to disappear. If it persists, a doctor may use ultrasound, X-ray or laparoscopy to learn about the cyst. A tissue sample will reveal if it is benign or malignant. Doctors disagree about the necessity of removing benign cysts, though most agree that cysts remaining after attempted suppression with oral contraceptives should be treated.

If your doctor advises removal of the ovary along with the benign cyst, get a second opinion. This practice is, in many cases, unnecessary. Ovaries perform many functions, even after menopause.

Recurrent cysts may indicate a hormonal imbalance or life stresses. Changing your diet, learning how to reduce stress, and alternative approaches to health and healing may help to get your system back in balance.

CANCER OF THE OVARY

Although cancer of the ovary is less common than cervical or uterine cancer, it accounts for 3,500 deaths a year in England and Wales – the greatest gynaecological cause of death.[35] The exact causes are unknown, but it is clear that women who have never had children, post-menopausal women and women who have breast cancer or cancer of the intestines or rectum are at increased risk for ovarian cancer. Women who work in the electrical, textile and rubber industries, have received extensive pelvic radiation or live in urban areas seem to develop it more often than others. Women with a family history of ovarian cancer and women who are very overweight are also prone to develop this cancer.* Recent evidence suggests that the regular use of talcum powder on genitals and/or sanitary towels increases the risk by as much as three times.[36]

*While removal of the ovaries (oophorectomy) is frequently suggested in order to protect women who are at risk of ovarian cancer, the possible risks and effects of this operation do not justify it.

DES

Rewritten by
JILL RAKUSEN

VAGINAL CANCER

Until 1970 vaginal cancer was one of the rarest human cancers, virtually unknown in women under fifty. Since that time, it has been identified in several hundred young women (including some pre-adolescents), almost all of whose mothers were given diethylstilboestrol (DES) during pregnancy to prevent miscarriage. Almost all reported cases were in the USA. Tragically, it was already known as early as 1953 that DES, a synthetic oestrogen, did not prevent miscarriage; but many obstetricians continued to prescribe it for this purpose, and indeed some did so right up until the first link between DES and vaginal cancer was demonstrated in 1970. Vaginal clear-cell adenocarcinoma is fundamentally a new iatrogenic (medically-induced) disease.

The link between this oestrogen, when given even in small doses during the first three months, and clear-cell vaginal cancer in female children is now clearly established. If you took DES, or suspect that you may have been given it and you have a daughter, insist that she be referred to a specialist for checks. If your mother was given DES (ask her!), you should be checked yourself. You cannot get access to your medical records in Britain, but your GP should have them; if s/he doesn't, s/he can get them and can also ask for information from your mother's records. It may be difficult to find out, but if you have the slightest suspicion (e.g. your mother had treatment for recurrent miscarriages), you should push for this important information.

If you suspect you are at risk, diagnosis involves not only smears and routine vaginal examinations but also examination by colposcope (see p. 527). This examination should be repeated at six-month intervals to detect any cancer cells as soon as possible. A second test involves painting the entire vaginal area with a stain (Schiller test) to reveal the presence of any abnormal cells.

These tests are vitally necessary, since most of the cases so far discovered have been fairly advanced at the time of diagnosis and *had not been picked up in previous routine gynaecological examinations.* Many women had been reassured that they were perfectly normal, only to have their cancers detected by these other techniques later.

Because this disease is so new, all treatments are by definition experimental. Some doctors believe it may be possible to stop or even reverse the progress of the disease with progesterone suppositories. Various types of surgery and cauterization as well as radiation have all produced some beneficial results. If part of the vagina is removed, it is possible that this can be followed by reconstructive surgery.

Obviously, treatment involves (or should involve) prevention of any additional exposure to oestrogen or DES specifically. This means avoiding all oestrogens until more is known. If DES or oestrogen is taken as a morning-after pill for a suspected pregnancy and does *not* bring on menstruation, an early abortion could be sought to avoid the possibility of cancer in female children.

OTHER PROBLEMS

DES causes other abnormalities of the reproductive organs, such as a 'T-shaped' uterus, which can make pregnancy difficult. As a result, DES daughters are at risk of *infertility* problems, *miscarriage, ectopic pregnancy* (Chapter 21) and *premature delivery.*

Abnormalities of the genitals have also been found in *male children.* They are: small testes; infertility; subfertility; and, in some subfertile men, damaged sperm. No one knows how this would affect offspring. Though malignancy has not yet appeared in males, other effects may be discovered in their female offspring. All DES children should be watched.

Finally, DES seems to be associated with an increased risk of *breast cancer* in women given the drug while pregnant, with a time-lag of ten to twenty years before onset of the cancer. Cancer of the uterus, ovaries and cervix may also be associated with it.

Early signs are often vague. They include mild stomach upsets, wind and abdominal pain. Sometimes there is tenderness and pain from a build-up of fluid within the pelvic and abdominal cavity caused by irritated gland cells.

Diagnosis

Your doctor may suspect ovarian cancer if during a pelvic examination your ovary feels enlarged or less mobile than normal, or if s/he feels unusual growths. Diagnostic tests may include ultrasound and X-rays of your stomach and bowel, and a CAT scan. You may also have a blood test to check for cancers which produce their own protein or hormonal substances. If you have surgery, a frozen section of cystic or solid tumour will indicate whether the entire ovary should be removed, as well as the need for further surgery. Ovarian cancer is more common in older women, and in women over forty an annual pelvic examination is often recommended, not least because it can pick up ovarian cancer. Screening tests for ovarian cancer, involving blood tests or ultrasound, are currently being investigated and may become available on the NHS – though, possibly, only if women campaign for them.

Treatment

The many types of ovarian cancer differ in their sensitivity to different types of therapy. Orthodox treatment involves radiotherapy, chemotherapy and/or surgery.* Cure rates are not good, however – 10–20 per cent. Please see Cancer, p. 567, for a discussion of treatments and prognosis (including complementary and alternative approaches), and Living with Cancer, p. 582.

CERVIX
Rewritten by JILL RAKUSEN

CERVICITIS

Cervicitis is a term used loosely to describe an inflammation or infection of the cervix. Cervicitis is often related to other infections, such as common vaginal infections, STDs and PID, and you should therefore be investigated for these. It can also result from an infection following an IUD insertion, abortion or childbirth. Untreated, chronic cervicitis can cause fertility problems by blocking the passage of sperm or altering the cervical mucus.

Depending upon the severity and length of infection, you may notice an increased vaginal discharge, pain with intercourse, an aching sensation in the lower abdomen and/or the need to urinate more frequently. Severe infections may also bring fever.

Diagnosis

When you touch your cervix, it may feel warmer and larger than usual. Movement of your cervix with your finger may be uncomfortable. If you examine yourself with a speculum, your cervix will look red and slightly swollen and you may observe a discharge. If only the cervical canal is affected, your cervix will look normal but you may see a yellowish discharge coming from within the cervical opening.

If you have an internal examination, be sure to tell the practitioner whether or not your discharge is normal. (Sometimes doctors mistake scar tissue and normal discharge for cervicitis.) A culture and wet mount will determine the cause of the infection. In some cases, a cervical smear will also be taken to rule out the possibility of cervical cancer.

*One particular form of chemotherapy – cisplatin – causes very severe nausea and vomiting which in some women cannot be alleviated and can carry on for two weeks after the chemotherapy. A new form of drug, called Carboplatin, has been developed which causes much less nausea and vomiting, and it also has less damaging effects on the kidneys. However, it is not freely available because it is expensive.

Orthodox Treatment

If tests show that an STD such as gonorrhoea, syphilis or chlamydia is responsible for the infection, you will get oral or injected antibiotics. For mild cervicitis caused by other infections or injury, doctors usually prescribe vaginal creams containing sulpha, antibiotics or iodine-based gels. For more severe cases, some doctors recommend cryosurgery or electrocautery (see pp. 526). While these treatments work well when all other methods have failed, use them only as a last resort, as they can be painful and it will take about six weeks for your cervix to return to normal.

Self-help

When symptoms are mild and not related to PID or STDs, the following remedies may help: goldenseal douche (a quarter of a teaspoon to one quart of water twice a day for two to three weeks), Vitamin C douche (500 milligrams in one quart of water daily for three to four weeks) or vinegar douche (see p. 490). For more information on herbal remedies, see Resources.

To speed healing and strengthen the immune system and for future prevention, you may want to try oral doses of Vitamin C (500 to 1,000 milligrams a day – but see p. 52 if you are on the Pill), zinc (25 milligrams a day) and Vitamin E (400 milligrams a day). You can also apply Vitamin E directly to your cervix with your finger.

No matter what treatment you use, try to combine it with extra rest and good nutrition.

CERVICAL 'EROSION'

Cervical 'erosion' is a common condition in which the tissue which lines the cervical canal is seen around the cervical os. This looks red with a bumpy-looking texture but it is smooth to the touch. It requires no treatment unless accompanied by infection. Those of us whose mothers took DES during pregnancy are more likely to have 'erosion'. Most women do not have any symptoms; in those who do, the most frequent sign is a slightly increased non-irritating vaginal discharge.

The term 'erosion' is misleading because it suggests there is something wrong when, in the vast majority of cases, it is a normal thing which happens at various phases of our lives (it tends to be governed by hormonal changes). A more apt term would be cervical 'eversion', as it is called in the USA.

CERVICAL CELL ABNORMALITY AND CERVICAL SMEARS
Rewritten together with CHRIS BENNETT

The cervix is unique in that a special test (a cervical smear) can diagnose so-called *pre*-cancerous changes of cells in the cervix. The 'smear' test means that suspicious cells can be watched, and treated if this is considered necessary, before they turn into cancer.* Such treatment is thought to be a very effective way of pre-empting the development of many cervical cancers. About sixteen women in every 100,000 will develop cervical cancer, which means 4,000 cases each year, resulting in just over 2,000 deaths. The lives of many of these women could be saved by an effective screening programme.

In this section we take you through having a smear, the results and treatment options (including what you can do to help yourself). The next section discusses cervical cancer and its treatment, and the final section discusses screening in more general terms.

Cervical Smear Test or Cyto-test

The cervical smear test can tell us about changes in the cervical cells, pick up infections and inflammations, and is a useful way to monitor our gynaecological health. This is not a 'cancer test'; it is a means of finding out if any surface cells are abnormal. Only if they are grossly abnormal is there suspicion that the underlying cells could be abnormal also. To find out you will need further tests (see below).

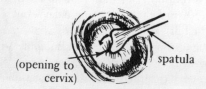

(opening to cervix)   spatula

Spatula scrapes cervix for cervical smear (see p. 33 for location of cervix).

The smear test involves taking a sample of cells from a particular point on the cervix called the *transformation zone*. (The outside of the cervix is covered with tough, water-resistant skin (*squamous epithelium*), while the cervical canal is lined with special glandular tissue which secretes mucus (*columnar epithelium*); where the two types of skin join is the transformation zone.) At the transformation zone the cells have the potential to develop into squamous or columnar cells and because of this unstable state it is here, at the *squamo-columnar junction*, where most abnormal cell changes occur and where cancer of the cervix is most likely to begin.

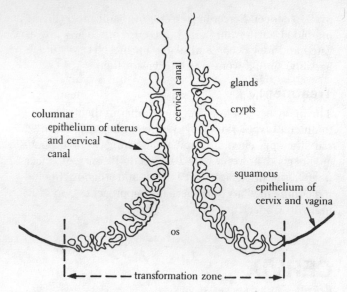

Diagram of a premenopausal woman's cervix, showing the transformation zone. After menopause, the transformation zone tends to move up the cervical canal.

A smear is usually taken when you are lying on your back with knees wide apart. There is no need to take off all your clothes. A speculum (see p. 594) is inserted to open the vaginal walls,* then a small wooden spatula or brush is gently rotated around the os to pick up cells which are smeared on a glass slide and 'fixed' with a solution to prevent them from deteriorating. The slide is sent to the laboratory for analysis.

You may feel nothing or a mild scraping sensation; it is unlikely to cause pain or discomfort unless the smear taker is insensitive. Procedures of this kind can be difficult for us psychologically: an intimate part of our body is being viewed and we cannot see what is happening. The attitude of those involved can help reduce any stress and anxiety. Relaxing helps – e.g. taking deep breaths. You can ask the practitioner to 'talk you through' the procedure, and even to insert the speculum yourself.

Getting a Smear

The government has recommended that all women between the ages of twenty and sixty-five should be invited to have a smear at least once every five years. However, it is not providing the money to finance this recommendation, and its decision coincides with relentless cuts in the NHS – which means that many districts have been obliged to *reduce* their smear-testing services. GPs are still paid for taking smears every five years only if the woman concerned is over thirty-five, or if she has been pregnant on three or more occasions (not necessarily had three children), so some GPs are likely to suggest that women outside these two categories go to a clinic for a smear. Nevertheless, some GPs run special sessions for taking smears and provide a

---

*The process by means of which pre-cancerous cells turn into cancer is poorly understood. Certainly it can take years, but, equally certainly, by no means all pre-cancerous changes will become cancer: indeed, only a tiny minority will. Currently, most treatment recommendations are made on the basis that since for some women the changes will become cancerous, all pre-cancerous smears should be regarded with suspicion. There is no way of predicting with accuracy in any individual case whether abnormal cells would have in fact become cancerous, although the risk of progression is thought to be increased in certain circumstances (e.g., if a woman has HPV – the wart virus – see p. 500.) See Cancer, p. 567, and Self-help, p. 525, for how we ourselves can intervene in the healing process.

---

*Because of the risk of contracting wart virus (see p. 500) it is important that the speculum is adequately sterilized (see p. 594).

service for younger women. Some also screen women at least every *three* years.*

Some health authorities do run special cytology sessions – usually with a woman doctor. Telephone your district health authority headquarters to find out. Family planning clinics usually ask when you had your last smear and are unlikely to refuse to do a smear when you are being examined, particularly if you fall into a high-risk category (see p. 530). STD clinics (see p. 489) often take a smear routinely unless you have had one recently.

If you are pregnant, you will probably have a smear early in your pregnancy or six weeks after the birth – ask when you are being given an internal examination. Smears are also available at most well woman clinics. Your employer or union could be encouraged to arrange for a mobile clinic to visit your workplace, e.g. one run by the WNCCC (see Resources). See p. 531 for suggestions on campaigning for adequate facilities.

To get the most accurate result from a smear, it should be done by a well-trained practitioner† and the cells should be 'at their best'. Ideally, the cervix should be undisturbed for at least twenty-four hours, so douching, sexual intercourse and even using tampons are probably best avoided. Do not have a smear while you are menstruating, as blood interferes with the reading. The best time is just before or at ovulation when the oestrogen level is high, as this makes it easier to 'read' the cells. It is unwise to repeat the smear before a new layer of cells has reached the surface of the cervix. This takes up to three months.

Getting the Result

There is no national system for informing women about their test's result. Usually, women are asked to telephone after a specified number of weeks, depending on the time it is currently taking the laboratory to process smears.

> I found out . . . that I'd been given a smear test three years ago when being examined for the NHS abortion I didn't get. They'd written to my GP about it, I saw the carbon copy of the letter, but *he's never told me*. Perhaps he never got the letter? It wasn't in my files at the surgery, and my then GP is dead now and can't be asked. Whatever the reason, I reckon I should have been informed as well by the hospital.[38]

This is not an unusual experience. The need for women to be notified directly of their smear test result has been highlighted after a thirty-two-year-old Oxford woman died

and two others were seriously ill after learning the result of smear tests three years too late. Studies of both NHS and private care suggest that almost half of abnormal smears may not be satisfactorily followed up.[39] Ideally, every woman should receive the result of her smear test in writing, and laboratories should not those which need following up or repeating and chase doctors when no action has been taken. A 'no news is good news' policy (where you are notified only if your smear test is abnormal) is not good enough. Until a better notification system exists, we would be wise to chase up the result to make sure both that the smear sample contained suitable cells for testing (see above) and that a satisfactory explanation about the outcome of the test is obtained.

For more discussion about the politics of cervical screening, see p. 529.

Understanding the Result of a Smear Test

Most smear test results are negative; this means that no abnormal cells were found. Only a tiny minority are positive. A positive smear test result does *not* mean cancer; it usually means that some abnormal cells were seen on the slide, and a repeat smear and possibly further investigation are needed. Even if you have a negative result, it may well be necessary to repeat the test because the first smear was inadequate. This may be because it contained no cells from the transformation zone* or because of the presence of substances like blood or spermicide.

Many suspicious smear test results will mention infection or inflammation. Make sure your infection or inflammation is treated before you have a repeat smear. Abnormal cells can return to normal when the cervix returns to a more hospitable environment: this may take six months.

Because of the large minority of false negative results (e.g. see Jordan 1988 in Resources), we recommend that, at the very least, a woman's first smear test should be followed by a second test six to twelve months later to confirm the negative diagnosis.

The medical term now used to describe abnormal cells on or near the cervical canal is *dyskaryosis*.** Dyskaryosis may be suggestive of a condition called *cervical intraepithelial neoplasia* (CIN). Although this condition is poorly understood, the abnormalities are believed to progress along a continuum, with normal cells at one end, followed by CIN I, CIN II and CIN III.† Micro-invasive cancer and frank invasive cancer (see p. 529) are thought to follow. CIN and cancer can be confirmed only by further tests (see p. 524).

The result of the smear may therefore come back as 'moderate dyskaryosis suggesting CIN II' or 'severe dyskaryosis suggesting CIN III', for example. Currently, orthodox treatment recommendations are made on the

---

*A new GP pay structure being discussed as we go to press will change this system – we hope for the better.

†It is best to go to a practitioner well trained and experienced in doing smears: errors, for example when taking smears, result in as many as 30 per cent of the smears taken by some GPs being useless. And a study in Glasgow reported that up to 12 per cent of smears gave a false negative result – many of these false negatives being due to doctors' poor sampling technique.[37]

*It is particularly important that a competent practitioner takes smears of women after menopause, because the transformation zone moves up into the cervical canal and is harder to reach.

**Until recently, the term *dysplasia* was more commonly used.

†CIN III includes abnormalities previously diagnosed as 'carcinoma-*in-situ*'.

WHO SHOULD HAVE A CERVICAL SMEAR AND WHEN

Although in 1988 the Department of Health recommended that all women have a smear test once every five years from twenty to sixty-five years, there is widespread agreement that testing every three years is desirable and even more often for some women. Many doctors do not consider this appropriate or have to follow a restrictive policy.* If you are refused a smear test by your doctor, the best place to try is an STD clinic (see p. 489) or a family planning clinic.

We believe that the following guidelines are in women's best interests. If local doctors or clinics disagree, you can contact WHRRIC and/or your CHC for support (see Chapter 28).

- If you have never had a smear, particularly if you are over thirty-five, have a first smear. Follow this by a second smear within the next twelve months.
- If you have reached menopause continue to have regular smears. You can safely stop at sixty-five as long as previous results have been consistently negative.
- If you have had a hysterectomy for cervical abnormality, you should continue to have vaginal vault smears.

- If you have ever had treatment for CIN or carcinoma-*in-situ* or a cone biopsy, you should be regularly recalled. Make sure that you are.
- Have a smear test within the first year of becoming heterosexually active and a second test six to twelve months later. You do not have to wait until you are twenty for a first smear.
- If you use oral contraception it is important to have regular smears (see p. 294).
- Lesbian women should have regular smears if you have had earlier heterosexual activity, or sexually transmitted infections.
- If you or your male partner have ever had warts or herpes you are strongly advised to have a smear test every year.
- If he has had cancer of the penis, regular smear tests are advised.
- If his previous partner had cervical cancer, then you should have annual smear tests.
- In addition, consider the risk factors discussed on p. 530; you may wish to have more frequent smear tests to take account of them.†

*See footnote on p. 528.
†If you have HIV, you may also wish to have frequent smear tests, as there is some evidence to suggest that HIV might be a risk factor for CIN.[40]

---

basis that, since for a few women changes will become cancerous, all pre-cancerous smears should be treated. However, if women – and doctors – were informed about preventive action that can be taken once a suspicious smear is diagnosed (see Self-help, p. 525, and Cancer, p. 514), then it is possible that fewer women might require treatment. Obviously, it is important that a woman who has had an abnormal smear is monitored.

If You Have a Suspicious Smear: Orthodox Treatment*

If you have a suspicious smear test result, you could start yourself on a self-help programme (see box) immediately while waiting for the second smear. Pre-cancerous changes, if they exist, mean that you do not have to rush for treatment and could usefully spend several months using self-help methods, which have been known to reverse abnormal changes.

You will need a repeat smear to confirm or challenge the result; you will usually have to wait three months to give a

new layer of cells time to reach the surface of the cervix. If the repeat smear is positive, you should ideally be referred for a colposcopy (see box, p. 527) so that further tests can determine what is going on and what treatment, if any, might be appropriate. (You may even be referred for a colposcopy straight away, or a *cervicography* (a new photographic screening technique), as both can aid diagnosis of suspicious smears.) If there is no colposcopy clinic in your area, you will be referred to an outpatient gynaecological clinic. You may decide after reading this section and the colposcopy box that you would prefer to go to a colposcopy clinic, and you can ask to be referred to one, although you may have to travel some way to get to one.

The aim of treatment is to remove all pre-cancerous cells. The treatment depends on the diagnosis, the extent of the abnormal area of cells (lesion) and how accessible it is, your age and desire for future pregnancies, how you feel about the various treatment options (treatment can be distressing), and the preferences and experience of the gynaecologist. For the early abnormalities there is little difference in the success of the different treatments. In 80 to 90 per cent of cases, one treatment will be sufficient. Any remaining abnormality usually shows up in the first year after treatment. It is, however, important to continue with regular smears.

*For a discussion of alternative and complementary approaches, see Cancer, p. 574, and Chapter 7.

SELF-HELP

While we wait for repeat smears or referrals for colposcopy, use of the following self-help strategies is very worthwhile and might help reversal of the abnormality.

- Check for and treat any infection or inflammation. You might consider going to an STD clinic for thorough infection testing (see p. 489), as there is evidence that dealing with infection on its own is associated with reversal of abnormal smears.

- Are you exposed to carcinogens – e.g. do you or your partner smoke? (both increase the risk of cervical cancer specifically, see p. 525); at the very least, cut down, but, better still, stop altogether. Read Chapter 5 for help with this. Are you or your partner exposed to substances such as machine oil (whether through your work or through doing activities such as car maintenance – see p. 530 for more about occupational hazards)? Can you reduce your exposure? Men are notoriously ignorant about how their lack of hygiene affects their female sexual partners. A frank discussion may be needed about the importance of cleanliness: men should always wash the penis before intercourse without a condom (especially under the foreskin if they have one), and partners should always make sure their fingers and fingernails are scrupulously clean if they have any contact with the vagina.

- If you are heterosexually active, consider using a barrier method of contraception. Condoms are a very effective way of protecting the cervix from carcinogens and infections. When a group of 139 women with dyskaryosis were advised as their sole 'treatment' to use condoms, in 136 (98 per cent) their diagnosis was subsequently reversed.[41] Even allowing for a considerable over-diagnosis at the initial smear stage, this represents an impressive percentage change.

- If you are on the Pill, current FPA advice is that there is no reason why you should discontinue it. We are surprised at this. For example, notwithstanding the study referred to above,* and evidence of diaphragm-users' lower relative risk of cervical cancer when compared with Pill-users,[43] there is evidence of an increased rate of cervical cancer with increased duration of Pill use.[44] Also, as we reported in our last edition, there is evidence that the Pill increases the risk of cervical cancer in women who already have abnormal cells before starting on the Pill.[45] And as Potts and Diggory themselves acknowledge in the most recent edition of *Contraceptive Practice*,[46] the rate of progression 'may possibly be accelerated by prolonged use' of the Pill. Although one study has recently been published which claims no role of the Pill in the progression of abnormal cells,[47] it fails to examine important variables. We remain sceptical of current FPA advice not only for the above reasons: in addition, the Pill seems to have a depressive effect on the immune system[48] (possibly this is connected with its effect on nutrient levels in the body – see Cancer, p. 574, for the role of the depressed immune system in the development of cancer).

Women with dyskaryosis may therefore see the wisdom of trying to pre-empt the need for unnecessary treatment by switching to barrier methods, even if their advisers don't.

- Read Cancer, p. 577, concerning the role of diet in relation to cancer. Certain nutritional deficiencies have been associated specifically with pre-cancerous and cancerous smears, and improved diets with regression – in particular diets which include adequate intake of beta-carotene, Vitamin C and folic acid.

- Emotional factors can play an important role in cancer, and according to Kinesis (see Resources) many women have noticed an abnormal smear test result came at a time of worry, problems in relationships, bereavement, difficulties at work. Read Cancer, p. 574, and Chapter 7 for more information and ideas on how you can use your mind to help you become well.

For more about self-help and cervical cancer, see Kinesis article.

*Unfortunately they did not establish women's use of the Pill.[42]

Below we describe the most usual approaches that doctors take to suspicious smears:*

- *CIN I/'mild dyskaryosis'*. Most likely a 'wait and see' approach with repeat smear in three or six months, as it may well revert to normal. Any infection or inflammation should be treated. Read the self-help box. If CIN persists, you may be referred for treatment.

- *CIN II/'moderate dyskaryosis'*. This might be considered as CIN I or might be referred for investigation depending on the doctor or the advice from the laboratory.

- *CIN III/'severe dyskaryosis'*. Further investigation is required (by colposcopy and punch biopsy, and

*Hysterectomy is rarely appropriate for any of these conditions, but it is occasionally necessary when further diagnostic tests (see below) are equivocal. For invasive cancer, see p. 529.

possibly cone biopsy; see pp. 527 and 528), to rule out invasive cancer. At least three-quarters of women with CIN III are suitable for simple local outpatient treatment. However, the abnormality could regress, and taking self-help measures improves the chances of regression.

Until the mid-1970s the standard treatment for cervical abnormalities was admission to hospital for a cone biopsy, cauterization* or hysterectomy. While outpatient treatments were being used occasionally, the development of the colposcope (see box, p. 527) has enabled them to be used more effectively and more widely. All the following treatments can in most instances be used instead of a cone biopsy or the other more radical treatments, *provided* that the colposcope has enabled the entire transformation zone to be examined, and that there is no suspicion of invasive cancer. These treatments are normally carried out on an outpatient basis, though as we indicate below, some women might prefer a general anaesthetic to be used.

Carbon dioxide laser. Laser stands for 'Light Amplification Stimulated Emission of Radiation'. The laser beam vaporizes the water that makes up most of the tissue, leaving a small charred crater. Because it can eradicate any abnormality up to a depth of about 1 cm, and can do so to a controlled depth and width, it tends to be used if it is available. *In experienced hands*, it is a very precise method. There is less discharge, fewer complications, minimal scarring, and healing is faster than with other treatments.

Cold coagulation. Contrary to what its name implies, this form of treatment is very hot. In fact, it is a more modern form of cauterization, simply not quite as hot as diathermy (see footnote). Unlike diathermy, which requires hospitalization and a general anaesthetic, cold coagulation can be done on an outpatient basis.

Cryocautery (cryotherapy, cryosurgery, cold cautery). This involves the use of a compressed gas, liquid nitrogen, which is released from a tank into a gun-shaped instrument. It expands rapidly to produce intense cold, freezing the tissue and destroying it. The destroyed cells slough off allowing other new cells to replace them. The sloughing may result in a watery discharge (which may be profuse at first) for two or three weeks, and possibly spotting or bleeding. Cryocautery can destroy cells to a depth of 3 to 4 mm and is therefore unsuitable if there are underlying abnormalities. It is becoming increasingly less used for CIN for this reason, but it is used to treat other conditions, such as chronic cervicitis or endometriosis of the cervix.

Discomfort from Outpatient Treatments

Although these treatments do not take long, you should take them seriously and give yourself time to deal with the physical and psychological effects. Take someone with you to the hospital for support and in case you feel shaky. You may feel fragile for a while. Take the day off work, have someone look after the children and/or have someone at home to fuss over you. You will need a supply of sanitary pads.

Contrary to what medical students are taught, the cervix can be very sensitive. Women vary quite a lot in how much we may feel. Doing anything to the cervix can result in uterine contractions, which we may feel as cramps. This is a common reaction with laser treatment, and a burning sensation is sometimes experienced too. With cryocautery, additional sensations may include hot flushing, dizziness or headache. In one recent study, approximately half the women experienced considerable distress during or after outpatient treatment by either cryocautery or laser.[49] There are wide variations in the provision of pain relief for outpatient treatment and you may want to discuss this before you embark on treatment, particularly if your cervix felt very sensitive during a smear or colposcopy examination. It is a scandal that women are not always offered pain relief for these treatments.

Other Negative Effects

Aside from pain during and immediately after the procedure, a possible negative effect is that an invasive cancer might be missed, either by inaccurate diagnosis, or by not treating sufficient area of tissue (hence the importance of a skilled colposcopist – see box). In addition, these treatments share with cone biopsy (see p. 528) the possibility that subsequent smears may be difficult to interpret. However, skilled practitioners can minimize tissue damage; laser tends to damage remaining tissue least.

For women who may wish to become pregnant in the future, these procedures appear to cause less potential problems than cone biopsy with regard to fertility, pregnancy and birth.

After the Treatments

The advice given to women seems to vary with each specialist, but basically you should not douche, use tampons or have sex involving penetration for ten to fourteen days, to minimize pain and the risk of infection.* It might be wise to use condoms for six weeks until the tissue has healed. Orgasms do not harm the healing and may well help, as well as helping you feel good about your body. Your next period may not be on time.

Some women recommend drinking raspberry-leaf tea and calendula tea to help the healing process, and eating foods high in potassium (bananas, dates, green leafy vegetables, citrus fruits), as a lot of potassium is lost in the discharge and needs to be replaced.

Your follow-up smear test or colposcopy appointment should be arranged four to six months later to check that all the abnormal area was treated and that the cervix has healed.

---

*The type of cauterization normally used then (called electrocautery or cervical diathermy) required a general anaesthetic and has largely been replaced by the treatments discussed here.

*Some people say avoid these for one month to encourage healing to take place.

COLPOSCOPY

A colposcope is a lighted magnifying instrument like a small pair of binoculars on a stand. It enables the colposcopist, who may be your gynaecologist, to view the cervix and vaginal walls very clearly while you are lying on your back with a speculum inserted, as if having a smear test. Some colposcopes allow two people to view your cervix at the same time, and to take photographs of your cervix, or to project a picture of it on to a large screen, so that you too can see what's going on if you wish. Colposcopy has revolutionized the diagnosis and treatment of CIN.* It can confirm whether there is any suspicion of invasive cancer and, provided there is none, *and* that the whole extent of the transformation zone can be examined, then 'conservative' (i.e., outpatient) treatment becomes possible.

However, colposcopy is not available in all areas. The Royal College of Obstetricians and Gynaecologists study group in 1982 concluded: 'ideally no patient with CIN should be treated unless there has been prior colposcopic assessment.'[50] It is worth insisting on this, particularly before agreeing to cone biopsy or hysterectomy. You may still need such an operation, but the area requiring surgery will have been clearly identified and assessed by colposcopy.

It is of course essential that you are seen by an experienced colposcopist. Find out your specialist's experience and reputation, if necessary by asking her/him.

COLPOSCOPY AS A DIAGNOSTIC TOOL

First of all, the colposcopist looks at the cervix and vaginal walls to see if s/he can see anything abnormal. Then a repeat smear is done and swabs may be taken. The area is cleaned with a mild saline solution, and then acetic acid (mild vinegar) solution and an iodine solution are applied to show up any abnormal tissue. As abnormal tissue does not take up the iodine stain, the areas needing further testing are obvious. (This is known as Schiller's test.)

One or more cervical biopsies are taken. This involves pinching out tiny samples of tissue from these abnormal areas with an instrument like a long pair of scissors. These are put in small containers and sent for examination. Some women feel a stinging sensation when the biopsies are being taken and there may be some bleeding and cramping.

Very occasionally an endocervical curettage may be done next if the transformation zone is hidden in the cervical canal. This involves inserting a sharp-bladed instrument into the cervical canal to ensure cells from your transformation zone are collected. Although it doesn't last long, the pain from an endocervical curettage can be intense. You may want to ensure adequate analgesia if an endocervical curettage is necessary (you can know this in advance by asking the doctor who takes your smear).

Having a colposcopy does not require analgesics or anaesthetics though the procedure can take up to half an hour, which some women find physically or psychologically uncomfortable. Visualizing something enjoyable or talking to the nurse can help. If your legs are in stirrups, you can ask for them to be adjusted if they are uncomfortable.

Despite all the grimness of the colposcopy examination, the most undignified aspect was being fitted with an NHS standard issue tie-on sanitary pad in case any iodine or blood escaped.

Staff bustled about the room in preparation for the next victim, and I stood staring at the doctor's back. He turned. 'Any questions?' Thousands! Timidly I shook my head, clasped the back of my gown with one hand, and gracefully made an exit. It appeared I had survived my first test for cancer.[51]

After the examination, my gynaecologist sat me and my friend down, drew diagrams to explain what he had done, and told us what he thought was happening to my cervix. This gave us the confidence to ask the many questions we had, and having my friend there meant we could remember more of what he said.

Note: The results may take at least three or four weeks to come through (not least because of NHS cuts which are affecting laboratories' workload), so you may want to check when – and how – you will be informed of the result. Some colposcopy clinics are using a process of frozen sections to speed up the diagnosis. Results are available in minutes and outpatient treatment can be given at the same appointment. This will not suit some women who want or need time to consider their diagnosis and treatment options, or who wish to try alternatives or self-help. Be wary of being offered immediate treatment unless you would rather it all be done at once. The first time you meet the colposcopist would be the time to tell her/him you would like to take things slowly and have time to ask a lot of questions. It helps a lot at this stage to have a friend with you (see WHRRIC leaflet *The Investigation and Treatment of Abnormal Cervical Cells* in Resources).

*Colposcopy is also used in connection with certain vaginal and vulval problems too.

CONE BIOPSY (CONIZATION)

Cone biopsy is both treatment and diagnosis. It involves removing a cone-shaped part from the cervix for detailed examination under a microscope to determine, more accurately than a cervical smear or colposcopy can, the abnormalities that exist in the cell and tissue structures and the depth to which these have gone. The aim is to remove all the abnormal cells and a clear area of healthy tissue beyond them.

It can be difficult to determine how extensive to make the cone; if you are keen to bear children, the surgeon may be prepared to be 'conservative'. If the edge of the cone shows abnormal cells, further treatment is required. Prior colposcopy can help with assessing the extent of the cone required.

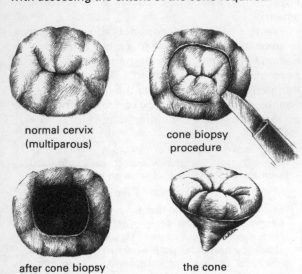

normal cervix (multiparous)

cone biopsy procedure

after cone biopsy

the cone

CONE BIOPSY

Cone biopsy used to be the standard treatment for abnormal cervical cells. Because of the range of outpatient procedures now possible for treatment of CIN, only a minority of women may need to be referred for cone biopsy.[52]

Cone biopsy is a major surgical procedure and you may be in hospital for three or four days. Under general anaesthetic, it takes about twenty minutes to remove the cone and depending on whether the cone is deep or shallow, the new edges of the cervix are either sutured (sewn back) or cauterized (burned) or sometimes left. A dilatation and curettage (D & C) should be done at the same time, to exclude other forms of cancer. (If you want to avoid an unnecessary D & C, you may wish to discuss with your doctor the reasons why s/he may feel that a D & C is necessary.)

You return to the ward with a 'pack' in your vagina to help reduce bleeding; this is removed after six to twelve hours, depending on the preferences of the surgeon or the depth of the cut. There is rarely any discomfort.

Bleeding, infection and inflammation are short-term complications. If the bleeding is heavy, you should contact your doctor. You may want to take two weeks off work and have help from relatives and friends. Follow the advice given for the treatments for CIN (p. 526). Any stitches will be removed at your follow-up appointment.

I didn't find the cone biopsy a problem as such, but I was surprised and appalled that they felt they had to shave me for the procedure. Maybe in retrospect I would have argued against it, as I'm sure it wasn't necessary – it isn't even necessary for childbirth!

Long-term complications do occur in a significant minority of women. Cone biopsy can make future smears unreliable; one study found that 46 per cent of women needed additional measures, including dilatation, endocervical curettage, or even hysterectomy.[53] Scar tissue can make the cervix stiff (cervical stenosis), which can mean that menstrual blood cannot get through the cervical canal. Lack of menstruation when it is due, plus pain and bloating are warning signs. Further surgery may be necessary to reopen the cervical canal. Cone biopsy can also lead to an increased risk of mid-trimester abortion and difficulties in delivery – either because of cervical stenosis, or because the cervix has been weakened (the medical term for which is 'incompetent cervix'). However, while of all the treatment procedures cone biopsy carries the biggest risk of long-term complications, pregnancy and labour do not appear to be affected in the majority of women.[54] In addition, there is very little evidence that cone biopsy adversely affects the ability to conceive.

A repeat cone biopsy is sometimes possible, but if further orthodox medical diagnosis or treatment were necessary, a hysterectomy would usually be considered the only option.

I did eventually with the help of friends find a sympathetic consultant who would do a third cone biopsy, but it meant being in an unknown town on my own and I was tired of being a patient so decided on the hysterectomy.

INVASIVE CANCER OF THE CERVIX

*When some people heard I had cervical cancer,
they implied that it was somehow my fault, I had
caused it. Then when I was cured, they considered
I hadn't had a 'real' cancer. These attitudes made
it all the more difficult to live with.*

If abnormal cells on the cervix spread into the underlying tissues, you have invasive cervical cancer. When it is very shallow, under 5 mm, it is called 'micro-invasive'. When it is more than 5 mm, it is a frank invasive cancer and the lymph system and other organs may be affected. Major deposits can be detected with general tests, but as tiny spreads may not be obvious in these tests, treatment decisions are made on the assumption that spread has occurred to ensure any possible cancer is treated.

Cervical cancer is graded according to the stage of its development from I (an early cancer) to IV (a very advanced cancer), and depending on whether it can be seen or felt by the consultant, and whether the tumour is restricted to the cervix, the pelvic area or has spread.

*It was very difficult to believe I had cancer. I
looked and felt well, I had no symptoms, no
irregular bleeding, no pain or bleeding with
intercourse, no discomfort in my pelvic region. But
I had an early cancer and it was successfully
treated.*

In the later stages of cervical cancer there would be symptoms such as bleeding between periods, chronic discharge, pain or bleeding on intercourse, pelvic discomfort, swelling of the legs, loss of weight, and problems with bladder function.

How good a recovery you make depends on a number of factors, including your age, general health, the stage of your cancer, the success of the treatment and your own inner resources. (See Cancer section, p. 567, for a discussion of 'cure' rates, orthodox, alternative and complementary therapies, a checklist of questions, and living and coping with cancer.)

Orthodox Treatment

The main treatments are hysterectomy (see p. 597), possibly including oophorectomy (removal of ovaries) and lymphectomy (removal of lymph nodes in the pelvic area); or radiotherapy; or a combination. These are frightening to face, particularly if you have not yet had children or would like more, and if you have not reached menopause. Removing both ovaries or radiotherapy would force an early menopause, and although hormone replacement therapy could be offered, it does have its own risks (see p. 456).

Because the above radical treatments are so successful, there has been little attempt to develop less damaging approaches which are less destructive to the woman. Considerable changes have been made in response to women's concerns about breast cancer treatment, so this could happen with cervical cancer too.

The treatment recommended will depend to some extent on the stage and type of your cancer, age and general health, as well as on the preference of the consultant and the hospital's facilities. No method has been shown to have a consistent advantage and it may be better to accept what the hospital does best.

A hysterectomy enables the extent of the cancer to be determined. In the early stages *all* malignant cells could be removed and you would be 'cured'. If examination of the tissue shows any spread, or even if it is not already proved to have spread, external radiotherapy (see p. 572) may be recommended after hysterectomy. Internal uterine or vaginal radiotherapy (involving the use of radio-isotope rods) may be used as well, or instead. The rods may need to stay in place for only a few minutes, but sometimes for a day or two, and the procedure may need to be repeated. Sometimes radio-isotope rods are placed inside the uterus while you are under a general anaesthetic. They can be extremely uncomfortable, so pain relief and sedation may be necessary while they are in place.

Side-effects of pelvic radiotherapy are: diarrhoea, cystitis, abdominal cramps and general tiredness. Although they can be severe, they usually settle down within four weeks. If after-care with douches is not advised, permanent scars can form in the vagina, which make vaginal penetration painful if not impossible. *If you have pelvic radiotherapy, make sure you are taught how to douche, and that you are given the equipment to do this.*

Chemotherapy (see p. 572) is sometimes offered as a treatment option. Given for relief of symptoms (including pain), it is said to have few side-effects. However, if it is offered to increase lifespan, the type of chemotherapy used is likely to result in fairly severe side-effects. Whether chemotherapy increases lifespan in relation to cervical cancer is a controversial subject and is currently being investigated in many centres. It is worth finding out the doctor's aims before embarking on any chemotherapy, and establishing whether you are part of a trial.

*Before my Wertheim's hysterectomy for an early
invasive cancer, I ate an extremely good diet,
increased my running, did relaxation exercises. I
also cried a lot, came to terms with the decision,
had good support from my partner and friends. I
made an excellent recovery and was running four
weeks later. The relief it is all over is tremendous.*

Whichever treatment you receive, you will be offered regular check-ups for at least five years. Please see p. 582 for a discussion on living with cancer.

CERVICAL SCREENING AND WOMEN AT RISK

Rewritten together with CHRIS BENNETT

Cervical screening is a political issue. Although it can prevent many unnecessary and premature deaths from cervical cancer, the government refuses to fund an effective screening programme. Eighty per cent of the women who die from this disease have never had a smear. Older, working-class women are less likely to be offered a smear by their general practitioner, and less likely to attend other clinics (such as family planning, ante-natal clinics) where smears are offered routinely.

Government policy aims to encourage screening programmes for women over the age of thirty-five every five years.* Yet even the government advises the inclusion of younger women and many experts advise shorter intervals between tests. You will also see from p. 524 and below that certain groups of women, whatever their age, should have smears *annually*. Needless to say, the government has not provided finance to enable health authorities effectively to carry out the minimal screening programme required.

While an effective screening programme is worth campaigning for, it must be remembered that screening is a limited preventive tool. Some cases, false negatives, are inevitably missed, particularly if diagnostic facilities by means of colposcopy have not been expanded. And true prevention involves tackling the causes – see below and Self-help box on p. 525.

Finally, screening programmes have their own costs. One cost which may be overlooked is the anxiety and damage caused to women who have positive smear results and then treatment for conditions which may never have had the potential to become life-threatening.

Women at Risk from Cervical Cancer

The reasons why some women develop abnormal cervical cells is not understood, but some women are at greater risk of developing this disease. We know that cervical cancer is a disease of women who are, or have been, heterosexually active, and that it is very rare in virgins. It is a disease primarily of poor women – cervical cancer is five times more common in social class V than it is in social class I. It is 40 per cent more common in the north-west compared to the south-east of England, and is the biggest cancer killer of women in the Third World.

Because cervical cancer appears to be a disease only of women who have been heterosexually active, the focus of medical interest has tended to be on women's sexual behaviour. This is damaging: we end up being 'blamed' for getting the disease, while the other possible causes of cervical cancer are completely overlooked in the obsession with uncovering our past sexual history.

In fact, a wide variety of factors is associated with increased risk of cancer of the cervix:

Age. Cancer of the cervix has always been a disease of older women, affecting predominantly women over fifty. There has, however, been an increase over the past ten years in younger women. Yet younger women make up 6 per cent of all cervical cancer deaths (about 120 a year). It is thought that early age of first intercourse may play a part in

predisposing women to cancer of the cervix later on, the theory being that the cells of the immature cervix are particularly vulnerable to carcinogenic agents (which might include sperm, chemicals, dust or other environmental hazards). *This means that the use of barrier methods of contraception is particularly important for younger women* (see Chapter 15).

Diet. Low levels of Vitamins A and C and folic acid have been found to be relevant to the incidence of cervical cancer. Both smoking and use of the contraceptive pill can reduce levels of these vitamins in the body (see Cancer, p. 577, for a discussion of the role of diet generally and suggestions for improving it).

Smoking. Women who smoke have an increased risk of cancer of the cervix. The risk may be three to seven times greater than for non-smokers and is particularly high at fifteen or more cigarettes a day. Other people's smoking also has an effect: nicotine has been found in the urine, breast fluid and cervical mucus of both smokers and non-smokers.

Contraception. Use of the contraceptive pill increases the risk (see p. 294); the use of barrier methods of contraception reduces it. One study suggested the risk for diaphragm-users was a quarter that of Pill-users, while use of the condom has been associated with the reversal to normal of abnormal cell changes in 98 per cent of women in one study (see p. 525).

Occupational risks. Women married to men whose work involves contact with substances such as dust, metal, chemicals, asbestos, tar, machine oil and coal have been shown to have an increased risk of cervical cancer. This risk may be reduced if adequate washing facilities are available (both at work and at home) and if men are educated about the importance of ensuring that their genitals and hands are kept clean. Women's occupation is also a factor: women who work in the textile industry, especially spinners, appear to be at increased risk. Again, hygiene may help, as may barrier methods of contraception.

Exposure to genital wart virus (HPV). Women with genital warts appear to have a greatly increased chance of developing CIN. Similarly, the woman whose male partner is infected with genital warts, especially penile, is at increased risk (see p. 500). We can protect ourselves from exposure to the wart virus to some extent by using barrier methods of contraception. We can also avoid other factors associated with the promotion of cervical cancer (particularly the Pill) and it has been suggested recently that women with visible warts should have a colposcopy even if their smear is normal.[55] *Annual smears are recommended if you have been exposed to wart virus, particularly HPV 16, 18, or 33.*

Exposure to genital herpes virus. This appears to be a risk factor too, although not as great as was originally thought – see Herpes, p. 496. An annual smear test may be reassuring. Again, barrier methods of contraception are likely to help prevent spread.

Sexual intercourse with a man who has a past history of sexually transmitted infections, especially warts or herpes,

*But see footnote on p. 523.

or with a man whose previous partner developed cervical cancer. Non-monogamous heterosexual relationships are also regarded as a factor, although it is important to see this in the context of the factors listed above. While statistically each additional male partner increases the risk, our male partner's sexual history, contraceptive use and the number of partners *he* has may be what puts us at risk. We can protect ourselves by insisting on using condoms or other safer sex practices (see p. 488).

Stress – and how we deal with it – also plays a role. See Cancer, p. 574, for details; see also Kinesis in Resources.

This list can seem frightening and demoralizing. *It is very important, however, to see 'risk factors' in perspective:* just because many risk factors might apply to you does not mean that you will get cervical cancer. And if knowledge about how to minimize our chances of cancer were widely available, there would be even less chance of our getting it, even if many risk factors applied to us – see Self-help, p. 525, and Cancer, p. 568.

The increase in cervical cancer in younger age groups has been blamed on the 'sexual revolution'. But it is unlikely that the so-called 'sexual revolution' started in the industrial towns of the north-west of England while London and the south-east lagged behind. Doctors defend the Pill by saying Pill-takers have more sexual partners than other women, but female mice get cervical cancer when they are exposed to synthetic hormones and nobody suggests it is their promiscuity that causes it.

Prevention of cervical cancer does not require a moral crusade but access to information about those factors which influence our health. Neither is more screening on its own the right answer. Real prevention means removal of the *causes* of ill health before disease starts.

Doctors are too ready to prescribe the Pill on the basis that preventing pregnancy now is worth the increased risk of cancer later on. Young women are advised to have smear tests when *real* prevention would mean the use of barrier methods of contraception and other safer sex practices, removing occupational risk factors, ensuring an adequate diet, etcetera. Young people need appropriate sex education so that they can enjoy their sexuality while protecting themselves from risk, whether of cervical cancer, HIV and other STDs, or unwanted pregnancy.

WHAT WOMEN CAN DO ABOUT CERVICAL CANCER

- If heterosexually active, use a barrier method of contraception or other safer sex practices.
- Be aware of the need for washing before sex – especially if you or your partner has a dirty or dusty job or hobby.
- Consider our other self-help guidelines on p. 525.
- Find out about the arrangements for screening and diagnostic follow-up in your area.
- Use your community health council to ensure that your health authority provides a truly effective service. To do so, it needs to ensure that

plenty of female staff are available to provide a screening service, open at hours to suit all women's needs; that all people who take and assess smears are adequately trained;* that staffing levels in laboratories are adequate; that an adequate colposcopy service exists; and that an efficient invitation and recall system is established.

For further information about prevention of cancer in general, see p. 568.

NOTES

1. *British Journal of Venereal Disease*, June 1981.

2. John C. Cutler. 'Venereal Disease Prevention', *Cutis*, vol. 27, March 1981, pp. 321–7.

3. Edward Brecher. *Journal of Sex Research*, vol. 11, no. 4, November 1975, pp. 318–28; see also John C. Cutler et al. 'Vaginal Contraceptives as Prophylaxis against Gonorrhea and Other Sexually Transmissable Diseases', *Advances in Planned Parenthood*, vol. 12, no. 1, Excerpta Medica, 1977, pp. 45–56.

4. Hershel Jick et al. *Journal of the American Medical Association*, vol. 248, 1982, pp. 1619–21.

5. See *American Journal of Obstetrics and Gynecology*, vol. 159, no. 1, July 1988, p. 32.

6. A. Blackwell et al. 'Anaerobic Vaginosis', *The Lancet*, 17 December 1983.

7. H. Hunter Hansfield. 'Nongonococcal Urethritis', *Cutis*, vol. 27, March 1981, p. 270.

8. 'Mycoplasma Infection Linked to Prematurity Risk', *Ob/Gyn News*, 1 August 1981; Ruth Kunsdin. 'Mycoplasmas in Humans: Significance of Ureaplasma Urealyticum', *H.L.S.*, vol. 13, no. 2, 1976, p. 144; Jan

Freiburg. 'Mycoplasmas, Ureaplasmas, Infertility and Abortion', *Fertility and Sterility*, vol. 36, no. 1, July 1981, pp. 88–91.

9. From a letter to *H.A. News*, journal of the Herpes Association (see Resources).

10. William Reeves et al. 'Risk of Recurrence after First Episodes of Genital Herpes', *New England Journal of Medicine*, vol. 305, no. 6, August 1981, p. 159.

11. *British Medical Journal*, vol. 291, July 1985, p. 7.

12. Mindel et al. 'Dosage and Safety of Long-term Suppressive Acylovir Therapy for Recurrent Genital Herpes', *The Lancet*, 23 April 1988, pp. 926–8.

13. John Grossman et al. 'Management of Genital Herpes Simplex Virus Infection During Pregnancy', *Obstetrics and Gynaecology*, July 1981, p. 159.

---

*Even consultant pathologists can have astonishingly limited experience in assessing cervical cytology.[56]

14. Singer Campion. 'Increased Risk of Cervical Neoplasia in Consorts of Men with Penile Condylomata Acuminata', *The Lancet*, vol. 1, 8435, 27 April 1986, pp. 943–6.

15. N. Robinson and V. Beral. 'Trends in Pelvic Inflammatory Disease in England and Wales', *Journal of Epidemiology and Community Health*, 35, 1981, pp. 265–70.

16. *New Scientist*, 20 September 1984 and 18 April 1985.

17. Adler et al. 'Morbidity Associated with Pelvic Inflammatory Diseases', *British Journal of Venereal Diseases*, 58, 1982, pp. 151–7.

18. US Department of Health and Human Services, Public Health Service, Centers for Disease Control, Center for Prevention Services, Venereal Disease Control Division. 'Sexually Transmitted Diseases Treatment Guidelines, 1982', *Morbidity and Mortality Weekly Report Supplement*, vol. 31, no. 25, 20 August 1982, pp. 435–45.

19. Information from Vancouver Women's Health Research Collective, 1501 West Broadway, Vancouver BC, Canada V6J 1W6.

20. Sandra K. Webster. 'Problems for Diagnosis of Spasmodic and Congestive Dysmenorrhea', in A. Dan et al., *The Menstrual Cycle, Vol. 1*. New York: Springer, 1980, pp. 292–304.

21. Sharon Golub. 'The Effect of Premenstrual Anxiety and Depression on Cognitive Function', *Journal of Personality and Social Psychology*, vol. 34, no. 1, 1976, pp. 99–104; Sharon Golub and Denise Murphy Huntington. 'Premenstrual and Menstrual Mood Changes in Adolescent Women', *Journal of Personality and Social Psychology*, vol. 14, no. 5, 1981, pp. 961–5.

22. Elizabeth R González. 'Premenstrual Syndrome: an Ancient Woe Deserving of Modern Scrutiny', *Journal of the American Medical Association*, vol. 245, no. 14, 10 April 1980, pp. 1393–6.

23. See, for example, G. E. Abraham and J. T. Hargrove. 'Effects of Vitamin B on Premenstrual Symptomatology in Women with Premenstrual Syndrome: a Double Blind Crossover Study', *Infertility*, vol. 3, 1980, pp. 155–65; and D. F. Horrobin. 'The Role of Essential Fatty Acids and Prostaglandins in the Premenstrual Syndrome', *Journal of Reproductive Medicine*, vol. 28, 1983, pp. 465–8.

24. Personal conversation with Penny Budoff MD, based on her clinical experience.

25. I. Brosens, I. and F. Cornillie. 'Peritoneal Endometriotic Implants'. Paper presented to the first International Symposium on Endometriosis, Clermont-Ferrand, France, 19–21 November 1986. Published in M. A. Bruhat and M. Canis (eds) *Endometriosis*, vol. 164 of *Contributions to Gynecology and Obstetrics* (series ed. P. J. Keller). New York: Karger, 1987.

26. J. L. Simpson et al. 'Heritable Aspect of Endometriosis', *American Journal of Obstetrics and Gynecology*, vol. 137, 1980, p. 327.

27. J. V. Meigs. 'Medical Treatment of Endometriosis and Significance of Endometriosis', *Surg. Gynaecol. Obstet.*, vol. 89, 1949, p. 317.

28. For example, D. L. Chatman. 'Endometriosis and the Black Woman', *Journal of Reproductive Medicine*, vol. 16, 1976, p. 303.

29. See, e.g., R. A. L. Low, A. D. G. Roberts and D. A. R. Lees. 'A Comparative Study of Various Dosages of Danazol in the Treatment of Endometriosis', *British Journal of Obstetrics and Gynaecology*, vol. 91, 1980, pp. 167–71.

30. W. P. Dmowski and M. R. Cohen. 'Antigonadotrophin (Danazol) in the Treatment of Endometriosis: Evaluation of Post-treatment Fertility and Three-year Follow-up Data', *American Journal of Obstetrics and Gynecology*, vol. 130, 1978, p. 41.

31. W. Matta. 'Preliminary Findings on Buserelin and Danazol', presented at an Endometriosis Society Workshop, London, 1986.

32. D. Horrobin. 'Findings on Evening Primrose Oil', presented at an Endometriosis Society Workshop, London, 1985.

33. O. Truss. *The Missing Diagnosis* (available from P.O. Box 26508, Birmingham, Alabama 35226, USA), 1983.

34. R. B. Greenblatt. *Recent Advances in Endometriosis*. International Congress serial no. 368, Augusta, GA. New York: Elsevier, 1975.

35. James Scott. 'How to Induce Ovarian Cancer and How Not to', leader in *British Medical Journal*, 29 September 1984.

36. See Brigham and Woman's Hospital Study reported in *Cancer*, 15 July 1982. See also D. L. Longo and R. C. Young. 'Cosmetic Talc and Ovarian Cancer', *The Lancet*, vol. 2, August 1979, pp. 349–51.

37. J. Laurence. 'The Cervical Cancer Scandal', *New Society*, 16 October 1987, p. 23.

38. Al Garthwaite. 'A Smear in Time . . .', *Spare Rib*, no. 68, March 1978. (What happens when a smear is positive: a personal experience with some medical details.)

39. See, e.g., J. Elwood et al. 'Are Patients with Abnormal Smears Adequately Managed?' *British Medical Journal*, 6 October 1984, p. 6449; and C. D. Ritchie and P. Last. Correspondence in *British Medical Journal*, vol. 289, 1984, p. 1224.

40. For example, see Spurrett et al. *The Lancet*, 30 January 1988, p. 237.

41. A. C. Richardson and J. B. Lyon. 'The Effect of Condom Use on Squamous Cell Cervical Intraepithelial Neoplasia', *American Journal of Obstetrics and Gynecology*, vol. 140, 1981, p. 909.

42. Personal communication from the authors of the study conveyed to Jean Robinson.

43. See, e.g., R. W. C. Harris et al. 'Characteristics of Women with Dysplasia or Carcinoma In Situ of the Cervix Uteri', *British Journal of Cancer*, vol. 42, 1980, pp. 359–69; and N. H. Wright et al. 'Neoplasia and Dysplasia of the Cervix Uteri and Contraception: a Possible Protective Effect of the Diaphragm', *British Journal of Cancer*, vol. 38, 1978, pp. 273–9.

44. See, e.g., M. P. Vessey et al. 'Neoplasia of the Cervix Uteri and Contraception: a Possible Adverse Effect of the Pill', *The Lancet*, 22 October 1983, pp. 930–4; leader article, 'Oral Contraceptives and Neoplasia', *The Lancet*, 22 October 1983, pp. 947–8; World Health Organization Collaborative Study of Neoplasia and Steroid Contraceptives, 'Invasive Cervical Cancer and Combined Oral Contraceptives', *British Medical Journal*, 30 March 1985, pp. 961–5; Harris et al, op. cit., note 43. See also Brinton et al. *International Journal of Cancer*, vol. 38, 1986, pp. 339–44; and V. Beral and C. Kay. 'Oral Contraceptive Use and Malignancies of the Genital Tract', *The Lancet*, 10 December 1988, p. 1331.

45. See E. Stern et al., 'Steroid Contraceptive Use and Cervical Dysplasia: Increased Risk of Progression', *Science*, vol. 196, 1977, pp. 1460–2; and leader article, 'Cervical Neoplasia and the Pill', *The Lancet*, 24 September 1977, p. 644.

46. Malcolm Potts and Peter Diggory. *Textbook of Contraceptive Practice* (2nd ed.). Cambridge: Cambridge University Press, 1983.

47. P. N. Bamford et al., 'An Analysis of Factors Responsible for Progression or Regression of Mild and Moderate Cervical Dyskaryosis', *British Journal of Family Planning*, vol. 11, 1985, pp. 5–8.

48. See, e.g., Royal College of General Practitioners. *Oral Contraceptives and Health*. London: Pitman Medical, 1974.

49. T. Posner and M. Vessey. *The Consequences of an Abnormal Cervical Smear: Women's Experiences*. London: King's Fund, 1987. See also I. E. Lowles et al. 'Women's Recollection of Pain During and After Carbon Dioxode Laser Treatment to the Uterine Cervix', *British Journal of Obstetrics and Gynaecology*, vol. 90, December 1983, p. 1157. The latter found that although most of the women who answered a postal questionnaire found laser caused only 'very slight' pain at worst, for almost half pain relief was necessary, and 5 per cent required a general anaesthetic to complete the treatment.

50. J. A. Jordan et al. *Proceedings of the Study Group*. London: Royal College of Gynaecologists, 1982.

51. Vonne Solis. 'My Story, Our Story', *Healthsharing*, Autumn 1981. About the experience of cervical cancer, colposcopy, etc. Available from WHRRIC (see Organizations).

52. J. A. Singer et al. *British Medical Journal*, 20 October 1984.

53. J. B. Trimbos et al. 'Reliability of Cytological Follow-up after Conization of the Cervix', *British Journal of Obstetrics and Gynaecology*, vol. 90, December 1983, p. 1141.

54. T. Weber and E. B. Obel. 'Pregnancy Complications Following Conization of the Uterine Cervix', *Acta Obstet. Gynecol. Scand.*, vol. 58, 1979, p. 3475.

55. N. G. Haddad et al. *British Medical Journal*, 2 July 1988, pp. 29–30.

56. See letter from I. G. Coulter, *The Independent*, 26 September 1987.

RESOURCES*
PUBLICATIONS

ENDOMETRIOSIS

Endometriosis Society. *Endometriosis: A Collection of Papers*, 1987 (available from the Endometriosis Society – see Organizations).

Fox, A. and B. **Fox**. *DPLA – an End to Chronic Pain and Depression*. New York: Long Shadow Books, 1985.

Graham, J. *Evening Primrose Oil*. Wellingborough, Northants: Thorsons, 1984.

Greenblatt, R. B. *Recent Advances in Endometriosis*. International Congress serial no. 368, Augusta GA, 1975. New York: Elsevier, 1976.

Grist, L. *A Woman's Guide to Alternative Medicine*. London: Fontana, 1986.

Hawkridge, Caroline. *Understanding Endometriosis*. London: Macdonald Optima, forthcoming.

Horrobin, D. F. 'Efamol and Efamol Marine in Endometriosis', in Endometriosis Society, *Endometriosis: A Collection of Papers*, 1987 (available from the Endometriosis Society).

O'Connor, D. T. *Endometriosis*, vol. 12 of *Current Reviews in Obstetrics and Gynaecology* (series eds A. Singer and J. Jordan). Edinburgh: Churchill Livingstone, 1987. A very good up-to-date summary.

Older, J. *Endometriosis: A Woman's Guide*. New York: Scribners (for information on how to obtain this – contact the Endometriosis Society).

Passwater, R. A. *Selenium as Food and Medicine*. New Canaan, CT: Keats, 1986.

Pleshette, J. *Cures that Work*. London: Century, 1986.

Sampson, J. A. 'Intestinal Adenomas of Endometrial Type', *Archives of Surgery*, vol. 5, pp. 217–80.

Weinstein, Kate. *Living with Endometriosis*. New York: Addison-Wesley, 1987 (available from the Endometriosis Society).

MENSTRUATION

Birke, Lynda and Katy **Gardner**. *Why Suffer? Periods and Their Problems*. London: Virago, 1982. By employing a feminist approach to period problems this book does not fall into the trap of treating periods as though they were a disease and women as though we were incapable. Needs updating, however.

Budoff, Penny Wise. *No More Menstrual Cramps and Other Good News*. London: Penguin Books, 1982. A medical approach to cramps and several other gynaecological problems.

Carpenter, Moira. *Curing PMT the Drug-free Way*. London: Century, 1985. Detailed advice on the role of nutrition, nutritional supplements and alternative remedies.

Dalton, Katharina. *Once a Month*. London: Fontana, 1984. This book is about progesterone therapy and is written by its greatest proponent.

Dan, Alice, et al. *The Menstrual Cycle: Volume 1: A Synthesis of Interdisciplinary Research*. New York: Springer, 1980. Good research papers covering a variety of topics.

Harrison, Michelle. 'Self Help for Premenstrual Syndrome', from Matrix Press, PO Box 740, Cambridge, Massachusetts 02238, USA. A self-help manual addressing the following: what is PMS? whom does it affect? where to start in treating PMS – diet, vitamins and minerals, progesterone, antiprostaglandins, diuretics, acupuncture, exercise, psychotherapy, stress reduction, peer support.

Kingston, Beryl. *Lifting the Curse: How to Relieve Painful Periods*. London: Sheldon Press, 1984.

Laws, Sophie, and Valerie **Hey**. *Seeing Red: the Politics of Premenstrual Tension*. London: Hutchinson Explorations in Feminism, 1984. A feminist critique of the concept of PMT and the way it has been used to put us down.

National Childbirth Trust, *Self-help with Period Problems*.

PMS Times, ed. Pat Britten, 19 St Stephen's Gardens, London W2 5QU; £2 for six issues. An excellent newsletter for PMS sufferers with news, views and debates about treatments.

Nazaro, Anne et al. *The PMT Solution*. Adamantine Press, 1986.

Sanders, Diana. *Coping with Periods*. Edinburgh: Chambers, 1985. A holistic approach to period problems from a feminist perspective.

Shreeve, Caroline. *The Premenstrual Syndrome*. Wellingborough, Northants: Thorsons, 1984.

Weidegger, Paula. *Female Cycles*. London: Women's Press, 1978.

WHRRIC, *Premenstrual Syndrome*, factsheet available from WHRRIC, (see Organizations).

Wright, Erna. *Periods Without Pain*. London: Tandem, 1966.

CERVIX

Barker, G. H. *Your Smear Test*. London: Adamson Books, 1987. May be useful if you are facing colposcopy.

Barnett, Robin. 'My experiences healing myself', in 'A Feminist Approach to Pap Smears'. *Kinesis* (see below).

Buckley, J. D., et al. 'Case control study of the husbands of women with dysplasia or carcinoma in situ of the cervix uteri.' *Lancet*, 11 September 1982.

Campion, M. et al. 'Complacency in Diagnosis of Cervical Cancer'. *British Medical Journal*. Vol. 294. 1987, pp. 1337–9.

DHSS. Health Services Management. Cervical Cancer Screening. Health Circular. DHSS. 12 January 1988.

Giles, J. A., et al. 'Colposcopic Assessment of the Accuracy of Cervical Cytology Screening'. *British Medical Journal*, vol. 296, 1988, pp. 1099–1102.

Jordan, J. A. 'The management of pre-malignant conditions of the cervix', in *Progress in Obstetrics and Gynaecology*, Studd, J. (ed.) Churchill Livingstone, 1982.

Jordan, J. A. 'Minor Degrees of Cervical Intraepithelial Neoplasia – Time to establish a multicentre prospective study to resolve the question'. *British Medical Journal*, 2 July 1988, p. 6.

Kinesis. 'A Feminist Approach to Pap Smears. *Kinesis* Supplement, February 1983 (Canada). Available from WHRRIC (see organizations). Excellent.

Robertson, J. H., et al. 'Risk of Cervical Cancer Associated with Mild Dyskaryosis'. *British Medical Journal*, 2 July 1988, pp. 18–21.

Robinson, Jean. 'Cervical cancer: a feminist critique'. *The Times Health Supplement*, 27 November 1981. On file at WHRRIC (see organizations).

Robinson, Jean. 'Cancer of the Cervix: Occupational risks of husbands and wives and possible preventive strategies', in *Pre-clinical Neoplasia of the Cervix*. Royal College of Obstetricians and Gynaecologists: London, 1982.

Savage, Wendy and A. **McPherson**. 'Cervical Cytology', in *Women's Problems in General Practice*, McPherson, A. and Anderson, M. (eds.) 1981.

Singer, Albert. Cervical Neoplasia and Young Women, *IPPF Medical Bulletin*, vol. 20, No. 3, 1986.

Skegg, D. C. G., et al. 'Importance of the male factor in cancer of the cervix'. *Lancet*, 11 September 1982, p. 581.

Trevathan E., et al. 'Cigarette smoking and dysplasia and carcinoma in situ of the uterine cervix'. *Journal of the American Medical Association*, vol. 250, 1983, pp. 499–502.

Walker, P. and A. **Singer**. 'Colposcopy: who, when, where and by whom?' *British Journal of Obstetrics and Gynaecology*, vol. 94, 1987, pp. 1011–13.

WHIC. *Women's Health and Cervical Cancer* and *An Abnormal Smear: What does that mean?* Two fact sheets, available from WHRRIC (see organizations).

MISCELLANEOUS

Adler, Michael. *ABC of Sexually Transmitted Diseases*. London: BMJ, 1984.

Barlow, David. *Sexually Transmitted Diseases: The Facts*. Oxford: Oxford University Press, 1981. Full of medical-school-type humour and nasty photographs, it is, however, a detailed guide to STDs, their symptoms and treatment.

Blanks, Sue and Carol **Woddis**. *The Herpes Manual*. London: Settle and Bendall (Wigmore), 1983. By two founder members of the Herpes

*For resources on HIV and AIDS, see Resources, Chapter 25.

Association. While nothing can be up to date in this field, this is a positive and supportive reader.

Chaitow, Leon. *Candida Albicans. Could Yeast Be Your Problem?* Wellingborough: Thorsons, 1986.

Clayton, Caroline. *Thrush*. London: Sheldon Press, 1984.

Duin, Nancy and Wendy **Savage**. *Hysterectomy: What It's All About*. London: Thames TV, 1982.

Kilmartin, Angela. *Cystitis: A Complete Self-help Guide*. London: Hamlyn, 1980.

Kilmartin, Angela. *Understanding Cystitis*. London: Arrow Heinemann, 1975.

Kilmartin, Angela. *Victims of Thrush and Cystitis*. London: Century Arrow, 1986.

Llewellyn Jones, Derek. *Herpes, AIDS and Other Sexually Transmitted Diseases*. London: Faber and Faber, 1985.

Nissim, Rina. *Natural Healing in Gynaecology*. London: Pandora, 1986. Plenty of self-help but hard to follow.

North, Barbara and Penelope **Crittendon**. *Stop Herpes Now! – a Self-Help Guide to Understanding and Controlling Herpes*. Wellingborough, Northants: Thorsons, 1983. Concentrates on nutrition and other complementary approaches.

PID, Information sheet available from WHRRIC (see Organizations).

Potts, Billie. *Witches Heal: Lesbian Herbal Self-sufficiency*. Hecuba's Daughter, 1981.

Smith, Carol. 'Vaginal Infections', *Spare Rib*, nos. 168–9, July and August 1986. Photocopies of this article and other leaflets on herbal remedies are available from WHRRIC (see Organizations).

FILMS AND VIDEOS

Chlamydia: Never Heard of It. Diverse Productions programme presented by Angela Phillips, April 1987.

Helping Yourself in Cystitis, UK, 1978, 20 mins. Distributed by Concord Films Council Ltd, 201 Felixstowe Road, Ipswich, Suffolk IP3 9BJ. Tel: 0473–726012.

Well Being: A Woman's Lot, Channel Four, 1983, 35 mins. Deals with premenstrual tension and painful or heavy periods.

Well Woman: Private Places, BBC, 1983, 25 mins. Deals with cystitis, and is recommended more highly than the above.

Well Woman – Rhythm and Blues, BBC, 1983, 25 mins. Women talk about periods.

ORGANIZATIONS

Endometriosis Society, 65 Holmdene Avenue, London SE24 9LD. Has a variety of publications, including an introduction to endometriosis in Asian languages. Enclose large sae.

Frontliners, 52–54 Gray's Inn Road, London WC1. Tel: 01–831 0330/01–404 4324 (answering machine). Self-help group for people with AIDS. Emotional and practical support.

Herpes Association, 41 North Road, London N7. Helpline: 01–609 9061. Runs a telephone counselling service and advice centre and can give you the name of your local group contact.

National AIDS Helpline, Tel: 0800–567 123.

National Association of PMS, 2nd floor, 25 Market Street, Guildford, Surrey GU1 4LB. Tel: 0483–572715. Helplines: 0483–572806 (day), 09592–4371 (night).

NHS PMS Clinics are available in some areas. Ask your GP or community health council. Some clinics, both NHS and private, are mainly concerned with hormone therapies. It is worth finding out first what approach is taken.

PID Support Group, c/o WHRRIC, 52–54 Featherstone Street, London EC1Y 8RT. Tel: 01–251 6580/6332. Groups of women who suffer from chronic PID share information and provide support to new sufferers.

Positively Women, Soho Hospital for Women, 15 Soho Square, London W1V 5TW. Tel: 01–734 1794 (day). Support group for women with HIV and AIDS.

PREMSOC PO Box 102, London SE1 7ES. For PMS sufferers and professionals interested in PMS. It assists self-help groups, runs seminars, answers general inquiries and provides some products at cut prices. (It does not recommend any particular form of treatment.) Send sae for information.

The Terrence Higgins Trust, BM AIDS, London WC1N 3XX. Tel: 01–242–1010. Provides support to AIDS sufferers and their friends.

Women's National Cancer Control Campaign, 1 South Audley Street, London W1. Tel: 01–499 7532.

Women's Health and Reproductive Rights Information Centre, 52–54 Featherstone Street, London EC1Y 8RT. Tel: 01–251 6580/6332.

CHOICE AND CONTROL IN BREAST DISEASE

Prepared by
THE TRANS-PENNINE BREAST CANCER GROUP*

Breast problems and breast diseases, particularly breast cancer, are a cause of great anxiety for many women. Many of us fear the possibility of losing a breast, and we may also have very mixed feelings about our breasts.

It is hardly surprising that we feel self-conscious when newspapers, cars, books and films are often promoted by displays of women's breasts, and men feel free to whistle or stare at our breasts or even to touch them uninvited.

It is common for us to associate our breasts with feeling womanly. Few of us like our breasts – they are too big or too small, not firm enough, the nipples are too large or small. This can affect how we feel about our own bodies and the way we assume others will view them.

Breast development is the most obvious outward sign of puberty, and likely to cause young women some anxiety and confusion. Many of us were self-conscious about our breasts – or lack of them – and several of us may have very vivid memories of this period, like the woman below:

Ann: *I was a late developer compared to the rest of my class at school and I was extremely aware of this. Fortunately my best friend was also, and when we did begin to develop breasts we would excitedly compare progress. For what seemed ages we both wore baggy jumpers to hide our flat chests and I clearly remember the day I first wore a bra, when I put on a tight jumper for the first time. We went on a family picnic and I think my mother had made my father aware of how important it all was for me. I remember him telling me how nice I looked. One advantage of waiting so long was that despite the fact that my breasts grew relatively large, this has never bothered me, in fact I rather like them.*

Society's image of women and our breasts is well illustrated by the focus on feminists as bra-burners. In the late 1960s, when women's liberation again became an active movement, this was the image perpetuated by the media. An important aspect of feminism in the last twenty years has been that women should decide for themselves how they want to dress, regardless of the dictates of fashion and male attitudes. Some women found that going bra-less was more comfortable and helped them to challenge male images of what is attractive. It should be said, however, that bra-less women are seen as being even more attractive by some men.

In contrast, the physiological importance of women's breasts receives little public attention. While we are told that breastfeeding is best, we are not supposed to do it in public, sometimes not even in front of friends and relatives. Some women enjoy breastfeeding and get sexual pleasure from their breasts. A few women can experience orgasm from breast stimulation alone.

Those mixed feelings which are likely to occur at puberty, when our bodies are changing so much, often continue with us throughout our lives because of society's attitudes. Our breasts do continue to change, maybe getting larger before periods, during pregnancy and breastfeeding and weight gain, and becoming smaller with loss of weight, after breastfeeding and at menopause and after. Our anxiety that people may not think we are attractive because of our breasts may be a reason why breast disease and breast problems, in particular breast cancer, can affect our confidence in ourselves to such a large degree. While all cancers are frightening, breast cancer seems to hold the most terror for us as women. The available research reports on causes and treatments are confusing, and experts often disagree. This makes it even more important that we become active participants in all stages of detection, treatment and decision-making.

---

*Judith Emanuel, Laura Potts, Lesley Thomson and Mary Twomey. The quotes in this chapter come mainly from interviews we conducted with seven women, whose autobiographical notes appear on p. 555.

FINDING SYMPTOMS OF BREAST PROBLEMS

Finding a lump or any kind of change in your breast can be a frightening and distressing experience, despite the fact that in the vast majority of instances the problem is benign – i.e. not cancerous. However, this is not particularly reassuring until an accurate diagnosis has been obtained. If a symptom cannot be accurately diagnosed as benign by a GP, many women will go through the anxiety of being referred for examinations to exclude breast cancer. Yet a large number of women who seek help about breast problems will not need a biopsy or surgical intervention to exclude the possibility of cancer. Although cancer is the breast disease that we fear most, it is not the most likely cause of breast lumps or discomfort.

I am stunned. Right under my fingers, as big as a wad of bubble gum, only harder, like the cap on a toothpaste tube. I feel it again, and my stomach jumps up into my chest.[1]

Most women find symptoms accidentally – in the bath or in bed, for example. Other women find them when doing self-examination, or they may be found through mammography (see p. 542).

Women react differently to finding a lump: trying to ignore it; telling a friend or relative who may be able to give support and then encourage us to take some action; or wanting to go to a GP as soon as possible. Some of us may decide to try to get rid of the lump by altering our diets or taking other self-help approaches (for example, see Things You Can Do Yourself, p. 538; see Cancer, p. 567, and Chapter 7). We may decide to get help from an alternative practitioner. If we do, we may also decide to have the problem diagnosed by having a biopsy – a medical procedure in which a section is removed and examined to find out what it is (see p. 537).

Making the decision to go to the GP can be difficult, partly because it means having to think about the possibility of having breast cancer.

Josephine: *It was like a shock . . . 'if I don't think about that and leave it for a while, it might go away, or maybe it's just a swollen gland' . . . think of a million and one things it can be rather than go have it out.*

Just as our reactions to finding breast symptoms differ, so do the reactions of GPs. You may find that your GP refers you to the local hospital immediately. Even though your symptoms may not be cancer, your GP may not have enough experience of breast diseases to detect this, so may refer you. An immediate referral can be very frightening.

Joan: *[My GP] just looked at it and said straight away that it needed checking. Well, then the rot set in. Then I worried, really worried.*

Not all GPs refer women so quickly, however. You may find that your GP tells you 'not to worry' or to 'keep an eye on it'. One woman described going to her GP for over three years with a lump:

Sue: *I still kept going to the doctor. He still kept patting me on the head, telling me it was nothing to worry about.*

Sue was eventually referred after she saw a different doctor who recognized that her anxiety was justified. It is important to remember that we have good reason to worry about symptoms of breast disease, as this can sometimes be undermined by GPs.

Laura: *[My GP said] 'Stop worrying about it because you're causing problems for yourself.' She made me feel really stupid for going in the first place.*

Laura eventually decided that she had been given bad medical advice and that she shouldn't take risks with her own health.

If you are not happy with your GP's response to your anxiety, you can try to see a different GP or go to a family planning clinic, well woman clinic, or well woman centre (see p. 630).

Once a referral has been made, a hospital appointment often comes quite quickly. This will involve attending the outpatient department where you will be 'clinically

---

SIGNS AND SYMPTOMS OF BREAST DISEASE

Breast
- Change in shape
- Change in size
- Puckering or dimpling of skin
- Enlarged veins
- Lump or thickening anywhere

Nipple
- Discharge (of any kind)

- Drawing in
- Rash on nipple or areola
- Lump or thickening
- Change in skin texture

Arm
- Swelling of upper arm
- Swelling in the armpit or above the breast

examined' by the doctor. This includes feeling for lumps (*palpating*), and comparing one breast with the other. After this examination the doctor may feel confident that the problem is benign and needs no immediate treatment, although this may be difficult for you to believe without concrete proof. Alternatively, the doctor may be fairly sure on your first visit that the problem is cancer – again this may be hard to believe, but this conclusion is based, for example, on the type of symptom, or the size, position and feel of the lump.

If a lump seems like a fluid-filled cyst (see p. 539), the doctor may try to 'aspirate' it immediately. If fluid is drawn off, the lump will immediately disappear, and that will be the end of your worries. However, whether you have an *aspiration* or not, you may be asked to go back in a few months, to see if the breast has changed or the lump recurs.

Another test that may be performed is *mammography* (X-ray of the breast), which can help with diagnosis and in pinpointing the exact position of the lump.

If you are anxious about the conclusions reached by the doctor examining you, ask for an explanation of how the conclusions have been reached. When you leave the hospital you should feel that necessary action is being taken, or feel reassured that you require no further help from the hospital at that time. If that is not the case, you will probably feel anxious and dissatisfied, with justification.

If you or the doctor is not convinced about the diagnosis (with or without mammography), a *biopsy* will probably be necessary. This does not mean you have cancer – in approximately 70 per cent of cases where a biopsy is performed, the symptoms are not caused by cancer.

BENIGN BREAST CONDITIONS

DISCOVERING THE SYMPTOMS ARE BENIGN

Helena: *I was on a high when I left the hospital. So much so that I almost knocked a man off his bicycle and mounted the pavement in my excitement at the realization that I had life ahead of me. I was also going to be released from the isolation of the unshared and unspoken-about experience. It was mid-June and everything looked glorious.*

Although the relief of being told we do not have cancer can be tremendous, we need information about our symptoms and explanations about the possible treatments. Too often this is forgotten by doctors, who assume that it is enough to tell us, 'Your lump is not malignant.'

Sometimes doctors refuse to take our symptoms seriously, even though they are benign. Yet some conditions, though benign, can be very painful. Women are often told that they must learn to live with such discomforts, with little recognition of the distress that this can cause.

The names which doctors give to benign breast problems are complicated and confusing, even among the 'experts', who find it hard to agree on the exact differences in classification between one condition and another. You

---

BIOPSY

Biopsy involves removing some breast tissue so that the cells can be examined under a microscope. It is the most accurate means of diagnosis. There are different types of biopsy; most are done under general anaesthetic. However, a *needle biopsy*, involving removal of a very small portion of tissue, can usually be done in an outpatient department. Results of a needle biopsy might be misleading because such a small portion of tissue is removed that cancer cells can be missed. The procedure can also be painful.

It may take a few days before the results of a biopsy are ready. However, some surgeons suggest taking a *biopsy under general anaesthetic* and examining the cells immediately, and then going straight on to further surgery if the diagnosis is cancer. This is called a *'frozen section' biopsy*. The advantage of this procedure is that it means that only one general anaesthetic will be necessary. The disadvantages include not only the fact that the diagnosis is less thorough (and therefore potentially less accurate), but also that we have no opportunity to consider treatment options.

Despite the problems with frozen sections, some of us may prefer to get all the surgery over in one go and avoid a second anaesthetic. But for many of us, the thought of having an operation without knowing whether or not we will wake up having lost a breast is very frightening. You do not have to agree to a frozen section and should find out what the surgeon's intentions are and clearly state your views before deciding whether or not to sign a consent form (see p. 631, Consent Forms).

You can have the operations separately, which means not only that the diagnosis of whether you have cancer or not is more accurate, but also that if you do have cancer, it is possible to obtain more information about the type of tumour, and to have greater opportunity to be involved in decisions about treatment. Remember that if you do have cancer, it has probably been there for a long time and so it is unlikely that a few more days or weeks will make any difference to the success of the treatment.

may hear the term *mastitis* used to cover any condition in which the breasts are generally lumpy and tender, although true mastitis is an inflammation of the breast, rarely found in women who are not breastfeeding.

Adenosis, Fibrosing Adenosis, Cystic Mastitis, Fibrocystic Disease, Mastodynia and Mastalgia

These are all terms used to describe tender, irregular, lumpy breasts. Some of us may only find changes in the texture of our breasts just before a period, while others find our breasts begin to change when we ovulate and become steadily more painful and lumpy until menstruation starts. This build-up of tenderness and unevenness in texture is so common that many doctors argue that it is not a disease at all but simply a normal, if uncomfortable, part of the menstrual cycle.[2] Some women find the discomfort severe enough to seek treatment, and for an unfortunate few the breast pain may be bad enough seriously to interfere with their lives. It may remain constant throughout the menstrual cycle, radiating from the breast, which may be agonizingly tender, down the arm. One or both sides may be affected.

All these lumpy, painful conditions are thought to be caused by a hormone imbalance, either over-production of oestrogen or lack of progesterone. Unfortunately, there is no one 'right' hormone balance. It is an individual system, unique to each person. In time the body corrects itself, usually as a result of a major hormonal change such as pregnancy, stopping the Pill, or menopause. All these may seem distant and out of the question for the woman in severe pain.

What helps? Conventional medicine has little to offer. Diuretics (pills which make you pass more urine) may help to relieve the build-up of fluid in the breasts before a period. Hormone treatment with prolactin or danazol (testosterone, see Endometriosis, p. 515) is more likely to be successful in relieving the pain but all these hormones have unpredictable and potentially serious side-effects.

Very painful breasts are usually more comfortable given day and night support from a well-fitting bra made from stretchy material, like most sports bras, and not underwired. Alternating hot and cold showers sometimes help relieve acute pain (a form of naturopathic water treatment – see p. 96). Some women find relief by taking Vitamin B6, 100mg daily throughout the month not just before a period; or evening primrose oil. Others are helped by various types of alternative medicine such as homoeopathy, herbalism or acupuncture (see Chapter 7). See also Things You Can Do Yourself, below, and PMS, p. 510.

Occasionally, the pain is so severe and goes on for so long that a woman or her doctor may suggest mastectomy for relief. Unfortunately, even after this drastic measure, some women may still get pain across the chest wall and down their arms so it is worth remembering that even this does not guarantee cure. Pain which originates in your neck or

---

THINGS YOU CAN DO YOURSELF

There are some ways in which you may be able to distinguish between lumps more likely to be benign and those which probably require medical attention. The following steps may be especially helpful to women with lumpy breasts.

First, if you are still having periods and have no previous history of either lumps or cancer, observe whether the lump disappears or fluctuates in size during your monthly cycle – a sure sign that it is not malignant. It is common medical practice, especially for younger women, for a doctor to recommend first watching the lump for a month or two. *There is no evidence that this will make any difference in length of life, even if the lump does prove cancerous.** Do not feel the lump every day or you may not be able to tell if there is any change. The best times to check are during the three or four days before and, for comparison, three or four days after the first day of your period.

You can also try changing your diet. Many women have found that they can reduce or totally eliminate certain non-cancerous lumps this way. Though not yet proven conclusively, many medical studies have supported links between diet and benign breast conditions. Here are some suggestions on diet that often help reduce breast lumps:

1. Avoid fatty and fried foods.
2. Reduce salt intake.
3. Eliminate foods and beverages containing caffeine – coffee, tea, most colas, chocolate and many brands of aspirin and cold remedies.[3]
4. Don't smoke.†

While dietary changes bring lump reduction in some women within just one cycle, others must continue the diet for up to six months to get improvement.** If after two months the lump has not definitely decreased, you will probably want to proceed to medical screening.

*Many experts agree with this statement, especially since we have so little evidence of treatment benefit. Certainly, if this active watching makes you anxious, seek a biopsy as soon as possible.

†One study found that all the women who got no relief from eliminating salt and caffeine were also smokers. The women who then stopped smoking subsequently found their lumps noticeably reduced.

**For a discussion of how dietary changes may reduce the risk of cancer, see p. 577. See also Get Well Diets, p. 52.

shoulders may also be felt in the breasts. Muscle strain around your chest or problems with your ribs may also cause breast pain.

Fibroadenomas

These are firm, smooth lumps of fibrous tissue in the breast which are most commonly found in women in their teens and twenties. They do not change in size with the menstrual cycle and are usually harmless and painless. Some women develop many fibroadenomas and occasionally they may grow big enough to distort the whole breast. The reason why fibroadenomas are usually removed by surgery is that it is impossible to be 100 per cent certain that a lump which feels like a fibroadenoma is not a cancer. They are not, in themselves, linked with breast cancer and do not turn cancerous. Some women, however, may go for surgery not knowing whether their lumps are fibroadenomas or not and not knowing whether further surgery will be performed (see Consent Forms, p. 631). This can be very distressing.

Sue: *I didn't know if I was going to wake up with a breast or without a breast, which is pretty awful, but I don't think it is quite as bad as thinking there is nothing wrong with you and then being told there is. And it was a very strange sensation, to be coming out of anaesthetic and although you are so drowsy, immediately looking to see if your breast is there. But it was a lovely feeling when it was.*

Cysts

Cysts are sacs filled with fluid or jelly and are by far the most common sort of breast lump, especially in premenopausal women over thirty. They may be large – as big as a plum – or very tiny. Some women have only one cyst, others are plagued by them for years. They are thought to develop under the influence of hormonal changes, and usually disappear with menopause. Chronic cystic disease is associated with a very slightly increased risk of breast cancer so most doctors take breast cysts very seriously. They will usually insert a needle into the lump and draw off the fluid. Once that has been done there should be nothing abnormal to feel in that area at all. If there is still a lump there, or if the cyst keeps refilling, many doctors will recommend surgery to remove it.

Helena: *The surgeon was able to aspirate one cyst in the outpatients' clinic, but said he would have to do a lumpectomy on the other. Would I come into the hospital next week? This all seemed a lot more dramatic than last time. I was not very happy. My husband was off on his business trip and I decided to tell my children and my brother the night before I went into the hospital – I thought it extremely unwise not to. I was asked to sign a form giving permission for further surgery to be done if seen to be necessary, which I refused to*

do. *I insisted that I would make my own decision once they had the result of the biopsy. I was making myself very unpopular. At that moment the surgeon walked into the ward and I explained how I felt. 'I never do a mastectomy,' he said. I was lucky – in the event he did not even have to do a lumpectomy; while I was under anaesthetic he was able to aspirate the cyst.*

Intraductal Papilloma

This is a tiny, non-cancerous tumour which grows in a milk duct. Often there is no lump to feel but the blocked duct may produce a nipple discharge – watery, green or blood-stained. The papilloma is removed in an operation called a *microdochectomy*. This gives only a very small scar and should not affect the ability to breastfeed.

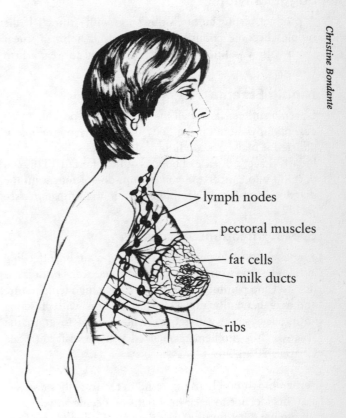

Christine Bondante

lymph nodes
pectoral muscles
fat cells
milk ducts
ribs

Breast showing structure of milk ducts, lymph nodes, and fat cells.

Duct Ectasia

Older women are more likely to get this chronic inflammation of the milk ducts and it can be in one or both breasts and sometimes the affected ducts can be painful. It affects all the ducts and there is often a sticky nipple discharge with inflamed areola and a hard, lumpy feeling under the nipple. The only cure is surgical removal of the nipple with the possibility of later plastic surgery to restore it. Duct ectasia is not cancerous or otherwise dangerous so there is no need to have treatment if you don't want such drastic surgery. Despite the fact that these two conditions occur in milk ducts they are not related to whether you have breastfed or not.

Lipoma

This is a harmless, fatty lump which may develop anywhere in the body including the breasts. There is not usually any treatment necessary, but mammography may be helpful in confirming diagnosis.

Fat Necrosis

This happens as a long-term result of injury to the breast. It is a rare condition but the hard lump of dead, fatty tissue in the breast may feel very like a cancer so it is unusual for a doctor to be able to tell you that you have fat necrosis without doing a biopsy first to exclude cancer. No treatment is necessary.

Jogger's Nipple

A product of our culture's obsession with 'fitness'! If the nipples become painful from friction, it helps to smear them with Vaseline before exercising, and to wear a firm bra.

Nipple Eczema

Eczema sufferers know all too well that it is possible to get eczema anywhere on the body, but if only one nipple is affected it may be a condition called Paget's disease of the breast. (Paget's disease of bone is quite different.) This can develop into cancer and you or your doctor may want the diagnosis confirmed by biopsy or a mammogram (see p. 542).

Breast Infections/Abscesses

These are most common in women who are breastfeeding although some women get repeated abscesses. The breast is hot, red and painful and you may have a high temperature and feel generally unwell. Most doctors will prescribe antibiotics, some will recommend surgery to drain the abscess. (For problems associated with breastfeeding see Chapter 20, p. 409.)

Benign breast problems may tend to recur. If they do, you may decide not to seek treatment or decide to go to an alternative practitioner rather than a GP. For some of us, finding further lumps or symptoms can be just as frightening as finding the first. One woman who had previously had breast cysts describes waiting for her hospital appointment after she developed further problems:

Helena: *Having experienced one breast lump I think it is not unusual to be far more apprehensive about examining your breasts. That is how it was with me. Some years later I knew my right breast was 'lumpy' but could not (or did not want to?) feel any distinct lump. However, in 1980 I went for a routine cervical smear and mentioned to my doctor that I thought there might be a problem. He could feel two lumps and said they should be looked at.*

BREAST CANCER

WHY DO WOMEN GET BREAST CANCER?

Eileen: *I was working nights. And I always did what I wanted to do, regardless of whether I had enough sleep or not. I never considered tiredness a reason for not doing something. But you can only go on so long like that, you do have to pay a price for all that. You have to restore your body's vitality or you're going to drain it away. Well, I think I drained it! I think the first time I got it, it was probably stress. My daughter had a fairly unhappy marriage and was going through a difficult time, and my sister-in-law died very suddenly, which was quite a shake-up in the family – all at the same time. I was working at the adolescent unit, which could be quite traumatic at times.*

Josephine: *For me, the two relationships I had with my two husbands, they were very, very demanding. And my girls growing up into teenagers. I knew they needed things and just didn't have the money to buy them for them. And paying for the mortgage, and having a full-time job, living from week to week for years and constantly having to count the pennies. And I had to cope with a new land, new environment, new traditions, new culture, new language, new way of life.*

The family comes first, and somehow or other Mum doesn't seem to belong in the family. She comes last. But you are a person and you need taking care of, and who else but you can take care of you?

Jo: *I was running on borrowed time, overworking and collapsing as a pattern, and never saying, sometime I've got to stop and take stock of it, because every time you get better and you say – oh well, I'll have another go at running my life . . . I don't want to stop working because I want to do political work . . . you don't get paid for the work that any of us do, it's purely what's in your head that's driving you on.*

Some women we talked to said they knew why they got breast cancer, often connecting it with a time of particular stress. While there is no one single cause, there are factors which increase the likelihood of developing the disease, and stress may be one of them.

There are forces outside us which affect our lives and we need those forces to change in order for our lives to be healthier. In recognizing how hard it is to bring about even the smallest personal changes, we can try to help and support each other in enjoying ourselves, relaxing and relieving stress. (See Cancer, Chapter 25, p. 568 for more on the role of stress and other psychological mechanisms, and p. 574 on ways of dealing with them.)

Hormonal and Environmental Influences

Women with breast cancer are more likely to have started menstruating early (before the age of twelve), to have reached menopause after the age of fifty; to have had their first or only child after the age of thirty-five, or not to have borne any children. Women who have had a full-term pregnancy before the age of twenty-two seem to have a reduced risk of breast cancer, as have women who have an artificially early menopause. This all suggests an association between cyclical changes of our bodies' hormones and susceptibility to the possible development of breast cancer.

It is not clear whether and in what way breastfeeding may offer protection against breast cancer.*

The Pill which contains synthetic versions of the female hormones oestrogen and progesterone is also linked with breast cancer. The evidence is conflicting, but increasingly still worrying – although it has been consistently played down by most of the medical and nursing professions, and particularly by the Family Planning Association. Studies which suggest an increased risk of breast cancer with Pill use link it with a woman's age when she started taking it (before age twenty-five) and the number of years of use (upwards of four or five years);[5] long-term use (eight years) is particularly implicated.[6] But other studies suggest that there is no greater risk.[7]

In trying to make a clear assessment of the evidence, it is important to bear in mind the following: we know that many breast cancers are hormonally dependent and that the Pill contains hormones that can promote cancer (see also Cervix, p. 525); secondly, much of the research suggesting no increased risk has not involved many women who started the Pill when young; and thirdly, breast cancer tends to have a long latency period (it can develop for decades before it is detectable). Klim McPherson et al., discussing this issue in 1986,[8] show how the question of latency may well be at the root of the apparently conflicting evidence produced by those studies which appear not to show an increased risk.[9]

The Pill, though the most widely-researched drug, is still an experiment – it has been called 'the largest uncontrolled experiment in human carcinogenesis ever known'.[10] We are still not in a position to evaluate its full effects on women's health, particularly in relation to cancer. Many of us are anxious about the risks we run by taking the Pill, and feel trapped into using it as it is promoted as the most convenient and reliable method of contraception available. See Chapter 15 for a discussion of other methods we can use.

Hormone Replacement Therapy (HRT). HRT, sometimes prescribed to women during and after menopause, has also been linked with breast cancer, and the evidence is again conflicting (see p. 457). Since research into HRT has not been as great as with the Pill, we are even less able to assess its risks at this stage. We may wish to consider non-hormonal approaches to the treatment of problems associated with menopause (see p. 458).*

Heredity. Having a close female relative (grandmother, mother, sister or aunt) who has developed breast cancer before her menopause also seems to increase the risk of developing the disease. Some women we talked to who had had breast cancer mentioned their fears that their daughters might have an increased risk of getting it. It is not, however, clear to what extent a family tendency to breast cancer is caused, for example, by purely genetic factors or by a shared lifestyle.

Diet. There seem to be some connections between breast cancer and what we eat, in particular with a Western-type diet which tends to include a lot of saturated fat, animal protein, dairy products and refined sugar. Differences in diet could account for the low incidence of breast cancer in Japan, Thailand and the Philippines in particular, and it has been noticed that when women from these countries emigrate to North America and change their eating habits, within a generation their incidence of breast cancer rises dramatically.

Explanations for these correlations vary: it may be that women eating a typical Western diet high in animal fat make more oestrogen, which seems to be related to the development of some breast cancers. Women whose diets include a high proportion of fresh whole foods (including vegetarians) are thought to have a reduced likelihood of breast cancer developing because their bodies are better at dealing with oestrogen.[11]

High alcohol consumption is also associated with breast cancer.[12] For more about diet in relation to cancer, see p. 569 and p. 577.

THE NATURE OF BREAST CANCER

Before we can begin to have any kind of understanding of the dilemmas that breast cancer poses for us, we need to look at the nature of the disease.

Breast cancer begins as collections of abnormal cells in the breast tissue. Sometimes abnormal cells are very like the normal tissue surrounding them, and they do not have the ability to invade surrounding areas or to travel (*metastasize*) to other parts of the body. Cells at this stage are known as *non-infiltrating, non-invasive* or *carcinoma-in-situ* (CIS). More often, however, the cells are clearly cancerous, i.e. they are invasive and able to spread even at an early stage.

An invasive cancer may lay down tiny deposits of cancerous cells in other places, which are too small to be detected by scans, X-rays or blood tests, and so are called *micro-metastases*. Thus, some women with breast cancers which are very small at the time of diagnosis may get

---

*Editors' note: however, two recent papers have suggested that breastfeeding for six months halves our chance of getting breast cancer in later life.[4]

*Editors' note: there is clear evidence that the hormone diethyl stilboestrol, when given to women to prevent miscarriage, exposes them to a higher risk of breast cancer in later life, as well as inducing vaginal cancer in some of the daughters exposed to DES in the uterus (see p. 520).

recurrence in other organs years later. For these reasons some doctors believe that breast cancer is nearly always a systemic disease – that is, one of the whole body – by the time it is detectable by any means.[13] Nevertheless, the smaller the cancer when treatment is started, the less likely it is to have spread extensively to other parts of the body, and so the greater the chance of successful treatment.

We might think that success means cure, or that our life expectancy is unaltered, but in fact what is meant by success in medical terms is survival for a given number of years after treatment, even though we may eventually die of breast cancer. Thus, specialists tend to talk about survival rather than cure, and their statistics are based on five-, ten-, twenty- and thirty-year survival figures, because it is so difficult to judge the success of treatment in a disease which may recur up to thirty years later. For this reason, some doctors consider that the aim of treatment is control rather than cure of the disease (see Living with Breast Cancer, p. 553). Nevertheless, other doctors believe it is possible to eradicate even invasive breast cancer before it has spread, by radical treatment to the breast, involving surgery and radiotherapy (see Treatment for Breast Cancer, p. 544). They do, however, acknowledge that they have no way of assessing the outcome until many years later.

The likelihood of CIS developing invasive characteristics and spreading to other parts of the body, and the time this process may take, varies greatly between individuals. The trigger factors which encourage it to become invasive are unknown (though see Why Do Women Get Breast Cancer?, p. 540 and Cancer, p. 567), and it is not a steady process which can be monitored. For women with CIS, treatment options vary from careful follow-up to radiotherapy or extensive surgery. If you have CIS diagnosed you may want to consider approaches which help strengthen the body's defences, because it could be many years before it becomes invasive and capable of damaging your health, and for some women it may never happen. See p. 574 and Chapter 7 for what you can do.

SCREENING FOR BREAST CANCER

In recent years there has been increasing emphasis on early detection and treatment of breast cancers, first because it may *sometimes* be possible to treat the cancer before it has spread, and second because smaller cancers mean that mastectomy – removal of the whole breast – may not be necessary for successful treatment. (Mastectomy may not always be necessary for larger cancers either.) Women with cancers of less than 2cm in diameter live longer after treatment than women with larger tumours – but see discussion on p. 545.

The two main methods of screening for breast cancer are *mammography* (X-rays) and *breast self-examination* (BSE).

Mammography

This method is the most accurate and more likely to save or extend a woman's life, as it may be possible to pick up early cancers before they can be felt, by detecting certain types of 'microcalcification' – tiny particles of calcium which show up on the mammogram.

Three large-scale studies in New York, Holland and Sweden[14] have shown that mammographic screening can lead to a reduction in deaths from breast cancer. So far it is only in women over fifty that this has clearly been shown to be the case. The Forrest Report[15] was commissioned to look into the feasibility of breast cancer screening in the UK, and as a result of its recommendations, a national mammographic screening programme, for women over fifty, began in certain health districts in 1988. The programme is planned to extend to all districts as from 1991.

Yet the issue of mammographic screening is not altogether straightforward. For example:

1. The discovery of carcinoma-*in-situ* can present us with the problem of whether to go ahead and have treatment for something that may not become invasive (see The Nature of Breast Cancer, p. 541).

2. With those tumours that spread very late in life, if at all, the likelihood of successful treatment would be unchanged. The only difference would be that if such a tumour were detected early, *treatment* would be performed early too, so that the time a woman lived knowing she had cancer, and the amount of treatment she received, would be extended, rather than her lifespan.

3. Of the tumours that have spread before they were picked up by mammography, treatment would be likely to be no more successful than if the cancer were detected by breast palpation (touch).

4. If suspicious microcalcifications have been found, and surgery is performed, the surgeon may find it difficult to remove the right piece of tissue.*

5. Although modern mammographic techniques have considerably reduced the amount of radiation a woman receives, many of us are wary of the carcinogenic effects of repeated X-rays and would therefore be unwilling to undergo regular mammography simply for screening purposes. Regular mammographic screening of young women is inadvisable, not only because it could lead to a high cumulative dose of radiation, but also because it is in any case difficult to detect abnormalities via mammography in women before menopause, and there is no clear evidence that mammographic screening reduces death rates from breast cancer in women under fifty.**

Nevertheless, mammographic screening can pick up cancer at an earlier stage than would otherwise be possible, and the smaller the cancer the greater the chance of successful treatment (see above).

---

*However, the use of a fine needle inserted into the breast under local anaesthetic can pinpoint the abnormality and help ensure that the right tissue is removed. Most hospitals also X-ray the removed tissue as an additional check.
**Editors' note: however, younger women at especially high risk (e.g. who had a late first pregnancy *and* whose mother or sister died prematurely from breast cancer) *may* benefit from regular screening, although no research has been done to establish this.

Breast Self-examination (BSE)

BSE is based on the idea that if we examine our breasts regularly for unusual lumps, thickening or skin changes, we are likely to pick up possible abnormalities earlier than if these were discovered accidentally. However, there is as yet no clear evidence that BSE reduces deaths from breast cancer and most of the issues discussed above also apply to BSE. Nor is there clear evidence that women practising BSE detect smaller cancers than women who find them by chance.

Yet one major difference between mammography and BSE is that BSE involves no physical risk and may give some of us confidence in understanding the normal changes our breasts go through.

If you are interested in doing BSE, it is usually recommended that you practise it as follows.

- Do it once a month or, if you are still menstruating, once during each menstrual cycle – usually after your period when your breasts feel less lumpy.
- First look carefully at your breasts in the mirror for any obvious change in shape, size, skin texture or discharge from the nipples.
- Then lie flat, perhaps with a folded towel under the shoulders on the side you are going to examine, and carefully feel each section of the breast with the flat of your fingers. Some women find this easier to do in the bath with soapy hands.

If this is practised regularly you should become familiar with the normal lumps and bumps in your breasts, and so pick up changes quickly. In order to practise BSE effectively it is important to be shown how, probably more than once, by someone who is experienced in teaching it. In theory this service should be available at family planning clinics and GPs' surgeries, but this is rarely the case. Leaflets are available from health education departments (see p. 627), family planning clinics and the Breast Care and Mastectomy Association (see p. 556).

The government and the medical establishment promote BSE in a very prescriptive way, suggesting that the onus is wholly on each individual woman to be sensible and check her breasts. But doing BSE forces us to confront the possibility of finding a lump which might turn out to be malignant, and so it can provoke a great deal of anxiety. Until it can be clearly shown that earlier detection of breast cancer by BSE gives us a better chance of survival or a better chance of an improved quality of life, then we can have quite rational reasons for choosing not to add the stress of regularly checking our breasts to already stressful lives.

Responsibility for our health is a double-edged weapon which can be used against us, making us feel it is our fault if we get breast cancer and guilty if we don't examine our breasts regularly.

It's one of those things I'm always meaning to do, that eventually, when I'm really sorted out about my life, will be part of a new wonderful routine! As it is, I remember occasionally at a convenient time – like in the bath, and I do it. But in fact it just makes me feel guilty for all the other times I don't make time or forget. And it also makes me feel anxious about what I might find.

Most campaigns to get women to come for screening tests or to learn and practise BSE are focused on us in isolation; and so we suffer our fears, anxieties and guilt in isolation too. Much of what we've learned over the years in the women's health movement has demonstrated the power of acting together and supporting each other, and the value of sharing experiences in relieving anxiety and loneliness.

So, in practice, this might mean learning BSE with other women, rather than from a leaflet. Well women centres may also provide this kind of support. We can try involving a lover, if we have one, in the regular check, so we aren't so isolated with the anxiety it may provoke.

In many respects, there are still no definite answers concerning screening. More emphasis on discovering *why* so many women get breast cancer may eventually help to reduce the number of women who develop the disease.

DISCOVERING WE HAVE BREAST CANCER

Breast cancer arouses a lot of fears in us – fear of death, of mutilation, of painful medical treatment, of losing control of our lives and our bodies. It threatens our sexuality and self-image and puts an added strain on financial, domestic and work responsibilities. We hope that the following sections will give women strength to decide what is best for each of us individually.

If we are told that our biopsy contained malignant cells, this can be devastating. The sensitivity of doctors and nurses is particularly important at this time, though unfortunately they often fail us.

Josephine: *And he came round to me and there was about five of them – I'll never forget. And they sort of stood round my bed and he sort of looked at me and he got a serious face and said, 'I'm ever so sorry, Mrs C., but it is breast cancer.' And I couldn't say a word. I just couldn't believe what I was hearing, and I just burst out crying because I couldn't say anything else.*

Being told that the diagnosis is cancer can be particularly devastating if you have been reassured beforehand that you are unlikely to have it. Some women may already have been told that their symptoms indicate cancer, and a biopsy may be confirmation of this. It is at this time that women may feel in particular need of support; we may want to arrange for a friend to be with us when the biopsy result is given, or we may have already made contact with a supportive group or individual (see Support, p. 552).

All too often doctors adopt an authoritarian attitude towards us which makes any kind of two-way communication based on mutual respect impossible. They may dismiss our fears as 'neurotic' or 'irrational'; in contrast, we may be rushed into hospital or bulldozed into treatment before we have had time to think; or if we have had time to collect some information and have ideas about what we want, we are accused of 'playing the doctor'.

Balancing how much information we want, and how much responsibility we can take on for ourselves are perhaps among the most crucial issues raised about health topics generally and about breast cancer in particular. Each of us needs to reach a decision we will feel most comfortable with. And while such decisions are very personal, we need help and support in making them. Having more information can make us feel frightened and anxious and not necessarily stronger. We may feel devastated and hopelessly powerless to learn that breast cancer is the main cause of death in women aged between thirty-five and fifty-four in the UK, and that England and Wales have the highest breast cancer rate of anywhere in the world; that one woman in twelve can expect to develop breast cancer; and that it is likely to affect our whole body. The medical profession's definition of factors putting women at a higher risk of developing breast cancer (see pp. 540 and 567) can make us feel guilty about aspects of our lifestyles, and helpless about our ability to change them. Such feelings do nothing for our mental well-being!

This situation seems to parallel our awareness of the nuclear threat. For many women it is paralysing, too large and frightening to cope with, and so we push the thoughts as far away as possible. But the experiences of women involved in anti-nuclear campaigning, at Greenham Common and elsewhere, have been that sharing fears and anger, and translating them into action, can be very empowering. Audré Lorde, who has had a mastectomy for breast cancer, vividly expresses this positive approach:

> I have been to war, and still am . . . For me, my scars are an honourable reminder that I may be a casualty in the cosmic war against radiation, animal fat, air pollution, McDonalds hamburgers and Red Dye no. 2, but the fight is still going on and I am still a part of it. [16]

We need the support of others around us and of skilled health workers, to engage in the fight against breast cancer. This is in marked contrast to the passive and mechanistic view of us held by many hospitals and doctors.

> Eileen: *It felt as though you'd left your personality behind, as though you got to the hospital door and turned your body over to the doctor, and 'you' were expected to wait with your clothes in the suitcase, wherever it was put, and to take it home again when they'd finished with you. I felt as a person they didn't want to know about you. I tried to tell the doctor this afterwards, that I felt depersonalized.*

TREATMENT FOR BREAST CANCER*

This is a very complicated issue and one on which many of the 'experts' disagree. Breast cancer is not one but a collection of diseases, and the treatment a doctor recommends should be influenced by the type and extent of breast cancer in any particular case; by whether or not the cancer is sensitive to hormones (see further explanation below); by the size and position of the tumour, and by how far s/he thinks the cancer may have spread. In an attempt to establish this information, further tests may be carried out.

Further Tests

We may feel that we need as much information as possible in order to be involved in making decisions. On the other hand, we may feel that we don't want to know the details of the disease at this stage, so it's important to be aware that we have a choice about what we ask. Perhaps we could think, 'What sort of person am I? Will having this information make me feel more powerful or increase my fear?' Often we can rely on our intuition or gut reactions when faced with such a situation, and someone to give sympathetic support and understanding can be helpful (see p. 552 for more on support).

The tests, which may be called *staging*, may include bone scans, X-rays, tests of the liver and blood, and urine tests. If you attend a hospital which carries out bone scanning, liver tests, etcetera, this does not necessarily mean that your cancer has spread, just that these procedures are part of the process of diagnosis. As a result of these tests, and following whatever surgery is done, the cancer will be 'staged' according to three criteria: size of the tumour, whether or not the lymph nodes are affected, and whether or not the disease has spread (metastasized) to another part of your body.

There is a lot of controversy about the use and accuracy of staging: for example, having 'negative' lymph nodes (i.e. lymph nodes with no cancer cells in them) does not rule out the possibility that the cancer has spread elsewhere (it could just be that the lymph node has successfully destroyed all the cancer cells present); however, positive lymph nodes do mean an increased likelihood of spread.

Staging also allows comparisons of groups of people for the international study of breast cancer. If you feel you would like your cancer to be staged and are referred to a hospital that does not offer it, you could ask to be referred to one that does. However, you may decide that you prefer not to undergo staging, and make decisions about treatment based on different criteria. Staging should not be the only factor which helps you decide about treatment. It may, however, help doctors to decide what to offer.

---

*This section concentrates mainly on the consideration of orthodox (allopathic) treatments. This is not because we believe that allopathy is preferable to complementary and alternative approaches but because such approaches are dealt with in the general discussion of cancer in Chapter 25.

WHAT DO THE STUDIES SHOW?

Studies that follow the course of breast cancer from diagnosis to death (whether from cancer or other causes) of a large number of women find that almost 80 per cent of women who develop breast cancer eventually die from it. This rate has not changed significantly since the 1930s. Some women, however, live with the disease for as long as twenty or thirty years; while they do eventually die of breast cancer, their lifespans have not been shortened.

Some groups of women tend to do better than others:

1. Women who are past menopause.
2. Women with no malignant lymph nodes. This is the most important single predictor found so far.
3. If the cancer is hormone dependent – has high levels of oestrogen and progesterone receptors.

These hormone-receptors-high (HR-high, also called 'positive') cancers tend to have fewer or later recurrences no matter what type of treatment is used. HR-high cancer is more common in post-menopausal women.

4. Types of cancers with cells that tend to grow and metastasize very slowly. They account for about 20 per cent of all breast cancers.
5. If the tumour cells are highly diffentiated; that is, they retain the characteristics of normal breast cells rather than the appearance of advanced cancer cells.

However, even with these indicators, it is impossible and inappropriate to make predictions for any specific woman. See What are Our Chances?, p. 570. In particular, our own role in the healing process may play a significant part – see p. 568.

Making Decisions about Treatment

Until recently, the majority of women with breast cancer had mastectomies (removal of the breast – see p. 546); it is now acknowledged that other, less mutilating treatment options, such as lumpectomy plus radiotherapy (see p. 546), can be equally effective in terms of survival. Some doctors, however, will favour one particular treatment and will deal with all women in the same way. Each treatment option has its own advantages and disadvantages, and may be more or less appropriate according to the condition of the cancer and an individual woman's own preferences.

Some women have strong feelings and opinions about the type of treatment they find acceptable. Others are confused and frightened at the prospect of having to make choices for themselves.

Sue: *There wasn't enough told to me before the operation. I didn't realize at the time that they could partially remove the breast, or that they could just remove the lump. There were no alternatives given to me. There was just the thing, you have it done and you live, or you don't have it done and you die, that was the choice I was given. What my choice would have been I don't know, but in retrospect I would have liked a wider choice.*

'Shopping around' among doctors may increase the difficulties, because you may be given several conflicting opinions. It may, however, be worth asking for a second opinion if you are unhappy with your doctor or if the only treatment s/he suggests is something which you find unacceptable.

It helps enormously to have a doctor whom you trust and who justifies, to your satisfaction, his or her proposed treatment plan so that you can fight your disease together.

Many women also find it helps them if they have someone present when they discuss treatment with their doctor, because it is so easy, under stress, to forget to ask important questions or to misunderstand what has been said. Unfortunately, staff in some places find this very threatening and may be obstructive.

Facilities and services for the treatment of breast disease vary enormously. In smaller towns women with breast lumps are likely to see a general surgeon, whose knowledge of breast cancer may not be as up to date as that of a surgeon specializing in breast disease.

A major criticism of hospital services that women have is lack of information about what treatments are available and their effects. The women we spoke to who had opted for private treatment had similar criticisms to those of women treated in the NHS, namely lack of information and emotional support.

If you are trying to make a decision about treatment, or support someone else in doing so, you may want to look at Chapter 7, Alternative and Complementary Approaches to Health and Healing, and also at p. 578, which looks specifically at such approaches in relation to cancer. Since these approaches best involve the whole person, body, mind, emotions and spirit, there is none specific to cancer of the breast. As breast cancer is often regarded as a systemic disease (see The Nature of Breast Cancer, p. 541), this may seem particularly appropriate. Most women choose a holistic approach for reasons relating to its nature and quality, rather than to try to increase their lifespan.

Jo: *At last someone was going to listen to you and he took into account your personality . . . I'm just trying to integrate the best that's around at what I can afford. And by best I don't mean that they have proven results and statistics, because the money isn't available for that, but actually at a gut level: what suits my personality best, what can I stand?*

In general, alternative and complementary approaches require us to take a much greater control over our health and illness than more orthodox approaches. However, taking on responsibility for our lives and health, particularly at such a stressful time, can be the last thing we want to do. And this can be especially true after a lifetime of having very little control.

We do not necessarily need to choose between 'orthodox' and 'alternative' approaches. Nearly all the women we spoke to underwent conventional treatment *as well as* using other approaches, including diet, yoga and stress reduction generally. If you want to consider a complementary or alternative approach to your therapy, see Cancer, p. 578, and Chapter 7.

Surgery

Orthodox treatment for breast cancer usually involves some form of surgery. It may seem as though this is inevitable because, although it isn't the only option, it is the one most commonly offered. The advantages of surgery are that it may prevent 'local recurrence', and that the removal of a mass of cancerous cells may decrease their spread. Untreated breast cancer could eventually ulcerate and fungate, which is distressing and unpleasant; the surgical removal of the growth is one very decisive way of halting that outcome.

It is important to find out what kind of operation you are agreeing to before you sign a consent form (see p. 631), and to ask exactly what part of the breast will be removed, what will be left, and whether further treatment will be necessary. You may also want to know if implants or plastic surgery may be possible (see p. 551).

Laura: *A doctor came along and said, 'Sign this form', and the form was saying if there's anything more, you give your consent for the surgeon to do what's necessary . . . I didn't know what 'radical mastectomy' meant and I can remember asking the surgeon about that and him saying, 'Now, don't you worry about that, it doesn't matter, it's not a concern of yours.' At which point I said, 'Well, I'd like to know, it does matter to me!'*

It is often easier to disguise a flat chest wall with an artificial breast (prosthesis; see p. 550) than to fill out and equalize a breast which is small and misshapen after extensive surgery – a factor which you may consider important. Some of the different operations which may be performed for breast cancer are:

1. *Lumpectomy*, or wide local excision of the tumour. This is removal of the lump and a small area of breast tissue around it. Since without radiotherapy there is a 30 per cent chance that the cancer may recur in the breast, additional (often called adjuvant) treatment with radiotherapy is usually recommended too (see p. 548).

The final appearance of the breast after treatment will depend on the size and position of the lump and how great a percentage of the breast tissue had to be removed to ensure adequate clearance of the tumour. In many cases where the lump is small (below 3cm in diameter) and there is no evidence that the disease has spread, lumpectomy plus radiotherapy has proved to be as effective as mastectomy in controlling breast cancer.

2. *Partial mastectomy* (may be called *tylectomy* or *quadrantectomy*). This is removal of a substantial part of the breast. It is quite a disfiguring operation and often means you will lose your nipple.

3. *Simple mastectomy*. This is removal of all of the breast tissue leaving the chest wall flat. If you have a mastectomy, you will have a long scar which usually runs across the middle of your chest wall but may be diagonal, from the bottom of your armpit to your breast bone. The nipple is removed with the breast but it is sometimes possible to leave a fold of skin at the breastbone end of the scar, which will give the impression of a 'cleavage' when you are wearing a low-cut top or swimsuit.

4. *Extended simple, Patey* or *modified radical mastectomy*. These are all stages between simple and radical mastectomy when the breast is removed with some other tissue – often lymph nodes from the armpit and perhaps some of the chest-wall muscle. These operations are likely to affect arm and shoulder movement more than a simple mastectomy, so they may be a bit more painful and you may need to work harder at arm exercises to restore full movement after surgery.

5. *Radical* or *Halsted mastectomy*. This involves removal of the breast as well as all the chest-wall muscles and all the tissue from the armpit (axilla). It is a very disfiguring operation which may leave the shoulder joint misshapen, the chest wall concave and the arm stiff and swollen. Because so little tissue is left covering the ribs, skin grafts may be needed to cover the area and the scarring will be extensive. Surgeons used to perform this operation in the belief that it would increase the chance of eliminating the cancer completely. However, long-term survival after less drastic operations is equally good, and cancer can still recur even after Halsted mastectomy.

The mastectomy scar goes across the chest and the tissue is removed from under the skin. Some hospital staff put pressure on women to look at the mastectomy scar. Don't try until you feel ready to look at it. It may be easy or it may be hard for you to accept the scar and the changes to your body.

Laura: *You wonder how someone with a thirty-two-inch bust can get such a big scar across the chest . . . but I can't think of any major changes in my life because of this visual appearance. My figure or my bust weren't important factors in my life before*

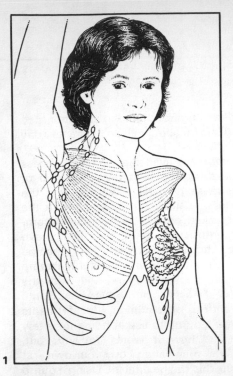

1 This illustration shows the underlying structures of the breast: the rib cage, pectoral muscles, lymph nodes, fat and milk glands. The right breast glands are transparent to show the entire pectoral muscle.
2 Lumpectomy: tissue affected by removal of a lump
3 Mastectomy
   a Modified radical mastectomy: breast removed together with lymph nodes
   b Simple mastectomy: breast only removed
4 Radical mastectomy: tissue affected by removal of the breast, lymph nodes and muscle
5 A scar from a radical mastectomy

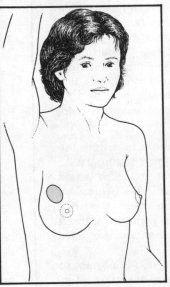

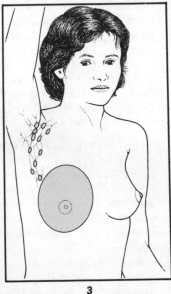

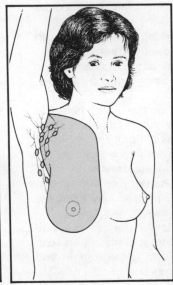

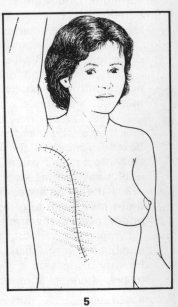

Pond/Giles

I had the mastectomy . . . it was more, the important thing is the person, not the bust measurements.

Josephine: *The girl next to me, she was a bit braver than I was. She was the first one to look at it. 'It's not so bad as I thought,' she said. So I went into a cubicle and took my top off, and I just looked at myself straight in the mirror, and I didn't feel sick and I didn't feel surprised. I just took it as – I've got stitches there and it's quite a big scar, but it doesn't look as awesome as I thought it would. I'd made up my mind to expect something really horrid and when I looked at it, it looked quite neat and clean. That was about the fourth day after the operation, when they took the*

bandage off and you had just a loose bit of gauze on it.

Sue: *When I first looked I threw myself on the bed and skriked [cried].*

After the operation, you may experience lymphoedema (see box).

Radiotherapy

Radiotherapy is treatment with high-energy X-rays – see p. 572. In breast cancer treatment it is usually given in the area of the breast itself and of its surrounding lymph nodes. Some doctors implant the breast with radioactive material. It is necessary to stay in hospital for this but otherwise most radiotherapy is given on an outpatient basis. Treatment

LYMPHOEDEMA

This may occur after the operation: the arm swells due to inadequate drainage of lymphatic fluid. Lymph is a clear fluid which circulates round the body in a similar way to blood, carrying various substances needed for repair and maintenance of cells to the tissues and removing the debris of normal wear and tear from them. Lymph has its own system of channels – the lymphatic vessels – throughout the body. Spaced along these vessels, rather like beads on a chain, are the lymph nodes, which act like filters for the lymphatic fluid and form a valuable barrier against infection by stopping unwanted substances from entering the bloodstream. There are many of these lymphatic vessels and nodes in the armpit area and it is here that cells which have broken away from a breast tumour may be stopped and harboured. This is why some surgeons remove the lymph nodes from this area as part of breast cancer treatment, while other doctors recommend radiotherapy to the armpit.

There are three ways in which lymphoedema can occur following breast cancer treatment.

1. If many lymph nodes are removed at the operation the lymphatic drainage may be left permanently inadequate.

2. Radiotherapy may cause the lymph nodes to lose their elasticity and they may gradually cease to be able to cope with the flow of fluid. This is often a slow process and you may not notice any swelling until many months after your treatment.

3. If the lymph nodes are harbouring cancer cells, these may begin to grow and gradually block the nodes, causing the arm to swell.

Lymphoedema is not, in itself, a dangerous condition but it is very difficult to treat medically and can be very distressing if the arm is large, tight and heavy. There are some things that can help:

- *Gravity* is often the best thing. Try to keep your arm as high as possible all the time, i.e. rest it along the back of a settee when sitting; prop it up on cushions in bed.
- *Elastic sleeves* (like elastic stockings) help some people. However, you must put the sleeve on when the arm is at its slimmest each day, as it works by stopping the fluid coming down, not by pushing it back.
- *Massage.* A firm massaging stroke of your raised arm moving from hand to shoulder may help. Doing this for about half an hour every day should be effective.
- *Electric pumps* are available which compress the arm, pushing the fluid back – a kind of automated massage. These work only if the lymph nodes are there but inadequate. If the nodes are blocked, or have been removed, compression pumps will make the fluid move upwards so that your back and side become swollen, or will simply be very painful. If a pump is appropriate it means sitting still, with the pump on, for at least two hours every day. Some hospitals and/or physiotherapy departments will lend you a pump to use at home for a few weeks to see how it works for you but, ultimately, you may have to buy your own – at around £100, this can be difficult. Using a pump can be dangerous to women with heart conditions or whose blood clots easily.
- *Exercise.* Some women find that exercise generally, and arm exercises in particular, reduce their lymphoedema; others find that exercise aggravates the condition. Check this out and do the best thing for you.
- *Diuretics* (water pills). These occasionally help, but not in many cases.

Unfortunately, it is not possible to restore the lymphatic drainage by any form of surgery.

Laura: No one ever said that your arm would never be back to what it was in the beginning, and that maybe forever you couldn't push a vacuum cleaner or clean the windows without feeling physically tired in that arm for days afterwards.

If you have lymphoedema it is important to remember that the affected arm has little protection against infection. Therefore, if possible:
- wear gloves for gardening and housework or any rough, dirty jobs;
- wear a thimble when sewing;
- be careful not to damage your cuticles and nailbeds;
- treat even small cuts or scratches with antiseptic and keep them covered;
- don't let anyone take blood samples or blood-pressure recordings from that arm.

may be given daily or two to three times a week, and a full course may be anything from one to twenty treatments. Each session lasts only a few minutes and is painless. Because of the word 'rays' people sometimes think they will feel heat coming from the machine but this is not so. Towards the end of the treatment course the skin may turn pink and flaky and some women develop a reaction that is very like a burn because of radiation damage to the skin cells. This usually reaches its peak about two weeks after the end of treatment and then heals gradually. You may develop a sore throat or difficulty with swallowing but this is a fairly transient effect. Nausea is much less of a problem with the more modern machines and it is now rare to feel nauseated.

Rita: *I was getting very, very low-spirited and tired, and then my skin started to break up . . . nobody said this is liable to happen or that is liable to happen . . . I took the cream they gave me home with me, and the burns started to come out and the skin dried off and it was really rather painful. That was when I began thinking, they ought to tell you about this; why wasn't I told about this?*

Radiotherapy does some degree of permanent damage to all the parts of the body which are treated. This means that it may not be possible to treat the same area again. Some women cannot see or feel any signs of this permanent cell damage, while others are left to cope with a permanent legacy of their treatment. These effects may include skin that remains discoloured or has visible, brittle blood vessels close to the surface (*telangectesia*) or a breast that becomes smaller, harder and less even in texture than the other following lumpectomy and radiotherapy. Occasionally, a breast may get larger rather than smaller.

Many women also lose the hair from the armpit on the treated side and the sweat glands there may never become active again. There may be serious long-term effects of radiotherapy, such as permanent damage to the part of the lung underneath the treated area and/or to the affected ribs (which may become brittle and easily broken), or a second cancer may develop elsewhere in the body. Although such side-effects *may* occur, most women who have radiotherapy after surgery do not appear to suffer severe long-term effects and, if the radiotherapy is carefully given, the skin should return to normal and the shape of the breast likewise.

Brenda: *It's now almost two years since I had the radiotherapy. I didn't seem to have any effects from it, although I did get fed up of going to hospital each day. My breasts don't look any different, although the one that was treated feels a lot firmer. I am very pleased with the result.*

Unfortunately, it is not possible to tell in advance how extensive or troublesome any permanent effects of radiotherapy will be in any particular woman.

Chemotherapy (see p. 572)

Chemotherapy involves the use of cell-poisoning drugs, usually to control cancer cells which have spread to other parts of the body, but which are not causing symptoms and may not be detectable. It may be given after surgery, in which case it is called 'adjuvant chemotherapy'. It may also be used to help stop symptoms in the breast, e.g. by helping to reduce tumours and swelling of the arm due to cancer in the lymph nodes. Unlike radiotherapy, it affects every part of the body, travelling through the bloodstream. It can have very unpleasant side-effects (see p. 572) but this is not always the case.* If you are considering whether or not to

---

*For example, when chemotherapy is used to help stop symptoms in the breast, it tends to be given in much smaller doses which cause very few side-effects.

have chemotherapy, it may help to get your doctor to go through the specific side-effects of the drugs s/he intends to use.

Josephine: *The doctor told me the disadvantages of chemotherapy are feeling sick, you might lose your hair and generally feel unwell. When he said lose my hair, somehow or other I just couldn't take that; I cried for two days and two nights. All I could see myself as, was having to go back to work with a wig. And I thought that was the most awful thing that could happen to me . . . My hair went much thinner and much limper, but then I washed it with coconut shampoo. I put all sorts of conditioners on and I used to treat it as if it was gold. I was very careful with it . . . It helped it.*
I had to cope with a year of chemotherapy treatment, on a twenty-eight-day cycle. On the first day you had injections, then take the tablets for fourteen days, injections again on the eighth day. Then you had fourteen days off. They made you feel very low. All the time a sicky feeling as if you wanted to be sick but you couldn't. And very depressed, like suffering from flu all the time.

Chemotherapy is sometimes used for women who are premenopausal with positive lymph nodes, because of the results of recent studies which seem to indicate an increase in long-term survival rates and time between treatment and recurrence in this group of women.[17] However, some doctors believe that the survival advantage is caused by the fact that a side-effect of the chemotherapy is suppression of the hormones produced by the ovaries.[18] Hormone therapy given directly would therefore produce the same results without many of the side-effects – see below.

Josephine: *Nine months on . . . two years post-mastectomy. I haven't started squash yet because with the year of chemotherapy I felt so tired all the time, but I'm beginning to get my strength back now. I'm almost the girl I was before.*

Hormone Therapy

It has been known for many years that changing the hormone balance in a woman's body could affect breast cancer, either by encouraging the cancer to grow or causing it to get smaller, but little was understood about how this works. The effectiveness of hormone therapy is not fully understood. The presence or absence of hormone receptors (HR) in the tumour gives some indication of how well the tumour will respond to hormone therapy. The test for the presence or absence of hormone receptors is still available only at larger breast cancer treatment centres, but this test will not necessarily indicate whether or not you will benefit from hormone treatment. None the less, the higher the level of receptors, the greater is the likely response to any form of hormone therapy. For younger women, this may mean a radiation- or drug-induced menopause to cut down the amount of oestrogen that is 'feeding' the cancer. Women may benefit from a drug called tamoxifen, which seals over the hormone receptor sites in the tumour cells and has few side-effects.* There are several other drugs used in hormone therapy which may be effective at controlling the cancer in hormone-responsive tumours, but they generally have more side-effects than tamoxifen.

PROSTHESES

After mastectomy, most women are offered an artificial breast, known as a breast prosthesis. This means that, when dressed, you *look* as if you have two breasts. It also helps your body feel better balanced. Some women, particularly those who dislike wearing a bra (necessary to hold the prosthesis in place) may prefer to be without a prosthesis. The only physical problem with this is that a heavy-breasted woman may find that, over a period of months, the shoulder on the operated side may rise due to the lack of weight, and cause pain in the neck and spine.

The pressure other people put on women to hide the effects of mastectomy is enormous. It means that they carry the additional burden of coping with scars and loss in isolation. Audré Lorde, in *The Cancer Journals* (see Resources), tells us that she has refused to wear a prosthesis, as she does not wish to hide her loss. One woman we interviewed did go without a prosthesis but later started wearing one:

Laura: *I felt guilty putting people through what I was putting them through . . . If I have accepted this why am I making other people suffer – they're still not accepting it by making them confront it. I wanted people to ask questions and I wanted people to talk about it, but somebody stopped me in my tracks one day and said, 'Well, you think you're so self-righteous and why, what are you trying to prove and why should everybody accept it?' And that really upset me then.*

The set-up for the provision and fitting of prostheses varies immensely between hospitals. A caring and sensitive service can be very helpful. Hospitals should issue women with a soft, lightweight, temporary prosthesis before they go home. If this does not happen, these can be bought from the Breast Care and Mastectomy Association (address in Resources). The permanent prosthesis is fitted when the wound has healed and the chest wall is comfortable enough for you to wear a bra for most of the day. There is no need for special bras, though these are available, but a prosthesis

will not usually fit very well into a half-cup bra, or one that is really too big or too small.

To get your prosthesis, you will need a note signed by the surgeon and this is generally taken, or sent by the ward, to the hospital's surgical appliances department.

The system for the provision of breast prostheses within the National Health Service is very complicated. Basically, each hospital contracts out the service to a private supplier so that the standards of care and service vary enormously between hospitals.[19] Women seldom complain about the service although many are unhappy with it, and this perpetuates the haphazard system. The Department of Health has approved twelve different sorts of breast prosthesis for free issue under the NHS. Each of these comes in a wide range of shapes, sizes and skin tones, but it can be very difficult to obtain a black prosthesis, although they are manufactured. The law states that women are entitled to be fitted with a 'suitable' breast prosthesis, and that this prosthesis should be renewed and replaced when necessary, for life. There should, therefore, never be any need for us to buy our own prostheses, but sadly, many women do so (at £50 plus) because the system in their area is woefully inadequate.

The informal support women give one another is invaluable.

Sue: *I was lucky that this friend came to see me, who'd had a mastectomy. She took the prosthesis out and let me see it and hold it. So that when I actually went to be fitted it wasn't a complete shock.*

A woman who was treated at a London teaching hospital was told by the fitter:

Josephine: *. . . if it ever happened to her [she said] she would want the best prosthesis available and with that frame of mind she did her job, she was getting the best for us . . . she let you try on various sizes until you were quite sure what you looked the best in, what you felt was your proper size. And then you take one home and then every two years you get a replacement on the NHS . . . she recommended us to wear bras with a criss-cross design (not mastectomy bras) and I haven't changed one bit of clothing like they tell you in books, you have to change your dresses . . . I'm still using the same bras.*

In contrast, another woman told us:

Laura: *I told her that I still wasn't my own weight and she told me that lots of women imagine they're bigger than they actually are after a mastectomy, it was psychological . . . They give you two covers for the prosthesis that is expected to last a lifetime, and they tell you if you want some more to make*

*Premenopausal women may find that their periods become irregular or cease altogether and that they have other menopausal symptoms such as hot flushes and vaginal dryness. (See p. 458 for non-hormonal measures that can help with these problems.)

your own . . . and they're supposed to be trying to make you 'normal', as they put it.

Women's attitudes to wearing a prosthesis vary, too: the woman who had a good experience at a London teaching hospital finds hers comfortable and is confident wearing it. Other women have more mixed or negative experiences.

We can work towards improving the provision and choice of breast prostheses in our area by talking to hospital appliance officers, surgeons and community health council officers (see CHCs, p. 642). Nationally, the Royal College of Nursing Breast Care Nursing Forum is putting pressure on MPs to improve and standardize the service and to increase the provision, so we can also write to our MP or the Minister for Health.

Finding prostheses and clothes which are comfortable can have an enormously beneficial effect.

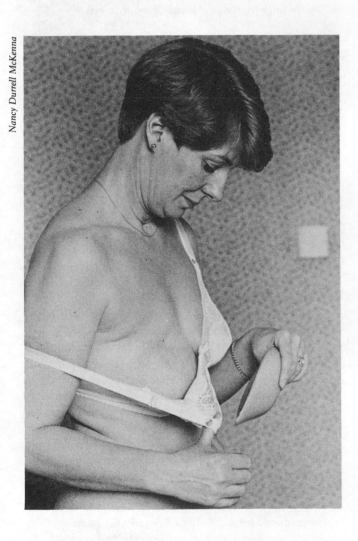

Nancy Durrell McKenna

Joan: *A huge turning point for me was the fact that I had a bra that I could do anything in. I could go and play badminton and nothing wobbled or moved and you didn't have to think about it. But there is no way I would go in a shower. Not because I don't want people to see me but I think it would upset them to see me.*

IMPLANTS AND PLASTIC SURGERY

Sue: *Billy Connolly, the comedian, was doing some song and he was going on about a woman with one breast. And it was just at a point where I was starting to feel very, very low about it and I was just devastated by it. All the audience laughing at the words and that. I don't think I could describe how I felt. I just verged on hysteria, I felt such a freak. And it was from that that I started mithering the doctors when I went for my check-ups for an implant.*

A *breast implant* is simply a prosthesis underneath the muscle of the chest wall. This can be done at the time of mastectomy or any time later. Women who wait some months after a mastectomy may be able to have a more elaborate *breast reconstruction* done by a specialist plastic surgeon. Reconstruction produces a larger, more realistic-looking breast, but usually two and sometimes three operations are involved and you may have to have your own 'good' breast reduced in size or firmed by plastic surgery to match the reconstruction, particularly if you are heavy-breasted or have a breast which has started to droop after menopause.

Unfortunately, the ease of obtaining implants and breast reconstructions often has more to do with the eagerness of the surgeons than the desires of individual women. One woman who was in her twenties was strongly encouraged by the surgeon to have an implant; he had done the mastectomy with a view to doing an implant.

Laura: *I didn't know if I wanted it done or not. The visible thing of having no breast didn't bother me at all, but the hassle of the prosthesis . . . and not being able to go swimming and wear certain clothes, that was a nuisance. I had questions I wanted to ask . . . The surgeon's idea of problems and mine were two different things. I was thinking along practical lines, he didn't have the kind of answers I wanted, and he was thinking along medical lines.*

Laura did eventually get her questions answered by a mastectomy counsellor from another health district.

Sometimes the professionals seem to have different priorities:

Laura: *They'd say, have you discussed it with your husband? I didn't think that was a consideration with my own body. They seemed to think it was a major factor, whether your husband would like you to have it. But no one would discuss it with you.*

Another woman told us:

Joan: *I hated the prosthesis. I thought, there is no way I'm going to go through life like this. But I can't say it bothered me that much at the beginning. I had to be convinced this cancer was going to go. At one stage I saw a psychiatrist and it was him who recommended the reconstruction. I started to feel better from then, with the reconstruction to look forward to.*

Her own surgeon was not very keen. She waited seven months to have the first operation, which involved taking a muscle from her back and was very painful; the second part, six months later, involved putting a nipple on and reducing the other breast. No silicone was used. She is delighted with the result and feels it is worth all the effort.

Breast reconstruction and implants are available on the NHS but are by no means offered to every woman. In some areas you may have to fight very hard for this option.

Some surgeons reconstruct the breast using a muscle flap taken from elsewhere in the body, usually the back (as in Joan's case) or the abdomen, to make a pouch. This may be large enough in itself, or may need to be filled out by the insertion of a silicone implant. Another technique is to insert a balloon called a tissue expander under the chest-wall muscle. The balloon is gradually filled with fluid by weekly injections and, as it grows, the skin and muscle over it expand, rather as the abdomen of a pregnant woman expands. When the new breast reaches the appropriate size, the tissue expander is taken out and replaced by a silicone prosthesis. At this second operation an artificial nipple is usually made on the reconstructed breast.

Women are sometimes concerned that further surgery may cause the cancer to recur. There is no evidence that this is so. Some women do get recurrences, but there is no higher incidence among those who have had plastic surgery than among those who have not. Another fear is that recurrence will be hidden by the reconstructed breast and, therefore, discovered later. This is most unlikely since it is very rare for the cancer to recur in the tissue underneath the breast; if it is going to reappear, it is more likely to be in the scar or the surrounding lymph glands, all of which are still visible after reconstruction.

Rejection of an internal silicone prosthesis is possible, but very rare. A more likely complication is that the body forms a fibrous capsule round the prosthesis, causing it to feel hard and uncomfortable. These fibrous bonds can be broken but it may be a painful experience and they can re-form, which causes some women to have the implant removed.

Another potential difficulty is that the implant can move, particularly during the first three months, so that the new breast ends up being much higher or lower than the other one, or even too near the centre of the chest or under the arm. This risk can be minimized by wearing a firm supporting bra day and night for several weeks after the operation, and not stretching or swinging your arms for the first month. Even the most experienced plastic surgeon cannot guarantee an exact match in size, shape or position with any breast reconstruction/implant, so if you want to have this done, you must be prepared to accept a compromise if necessary. Some women may have had such drastically radical surgery or have tissue which has been damaged by radiation so badly that it is very difficult for the surgeon to do anything at all to reconstruct the breast. Each case is different. It is important to have a clear idea of what the surgeon thinks can be done for you so that you know what to expect from the operation.

SUPPORT

In a few hospitals there are now *nurse counsellors* for women with breast cancer, who may help.

> Rita: *She had seen breast cancer of all sorts. She would describe what to anticipate . . . it was enlightening because I could ask her things and tell her what was happening to me, and she could tell me plainly from her experience what it was.*

Their role can be seen as humanizing the NHS, as 'helping women clarify the meaning of the experience of breast cancer to themselves', as one liaison nurse with a breast unit told us. Women can ask her a whole range of questions, particularly if they are not sure who to ask about something, or where to start.

> *Lots of women want me to change appointments for them, or give advice about bras and prostheses and so on – not telling them what to do, but sorting out what they want and what their priorities are.*

Nurse counsellors also cope with questions like, 'Am I going to die?', not necessarily by using their access to clinical records, but by giving a woman space to talk then and there about the possibility of dying.*

There are also *self-help groups* for women with breast cancer. *CancerLink* keeps a directory of these – see p. 592. They can tell us about the treatment options available and how these are likely to make us feel; they may provide contacts for alternative or complementary therapies; offer a point of contact to talk with other women about mastectomies and prostheses; and generally help to break down the social stigma which is all too often associated with cancer. They may also be able to give support to friends and relatives of women with breast cancer. For more about support groups, see p. 585.

Support need not, however, be so formalized.

> Josephine: *This old lady in her seventies came along; she had a radical mastectomy and she looked a picture of health. This was about four days after her operation. It cheered us up. It was a real booster. And I think I felt, if she can do it, I can.*

*See also Confronting Our Own Mortality, p. 581.

I got so much moral support from the nurses, I can honestly say they pulled me through . . . they were all so supportive and encouraging. It was almost like having your friends looking after you . . . when they did something, you felt they were doing it for you. And they were doing it with care, for your physical needs and also your mental needs.

We can all, through our own experiences, through the information we have, and through caring, give very real help to each other.

Sue: *I felt very very strongly at the time that I wished there had been some way I'd been able to help other women . . . just to say it's not the end of the world. It's bad and it's upsetting but it's not the end of the world . . . I was lucky that this friend came to see me who'd had a mastectomy – I didn't know she'd had it done, actually. She'd had it five years before me and she'd had radiation treatment and was very badly scarred. She was very, very strong. Talking to her helped.*

We can support each other by demanding that doctors communicate with us in a way that is easily comprehensible and sympathetic.

Laura: *There's a lot of things that cropped up later on that if they'd explained beforehand it would have been better, such as after-effects that caused problems, because twelve months later you can still be worrying . . . and you have to keep badgering doctors and they say, 'Well, we didn't actually tell you that because it doesn't happen to all patients' . . . but that makes you feel maybe something's going wrong again.*

Rita: *I felt he was the surgeon and I was moving into someone else's hands, and therefore I wasn't supposed to ask him, which isn't like me . . . But somehow, with doctors, they are very, very good at putting themselves in compartments; a curtain comes down and they are very good with phrases which shut the door.*

All of us should have the information we want, and the appropriate care and help, to make us stronger and to cope with breast cancer in our own way.

LIVING WITH BREAST CANCER*

Women often live for many years after their initial treatment for breast cancer. During these years they may be free

*Issues affecting women living with any form of cancer are discussed in the general section on cancer in Chapter 25. Here we discuss aspects which relate specifically to breast cancer. This section should be read in conjunction with the general section on p. 567.

from disease or may have to cope with recurrences or secondary spread. Breast cancer is not a disease that can be treated and then easily forgotten about but is one which can affect our lives in a number of ways.

Uncertainty about the possible progression of the disease, and about the success of treatments, can be very difficult to cope with. We may become very angry because we cannot get anyone to give us the reassurance we want. There is also the continuing anxiety about possible recurrence or the spread of cancer to other parts of the body.

It may help us to see breast cancer more as a chronic disease, like asthma or diabetes, than a make-or-break medical emergency (see The Nature of Breast Cancer, p. 541). Many women never have any further trouble after the initial treatment, though whether they are actually 'cured' or not is impossible to say. Others who do get a recurrence live for many years with their disease, having treatment as and when required, as they would for any other chronic disease.

Jo: *There's the cycle of the cancer itself which makes you seasonally ill, or ill in relation to your environment, or from working too much, or being under stress . . . it's not a cycle in the sense that the seasons come regularly, it's something that moves and shifts.*

There does seem to be some connection between psychological mechanisms and cancer (see p. 568), and it is certain that stress and constant worry about recurrence will impair the quality of our lives. It is important, therefore, to find a way of handling the uncertainty that leaves us free to get on with living (see p. 582).

Jo: *When you have a potentially killing disease you have to live in hope . . . you need the confidence to go on. I had to be convinced that this cancer was going to go. And then you realize that it takes years, anyway, before anybody's going to say, 'Well, you've probably cracked it.'*

Different women use different approaches to help them live with their disease. Some get angry and fight it:

Laura: *Anger. Why should I have this? I still associated cancer with smoking and that sort of thing, so why should I have cancer.*

Some take steps to change their diet and try to cut down stress in their lives, for example by doing yoga or meditation. Others fill their lives, living every minute, so they have no time to think of a gloomy future.

Eileen: *You either accept that you're going to carry on in the same way and perhaps go out with that, or you're going to change your pattern. So now I'm in the process of trying to change my pattern a bit, but it's very hard.*

AFTER BREAST CANCER: PREGNANCY, THE PILL AND HORMONE REPLACEMENT THERAPY

The exact relationship between breast cancer and pregnancy is still unclear but there is no doubt that the large volume of hormones in the bloodstream during pregnancy and breastfeeding does have some effect, particularly on hormone-dependent cancers. Breast cancers which develop during pregnancy often grow very fast, though they do not necessarily spread to other parts of the body more quickly than in non-pregnant women. Some women worry that their baby may get cancer from sucking milk from a breast which turns out to have a cancerous lump in it, but there is no danger to the baby. The cells are most unlikely to get into the milk and, if they did, could not get into the baby's bloodstream.

Most doctors advise women not to get pregnant within two years of having treatment for breast cancer. Many women have later become pregnant and breastfed the baby from the remaining breast. It would be unwise to use the Pill for contraception and likewise hormone replacement therapy if you have had a natural or artificial menopause. See p. 541 for discussion on these points.

WITHOUT

Without breasts
a woman's heart
rounds and softens her body,
bears her milk.

Without hair
a woman can fully
receive sunlight,
is crowned with the smoothness
of her scalp.

Without legs
a woman moves
with song and thought.

Without ears
she hears
what words
obscure.

Without eyes
she is not limited
by the confusion
of objects, colour.

Without uterus, ovaries,
she spawns wisdom
with the turn of the moon.

Without her life's breath
a woman becomes earth,
the bearer of herb and seed,
rock and ground root.

© ELANA KLUGMAN

Breast cancer and any recurrences are likely to have many causes, and any steps we can take that help build up the immune system and the body's defences are likely to be of benefit. See Cancer, p. 574, for ways of doing this.

Doctors are currently uncertain of the usefulness of regular check-ups and screening tests for women who have had breast cancer treatment; they don't *prevent* you getting breast cancer again. If you find the check-ups reassuring then they are obviously worthwhile for you. If, on the other hand, you find they increase your anxiety and threaten the control that you feel you could have, then you may decide that they are not helpful.

The risk of developing benign breast lumps is the same for all women, whether or not we have or have had breast cancer. There is a slightly increased risk of getting cancer in the other breast if we've already had it in one. When this happens it is usually a completely separate primary tumour, not a spread from the first one, and treatment is as likely to be successful as it was the first time round.

We need to translate our fears of breast cancer, fatalism about our survival chances, frustration at the limitations of our personal situations, and anger at the nature of our lives and the environment – all which make us vulnerable – into strategies and campaigns for better health in all respects, for the treatment we want, for research into the causes and action to limit their effects.

AUTOBIOGRAPHICAL NOTES ABOUT MOST OF THE WOMEN QUOTED IN THIS CHAPTER.

Rita: I am over sixty, live alone, have no dependants and am healthy, free-thinking, filled with curiosity and practical. An acceptance of authority dating from childhood and ignorance about cancer and treatments made me accept the consultant's decisions unquestioned – partly because I wanted the cancer dealt with quickly. But I 'came out' very critical of the lack of advice, of information and of counselling. I haven't forgotten that a surgeon has removed a part of me that was stated to be cancerous (the Doubting Thomas in me would like to have seen the path. report!) but the experience has not greatly changed my way of living and thinking over the past four years – though it has confirmed my philosophy of life and death.

Sue: I am now thirty-seven and married with a twelve-year-old daughter. I was twenty-eight when I had the mastectomy. The breast implant was done when I was thirty. The important things in my life now are obtaining my degree in English language and literature and being my own person – not what other people expect or want me to be.

Joan: I am forty-seven, married with two teenage daughters. I was found to have cancer of the breast when I was forty-three and underwent a mastectomy. I had reconstruction surgery approximately two years later, which for me was a success. I am now in excellent health and live my life to the full and scarcely give breast cancer a thought.

Josephine: I was born in Belgium and came to England when I was twenty-one to be married and to stay for good. Now I am fifty-three and work as an assistant underwriter for a reinsurance company. I have been married twice and have two grown-up daughters. I am legally separated and have lived by myself for the past twelve years. My cancer treatment finished a year ago. I am in very good health once again and just as active as before. I am playing squash which I thought I would never be able to play again. I also have changed to a much healthier diet.

Jo: I am aged fifty-two and work as an educational photographer and writer concerned with issues relating to our bodies as women – both in the sphere of visual representation and, of course, health. My experience of orthodox breast cancer treatment traumatized me so much that I moved to Traditional Chinese Medicine as a more gentle system of healing.

Helena: I am fifty-seven and work as a freelance editor and researcher. I have been married for thirty-three years and have three grown-up daughters. I am very much a 'home' person enjoying my work, music, books, gardening and cooking. I discovered cysts when I was forty-five and again at fifty-two. My health is excellent.

Laura: I first noticed a breast lump after watching a television programme about breast cancer when I was in my early twenties. It took twelve months before I managed to get a GP to refer me to a hospital. I had a biopsy and a frozen section followed by a radical mastectomy. Three years ago I had a breast implant. My life is a bit like a juggling act with bringing up my two sons and developing my career as a community worker. My cancer tends to take a back seat, surrounded by silence.

Eileen: Eileen got breast cancer in her late fifties, she believed because she had completely drained her body's vitality. She took a very active role in her treatments after a mastectomy, choosing to follow a macrobiotic diet as far as possible and to practise yoga. She had a great deal of loving support from friends and family to help her in her choices and to sustain her when she was dying – something which she never feared but regarded with curious interest.

NOTES

1. Dorothea Lynch and Eugene Richards. *Exploding into Life*. London: Phaidon, 1986.
2. S. Love et al. 'Fibrocystic "Disease" of the Breast – a Non-disease?', *New England Journal of Medicine*, no. 307, 1982, pp. 1010–14.
3. U. Ernester et al. 'Effects of a Caffeine-free Diet on Benign Breast Disease', *Surgery*, vol. 10, no. 91, 1982, p. 263.
4. See A. McTieran and D. Thomas. 'Evidence for the Protective Effect of Lactation on the Risk of Breast Cancer in Young Women', *American Journal of Epidemiology*, vol. 124, 1986, p. 353; and J-M Yuan et al. 'Risk Factors for Breast Cancer in Chinese Women in Shanghai', *Cancer Research*, vol. 48, 1988, p. 1949.
5. See, e.g., M. C. Pike et al. 'Breast Cancer in Young Women and Use of Oral Contraceptives. Possible Modifying Effect of Formulation and Age at Use', *The Lancet*, vol. ii, 1983, p. 970; K. McPherson et al. 'Early Oral Contraceptive Use and Breast Cancer: Results of Another Case-control Study', *British Journal of Cancer*, vol. 56, no. 5, November 1987, pp. 653–60; C. R. Kay and P. C. Hannaford. 'Breast Cancer and the Pill – further report from the RCGP's oral contraceptive study', *British Journal of Cancer*, vol. 58, 1988, p. 657; and D. R. Miller et al. 'Breast Cancer before Age 45 and Contraceptive Use: new findings', *American Journal of Epidemiology* (in press).
6. O. Mirik et al. 'Oral Contraceptive Use and Breast Cancer in Young Women', *The Lancet*, 20 September 1986, pp. 650–4; and McPherson et al., op. cit., note 5; and UK National Case-Control Study Group. 'Oral Contraceptive Use and Breast Cancer Risk in Young Women', *The Lancet*, 5 May 1989, p. 973. This latter study is the first to show a link with dosages: pills with less than 50mcg of oestrogen appearing to carry less risk. It also suggests for the first time that the *progestogen-only* pill might possibly have a protective effect.
7. One such study, widely regarded as providing strong evidence as to the safety of the Pill with regard to breast cancer, is the CASH Study (B. Stadel et al, 'Oral Contraceptives and Breast Cancer in Young Women', *The Lancet*, vol. ii, 1985, p. 970: and B. Stadel et al, 'Oral Contraceptives and Premenopausal Breast Cancer in Nulliparous Women', *Contraception*, 1988, vol. 38, p. 287. This study looked only at women under the age of 45 and its conclusions have recently been thrown into serious doubt by Julian Peto ('Oral Contraceptives and Breast Cancer: Is the CASH Study Really Negative?' *The Lancet*, 11 March 1989, p. 552). He went back to the original figures and found that the study appears to show an *increased* risk for certain groups of young women, thus making it in line with other studies after all.
8. K. McPherson et al. 'Early Contraceptive Use and Breast Cancer: Theoretical Effects of Latency', *Journal of Epidemiology and Community Health*, vol. 40, 1986, pp. 289–94.
9. Julian Peto (see note 7) concludes that 'The results of all major studies . . . appear to be consistent with some increase in risk in women aged up to about 35 or 40'. We do not yet know how the Pill may affect women in older age-groups.
10. Samuel Epstein. *The Politics of Cancer*. New York: Anchor Books, 1979.
11. For example, see C. Fredericks. *Breast Cancer: a Nutritional Approach*. New York: Grosset and Dunlap, 1978; B. R. Goldin et al. 'Effect of Diet on the Excretion of Oestrogen in Pre- and Post-Menopausal Women', *Cancer Research*, vol. 41, 1981, p. 3771.
12. See, e.g., D. C. G. Skegg. 'Alcohol, Coffee, Fat, and Breast Cancer', *British Medical Journal*, 24 October 1987, pp. 1011–12.
13. See, e.g., W. Duncan and G. R. Kerr. 'The Curability of Breast Cancer', *British Medical Journal*, 2 October 1976.

14. S. Shapiro et al. 'Ten to Fourteen Year Effect of Screening on Breast Cancer Mortality', *Journal of the National Cancer Institute*, vol. 69, no. 2, 1982, pp. 349–55; A. L. Verbeek et al. 'Reduction of Breast Cancer Mortality Through Mass Screening with Modern Mammographs', *The Lancet*, vol. i, 1984, pp. 1222–6; L. Tabar et al. 'Reduction in Mortality from Breast Cancer After Mass Screening with Mammography', *The Lancet*, 13 April 1985, pp. 829–32.

15. P. Forrest et al. *Breast Cancer Screening: Report to the Health Ministers of England, Wales, Scotland and Northern Ireland* (The Forrest Report). London: HMSO, 1986.

16. Audré Lorde. *The Cancer Journals*. London: Sheba, 1985, p. 52.

17. G. Bonadonna et al. 'Adjuvant Chemotherapy in Breast Cancer', *The Lancet*, vol. i, 1983, p. 1157.

18. N. Padmanabhan, A. Howell and R. D. Rubens. 'Mechanism of Action of Adjuvant Chemotherapy in Early Breast Cancer', *The Lancet*,

19. Grace Simpson. *Senior Nurse*, February 1985.

RESOURCES
READING

Boston, Sarah and Jill **Louw**. *Disorderly Breasts*. London: Camden Press, 1987. Written by a woman who has breast cancer and her friend, this book covers the diagnosis and treatment of both malignant and benign breast conditions.

Brohn, Penny. *Gentle Giants*. London: Century, 1986.

Forrest, P. et al. *Breast Cancer Screening: Report to the Health Ministers of England, Wales, Scotland and Northern Ireland* (The Forrest Report). London: HMSO, 1986.

Guide to Breast Self-examination, available from clinics and health education departments.

King's Fund. *The Treatment of Primary Breast Cancer – Consensus Statement*, 1987. Available from King's Fund College, 2 Palace Court, London W2 4HS.

Kushner, Rose. *Breast Cancer: A Personal History and Investigative Report*. New York: Harcourt Brace Jovanovich, 1975.

Living with Breast Surgery. Leaflet produced by the Health Education Authority and available from clinics and health education departments.

Lorde, Audré. *The Cancer Journals*. London: Sheba, 1985. A black feminist's sensitive description of the loss of her breast. She challenges many of society's attitudes to women, attitudes which also influence the approach of the medical profession to breast cancer.

Lynch, Dorothea and Eugene **Richards**. *Exploding into Life*. London: Phaidon, 1986. A moving account of Dorothea's experience of breast cancer and secondaries with photographs by her lover. As well as telling Dorothea's story, they write about and photograph other people with cancer.

Manchester Breast Cancer Study Group. *Thinking About Breast Cancer*. Cambridge: National Extension College, 1988. Several of the women who prepared this chapter were members of the collective which wrote this pamphlet.

Skrabanek, P. 'False Premises and False Promises of Breast Cancer Screening'. *The Lancet*, 10 August 1985.

Watts, G. T. 'Some Aspects of Primary Reconstruction of the Breast Following Mastectomy for Carcinoma in Yorkshire Breast Cancer Group', Breast Reconstruction after Mastectomy Symposium Paper, 1978.

Women's Health and Breast Cancer, factsheet available from WHRRIC (see p. 334).

MODEL

Breast self-examination silicone model breast with lumps for teaching self-examination. Available from WHRRIC (see p. 638) for returnable deposit.

ORGANIZATIONS
See also Organizations on p. 592.

Breast Care and Mastectomy Association, 26A Harrison Street, London WC1 8JG. Tel: 01–837 0908. The association provides practical, non-medical advice and support to women who have had breast surgery of any kind. They also run a one-to-one contact service using volunteers who have had breast surgery, who will visit women in hospital or at home.

Women's National Cancer Control Campaign, 1 South Audley Street, London W1Y 5DQ. Tel: 01–499 7532.

CERTAIN DISEASES OF THE WHOLE BODY, CANCER AND FACING DEATH*

Rewritten by
JILL RAKUSEN
(*unless otherwise indicated*)

ANAEMIA

Prepared by ANGELA PHILLIPS

Our blood carries oxygen to every part of our bodies in the haemoglobin (part of the red blood cells). When there is not enough oxygen in the blood, we become anaemic. *Deficiency anaemias* tend to cause vague symptoms such as tiredness, irritability, dizziness, shortness of breath, headaches, bone pain and vulnerability to infection. Dark-skinned women may look grey, light-skinned women get very pale. Deficiency anaemias are four times more common among women than men as we lose iron through menstruation and childbirth. The *hereditary anaemias* are far more severe (see below). Anaemia can also be caused by chronic illness, such as kidney or thyroid disease, arthritis or cancer, exposure to certain drugs, chemicals and metals or radiation (see p. 345 for Anaemia in Pregnancy).

TESTING FOR ANAEMIA

Deficiency anaemias can be checked by a simple blood test to check the haemoglobin content. The normal range lies within Hb 11–13. It is possible to tell whether the anaemia is due to iron or vitamin deficiency by checking the size and shape of the red blood cells. Hereditary anaemias cannot be identified with this test. A special blood test (haemoglobin electrophoresis) is required. This test should be routine during pregnancy and newborn babies should also be checked. However, routine screening is not available in this country and policies for screening vary.

IRON-DEFICIENCY ANAEMIA

Iron-deficiency anaemia is by far the most common form in women, often caused by heavy menstrual periods as well as

*See Chapter 23, pp. 502 and 503 for Hepatitis B and Scabies.

bleeding associated with miscarriage, abortion, childbirth or surgery for fibroids. The best preventive is an iron-rich diet (including meat, dried fruit and green vegetables). Cooking foods in iron pots increases their iron content. If despite eating an iron-rich diet you are still anaemic, you may want to take supplements. (Some practitioners recommend that pregnant women routinely take iron supplements.) Ferrous gluconate and chelated iron are the most easily absorbed forms of iron. They work best on an empty stomach, but if they cause nausea or cramps take them with food. Eating food high in Vitamin C at the same time will increase absorption. Even so, some women find through subsequent blood tests that they cannot absorb iron pills. In that case, try blackstrap molasses. Iron pills can cause tarry stools or constipation, which can be remedied by eating more whole grains and fruit and drinking lots of water. Iron interferes with the absorption of Vitamin E. If you are taking Vitamin E supplements, be sure to take them at least six hours before the iron.

VITAMIN-DEFICIENCY ANAEMIAS

Pregnant women, women who have had many children, women on oral contraceptives and malnourished women can become anaemic due to a lack of folic acid (an essential B vitamin). You can prevent or treat this deficiency by eating whole grains and dark green vegetables and/or taking folic acid supplements. (One caution: too much folic acid may contribute to the development of breast cysts.) Vegetarians who eat no animal or dairy products sometimes suffer from pernicious anaemia caused by lack of Vitamin B12 (present in all animal products). Symptoms may include burning or weakness in the legs. Adding brewer's yeast (which often contains B12), a fortified cereal like Grape-Nuts, or fermented foods like miso, tempeh or fermented sprouts to the diet will help. Women who lack a protein called the 'intrinsic factor', necessary for oral absorption of Vitamin B12, will need monthly injections of this vitamin.

HEREDITARY ANAEMIA

In Britain the most common forms of inherited anaemia are sickle-cell anaemia (which mainly affects African and Caribbean people) and thalassaemia (which is mainly suffered by people from the Mediterranean and Asia). Some black and Mediterranean people also inherit a deficiency of the enzyme G6PD (glucose-6-phosphate-dehydrogenase). People with this deficiency cannot take sulpha drugs, aspirin or anti-malarial drugs, as they trigger haemolytic anaemia (which can be fatal).

Screening and specialist centres for these diseases are patchy and rely heavily on voluntary work and fund-raising. Compare this to the 110 specialist clinics provided for haemophiliacs (a disease of white males). Yet three times as many babies are born each year with sickle-cell disease and thalassaemia.

Sickle-cell anaemia is a disease of the haemoglobin. When the red blood cells become short of oxygen (which can be caused by over-exertion, infection or even changes in temperature), they become sickle shaped (known as sickling) and block small blood vessels. This leads to severe pain.

Sickle-cell anaemia develops only if both parents have what is known as a trait. (See Chapter 18, p. 343, for genetic screening.) The trait itself rarely causes health problems. Sickle-cell disease varies in severity. It may cause general ill health and exhaustion and can be life-threatening if sickling crises (see above) are not properly and promptly dealt with. With enough information and support, the disease can be controlled.

Though men and women suffer in equal numbers from the disease, women, as mothers, are usually faced with setting the patterns of care in childhood which will keep the disease in check. It can be a frightening and lonely task. Self-help treatment includes rest, plenty to drink, a good diet, warm living conditions, plenty of sleep and no strenuous exercise. Anaesthetics can be dangerous; infections of any kind must be dealt with promptly. During pregnancy, crises are more common so special care is needed. Oestrogen in the combined Pill, or hormone replacement therapy, should be avoided (see Chapter 15).

The **Sickle Cell Society** and **Thalassaemia Society** provide information about these conditions and how best to cope with crises (see Resources). For information on sickle-cell screening in pregnancy, see p. 343.

ACQUIRED IMMUNE DEFICIENCY SYNDROME (AIDS)*

By VICKY WHELAN, CO-ORDINATOR OF MANCHESTER AIDSLINE

AIDS is a syndrome not a disease, in which a person's body is weakened and cannot cope with a specific range of infections it would ordinarily be able to deal with. The body is weakened by HIV (see p. 501) entering a person's blood-stream and damaging the immune system. The way the virus damages the immune system is complex and not completely understood. HIV is a retrovirus – a rare type of virus which has only recently been discovered. Unlike other viruses, such as those which cause the common cold, which you can overcome, HIV enters particular cells (T4 cells) in the immune system. Once it is inside these cells the virus inserts its own genetic code in place of those of the T4 cell so that the cell actually produces more virus instead of more T4 cells. The virus becomes part of the structure of the body's cells and is there for life. The T4 cell can now make more virus, which can enter other T4 cells for the process to be repeated. However, what is unknown is what triggers or checks this process so that some people go on to develop AIDS and others stay well. What is becoming clearer is that factors such as previous medical history (sexually transmitted diseases, e.g., syphilis), drug use (including alcohol and nicotine), poverty, repeated exposure to HIV, a person's genetic characteristics, or stress can have influences – from initial exposure, coping with repeated exposure, or going on to have AIDS.

Current research among people who have gone on to develop AIDS or other related conditions is showing an incubation period of five to ten years. It is not yet certain whether everyone carrying the virus will go on to develop AIDS. This uncertainty is a high-stress factor for those who know they are infected with the HIV (people who have had an HIV antibody test which has given a positive result). Stress itself can be a trigger for people to go on to develop AIDS or other related conditions. People who are HIV positive, in the present state of knowledge, have to assume that they are infectious, and need to protect themselves and others by using safer sex (see p. 488). However, there are many recorded cases of gay and straight relationships where one partner is HIV negative and one is HIV positive so it is possible to be exposed to HIV without becoming infected. What is clear is that repeated exposure to HIV means that you are more liable to be infected. Women who are HIV positive and who are considering pregnancy need to seek early, sympathetic medical advice. At present it appears that there is a 50 per cent chance that the virus can be passed on to the fetus. It is still unclear whether pregnancy itself is a trigger for a woman with HIV infection to go on to develop AIDS. What does seem clearer is that poor diet, inadequate housing and other consequences of poverty can precipitate AIDS. Early or mid-term abortion does *not* seem to halt the progression to AIDS. There are HIV-positive mothers in Britain at present who are now considering whether to have a second child.

*When the most recent American edition of *Our Bodies, Ourselves* was written, AIDS had not yet been seen as an issue for women and was not discussed. Things have moved so fast since then that this section has already been rewritten three times, and will be out of date by the time you read it. Please see Organizations in Resources for up-to-date information.

The symptoms of AIDS mimic many things which happen to people when they are under stress. Experience has shown (via breakdowns of AIDS Helpline calls) that listing a range of symptoms only raises anxiety. The important points are that symptoms are severe and prolonged (of more than three months' duration for which no other medical explanation can be given). The two most common symptoms associated with AIDS are a skin cancer known as Kaposi's Sarcoma and pneumocystis carinii (a severe pneumonia). Medical treatments are available, and improving, for AIDS-related infections, and people in Western countries can live for years with AIDS (in Africa very little treatment is available). However, because people's immune systems have been weakened, they will never recover and will eventually die – so AIDS is a life-threatening illness. Anecdotal evidence is showing that coming to terms with a diagnosis of AIDS is easier than an acceptance of being HIV positive, because of the uncertainty of the latter state. See Chapter 7 for approaches which can help us live with HIV and AIDS. See also Resources, p. 592.

There are many local AIDS groups and Helplines in the British Isles at present and the National AIDS Helpline telephone can put you in touch with your nearest one. Many of them have support groups specifically for women with concerns about HIV and AIDS and many are waiting for the need to be shown to help set up such a group.

CIRCULATORY DISEASES

Heart attacks and strokes are second only to cancer as the leading cause of premature death in women in the UK. We can be forgiven for being ignorant of this – although it has been known for years – because health education programmes and literature have focused almost exclusively on men and tended to ignore the importance of circulatory diseases (particularly heart disease) in women. Where women have been considered at all, this has usually been as key people in the prevention of heart disease – not of our own, but of men's. Not surprisingly, therefore, most people typically think of men, not women, as having heart attacks, and most research on the subject has been on men.

POLITICS AND CIRCULATORY DISEASES

Circulatory disease is a major political issue: first, because of the inadequate amount of resources directed towards its prevention when compared with the increasing amount expended on high-technology treatment; second, because of the derisory amount of research concerned with women – as opposed to men; and third, because so little attention is paid to socio-political causes and solutions – whether in relation to women *or* men.

In the following pages we try to draw out these issues, particularly the two latter points. This has not been an easy task since so little suitable research has been done. The political issues surrounding circulatory disease are most clearly described in Prevention, below.* A similar understanding is required, both of strokes *and* high blood pressure, but while much of our analysis concerning heart disease is broadly relevant to these health problems too, more work is needed in these areas. It is only in the last few years that feminists have begun to get to grips with the political issues underlying medical approaches to heart disease; we hope that in the next few years, equal attention will be paid to strokes and blood pressure.

HEART DISEASE

Heart disease accounts for about 22 per cent of all deaths among women (and about 30 per cent among men). In 1983 over 75,000 women in the UK died from coronary heart disease.

The most common form of *coronary heart disease* (CHD; also called *coronary artery disease* or *ischaemic heart disease*) is caused by *atherosclerosis* or *atheroma*. This is a slowly developing disease process in which the passageway through the arteries becomes narrowed and roughened by fatty deposits called plaque. The development of plaque then blocks one or more of the arteries that supply the heart muscle with blood. When sufficient blood can no longer reach the heart, part of the heart dies from lack of oxygen and other nutrients. This is a *heart attack* (or *myocardial infarction*, *coronary thrombosis* or *coronary occlusion*). When the artery blockage is partial it may cause chest pain, a condition referred to as *angina*.

Atherosclerosis can also lead to a narrowing of the blood vessels which supply blood to the brain, causing a stroke (see p. 563).

Prevention**

While most people assume that heart disease is a 'disease of affluence' in industrialized countries, it is in fact a disease of the poor. Working-class people suffer from it more than middle-class people, and for women the class difference is greater than the class difference in relation to men.

The British Regional Heart Study, which investigated the causes of heart disease among men, found that among the factors most closely associated with (high) heart disease rates in any area of Britain were how many people in each area were unemployed, did not have cars and lived in council housing. Yet, instead of focusing attention on the hazards of the environment in which people live and work and these kinds of social risk factors, medical researchers

---

*Mel Bartley, Wendy Farrant, Linnie Price and Jill Russell have helped greatly in clarifying the issues in so far as it is possible to do so at the present time. Since feminist analysis (mainly their own) has in the main concentrated on coronary heart disease, this is reflected in the text – which relies heavily on their work (with their consent!) – see Resources (Publications) for further details.

**After this chapter was written, a new study was published that indicated the value of taking aspirin as a means of preventing heart attacks. While this is obviously a valuable discovery (see box, p. 561), it does not *per se* provide the answers to the prevention of heart disease. To do that, we need to look at the underlying causes of the disease.

and health educators have chosen to concentrate on people's individual behaviours, such as 'over-indulgence' and 'slothfulness'.

Nowadays most studies of heart disease concentrate on three standard risk factors (i.e. factors that are considered by medical researchers to be associated with an increased risk of developing the disease): smoking cigarettes, raised blood pressure, and a raised level of cholesterol in the blood. Although only a minority of medical and health professionals are prepared to admit it publicly, there are still scientific doubts over these risk factors, particularly the latter two.

Only a small part of the difference in deaths from heart disease between working-class and middle-class people can be explained by differences in the conventional risk factors. Even in so far as working-class people do, for example, tend to smoke more than middle-class people, this only accounts for a part of the class difference, and this still begs the question of what it is about our society that makes it harder for some people, for example, to give up smoking than for others. Furthermore, if we start to look at heart disease as it affects both men *and* women, white *and* black people, middle- *and* working-class people, then the accepted explanations of what causes the disease seem unconvincing. For example, women, on average, have similar or higher blood pressure and cholesterol levels than men but lower rates of coronary deaths. Asian men and women in Britain appear to have the highest rates of heart disease of all ethnic groups, but in terms of conventional risk factors, they would not seem to be at high risk.*

If we look at the role of fat in the diet, evidence for this is based mainly on epidemiological research which indicates that the *overall* level of saturated fat in the diet of *populations* is related to the incidence of CHD. This does *not* mean that reduction of fat content in diet *necessarily* reduces the risk in any individual, and indeed, is unlikely except in a minority of cases. A major reason for this is because of the limitations of the concept of being 'at risk', or 'risk factors'. Atherosclerosis, for example, is present to some extent in everybody, at least in the West, and advanced atherosclerosis does not necessarily lead to heart attack or premature death. Equally, people die from coronary heart disease who are subsequently found to have little or no atheroma.

The data have been consistently misrepresented because of a simplistic notion of cause and effect that is prevalent in medicine; a notion which fits in with the views of many health promotional strategists (it makes promoting health so much easier if you have a simplistic strategy that fits within traditional medical concepts). But more than that, any approach which lays the blame for a widespread health problem firmly at the door of the individual leaves the status quo intact and lets the government off the hook. Successive governments (and governments in many parts of the

world) have been quick to grasp this – and hence we, via the government-funded Health Education Authority, are at the receiving end of such clear victim-blaming propaganda.

Let us now look at one important socio-political factor in the cause of heart disease.

Women's Work and Heart Disease

The vast majority of research studies on heart disease have focused narrowly on the conventional risk factors. Two studies that have taken the environment seriously found that knowing what sort of job a person does can tell us more about that person's risk of heart disease than knowing about their smoking habits. One of these studies was done in England and is about men only but has important implications for women.[3] The other is American and looked at both men and women.[4] The results of these two very different studies are very consistent.

The English study (called the Whitehall Study) found that male civil servants in the lowest grade jobs (incidentally, of course, the sorts of jobs that women are most likely to be doing as well) had nearly four times the death-rate from heart disease than men in the highest, best-paid grades (i.e. the jobs that are generally occupied by men).

In attempting to explain what it might be about poorly paid, routine work that increases these workers' risk of heart disease, the authors of this study observed:

> More of the men in the lower grades reported that they had little or no control over their work, and that their work contained little or no variety . . . lower grade men [also] have fewer social contacts with workmates, neighbours and with relatives and other friends.

The lack of variety and control, and the social isolation that men in the above study complained of characterizes not only women's work outside the home, but, even more so, women's work within the home. Also, many women experience feelings of lack of control not only over their work, but over their whole lives.

The American study which shows such similar results is a long-running study of men and women (mostly middle class) in a small town called Framingham. All the people in this study were examined at regular intervals as they grew older, to see what it was about their physical health and lifestyle that related to their eventually getting heart disease. One factor that the Framingham team looked at was people's jobs. They found that women with children *and* doing worse paid, more repetitive and routine jobs, such as clerks and secretaries, were twice as likely to get heart disease as women who worked only in their homes. Women with better paid, professional jobs had no excess risk. Having few promotion opportunities and a difficult boss also increased the women clerical and secretarial workers' risk. When the Framingham investigators looked at things like blood pressure, smoking and blood

*The death-rate from coronary heart disease for Asian women in the UK is 30 per cent higher than the UK average, and that for Asian men is 29 per cent higher.[1]

cholesterol, these were found to be no help in predicting which women would get heart disease. Another factor predicting heart disease among these women was having a husband in a lower-paid job. In summing up what the results of this study can tell us about women's risk of heart disease, Mary Ann Haw says that they:

> provide the most convincing evidence that the combination of certain job conditions and family responsibilities may lead to structural and functional damage [to the heart].[5]

This combination of certain job conditions and family responsibilities is a particular source of stress for working-class women, and this must be especially true at the present time of increases in family poverty, reduction in social support services, etcetera. We can only speculate why Asian women (as well as Asian men) seem to be at such high risk; we wonder if sufficient account is being taken of the added stress of racism.

Alternative Strategies

You may wonder, in view of the research we have mentioned, why more attention is not paid to avoiding heart disease by means of improving the work and home environments of men and women. Obviously, this kind of prevention raises political issues about the nature of work and family roles with which most doctors and health educators feel uncomfortable. They tend to argue that we *know* it's good for you to reduce your weight and stop smoking and take more exercise, and this is simpler to address than 'political' issues; that people should be given simple advice about things it is possible for them to change as individuals. And no one is denying that changes of this sort are good for health.

But there are many reasons why women find it particularly difficult to take this kind of preventive action. And these difficulties *themselves* are related to our work and family responsibilities. So it seems that by tackling these we might at the same time make other kinds of healthier life choices easier for ourselves. By failing to take on the issues of work and family stress, health educators and doctors only make it less likely that women will be able to make those changes we are supposed to be 'individually' responsible for. *Improving women's health, in other words, cannot be separated from improving the quality of women's lives.*

For example, a more interesting job would make over-eating out of boredom less likely. There is a great deal of evidence that availability of work which women with children at home can fit into our lives protects against depression. Less stress caused by sexism and racism would make it easier for some of us to relax at home and at work. Shorter hours of work for men *and* women, and shared child care would give us the time to get out and about and increase our 'levels of physical activity' and so on.

Some trade unions are beginning to take up work on stress as a major health and safety issue. (See Stress, p. 20.)

The trade union ASTMS (now MSF) has issued a policy document on stress,[6] and others could be encouraged to do the same. Recognition of a woman's work responsibilities by her family, and of family responsibilities of both men and women by employers should be taken equally seriously by unions and women's organizations. Health education and health promotion workers are also beginning to take up the question of the way in which women's lack of control over our lives at home and at work makes it naive and complacent for them simply to tell us to slim or stop smoking or 'relax'. After all, eating or smoking may be our 'coping behaviour'. As Arabella Melville and Colin Johnson say:

> Cutting off support in the form of coping behaviour could be like taking the lid off a pressure cooker without cooling it first . . . removing a coping mechanism, no matter how understandable, will increase your stress. Dealing with a cause, no matter how difficult, will decrease it.[7]

A strategy for preventing heart disease among women needs to build our confidence to take collective action to change our environment.

Following research that strongly suggests that aspirin can significantly reduce the risk of heart attack,[2] many doctors are now suggesting taking the equivalent of a 'junior' aspirin every two days as a preventive measure.

If you want to consider this form of prevention please discuss it first with your doctor. It is never a good idea to take drugs, including aspirin, on a regular basis without a very good reason; aspirin can interact dangerously with certain prescription drugs as we get older.

Recognizing the Signs of Heart Attack

Unfortunately, the first sign of heart disease can be sudden death from heart attack. One quarter of all people who have heart attacks had no previous 'warning' or knowledge of heart disease, and 60 per cent of heart-attack deaths occur before the person reaches the hospital.

The symptoms of a heart attack are pain in the chest, which may also be felt in the arm, shoulder, neck or jaw (occasionally worse in these areas than in the chest), accompanied by shortness of breath, sweating, faintness or an irregular pulse. Some people describe the pain as vice-like or constricting, like a rope being pulled around their chest. Others describe the pain as feeling like a heavy weight crushing their chest. It is useful to know that chest pain can also come from conditions other than heart

RISK FACTORS

As we show in our discussion under Prevention (see p. 559), the concept of risk factors in relation to heart disease is fraught with confusion and open to misinterpretation and abuse. What we have listed here are all the risk factors known to date where there is considerable evidence for them to be taken seriously. How seriously, and how seriously relative to each other, is a moot point. At the very least, they cannot be taken as being able to *predict* heart disease, and though the more risk factors that a person has the greater the risk is likely to be, they would still have a higher chance of *not* having heart trouble than of getting it – even if all the risk factors applied to them. However, we must emphasize that leading a healthy life – and having the opportunity and resources to do so – are far more important for our health generally than being seen solely as ways of preventing even heart disease.

- *Social class.* As with virtually all causes of death, working-class people are at highest risk of getting coronary heart disease. This may be due to stress in relation to poverty, housing, poor quality of life in general, and/or in relation to work, and/or to dietary effects of poverty. Action through community groups and trade unions may help: use this text and the WHRRIC broadsheets (see Resources) as educational material. See also Women's Work and Heart Disease, p. 560; Stress, p. 20, and Chapters 4, 9 and 7.
- *Smoking.* For help on giving it up, see Chapter 5.
- *High blood pressure.* See p. 564 for how to reduce it.
- *Diet.* Cutting back on saturated fats (see p. 48 in Chapter 4) may help prevent heart disease. However, the food industry has been capitalizing on the low-cholesterol issue by promoting highly processed foodstuffs as beneficial because they are 'polyunsaturated'. Many scientists now question the value of eating more polyunsaturates and are increasingly concerned about the negative health effects of highly processed foods. (It may well be that Essential Fatty Acids, see p. 46, are necessary to prevent heart disease and that lack of fresh greens, fish and vegetable oils may be far more important than too much saturated fat.)

  Current medical advice to avoid foods high in cholesterol and saturated fats may pose special problems for women. In an effort to reduce fat intake, some women may eliminate or cut back on dairy products, which may be their main source of calcium. (Inadequate calcium is a factor in the development of osteoporosis and hypertension.) See Chapter 4 for a discussion on this.
- *Lack of exercise.* Regular exercise is believed to reduce the risk of heart attack and can definitely lower blood pressure (see Chapter 6).
- *Excess weight.* A combination of general weight reduction, associated with dietary improvement, and exercise can be an important strategy for reducing the risk of cardiovascular and circulatory disease in some women.
- *Taking oral contraceptives* (particularly if the woman also smokes). (See Chapter 15.)
- *Removal of the uterus and/or ovaries before menopause* may be a risk factor (see p. 60).
- Some studies have indicated that certain behavioural factors (habitual impatience, hostility, high competitive drive, for instance) may predict heart attacks and can be minimized by stress-reduction techniques. However, these studies have been done almost exclusively on men, and as the WHRRIC broadsheet shows (see Resources), these types of studies are too male-orientated to be of much ultimate benefit to women.
- *Impaired thyroid function* and *diabetes* are also risk factors in relation to heart disease.

attack.* Heart pains that occur with exertion but go away with rest indicate angina, a condition which may not be immediately life-threatening, but which should be evaluated by a doctor.

*Chest pain is often due to indigestion. It can also come from muscles in the chest, lungs, diaphragm, spine or organs in the upper abdomen. Often it is difficult even for practitioners to determine the pain's precise origin. Shooting pains that last a few seconds are common in young people, and a 'catching' sensation at the end of a deep breath does not need attention. Chest-wall pain, rarely present at the same time as a heart attack, can often be identified by pressing a finger on the spot, which would increase the pain. Hyperventilation (too rapid breathing which changes the carbon dioxide balance in the blood) can lead to both dizziness and chest pain, and it is now believed that many people wrongly diagnosed as having heart disease are in fact suffering from the effects of anxiety.

Getting Help

If you, or anyone you are with, experience heart-attack symptoms, CALL YOUR GP. IF S/HE IS NOT AVAILABLE, DIAL 999 OR GO TO A HOSPITAL IMMEDIATELY. DO NOT WAIT TO SEE IF THE SYMPTOMS GO AWAY! As women, we may be afraid of being seen as 'hysterical' or feel that we will be ridiculed for going to the hospital unless we have something 'really serious'. To ignore heart-attack symptoms is to risk our lives.

Most major hospitals have special coronary care units where the rhythm of the heart can be continuously monitored and an infusion of *streptokinase* can be given.

This drug has been found to be phenomenally successful at saving lives, particularly if it is given with *aspirin*; the sooner after a heart attack it is given, the better. This means that hospital casualty departments need to refer on quickly, or to be well-versed in its use. An aspirin on its own (chewed while waiting for the ambulance, for example) can also be a life-saver, but it is important to be clear about the diagnosis and whether there are any contraindications (such as a history of gastrointestinal bleeding or stroke) before embarking on this course of action. While some doctors think the possible benefits of monitoring can be outweighed by the damage done by the journey and hospital admission, preferring home care for some people, they need to take into account the importance of streptokinase treatment, which normally requires admission to hospital. We wonder if the emergency services, already overstretched, will be able to play their part in saving thousands of lives with this now internationally accepted treatment.

FIRST AID

When someone collapses with a heart attack, cardiac resuscitation may be life-saving in keeping the circulation going until expert help is available. The more people who learn to recognize the signs, start mouth to mouth respiration and give external cardiac massage, the more lives can be saved, as most deaths occur in the early minutes or hours before the doctor or ambulance arrives.

To learn about first aid for heart attacks, contact your health education department (see p. 627) or your local branch of the Red Cross. See also our discussion on aspirin above.

Treatment

For women who have had a heart attack or who have been diagnosed as having coronary artery disease or angina, there are two approaches to treatment: medical and surgical. Within the medical and scientific communities, there is considerable controversy over the relative effectiveness of these two approaches.

Coronary bypass surgery, popular in recent years, is done primarily to relieve chest pain which persists in some people after a heart attack. Coronary bypass surgery involves removing a vein from the leg and attaching it to the coronary artery to 'bypass' the obstructed area. Some people experience dramatic relief of pain and can lead physically active lives after surgery. There is no evidence, however, that surgery increases life expectancy.[8]

Several excellent studies have shown that more conservative treatment is equal or superior to bypass surgery for most people. The medical approach is aimed at preventing a further heart attack. In the USA the method is called *heart conditioning* – a programme of progressively more strenuous exercise combined with a low-fat diet, relaxation techniques and drug therapy. Blood pressure is lowered and participants are urged to stop smoking. (For some people, any exercise at all is dangerous.)

In the UK, Dr Peter Nixon has pioneered an approach to coronary care which, though ridiculed by many of his colleagues, has a lot in common with a holistic approach to health and disease generally. His approach is as relevant to treatment as it is to prevention; it takes as its starting point the belief that heart disease is a biological response to circumstances. Since it is a *response* rather than a primary *disease*, it is possible to consider ways of helping the individual to 'outwit the destructive changes and to reinforce his [sic] coping and surviving skills'.[9] The Nixon approach, which is really no different from *any* holistic approach to *any* disease, involves paying careful attention to the person's life and how s/he feels about it, and helping her/him to make changes. The tools he uses towards this end range from counselling and massage to meditation. For more about his approach, and for books which promote self-help following cardiovascular problems, see Resources. See also Chapter 7.

STROKE

Women are more likely than men to have strokes, despite the fact that overall stroke deaths have been declining for some years. Stroke is directly related to high blood pressure, which becomes much more common after menopause.

Since high blood pressure is the major cause of strokes, it is clear that many are easily preventable (see p. 564). Some strokes are also the result of atherosclerosis, and some of these may also be preventable – but see p. 559 for the complexities surrounding prevention of atherosclerosis and heart disease.

Strokes may be very mild, so mild that you or your practitioner may not recognize them. They may cause only minor or temporary impairment. These are called *transient ischaemic attacks*, or TIAs. When an artery bursts because of high blood pressure, either damaging part of the brain or impairing its function due to the pressure of pooled blood, the result is a *cerebral haemorrhage*. Depending on the type of stroke you have, if you survive you may experience speech loss, paralysis or other loss of mental and physical function.

> Everything was there, but I couldn't speak. I was conscious that I was speaking but I couldn't speak, if you see what I mean. That was a miraculous thing. I did everything but I couldn't speak. It was awful.[11]

---

*For only one group, those with obstruction of the left main coronary artery, does surgery improve chances of survival.

*Dr Nixon appears to spend most of his time and energy working with, and considering the needs of, male patients. As yet, we are not aware of anyone focusing similarly on the needs of female patients.[10]

Rehabilitation and therapy can often help you to recover certain functions, but it is important that this is begun as soon as possible. (Contact the Chest, Heart and Stroke Association for advice on the type of help that might be available. Some people find that practices like yoga can aid recovery too.) Geriatric wards, often considered to be depressing places, can be the best places for people with strokes, for they are usually geared to rehabilitation far more than general medical wards.

Despite the unavoidable sadness of a ward full of elderly, frail and sometimes confused women, there was a busy, cheerful and optimistic atmosphere.[12]

Signs of Stroke or TIA

These include intense, mounting headache lasting many hours; sudden or gradual blackout; dizziness or vision problems; sudden weakness or numbness in the face, arms, fingers, toes; slurring of speech; difficulty in walking. Any one or more of these symptoms call for action, even though they may happen over several hours. Call your GP or go immediately to a hospital casualty department.

Prompt treatment may reduce impairment, prevent another stroke (several may occur in quick succession) and maximize future functioning.

HIGH BLOOD PRESSURE

High blood pressure (hypertension) is sometimes called 'the silent killer' because it is often symptomless and, when untreated, can lead to strokes and is thought to be related to heart disease too. Untreated, it can also affect the brain, kidneys and eyes and cause serious problems during pregnancy.

About 20 per cent of women of all ages in this country develop high blood pressure at some point in their lives. (Even children may do so.) No one yet knows how high blood pressure in women of thirty-five and under ultimately affects life expectancy. See Chapter 15 for the relationship between the Pill and high blood pressure.

Black women of African descent seem to be particularly at risk of hypertension. This is probably due to a combination of factors, of which the most important is likely to be economic (the incidence of high blood pressure seems to increase in inverse proportion to income).[13]

Symptoms

Severe high blood pressure may be accompanied by warning symptoms such as headache, dizziness, fainting spells, ringing in the ears and nosebleeds. However, most people with high blood pressure have absolutely no symptoms and feel quite well.

Diagnosis

Blood pressure is described by two numbers (for example, 120/70). The first number is the systolic pressure (the force of the blood in the arteries when the heart is pumping blood out). The second number is the diastolic pressure (the force of the blood in the arteries when the heart is filling with blood). In general, a systolic pressure of above 140 or a diastolic pressure above 90 are considered signs of hypertension.

Blood pressure varies with the time of day, activity and stress. Different observers and different machines also can give wildly different readings.[14] Only a *consistent* elevation of the blood pressure on at least three separate occasions can enable hypertension to be diagnosed with any accuracy. Even then, some researchers think that a diagnosis of mild or borderline hypertension should be delayed until consistent readings have been obtained over a period of years, since slightly elevated blood pressures fall by themselves within a few years in a majority of cases.*

Prevention and Self-help

Approximately 5 per cent of all cases of high blood pressure can be diagnosed as due to glandular or hormonal abnormalities. All other cases are referred to as 'essential hypertension': this may be due to oral contraceptives, diet, properties of the water supply, the person's size, stress and heredity. Many of these factors may interact to cause hypertension. They may also interact with other as yet poorly investigated factors, such as exposure to lead.[15] However, as with heart disease, the socio-political causes of hypertension may well be the most significant – see our discussion on p. 559.**

You can often prevent hypertension in a number of simple ways, and also lower mildly raised blood pressure – enough, in many cases, to eliminate the need for potentially risky drug treatments.

1. *Stress*. When our lives are continually stressful, we have a greater chance of developing high blood pressure. We can try to tackle both the external and internal causes of stress in our lives. The checklist on p. 21 may help you identify external ones, and various chapters in the rest of this book will, we hope, provide ideas and support for dealing with them. With regard to our *responses* to stress, meditation and relaxation have been shown to be effective in reducing blood pressure. See Appendix to Chapter 7 for information about these and other approaches to stress reduction. But remember that there are usually social and political reasons why our lives are stressful: concerted political action to change these is just as important. For more on stress, see p. 20.

2. *Diet* is thought by many to be the single most important factor in preventing and treating mild hypertension, in particular, diets that involve limited salt

---

*In Western societies, average blood pressure readings rise with age. This may be due to the amount of salt in the diet, as this rise with age is not found in societies where people don't add salt to their food.

**J. Eyer, who has studied the socio-political causes of high blood pressure, concludes that his data 'imply that major social changes are necessary to prevent modern hypertension', and in particular stresses the need to redefine 'the nature of production and productivity, and major reorganization of lifetime work patterns'.[16]

intake,* sufficient calcium, and/or sufficient potassium. While the role of diet remains controversial, the following recommendations are likely to be beneficial to your health generally, and possibly to your blood pressure as well: gradually restrict salt intake by avoiding processed foods and eliminating salt during cooking and at the table, replace white flour with whole grains whenever possible and make sure to include enough protein, potassium and calcium in your diet (see Chapter 4). Improving potassium intake by a moderate increase in fresh fruit and vegetable consumption may alone improve blood pressure. Supplements – e.g. of Vitamin B, potassium and calcium – can also be helpful[17] but you would be wise to consult your doctor about this. If there are no contraindications you may even manage to obtain them on prescription. Eating garlic is thought to help prevent or reduce slightly elevated blood pressure.

3. Avoid *smoking* and keep *alcohol* consumption down. (See Chapter 5 for hints on how to do this.)

4. Get together with people in your community to investigate the *water supply*. A high salt level may call for changes in winter road maintenance, or in wetlands development. If the water is soft, it may contain cadmium (which has been linked to hypertension) and too little calcium – another risk factor. You can reduce your cadmium intake by eating less white flour products. For how to increase your calcium intake, see p. 49.

5. If you take *combination oral contraceptives* and other oestrogens, insist on finding out your blood pressure both before and a few months *after* starting, and then regularly every six months. If it is initially high, don't take the Pill; if it rises, switch to another contraceptive.

6. *Regular exercise* may help to reduce blood pressure in several ways: many people find gentle exercise relaxing, thus reducing their level of stress; more strenuous exercise, to the point where heart and breathing rates are increased, helps to tone up the heart and lungs.

7. *Losing weight* if you are overweight by 15 per cent or more can prevent or lower high blood pressure. It is most effective in conjunction with exercise. Crash dieting, however, is *not* recommended.

Orthodox Treatment

When the above methods do not work or hypertension becomes severe, you may need drugs. Diuretics (which eliminate water from the tissues) are often used. The other major group of drugs used for high blood pressure is the 'betablockers', which block some of the effects of adrenalin on the heart and blood vessels and slow down the heart. Often a combination of the two is used, sometimes in a single daily tablet – which reduces the cost of the prescription. Hypertension drugs treat only the symptoms of the disease; they do not cure it. You will probably have to take medication for life. Be cautious when doctors recommend drug therapy without attempting less risky methods first.

SYSTEMIC LUPUS ERYTHEMATOSUS (SLE)

Rewritten by ANGELA PHILLIPS

In Britain, SLE is a largely unrecognized problem which is probably massively under-diagnosed. It affects ten times as many women as men and is much more frequent among black (including Asian) people. In the USA the disease hits one in every 250 black women and there is no reason to suppose the figures differ in this country. No studies have been done to confirm this.

The disease attacks the auto-immune system, which then produces antibodies against parts of the body, causing tissue injury. A hallmark of the disease is often unusual fatigue, a sign of generalized inflammation. People with SLE have both flare-ups and symptom-free periods.

SYMPTOMS

Since SLE is so often misdiagnosed and therefore mistreated, it is important for women to learn about its characteristics and symptoms. Any four of the following could indicate the presence of SLE:

1. facial rash ('butterfly' across the cheeks);
2. other disc-like lesions or rash marks (discoid lupus);
3. whitening of fingers after exposure to cold (Reynaud's phenomenon);
4. hair loss;
5. mouth or nasal ulcers;
6. arthritis *without* deformity;
7. kidney damage;
8. inflammation of the lining of the lungs or heart (pleuritis or pericarditis), often indicated by shortness of breath and/or chest pains;
9. light-sensitivity;
10. convulsions;
11. migraine;
12. major psychiatric states;
13. anaemia, low white-blood or platelet count;
14. chronic false-positive tests for syphilis;
15. excessive protein or cellular casts in the urine.

Other characteristics include fever, muscle weakness, joint pains and/or redness as well as the fatigue mentioned above. While many women with lupus have these symptoms, others simply don't feel well but can't put their finger on a specific problem.

DIAGNOSIS AND TREATMENT

A blood test identifying antibodies provides a 95 per cent positive diagnosis. However, there are very few specialist

---

*There is evidence that salt intake in early childhood has an effect on cells in the kidney which are involved in the control of blood pressure. It may be that the most important preventive action we can take is to stop salting our children's food, and stop giving them highly salted snacks such as crisps, as well as take action to cut their manufacture, distribution and promotion. There is, however, a small group of people for whom salt reduction *increases* blood pressure.

lupus clinics in this country. In other places you will be treated by whichever specialist is dealing with your major symptom. If you suspect you may have undiagnosed SLE you should ask to be referred to a specialist clinic.

Mild SLE is usually treated with anti-inflammatory and anti-malarial drugs (these can cause eye damage so regular eye examinations are important). More severe cases will require steroid treatment, which should be started in small doses. If the disease is regularly monitored, it should be possible to control it without staying permanently on these drugs, which can have other severe side-effects and predispose you to infections of other kinds. In the most severe cases it is possible to do a plasma exchange which clears the blood of affected plasma and can control the disease for months at a time.

At University College Hospital in London a controlled trial is being set up to investigate the effect of a low-fat diet, which is thought to be beneficial. In most cases it helps to get plenty of rest, avoid the sun and eat well (see Chapter 4). SLE is not usually life-threatening and tends to burn itself out after menopause. However, uncontrolled kidney involvement can prove fatal. For women with a particular form of the disease, recurrent miscarriage is a problem but, otherwise, provided the disease is well controlled, pregnancy should not be a particular worry and the disease is not likely to be passed on.*

Because symptoms are often invisible, vary a lot in severity and usually come and go (as with many chronic diseases), women with lupus are often accused of being hypochondriacs. Medical ignorance, job discrimination, lack of support from family and friends and the need to restrict activities are just some of the problems experienced by women with SLE.

Support groups are a key resource for women coping with lupus. If you have lupus, contact the British Rheumatism and Arthritis Association (see Resources) to put you in touch with a local lupus group. (See also Chapter 7 for approaches that might help.)

When I first found out I had SLE ten years ago, I was immediately faced with many changes: I had to drop out of college, was hospitalized three times that summer, gave up running five miles a day and lost twenty pounds by autumn. In the years that followed I learned to cope with my limitations and regain my strength. When my ninety-year-old grandmother complains about not being able to do what she used to, I sympathize. For me that happened at twenty-five. Today, after returning to complete a second graduate degree, I work full time. I control my illness by taking medication daily but I am still afraid to tell my employer and hate to miss days because of flare-ups. I maintain my health with regular exercise (I swim three-quarters of a mile a day), a good diet and rest. Acquaintances and even good friends don't always understand when I cancel plans, leave early or wear long sleeves in summer. But the other lupus patients in a support group I attend understand me; we speak the same language.

TOXIC SHOCK SYNDROME (TSS)

Prepared by ANGELA PHILLIPS

Toxic shock syndrome (TSS) is a rare but serious disease which mainly strikes menstruating women under thirty who are using tampons. Menstrual sponges, contraceptive sponges and diaphragms used during the menses have also been associated with TSS (see Chapter 3, p. 36, for ways of minimizing the risk). Although only a small number of menstruating women have developed TSS (6 to 15 per 100,000 menstruating women), a few of them have died. An increasing number of non-tampon-related cases are showing up in post-operative (male and female) and post-partum patients in hospitals.

TSS is probably caused by a new strain of the bacterium *Staphylococcus aureus* (*S. aureus*), which infects some part of the body, often the vagina, and produces toxins (poisons) which go into the bloodstream, causing a bodily reaction. No one yet knows why some women with *S. aureus* bacteria in their vaginas get TSS and others don't. We wonder if a woman's vaginal secretions and the type of birth control she uses, which significantly affect the vaginal pH, are factors. Higher-absorbency tampons are more likely to be associated with TSS.

This disease is a syndrome, or group of symptoms. At present, only those people who have *all* the symptoms are officially counted as having TSS. However, there are reports of people with a few of the symptoms who may have a milder form of the same disease. The symptoms are:

- a high temperature, usually over 102 degrees;
- vomiting;
- diarrhoea;
- a sudden drop in blood pressure which may lead to shock;
- a sunburn-like rash which peels after a while. The rashes are easiest to see on a person's trunk and neck, and the peeling is obvious on the palms of the hands or the soles of the feet.

TREATMENT

If you get any of the aforementioned symptoms during your period and you are using a tampon, remove it immediately. Do not use tampons or any other internal method for catching menstrual blood until you get a culture showing that you have no *S. aureus* in your vagina. TSS can progress extremely rapidly, within hours. Contact your

---

*In a recent trial, pregnant women with SLE were treated successfully with a low dose of aspirin. The number of miscarriages dropped and pregnancy outcome improved.[18]

doctor or go to a casualty department immediately.

> *I thought I had food poisoning so I waited far too long before going to hospital. For a while they didn't think I would make it. My body was barely alive when I got to casualty.*

For a mild case, the most important thing is to drink lots of fluids and rest if possible.

TSS involving severe dehydration or very low blood pressure may require hospitalization. Although antibiotics do not seem to affect the symptoms once the disease has started, they can still significantly reduce the chance of recurrence. Since this type of *S. aureus* is penicillin- and ampicillin-resistant, other antibiotics must be used.

CANCER*

Women develop less cancer, and die less frequently from it, than men do, but the gap between the sexes is narrowing. Women's lung cancer rates in particular are increasing very rapidly. Yet most of us (about two-thirds) will never get cancer. Many who do are cancer-free years after their original diagnosis. Why does this illness hold so much terror for us? It is partly because of the relative ineffectiveness and unpleasantness of Western medical treatments for many cancers,** partly because of the constant media search for medical 'breakthroughs', and partly because of health educators' emphasis on early diagnosis – which in itself unwittingly promotes and fosters the fear of cancer even further. For women, there is the added factor that cancer often develops in our sexual or reproductive organs. Since the conventional treatment, for example, in breast cancer, has been surgical removal, we may fear losing our attractiveness or 'womanliness' in a society which so often locates a woman's identity in her physical attributes. We may also face the loss of certain sexual pleasures; see the discussion of hysterectomy on p. 597, for example.

Then there is the shame, the 'What have I done to deserve this?' feeling which so often sweeps over someone who has cancer. And no wonder! All around us, the word 'cancer' is used to describe any particularly immoral or illegal situation. This fear and shame means that many of us avoid thinking about cancer even when we ourselves have it. Because of this avoidance, we do not always make the best medical decisions or live as full a life as possible.

HOW DOES CANCER DEVELOP?

Through a process not completely understood, normal cells sometimes become abnormal and then multiply out of control. These abnormal cells may spread (metastasize) to different parts of the body, entering organs and preventing them from functioning. The process of how cells become cancerous is thought to involve several steps and may take years. During that time, the process is subject to intervention by the body's immune system – so that cancer may in fact never appear (see Complementary, Self-help and Alternative Approaches to Cancer Treatment, p. 574).

There are many different kinds of cancer; some for example are fast-growing, others slow. Each type of cancer tends to have its own particular pattern of growth and spread. Yet two people who develop the same kind of cancer may respond in very different ways – both to the disease and to treatments.

CAUSES

Although the causes of cancer are not clearly understood, it is widely acknowledged that there are many factors involved, and that they are interlinked. Environmental and hereditary elements appear to play an important role. Heredity means traits and tendencies passed on to us by our parents in our genes, and they may mean we possess certain biological ways of responding to carcinogens (cancer-inducing agents) in the environment which make us more (or less) susceptible to the development of cancer. However, we also have certain patterns of behaviour (such as ways of responding to stress, or dietary habits), perhaps some of them inherited. But such patterns, even if 'inherited', can be changed (which we discuss later on).

Environment includes all that we eat, breathe or come into contact with. Some apparently inherited effects may themselves originally be caused by environmental factors,* though this is seldom recognized. Some researchers believe that carcinogens are responsible for 85 to 95 per cent of all cancers.[19] While this figure is disputed, there is no doubt that cancer rates increase with exposure to carcinogens – in the environment at large, in the home or in the workplace. This brings cancer into the political arena, and it is important to bear in mind that political considerations play a large part in how the causes are discussed.**

Viruses have also caused cancer in laboratory animals and there is good evidence for the role of viruses in relation to Burkitt's lymphoma and cancer of the cervix (see p. 530), but as yet not for other human cancers. On the

---

*Here we take an overview of cancer, concentrating on those aspects of the subject that are least accessible. Please see Chapters 24 (breasts) and 23 (cervix, etc.) for specific cancers covered in this book.

**Survival rates for most of the common cancers have improved very little over the last thirty years. Cancer is the cause of about one in five of all deaths and is the most common cause of death in the age group thirty-five to fifty-four; in the age group fifty-five to seventy-four it's the next most common cause of death after heart disease; and in the age group five to thirty-four, it is the next most common cause of death after accidents.

---

*For example, due to eggs or sperm being damaged at some stage by chemicals, the effects of which are not apparent until subsequent generations are born.

**Cancer in Britain by Lesley Doyal et al. discusses many of the vested interests and political considerations which impinge on the cause-of-cancer debate. They show, for example, that premature death from cancer in men is clearly linked to class inequalities, though there is less of a link with regard to women, probably because breast cancer – the most common cancer in women – is more common among women who are affluent.

environmental side, sunbathing appears to play an important part in the steep rise in malignant melanoma among white women – a particularly virulent form of skin cancer which is now twice as common in women than men. The reduction of the ozone layer in the upper atmosphere, due to pollution, has meant that our skins are less protected from harmful rays.

Yet exposure to a particular carcinogen or virus does not necessarily mean one will get cancer, and it is not clear how carcinogens or anything else induce or promote the disease. It is becoming increasingly recognized, however, that our response (in medical jargon the 'host response') is crucial concerning whether we fight off or succumb to cancer. In particular, this means the state of our immune system. This may be in dire straits following years of poor nutrition, for example, or exposure to environmental chemicals. We discuss the role of diet in relation to cancer on p. 577 (see also Chapter 9). Our immune system can also be affected by the stress we experience in our lives, and by the way we respond to this stress, and to feelings in general.[20] (See also Breast Cancer, p. 540, where several women talk about the role of stress in their disease.) This is an area where little good-quality research exists, and such good-quality research that has been done has largely been ignored,[21] but there is increasing scientific evidence, for example, that people with cancer:

- tend to bottle up their feelings and not express anger.[22] They may not necessarily even be aware that they ever feel angry, though research suggests that in people whose minds may not be aware of negative emotions, their bodies often are.[23] In other words, if we don't acknowledge our emotions, our bodies end up having to deal with them instead.

- may have a high potential for feelings of hopelessness, so that the cancer, at least in part, can represent a logical response to the person's despair and lack of will to live. This may have been suppressed or latent for a long period of time.[24] (We discuss psychological mechanisms in relation to survival – and the possibility of ameliorating them – on p. 571.) This supports the theories, practice and clinical experience of many holistic practitioners (see p. 574).

We should, however, guard against these psychological theories being used to 'blame the victim' for the disease. This may be easier said than done – as Penny Brohn says:

I hated being just like they said in the textbooks – unable to express negative emotions. I seethed with resentment and sulkiness.

But she describes in her book how learning to find a different way of being – and of expressing – has helped her, and not only with her cancer.[25]

It is important also to remember that even if we do manifest certain personality traits this does not mean that we are necessarily prone to any particular disorder: as Kenneth Pelletier says, carcinogenic factors are influences and predispositions, not certainties.[26] Moreover, it is difficult, if not impossible, to prove the role of psychological mechanisms because it is so difficult to conduct research in this area; it is also difficult to categorize people into crude 'personality types', which so much research has tried to do. Lawrence Le Shan's approach, based on his deep and intensive work with cancer patients, has led him to draw up a checklist of what seem to him to be important psychological variables – all of which are open to change. If you're worried about any predisposition you might have to cancer, read his book *You Can Fight for Your Life* (see Resources).

There are reasons why our emotional patterns may play such a large part. Stress often induces the release of corticosteroids, which can in turn suppress the immune system – rendering the body less able to fight off disease, including cancer.[27] It has been found that women who habitually suppress anger have raised levels of the immunoglobin IgA in the blood[28] and that this is related to breast cancer and metastatic spread. This supports the theory that bottling up feelings, even if we are unaware of doing so, stresses the body and ultimately may lead to disease. As Watson et al. say:

Personality traits, such as emotional control and repression . . . may represent a risk factor in cancer because the degree of somatic [i.e. bodily] stress experienced may be abnormally augmented or prolonged by those typical responses to stress.[29]

It follows, then, that if we were to change our responses to stress (what are regarded as personality traits are by no means unalterable), we could not only enhance our well-being but possibly also increase our resistance to disease generally.

While rigorous scientific proof is lacking, the kinds of approaches promoted by those who help people to heal themselves (see p. 574) are clearly valuable. They are concerned with each person's emotional and spiritual health, with enabling them to break free of past hurts, resentments and anger, to embrace their innate creativity, to embrace life. Few would deny the inherent value of this approach to humanity. Perhaps if it were taught in schools, we'd have a much happier population, emotionally healthy, and any reduction in cancer- and other disease-rates would be an added bonus.

Having discussed all the possible causes of cancer we must emphasize what Kissen, one of the early pioneers of rigorous psychological research in this area, suggested: it is when a risk factor such as smoking is combined with a risk factor such as 'restricted outlet for emotional discharge' that cancer is more likely. More often, then, it seems to be a *cumulation* of risks that seem to result in cancer rather than isolated risk factors.

PREVENTION

Cancer is a big money-spinner. The total cost to the US economy of cancer research and treatment is said to be

CARCINOGENIC FACTORS

The following are well recognized as being carcinogenic, though this does not mean that they will necessarily cause cancer in any one individual.

Factors that seem to be especially – but not necessarily solely – related to breast cancer are marked thus* and factors related to cervical cancer are marked thust.

- *Smoking.*†[a]
- *Heavy alcohol consumption.**[b] Both together combine to increase the risk disproportionately.
- *Certain pollutants* in the workplace, home or environment at large, e.g. asbestos, radiation.[c]
- *Certain substances in food* such as nitrites and nitrates which may encourage formation of nitrosamines in the stomach. Nitrates mainly get into water through the use of artificial fertilizers, occur naturally in foods, especially vegetables, and along with nitrite are also used to 'cure' and preserve meats and meat products, including ham, bacon and corned beef. Smoked foods such as smoked meat, fish and cheese also contain nitrosamines. Certain natural substances present in food are also carcinogenic. As Creasey says: 'An astonishing variety of compounds occurring naturally in foods ... have been shown to be carcinogenic or mutagenic in experimental systems.'[30] Little is known about what contribution they play in relation to cancer in humans because they have not been adequately assessed.[d]
- *Excess fat* intake.*[e]
- Being 20 per cent or more *overweight*.*
- *X-rays*.[f]
- *Wart virus.*† (See p. 500.)
- *Herpes virus* Type II.† (See p. 499.)
- *Hepatitis B virus.*
- *Hormones,*†[g] e.g. in the Pill[g] (see p. 294); hormone replacement therapy (see p. 456); DES (see p. 520) and in cattle feeds.
- *Ultraviolet light*[h] – in sun, sunbeds.

Notes

a. Including other people's smoking. Women whose partners smoke are also at increased risk of lung cancer and cancer of the cervix, and there is tentative evidence that people who as children lived with parents who smoked are at increased risk of developing cancer in adulthood (see Sandler et al. 1985 in Resources).

b. E.g., about four pints of beer a night or more. However, even mild drinking can lead to liver disease, which can sometimes lead to liver cancer.

c. The main problem about identifying carcinogenic substances is that, for so many of them, little or no suitable data are available. For up-to-date information, the Chemical Cancer Hazard Information Service can help (see Resources). See Resources also for other organizations and references.

d. They include: various *moulds* that may be present in certain foods such as peanuts, corn, cheese, fruit and apple juice (*aflatoxins* found in peanuts and corn are among the most potent animal carcinogens known); *cooking* that results in burnt or browned food produces potential carcinogens too; heat processing of foods may also produce mutagens. *Old, diseased, mouldy* or *bruised plant food* tends to be more likely to contain harmful substances (plants make their own pesticides and other toxic substances to resist attack and disease). For more about carcinogenicity of natural substances, see Creasey 1985 and Ames 1983 in Resources. See p. 577 re natural anti-carcinogens present in food, which may well cancel out the carcinogenic potential of these substances, if consumed in adequate amounts.

e. This may be most important during our early years rather than during adulthood (e.g. see Creasey). For more on diet and cancer, see p. 577.

f. Unnecessary X-rays should be avoided, including dental X-rays. In 1983 the World Health Organization reviewed X-ray practices worldwide and concluded that many X-rays are unjustified. If you are having a dental X-ray, a protective apron should be provided. In 1988 the National Radiological Protection Board warned of old equipment being used, which is exposing people to unnecessarily high doses as well. The Institute of Physical Sciences in Medicine has estimated that the government needs to spend at least £10 million a year to replace this equipment. The risk of excess radiation is particularly great for children.[31]

g. Some studies also indicate that the Pill may lower women's chances of developing uterine and ovarian cancer.

h. Sunscreen lotions and creams offer some protection: the higher the 'sun protection factor', the more protection it gives. (It may be best to avoid preparations containing psoralens such as 5-methoxypsoralen, which has itself been shown to be carcinogenic.)

---

about 15 to 20 billion dollars a year. But of the money that goes into research, most of it is directed towards cures rather than prevention. (Only 2 per cent of cancer charities' funds are spent on research into causes and prevention.)[32] The cancer industry stands to profit from the use of high technology, so much of the money goes into researching the development of technological approaches to both treatment and prevention.* Expensive drugs, body scanners and screening machinery have, for the most part, minimal effect on the incidence and death-rates for cancer. Meanwhile, government and industry do little to clean up the environment, the workplace or hazardous consumer products, or to discourage the profitable dietary and smoking

---

*Screening represents a technological approach to prevention. Misleadingly, the term 'screening' is frequently used synonymously with the term 'prevention'. Of course, screening for the *presence* of cancer has nothing to do with the *prevention* of cancer; screening in this country, with the singular exception of cervical screening – see p. 521 – is concerned for the most part with early diagnosis.

habits that contribute to cancer. A big part of the problem is that so many people depend on cancer for a living – people who range from shareholders and workers in tobacco companies to Third World countries forced to grow tobacco for the cash it brings in from the 'developed' world.

It is obvious that the prevention of cancer requires political will to change the social, political and economic conditions that play such an important part in its causation. Increasingly, environmental groups are campaigning in this area, as are some trade unions – MSF (formerly ASTMS), GMBATU (formerly GMWU) and NGA in particular. We can join them, give them our support, form new groups, and speak out against any attempts by government or health educators to relegate the prevention of cancer solely to the individual or technological arena. In *Cancer in Britain*, Doyal et al. make useful suggestions for strategies we can adopt, for example campaigning for an effective system for the control of all chemicals, for freedom of information and access to knowledge about carcinogens and the monitoring of them.

Yet at the same time, there are things we can do on a personal level: by not smoking we are protecting ourselves *and* those with whom we live and spend time – and not just from cancer either (see p. 66). We can learn to understand our responses to stress; we can learn to acknowledge our bodily, emotional and spiritual needs, recognize them and feed them (see p. 574 and Chapter 7 for more about this). We can work on our own resistance to improving our diet and that of our family and friends: any change can be threatening to them, and resisted by them. Once *we* decide to respect ourselves and our bodies more, we represent a challenge to them to look at their own lives, their own lack of respect for themselves.

> *I changed my diet when I was told I had cancer. After being treated like a freak at first, I'm pleased to say that countless people have changed their own eating habits after coming into contact with me!*

A healthy diet is not necessarily very expensive. The following quote is from a woman with cancer living on supplementary benefit.

> *I costed my change of diet and it didn't cost me more. And in the long term, not only do I eat less (because a healthy diet is more filling) but I also feel much better. I actually keep well! Eliminating sugar, reducing salt and fats doesn't cost anything, and changing to wholemeal flour is more filling. Fresh fruit, even unsugared dried fruits and plain nuts are no more expensive than chocolate bars.*

Cancer prevention means restructuring both our personal lives and society at large so that a clean environment, safe jobs, healthy food and less stressful living become top priorities.

IF WE DISCOVER WE HAVE CANCER
What Are Our Chances?

Many of us regard the diagnosis of cancer as a death sentence. But while the cancer statistics may seem depressing, *it must be emphasized that statistics provide a very partial story, from which very few useful conclusions can be drawn – particularly for those of us who have cancer.* They are based for the most part, for example, on approaches to cancer treatment that fail both to harness our inherent abilities to heal ourselves, and to recognize the role that medical help should play in promoting and facilitating these abilities. Far from the diagnosis of cancer being a death sentence, many people are discovering that it can mark a new beginning – as will be seen in the rest of this section.

Unfortunately, the efforts of many so-called cancer educators do little to help us. Partly no doubt because of their own anxieties, they skate over the unpalatable facts, and promote myths and half-truths:

1. They suggest, for example, that all we have to do is go for early diagnosis and we'll be all right. While early diagnosis may be very helpful for a limited number of types of cancer, e.g. some bowel, bladder and skin cancers, this is by no means necessarily the case for many (we show on p. 542 how, in relation to breast cancer, early diagnosis is a problematic area).*

2. In telling us that many cancers are curable, they on the one hand conceal the fact that most – and particularly the most common – have very poor cure rates on past experience, *and* on the other hand deny us the possibility of seeing how we can come to terms with cancer and how we can play a role in fighting it ourselves. This can easily foster feelings of confusion, guilt, self-blame and hopelessness if we develop cancer, and it actively undermines the possibility of self-healing taking place (see p. 574).

3. They distort the meaning of the word 'cure'. Elements of this distortion are clear-cut, others are more subtle: the clear-cut distortion relates to what 'cure' rates actually mean. They are often based on five-year survival rates. In other words, the proportion of people who are regarded as 'cured' may in fact be the proportion of people who simply live for five years after diagnosis. With breast cancer, for example, doctors often consider five-year survival as a cure, even though women may die from the disease in the sixth or seventh, tenth or fifteenth year. Cure rates may also be used as a way of describing *remission* – sometimes defined as improvement, other times used in a more technical sense with regard to specific changes (for example in tumour size or in the blood). Technical remission does not necessarily improve survival rates. Long-term remission, however, is a more accurate word than cure – as people with cancer more often have the cancer under control rather than entirely eliminated.

*However, re cervical smears, early diagnosis of so-called *pre*-cancer of the cervix is a different matter (see p. 521).

The more subtle distortion is to do with the concept of cure itself. Many of us have absorbed a crude concept of cure, whereby we, as passive victims, submit ourselves to various medical interventions which either cure us – or not. Yet this leaves no room for other types of intervention, and in particular what we ourselves can do. Here, a woman who has recently been pronounced cancer-free speaks:

It seems to me that saying anyone is 'cured' is misleading (for any illness) as unless we also do something about the causes and our own contribution to our ill health, we have only dealt with the end result. Without looking at the factors which promoted the cancer, it would surely be surprising if recurrence did not occur! Preventing recurrence or progression takes a lot of change and hard work – hard work which, in my case, seems to have paid off. But I don't feel I can ever say that I am 'cured', as the factors which led me to develop cancer will probably never be eliminated – maybe in twenty to twenty-five years when I'm exceedingly fit, ultra-healthy, blissfully calm, a wizard at coping with life, psychologically sorted out, and spiritually tuned in – but then my whole life will have changed. It is a continuous process for my life. And actually, I rather like it! I think the concept of cure is a con.

If we simply look for someone, some technique, to cure us, and act accordingly, we not only limit the quality of our experience, but also the possibility for a more satisfactory conclusion – involving *healing* rather than *curing* to take place.

So, while Western medicine has so far been of limited value with regard to the majority of cancers, we should keep in mind that statistics *cannot* predict what will happen to us as individuals. In particular, how we feel about ourselves and the illness, and what we want can play a crucial role, which we discuss on p. 574.*

Some Suggestions on What to Do

1. *Inform yourself.* If you read the rest of this chapter you will have an idea of what you do or don't want to find out more about. You may then want to follow up some of the resources we have listed on p. 591. It helps to be persistent in seeking up-to-date information and to have someone you trust do it with or for you. Whatever you are considering –

whether it is conventional medicine, alternative approaches, or a combination of the two – we urge you to study carefully what can reasonably be expected in your particular case.* (See Resources, p. 592, for organizations that can be of use.)

2. *Resist any pressure to rush.* Most cancers have been developing for two to twenty years before being discovered. A short delay of three or four weeks while you adjust to having cancer, seek out information and get second or third opinions won't do any harm; in fact, all it can do is good – enabling you to take your next step more knowledgeable, more confident. If, having explored and reflected, you decide to do what you were originally advised, you will feel much better about the decision. If you decide to take another course of action, you may have saved yourself unnecessary treatment or considerable regret at not having made your own choice.

3. *Talk to others with cancer.* Being with those who understand and have faced similar problems can provide invaluable practical information and emotional support. Try joining (or starting) a group for people with cancer (see Support Groups, p. 585).

I never thought I would want to join any kind of self-help group, but it has been reassuring and interesting to hear how others are coping with their cancer and to have others listen to me. No matter how supportive family or friends are, other people with cancer know and understand much better what I am going through, and it is easier to share with them the many thoughts and concerns I have that would only worry my family.

If you can't find or create a group, talk with individuals – people in medical waiting rooms, people suggested by your doctor, friends or clergy. Don't hesitate to phone people you haven't met. Many people with cancer are glad to talk about their experiences.

CONVENTIONAL MEDICAL TREATMENT**

There are three main approaches in the conventional treatment of cancer: surgery, drug treatment (chemotherapy) and radiotherapy. Depending on the type of cancer and its stage, and the interests of those treating you, either one or a combination of these treatments will be offered.

Nowadays you will usually be seen by a team of specialists including a surgeon, radiotherapist and either an oncologist (specialist in chemotherapy), haematologist (specialist in blood disorders) or gynaecologist. You may be seen in a general hospital or referred to a specialist cancer unit or hospital, depending on your local facilities.

There are many different regimes for treatment, especially in the area of chemotherapy. While a few have been

---

*Partly for reasons which will become apparent if you read Chapter 7, there is precious little research that we can draw on concerning the effect of so-called alternative medicine on survival rates. In addition, since in the UK alternative practitioners are forbidden by law from claiming that they can treat cancer, this makes the likelihood of suitable research ever being conducted even more remote. However, for alternative approaches used *in conjunction* with orthodox medicine it is possible to conduct research, and one such project looking at the overall effect of the Bristol Cancer Help Centre's approach in terms of survival rates is, at the time of writing, about to get under way, comparing the BCHC approach with that of the Royal Marsden Hospital in London. It will take at least five years to complete.

---

*See also Chapter 27.
*Virginia Laurence was a great help in rewriting this section.

found to be completely curative,* e.g. in the treatment of Hodgkin's disease, in most cases, treatment can be expected to have two aims: to improve life expectancy, or to improve quality of life remaining (e.g. through symptom control and pain relief). While it is often possible to do both, this is not always so. We may therefore want to know if we need to make a choice.

Some regimes are controversial and many have yet to be fully tried and tested. Doctors involved in trials can have differing motives: some are genuinely keen to find cures; others may be more interested in furthering their own careers by being able to publish a paper in a medical journal. If you are asked to take part in a trial, you may want to ask for as much information as possible, to find out what the treatment options are; whether the treatment being researched is new, and what the aims of your doctor are. You may be given the impression that the new regime is a breakthrough. While this may be the case, there have only been a few real advances despite many years of research. It is worth finding out whether you are part of a trial because it is possible you may not be asked. We think this is unethical (see Chapter 27 for more discussion about trials).

Surgery

Surgery involves removal of much or all of the tumour and surrounding tissues involved. In some cases, surgery can provide a cure – for those cancers in the early stages which have not spread and are known to grow slowly; such cancers may include localized lung and bowel cancers and cancers of the mouth and salivary glands, as well as certain skin cancers. When surgery cannot cure, it may be helpful in prolonging life, and/or providing control of symptoms (such as preventing bowel obstruction).

Before surgery, various tests may be performed, including blood tests, scans and X-rays, to give the doctor(s) an idea of whether the cancer has spread. Sometimes, however, surgery is necessary in order to establish the full extent of the spread, if any. The local lymph glands may be removed, for example, to see if they have been affected. After surgery, radiotherapy or chemotherapy may be considered in order to treat any remaining cancerous cells.

Radiotherapy

Radiotherapy via high-power X-rays or internal implants aims to damage growing cancer cells. On its own it is rarely 'curative' but in combination with surgery or drugs, radiotherapy can control local disease and help to prevent recurrence. In certain cancers it is also highly effective in curing pain.

A course of treatment is usually given over several days or weeks. Sitting or lying under the machine can be frightening at first but is completely painless (like an ordinary X-ray) and lasts only a few minutes. The treatment may be given on an outpatient basis, or sometimes it is more appropriate to stay in hospital.

*See discussion of cure on p. 570.

Nowadays most people don't feel unwell with radiotherapy but side-effects do occur. The commonest is tiredness. Nausea can occur but can be helped by certain drugs. Permanent loss of periods – and fertility – occurs if the area surrounding the ovaries is irradiated. Other side-effects depend on the area treated (radiotherapy damages healthy cells too) and can include lung fibrosis (inflammation of the lung) with subsequent scarring and therefore breathlessness, hair loss, cystitis, diarrhoea, and skin reactions (which can sometimes be like burns). The radiotherapist should be able to tell you what to expect and you might wish to discuss this with the radiotherapist before even deciding to have radiotherapy.

For the experience of radiotherapy in relation to breast cancer, see p. 548.

Chemotherapy

Chemotherapy consists of courses of tablets and/or injections usually given for several days every three or four weeks, possibly for six months or longer. The aim is to kill off dividing cancer cells and most of the side-effects occur because of damage to healthy cells. There are many different types of chemotherapy and new combinations are constantly being tried. Planning suitable regimes for people with particular cancers is a skilled task, and although chemotherapy has been found to be very useful in some circumstances, it has often been used inappropriately, where it cannot be expected to be of benefit.

While, in some instances, chemotherapy requires an overnight stay in hospital, in many cases it is possible to have it on an outpatient basis and, provided someone can take us there and back, this can even be done when we're unable to travel without help. Chemotherapy can cause severe side-effects depending on the drug(s) used and how they are given. Nausea and vomiting may occur within twenty-four hours of the injections; certain drugs, if effectively prescribed, can prevent this; you may wish to discuss with the oncologist their success rate with preventing nausea and vomiting: some centres and some individual doctors are very good at this; others not. Relaxation techniques and counselling have also been found to be helpful too.[33] Hair loss, including on the head, eyebrows and eyelashes, often occurs but is not permanent; menstruation may become erratic and if you are close to menopause, chemotherapy may bring it on. Some drugs cause increased susceptibility to infection.

While chemotherapy can be very unpleasant and disabling, many women find that they can continue working and only require a day off each month or so.

Because of the potential and actual side-effects, deciding whether or not to have chemotherapy can confront us with a serious dilemma: are we prepared to risk having the treatment and feeling very unwell for six months or so, with possibly little gain? Or should we decide against it and instead focus on enjoying life? Being informed about the potential benefits, and how great or small they are, can enable us to make this decision. We need the help of supportive and sensitive oncologists, and to be free of try new and untested regimes. Organizations like BACUP (see Resources) can be very helpful, particularly if we are faced with doctors who want to keep trying new drugs as each one fails.

There is hope of new forms of treatment becoming available which will enable chemotherapy to be directed towards cancer cells only. This is likely to reduce problems with side-effects dramatically and would revolutionize cancer treatment.

See pp. 549 and 521 for chemotherapy in relation to breast cancer and ovarian cancer respectively.

The field of conventional treatment is complicated and sometimes controversial. It is not easy to find out about the most up-to-date treatments while trying to cope with the knowledge of having a potentially fatal disease. We all need time and support to adjust to the diagnosis of cancer, and to reach decisions about if and how we want to be involved in our treatment. The checklist of questions below may help, and the organizations listed on p. 592 can help with up-to-date information and support. See also Support, p. 552, and Living with Cancer, p. 582.

Whatever treatment we may choose, if we choose one at all, there is a lot that we can do to help ourselves, and in particular to bolster our immune system so that it can fight the cancer. Indeed, the 7 to 8 per cent of cases which go into what doctors regard as 'unexplained remission' – where people with terminal cancer suddenly recover and live out their lives apparently free from disease – may well be explicable in terms of that person wittingly or unwittingly

---

A CHECKLIST OF QUESTIONS

Questions may be the last thing we're interested in.

What I wanted was someone to spend time with me – to slowly and carefully, with quite a bit of detail, tell me about my cancer and the treatment they proposed.

Yet having a checklist can be useful. Here is one checklist of questions which you may want to try to find out the answers to. You may want to make your own list.

- Exactly what form of cancer do I have? Is it slow- or fast-growing?
- What therapies are available? Here? Elsewhere?
- What benefits can I expect from the various possible therapies? Cure? (In which case, what definition is used?) Longer life? (By months or years?) Reduced symptoms? Reduced pain, etc.?
- What kind of research has been done with regard to the recommended treatment for the type of cancer I have?
- How many people get recurrences after this treatment, and how soon?
- Will I be able to continue my regular activities during the therapy? What about working? Exercise? Sex?
- Will the doctor(s) agree to discuss the therapy with me so that at any stage I can reassess what's happening and make alternative choices?
- Will the therapy require overnight stays in the hospital or can it be done on an outpatient basis?
- What are the potential negative effects? How serious are they? What percentage of people get them? Are they permanent? How can they be minimized/alleviated? How long does any symptom usually last? How soon after receiving treatment are symptoms likely to begin?

- How long will the therapy last? Each session? How many sessions?
- May I speak with some of the practitioner's other patients?
- Do they know of any local groups for people with cancer? Any groups for family members and friends?
- Am I part of a trial? (You may wish to be in a trial; you may not. You have a right to know and to opt out.)

Doctors and practitioners of any kind aren't used to being asked many questions, nor are they used to our being informed enough to know how to follow up their answers. It may require patience before you get what you want.

We went with a lot of questions. The specialist was quite taken aback. My husband was incredibly tense, trying not to cry, and he came across very stiffly as a result. The doctor didn't understand this and was very uncaring. He was prepared to talk about certain things, but utterly unaware of what we – and I believe anyone in our position – were going through. Ironically, one thing he seemed to feel able to mention was sex (he told us that we couldn't have intercourse for six weeks after radiotherapy): not exactly the most important question at that time. We were concerned about my LIFE and the side-effects of radiation therapy.

Bear in mind that the answers you may want aren't always available and that a practitioner who admits ignorance is someone with whom you can at least begin to form an honest relationship. With cancer treatment, as with much else in medicine, there are far fewer answers than questions.

harnessing her/his immune system. Many complementary and alternative approaches work on this level, and this is what we shall look at next.

COMPLEMENTARY, SELF-HELP AND ALTERNATIVE APPROACHES TO CANCER TREATMENT (AND PREVENTION)

Everything you can do to relieve your body of stress, in the form of grief, worry or even junk food, will enable your immune system to do more to help you get well again.[34]

So much of the course of illness is to do with *how we respond to it.*[35] We, therefore, are potentially our best allies. We can learn how to work with our body, our mind, our emotions, our soul. This is the aim of complementary, alternative and self-help approaches: to tap our innate self-healing potential, to liberate and nurture it on every level. We need a combination of approaches that support us in this venture, which we discuss below.*

All the approaches we discuss can be enormously helpful in enabling us to live with the disease, to live our lives to the full, and also in helping us to die. (We all have to come to terms with our mortality, whether we have cancer or not.) They also may limit the need for more orthodox treatment. Alternative and complementary approaches can sometimes appear to be responsible for cure, too; as yet, no research has been done which can scientifically prove the value of these approaches, but reports from complementary cancer clinics are promising – even for 16 to 18 per cent of 'terminal patients'.** But the primary focus of these approaches is *you*: how can you, *all* of you – mind, body, emotions, spirit – be really listened to, helped, encouraged, strengthened; how can *you* find nurturance and love (both outside, and most importantly within yourself), how can *you* tap the loving and joyful and creative part of you which will help you grow (and conversely, many believe, the cancer recede) and become more of who you are, enjoying life and feeling fulfilled?

Affirmations

To tap our healing and creative potential, first we have to recognize our own importance, our own inherent value, on a deep level. This can be a struggle for many people with cancer,† particularly women, since often we have felt deprived, and deprived ourselves, of nurturing.

---

*All of them, to a greater or lesser extent, have been pioneered at the Bristol Cancer Help Centre. Please bear in mind that we can provide only a glimpse of them in this book, as we can provide only a glimpse of complementary and alternative approaches generally. If you use them, please follow up some of the material we recommend, and it helps too if you can find at least one practitioner who can support, guide and encourage you in your healing journey.

** See Alec Forbes, 'Cancer and Its Non-toxic Treatment'. It is also worth remembering that the statistics we have on conventional medical treatments do not themselves show significant improvements in overcoming cancer.

† Lawrence Le Shan has found this to be a particularly problematic area for people with cancer – see his book *You Can Fight for Your Life*.

What do you do if you've neglected your health all your life and at forty-eight you realize you've got a potentially killing disease? How do you take account of the fact that you've never cared for yourself?

I feel a bit guilty, taking time off to look after myself, visit the healing centre, and so on. But as a friend said to me, which is better, your job or your health?

Affirmations, therefore, can be particularly useful. These can be said like mantras, and they can affect our view of ourselves profoundly (on the same basis that anything negative that we believe about ourselves can affect us profoundly). Affirmations quite simply recognize and tap the power of positive thinking. (See reference to Coué in Chapter 7.) Here is an example of an affirmation:

I am an important person, a worthwhile person. My personal needs and desires are important. I take them seriously. I am willing to love and nurture my way back to health, and I will remember to affirm this every day.

Affirmations, said regularly, can help us make more positive decisions in our lives, and take risks with helping ourselves to heal.

I'm not the sort of person who goes in for this sort of looking-after-yourself game. But since I've had cancer, I've been to a healer, I've been to groups, I've begun meditating and relaxing, and I'm learning a lot. I suppose I take myself and my health more seriously now.

For more about affirmations and other positive approaches to self-healing, see Louise Hay's publications, particularly *You Can Heal Your Life*.

Healing through self-discovery and self-expression.*

I have an interest which I may have had before but in some ways has been stimulated . . . and that is dealing with one's body through one's mind. I started thinking about this in connection with cancer.

When I attended the Centre, I saw a counsellor for an hour. It was the best hour of my life. I felt transformed.

---

*This is possible to do on our own but, as is shown in this section, a skilled therapist can help enormously. Indeed, staff at the Bristol Cancer Help Centre recommend that *everyone* works with a counsellor/therapist, *and* a healer. (See Chapter 7, Psychotherapeutic and Creative Approaches, and Chapter 8, particularly Psychotherapy and Healing, for more information. See also Le Shan in Resources on the special attributes required of a therapist working with cancer, particularly the ability to show love.)

This may involve looking at what may be preventing us from enjoying the present, or at what may be encroaching on it from the past. Expressing negative emotions about the disease seems to help.[36] Bringing painful memories to the surface so that feelings can be expressed and hurts healed can also be helpful.

> *I had one session where repressed emotions came up I never knew I had. My depression went. I felt alive. And what's more I wanted to remain alive. I stayed there.*

One woman is reported to have gone into total remission following emotional expression for twenty minutes about her rape at the age of seven by her father.[37]

Anger, when not allowed out, ferments into resentment and bitterness.

> *The surgeon put me in touch with my anger. I asked my counsellor to help me release it.*
>
> *It was all very well feeling how good my cancer was for my spirit. But I had to express anger too, otherwise I'd be the perfect host for it. I started by just shouting. Eventually, after some time, I managed to get angry. It took me some time to allow myself – really allow myself – to be angry, and I know that tears or anger have to be allowed to be beneficial.*

Grief is another emotion that may be dominating us to our detriment.

> *I felt it was really unfair that I got cancer because I thought my lifestyle and approach were exemplary. Then I began to realize that it was grief that was the problem for me. I asked for time to think before the operation and went through a lot of grieving – for both my father and mother, who died in quick succession not long before the cancer was diagnosed. I found some books particularly helpful too – e.g. the Scriptures, and Eliot's* Four Quartets.

Likewise *fear*. Groaning can help us to express fear. Confronting our fears about death may also be important (see p. 581).

The important thing with expressing emotion is to give ourselves total permission for it, not to mind crying, raging, stamping, trembling. If we don't fully allow it, then it still niggles and festers. We may have a strong fear of giving in to it, that there'll be no end – but if *really* allowed, the feelings do dissipate much quicker than we imagine. Co-counselling techniques can be a great help – and they don't cost much to learn (see p. 121). Autogenics too is a technique which is very effective for releasing emotions (to find out more about this, see the Centre for Autogenic Training in Resources).

Lack of forgiveness fosters bitterness and resentment,

neither of which is conducive to healing. Forgiveness allows love and healing energy to flow – to us and from us. By practising forgiveness – both of ourselves and our loved ones – for all the mistakes we have made, resentment, bitterness and fear can be banished and replaced by love and joy. Jerry Jampolski, who has worked wisely with cancer patients for years, has written a book, *Love is Letting Go of Fear* (see Resources), which many people with cancer have found helpful in this area.

Laughter is another, crucial form of self-expression, increasingly being recognized as essential to the healing process (and of course joyful living too!). Norman Cousins' book *Anatomy of an Illness* (see Resources) is primarily about how he laughed his way back to health. Some of us may need to relearn, or perhaps learn for the first time, how to play. We may need support in doing this – and friends and family can benefit from it too!

> *I needed an excuse to play. Everyone I knew was too busy being serious. I became like a 'child', infantilized through illness: I went round really wanting to play, and people kept saying 'I'm busy', 'I can't', 'Come back on Saturday'. But my partner and I have great fun. We often play 'mummies and daddies' (which, since I've been told I need to learn to 'parent myself', is a good 'education' for me too!).*

Healing through self-expression may also involve *looking at the links* between the site of the cancer, its literal meaning and emotional patterns. With stomach cancer, for example, is there anything you can't stomach? Or with the breast, there might be grudges being nursed which, once let go can mean you feel much better, and have more energy and commitment available for healing.

Discovering or *acknowledging* why we think we have cancer can also be important for some of us.

> *I wasn't shocked at the diagnosis. I was relieved, because I was so busy I couldn't see how I could get time to myself.*
>
> *I'm sick with grief, that's why I've got cancer.*
>
> *The price I've paid for being a strong and independent woman (a typical feminist in fact!) has meant that the side of me that needs looking after has lost out. Another reason for my being ill.*

Indeed, the therapists find at Bristol that many people who visit them 'know' why they had cancer. In their experience, it is *only* women who say they felt they had to have cancer in order to get the attention they needed.

We can use these insights, however crazy it may sound, to fight the disease. Some people come to realize that their will to live was so in abeyance that getting an illness believed to be incurable was a way of opting out of life – a 'socially acceptable form of suicide', no less.[38] Though this can seem an awesome revelation to be confronted with, it is also the key to change, as Le Shan shows so graphically in his book, for example, and as others also attest.

> I learned that by my sense of helplessness and deprivation I had unconsciously acquiesced in the onset of cancer . . . somewhere in the recesses of my mind I still wanted to turn away from life. The thought of shouldering all my old responsibilities so soon was appalling to me, and in November a lump appeared in the other breast. With the discovery of that lump a profound change had taken place in my mind. I decided totally that I would not allow this tumour to survive, it simply wasn't the answer to my problems. Far from being afraid, that week was the most exhilarating experience of my life . . . the sense of power was indescribable. There was no need to do the exercises, energy poured through me like champagne, and by the time I arrived back in hospital, feeling like visiting royalty, my breast was back to normal. The surgeon, a brilliant and humane man, not scalpel-happy, was concerned that a tumour could have broken up and dispersed, and recommended surgery. A short exploratory operation revealed nothing . . . There was no cancer present.[39]

Recognition of our spiritual needs may also be very important in providing the right conditions for recovery, and in enabling us to find strength and purpose. We are all spiritual beings,* whether we recognize this or not, and some of us may discover this for the first time through the experience of having cancer. This can open us up to universal love and great inner strength and guidance – and, for some of us, confusion. Some therapists can be very helpful in enabling us to make sense of the experience (see p. 135). (See also Spiritual Healing, p. 87.)

For more about how you can work on self-discovery and self-expression – and the value of it – see, in particular, books by Louise Hay, the Simontons, Lawrence Le Shan, Beata Bishop and Penny Brohn listed in Resources. By dealing with the anxieties that cancer has raised, either on their own or with help, many people have found the freedom to be themselves (having previously been only who they thought they were supposed to be), have found great inner strength and discovered what is most important in living, and led their lives accordingly.

> Alongside my physical recovery, I have . . . undergone an inner transformation that has stripped away many of my fears, burdens and obsolete values, leaving me with a sense of increased freedom and wholeness. I worry much less and laugh much more . . . But once you have travelled to the edge of death

and then returned to a life more abundant, your ability to worry simply melts away.[40]

Visualization

This involves using our imagination to heal ourselves. It is essentially creative, and since untapped or thwarted creativity has been found to be a major issue for many people with cancer, creating our own healing symbols and inner journeys can be particularly valuable for us.* It is possible to learn to visualize on our own (see Resources, p. 112 and p. 108), but some therapists or counsellors can be particularly skilled through their own sensitivity and inner strength (and through having faced their own terrifying realities) at helping us reach – and free – aspects of ourselves that we never knew existed.

> Through learning to visualize at Bristol, my whole life has changed. My whole attitude to my illness has changed. I now have a peace, a sense of purpose, and – yes – joy in living.

Visualization can be used as a protection against the harmful effects of radiotherapy – e.g. visualizing the radiation going directly to the cancer cells while protecting the rest of the body.

Other forms of creativity

It has been found by several therapists, in particular Le Shan, that people with cancer have needs to be creative in ways they may not even be aware of. Le Shan believes that finding our 'special rhythm', our unique 'unsung song', is of major importance for people with cancer – liberating our energy, for ourselves, counteracting despair. Many people have discovered, often with the aid of a counsellor or therapist, creative abilities that have been denied or lain dormant for years, possibly even all their lives. Creativity can be the key to tackling cancer. You may find a particular approach of your own is right for you. Jo Spence, a photographer, uses photography as an aid to the healing process (see Resources). For more about creativity and healing, see Chapter 7, p. 98 and Chapter 8, p. 135.

Deep relaxation and meditation

These are two important ways in which the body – and the rest of us – can be helped, restoring harmony, a deep sense of calm and promoting the healing process. It can also result in a new sense of purpose and meaning to life, both of which are essential for survival and can lead to a turning point. There is evidence that meditation can improve the immune system,[42] and that relaxation can help with nausea and vomiting associated with chemotherapy.[43] Ainslie Meares, an Australian psychiatrist, claims that intensive meditation and concomitant reduction of anxiety

---

*Spirituality means different things to different people. To some, for example, it means belief in God or Goddess, for some it's about Light, and for others of us it is simply a deep source inside ourselves that is greater than who we (think we) are.

*It has been claimed that the ability to perform visualization is a much better predictor of survival than either laboratory or clinical investigations.[39]

and development of a positive attitude, can lead to astonishing remissions.[44] Many practitioners specializing in cancer recommend three fifteen-minute periods of deep relaxation, meditation or visualization a day. Read Chapter 7 for more about them; see also Resources for further reading.*

Breathing

Many of us don't give our bodies a chance because we take in so little oxygen. At Bristol, training in breathing has been found to make an enormous difference to some people for whom all other approaches have failed. Many therapists, ranging from bioenergetics (see p. 132) to naturopaths (see p. 96), may teach breathing, as do therapists specializing in 'conscious connected breathing' (more commonly known as 'rebirthing'). To find out about rebirthing, contact the British Rebirth Society or read Leonard and Laut (see Resources).

Diet

Eating a good diet is probably one of the best ways of protecting ourselves against cancer and in enabling the body to fight it. There is no *scientific* proof that diet cures cancer, not least because the research hasn't been done, but there is plenty of evidence to support the theory, some of which we discuss below.

Laboratory workers have known for decades that tumour incidence in animals can be affected by the food they are given, and Bruce Ames – a leading researcher into the chemical causes of cancer – has concluded:

> [High cancer rates] may be due in good part to less than optimum amounts of anti-carcinogens and protective factors in the diet.[45]

Indeed, it has been claimed that half of all cancers in women and one-third of those in men are associated with dietary factors.[46]

We discussed briefly on p. 569 substances in food which are potentially carcinogenic. Many nutritionally-orientated practitioners recommend to cancer patients that they avoid these foods, if only on the basis of theoretical knowledge about carcinogens.** The diets that such practitioners recommend are many and varied. The most easily accessible and perhaps least demanding dietary approach to cancer is that currently used at the Bristol Cancer Help Centre. See Penny Brohn, *The Bristol Programme* and Sadhya Rippon, *The Bristol Recipe Book* (in Resources). The Centre provides leaflets on the diet, with recipes and suggested menus for a week at a time, suggestions for how to begin, and on what they consider to be appropriate supplements. People who visit the Centre are given a personal dietary appraisal.*

I'm really enjoying the diet I learnt at Bristol. It's nothing like as difficult as I expected, and I find sunflower sprouts absolutely delicious! I go out to work and just take the stuff in a sealed container.

Many diets include a period of 'detoxification' involving a cleansing of the digestive tract, either by the administration of certain herbs, or coffee enemas; this is thought to play a major role in enabling the body to become free of toxins and to absorb a high-quality diet. Many nutritional therapists believe it is dangerous to convert to a 'get well' diet without undergoing detoxification – believing that the poisons accumulating in the body over many years have prevented the system (particularly the kidneys, liver and pancreas) from functioning properly. For more about get well diets, including women's experiences, and the need for support, see Chapter 4, p. 52. For help in finding support, contact New Approaches to Cancer or the Bristol Cancer Help Centre (see Resources). Detoxification and get well diets should never be attempted without experienced supervision.

While few doctors support the nutritional approach as a major treatment for cancer, more doctors are beginning to recognize that nutritional support is important. People with cancer are often poorly nourished, and being poorly nourished makes it more difficult to tolerate and recover from orthodox treatment.**[47]

Anti-cancer Substances in Food

Here we have included only those substances in food where there is a reasonable amount of evidence concerning their anti-cancer properties, although the evidence with regard to the mechanisms involved is still poorly understood. The first four are substances classed as 'antioxidants' – substances which appear to enhance immune mechanisms in some way.

Vitamin A (particularly beta-carotene, which is converted to Vitamin A by the body). 'Vitamin A' covers a wide variety of related substances, the most important of which as far as cancer is concerned appears to be beta-carotene, which becomes partly converted to Vitamin A by the body. There is considerable evidence from both animal and human studies that Vitamin A and/or beta-carotene in food

---

*Some people use *biofeedback machines*, which can monitor one's state of arousal and help one relax, as an aid to learning relaxation. This is not essential, but it can speed up the process for some people. If you want to try this, contact NAC (see Resources) for where machines can be obtained. Occasionally, you may find biofeedback available on the NHS. Some psychology departments are interested in it, as are some holistically-orientated doctors (contact BHMA – see p. 174).

** Alec Forbes in *The Bristol Diet* recommends avoiding foods such as celery, parsnips and parsley for this reason. However, the Bristol Cancer Help Centre is now far less rigid about which foods one should not eat.

*There are many different approaches to nutritional supplementation (sometimes called 'metabolic therapy'). The Bristol approach tends to be the least rigid. Do not take supplements without consulting a reputable organization or an experienced practitioner. If you do wish to take them, a discussion with your doctor *could* be helpful – and increasing numbers of doctors are prescribing them on the NHS for cancer patients. A form P 11 will enable you to get a season ticket for NHS prescriptions if you are likely to need more than fifteen a year – this saves money.

**Nutritional requirements for people undergoing chemotherapy and radiotherapy are also thought to be increased – in the case of Vitamin C, threefold.

has anti-carcinogenic action.[48] The human studies include cervical dysplasia,[49] breast cancer,[50] lung cancer,[51] and many cancers among smokers.[52]

Of twenty epidemiological studies, eighteen have indicated a link between high beta-carotene intake in food and low incidence of cancer.[53] Many studies have shown a correlation between various cancers and low intake of green and yellow vegetables – foods high in this substance.[54] Beta-carotene is widely available in dark green leafy vegetables, carrots and certain yellow and red fruits and vegetables.

Vitamin A supplements should be avoided: they are not a substitute for beta-carotene and can be toxic.

Vitamin C is also considered important, partly because it enhances immune mechanisms, and also because it protects against infection. It appears to play an important role in maintaining skin tissue, including in the cervix, and in wound healing generally. It blocks conversion of nitrates to carcinogens in the stomach and may therefore be particularly important with regard to gastric cancer. And it is claimed by some (most notable of whom is Linus Pauling) that Vitamin C supplements are effective in cancer treatment.[55]

While *hard* data on Vitamin C's value are limited because so little research has been done, some data do exist; for example, that low C levels are associated with a risk of gastric cancer,[56] and cervical dysplasia (now referred to as dyskaryosis, see p. 523).[57] In this latter study, about 30 per cent of women with dysplasia consumed less than 30 mg of Vitamin C per day, versus only 3 per cent of controls; women with the lowest incomes appeared to be three times as likely to have low C intake. A Russian study[58] has also found decreased levels of Vitamin C in cervical tissue that is cancerous compared with normal cervical tissue.

Foods high in Vitamin C include citrus fruit, red and green peppers and potatoes. When eating citrus fruits, it is important to make sure that the pith is consumed as well as the flesh of the fruit: this contains biflavanoids which make absorption easier; pith is also thought to have a specific anti-carcinogenic action.[59] *Please note*: if you are on the Pill and decide to take extra Vitamin C, please see p. 294.

Vitamin E. This is particularly difficult to research because of the sensitivity of Vitamin E to storage and cooking. However, there is evidence that low intake when combined with low selenium intake (see below) appears to increase the risk of fatal cancer, and it is possible that the importance of Vitamin E, apart from being a major antioxidant, is its role in enhancing the value of selenium[60] as well as other antioxidants.[61] With regard to specific cancers, it has been found that Vitamin E levels tended to be lower in women with breast cancer compared with other women:

> Vitamin E levels showed a statistically significant trend in risk – those with the lowest vitamin E levels having the highest risk of breast cancer.[62]

Foods high in Vitamin E include whole grains, broccoli and eggs.

Selenium is a mineral and is considered by some to be the 'antioxidant par excellence'. While research on selenium is by no means definitive, selenium deficiency is thought by some to increase the risk of cancer, possibly irrespective of site,[63] and this effect seems to be made worse by low Vitamin E intake, and possibly low beta-carotene as well.[64] Cervix dysplasia and skin cancer seem to be implicated specifically with low selenium intake.[65] Selenium is toxic in high doses and may itself even promote cancer in such circumstances, so it is best to get it from food.

Foods high in selenium include: tuna, liver, kidney, whole grains, onions, garlic, tomatoes, broccoli, mushrooms, brewer's yeast and eggs. If supplements are taken, 400 mcg of the organic form is considered reasonable and safe. The inorganic form is less well absorbed and is possibly more toxic.

B vitamins. These are vital for recovery from illness, and requirements are increased for people having chemotherapy or radiotherapy. Folic acid deficiency has been implicated with regard to cervical dysplasia in women on the Pill; supplements appeared to reverse the cell changes. * Foods high in B vitamins are whole grains and green vegetables.

Certain plants are also thought to have anti-cancer properties. Those for which there is some evidence include garlic, mistletoe (in the form of iscador – a homoeopathic remedy which some doctors are prepared to prescribe) and periwinkle, which is the source of several anti-cancer drugs. Evening primrose oil is sometimes prescribed to promote healthy cell growth, and ginseng to improve immunity. Laetrile (more accurately called amygdalin), which is a substance found in various fruits, including almonds and apricots, has been under much debate for many years. The evidence for its value is confusing and, like chemotherapy and radiotherapy, it is toxic. The medical establishment now considers it ineffective on the basis of a poorly-conducted trial.[66] Further trials are unlikely to take place so the issue remains unresolved. The Bristol Cancer Help Centre has not used it for years, not least because of difficulties of maintaining high-quality supplies.

For practical information about get well diets, see Chapter 4.

Choosing Alternative or Complementary Approaches

Virtually all these approaches can be used in conjunction with orthodox medicine, so it is not necessarily a question of 'either–or', but more often 'what to do *as well*'.

The best thing to do is follow your instincts, choose what feels right for you, and do it with a positive belief in its

---

*Since taking folic acid supplements may lead to zinc deficiency, particularly in Pill-users (since the Pill reduces zinc levels anyway), it might be best, at least for those contemplating self-help, to take brewer's yeast; this enables B vitamins, including folic acid, to be taken in a balanced way. (Zinc is necessary for the functioning of the immune system, among other things.)

value. Don't push yourself beyond your limits, but try to make sure you are taking notice of the self that is you, that goes beyond your body, or your mind, or your emotions even. Penny Brohn, who speaks from personal experience as well as being a counsellor, believes strongly that we always know what is best for ourselves, though we may not always have had the opportunity to discover it, or the support to act on it. Choosing a type of treatment/approach can be extremely difficult.

You're told by the hospital that if you don't do this, you'll die. On the other hand you get home and in the alternative literature you are told if you do do that, it can spread disease. That's the kind of information I was picking up at that point. It's like being in a war, really.

Ever since I've been in the hospital, well-meaning friends and people I barely know have flooded me with Bibles, tracts on holistic therapy, macrobiotic diets, each wanting to be the one with the answer, the cure. They made me hopeful at first, then tired, tired.

It isn't made any easier by the attitudes of many doctors. A few may support us in using alternative approaches to complement more orthodox medicine, albeit grudgingly.

[The consultant] told me I should have a mastectomy. I would not agree to this but did agree to have the lump removed . . . I had already made up my own mind as to the treatment I was prepared to accept . . . I wanted to go to the Cancer Self Help Centre . . . He said that as I felt strongly about it he would agree, provided he could keep me under supervision.[67]

However, more commonly, they feel threatened and hostile.

The consultant said he didn't agree with what I was doing, which was going to the Bristol Cancer Help Centre . . . seven of his patients had died as a result of going there, that's what he actually said to me . . . If that was what I wanted to do, it was up to me, but he didn't want anything to do with it. There was no question of collaboration at all.

This can leave us feeling scared, abandoned and paralysed with indecision. It is important to remember that most alternative approaches can be used in conjunction with orthodox treatment, so you do not *have* to choose between the two. However, some alternative practitioners believe that orthodox treatment, particularly chemotherapy and radiation, can prejudice your chances by undermining the immune system. Some women decide, for this and other reasons – including despair at

---

CANCER HELP CENTRES

At diagnosis the patient is supported by the hospital, at their death it is the turn of the hospice. But we occupy the middle ground – the weeks, years, decades when the person knows they are a cancer sufferer. (Pat Pilkington, Bristol Cancer Help Centre.)

Many people have now heard of the Bristol Cancer Help Centre, set up in 1980, which continues to pioneer a holistic approach to cancer. It is as yet unique, but is influencing many people, within and outside the NHS, so that by the time you read this, there may well be several other places which might offer at least some of the type of care offered at Bristol.

What the Centre aims to offer primarily is love, and the kind of focus on each person who goes there that acknowledges their essence, their unique, personal, deeply-felt needs. These may be spiritual or emotional, often with a practical tinge (e.g. how to handle rude and/or undermining doctors). The Centre does not espouse any rigid rules and visitors are encouraged to formulate their own needs. Staff are chosen 'especially for their gifts of total commitment and loving service'.

Female energy got the Centre going, and it has helped a lot of people.

I just handed my body over when I was first diagnosed, and expected the doctors to get on with it. When I got it again, I began to question what was going on. Why I got it again, thinking about my stressful life, etc. Coming here is the best thing I ever did. I wouldn't have missed it for the world. It confirmed me in my line of thinking and really helped me look at myself and what I was doing and see how/what I can change. For one thing, my relationship will: there's no nurturing in it.

You really felt like you were an important person. At last someone was going to listen to you and he took into account your personality, as he called it.

Everyone who goes there sees a counsellor and a healer, and takes part in group activities ranging from relaxation and meditation to movement and art. When they leave, everyone is encouraged to find themselves a local healer and counsellor where they can continue the work they began at the Centre.

The Centre is a charity, and has to charge fees, but no one has been turned away because they couldn't afford it. It offers residential care for short periods, and also runs day sessions; close relatives are encouraged to attend as well. *Turning Point*, its journal, is published quarterly.

doctors' attitudes and behaviour – against any form of orthodox treatment.

Choosing the Alternative Route

The doctor wanted to remove my vulva for what he said was pre-cancer. What a nerve – just because he thought it may become cancer! I said no thanks. I'm into alternatives, cured my own arthritis etc. by being vegan, getting rid of my husband and all the usual things. It got better on its own – or rather with my help.

Why didn't I have surgery or radiotherapy? Because it would involve putting so much energy into doing that and coping with it, there'd be nothing left for doing all the other stuff, that I had to do . . . Of course, this was my decision. It doesn't necessarily mean it's right for others.

Choosing the alternative route can require enormous courage and strength in the face of medical opposition. The woman quoted immediately above continues:

It was very, very lonely in hospital, because I was trouble and had refused the recommended treatment. Nobody came to talk to me. Everyone else who was upset got chummy chats . . . Although I chose the alternative route a long time ago, I still visit the consultant because I still haven't weaned myself off the need for this authority/approval figure. I haven't had any treatment from him (yet).

Doctors aren't always negative. Dorothy Hollinrake's consultant, for example, responded very positively to her progress, which she mainly attributed to her regular visualizations.

My consultant was delighted with my progress and said everything seemed to be in order. I think he was so impressed that he asked me, if any future patient of his wished to follow a similar course, could he refer them to me for information: I readily agreed.[68]

Some doctors change their minds.

In fact, I did waver at one stage, and decided I'd have radiotherapy after all, because I realized my resistance was based on prejudice – an ego trip. I went to see the consultant who'd been trying to persuade me to have it, and he turned round and said he didn't want me to have it because he didn't think I needed it any more!

And some doctors even decide against orthodox treatment themselves.

I decided against radiotherapy and instead worked out my own approach, based on the Simonton method [see Resources], plus biofeedback and homoeopathy.

This was a long time ago, and she's still working.

Finding a good practitioner is particularly important if we opt for the alternative route. Since alternative practitioners aren't allowed to say they can treat cancer, they can be difficult to find. NAC keeps lists of practitioners throughout the country who deal with cancer (see Resources; they also have a list of doctors sympathetic to alternative treatment).

Because of the cost involved, you might decide that instead of paying for counselling or psychotherapy, you can do co-counselling, which requires very little money if any (see p. 121). You can enlist the support of friends and colleagues if need be. Most are only too grateful to be told how they can help.

Several friends have helped me pay for my health costs.

My husband said 'Where are we going to get the money?' And he was right. We couldn't possibly afford it. But I knew we'd get it somehow. And we did. Family, friends, everyone in the village was wonderful. They organized sponsored walks, football matches, pub crawls, the lot – all to raise money!

For more about choosing a therapist, see Chapters 7 and 8.

Whatever therapy you choose or don't choose, it helps a lot if you feel good about your decision. Remember that you can't do everything (no one can), and that while you can help yourself your aim is not so much cure as peace of mind, being able to be in charge of your life, happiness, etcetera, for whatever remaining life you have. (It may help to remember that *anyone* can be run over by a bus tomorrow.)

I am not better, in spite of beginning to take responsibility for my own health, and working out an integrated programme of health care with others. On the other hand, although I still have active cancer, and my general health is not good, I feel more in control of my life than at any other time previously. This has come about because of the questions I have been forced to ask myself about my belief system, my lifestyle and my attitude to my mind and body. As a result I see myself neither as 'heroine' nor 'victim', but merely as a person in struggle, changing and adjusting daily, and trying to keep a state of

CONFRONTING OUR OWN MORTALITY

Dying is having to face the unknown in a world controlled so thoroughly that unknowns are only fearful experiences.[70]

Having cancer confronts us with our own mortality.

It was the cancer. I couldn't convince myself that it was going to go. I just couldn't. I was waking up in the night panic-stricken, totally panic-stricken, which was all a part of not wanting to die.

What having had a cancer operation has done to me most positively is to inform myself of mortality, my mortality or anybody else's mortality . . . In many ways I feel that lots of doors have been opened to me. I can talk about mortality much more easily than I used to, recognizing what it means, and I've also become a bit more positive about my spiritual beliefs.

After I came out of hospital I went through two months' grieving for my own possible death. I managed to work during the week, and stayed in bed every weekend.

It can make us want to give up when it might be more appropriate to fight for our survival. Often giving up is a stage we go through.

I don't want to die now, but I do believe I did want to – unconsciously. I even wrote off to the Euthanasia Society.

If we are alone with our feelings, we can find it very hard to deal with the awesome prospect of our death, even if it's upwards of twenty years away. We can feel isolated and cut off from friends and family, and bewildered by the sheer enormity of what is happening to us. A support group might help (see p. 586), or a good counsellor or psychotherapist can help us unburden our feelings and enable us to find our way through them to a sense of freedom. We may have unfinished business they can also help us complete* and, in addition, they can help us consider the issue of *how* we might die.

My fears are not of dying but of pain and being helpless in the hands of careless people.

As Elisabeth Kubler-Ross and several others have shown, dying need not be torture or agony. Indeed, far from it (see, for example, p. 89). One recent study[71] involved interviewing people after the deaths of their relatives from lung cancer and most reported that the illness was not as bad as they had feared; 40 per cent of the relatives died with no pain at any time. (For a discussion of pain relief during terminal illness, see p. 587.)

An important part of any good counsellor's work is to help people find out what their fears are and what they want: where to die, with whom, what our needs are. This is how Penny Brohn, in a seminar for health practitioners, described her own needs as a woman living with cancer.

If I were to die in this room, I'd want forgiveness from all of you – for being a bore, for talking too much . . . I wouldn't want to be told 'Don't worry, you're not like that at all.' I'd need to know you knew what I was like and you still loved me.

Please see p. 574 for how self-discovery and self-expression among other things can help us deal with our cancer, as well as our mortality.

I really think it's the most interesting thing that happens to you in life, is dying. I have this great curiosity to know how it feels and what happens. I'd like to be conscious enough to say 'This is me dying, this is how it feels.' But if I tell the consultant that, he thinks I'm being morbid. What I'm trying to say is, because I have this great interest in dying, I have no fear of cancer at all. I've felt anxious about death for a long time, before cancer, without wanting to go bursting into it – I'm not in any rush to get this experience! It casts out fear. If you haven't got fear, you stand a better chance of conquering the disease.

I don't want to die, but since I accepted the fact that I probably will, I am more at peace. It's as if my energy had been used up denying the reality of my own impending death and, when I stopped struggling against the idea, I suddenly felt free. I could begin to think about living again, about what to do with the time I do have. I have my down days, when I ask, 'Why me? Why can't I die twenty years from now? Why can't I live to see my children grow up, my grandchildren born?' But these days are fewer and fewer. In a sense, I'm lucky to know about my death in advance. I won't be like those who die unexpectedly with things left unsaid and undone. I've planned what I want to do, who I want to see. I've started working on projects that I had always wanted to do but was too busy for. I can't afford to travel or do much special, but then anything I do now seems special.

*See Elisabeth Kubler-Ross's books in Resources for importance of unfinished business.

equilibrium which will allow me to function optimally, at the same time as I strive to regain my health.[69]

Dealing with cancer is a continuous process. While willpower can do extraordinary things, including apparently banish cancer, the concept of our being able to *control* whether we live and when we die implies an omnipotence that no one has. Self-help and alternative approaches to cancer treatment are about *living* with cancer. They are about life – our lives and every aspect of them. Having cancer can provide us with a reason for living *or* dying.

Warning. Alternative medicine, like all medicine, needs to be practised with care and sensitivity. Alternative practitioners do not have a monopoly on these virtues (see Chapter 7), and we need to be careful to avoid people who make us feel guilty or inadequate or helpless. Cancer stirs up a lot of emotions in alternative practitioners, just as with doctors, and they can end up manifesting the same rigidity, dogmatism and sense of their own omnipotence.

Alternative approaches, not least because they allow and actively encourage us to take responsibility for ourselves and our health, can also lead us to feel guilty, to blame ourselves, or to being blamed (see Blaming the Victim in Chapter 3). A good practitioner needs to be acutely aware of this syndrome, and to be clear that although there are ways in which we are all responsible for our lives, and our illnesses – whatever they are – this is not to say they are *our fault*. We may need help to learn not to blame ourselves – or others. If we need this, the last thing we need is an alternative practitioner who is into 'guilt-tripping'. For example, if we are recommended a particular diet and we sometimes fail to stick to it, we need support and understanding, and even perhaps recognition that the diet may not be that important or helpful.

Having cancer makes me think a lot about my past. For example, I'm very aware of the way I get tense in a lot of situations. But I look for ways of reducing the tensions rather than saying it's because I'm tense that I've got cancer. It's an opportunity to change and this includes changing situations and working towards political change.

Finally, having cancer can not only make us prey to our own fear and desperation, it can also leave us open to unscrupulous and/or ignorant practitioners. It is particularly important with cancer that we find a therapist who is sufficiently self-aware and sensitive to handle their own anxieties, let alone ours.

LIVING WITH CANCER

In 'Complementary, Self-help and Alternative Approaches' we showed how *living* with cancer – like treatment – is a continuous process. Getting to that point of realization is

itself a journey. How do we get there after those early months when we're reeling and coping and reeling and coping?

Initially, we may have feelings about giving up and dying, or they may be mixed up with appreciating life.

The first day I got up [after the operation], I can remember it was an absolutely gorgeous day, very blue skies, it was beautiful and it felt good to be alive . . . while my body was getting over it my mind wasn't too bad. It was when my body was recovered that my mind started to dwell on it.

Nothing is what I thought it would be, I tell him, not cancer, not dying, not being alive. I feel I've been given a reprieve . . . the sound of my own heart is a miracle. The feel of clean sheets against my skin is . . . Dr Oates interrupts to say I am experiencing a medical phenomenon called euphoria, quite common after a major operation. What I should expect, he says, is to have sexual difficulties, be short-tempered and more impatient with people. After Dr Oates leaves, I close the door and do twenty-four sit-ups and leg raises, carefully not to crush my swollen arm, working against being a textbook cancer patient, I suppose. I keep wishing he would come back and catch me at it.[72]

Coming home from hospital may bring to the forefront how everything has changed.

It's funny, you know, one of the things that was very hard to cope with was actually coming home. When you are in the ward you are in this close-knit community where you are being supported by staff and by other patients and everybody has got something wrong with them. You are one of a group. And all of a sudden it's like being pushed outside the rest and you suddenly realize you've got to face the world now. It was terrible, coming home, I cried all the way home. I wanted to come home, yet at the same time the world seemed so big when I came outside. I was shaking all the way.

We may feel a desperate need to be able to withdraw for some time.

When I came home I was really exhausted. All I wanted to do was crawl into my own house and stay there and be alone.

There may also be the frustration of not being able to do ordinary, simple tasks.

I wanted things done and I couldn't do them and I had to depend on someone else . . . I wanted things to go on as they were before, and a home help would just be such a difficulty although I did need helping.

Friends and Family

Coping with other people's feelings about our having cancer can be difficult at first.

Although I accepted it, the family didn't, and everyone around at the time when I needed some back-up was falling to pieces.

We may need to learn how to cope with other people's reactions to us, including the possibility of acquaintances crossing the road, close friends and even family disappearing or displaying incomprehension or anxiety.

I show her my notebooks, explaining that I am writing what it is like to have cancer. Why? Because writing is what I do. It helps me sort out ideas and emotions and find out what I really feel . . . Slowly, deliberately, Helen nods her head, not saying a word. I want her approval, so I keep talking. Surely having cancer is as important as having a baby or getting married, or sleeping with a man. Women write about these experiences all the time.[73]

Other people are my problem. The mastectomy is not my problem any more, it's other people's problem . . . nobody else can accept it, no one else can actually just take today, everybody else wants to know if you're going to be here tomorrow.

Since the fact of our disease threatens other people too, we may need to help them to cope with it. When Pam Smith became ill with cancer, she asked her colleagues at the Women's Therapy Centre for their help, and she helped them see how they could give it.

She took charge of getting support and help for herself. She found herself a Gestalt therapist. She chose to become more open with us, but she set the terms . . . She told us how she would like to deal with [the cancer] and asked for our help and cooperation . . . she was very specific about what she needed from us. Ironically, it seemed that she managed to ask us then for the emotional care we would have been happy to give much earlier.[74]

It can be particularly hard for friends and family to cope with our disease if we pursue complementary or alternative approaches.

I found it a great shock to discover the various negative reactions of my family and friends, both to the fact that I had cancer and that I chose to deal with

it in a particular way. I was much comforted by being able to talk about this to others who had known similar experiences.[75]

I was given six months to live, and I had to tell my grown-up son to go, even though we loved each other dearly: he couldn't cope and all he wanted was for me to die quickly. It was an enormous relief when he went, because I could then concentrate on getting better – which I did.

This is often because by doing so, we are keeping the fact of our illness alive in them, daily. We're not allowing them to forget it.

A major part of the work of the Bristol Cancer Help Centre is with friends and family, helping them find helpful and healthful ways of coping with their loved ones, and vice versa.

Some people can handle our illness only if we play the 'sick role' and lie floppy in bed – this helps them to live with *their* feelings, and can force us into a role that is not of our choosing. They may resist our getting better – as if *they* have given up hope and are waiting for us to die. It can be seen as eccentric behaviour if we don't just lie down and die. Indeed, partners may find our cancer harder going than we do.

There's the problem of having to be strong for him. Sometimes I think it seems easier to cope being the person with the cancer than the other person. And I do recognize how much easier it is for another cancer patient to give you some criticism, say about the way you may be using the cancer to get back at someone . . . rather than family trying to tell you!

Yet cancer can make friendships and partnerships blossom and deepen – perhaps *because of* going through some of the difficulties we've described. Here some women with cancer speak of how lovers and/or husbands, friends and even acquaintances helped them.

Cancer gives you that opportunity for love. Our relationship moved light-years. My husband gave so much unconditional love.

I was using a macrobiotic diet and yoga, and my friend gave me invaluable support by saying 'We'll go on a ten-day brown rice fast and really begin this thing properly, and I'll go on it with you.'

The friend who entered into my pain was a treasure. She came after she heard about the diagnosis, said 'God how awful,' put her arms round me and cried. That was where I was at and it was wonderful. About three minutes later, we stopped and then chatted about books we'd bought. It was perfect.

So many times someone would just take my hand, hold my hand, it would be the right thing. So many times people just brought flowers, or good books, or happy stories about their own lives. Women I didn't always see sent me letters, cards – women who were on the fringe of our immediate circle of friends, who cared. They were sending me all these wonderful vibes.

Tierl wasn't allowed to touch me but she would put her plastic covered hand on top of my hand which lay under the blankets. It meant so much to me; the slight pressure of her hand was the only time I felt. It was like a morsel of food to a starving person. Physical nourishment wouldn't stay down. But this person wanted me to live and was communicating that to me in the most tangible way.[76]

I had a very good neighbour across the road, able and understanding, who didn't know anything about cancer at all . . . Without her, without that woman, I know I would have become very, very depressed.

The experience of having cancer, shattering though it is, often leads us to make changes in our lives – changes for the better. In fact, all the women we have spoken to have grown and developed. Sometimes it can seem close to the best thing that ever happened to us.

I'd never have wanted or wished I'd had cancer but I'm glad I've been through it for this, for the joy and happiness I've discovered through having cancer.

I know a lot of women with cancer who've said they wouldn't have not had it – because of what they've learned – and I'm almost getting to that point myself. A friend now has just had a mastectomy and it's changed her whole life. She's much happier.

It has put my priorities right. Now I'm definitely looking after myself first, and what's good and healthy for me . . . instead of always first thinking of what's good for other people I had to look after . . . Since this has happened I certainly don't work myself to death any more.

One woman has started university, having done 'O' and 'A' levels, one no longer has problems with her nerves, one has retired early, and another has started doing paid work. They made these changes in spite of frequently being discriminated against by others. Having cancer usually means you are no longer a good risk for life insurance and mortgages; employers can decide you are unsuitable for

jobs because of your medical history.* As a result, we may want to be careful whom we tell about our experience of cancer. You may feel it is important to tell people whom you can trust, as you need support, but it may be equally important to avoid telling people who might abuse the information. This can be a particular problem at work. Some women have got a lot of support from employers or workmates.

My doctor, generous employers and the DHSS agreed that I should have six months off work and I took my son to Spain for five of them. He went to the village school while I, for the first time in my life, was housewife; cooking, cleaning and catching up with the daily gossip in the shop. There I found peace of mind and a return to health.

At work they were very good. On the days when I had the injections I had to go home and straight to bed.

However, this is not always the case.

My job wasn't very secure and should have been coming to an end a couple of weeks after the [breast] implant was done. It was suggested that maybe there would be some problems. I'd had this mastectomy and I wouldn't be required, which I thought was most unfair.

When I was looking for another job my boss said 'There is a possibility you won't get this job because of your illness.' It was like waving a red flag at a bull. I don't get coughs, colds, sore throats and I don't do quite a lot of things people do to get time off, and it's just discrimination.

Judging the situation can be very difficult.

I didn't feel I could go to the interview and say 'By the way, I've had a mastectomy', although part of me felt it shouldn't make any difference, but if I did say it, it would make a lot of difference. So that's another person you can't be yourself with. Little things do come up which need explaining. It involves saying you've had a mastectomy and you don't feel you can do that.

Educational institutions can also be discriminatory.

The application form for the poly asked the question 'Have you had any serious illness in the past five years?' and then pretended it's in case you have hay fever and want to do agriculture!

*One psychiatrist advises people who have either had cancer or psychiatric problems not to admit it – to minimize the chances of being discriminated against. Contact BACUP for up-to-date information and advice on issues involving mortgages, life insurance, etcetera.

But one woman describes being helped by a sensitive lecturer.

'Well, I can't carry these books and I don't think I should come here any more . . .' and he said 'Have you had a hysterectomy?' and I said no, and he said 'Well, have you had a mastectomy?' and I was really surprised, somebody using this word, and then I had this long conversation with him. He was really supportive, a real help, but he was the only one.

Some equal opportunities units are now demanding that questions about medical history on application forms be removed if they have little bearing on the specific course or job. This is something we should raise with all employers and educational institutions through trade unions, equal opportunities committees, etcetera. As one woman asks: 'Is it really that they think you can't cope with the work, or that they can't cope with you?'

Dependants

Women who get cancer when their children are young have a multitude of extra problems to cope with.

When you've got a child and you've got to come home and start coping, it's difficult and nobody gives that any consideration. You don't get a health visitor, a nurse, nobody comes. Two days after the operation my daughter was taken ill and I wasn't up to nursing her and that was upsetting. And when I went in for the [breast] implant she was actually taken ill again . . . and that made me feel so guilty, that I wasn't there to look after her when she was ill and I began to feel it was a purely selfish operation.

You may be able to get some extra help if you want it, for example a home help to do some housework, or a nursery place for a child, so it is worth asking for this before you leave hospital, or once at home apply to the local social services. Children are often affected by the disruption in their routine and others have to face this at a time when they have a lot of needs of their own.

When I came home from hospital after having the mastectomy she was only eight. I was a bit tearful. It was too much, and she cannot stand me looking miserable. Her Dad said to her, 'Just leave your Mum alone, she needs time to get used to being back at home again.' She, my daughter, said, 'She's had a bit of time, she's been in hospital two weeks.'

One woman mentioned her children's needs as an important motivator in her will to live.

That is an incentive, though, they're still young and my younger daughter especially, she'd be totally devastated. I think she'd have problems for the rest of her life if she lost her mother early . . . the responsibility of this weighs heavily sometimes and then again it makes you feel 'No way, I've got to get to an age where she is not as dependent on me.' And I still won't give up then.

Sharing the experience with children differs. One woman whose daughter was four when she had the cancer diagnosed said:

We told her when I came out of hospital what had happened. We'd also brought her up not to worry about seeing us with no clothes on and I did try it and I couldn't face the way she stared at me, so I never let my daughter see me undressed again to that extent. But she does know and we explained to her what happened when I had the implant done, so she understands that as well. She has just accepted it, and just now and again if anything comes on about cancer she'll say 'That's what you had, isn't it?' And I don't really talk, just leave it, try and treat it as something that has happened and is there.

The children knew everything. My younger daughter took it better than my older daughter. I knew inside my older daughter was feeling it but just ignored it, felt for me but couldn't show the affection the same as the younger one can. Now the younger one, she wanted to see the [mastectomy] scar straight away, the elder one didn't, really. I never used to hide myself before and I didn't know what to do, I was in a quandary. But she wanted to see the scar, so she looked and went, 'That's awful.' And I said it will get better. Well, she had to inspect my scar every night . . . one night she came in the bathroom and she said 'Most Mummys would be upset if that happened to them, wouldn't they? You are not, are you?' And I said 'No, because it's made me better.' And she said, 'Anyway you've still got two, one like you and one like me' which I thought was lovely.

FACING DEATH

At all ages we struggle with the reality of death. We lose our parents; as parents we may lose infants or children. People we love die. If we become ill with a life-threatening disease, or terminally ill, we have to cope with our imminent deaths.* But the impetus to accept this reality for ourselves comes for most of us as we grow older.

*On the immediately preceding pages we discuss women's ways of facing their own mortality following the diagnosis of cancer.

SUPPORT GROUPS

There is no compulsion to keep up a false front of optimism. Yet, surprisingly, this is not a depressing group. Telling the truth about your fears is releasing. There is a great deal of laughter when we meet.[77]

There are now over 200 support groups throughout the country for people with cancer. Some of them are very well run, others can leave us feeling more anxious or provide us with inappropriate help. Some groups are run in hospitals or with hospital support, others are based in health centres or community centres. Some are run by professionals; others by the members themselves. CancerLink (see Resources) can put you in touch with a group in your locality (if one is federated to it), and NAC can do the same for groups taking a complementary or alternative approach. If you can't find a suitable group for you in your locality, try advertising, say in a local health food shop, health centre, or even a national magazine like *Here's Health*. Remember that if you are taking an alternative or complementary approach, you may be better joining with others fighting similar degenerative diseases – such as MS or arthritis – rather than joining a group where everyone is 'accepting' their illness and terrified or ambivalent about taking an active stance in relation to it.

Not all of us survive. Greta did not. She was a lively lady who didn't look her sixty years. She loved the group and had a special relationship with each of us. 'I'm glad I had cancer,' she told us. 'How else would I have met such a group of people? How else would I have learned to know so much about myself or how to appreciate myself?'[78]

We have the fear that if a person faces death that means she does not participate in life. Actually, it works the other way. The more we acknowledge and recognize death, the more we can live in the present. [A fifty-two-year-old woman]

I am more aware of a mystery and beauty in life since I have accepted death as a personal eventuality for me. Before then, I had thought of death out there; now I know that I am going to die. That has released me for more vivid living. I reach out more. Almost everything reminds me of its connections with other things; my present is many-textured. I do not look to the future with dread. It has to be shorter than my past but it does not have be less rich. [A seventy-eight-year-old woman]

Discussion of death is still relatively taboo, particularly for those of us brought up in a European culture. Allopathic medicine often distorts our ideas of death. Many doctors, particularly hospital doctors working in acute specialties, view it as an adversary, an evil, a visible defeat. They often use every medical means possible to prolong life for its own sake without considering its quality or whether there is any hope of recovery, and without taking into account the ill person's wishes. Some doctors disregard our wishes to such an extent that they withhold information about our state of health even when we ask for it.

In response to the medicalization of death, and to the gross suffering such medicalization has caused countless people, Cicely Saunders pioneered the hospice concept, a way of caring for seriously ill and dying people that has challenged the very core of medical practice, and led the way for all those caring practitioners looking for a better approach. The aim of a hospice, or hospice unit, is to care for people on every level. As Cicely Saunders says:

A hospice today forms a community fully committed to the care needed not only for those with persistent and terminal cancer but also for those with long-term illness, chronic pain and, in some cases, frailty and old age.

She tells people:

You matter to the last moment of your life, and we will do all we can not only to help you die peacefully, but also to live until you die.

What many of us fear is not knowing. This is what the parents of Jane Zorza wrote after her sudden illness and death, aged twenty-five:

The time of greatest suffering was when the doctors were refusing to tell [our daughter] what her chances of survival were. Once she was told, after several months of uncertainty . . . she cried a little, and then smiled through her tears. 'Now that I know,' she said, 'I want to enjoy every day I have left. I want to be happy – and I want you to help me be happy.' . . . At the hospital, Jane could never be sure that they were telling her the truth. At the hospice, she knew they would never tell a lie.[79]

Many of us also fear prolonged and unmanageable pain. Hospice workers play a vital role in dealing with this.

At the hospital, Jane had to beg for painkillers. At the hospice, the doctors had studied carefully the source of her pain – they identified eight of these – and treated each of them separately . . . They made sure that the drugs would be administered . . . before the pain had a chance to start clawing at her again. They didn't make her into a zombie filled with drugs.[80]

Hospice workers assist many people to live and die at home. Of those who enter a hospice, about 80 per cent leave, and eventually die at home. Both the ill person and her family and friends together are the focus of hospice workers' attention. They offer support, understanding and respite to everyone involved. (Most people in fact go into hospice units so that their relatives can have some respite themselves.) The support may continue well beyond the death of the 'patient'.

Since 1967, mainly as a result of Cicely Saunders' work, the numbers of hospice beds have increased from 120 to nearly 2,000. But there is still a long way to go. Only about half are funded by the NHS; many hospice units have sprung up in inappropriate places and with inadequate funding. At the time of writing, the Conservative Government is urging health authorities to take on more responsibility for the care of the dying but promising no extra resources with which to do this.

However, more hospices is not necessarily the answer. What is needed is an awareness of the hospice concept – so that health workers in hospitals and in the community can develop it in all their work. There is no valid reason why a good GP or district nurse cannot enable us to live and die in the way we want.* To that end, we also need more home care and hospital support teams which can advise their colleagues and support people in the community. But perhaps, ultimately, we need better training of all health workers which takes into account their own fears and anxieties about death and dying. For it is only when people have been able to confront these that they can really put into practice the kind of caring that we all need. See Resources, p. 592, for where you can find out about hospices and hospital support teams. See also Healing and Dying on p. 89.

Making Decisions Concerning Our Own Death

We know we cannot control whether we die, so we often jump to the conclusion that there is *nothing* we can do about it – no control, no choice. Yet we do have elements of control. As long as we are able, we can fight for the right to choose our place of death, and for medical care that allows us to keep our dignity, instead of accepting care

which is inappropriate for extreme pain* and terminal illness. Some doctors – and their numbers are increasing – are encouraging us to take the decisions about how we want to live our dying.

What did Jane want, the doctors asked her. She wanted one of us, her father or mother, to be with her – always until she died. That was easy. The nurses wheeled another bed into Jane's room, and from then on one of us was with her day and night – except once or twice, when we were talking to the doctor. Then a nurse – or once, when the nurses were busy, the hospice porter – came to hold her hand and talk to her.[81]

Yet economic and social constraints can still make it difficult for us, and our friends and families. Jennifer FitzGerald wrote to the *Sunday Times* concerning the deaths of two people close to her:

We were in a position to make arrangements with employers to be free to be by the bedside night and day for weeks or months. But there were [others] dying in adjacent rooms, equally confused, whose relatives could not make such arrangements. As long as our society makes rigid divisions between work (total dedication to an employer for so many inflexible hours per week) and emotion (what happens privately behind closed doors), it will not be possible for the dying to receive the love and company they need.**

Though legal, medical and theological controversies abound, some of us would also like to participate fully in decisions about when we will die. We may want to be able to define for ourselves what we consider a tolerable quality of life, a worthwhile existence.

I've had a lot of things done to my body and I'm seventy-three. I've made up my mind that enough has been done to me. If something bad happens, something major, I'm not sure I want to be repaired again.

An elderly friend of mine had had one stroke and was on strong medication to prevent another. One day, despite a warning sign, she did not call her doctor. 'He'd just put me back into hospital.' The

---

*Indeed, many GPs are very good at terminal care – even those who are quite reactionary in other ways. Those few district nurses that exist can also, if allowed to, give excellent care to dying people.

*Fortunately, mainly through the work of such people as Dame Cicely Saunders, increasing numbers of doctors and nurses are now reassessing the inappropriate and even cruel approaches that have for decades been the norm concerning the relief of pain.

**Understaffing in NHS hospitals means that nurses don't have time to 'be with' dying people – or indeed to just 'be with' anybody. Our society also fails to value people when they aren't serving the needs of capitalism – either as workers or consumers.

next day she died peacefully in her bed, having remained active to the very end. I call that a good death.

We may even want to play an active part in our own death.

I have for years kept a precious bottle somewhere. I talked with my daughter about it and she asked me, 'Please, if you are ever ready to do this, tell me first.' But I said I couldn't do that because I would be laying too heavy a burden on her; she would certainly feel that it was her job to dissuade me.

Yet people who receive the type of care they really need, even though their lives have been devastated by disease, rarely tend to even consider euthanasia. It is a scandal that this kind of care, which places equal emphasis on the physical, emotional, social and spiritual needs of the person and her family is so rarely available.* The chairperson of the Voluntary Euthanasia Society (a pressure group for the legalization of voluntary euthanasia – see Resources) wrote the following to Cicely Saunders after visiting a hospice:

There would be little or no problem with euthanasia if all the terminal disease folks could end their lives in that atmosphere you have done so much to create – but alas that can hardly be the case for many a long year.

That was written in 1961. Since then, the hospice movement has gained a firm foothold in Britain and a snowball effect has begun. With increasing, informed pressure** from all of us concerned about the living and the dying, we can hopefully ensure that a 'good death' will before long become the rule rather than the exception, and that friends and relatives of the ill and dying receive the support and help that they need.

Please see p. 592 for organizations and further reading concerning death, dying, bereavement and mourning.

SONG

We always said there'd be some
                            time for caring
            for all the caring that we didn't do
that we put off rushing places
meeting faces, meeting deadlines
holding on until there'd be some time

now we sit and snatch the hours
with faces staring
press the minutes to our hearts
that seem to be breaking
not planning or waiting or dreaming
just sitting wondering if there'll be
                            some time

© TIERL THOMPSON

NOTES

1. See Health Education Authority and Coronary Prevention Group. *Heart-Health and Asians in Britain – Report of a Workshop*, November 1987 (available from HEA, see Organizations); Coronary Prevention Group and the Confederation of Indian Organizations. *Coronary Heart Disease and Asians in Britain*. Coronary Prevention Group, 1986.
2. Steering Committee of the Physicians' Health Study Group. 'Preliminary Report: Findings from the Aspirin Component of the Ongoing Physicians' Health Study', *New England Journal of Medicine*, 28 January 1988, p. 262.
3. M. G. Marmot et al. 'Employment Grade and Coronary Heart Disease in British Civil Servants', *Journal of Epidemiology and Community Health*, vol. 32, 1978, p. 244.
4. See, for example, S. G. Haynes and M. Feinleib. 'Women, Work and Coronary Heart Disease: Prospective Findings from the Framingham Heart Study', *American Journal of Public Health*, vol. 70, 1980, pp. 133–41.
5. Mary Ann Haw. 'Women, Work and Stress: A Review and Agenda for the Future', *Journal of Health and Social Behaviour*, vol. 23, June 1982, p. 132.

6. ASTMS. *Occupational Stress: an ASTMS Policy Document*. December 1983 (available from HSF, 79 Camden Road, London NW1 9ES).
7. Arabella Melville and Colin Johnson. *The Long-Life Heart: How to Avoid Heart Disease and Live a Longer Life*. London: Century, 1985.
8. For an excellent discussion of the controversy with reference to the medical literature, see Marcia Millman, *The Unkindest Cut: Life in the Backrooms of Medicine*. New York: Morrow, 1978, pp. 215–52; see also Office of Technology Assessment, US Congress. 'Assessing the Efficacy and Safety of Medical Technologies' (GPO Stock no. 052–003–00593–0), September 1978.
9. Peter Nixon, 'Cardiovascular Disease: Drugs and Risk Factor Control are Not Enough', leader article in *Geriatric Medicine*, November 1985, p. 8.
10. See also Neville Hodgkinson. 'When the Heart Surgeon's Scalpel Misses the Point', *Guardian*, 17 April 1985, p. 13; and Peter Nixon. 'The Human Function Curve: with Special Reference to Cardiovascular Disorders', *The Practitioner*, vol. 217, 1976, p. 935.
11. Julian Arloff, 'My Mother's Stroke', *Changes*, July 1984.
12. Ibid.

*Of course, anyone who is an active member of a religious group will have potentially more opportunity for *spiritual* comfort. And it is perhaps fair to say that hospital chaplains and ministers of many religions can have something to offer anybody . . . if they have that rare quality of acceptance of whoever we are, which overrides any rigid adherence to doctrinal views.

**Without that pressure, it is likely that if and when voluntary euthanasia becomes legal, then incurably ill and elderly people will feel under increasing pressure to end their lives.

13. D. G. Beevers, 'Hypertension', *Update*, Postgraduate Centre Series, London, 1982.

14. Eoin O'Brien et al. 'Blood Pressure Measurement: Current Practice and Future Trends', *British Medical Journal*, 9 March 1985, p. 729.

15. See, for example, V. Batuman et al. 'Contribution of Lead to Hypertension with Renal Impairment', *New England Journal of Medicine*, 7 July 1983, p. 17; and A. G. Shaper and S. J. Pocock. 'Blood Lead and Blood Pressure', *British Medical Journal*, 26 October 1985, p. 1147.

16. J. Eyer. 'Prosperity as a Cause of Death', *International Journal of Health Services*, vol. 7, no. 1, 1977, p. 125.

17. See Jose Beliza et al. 'Reduction of Blood Pressure with Calcium Supplementation in Young Adults', *Journal of American Medical Association*, vol. 249, no. 9, 1983, p.1161; and Graham MacGregor et al. 'Moderate Potassium Supplementation in Essential Hypertension', *The Lancet*, 11 September 1982, p. 567.

18. M. G. Elder et al. 'Low Dose Aspirin in Pregnancy', *The Lancet*, 20 February 1988, p. 410.

19. See, for example, Lesley Doyal et al. *Cancer in Britain: the Politics of Prevention*. London: Pluto Press, 1983.

20. For example, see Tom Cox and Colin Mackay. 'Psychosocial Factors and Psychophysiological Mechanisms in the Aetiology and Development of Cancers', *Social Science and Medicine*, vol. 16, 1982, p. 381; Basil Stoll (ed.). *Mind and Cancer Prognosis*. London: John Wiley, 1979; Lawrence Le Shan. Lawrence. *You Can Fight for Your Life – Emotional Factors in the Treatment of Cancer*. Wellingborough, Northants: Thorsons, 1984.

21. S. Greer. 'Psychological Enquiry: a Contribution to Cancer Research', *Psychological Medicine*, vol. 9, 1979, pp. 81–9.

22. Ibid.; Tina Morris et al. 'Patterns of Expression of Anger and Their Psychological Correlates in Women with Breast Cancer', *Journal of Psychosomatic Research*, vol. 25, no. 2, 1981, p. 111; Maggie Watson et al. 'Emotional Control and Autonomic Arousal in Breast Cancer Patients', *Journal of Psychosomatic Research*, vol. 28, no. 6, 1984, p. 467; Caroline Thomas et al. 'Family Attitudes Reported in Youth as Potential Predictors of Cancer', *Psychosomatic Medicine*, vol. 41, 1979, p. 287.

23. For example, C. D. Anderson. 'Expression of Affect and Physiological Response in Psychosomatic Patients', *Journal of Psychosomatic Research*, vol. 25, 1981, p.143; G. H. Gudjohnsson. 'Self-reported Emotional Disturbance and Its Relation to Electrodermal Reactivity Defensiveness and Trait Anxiety', *Journal Pers. Ind. Diff.*, vol. 2, 1981, p.47.

24. For example, see Le Shan, op. cit. note 20; and Stoll, op. cit., note 20. Research by A. H. Schmale and H. Iker. ('Hopelessness as a Predictor of Cervical Cancer', *Social Science and Medicine*, vol. 5, 1971, p. 95); and Donald P. Spence et al. ('Lexical Correlates of Cervical Cancer', *Social Science and Medicine*, vol. 12, 1978, p. 141) focuses solely on women with cervical cancer in this respect.

25. Penny Brohn. *Gentle Giants*. London: Century, 1986.

26. Kenneth R. Pelletier. *Mind as Healer, Mind as Slayer*. London: Allen and Unwin, 1978.

27. For example, see Stoll, op. cit., note 20, in which the role of stress is discussed at length.

28. K. W. Pettingale et al. 'Serum IGA and Emotional Expression in Breast Cancer Patients', *Journal of Psychosomatic Research*, vol. 21, 1977, p. 395.

29. Watson et al., op. cit., note 22.

30. W. A. Creasey. *Diet and Cancer*. Philadelphia: Lea and Febiger, 1985.

31. See Richard Danwood and Christine Hall, BMJ, 7 May 1988.

32. A. Mackie in T. J. Deeley (ed.). *Communication and Cancer Education*. Cardiff: Alpha Omega Publications, 1981.

33. Gary Morrow and Christine Morrell. 'Behavioral Treatment for the Anticipatory Nausea and Vomiting Induced by Cancer Chemotherapy', *New England Journal of Medicine*, 9 December 1982, p. 1476.

34. Penny Brohn. *Working Your Way Back to Health*. Pamphlet published by the Bristol Cancer Help Centre (see Resources).

35. See, for example, Le Shan, op. cit., note 20; S. Greer et al., 'Psychological Response to Breast Cancer: Effect on Outcome', *The Lancet*, 13 October 1979, p. 785; Stoll op. cit., note 20; K. W. Pettingale. 'Coping and Cancer Prognosis', *Journal of Psychosomatic Research*, vol. 28, no. 5, 1984, p. 363; Cox and Mackay, op. cit., note 20; Cary L.

Cooper, (ed.). *Psychosocial Stress and Cancer*. London: John Wiley, 1984.

36. See, for example, P. Maguire, 'The Will to Live in the Cancer Patient' in Stoll, op. cit., note 20.

37. Personal communication to Jill Rakusen from Ludi How.

38. Some research supports the importance of the will to live. See, for example, Maguire, op. cit., note 36.

39. Gillian Barnett. 'Saying No to Cancer', *Guardian*, 30 September 1982.

40. Beata Bishop. A *Time to Heal*. London: Severn House, 1986.

41. C. Holden. 'Cancer and the Mind: How are They Connected?', *Science*, no. 200, 1978, pp. 1363–8.

42. See Gar Hildebrand. 'Immunity Can be Improved by Medication', *Journal of Alternative Medicine*, February 1986.

43. Morrow and Morrell, op. cit., note 33.

44. Ainslie Meares. 'Meditation: a Psychological Approach to Cancer Treatment', *The Practitioner*, vol. 222, January 1979, p. 119; 'Cancer, Psychosomatic Illness and Hysteria', *The Lancet*, 7 November 1981, p. 1037.

45. Bruce Ames, 'Dietary Carcinogens and Anticarcinogens', *Science*, vol. 221, 23 September 1983, p. 1256.

46. Creasey, op. cit., note 30.

47. See, for example, R. Morton and I. Campbell. 'Nutritional Support and Cancer Chemotherapy', *The Lancet*, 17 September 1983, p. 687.

48. See Creasey, op. cit., note 30; 'Vitamin A and Cancer', leader in *The Lancet*, 11 August 1984, p. 325; De Witt S. Goodman. 'Vitamin A and Retinoids in Health and Disease', *New Engand Journal of Medicine*, 19 April 1984, p. 1026.

49. E. B. Dawson et al. 'Serum Vitamin and Selenium Changes in Cervical Dysplasia', *US Fed. Proc. Reports*, vol. 43, no. 1914, 1984.

50. N. J. Wald et al. 'Plasma Retinol, β-carotene and Vitamin E Levels in Relation to the Future Risk of Breast Cancer', *British Journal of Cancer*, vol. 49, 1984, p. 321.

51. R. B. Shekelle, et al. 'Dietary Vitamin A and Risk of Cancer in the Western Electric Study', *The Lancet*, vol. 2, 1981, p. 1185.

52. J. T. Salonen et al. 'Risk of Cancer in Relation to Serum Concentrations of Selenium and Vitamins A and E: Matched Case-control Analysis of Prospective Data', *British Medical Journal*, 9 February 1985, p. 417.

53. R. Peto et al. 'Can Dietary β-carotene Materially Reduce Human Cancer Rates', *Nature*, vol. 290, 1981, p. 201.

54. Creasey, op. cit., note 30.

55. E. Cameron and L. Pauling. 'Supplemental Ascorbate in the Supportive Treatment of Cancer: Re-evaluation of Prolongation of Survival Times in Terminal Human Cancer', *Proceedings of the National Academy of Science* (USA), vol. 75, 1978, p. 4538. This research has been challenged by C. G. Moertel et al. 'High Dose Vitamin C Versus Placebo in the Treatment of Patients with Advanced Cancer Who Have Had No Prior Chemotherapy', *New England Journal of Medicine*, 17 January 1985, p. 137. For a critique of Moertel, see Leon Chaitow. 'Vitamin C Study on Cancer Patients Seriously Flawed', *Journal of Alternative Medicine*, April 1985, p. 18.

56. As reported in W. C. Willett and B. MacMahon. 'Diet and Cancer – an Overview', *New England Journal of Medicine*, 8 March 1984, p. 633 and 15 March 1984, p. 697.

57. S. Wassertheil-Smoller et al. 'Dietary Vitamin C and Uterine Cervical Dysplasia', *American Journal of Epidemiology*, vol. 114, 1981, p. 714.

58. G. C. Autandilou et al. 'The Microspectrophotometric Research of the Content of Ascorbic Acid in the Carcinomas of the Uterine Cervix', *Acta Histochem. Bd.*, vol. 59, 1977, p. 254.

59. Creasey, op. cit., note 30.

60. Salonen et al., op. cit., note 52.

61. Willett and MacMahon, op. cit., note 56.

62. Wald et al., op. cit., note 50.

63. See Creasey, op. cit., note 30. See also W. C. Willett and M. J. Stampfer. *British Medical Journal*, 3 September, 1988, p. 573, for a slightly more sceptical view.

64. Salonen et al., op. cit., note 52.

65. Dawson et al., op. cit., note 49; 'Plasma Selenium and Skin

Neoplasms: a Case-control Study', *Nutrition and Cancer*, vol. 6, no. 1, 1984, p. 13.

66. C. G. Moertel et al. 'A Clinical Trial of Amygdalin (Laetrile) in the Treatment of Human Cancer', *New England Journal of Medicine*, 28 January 1982. pp. 201–6.

67. D. Hollinrake. 'Imaging', *Centrepage* (newsletter of Bristol Cancer Help Centre), Autumn 1984.

68. Ibid.

69. Jo Spence. 'The Picture of Health?', *Spare Rib*, no. 163, February 1986, and no. 165, April 1986.

70. Stanley Keleman. *Living Your Dying*, New York: Random House, 1974.

71. *British Journal of Diseases of the Chest*, vol. 78, 1984, p. 388.

72. Dorothea Lynch and Eugene Richards. *Exploding into Life*. London: Phaidon, 1986, p. 40.

73. Ibid.

74. Esther Green et al. 'Dealing with Dying', *Spare Rib*, no. 144, April 1984. p. 8.

75. Brohn, op. cit., note 34.

76. Nicolle Freni and Tierl Thompson. 'Surviving Cancer, Facing Death', *Spare Rib*, no. 100, November 1980, p. 65.

77. Pat Kitto. 'Running a Cancer Support Group', *Self-Health*, June 1985, p. 25.

78. Ibid.

79. Rosemary and Victor Zorza. *A Way to Die: Living to the End*, London: Sphere, 1981.

80. Ibid.

81. Ibid.

RESOURCES
PUBLICATIONS

HIV AND AIDS

Ardill, Susan. 'AIDS – Getting the Story Right', *Spare Rib*, no. 175, February 1987, pp. 10–11.

Ardill, Susan and Sue **O'Sullivan**. 'AIDS and Women', *Spare Rib*, no. 177, April 1987, pp. 14–19, and no. 178, May 1987, pp. 40–43. Excellent articles exploring the issues for women.

Chirimuta, Richard and Rosalind. *Aids, Africa and Racism*, 1988, available from Bretby House, Stanhope, Bretby, Burton-on-Trent DE15 0PT.

Frontliners. *Living with AIDS*. London: Terrence Higgins Trust, 1987. Written by a self-help support group for people with AIDS. Available from Terrence Higgins Trust (see Organizations), free to anyone with AIDS.

Mars-Jones, Adam and Edmund **White**. *Darker Proof*. 2nd rev. edn. London: Faber & Faber, 1988. Selection of short stories about people living and coping with AIDS and HIV infection.

Peabody, Barbara, *The Screaming Room*. San Diego: Oak Tree, 1986. Moving account of a mother caring for her son who is dying.

Richardson, Diane. *Women and AIDS*. London: Pandora Press, 1987.

CIRCULATORY DISEASES

Items which can be used on a self-help basis are marked with a star.

Anon. 'Diet and hypertension', *The Lancet*, 22 September 1984, p. 671.

Anon. 'Should People with High Blood Pressure Avoid Sodium?' *Drug and Therapeutics Bulletin*, vol. 24, no. 7, 7 April 1986.

Arloff, Julian. 'My Mother's Stroke', *Changes*, July 1984.

Bartley, Mel. 'Coronary Heart Disease and the Public Health', *Society, Health and Illness*, vol. 7, no. 3, November 1985.

*****Cousins**, Norman. *The Healing Heart: Antidotes to Panic and Helplessness*. New York: Norton, 1983. Takes a holistic approach.

Eyer, J. 'Prosperity as a Cause of Death', *International Journal of Health Services*, vol. 7, no. 1, 1977, p. 125.

Farrant, Wendy and Jill **Russell**. *Beating Heart Disease: a Case Study in the Production of Health Education Council Publications*. Bedford Way Paper, University of London Institute of Education, 1986.

Gibney, Michael. 'When A is for heart attack', *Guardian*, 22 November 1984, p. 13.

Haw, Mary Ann. 'Women, Work and Stress: a Review and Agenda for the Future', *Journal of Health and Social Behaviour*, vol. 23, June 1982, p. 132.

*****Health Education Authority**. 'Beating Heart Disease', booklet available free from HEA and local health education departments.

Heller, R. F. et al. 'How Well Can We Predict Coronary Heart Disease? Findings in the UK Heart Disease Prevention Project', *British Medical Journal*, 12 May 1984, p. 1407.

Johnson, J. L. et al. 'Cardiovascular Risk Factors and Mortality in Black and White Women aged 40–64 Years in Evans County, Georgia', *American Journal of Epidemiology*, vol. 123, 1986, p. 209.

*****McCormick**, Elizabeth Wild. *The Heart Attack Recovery Book – a Look at the Emotional and Practical Problems Encountered during Rehabilitation, for Patients and Their Families*. rev. edn. London: Unwin, 1987. Takes a holistic approach, but unfortunately considers men as the patients and women as the carers throughout.

Marmot, M. G. et al. 'Employment Grade and Coronary Heart Disease in British Civil Servants', *Journal of Epidemiology and Community Health*, vol. 32, 1978, p. 244.

Marmot, M. G. 'Socioeconomic and Cultural Factors in Ischaemic Heart Disease', *Advances in Cardiology*, vol. 29, 1982, p. 68.

*****Melville**, Arabella and Colin **Johnson**. *The Long-Life Heart: How to Avoid Heart Disease and Live a Longer Life*. London: Century, 1985. A practical book, taking a holistic view. Particularly good in relation to strategies for stress and life management, and recognizes the importance of spontaneity and fun!

Nixon, Peter. 'The Human Function Curve: with Special Reference to Cardiovascular Disorders', *The Practitioner*, vol. 217, 1976, p. 935.

Open University Health and Disease Course Team. *Caring for Health: Dilemmas and Prospects*. Milton Keynes: Open University Press, 1985. Contains a useful chapter ('A Cautionary Tale') discussing the value of current curative and preventive strategies.

Ruberman, William et al. 'Psychosocial Influences on Mortality after Myocardial Infarction', *New England Journal of Medicine*, 30 August 1984, p. 552.

Sarton, May. *After the Stroke*. London: Women's Press, 1988. An inspiring book.

Tunstall-Pedoe, Hugh. 'Paunches and the Prediction of Coronary Heart Disease', *British Medical Journal*, 2 June 1984, p. 1629.

*****Warlow**, Charles and Barbara **Woodhouse**. *Stroke and Living with a Stroke*. Rickmansworth: B. W. Campions, 1987.

Women's Health Information Centre. 'Women's Health and Heart Disease' 1986. Broadsheet available from WHRRIC (see Organizations).

CANCER: GENERAL READING

ASTMS. *The Prevention of Occupational Cancer*. ASTMS policy document, 1980. (Available from MSF, 79 Camden Road, London NW1 9ES.)

Bertell, Rosalie. *No Immediate Danger: Prognosis for a Radioactive Earth*. London: Women's Press, 1985.

Brown, Wilmette. Black Ghetto Ecology. Pamphlet about the politics of cancer in relation to black women, by a cancer survivor. Available from King's Cross Women's Centre, 71 Tonbridge Street, London WC1.

Cook, Stephani. *Second Life*. London: Michael Joseph, 1982. One woman's story of how she came through life-threatening disease despite painful and sometimes incompetent medical treatment.

Doyal, Lesley et al. *Cancer in Britain: the Politics of Prevention*. London: Pluto Press, 1983. Focuses on occupational and environmental causes of cancer, though only discusses diet in relation to chemical additives and pollutants.

Farber, Emmanuel. 'Chemical carcinogenesis', *New England Journal of Medicine*, 3 December 1981, p. 1379.

Freni, Nicolle and Tierl **Thompson**. 'Surviving Cancer, Facing Death', *Spare Rib*, no. 100, November 1980, p. 65.

General and Municipal Workers' Union. *A Preliminary Cancer Prevention Campaign*, 1980. (Available from GMBATU at Thorne House, Ruxley Ridge, Claygate, Esher, Surrey KT10 0TI.)

Harrison, Shirley. *New Approaches to Cancer*. London: Century Hutchinson, 1987. About orthodox and complementary methods.

Leonard, Jim and Phil **Laut**. *Rebirthing: the Science of Enjoying All of*

Your Life. Hollywood, CA: Trinity Publications, 1983. A clear and comprehensive guide, though somewhat prescriptive at times.

Le Serve, A. et al. *Chemicals, Work and Cancer*. London: Nelson, 1980. A good guide for workers.

National Graphical Association. *Occupational Cancer in the Printing Industry*, 1980. (Available from NGA, 63–7 Bromham Road, Bedford M40 2AG.)

Piff, Christine. *Let's Face It*. London: Gollancz, 1985. One woman's story about how she dealt with cancer which attacked her face. The author has since set up a support network for facially handicapped people. They can be contacted at PO Box 4000, London W3 6XJ.

Sandler, Dale et al. 'Cancer Risk in Adulthood from Early Life Exposure to Parents' Smoking', *American Journal of Public Health*, vol. 75, no. 5, 1985, p. 487.

Sarton, May. *A Reckoning*. London: Women's Press, 1984. Novel about a woman's reconciliation with her own life once told she has cancer.

Smith, Tony. 'Consensus on Overtreating Cancer', *British Medical Journal*, 13 August 1988, p. 438.

Tait, N. *Asbestos Kills*. Spaid 1977. Available from Spaid (see Organizations). Exposes the dangers of asbestos.

CANCER: HOLISTIC APPROACH

Bishop, Beata. *A Time to Heal*. London: Severn House, 1986.

Brohn, Penny. *Working Your Way Back to Health* (pamphlet). Bristol Cancer Help Centre.

Brohn, Penny. *Gentle Giants*. London: Century, 1986. Describes her feelings about having cancer and how she pursued treatment that helped her emotionally and spiritually as well as physically.

Brohn, Penny. *The Bristol Programme*. London: Century 1987. Describes the current approach of the Bristol Cancer Help Centre.

Cousins, Norman. *Anatomy of an Illness*. New York: Bantam, 1981.

Kidman, Brenda. *A Gentle Way with Cancer* (rev. ed.). London: Century, 1985.

Mouat, Kit. *Fighting For Our Lives: an Introduction to Living with Cancer*. London: Heretic Books, 1984.

Pearce, Ian. *The Holistic Approach to Cancer*. ANAC 1983. Available from ANAC (see Organizations).

Spence, Jo. 'The Picture of Health?' *Spare Rib*, nos. 163 and 165, February and April 1986.

PSYCHOSOCIAL FACTORS AND CANCER

Starred items denote resources which may be of practical help; for further practical materials, see 'alternative approaches' above.

Blohmke, Maria et al. 'Psychosocial Factors and Smoking as Risk Factors in Lung Carcinoma', *Journal of Psychosomatic Research*, vol. 28, no. 3, 1984, p. 221.

*****Cade**, Max. *Self Awareness and ESR* [Electrical Skin Resistance]. About biofeedback. Available from Bristol Cancer Help Centre.

Cooper, Cary L. (ed.). *Psychosocial Stress and Cancer*. London: John Wiley, 1984.

Greer, S. 'Psychological Enquiry: a Contribution to Cancer Research', *Psychological Medicine*, vol. 9, 1979, p. 81.

*****Hay**, Louise L. *You Can Heal Your Life*. Santa Monica, CA: Hay House, 1984. (Available from Heaven on Earth Books, 126 Elms Crescent, London SW4 8QR.)

*****How**, Ludi and Michael **Brookman**. *Relaxation and Meditation* (pamphlet). Bristol Cancer Help Centre.

*****Jampolski**, Gerald. *Love is Letting Go of Fear*. Millbrae, CA: Celestial Arts, 1979.

*****Le Shan**, Lawrence. *How to Meditate*. Wellingborough, Northants: Thorsons, 1983.

*****Le Shan**, Lawrence. *You Can Fight For Your Life – Emotional Factors in the Treatment of Cancer*. Wellingborough, Northants: Thorsons, 1984.

Morris, Tina. 'A "Type C" for Cancer?' Paper delivered at the Royal Society of Medicine, Clinical Oncology Study Course, London, September 1977.

*****Pelletier**, Kenneth R. *Mind as Healer, Mind as Slayer*. London: Allen and Unwin, 1978. (Not just about cancer.)

*****Rainwater**, Janette. *You're In Charge*. Wellingborough, Northants: Twinstone Press, 1981.

*****Simonton**, Carl and Stephanie **Matthews-Simonton**. *Getting Well Again – A Step-by-Step Self-Help Guide to Overcoming Cancer for Patients and Their Families*. London: Bantam, 1978.

Stoll, Basil A. (ed.). *Mind and Cancer Prognosis*. London: John Wiley, 1979.

*****Wheelwright**, Jane Hollister. *The Death of a Woman – How a Life Became Complete*. New York: St Martin's Press, 1985 (UK distributors: Element Books). A deeply moving and at times inspiring book written by a therapist who worked with a woman who eventually died of cancer.

CANCER AND DIET

Starred items denote resources which may be of practical help.

Ames, Bruce. 'Dietary Carcinogens and Anticarcinogens', *Science*, vol. 221, 23 September 1983, p. 1256.

*****Brookman**, Ute. *The Diet* (pamphlet). Bristol Cancer Help Centre.

*****Cameron**, E. and L. **Pauling**. *Cancer and Vitamin C*. New York: Warner, 1979. (See also note 55.)

Creasey, W. A. *Diet and Cancer*. Philadelphia: Lea and Febiger, 1985.

Forbes, Alec. *Non-Toxic Metabolic Therapy* (pamphlet). Bristol Cancer Help Centre.

Forbes, Alec. *The Bristol Diet*. London: Century, 1984. (NB This has been superseded by Penny Brohn's *The Bristol Programme*.)

*****Gear**, Alan. *The Organic Food Guide* (available from health food shops).

*****Gerson**, Max. *A Cancer Therapy: Results of 50 Cases*. CA: Totality Books, 1977.

Passwater, R. *Cancer and its Nutritional Therapies*. New Canaan, CT: Keats Publishing (rev. ed.), 1983.

*****Rippon**, Sadhya. *The Bristol Recipe Book*. London: Century, 1987.

Stafford, Julie. *Taste of Life*. London: Souvenir Press, 1985. Cookbook for people with cancer.

DEATH

du Baclay, Shirley. *Cicely Saunders*. London: Hodder and Stoughton, 1984. Biography of pioneering spirit who has done so much to improve care of people who are dying. An inspiring book that also challenges the concept of euthanasia.

Downing, A. B. and B. **Smoker** (eds). *Voluntary Euthanasia*. London: Peter Owen, 1986.

Green, Esther et al. 'Dealing with Dying', *Spare Rib*, no. 144, April 1984, p. 8. About the death of a colleague and friend, and how she and the authors dealt with it.

Humphrey, Derek with Ann **Wickett**. *Jean's Way*. London: Fontana, 1978. About choosing when to die.

Keleman, Stanley. *Living Your Dying*. New York: Random House, 1974. Written for 'all of us who one day will die'. An inspiring and enlivening book.

Kubler-Ross, Elisabeth. Kubler-Ross has brought death out of the closet for many people world-wide. Her works are classics. They include *On Death and Dying* (London: Tavistock, 1970), *Death, the Final Stage of Growth* (New York: Touchstone Books, 1986), *To Live Until We Say Goodbye* (Englewood Cliffs, N.J.: Prentice Hall, 1978), *Living with Death and Dying* (London: Souvenir Press 1982) – about how to cope with dying children, and *Life, Death and Life After Death* (1980) – an audiotape, available from Friends of Shanti Nilaya, PO Box 212, London NW8 7NW.

Lewis, C. S. *A Grief Observed*. London: Faber & Faber, 1966.

Lunt, Barry and Richard **Hillier**. 'Terminal Care: Present Services and Future Priorities', *British Medical Journal*, 29 August 1981, p. 595.

Moody, Raymond. *Life After Life*. New York: Bantam, 1984. Presents details of a variety of near-death experiences.

Pincus, Lily. *Death and the Family – The Importance of Mourning*. New York: Vintage Books, 1976. Particularly good on helping us to recognize the patterns of our lives, our resentments, our needs, and how they interact with facing death – our own or a loved one's. Includes a chapter on how to help the bereaved.

Rachels, James. *The End of Life*. Oxford: OUP, 1986.

Robertson, John A. *The Rights of the Critically Ill*. New York: Bantam, 1983. American but still relevant. Sponsored by the American Civil Liberties Union.

Saunders, Cicely (ed.). *The Management of Terminal Disease*. London:

Edward Arnold, 1979. Written for professionals; includes excellent chapter on pain relief.

Zorza, Rosemary and Victor. *A Way to Die: Living to the End*. London: André Deutsch, 1980. Written at the request of their daughter Jane, who died of cancer aged twenty-five, in order that others might benefit from the mistakes and triumphs she and her family experienced, and in particular what a hospice can do for those who are dying, their friends and families.

ORGANIZATIONS

See also Resources listed in Chapters 7 and 8.

BACUP (British Association of Cancer United Patients – and their families and friends), 121/3 Charterhouse Street, London EC1M 6AA. Tel: 01–608 1661 or free from outside London on 0800–181199. Orthodox in orientation, but committed to providing information (not only on medical issues), facilitating people with cancer learning from each other, and improving doctor–patient communication.

Brent Sickle Cell Centre, Willesden Hospital, Harlesden Road, London NW10 3RY. Tel: 01–459 1292 ext. 235. Clinic open Monday to Friday, 9.00 am to 5.00 pm.

Bristol Cancer Help Centre, Grove House, Cornwallis Grove, Clifton, Bristol BS8 4PG. Tel: 0272 743216.

British Colostomy Association (formerly Colostomy Welfare Group), 38–9 Eccleston Square, London SW1V 1PB. Tel: 01–828 5175.

British Heart Foundation, 102 Gloucester Place, London W1H 4DH. Tel: 01–935 0185/7491/9333. Can, among other things, provide information about orthodox treatments and recovery, emergency pacemaker centres and heart attack resuscitation cards.

British Rebirth Society, Robert Moore, Secretary, 18a Great Percy Street, London WC1X 9QP. Tel: 01–833 0741.

British Red Cross Society, 9 Grosvenor Crescent, London SW1X 7EJ. Tel: 01–235 5454. Loan practical items for help in home nursing, and some areas provide other forms of help such as a 'beauty care and cosmetic camouflage service'.

CancerLink, 17 Britannia Street, London WC1X 9JN. Tel: 01–833 2451. Provides information about cancer and about forms of practical and emotional support available to people with cancer, their friends and their relatives. Promotes formation of support groups and provides back-up and training for such groups. CancerLink groups tend to be orientated towards orthodox medicine, but the central organization does try to provide a directory of *all* support groups throughout the country.

Cancer Relief Macmillan Fund, registered as **National Society for Cancer Relief**, Anchor House 15–19 Britten Street, London SW3 3TZ. Tel: 01–351 7811. Provides 'Macmillan' homes for inpatient NHS care and trains community nurses in cancer care. Also gives grants to 'needy patients and their families'.

Cancer Support West London (A Black Cancer Support Group), Acton Hill Church Centre, Woodlands Avenue, London W3. Tel: 01–993 3331.

Centre for Autogenic Training, 12 Milford House, 7 Queen Anne Street, London W1. Tel: 01–637 1586.

Chemical Cancer Hazard Information Service, Department of Cancer Studies, The University Medical School, Birmingham B15 2TJ. Tel: 021–472 1010.

Chest, Heart and Stroke Association, Tavistock House North, Tavistock

Square, London WC1 9JE. Tel: 01–387 3012. An advisory service, including a volunteer stroke scheme that aims to involve volunteers in helping people who have been disabled in some way following a stroke.

Coronary Prevention Group, 60 Great Ormond Street, London WC1N 3HR. Provides general information, including various publications.

Cruse, 126 Sheen Road, Richmond, Surrey. Tel: 01–940 9047. Provides help and support for women who are bereaved.

Heart to Heart, c/o Mike Preston, 60 Barry Road, Netherhall, Leicester LE5 1FB. Tel: 0533–431194. Also at 7 Dineley Road, Peopleton, Pershore, Worcs. Tel: 0905–840446. An informal network for women and men about to undergo heart surgery or recovering from it.

International Society for Humanism in Cardiology, 43 Weymouth Street, London W1. Tel: 01–486 4191.

Marie Curie Memorial Foundation, 28 Belgrave Square, London SW1 8QG. Tel: 01–235 3325. Advisory and counselling service and provides short- and long-term care in eleven Marie Curie homes, and nationwide domiciliary care.

National AIDS Helpline. Tel: 0800–567 123.

New Approaches to Cancer, The Seekers Trust, Addington Park, Maidstone, Kent, ME19 5BL. Tel: 0732–848336. Can supply relaxation and meditation cassette tapes, a video and books specifically designed for people with cancer; also keeps a list of non-orthodox practitioners willing to work with people with cancer.

Organization for Sickle Cell Anaemia Research (OSCAR), 22 Pellate Grove, London N22 5PL. Tel: 01–889 4844.

Positive Health Centre, 101 Harley Street, London W1. Does autogenics and 'creative mobilization'.

Positively Women, c/o Soho Hospital for Women, 15 Soho Square, London W1V 5TW. Tel: 01–734 1794 (day). A support group for women who have HIV.

Sickle Cell Society, Green Lodge, Barretts Green Road, Park Royal, London NW10. Tel: 01–961 7795/8346.

Society for the Prevention of Asbestosis and Industrial Diseases (SPAID), Nancy Tait (secretary), 38 Drapers Road, Enfield, Middx. EN2 8LU. Tel: 0707–873025/01–366 1640 (weekends, evenings).

Springhill Cancer Centre and Hospice, Cuddington Road, Denton, Aylesbury, Buckinghamshire HP18 0AD. Tel: 0296–748432/748278. A day and residential centre, which does not charge a fee.

Terrence Higgins Trust, BM AIDS, London WC1N 3XX. Tel: 01–242 1010. Provides support and information for people concerned about HIV or AIDS.

Thalassaemia Society UK, 107 Nightingale Lane, London N8 7QY. Tel: 01–348 0437.

Urostomy Association, Central Office, Mrs Angela Cooke, Buckland, Beaumont Park, Danbury, Essex CM3 4DE. Tel: 024–541 4294.

Voluntary Euthanasia Society, 13 Prince of Wales Terrace, London W8. Tel: 01–937 7770.

Volunteer Stroke Scheme of the Chest, Heart and Stroke Association, Tavistock House North, Tavistock Square, London WC1. Aims to involve volunteers in helping people who have been disabled in some way following a stroke.

Women's National Cancer Control Campaign, 1 South Audley Street, London W1Y 5DQ. Tel: 01–499 7532/3. Also runs a helpline during office hours, Monday to Friday. Tel: 01–495 4995.

COMMON TESTS, PROCEDURES AND OPERATIONS*

Rewritten by
JILL RAKUSEN

In this chapter we discuss some of the most common procedures used for general diagnostic or surgical reasons. Since they can sometimes be invasive, upsetting and even unnecessary,** it can be useful to have a checklist of questions to ask your doctor (the answers can help you decide whether you want to go ahead with her/his recommendations).

1. Why does s/he think you need the procedure?
2. What are the benefits of this procedure over others?
3. How is it done?
4. What are you likely to feel during and after the procedure?
5. What are the risks involved?
6. What are the negative effects, including possible effects on future fertility?
7. What may happen if you have no procedure done?
8. Who will be doing the procedure and how experienced and skilled is s/he? For instance, how many does s/he perform in a year?†
9. Will I have to go into hospital? If so, how long am I likely to be there, and how soon afterwards can I expect to return to normal life?

While no health practitioner can guarantee the outcome of any examinations, tests or procedures, s/he has a responsibility to give you all the available information. If you have doubts or feel you need more information, seek another opinion.

During any procedure, a practitioner should take the time to explain exactly what s/he is doing and why. This enables us to learn more about our bodies and ask questions if we are unsure about anything. Bring a friend along to act as your advocate if that is what you want. With a practitioner who is respectful, gentle and informative, you will be able to relax more easily during the procedure.

GYNAECOLOGICAL TESTS AND PROCEDURES

VAGINAL EXAMINATION
Rewritten together with MAGGIE EISNER

Ask if you should empty your bladder before being examined, and check if you should save a specimen of urine for testing. The examination is more comfortable with an empty bladder, and it is also much easier for the examiner to feel your uterus. But, in a VD or genito-urinary (GU) clinic, the doctor may want to examine you and take a urethral swab (see overleaf) before your urine has 'washed out' your urethra.

It also helps if you say if you feel nervous about the examination, for example, if it is the first one you've had.*

In Britain the woman usually lies on an ordinary examination couch, with her knees bent and legs apart. You may find it most comfortable to put your feet together, and then let your bent knees drop apart, but if your hips are stiff for any reason, this will be difficult and you'll need to put your feet apart. Vaginal examination is also possible with the woman lying curled up on her side with her knees drawn up; the practitioner then approaches the vagina from behind the woman. (One doctor says she suggests this position for women who are very shy or embarrassed, perhaps because of their upbringing, culture or religion.)

In the US, and in some hospital clinics in Britain, women are examined on a special couch with stirrups to hold their feet.

---

*For procedures performed in connection with specific conditions, see appropriate section (e.g., cervical smears: cervical cancer; blood pressure readings: blood pressure, etc.). Here we discuss general procedures performed for a variety of reasons.

**In the USA some doctors order tests simply to try to protect themselves against potential law suits – a practice which is becoming more common in the UK.

†One doctor, writing in the 'Minerva' column of the *British Medical Journal* (19 April 1986), asked in relation to a study exposing complication rates of junior doctors: 'How much longer will informed consumers sign the sort of consent form that requires them to agree to any surgeon carrying out the operation?' It may take a long time before we change, but it's about time we started!

*You could also ask for a 'running commentary' explanation of the examination. Some women find this very helpful – others might prefer a chat to distract them.

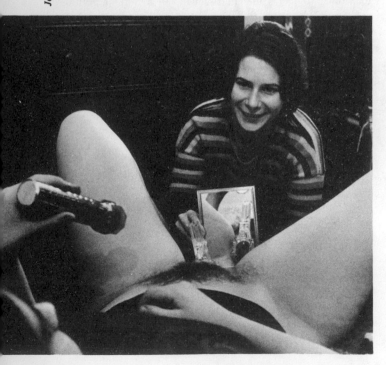

Virginia Coudron

Jean Raisler

There are three parts to the examination:

1. *Inspection of the vulva*: this means looking for signs of problems such as skin rashes, discharge, warts, pubic lice (crabs), etc.

2. *Speculum examination*: the practitioner slides a closed speculum into the vagina, and opens it slightly to hold the vaginal walls apart, so that s/he can see the cervix

(neck of the womb). The speculum may be made of metal (reusable) or plastic (disposable). It is important that a reusable speculum is properly sterilized by boiling. Anti-bacterial solutions do not kill viruses and a wart virus (which increases the risk of cervical cancer) could be passed on. Clinics may not always sterilize properly so it is worth checking. The part of the speculum which goes into the vagina consists of two curved blades which open like a duck's beak. There is an outside handle with a screw or ratchet arrangement to hold it open (see diagram).

A considerate practitioner should warm the speculum, and may lubricate it with a clear jelly. Many women find a speculum uncomfortable inside them, but it shouldn't actually be painful. It helps a lot if you can relax – if you are tense, the vaginal muscles may tend to grip the speculum, and this feels painful. When the speculum is in place, the practitioner can see the vaginal walls and the cervix. S/he can take a *cervical smear* to check for pre-cancerous changes in the cells of the cervix (see p. 521). S/he can also take *swabs* from the cervical opening or from the top of the vagina, to check for infection. This is done by dipping a cotton-tipped stick (like the 'cotton-buds' sold in chemists) in the mucus or discharge, and putting it in a pot of special jelly which will preserve any abnormal organisms present. It is then sent to the bacteriology laboratory to see if any organisms can be grown. In a GU clinic, the swab may be smeared directly on to a glass slide which is examined under the microscope in the clinic. A swab may also be taken from the urethral opening.

Some practitioners will let you look at your cervix in a small hand-mirror while doing a speculum examination. This is more useful if you have seen pictures of cervixes before, or if you have done self-examination – see p. 32.

3. *Bimanual examination*: wearing a clean polythene glove, the practitioner slides two fingers into the vagina (this is much less uncomfortable than a speculum), and puts the other hand on the bottom of your abdomen. Feeling between the two hands, s/he can usually feel the size, position and shape of your uterus, and can feel if your tubes or ovaries are enlarged or tender.

Many women's ovaries are slightly sensitive when squeezed (like men's testicles – for once, women are better protected), and some women experience an unpleasant sensation when the cervix is manipulated: both of these reactions can be normal.

The examination will be more difficult if your abdominal muscles are tense, which happens if you are feeling tense in yourself, or if you aren't lying with your head relaxed. It is also more difficult for the practitioner to be sure of what s/he is feeling if you have a thick layer of fat on your belly, and if you have a full bladder.

DILATATION AND CURETTAGE (D & C)

A D & C is often used to find the cause of uterine bleeding or to treat it, especially in emergencies. It is also used to diagnose uterine fibroids, endometrial polyps and uterine cancer. In addition, it may be part of the investigations for

PLACEMENT OF SPECULUM FOR A PELVIC EXAMINATION

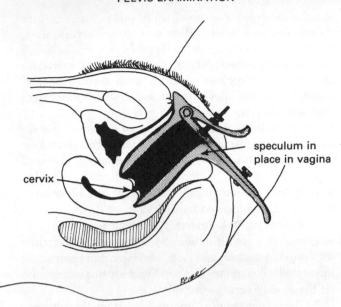

speculum in place in vagina

cervix

BIMANUAL PELVIC EXAMINATION

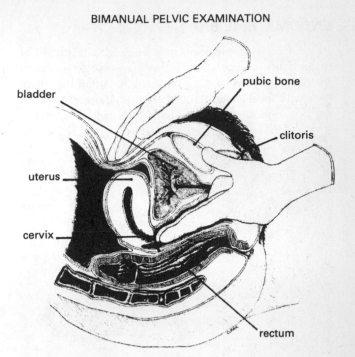

bladder

pubic bone

clitoris

uterus

cervix

rectum

cervical cancer. It is often performed to prevent infection following an incomplete abortion or after delivery, if part of the placenta is left in the uterus. The diagnostic D & C is rapidly being replaced by vacuum (Vabra) aspiration or endometrial biopsy (see p. 596).

Many doctors still prefer to do a D & C using general anaesthesia, which creates total relaxation of the pelvic muscles and allows a more accurate pelvic examination. If you are able to relax well, this is usually unnecessary, and you may wish to consider an outpatient procedure with a local anaesthetic (see Anaesthetics, p. 596).

DILATOR AND CURETTE INSTRUMENTS FOR A D & C

Nina Reimer

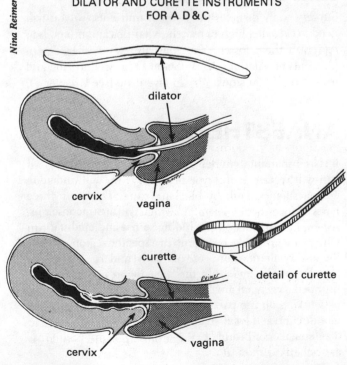

dilator

cervix

vagina

curette

detail of curette

cervix

vagina

D & C involves enlarging (dilating) the opening of the cervix by inserting a series of tapered rods that become progressively wider in diameter. A few doctors favour inserting laminaria (long stems of kelp) twenty-four hours before the D & C to dilate the cervix gradually and painlessly. The doctor then inserts a long, thin metal instrument with a spoon-shaped end (curette) through the cervix into the uterus to scrape out some of the uterine lining. (The doctor sometimes takes a tissue sample from the cervical canal.) The procedure should take five to fifteen minutes.

Most women have some bleeding following a D & C and may also pass small clots and/or have cramps for a couple of days. The main risk of a D & C, as with most operations, is having a general anaesthetic (see p. 597). Other risks include infection, excessive bleeding and, very rarely indeed, perforation of the wall of the uterus, causing possible damage to other organs such as the bowel. For symptoms to look out for following a D & C, see Chapter 17, p. 330.

VABRA ASPIRATION*

A newer alternative to the D & C for diagnostic purposes is Vabra or endometrial aspiration, which involves inserting a small tube into the cervix and removing the uterine lining by means of low-pressure suction. This procedure can be done on an outpatient basis under local anaesthesia, thus eliminating the risks of general anaesthesia. It usually causes the same mild to moderate cramping as a D & C.

*Regular Vabra aspiration or endometrial biopsy is sometimes recommended for women using hormone replacement therapy, unless they are having regular vaginal bleeding.

ENDOMETRIAL BIOPSY

In a biopsy, a sample of tissue is removed to be examined under a microscope as an aid in diagnosis. In an endometrial biopsy (which can also be done on an outpatient basis with local anaesthesia, if necessary), usually a scraping instrument (curette) is inserted through the cervix to

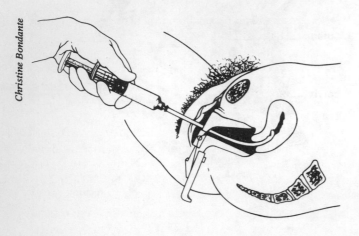

Christine Bondante

obtain a sample of the uterine lining. The procedure may be part of an infertility investigation. It has a fairly high accuracy rate when used to diagnose cancer of the uterine lining (endometrium) but the Vabra technique is generally thought to be more accurate for this purpose.

LAPAROSCOPY

The laparoscope is a lighted tubelike instrument which, when inserted through a small incision made close to the navel, allows the uterus, tubes and ovaries to be seen.

Laparoscopy is useful in the diagnosis of ovarian cysts, ectopic pregnancy, infertility caused by blocked tubes, unexplained pelvic pain or masses, endometriosis, and in the recovery of an IUD which has perforated the uterus. It is also used in some female sterilization techniques. Laparoscopy is usually done in hospital under either a general or local anaesthetic (see below). Before inserting the laparoscope, the practitioner will inflate your abdomen with carbon dioxide gas to move the intestines out of the way and expose the pelvic organs to better view. The gas is introduced through a tube in another tiny incision at the lower end of the abdomen, so a laparoscopy leaves two tiny scars about 1cm long. With a local anaesthetic, you may experience an uncomfortable pressure or fullness. After the operation you may feel mild to severe pain under your ribs for the first few days as your body gradually absorbs the excess gas. You may also have discomfort due to manipulation of the internal organs. Many doctors promote laparoscopy as a minor procedure, though many women find it takes several days to get over it.[1]

SURGERY

In countries with a predominantly private medical care system, unnecessary operations are commonly performed, because profits are made from them. In Britain this has up till now been less of a problem, but unnecessary operations are carried out because of the surgical mentality: 'If in doubt, cut it out.' They may well increase with the current expansion of private medicine.

It is important for us to consider carefully when we are told we need an operation, and not automatically to assume that the surgeon who suggested it is right. (We may well have plenty of time to think, while we are on an NHS waiting list – the only possible advantage of waiting lists!)

Some steps you could take include:

1. *Discussing the surgeon's opinion with your GP*: surgeons often find it difficult to communicate helpfully with ordinary people, and GPs, who have more practice at this, usually do it rather better. (Obviously this will depend on the kind of person your GP is.)

2. *Asking for detailed information* (from the surgeon, your GP or from books). Look back at the questions at the beginning of this chapter (p. 593) and apply them to your particular operation.

3. *Talking to other people*: there may be a relevant self-help group, or you may be able to get in touch with others who have had the operation. Remember, though, that everyone's life and health are different; what applies to them may not be the same for you.

4. *Asking for a second opinion*: if you don't feel happy with the advice you have had from the surgeon, ask your GP to refer you to another specialist.

For a discussion of consent forms, see Our Rights, p. 631.

Before and After Surgery

Surgery badly depletes the body of nutrients, so you will need to eat a diet high in protein, vitamins and minerals to replenish these losses. You may also want to take supplements of Vitamins A, B, C and D, as well as zinc and iron. And if you smoke, try to give it up (see Chapter 5).

ANAESTHETICS

It is as important to understand the type of anaesthetic that you will receive as the type of surgery you will undergo.

Anaesthetics work by blocking pain. There are three types of anaesthetic: *general*, in which you are unconscious; *regional* or *conduction* (including spinal and epidural), in which you are awake but numb in a specific region, usually the lower half (or a zone) of your body; and *local*, in which you are awake and only the area being operated on is numbed. A general anaesthetic makes you unaware of pain by working on the part of the brain that recognizes pain. Conduction and local anaesthetics block the signals sent to the spinal cord and brain from the site which is anaesthetized.

General anaesthetics are administered by needle into a vein (intravenous), by inhalation or by a combination of both. With the intravenous approach, you will probably first be medicated with sodium pentothal (to induce deep sleep). * If you receive gas, this involves inhaling it directly into the lungs via a tube inserted down your throat. Most types of anaesthetic are administered after you are given pre-medication to help you relax. If you are given gas (such as halothane or nitrous oxide), adequate oxygen must be mixed with the gas, to maintain blood pressure and respiration rate. You may experience nausea, confusion or dizziness for several hours or days after having either type of general anaesthetic. Rarely (about once in 10,000 to 20,000 cases) there is a death or paralysis as a direct result of the anaesthetic. Because anaesthetists are usually trained to watch for changes in skin colour in white people only, black women may face additional risks when undergoing a general anaesthetic, due to medical ignorance, so it is particularly important to make sure your anaesthetist is experienced if you are black.

An epidural or caudal anaesthetic is injected continuously into the space near the base of the spinal column but not into the canal itself. It works by bathing the nerve endings leading to large areas of the body, such as the perineum and legs, with anaesthetic solution, and is most frequently used in childbirth. For more on epidural and caudal anaesthetics (similar to epidural, sometimes used for rectal and genital surgery), see Chapter 19. You may ask whether a regional rather than a general anaesthetic is possible in your case, especially if you are black and/or have a history of respiratory problems.

With a *local anaesthetic* a solution or jelly which numbs the nerve endings is applied to the mucous membranes, followed by an injection which blocks specific nerves (e.g., an injection of lignocaine given by the dentist).

> *Having heard about what can go on in operating theatres, I decided I wanted to have a local anaesthetic when I had my vulval and vaginal warts removed. The request was regarded as very unusual. It wasn't painful, but seeing the smoke rise from between my legs was unexpected!*

Before surgery, you may want to ask the anaesthetist about the type of anaesthesia they are planning to use, what the risks are, what you can do to minimize them, and what to expect after the operation. (It is also important to tell them about any allergies to medication, prior anaesthetic reactions, current drugs you may be taking and information about your past and current health.) Your life is in the hands of the anaesthetist and her/his back-up staff perhaps more so than in the surgeon's hands. It's the anaesthetist who keeps you breathing. While people rarely die under a

general anaesthetic, short staffing and other pressures, together with our own ill health certainly increase the risk. If you choose a local anaesthetic, however, remember that the staff aren't used to having a conscious 'patient' on the table, and may not remember to put you at your ease during the procedure.

HYSTERECTOMY AND OOPHORECTOMY

Hysterectomy means surgical removal of the uterus. There are several types of hysterectomy.

1. Removal of the uterus alone, leaving the cervix in place (*sub-total* or *partial hysterectomy*): this operation is uncommon, largely because few doctors consider why leaving the cervix might be important for some women (see Sexual After-effects, p. 602). *

2. Removal of the uterus and cervix (*total hysterectomy*): this is the most commonly performed type of hysterectomy in the UK.

3. Removal of the uterus plus fallopian tube(s) and ovary(ies) (*unilateral* or *bilateral salpingo-oophorectomy*): unilateral means one side, bilateral means both sides – i.e. the latter means removal of *both* ovaries and *both* tubes. It is often possible to keep one ovary, or even part of an ovary – which means that your body can still secrete important hormones (see Oophorectomy, p. 600).

4. Removal of the uterus plus the upper portion of the vagina and sometimes some lymph nodes too (*Wertheim's* or *radical total hysterectomy*): this is relatively rare, and is usually used in the treatment of cancer.

The term 'hysterectomy' is often used very loosely. As will become clear in this section, it is important that we – and our doctors – are precise about exactly what types of hysterectomy might or might not be appropriate in each case.

If the uterus is removed together with both ovaries (hysterectomy plus oophorectomy), and you have not stopped menstruating, then you are likely to undergo the symptoms of oestrogen withdrawal (see Menopause, p. 453) as well as ceasing to menstruate, because no more ovarian hormones can be produced. If the ovaries remain, and you have not yet had your menopause, this usually means that you will continue to ovulate and most likely continue to experience any premenstrual symptoms that you experienced previously and other symptoms associated with the hormonal cycle even though you will no longer menstruate.

Whatever the type of hysterectomy, it is a major operation. As such it should not be undertaken lightly. While it

---

*However, you are not truly 'asleep', and you may hear or even remember conversations of those around you.

*If hysterectomy is recommended for you, you may want to consider the possibility of keeping your cervix – provided, that is, that there are no medical reasons for its removal. Retaining the cervix obviously means that you will remain at risk from contracting cervical cancer, so please see Cervical Smears, p. 521.

HYSTERECTOMY PROCEDURES

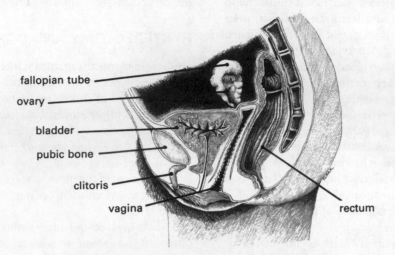

Peggy Clarke

fallopian tube
ovary
bladder
pubic bone
clitoris
vagina
rectum

TOTAL HYSTERECTOMY. Removal of uterus, including cervix (ovaries and tubes are then attached to top of vagina).

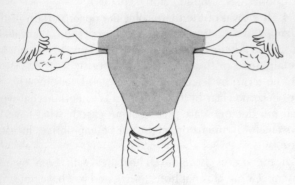

Sub-total or partial

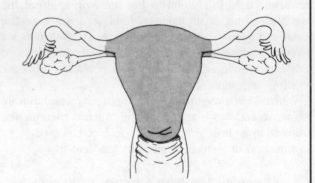

Total or complete

Christine Bondante

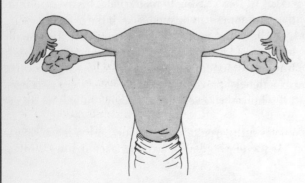

Total with bilateral salpingo-oophorectomy

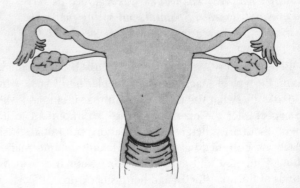

Wertheim's or radical

can save lives and restore health for many women, it also involves risks and possible complications (see below).

When is Hysterectomy Necessary?

Although in the UK our hysterectomy rate is roughly half that in the USA, there is still evidence that a considerable number of hysterectomies are performed unnecessarily. In one recent study, the hysterectomy rate was found to have doubled in ten years, yet in nearly half of the women involved, microscopic examination revealed no abnormality – and so in at least some of the cases, the operation would have been unnecessary.

A hysterectomy is usually considered essential in the following situations:

1. invasive cancer of the uterus (see p. 519), cervix (see p. 529)*, vagina, fallopian tubes and/or ovaries (see p. 519). Eight to 12 per cent of hysterectomies are performed to treat cancer;

2. severe, uncontrollable infection (PID);

3. severe, uncontrollable bleeding;

4. life-threatening blockage of the bladder or intestines by the uterus or growth in the uterus;

5. severe uterine prolapse, when the uterus drops out of the vagina;

6. conditions associated with rare but serious complications during childbirth, including rupture of the uterus, which is technically impossible to repair.

If you have any of these conditions, hysterectomy may free you from significant pain and discomfort and even save your life.

Some conditions which are not life-threatening but may justify hysterectomy include:

1. pre-cancerous changes of the endometrium (hyperplasia);

2. severe, recurring pelvic infections (see STDs and IUDs in Chapter 15, and PID in Chapter 23);

3. extensive endometriosis, causing debilitating pain and/or involving other organs (see Endometriosis, p. 515);

4. fibroid tumours which are extensive, large, involve other organs or cause debilitating bleeding;

5. pelvic relaxation (uterine prolapse).

Depending on their severity, many of these conditions can be treated without resorting to major surgery.† Fortunately, diagnostic techniques now make it possible to avoid or delay many hysterectomies that might have been done in the past. And by delaying the operation, this can give us time to prepare ourselves for it – or find ways of avoiding it; if the problem is heavy bleeding, it may even go away! Unfortunately, some gynaecologists believe that

there is no advantage to saving a uterus, especially if a woman is past her childbearing years, so we may have to be forceful if we disagree.

Why do doctors sometimes perform unnecessary hysterectomies? This quote from an American doctor, Ralph C. Wright, could equally apply to some British doctors.

> The uterus has but one function: reproduction. After the last planned pregnancy, the uterus becomes a useless, bleeding, symptom-producing, potentially cancer-bearing organ and therefore should be removed. If, in addition, both ovaries are removed . . . another common source of inoperable malignancy is eliminated. *[2]

Indeed, as one British doctor writes in a medical magazine:

> Most gynaecologists . . . will advise hysterectomy in women in their forties, because of an estimated risk of 20 per cent of the later development of endometrial cancer.[3]

This sort of reasoning does not stand up to examination. It is illogical to carry out a major operation on hundreds of women to prevent the occurrence of cancer or further complications in a few.** One cannot imagine similar logic being applied to the removal of any part of the male sexual anatomy. Given the severity of the possible side-effects of the operation, it is a particularly worrying argument.

If a GP does not take the trouble to explore a woman's problems before referral to a gynaecologist, it is possible that she will be operated on simply because the consultant does not have the time (or the inclination?) to discuss the matter fully.

> Examination over, the Presence [the gynaecologist] explained that it was necessary for me to have my uterus removed soon, 'the thing anyway would be useless to you, quite useless' . . . at that time I had no idea what a uterus was. A womb was a womb, but a uterus? I thought, perhaps some odd little organ like an appendix which one could take or leave. He enquired about my having a child and my lame 'no . . . but . . .' was interrupted by his observation that if I had really wanted 'em I would have had 'em by now . . . So that was that.[4]

---

*For early invasive cancer of the cervix a radical (Wertheim's) hysterectomy is performed, see p. 597.
†See individual sections for alternative treatment.

*The removal of ovaries as a form of cancer prevention is a particularly spurious argument, since ovarian cancer is rare.
**See also endometrial cancer, p. 519 – which has a good survival rate.

OOPHORECTOMY: REASONS AND RISKS

Oophorectomy means removal of one or both ovaries; the fallopian tube(s) may be removed as well. Common reasons for oophorectomy include ectopic pregnancy, endometriosis, benign or malignant tumours or cysts on the ovary and pelvic inflammatory disease.* An enlarged post-menopausal ovary may be cancerous and urgently requires a check-up.

If only one ovary is removed and not your uterus, you will normally continue to be fertile and have menstrual periods. If one or both ovaries or even *part* of one ovary are retained after hysterectomy, you are unlikely to be plunged into menopause (see p. 453), although you may experience some symptoms of hormonal loss because of loss of blood supply to the ovaries. If both ovaries are removed, however, you will probably experience menopausal symptoms – though not necessarily.

> *I've suffered no effects (apart from much improved general health), except some irritability, and even that has been almost banished by taking ginseng!*

The routine removal of the ovaries during hysterectomy, whether or not the ovaries are diseased,** if the woman is past forty-five or so, is now less common but is still practised by some doctors. They argue that oophorectomy prevents the possibility of future ovarian cancer, which strikes 1 in 100 women over forty and has a cure rate of only 10 to 20 per cent. On the other side, studies show that the actual risk of developing ovarian cancer following hysterectomy is very small (about 1 in 1,000). Other doctors think the cancer risk is insignificant compared to the risks involved in losing ovarian function: possible circulatory disease, premature osteoporosis and sudden menopause, all of which raise the difficult question of HRT. (See the sections on Menopause, p. 453, and HRT.)

Oophorectomy affects the hormonal balance of both post-menopausal and premenopausal women, since the ovaries usually continue to produce significant amounts of hormones after menopause (see Risks and Complications, below). Many women may therefore prefer to keep their ovaries if at all possible.

> *A friend of mine had both her ovaries removed at nineteen, apart from a tiny bit (about an eighth) of one which they managed to save. She continued to have periods and got pregnant twice.*

Indeed, if your ovaries are removed without good medical reason, some doctors consider you may be justified in taking legal action.

*Rarely, ovaries were removed in cases of cancer of the uterus, breast, cervix or abdominal cavity because ovarian secretions can increase the chances of developing recurrent cancer in these areas. This strategy is now outmoded and has been replaced by chemotherapy (see Chapter 23 on cancer).

**The terms 'diseased' and 'healthy' are frequently used carelessly by surgeons when referring to ovaries. Given the rarity of ovarian cancer, ask carefully in advance whether an ovary with a cyst or mild fibrous involvement would be removed as 'diseased'.

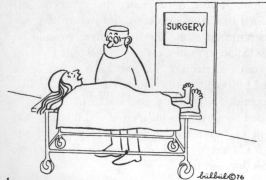

I hope you can justify this hysterectomy to my women's health group.

Risks and Complications

Surgical complications. These may occur in up to 50 per cent of cases. They may include:

- *Infections.* Most can be treated successfully with antibiotics, but some infections can be severe or even uncontrollable. Some gynaecologists now use antibiotics routinely before surgery.
- *Urinary tract complications.* Kidney or bladder infections are very common. In most cases the problem is not serious, but sometimes additional surgery is necessary. In radical hysterectomy, sensory nerves may be cut (sometimes unnecessarily) and women can lose both the sensation of having to urinate and control over bladder functions. Injury to the ureters or urinary tract has been found to occur in 5 in every 1,000 cases.[5]
- *Haemorrhage.* Sometimes requiring a blood transfusion.

Less common surgical complications include:
- *Bowel problems,* which can occur if there is damage to the intestines during surgery; in 2 per cent of cases further surgery to remove scar tissue from the bowel may be necessary.

ABDOMINAL VS VAGINAL HYSTERECTOMY

Removal of your uterus can be done either through an abdominal incision or through the vagina. The surgeon will have to recommend an abdominal incision if your ovaries are to be removed, if there is a large tumour in your uterus or if you have chronic pelvic disease. (Surgeons usually prefer an abdominal approach because it enables them to see the pelvic cavity more completely.) The incision is made either horizontally across the top pubic hairline (called a pfannenstiel or 'bikini' incision) or vertically between the navel and pubic hairline. Vertical incisions (across the grain of the muscle) tend to heal more slowly. Discuss with your doctor whether you can avoid one.

Vaginal hysterectomy, useful in cases of prolapsed uterus (when the uterus bulges into the vagina) and for a number of other conditions, has the advantage of a shorter recovery period and faster healing. In addition, because the incision is made inside the vagina, you will have no visible scar. However, since vaginal hysterectomies are performed less frequently and require greater skill, it is important to find a surgeon who does this procedure regularly. Mistakes during surgery can result in permanent urinary tract difficulties. Other disadvantages include a possible shortening of the vagina, which can result in painful intercourse afterwards.

- *Other complications* can include improper healing that can cause narrowing of the vagina and heavy discharge.
- *Death*. Between one and two women out of 10,000 may die as a result of the operation, e.g. because of uncontrollable infection, haemorrhage or blood clots.

Possible long-term risks. Some recent studies suggest that if you are premenopausal at the time of hysterectomy, with or without oophorectomy, you have a greater risk of later developing *coronary heart disease*. According to one of these studies, 'there are more deaths from coronary heart disease following hysterectomy than deaths from uterine cancer.' It is not as yet possible to assess whether this is a real risk, and, if so, whether the factors leading to the operation *also* predispose to heart disease. For example, it may be connected with the strain women may have been under beforehand, and/or the emotional effects of having to come to terms with a prematurely induced menopause. If hysterectomy is performed, then it is important that we are given the help we need to come to terms with it. In this way, one of the major risk factors associated with heart disease may be avoided (see p. 560).

Even if your ovaries are *not* removed, there is a slight chance of sudden or *premature menopause*. Most doctors assure us that we can avoid these risks and symptoms by taking HRT. But this has its own risks (see p. 456).

Hormonal responses vary from one woman to the next, for reasons not yet established. Some women suffer severe hot flushes and lack of lubrication. Others are more fortunate.

After my hysterectomy-oophorectomy, I went home with my prescription for HRT. I started to read a lot about it. The reasons for not taking it seemed to be a lot stronger than my fears of menopause, so I stopped. Lubrication was a problem at first after discontinuing the oestrogen. We kept the tube of K-Y jelly by the bed. My own glands took over and lubrication is rarely a problem now.

Some women continue on HRT while still others may wish to follow the more gradual reduction suggested by Suzanne Morgan in *Coping with Hysterectomy* (see Resources; see also Vaginal Changes, p. 455).

Psychological after-effects. Some women feel only relief following hysterectomy or hysterectomy-oophorectomy, especially when the operation eliminates a serious health problem or chronic, disabling pain. But even if we were prepared for hysterectomy and did not expect to feel depressed, we may cry frequently and unexpectedly in the first few days or weeks after surgery. This may be due to sudden hormonal changes – whether we had an oophorectomy or not.* It is also more likely to occur if we have not had sufficient information or sufficient emotional help both before and after the operation, though some hospitals are beginning to recognize the importance of counselling (see also Recovering from a Hysterectomy or Oophorectomy, p. 603). Many women are upset. Losing any part of ourselves, especially a part that is so uniquely female, is bound to have an impact. Those women who have seen their roles primarily as mothers tend to react more strongly than those of us who have a variety of roles. We may feel robbed. If we are premenopausal we may bitterly resent the fact that we cannot have children. Acknowledging feelings of anger and grief after losing a part of ourselves is an important part of the recovery process.

My hysterectomy was the best thing I've ever done. But I did have counselling to help me come to

---

*In two separate studies,[7] Dr Montagu Barker and Dr D. H. Richards found that women for whom hysterectomy solved a previously serious condition were far less depressed afterwards than those in whom no physical abnormality was found. Overall, these studies indicated that there is an increase in depression among women who have hysterectomies as opposed to other major operations. Dr Richards speculates that this could be due to a formerly unsuspected interruption of normal hormone flow even when the ovaries are left intact. This theory is still speculation and has not been confirmed by more recent studies. However, if the depression is hormone-connected it could be treated in a similar fashion to menopausal depression.

terms with not being able to have any more children.

Sexual After-effects

Many women are concerned about the effect that hysterectomy with or without oophorectomy will have on sexual response. Doctors and popular literature tend to be blandly reassuring and state that any sexual difficulties we may experience are 'all in our heads'. Only recently has the physiological basis of women's sexuality begun to be understood. In fact, from 33 to 46 per cent of women have difficulty becoming aroused and reaching orgasm after this surgery.[8] Moreover, we now know why these changes occur.

First, many women experience orgasm primarily when a lover's fingers or penis push against the cervix and uterus, causing uterine contractions and increased stimulation of the abdominal lining (peritoneum). Without the uterus or cervix, there may be much less of this kind of sensation. Yet doctors may not always be sympathetic:

> Occasionally a patient complains that the loss of the cervix has affected her libido during coitus but an assurance that a possible cancer-bearing area has been removed should be enough to satisfy her.[9]

Second, if the ovaries are removed, ovarian *androgens* which affect sexuality may be greatly reduced, thus lowering sexual response (but see androgen replacement below). Even when the ovaries are not removed, this hormonal change may occur because the surgery may interfere with the blood supply.

> *I had a hysterectomy two years ago at the age of forty-five. I went from being fully aroused and fully orgasmic to having a complete loss of libido, sexual enjoyment and orgasms immediately after the surgery. I went to doctors, all of whom denied ever having seen a woman with this problem before and told me it was psychological. Before surgery my husband and I were having intercourse approximately three to five times a week, simply because we have an open and loving relationship. Now I find that I have to work at becoming at all interested in intercourse. And I no longer have the orgasm that comes from pressure on the cervix, though I still have a feeble orgasm from clitoral stimulation.*

Third, vaginal lubrication tends to lessen after oophorectomy.

Fourth, local effects of surgery may occasionally cause problems. If your vagina has been shortened (see box, Abdominal vs Vaginal Hysterectomy, p. 601), intercourse may be uncomfortable. Scar tissue in the pelvis or at the top of the vagina from either the vaginal or abdominal procedure can also cause painful intercourse.

Some of us will find sex unchanged or more enjoyable after hysterectomy, particularly when the operation helps to relieve a painful condition such as infection, endometriosis or heavy bleeding. In the words of a woman who had a hysterectomy because of huge fibroids:

> *I had terrible cramps all my life and genuine feelings of utter depression during my periods. My ovaries were not removed and my libido was not affected. My sexual response, if anything, improved. I also had for the first time no fear of unwanted pregnancy and more general good health.*

If you have any sexual after-effects after a hysterectomy, you may find some of the following suggestions from other women helpful. *

- More strong and deliberate 'turning on' by themselves or their partner, e.g. through reading, pictures;** through verbal love-making; through massage, 'sexy' clothing, candlelight, change of location or partners or techniques, dancing, (play) wrestling and activities which physically move the pelvic area.
- More effort in love-making to push hard against the far end of the vagina in order to stimulate the peritoneum. Deep penile penetration is helped by the female-astride position or the man-on-top position with the woman's legs on the man's shoulders and pillows under her hips.
- Use of coconut oil or K-Y jelly to lubricate the clitoris and vagina.
- Doing pelvic floor exercises (see p. 31).
- More experimentation with oral sex or delicate manipulation of the clitoris.
- Pacing love-making slowly, respecting the fact that arousal may take longer.
- Trying the testosterone pellet to restore the ability to become aroused. This is at least partially effective in restoring sexual response. Testosterone is an androgen that is normally secreted by the ovary, along with oestrogen. If it is administered orally or through injection in a dosage sufficient to restore libido, 'masculinizing' effects may occur, such as lowered voice, acne and facial hair. However, another way of administering testosterone, with greatly lowered side-effects, is through a small slow-release pellet inserted under the skin in the hip region by a simple outpatient procedure every six months.[10] This procedure may not be readily available unless you press for it. One woman who has received this kind of therapy says:

> *In the last week we've made love oftener than in*

---

*See also Chapter 14, and Sexuality and Menopause section in Chapter 22.
**Most erotic material is produced by men for men, and much of it is degrading to women. However, one book that many women have found a turn-on, written by women, is *Pleasures – Women Write Erotica* edited by Lonnie Barbach (London: Futura, 1986).

the past two months. It's a great feeling. We've giggled and rolled on the floor like a couple of kids. Previously, I'd shied away from physical contact that would end up in bed. My body is much more sensitive, though I don't have the same deep internal orgasms as before. Sometimes I think if I'd had the help of hormones a few years ago, I'd never have appreciated the feelings I have now. I know there will still be times when I am depressed and longing for the deep orgasms I once had, but I'll be able to remember the three years when I had no feelings at all and it won't seem bad.

We have our doubts regarding *any* hormone therapy. Keep looking for new information about it.

● Finally, remember that with time, your body and your sex life may adjust. As one woman found:

After eight months I now find the quality of orgasms is just as good as before. I think that a considerable period of time needs to elapse for the sensations to return to the whole pelvic area.

Recovering from a Hysterectomy or Oophorectomy

You may be in the hospital for five to seven days, depending on the kind of procedure and the amount of anaesthesia you had. For the first day or two you will probably have an intravenous drip and a bladder catheter inserted. You will usually be given medication for pain and nausea. Within a day you will be on your feet and encouraged to do exercises to get your circulation and breathing back to normal. You may also be told to cough frequently to clear your lungs. (Holding a pillow over an abdominal incision or crossing your legs if you had a vaginal incision will help to reduce pain.) When your bowels become active again (usually on the second day) you may also have 'wind' pains to contend with. Walking, holding on to a pillow and rolling from side to side in bed and slow deep-breathing exercises will help.

After you go home, you will have light vaginal bleeding or oozing that gradually tapers off. You may also have hot flushes caused by oestrogen loss. You will probably continue to have some pain as well which pain-killers may not relieve entirely. Consult your GP if you have excessive pain accompanied by fever or discharge, as this may signal an infection.

Try to arrange for someone to take care of you for the first

few days.* For at least the first few weeks, ask family and friends for help with household chores and children. If you live alone, you may be able to get a home help for at least a few hours a week, from the social services. Contact them directly or via your GP or health visitor, as soon as you know your admission date.

Your GP may tell you to avoid baths, douches, driving, climbing or lifting heavy things for several weeks. If you have to drive or have small children at home who need to be carried, ask for suggestions as to how to do these tasks safely. Most doctors also recommend waiting six to eight weeks before resuming intense physical activity. Some women start much earlier, e.g. with light exercise (such as walking) and gradually building up the pace and range of activities.

With regard to sex, doctors usually recommend that 'intercourse' or 'sex' should not take place until six weeks after the operation. Unfortunately they are rarely, if ever, clear about what they mean. As Val Wilmer points out:

It can be assumed that they are referring to intercourse, but this interpretation totally ignores the many other ways in which people can have sexual relations.[11]

She later discovered that after masturbating she started to bleed, and felt very sick and frightened by this, because she had been so badly informed. In fact, orgasms as such are unlikely to cause harm and, if they cause a little bleeding, this too is unlikely to be a problem. However, it is wise to avoid putting anything in your vagina until your body has had a chance to heal.

If you are depressed after your operation, try to find a women's support group where you can talk about your feelings in a supportive atmosphere. If you can't find a group through a local women's centre, GP or health visitor, consider starting a post-surgery group of your own, perhaps with the help of your district nurse or health visitor. (For information about support groups, see Resources.) Visualizing yourself as healthy and active can help enormously with the healing process (see Chapter 7 for more ideas). Full physical recovery generally takes four to six weeks, but some women feel tired for as long as six months or even a year after surgery.

For more information on recovery, see the books listed in Resources.

Note: If you have had a hysterectomy for cancer, it is still important that you have regular smear tests, even if the cervix has been removed.

NOTES

1. See, e.g., Betty Cuthbertson. 'Only a Quick Look Round?' *Healthsharing*, Winter 1981; and Annals of the Royal College of Surgeons of England, vol. 67, 1985, pp. 103–4.
2. Ralph C. Wright. 'Hysterectomy: Past, Present, and Future', *Obstetrics and Gynecology*, vol. 3, April 1969, pp. 560–3.
3. Louis Goldman. 'Managing Patients with Abnormal Vaginal Bleeding', *Doctor*, 31 July 1980, p. 16.

4. Margaret Danks. *British Journal of Sexual Medicine*,
5. See, e.g., Charles L. Easterday, David Grimes and Joseph Riggs. 'Hysterectomy in the United States', *Obstetrics and Gynecology*, vol. 62, August 1983, pp. 203–12.

---

*Ten years ago, it was common practice for women to be sent for two weeks' 'convalescence' after hysterectomy, subsidized by the NHS.

6. Brandon Centerwall. 'Pre-Menopausal Hysterectomy and Cardiovascular Disease', *American Journal of Obstetrics and Gynecology*, vol. 139, 1981.

7. Montagu Barker. *British Medical Journal*, vol. 2, 1968, p. 91; D. H. Richards. 'A Post-Hysterectomy Syndrome', *The Lancet*, vol. 2, 1973, p. 430.

8. L. Zussman, S. Zussman, R. Sunley and E. Bjornson. 'Sexual Response After Hysterectomy-Oophorectomy: Recent Studies and Reconsideration of Psychogenesis', *American Journal of Obstetrics and Gynecology*, vol. 40, no. 7, 1 August 1981, pp. 725–9.

9. Doctor quoted by Jean Robinson in *Spare Rib*, no. 30, December 1974.

10. J. W. Studd, and Margaret H. Thom. 'Hormone Implantation', *British Medical Journal*, 22 March 1980, pp. 848–50; also Thom and Studd. 'Ovarian Failure and Ageing', *Clinics in Endocrinology and Metabolism*, vol. 10, no. 1, March 1981, p. 105. The latter has a long and useful bibliography.

11. Val. Wilmer. 'No Sex Please, You're Female', *Time Out*, March 1980.

RESOURCES
PUBLICATIONS

Dennerstein, Lorraine et al. *Hysterectomy: How to Deal with the Physical and Emotional Aspects*. Oxford: Oxford University Press, 1982.

Federation of Feminist Women's Health Centres. *How to Stay Out of the Gynaecologist's Office*. USA: Peace Press, 1981. Available from feminist bookshops or on loan from the Women's Health and Reproductive Rights Information Centre (see below).

Henriques, Nikki and Anne **Dickson**. *Women on Hysterectomy, or How Long Before I Can Hang-glide?* London: Whole Woman Books, 1986.

Morgan, Suzanne. *Coping with Hysterectomy*. New York: Dial Press, 1982.

ORGANIZATIONS

The Hysterectomy Support Group c/o the **Women's Health and Reproductive Rights Information Centre** (WHRRIC), 52–54 Featherstone Street, London EC1Y 8RT. Tel: 01–251 6580/6332.

PART VII

WOMEN AND
THE MEDICAL SYSTEM

THE POLITICS OF WOMEN AND MEDICAL CARE

Rewritten by
ANGELA PHILLIPS
(unless otherwise indicated)

Two ideas in particular seem to be basic to contemporary medical definitions of women and can be found in medical textbooks and in the attitudes and pronouncements of individual doctors. The first is that men are normal whereas women are abnormal. The second is the belief that this abnormality stems from the fact that a woman's natural role is motherhood. The capacity to have children continues to be seen as the central characteristic of woman's nature and it is assumed to make her intellectually and emotionally different and, by implication, inferior.

Little attention is paid in the medical curriculum to problems suffered by women unless they relate directly to childbearing, so common problems such as thrush, cystitis and other vaginal infections are not taken seriously either by researchers or by most doctors. Textbooks which form an important part of medical training include so-called facts which turn out, on closer examination, to be little more than blatant prejudice. Such books almost always emphasize the inevitable superiority of the doctor's clinical experience over a woman's subjective experience, even when it is the woman's own experiences that are under discussion.

Take the portrayal of female sexuality in a standard textbook produced twenty years after the Kinsey Report and ten years after work published by Masters and Johnson:[1]

In the woman sexual feelings are dormant compared with those of the man and only develop gradually with experience . . . Some women never achieve vaginal orgasms and always depend on stimulation of the clitoris, vulva and extra-genital erogenous zones for satisfaction. Indeed, one current view denies the existence of the phenomenon of the vaginal orgasm . . . but most women with satisfactory sex lives have no doubt that vaginal orgasm is real and much more powerful than that induced by superficial stimulation . . . The above views, long established and confirmed by nearly all normal women, are an anathema to small pressure groups, agitating for the liberation of women and equality of the sexes in all matters. They protest that the concepts of masculine initiation of sexual activity . . . reflect the prejudice of males in general and of male gynaecologists in particular. And such protagonists maintain that the sex drive and desire are spontaneously just as strong in girls and women as they are in boys and men, being motivated by personal pleasure rather than by a procreational instinct or anxiety to satisfy their lover. If this is what they really believe to be true in general, rather than in isolated cases, they deceive themselves, but not others, not even the majority of women. Sex equality in many respects is desirable; but equality in sex desire is unattainable, being contrary to an all-powerful inherent law of nature.[2]

The assumption of women's sexual passivity pervades medical training. According to Jean Robinson, a patients' rights advocate:

Doctors are still taught gynaecological exams on unconscious patients who have not consented. I think that is wrong for patients, but it is just as wrong for doctors because again they are learning that patients are there to be used.

It is against this background that women receive treatment from doctors.

I sat down and actually worked out how many doctors I had seen over a five-year period. Actually I had seen fifteen. Five gynaecologists, two privately; five GPs and I had been through two hospital operations and seen about five doctors during that period of time as well. Not one of those doctors even suggested to me that my partner was causing the infection.

This woman was suffering from pelvic inflammatory disease (PID) and being continually reinfected by her partner.

My doctor said the pains were caused by anxiety. I believed her and every time the apparently random attacks came I searched my mind for the lurking fears which could be triggering such devastating pain. One night I could stand it no longer and went to my local casualty department. The doctor immediately diagnosed gall-stones. He said he couldn't understand how I had stood the pain so long and gave me strong pain-killers to tide me over till I could see another doctor.

Group gathers at end of bed. Consultant surrounded by registrars, students, ward sisters, etc. I am not consulted. How old is she? (to sister). Get that thing off her (my nightie). What does she want to wear those for? (cotton briefs under my short nighties to protect their blasted sheets from menstrual leakage). No wonder she's got a rash. The group then continued to waffle, each airing their pet theories including the psychosomatic bit (from the registrar) and the assumption that I had been self-medicating (the consultant). Why not ask me? I knew what caused the reaction and my subsequent refusal of the suspect drug and consequent improvement justified my conviction.

It is therefore unsurprising that many women are angry about doctors who have

- not listened to them or believed what they said;
- withheld knowledge;
- lied to them;
- treated them without their consent;
- not warned them of risks and negative effects of treatments;
- experimented on them or used them as 'teaching material';
- treated them poorly because of their race, sexual preference, age or disability;
- offered them tranquillizers or moral advice instead of medical care or useful help from community resources (self-help groups, battered women's services);
- administered treatments which were unnecessarily mutilating and too extreme for their problem, or treatments which resulted in permanent disability or even death (*iatrogenesis*);*
- prescribed drugs which hooked them, sickened them, changed their entire lives;
- performed operations they later found were unnecessary, and removed organs that were in no way diseased;
- abused them sexually.

*Iatrogenesis is the process by which illness, impairment or death results from medical treatment. Some examples are cancers caused by DES, pelvic inflammatory disease (PID) or hysterectomy caused by an IUD, death or disability due to anaesthetic accident (particularly when the surgery may not have been necessary), electrocution or burns from hospital equipment, infection from respirators, crippling or fatal strokes due to the birth control pill, addiction to tranquillizers and illness or death resulting from infant formula feeding in hospitals.

WOMEN IN THE HEALTH CARE SYSTEM

Women are part of the health care system. We care either for ourselves or our children, spouses or ageing parents. In a survey from the Women's National Commission nearly one-third of women questioned had made their last medical consultation on behalf of another person. While ailing men do report many of the same problems with the health care system as women, men use the system less. They do not, like women, have to consult doctors for normal events in the reproductive cycle; men tend to come into the system only during crises. Many different studies have shown that medical care providers treat men with more respect than women and offer fewer tranquillizers and less moral advice.[3] Also, since only a minority of doctors are women, most women see male physicians, a situation which severely exaggerates male–female power imbalances.

Women are also 75 per cent of the workers in the National Health Service. We carry out most doctors' orders – treatment regimens like special diets, medications and bed rest – either as unpaid workers at home or as paid workers. We teach about health both in the home and in the system – what is 'good' and 'not good' for you. At home we are usually the first to be told when someone doesn't feel well, and we help decide what to do next. Some health-care analysts even call us 'primary health-care workers' or the 'layperson on a team'. Most 'patient' communication for and about family members flows through women: we report signs and changes, symptoms, responses to treatments. The system also depends on women: our direct reporting forms the basis of much of what medicine calls 'scientific results', and our bodies provide the raw material for experimentation and research (e.g. the birth control pill), often without our knowledge and consent.[4]

Yet despite our overwhelming numbers and the tremendous responsibility we carry for people's health, we have almost no power to influence the health-care system. Few women serve on health authorities and male policy-makers have designed the system primarily for the convenience of doctors, hospitals and the medical industries. *We believe that women, as the majority of consumers and workers, paid and unpaid, should have the major voice in health and medical care policy-making in this country.*

The last edition of *Our Bodies, Ourselves* expressed considerable optimism that women would be able to work together to change medical care. Indeed, women have joined together in local communities and nationally as consumers and, as workers, through their unions. There has been a significant change in the way in which many women look at medical care, and there has been some response to our needs from the medical system. Yet the medical care system remains basically unresponsive, deeply entrenched as it is in British social and political structures. In the last ten years the remaining British general hospital catering solely for women has been closed, many smaller maternity units have disappeared, the system for cervical smear testing has further deteriorated and doctors are still among the least accountable of all professionals. At the same time, the influence of medicine on people's lives continues to grow* and the present government has set its sights on encouraging the private sector – which will, of course, serve only to reinforce doctors' power.

Our critique of medicine has taken on a new dimension. We see basic errors in its fundamental assumptions about health and healing. Although conventional medical care may at times be just what we need, in many situations it may be bad for our health because it emphasizes drugs, surgery and crisis action rather than prevention. It is not enough to provide or improve medical care, to have more women doctors to stop the abuses or to equalize access to existing health and medical care for all groups. We want to reclaim the knowledge and skills which the medical establishment has inappropriately taken over. We also want preventive and non-medical healing methods to be available to all who need them.

Pessimistic as we are about the present system – about its dominance by doctors and about the latest government plans to ensure the NHS cannot survive – we believe in the healing powers within all of us and in the power of small groups as sources of information-sharing, support and healing. We still believe that we, as women, are the best experts on ourselves. The more we understand how vulnerable we become – both to disease and to dependency on experts – when isolated from one another, the more we see group experience and action as essential resources for health, from small consciousness-raising or self-help groups to large numbers of women organized for political action.

In this chapter we discuss some of the dangers of this system and offer strategies to make it work for you as well as possible.

THE POWER OF MEDICINE IN SOCIETY**

Why do so many people have an almost religious belief in medicine? Despite numerous bad or disappointing experiences, so many women say, 'It must be my fault', or 'I must just have had the wrong doctor', and fail to see that the system itself has serious faults. The institution and ideology of medicine have penetrated so totally into the fabric of our lives over the past fifty years that most of us aren't even

---

*We use 'medicine' to mean both the *tangible* personnel and institutions of the medical system like doctors and hospitals, and the discipline, field or profession of medicine. We also mean the *intangible* institution of beliefs, ideology and assumptions which influence or control our daily habits in ways most of us are not aware of (as do 'the family' and 'religion').

**In this chapter, unless otherwise stated, the term 'medicine' is used to mean 'orthodox' or 'allopathic' medicine, since that is the term's common usage. Please see Chapter 7 for more discussion on this.

aware of their influence. Their power rests mainly on several widely held myths. Brought up as most of us were to 'believe' in medicine, it is hard at first to realize how influenced (even at times manipulated) we have been by it.

MYTH: MEDICAL CARE HAS BEEN RESPONSIBLE FOR THE MAJOR IMPROVEMENTS IN WORLD HEALTH

Fact: Many dreaded infectious diseases* were 'conquered' in the past century, but this was most likely because of improved nutrition and sanitation, not medical care. *Their incidence rates were already falling* when medical treatments and vaccines were introduced. With the exception of smallpox, vaccines helped speed the decline of these diseases only minimally. *The disappearance of these diseases is the major source of our greater life expectancy in this century, leaving the chronic diseases, for which medicine has provided no cures.*

Careful studies reveal that medical care has *not* been the most important factor in improving infant mortality rates. *General improvements, especially in nutrition and fertility control, have contributed most to improvements in neonatal mortality rates.*[5]

In Britain today class is still the major determinant of health. Those in low-income jobs or surviving on state benefits suffer from all the attendant disadvantages: poor housing, overcrowding, damp, poor nutrition, workplace hazards leading to depression and a greater reliance on such solace as cigarettes. Women alone with children and women pensioners make up a significant proportion of society's poorest.

A child born to unskilled manual workers is still twice as likely to die in the first week and four times as likely to die before its first birthday than a child born to professional parents and can expect a lifespan, on average, five years shorter. A child with only one parent is at even higher risk. Women and men in unskilled occupations suffer three times more chronic illness than their professional counterparts and, according to one report, suffer four times as much chronic bronchitis.

While working-class people suffer more ill health than do professionals, they do not receive a matching proportion of care. As the Black Report documents, services in working-class areas are poorer and less accessible; GPs are more likely to be older, and to run single-handed practices with fewer diagnostic services.[6] Working-class people tend also to have shorter consultations than middle-class people.

In fact, our health is primarily the result of the food we eat, the water we drink, the air we breathe, the environment we live in, the work we do and the habits we form, which in turn result primarily from the education we have, the money we are able to earn and the other resources we

---

*The diseases were typhoid, smallpox, scarlet fever, measles, whooping cough, diphtheria, influenza, tuberculosis, pneumonia, diseases of the digestive system and poliomyelitis.

are able to command. Still other factors contribute to good health and long life: control over one's personal life, influence over the larger forces that affect all our lives, loving friendships and a supportive community.

Drugs, surgery and medical technology (kidney dialysis machines or blood transfusions, for example) are invaluable tools, and many people would not be alive today without them. While few of us would want to live without these skills and emergency resources available to us and our families, it is not emergency intervention which creates good health.

By focusing on crisis-care after people get ill rather than using its tremendous resources to help us prevent illness before it happens, the medical establishment shows itself unwilling to consider what really can and must be done to keep people healthy. This is a political issue, not simply a medical one, although many medical spokespeople argue that medicine is apolitical, 'scientific' or politically neutral. The Thatcher Government, while paying lip-service to prevention, sees it as an issue of *individual* responsibility. In fact, current Government policies of cutting resources to local councils, abolishing free school meals, charging for eye tests, presiding over the dismantling of low-cost housing, all promote ill health. At the same time, the promotion of private health care will further overemphasize crisis intervention at the expense of prevention. *To consider reallocating the money available would force all of us to confront our economic, political and social system as major contributors to our ill health.*

MYTH: MEDICINE IS A SCIENCE

Fact: Medicine has prestige largely because it claims to be 'objective' and 'neutral' as opposed to the so-called 'super-

---

RACE AND HEALTH

Few UK statistics are kept to show the differing experience of black people. There are very few conditions which affect black people specifically. Sickle-cell anaemia is one of them (see p. 558) but even though it is a serious disease which deserves better care than it often receives, it is responsible for only a tiny percentage of the ill health suffered by black people as a whole. In general, the black population suffers from the same diseases as the white population; however, it is more severely affected by diseases of poverty such as tuberculosis, and diseases of stress such as high blood pressure (black people suffer between four and six times as often). The discrimination which keeps black people in the worst jobs and housing and among the lowest income groups ensures that we share, disproportionately, the ill health experienced by the least privileged in society.

In addition, black people encounter the health service as a racist institution which often ignores our own analysis of our condition and our needs.

> There is no standard procedure for dealing with sickle-cell diseases in crisis and there are many instances where doctors presented with cases have not known what to do or have even accused sufferers of malingering.[7]

> I used to spend ages waiting for a bus, ages waiting to see the doctor ... I never used to ask anything because they used to make out because you are black you are stupid.[8]

Some attempts have been made to close the gap between need and provision. A few examples are highly successful (see City and Hackney advocate scheme on p. 643) but many appear to be there more for the convenience of hospital staff than patients. Provision of translators is important for those of us who do not speak English. However, if they are randomly appointed volunteers or young people on Youth Training Schemes, they are unlikely to have the sensitivity and understanding to provide appropriate support and may end up simply as a means of passing on doctors' orders. The use of health workers who happen to speak another language is no solution either. For a start it is exploitative of the (usually low-paid) workers who are expected to perform a skilled task without pay; secondly, it fails to recognize the importance of confidentiality in medical matters.

The concentration on the need for interpreters has the added effect of blaming those who do not understand English for the failure of the health service to provide adequately for the black community. After all, communication failures with those people who have been brought up in Britain cannot be blamed solely on language.

When as black women and working-class women we are badly treated we may hesitate to complain because we feel powerless against the institution which is supposed to be providing our care. We may feel that if we complain the treatment will get worse. At times we may protest by avoiding the health-care services. As a result we are often blamed for non-attendance and therefore for causing our own ill health. Black people, most of whom live on low incomes, are turning in increasing numbers to private medicine as a means of buying the reassurance that the health service fails to provide – an indictment indeed of a service which set out to provide free, equal care to all.

stition' of empirical healers. In fact, medical research is riddled with value judgements and inappropriate conclusions from research. For example, the research finding that women who do not attend ante-natal care are more likely to have low birthweight babies has led to the conclusion that ante-natal care prevents low birthweight. In reality there is no evidence that this is so.

Most non-reproductive medical research is done only on men and the results are applied to women. Such a process is also far from 'scientific'. Despite the fact that women make up the greater number of patients, most research, in nutrition and drugs, for example, is conducted on men.[9] One result: women do not know the real benefits and risks of drugs they take.

Most accepted treatments, therapies and medical technologies today have never been *scientifically* evaluated in terms of benefit by randomized, controlled trials, or clinical controlled trials (RCTs and CCTs).* For these trials very large numbers are required. Such trials also require one group receiving treatment to be compared with another (control) group receiving different treatment, or no treatment. This poses a dilemma for a practising doctor for whom the withholding of treatment is abhorrent, and for us when we have to decide whether or not to be placed in a trial. However, without evaluation there is no way of proving that a certain type of medical treatment is effective even if some people do seem to get better.

> Only 10–20 per cent of all procedures used in medical practice have been shown by Controlled Clinical Trials to be of benefit.[10]

Most doctors have little or no training in how to evaluate medical treatments and technology. They often base their recommendations simply on what they think may work. As an assistant professor of medicine at Harvard Medical School told *Our Bodies, Ourselves*:

> *Too frequently, practising physicians indulge in 'cookbook medicine': they open the latest medical journal and inflict the latest recipe on patients, assuring their patients that on the one hand they are receiving 'the latest thing' and on the other hand that they are 'not guinea pigs' . . . In fact, the practising physician is often extending some scientist's last experiment into the community setting – and without obtaining the patient's informed consent! At the same time, the scientist who performed the original experiment five years ago and who wrote the paper two or three years ago has long abandoned that approach.*

Many practising GPs are guilty of not reading about new treatments at all. They may depend on drug company handouts for information without seeking any independent scientific evaluation.

TECHNOLOGY AND HEALTH
Rewritten together with JILL RAKUSEN

While the development of medical technology may at first sight be in our interests, we have shown many times in this book how women can suffer from it. This is connected with doctors' and scientists' inflated belief in themselves, and often, too, with the male antipathy towards women – conscious or unconscious – both of which can prevent them from seeing the potential their developments have for doing harm, either medically or socially. As Ann Oakley writes concerning ante-natal care:

> The process of technological innovation in ante-natal care has enjoyed a career spectacularly unhampered by the potential brake of clinical evaluation; new technologies have been dreamt up, introduced experimentally, and then rapidly non-experimentally into clinical practice. At times it has seemed that the nature and limits of technological innovation have been inspired 'simply' by a global impulse to expose as much of the foetus's intrauterine life to the physicians' gaze as is both technically and humanly possible.[11]

And, as a young doctor informed at the 1985 conference of the Association for Improvements in Maternity Services, the invention of an artificial placenta is only years away and its development is in the hands of at least one man who entered his specialty because he was 'funny about women'.

It would be naive to suggest that technology is never in our interests. However, the uncontrolled growth of expensive technological 'solutions' to problems that are often social rather than medical in origin is a matter of serious concern.

- If, say, in relation to infertility, there were official commitment to the genuinely social use of technology, we could be spending money on such things as screening services for the sexually transmitted diseases which are so often responsible for the tubal blockages which IVF, for example, seeks to circumvent. However, looking down a microscope for evidence of a bacterium which can then be killed with a prescription for antibiotics attracts neither fame, fortune nor the warm glow of gratitude experienced when a doctor is able to hand a woman a baby.

- Similarly, in relation to ante-natal care, a report on the perinatal mortality rate broken down into geographical areas produced a spasm of activity by local health authorities. These 'local variations' happened (not surprisingly) to coincide with areas of high unemployment and social disadvantage. Nevertheless, the response was to increase expenditure on machinery, not on the root causes of the

---

*For example, chorion biopsy sampling (see p. 371) is gradually gaining popularity but it has not yet been evaluated. Childbirth and maternity groups have put their name to a leaflet urging women to participate in a RCT in order to evaluate it before it becomes yet another routine weapon in the obstetric armoury.

problem. A local health education official in the north-east of England reported two years later, in May 1982:

Now they've got every conceivable gadget, superb resuscitation and sick-baby services. In the last two years inductions shot up to about 80 per cent with routine ultrasound, routine electronic fetal monitoring, and a tremendous amount of caesareans. The perinatal mortality rate has dropped slightly but the infant mortality rate has risen and so, alarmingly, has the number of handicapped survivors.

● And, on the subject of handicap, if we unquestioningly promote screening for it, knowing that it cannot be totally eliminated before birth, let alone afterwards, this carries extremely oppressive connotations not only for handicapped people but also for any of us who differ from the white ethnocentric and homophobic norms of our society.

Fetoscopy, which could herald surgical interventions on the fetus while in the uterus (*in utero* surgery), also raises difficult ethical and legal issues.

Legally speaking, a fetus of 20 to 22 weeks is not considered a viable human being. If, however, an operation could save its life, viability could become a very flexible concept, and decisions about abortion could become even more fraught than they already are. How could viability be weighed against the possible hazards to the mother, and against her rights? The development of medical techniques such as *in utero* surgery impinges directly on a woman's rights over the control of her own body. Her own needs are intermingled with those of the fetus, her partner and her role as mother.[12]

For some time scientists and doctors have been working on technologies that could substantially change our relationship to reproduction. This has already been seen to some extent with IVF – particularly where egg donation and embryo freezing are concerned. In the box, however, are some examples of current avenues being pushed – reproductive engineering – which seem to be removed from any kind of social need at all.

One source lists as the future goal of reproductive engineering 'the ultimate manufacture of a human being to exact specification'.[13] Whose specifications are they talking about? What would be the implication for minority groups? It is a goal that raises horrific spectres of eugenic manipulation, which would be certain to have consequences for all of us.

Yet it is not only doctors and scientists who suffer from an inflated belief in technology. We too can be seduced into believing that technology may be the ultimate solution. What happens if we believe that technology could, or should, have the answer to everything? We may so easily feel cheated if things don't turn out right and we may find it even harder to accept the pain, for example, of infertility after pinning our hopes on a cure (for further discussion of this point, see p. 431). In the end we may blame our doctors for failure when we are simply suffering from a misguided belief in their capacities and the capacity of technology to deal with life's realities.

A society which is still in thrall to doctors is in no position to direct them. But technology must be directed if it is to serve us rather than oppress us. We must learn to judge all technology in the context of the social, political and economic setting in which it is produced and used. We must look at who profits from it and whether it increases the power of professionals over us or increases our power and self-sufficiency. We must assess its social cost and whether we have equal access to any benefits it brings. We must learn to understand the implications of any tendency we may have to put our faith in technology, as well as the differences between genuinely valuable advances and dubious self-seeking innovations. In working to demystify medicine and technology, we may come closer to controlling its development in ways which are genuinely useful.

Significantly, the most vociferous opposition to new reproductive technologies comes from reactionary forces whom we have been used to fighting over abortion and other feminist issues. Feminists have only begun to develop our understanding in this area and to insist on a feminist perspective being heard. However, we have yet to clarify what an appropriate feminist perspective is – on past developments, let alone future ones.*

Nevertheless, we hope that more and more women will assert their right to participate in public debate about technology and the priorities and application of research, and in a way that recognizes the social, political and historical issues involved. Few of us can claim to have no need of technology. What we need now is a way of controlling it rather than being controlled by it.

MEDICALIZATION AND SOCIAL CONTROL OF WOMEN'S LIVES

Everywhere one turns, medical professionals are claiming expertise in matters never before considered medical: in criminality, adolescence, overactivity in children, sex, diet, child abuse, exercise and ageing. In this takeover, called *medicalization*, medical people become the 'experts' on normal experiences or social problems.[15] Surely the most striking example of this process is the medicalization of women's lives.

Consider how often we are expected to go to doctors for normal life events. When we embark on our sexual life we see a doctor about contraception. When our bodies tell us

*The following publications (listed in Resources) give a variety of perspectives: Rita Arditti et al. (eds), *Test Tube Women*; Debbie Cameron et al., *Reproductive Rights and Wrongs – Male Power and the New Reproductive Technologies*; Gena Corea, *The Mother Machine*; Helen B. Holmes et al. (eds), *The Custom-Made Child*; Jill Rakusen and Nick Davidson, *Out of Our Hands*; Michelle Stanworth (ed.), *Reproductive Technologies*.

REPRODUCTIVE ENGINEERING: BRAVE NEW WORLD?

The following developments involve serious issues for women, for our future children, and for society as a whole.

In *cloning*, the nucleus of an *in-vitro* fertilized egg would be replaced with the nucleus from a skin or other body cell of a chosen person. Since it is the nucleus that contains the genetic material, the resulting baby would be genetically identical – and would therefore look identical with the chosen person, no matter who furnished the egg or the sperm or in whose body the fetus grew. Many types of animal have been cloned. Of course, there is no way to know what this would mean for a human baby genetically identical to one of its parents.

With *parthenogenesis*, a woman would produce a child entirely by herself. This would involve stimulating an egg to divide spontaneously and to implant in her womb. Since all her eggs are X, all such embryos would be female. Parthenogenesis would involve serious risks. To round out the normal human complement of forty-six chromosomes per body cell, each of the twenty-three chromo-

somes in the egg would have to double itself. Each woman's eggs carry any number of genes that could produce abnormalities or diseases in our children, though we ourselves are not ill. Since in parthenogenesis all the genes, including the problem ones, would be duplicated, the chances of producing a genetically damaged child would be very high.

Egg fusion would involve joining two eggs *in vitro* and then implanting the conceptus in a woman's womb. The eggs could both be from the same woman or one each from two of us. As yet it has not been done, even with mice.

Still more speculative, but doubtlessly not too far away is the *artificial placenta* ('glass womb'). If and when this is perfected, the production of children could be entirely removed from women. Some of us wonder what women's fate would be if the glass womb were to be perfected.

On past record, we must question seriously and loudly whether our society can handle any such developments. While a few of us might welcome some of them. . .

I have a real longing for egg fusion because I am in a deep and long-term partnership with a woman and would love to have a child which comes truly from both of us. I know if we use AI or if we manage to adopt, I will love our child tremendously, but I do yearn to create a new being with her from the start.

. . . we need to remember that:

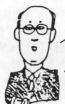 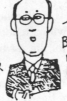

RESEARCHERS IN AUSTRALIA SAY THAT IT WILL SOON BE POSSIBLE FOR MEN TO BEAR CHILDREN.

AN EMBRYO FERTILIZED IN A LAB COULD BE IMPLANTED AND WE COULD DELIVER BY CAESAREAN SECTION.

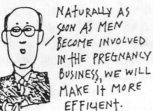 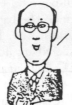

NATURALLY AS SOON AS MEN BECOME INVOLVED IN THE PREGNANCY BUSINESS, WE WILL MAKE IT MORE EFFICIENT.

WE CAN PROBABLY DO THE WHOLE DEAL IN 5 OR 6 MONTHS.

There may be very good reason for future developments in IVF, and even for artificial placentas and other technologies, which would be properly described as moving towards 'test-tube babies'. However, as with other dramatic technological developments . . . the pace of technological change is way out of touch with the social, political and moral framework into which it must fit.[14]

we are pregnant we still seek a doctor's confirmation before we believe it. During pregnancy we are urged to see obstetricians to be sure all is proceeding normally, and few of us have any alternative but the hospital for giving birth. (See Chapter 19.) The medicalization of childbirth has become so complete that it resembles treatment for a severe, life-threatening illness. When birth goes well we are often grateful to the doctor, and give her or him the credit for our success; when it goes badly, we are even more grateful for the interventions we believe saved us and our babies. When we are depressed or having difficulties in a personal relationship we may even talk to our doctors rather than our friends.[16]

Menstruation, from onset to menopause, is now often

discussed as though it were a disease. In a sense the medical world defines women as inherently defective throughout life in that we 'require' a doctor's care for all of our normal functions.

Medical care often extends to value judgements about our behaviour and sexual orientation.

After advising me when to put in my diaphragm ('Dinner, dishes, diaphragm,' he said), my doctor went on to speak about the fairly serious postpartum depression I was experiencing. 'I like to tell my new mothers to get out to the library once in a while to keep their minds alive, but basically to find their happiness in the fact that they are taking care of their husbands and bringing up a new generation.'

When I told my doctor (foolishly) that I'm a lesbian, the whole visit turned into a moral lecture and he never really paid attention to my problem. I walked out when he recommended a psychiatrist.

Gordon Bourne, obstetrician, gynaecologist and author of a widely read guide to pregnancy, comments:

From a purely biological aspect the masculine type of female and the effeminate type of male are not good vehicles for reproduction and the procreation of the human race. Nature caters for these phenomena by introducing female homosexuality, or lesbianism . . . Associations of this nature are, of course, reproductively sterile, which is the obvious biological solution to the problem in so far as it automatically eliminates such particular human types from procreation.[17]

These moral judgements carry a weighty power, though they are no more 'scientific' than the judgements of a priest or rabbi.[18]

We don't question the role that the doctor has taken in our lives because, for one thing, our exposure and acceptance began early. When we were little, our mothers took us to 'the doctor', an extremely busy and important person, who may have ignored what our mothers said, and certainly what we said, and had his own answers.

Through these many medical encounters in the course of our normal life experiences, doctors gradually initiate women into the medical belief system, warning us against listening to other women, belittling the advice of mothers, aunts, grandmothers and midwives – female lore – by calling it 'old wives' tales'.

Probably more is done by wicked women with their malicious lying tongues to harm the confidence and happiness of a pregnant woman than by any other single factor.[19]

In this way, doctors prepare us to be their disciples. As we carry their message into our families and communities, we further contribute to the medicalization of society and a narrow, biological/technological perspective on the solution of human problems.[20]

It is difficult for most of us to recognize how 'allopathic' (Western) medicine's proponents historically used women and women's central life experiences to initiate our entire society into a belief in, and dependency on, medicine. Despite much evidence to the contrary, most doctors believe sincerely that modern medicine has always helped women and that it deserves credit for society's overall health improvements since the turn of the century. Thus they tend to feel it is women's moral duty to teach children to place their faith in medicine.

All these factors together have brought us into an extreme and enforced dependency on professional experts – usually male doctors or those trained by them.[21]

THE MAKING OF A MALE MEDICAL MONOPOLY
Rewritten together with MARY CHAMBERLAIN

Medicine, like war, is an extension of politics. The story of the old wife is not the story of an inferior practice losing ground with the advances of medical science and technology; rather, it is a story which concerns the politics of medicine – a story of control and access.[22]

There are two histories of healing. The first of official medicine, in which caring has been mixed with controlling, and the second of popular medicine, in which skills have been shared among equals for the good of the community. Official medicine has almost always been closely allied to religion: the power of God (or gods) over life and death, vested in the hands of their representatives on earth. In 3000 B.C. the gods were often women.

In nearly all areas of the world, goddesses were extolled as healers, dispensers of curative herbs, roots, plants and other medical aids, casting the priestesses who attended the shrines into the role of physicians for those who worshipped there.[23]

The spread of male-dominated religions swept away the old religions of the West, and the male representatives of the one all-powerful God took over official responsibility for medicine. The battle of Church-led medicine versus popular healing was a long and bloody one. Since healing was considered magical and women could not be the officers of God, their powers, it was assumed, must come from the devil. During the Middle Ages thousands of women were burned at the stake as witches. Middle-class women attempting to learn medicine officially were turned away by universities because they were thought to be 'governed by the senses rather than by reason'.

The Church failed to suppress women healers. The community needed them. So, in spite of attempts by the Royal College of Physicians in the sixteenth century to establish a monopoly which excluded their rivals, at the end of the eighteenth century women were still part of a broad spectrum of healers which included physicians, surgeons, apothecaries, 'old wives' and midwives.

[The old wives] were the custodians of communal and community medical knowledge. But this knowledge was free and freely given. With no money at stake there was no need to preserve a 'closed' profession in terms of entry, training dissemination and knowledge.[24]

It was the social and economic changes of the eighteenth and nineteenth centuries which laid the conditions for the establishment of a medical profession, and its monopoly over medical practice. On the one hand the emerging middle classes derived status from employing professionals to care for them. On the other, the working classes, now the growing masses of the urban poor, suffered from sickness caused by overcrowding and insanitary conditions which were, for the most part, beyond the scope of traditional healers, whose practices had evolved under very different, rural, circumstances. Medical doctors could not control these diseases either but they held out the promise of a superior, 'scientific' knowledge.

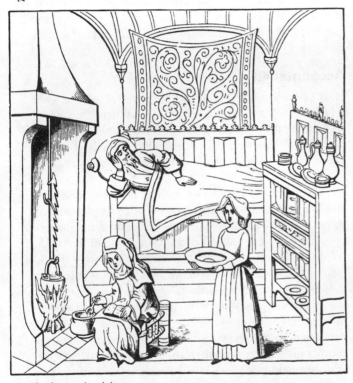

The Feminist Press

Lady as physician

With the growing organization of the industrial working classes, campaigns were launched for public health care to give working people the supposed benefits of middle-class medicine. Ironically, the very movement which sought to improve the health of working-class people through free access to medical care has also been the most powerful weapon against women's traditional practice.

Laws to control sanitation, water supplies and working conditions in fact brought the major benefits to the health of ordinary people but it has been the medical profession which has taken the credit. Under the 1858 Medical Act doctors were awarded a monopoly of practice under the Poor Laws and the Friendly Societies (early insurance agencies). However, unlike their counterparts in the USA, they did not succeed in establishing a total monopoly of health care. Doctors in the private sector were still forced to compete with alternative practitioners.

Midwifery was the area in which women remained strong. Midwives were cheap, and understood well the social and economic conditions of their patients. They were of the same class, and offered services which extended beyond the time of birth, into caring for the woman's home and family for the duration of her confinement. Many midwives were also prepared to offer other services, such as birth control advice and abortion – services which doctors in the nineteenth century avoided for fear of damaging the image of respectability which they had been carefully cultivating. (Many doctors were prepared to practise obstetrics only among middle-class patients or in hospitals and institutions where their integrity could be assured.)

Campaigns for better public health care bore fruit in the 1911 National Health Act, which was vociferously opposed by doctors through the British Medical Association although, for once, they proved to be its major beneficiaries. Maternity care was one matter which was not covered

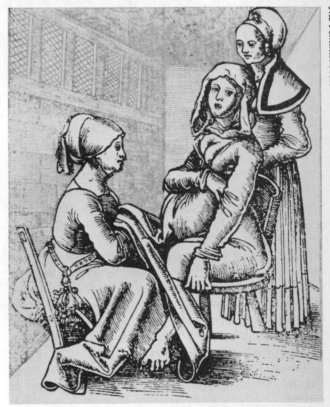

The Feminist Press

Midwife attending childbearing woman seated on obstetrical stool, 16th century

by the Act, which established an accessible personal health-care service built up from the friendly societies and provided by a range of charitable and commercial institutions. Only those in work could benefit from the sickness insurance and subsidized medical services. However, even these modest fees were beyond the means of the poorest families and the illness of a dependent woman or child could still be a crippling financial blow. It took several more years of campaigning before women won the right to a

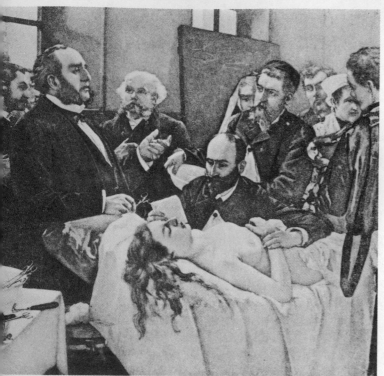

Male doctors teaching about woman patient

small maternity grant – which has just been abolished by the Thatcher Government. Maternity care was not included and was still supplied mainly by midwives.

With so many people uninsured there was still room, in the inter-war period, for traditional medicine – in the home or with the aid of herbal remedies. The emphasis on such care was necessarily on nursing. By the 1930s, demands for free and universal medical provision had increased. Socialist health campaigners wanted a system based on local health centres with salaried doctors; a model which would have emphasized primary care and provided a degree of community control over its delivery. However, the powerful BMA once again opposed the principle of free health care and their opposition was broken down only by the promise that doctors would retain control over health care and the right to practise privately.

So, in 1947 the National Health Service was born and the doctors had finally achieved a virtual monopoly of health care. Under these conditions the role of traditional medicine and traditional healers was usurped. The economic reasons for their continuation had been eroded, and medical 'science' itself was perceived to be a superior form of practice.

In their rise to power, men finally won supremacy not only over women and popular healers but also over the Church itself. In Britain and many other developed countries, doctors have taken over the role of the Church as the principal institution of social control. It is doctors who regulate female sexuality by their pronouncements, their control of contraception and abortion, and their treatment of mental illness. They have even been used to give

nationality checks a 'scientific' stamp of approval with the outrageous use of virginity tests and bone X-rays.

Women, still a majority of health workers, now work for doctors rather than for themselves – though the midwife, defined in law as an independent practitioner, is still fighting a rearguard action against total absorption. The mechanistic and interventionist nature of medical practice, developed in the period when doctors defined their approach as 'scientific' to distinguish it from the holistic and caring approach typified by traditional healers, has become the dominant medical model.

The NHS was created as a monolithic structure dominated by doctors against which the individual feels powerless. The great struggle which feminist health activists face today is to preserve the ideal of free care 'at the time of need' (as it was first established by the 'wise women'), while at the same time altering the nature of that care. (See also Chapter 28.)

Accountability

It is often argued that it is the removal of the cash relationship between doctors and patients that has allowed them to treat us as objects rather than people. The argument goes that if we paid our doctors directly, then we could use the withdrawal of patronage as a sanction against them.

This argument is put forward not only by those who would like to see our health service dismantled, but also by some people who are genuinely concerned to improve consumer choice. Sally Withington, president of AIMS, has publicly recommended to members that they should 'vote with their feet' and go to the private sector if the NHS fails to respond to their demands. While it is not beyond the wit of private practitioners to make cosmetic changes – birthing chairs and music in delivery suites – as the American system shows, a free market also produces the most crudely interventionist form of medical care. Doctors who are paid per procedure have no vested interest in preventive or conservative care.

At a more basic level such arguments fail to recognize that the people who are most badly treated by doctors are least able to go private. They also fail to take account of the power of the medical profession. Doctors' associations are there to protect doctors and even when there is a cash relationship this professional solidarity operates to protect them from complaints. This quote comes from the US edition of this book:

I reported a psychiatrist who had sex with two of his patients to the medical society. I called back two months later to find out what had been done. They told me that the doctor denied everything, and it was his word against the patients so they were dropping the matter. When I persisted, the chairman of the ethics committee told me, 'You know, my dear, we are not a consumer organization.'

Accountability should be about public *involvement* in health care. Yet, as Tom Richardson writes:

> Private for-profit industry and services as well as centralized state-run services and industries tend to force out public and community involvement to the point of elimination, although both forms of organization have a fundamental need for that public.[25]

Any strategy for improving accountability must include a return to a situation in which doctors work alongside other professionals and lay workers rather than over them, and in which patients are partners in health care rather than the passive recipients of it. But in demanding more accountability from doctors we must be prepared to take more responsibility for ourselves. Strategies for improving the accountability of medical services are discussed in the section on complaints, p. 633, and in the final chapter.

THE THREAT OF PRIVATIZATION

> Opportunities are especially bright in countries with ailing national health systems, such as England. Government support for private sector build-up has been especially encouraging for the American companies operating there.[26]

The Conservative Government of the 1980s is heavily committed to privatization in all fields. As we go to press, the NHS is facing unprecedented threats in spite of the fact that it is actually the most efficient and economical way of delivering health care. Indeed, the Government itself has stopped claiming that a private, insurance-based health service would be more economically efficient. While former Tory health minister Norman Fowler was forced to admit that:

> The advocates of compulsory [medical] insurance have to show that it is a more efficient way of providing patient care at a reasonable cost. I do not believe that case can be sustained.[27]

Nevertheless, the Conservatives are *ideologically* committed to private care and have done all they can to stimulate private investment and to bring private-sector methods into the NHS. Underfunding of the NHS and the creation of ever-longer waiting lists for treatment, creates an ever-larger potential market for health insurance companies and profit-making hospitals. Employer-purchased insurance now accounts for the major slice of the insurance market and tax relief on health insurance is now being actively considered. But it is senior management, not the shop-floor workers, who usually benefit, and few companies continue to pay premiums after retirement. Private care thrives on the subscriptions of the healthy. The old, the chronically ill and the fertile are not good risks and often

cannot be insured at all, and insurance premiums go up all the time. As a letter to the *Financial Times* observed:

> There are many elderly subscribers to health care who have been paying their premiums for years with little or no claims for benefits, and who find it difficult to maintain the higher subscriptions in their retirement, just the time of life when they are most likely to need treatment.[28]

Even within the NHS the Government is imposing crude measures of efficiency. The old 'consensus management' has given way to a centralized management structure. The power of doctors has, to some extent, been tempered, but in some cases by putting decision-making into the hands of people who may have no experience of health care and healing at all. In the process nurses have often been entirely excluded from management. The emphasis on 'patient through-put', 'income generation', minimum staff levels and false economies seems many light years away from the caring which is at the root of healing.

When the NHS is considered to be overspending, it is not the higher-paid workers who suffer wage cuts but the very lowest paid, who can least afford it. When cleaning is put out to private companies to cut spending, the savings come out of the wage packets of the cleaners themselves (the contractors still manage to make profits at their expense). (See Organizing for Change, p. 648.) For them, privatization means much lower pay and worse working conditions, precisely the sort of living conditions which create ill health.

Women in the community also have to pick up the tab for the work of caring that the NHS no longer has the staff to provide. People who leave hospital early (to improve patient through-put) do not evaporate; they return to a home where a woman, often having to give up paid work to be there, cares for them for free (see p. 619).

Privatization for many doctors means high wages (moonlighting in the private sector is not only sanctioned but actually encouraged for salaried NHS doctors) but for nearly everyone else it means lower wages, worse conditions and, in the long run, a two-tier standard of health care in which the poorest will get the least. So far it has been the low-paid ancillary workers who have put up the most sustained and effective fight against privatization.

THE DRUG INDUSTRY[29]

At the very heart of our nationalized health-care service lies the pharmaceutical industry producing, at the expense of the NHS, highly profitable drugs. The link between the NHS and the industry is direct. The Department of Health is actually responsible for protecting and promoting it as a valuable source of exports. The profit margins are extremely high because, according to the industry, the cost of research and development is high. However, the industry spends an average of £4–5,000 per doctor per year simply on *promoting* drugs; as for research, government officials, commenting on drug licences issued between 1971 and 1980, concluded that UK drug innovation was 'directed towards commercial return rather than therapeutic need'.[30]

Although there are no good drug treatments for over half the diseases of the Third World, only 1 per cent of the industry's research and development money, internationally, is spent on researching these diseases. Many apparently new drugs are just old ones with an often inappropriate or unnecessary added ingredient. Many are considered positively useless. For example, some 20 per cent of those listed in the *British National Formulary* (1984) are rated 'less suitable for prescribing'.

This dressing up of existing products is a way of 'adding value' which allows the drug to be heavily promoted under a brand name. Since little research and development is necessary, and the ingredients are reasonably cheap, the rest is pure profit. When truly innovative drugs are developed they get patent protection for twenty years, by which time heavy promotion has turned them into a money-spinning brand leader. Even when the patent has expired and other identical drugs are on the market, the branded product can be sold for much higher prices and will still command much of the market. Valium, for example, costs £13.62 per 1,000 tablets compared to £1.60 for an identical unbranded product. Nevertheless the makers, Hoffman La Roche, continue to hold 75 per cent of the market for diazepam (its generic name).

The Greenfield Report on prescribing costs suggested that, if pharmacists were simply to provide the basic 'generic' product for every prescription (unless the doctor specifically states a branded product), the NHS drug bill (of around £2,000 million a year in 1984) could be reduced by anything up to £200 million a year.[31] Nevertheless, this suggestion has never been accepted, even by the cost-cutting Conservatives, because the NHS has its hands tied by the industry. The government cannot on the one hand promote the profits of the industry and encourage multinationals to operate in Britain, and at the same time use its monopoly position as a customer to cut profits. So while staff cuts continue in the NHS, the private, multinational drug companies thrive on our subsidies.

High costs are not the only problem associated with the inefficiently-regulated drug industry. Doctors cannot possibly be expected to remember the side-effects and possible interactions of thousands of different products. Nor do they need to. The World Health Organization (WHO) suggests that a list of 250 drugs would cover 'essential' needs. In some countries restricted lists of drugs have been developed covering all basic needs. This simplifies prescribing and makes it far easier to monitor side-effects on a national scale. Such a system could only improve our safety. A partial system has recently been introduced in Britain but the 'limited list', which specifies which drugs may be prescribed on the NHS, covers few categories. Most can in any case be obtained without prescription and, combined with the ever-increasing prescription charges, it is clearly

an attempt to encourage people to go direct to chemists for minor illnesses. In spite of agitation from the drug industry, their profits are unlikely to be much affected.

Drug Regulation

The licensing of drugs is new in Britain. Before 1971, when the 1968 Medicines Act came into effect, drug companies could, according to the then health minister Kenneth Robinson, 'market any product, however inadequately tested, without having to satisfy any independent body as to its efficacy or safety'.[32] At that time there were 55,000 separate products on the market. They were licensed 'as of right' and are being reviewed, gradually, by the Committee on the Review of Medicines. It is unlikely that all of them will have been assessed by 1990. However, new drugs coming on to the market do now have to satisfy the Committee on the Safety of Medicines (CSM) that they are safe and of a reasonable quality. They do not have to be better than, or even as good as, other existing products and their prices are not considered by the committee. The CSM, in common with most other British regulating authorities, meets in secret. The reasons for its decisions are not made public. The secrecy is maintained to protect business interests.

Manufacturers are supposed to keep the CSM informed of adverse drug reactions. Doctors are also expected to report any problems through the 'yellow card system'. The average return of yellow cards is about one per GP every two years, so it often takes very many years for significant problems to come to light, and longer still for action (if any) to be taken. Unlike the US system, there is no avenue through which individuals can report suspected side-effects directly. Indeed, consumer interest in drug side-effects is not encouraged. The Coordinating group on Depo-Provera had to fight for the right to give evidence when a general licence was being considered for this drug (see p. 296). They were not, however, allowed to give verbal evidence at the hearing where their written evidence was discussed, even though it was clear that their submission formed the major evidence against the drug. However, it established an important precedent. For the first time, the health minister overruled the CSM and refused to allow a general licence. Though the drug has not been banned in Britain, higher standards have been set for 'informed consent', without which Depo-Provera should not be used. Although there is still evidence that the drug is used without proper informed consent (it tends to be prescribed disproportionately to women whose English is limited), its use without such consent would be sufficient grounds for a charge of 'assault'.

TRIALS AND ETHICS COMMITTEES[33]

While drugs are regulated, medical appliances and medical and surgical techniques are not. It is perfectly possible for a doctor to try out new techniques or appliances without setting out to evaluate them systematically. Techniques like ultrasound scans can be used routinely on pregnant women without any large-scale or long-term trials. (It is ironic indeed that obstetricians then feel free to turn round and demand proof that 'natural childbirth methods' are safer than their 'scientific' methods.)

Even when trials are established (usually to evaluate a drug) there is no adequate control of the research methods. Experimental work in hospitals is supposed to be regulated by ethics committees. However, there is no legal obligation to inform an ethics committee and no system for monitoring them. The BMA guidelines suggest that two lay members, GPs and junior medical staff should be included but many committees include none of these; some do not even meet but deal with research submissions by post.

Even when trial protocols are submitted to ethics committees, the interests of the consumers are often sacrificed to the supposed interests of science. Where doctors fear that people will not wish to be included in a trial, it is not hard for them to get permission to allocate people randomly to treatment groups *without obtaining their consent*, p. 631.

WOMEN AS HEALTH WORKERS

Consider a patient in his bed on a ward in a modern general hospital. Every member of the staff in the hospital must successfully perform his or her function. The patient's food has to arrive at the right time (cooks, porters), it must be of the right sort (dieticians), clean linen must be available (launderers, porters), supplies of drugs must come up to the ward (pharmacists, porters), materials must be sterilized (porters, sterilizers), laboratory tests must be completed (technicians, pathologists), X-rays must be taken (radiographers), records of the patient's past treatment must be available (clerical staff), orders for food and equipment must be prepared (administrators), nurses must be available night and day to monitor his condition and tend to him in emergencies. In order to carry out his role in the way he expects, a doctor in a modern hospital needs all these different workers to be functioning effectively.[34]

This is an extract from a textbook on sociology for medical students, which seems to suggest that all the other workers (male and female) do their work in order that the doctor (male) can get on with his work. In this complex division of labour there is a high degree of occupational segregation by sex, and men are more likely than women to be in positions of control. Most female health workers are found low down in the occupational hierarchy, particularly in nursing and ancillary work. Much of women's work is done part-time. Ninety per cent of nurses and most catering staff, launderers, cleaners and sterilization workers are women.

Women perform the traditional female task of caring for the intimate needs of the sick and the domestic duties of cooking, cleaning and laundering; thus the sexual division of labour in health-care reflects that of the wider society. The relationship between doctors and nurses, for instance, mirrors the relationship traditionally found between the sexes. The (usually) male doctor makes the 'hard' intellectual decisions while the (usually) female nurse carries them out and provides 'tender loving care' for the patient. Most NHS work is therefore 'women's work' and this is reflected in the inferior status, low pay and often unpleasant conditions that characterize many jobs in the health service as well as women's work in other sectors of the economy.

WOMEN AS UNPAID HEALTH WORKERS
Rewritten together with LESLEY DOYAL AND MARY-ANN ELSTON

Women's role in caring for the sick is by no means confined to the NHS. Women also provide a vast and largely invisible reservoir of care for those people who are in need but who are not deemed to be the responsibility of the health-care system. In practice, most of the chronically sick and disabled, the mentally handicapped and the elderly are not cared for by paid workers either in institutions or in the community, but by individual women who feel morally bound to do so – usually by ties of kinship or marriage.

Women have always been held responsible for maintaining the health of their families. 'Health-keeping' is part of women's normal domestic work. For some women (and some, but fewer, men) this health work goes much further.

My daughter has a muscle complaint which affects all her muscles . . . She is in the house all the time, and can only go out when I take her. We can't lay her down; if we did, she can't breathe, so she has to be propped up.

I get up at six o'clock and by the time I get her downstairs and have attended to her, it takes about two hours. It's a full-time job for me . . .

I have to cut her food up very fine and I have to make different food for her . . . I do all the washing. I couldn't afford to go to the laundrette. Well, she wets the bed because she can't get up.

I am caring for her because there is no one else to do it for her . . . My family life has been affected a lot. My husband and I have to go out separately. Caring has caused tensions in the family. We fall out. The other kids say 'You'll do it for Jill, but you won't do it for me' . . . I can't go out and leave her, I take her with me, but only to the shops and back. I don't have friends coming to the house. I used to have a lot of friends but they don't come now . . . I work picking and counting cones in a mill. I used to work thirty hours a week, but they said, even if it's only an hour a day to come in, as long as I don't leave. The doctor says I should be at home with her all the time, but I need the money . . . I've never asked for help from the Social Services, I have no help at all, I don't know about any help. I only get her tablets for nothing. I would like financial help so that I can pack in work. When I asked the doctor if I could get night allowance he said I hadn't been looking after her long enough. If she gets worse I couldn't do my job. I'd have to give that up – but I do everything as it is.[35]

According to Hilary Land, a researcher into social policy, services for the long-term sick are organized around two assumptions: that most people have female relatives to care for them; and that women have no other competing claims on their time.[36] However, the experience related above is shared by thousands of women. In 1981 the EOC estimated that there were about one and a quarter million 'carers' in Britain, most of whom were women.

The number of carers in the population is likely to grow as the number of very elderly people increases over the next thirty years. Most elderly people live at home or with family members, not in institutions. The welfare state provides for those without families, or where relatives can no longer cope. These services, such as home helps, always in short supply, have been further reduced in recent years.

A reduction in institutional provision is an explicit aim of current government policy. The reasons behind this are complex. One factor is that during the 1960s and early 1970s, research and a number of public inquiries showed that conditions in some of the large institutions for the long-term sick, handicapped or elderly were nothing short of scandalous, often exacerbating rather than relieving the suffering of their patients. 'Community care' has since been promoted as an alternative. But what exactly is meant by community care? As Janet Finch and Dulcie Groves[37] have pointed out, there has been a subtle shift in policy emphasis since the early 1970s from care in the community to care by the community. Care in the community focused on the establishment of small homes and hostels with care provided by paid workers. Care by the community means care by family and neighbours, usually care by women for love. In 1982 the EOC described the present policy of community care as a euphemism for an under-resourced system which places a heavy burden on individual women.

In the recent past, many individual women have been faced with two alternatives: placing a loved relative in an institution lacking in care, comfort and stimulation; or devoting their lives to the care of someone else, involving much personal sacrifice and loss. Policy-makers concerned with eliminating the first unacceptable alternative seem to give less consideration to the unacceptable aspects of the second (see p. 637 for support organizations for carers).

WOMEN AS PAID HEALTH WORKERS
Prepared together with LESLEY DOYAL AND MARY-ANN ELSTON

Ancillary Staff

The snobbery is horrific, real upstairs downstairs. There was one consultant who a few years ago walked on a woman's hand as she was scrubbing the floor. He never even apologised. She got her own back though when she tripped him up with her mop. The sister and the doctors on the ward usually expect the auxiliaries [untrained nurses] to make them cups of tea or coffee, endless cups served in the middle of whatever she is doing. The consultants and most doctors walk around as though no one else exists – walking over floors we're cleaning without a murmur.[38]

The NHS is maintained by the part-time employment of large numbers of working-class women, many of them black. 'Ancillary workers' occupy the lowest echelons of the health labour force. About one-third of all hospital workers (some 240,000 people) fall into this category and about 75 per cent of these are women, the majority part-time. These jobs are sex-differentiated, with men doing portering and maintenance jobs while women are involved in catering and domestic work. As a group these workers are badly paid with few opportunities for advancement. Since most

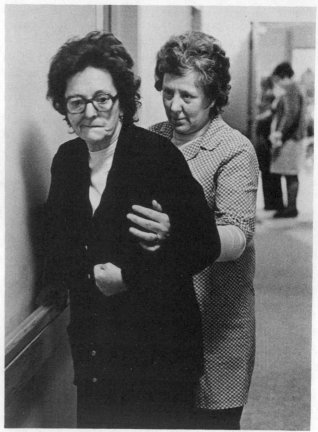

Angela Phillips

women work part-time in the jobs with lower earnings, there is also a marked sex differential in earnings. One of the few government reports to examine this group of workers suggested that in 1971 about 14 per cent of male and 21 per cent of female ancillary workers were born abroad. In some London hospitals the vast majority of ancillary workers, including over 80 per cent of domestic and catering workers, were born outside the UK. Discrimination and immigration controls are an effective bar from better work so they provide an important source of cheap labour while themselves suffering the deprivation of work in a low-paid, low-prestige sector.

Nurses

The following quotes are from the newsletter of the Radical Nurses' Group (see p. 638).

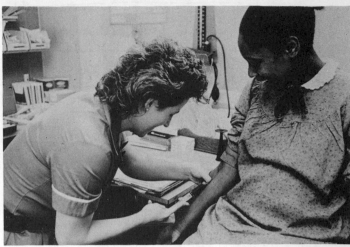

Sally & Richard Greenhill

> *There were many times when I loved our patients . . . But what they did to make me sometimes hate them was to bring their stereotypes of nurses into hospital with them. To some men, the ideal nurse seemed to be Barbara Windsor in a 'Carry On' film. Pert, pretty, always good for a naughty giggle, but at the same time, chaste little servants without too many brains. The women were more apt to play up the 'blessed virgin' aspect, sometimes almost extolling us as saints minus our haloes.* [J. Wilson, 1981]

> *There is no concept of our nurses' role as anything distinct in its own right, and therefore men can and do define our role for us to suit their own needs. They can define us as their skivvies. As a result, nurses carry on the bulk of doctors' work, implementing their orders, gathering information about their patients, etc., so that doctors can swoop in on their rounds, rush around the ward, while still believing that they are in control. All nurses, as all women, know that the men they service (their husbands, doctors, etc.) could not cope without them and yet, despite this knowledge, there is a conspiracy of silence, a fear of saying outright, 'You couldn't survive without me'.* [Kath, Report of a Workshop, 1981]

There are about 400,000 nurses in the NHS, of whom about 90 per cent are women. Historically, the nursing profession has been unique in having women dominant in both junior and senior positions, but this has not always brought the advantages that might have been expected. In the first place nurses have usually been thought of as the 'handmaidens' of doctors, with 'femininity' built into the very definition of what it is to be a nurse. As a result, nurses have always been closely controlled by doctors both at an inter-professional level and also in their everyday practice. They have been trained to obey their superiors unquestioningly and to dedicate themselves to their patients and their 'calling', a vocational ethos that has traditionally encour-

aged them to accept low pay and difficult working conditions.

In the 'caring versus curing' dichotomy which fragments medical care today, nurses traditionally do the caring – the day-to-day hands-on work with patients and their families, the listening, soothing, teaching, with a special emphasis on prevention. Nurses who want promotion and higher pay have to move into supervisory or administrative roles. Nurses active in working for change stress that they want to be able to care directly for patients, and to be valued and paid well for this work. They believe medical care will improve dramatically with this shift, since caring plays a far greater role in curing than medicine has been prepared to admit.

Those nurses who do want to progress through the hierarchy are in any case disadvantaged. Increasingly, female nurses work part-time to accommodate family commitments – a shift which has facilitated the growing power and prestige of that 10 per cent of nurses who are male. About 25 per cent of senior nursing posts (above staff nurse level) are now occupied by men, yet they provide only about 5 per cent of untrained auxiliary nurses. Much of this can be traced to an underlying belief that men are more competent in 'tough' managerial positions but it is also a reflection of the status of caring in medicine.

While nursing is relatively high in the hospital hierarchy of prestige and skill, it involves unsocial hours, disagreeable working conditions, and low pay as well as unquestioning compliance with authority. Because of their isolated situation in a strange country, foreign-born women are especially vulnerable to exploitation. The continuation of their status as overseas students is always dependent on their satisfactory performance in whatever tasks are allotted to them. After qualification they must obtain a job in order to remain in this country. They are therefore under considerable pressure to accept long hours, low pay and difficult working conditions that may well be compounded by racist attitudes from other staff or patients.[39]

Twelve per cent of nurses come from outside the UK. The percentage of students from abroad is 17 per cent. However, hospitals are discriminatory and selective. Only

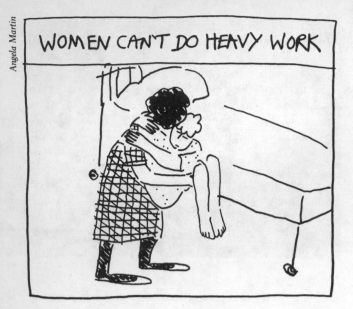

WOMEN CAN'T DO HEAVY WORK

Angela Martin

4 per cent of nursing students in the prestigious London teaching hospitals are born abroad.

Generally, overseas students are concentrated in the less popular psychiatric and geriatric hospitals caring for patients who the British-born nurses are less willing to look after. These nurses are also more likely to be channelled into the very courses, such as State Enrolled Nurse (SEN),* which are least likely to qualify them for work in their own countries: SEN training is not internationally recognized.

Midwives

The word 'midwife' means 'with women'. It has always been the role of the midwife to stay with women in labour and help them during the delivery and afterwards. The job of midwife is an old one (see p. 614), much older than that of obstetrician, yet in Britain today midwifery, in its full sense of providing birth control, abortion and pregnancy care, has been taken over by doctors. It is now rare for one midwife to be with a woman through ante-natal care, childbirth and postpartum, and their involvement in birth control is very limited. Although midwives still deliver most babies, they do so under the authority of obstetricians in hospitals. Their job has been divided up into its component parts and, increasingly, de-skilled. Many student midwives complete their training without learning how to deliver without tearing the perineum. They learn instead to cut the perineum and then wait for a doctor to come and sew it up. They are, as one midwife put it, 'learning to help doctors cure ladies of pregnancy'.[40]

Many midwives are now fighting back against this fragmentation of their job and erosion of their independence. The Association of Radical Midwives (ARM, see Resources) has put forward a plan, 'The Vision', for reorganizing the work of a midwife. It suggests that the majority of midwives should be divided into groups of between two and six and moved out of the hospitals into community practices. Here they would be able to provide ante- and post-natal care to the 85 per cent of women who have uncomplicated pregnancies, delivering their babies either in hospital or at home and getting to know the women they care for. Women would see an obstetrician only if the midwife diagnosed a problem which required further help. Those with complicated pregnancies (or those who prefer to see a consultant) would still go direct to a hospital, where midwives would also be divided into teams providing care but in closer relationship with the consultant. Caroline Flint, one of the authors of the document, explained:

> Midwives provide ante-natal, delivery and postnatal care to most women but they are giving it to strangers. The idea of our plan is that women should be looked after by people they know. The relationship between midwife and woman is fundamental but you cannot build up a relationship without meeting someone.

Over the next ten years the ARM hopes to get health authorities to adopt the plan. We can help them by making our wishes for sensitive maternity care known to directors of midwifery, unit general managers, maternity liaison committees and anyone else who will listen.

Doctors

One of the things which has worried me in speaking to medical students in various parts of the country is that a number of them have come up to me afterwards and said: 'We are very worried. We do not like what is happening to us as people during the course of our medical training; because of the pressures, because of the things we are expected to do, we feel ourselves turning into the kind of people we do not actually want to be. We can see what is happening to us but we feel we are powerless to prevent it. Certain ways of behaving are expected of us. Doing certain things is expected of us. We do not all think it is right but we have to get good reports. Sometimes we feel that our own values are being undermined.'[41]

Glaringly absent from medical training are most of the values, concerns and skills often thought of as 'feminine': nurturance, empathy, caring, sensitive listening, encouraging others to take care of themselves, collaboration rather than competition. The medical hierarchy relegates these values and skills to the domain of nurses, other helpers and (female) family members of the patients – doctors have 'more important' things to attend to. Patients deprived of these elements of caring may not be as quick to recover, may miss absorbing important information about after-care or preventive care and may end up feeling depressed about their experience because no one has paid attention to the emotional impact of their health problems. Similarly, vital

*SENs are being phased out, but it is probable that, if a new nurses' support grade is evolved, the same problems will emerge.

knowledge needed for optimum patient care – how to evaluate studies and risks accurately, how to recognize a patient's rights and identify the ethical issues involved in medical decisions, what patients could do for themselves to prevent illness – is either absent altogether or seen as peripheral to *real* learning. Most students get the message: this material is not important.

The oppressive view of women outlined earlier in this chapter is reflected both in the way medical education is carried out and in the content of what is taught. In lectures and seminars women can be treated by teachers as objects of ridicule, as a means to entertain male students. Feminist students frequently report the use of educationally irrelevant but sexually titillating slides, as well as the general denigration of women. Recent examples include menopausal women being referred to as 'prunes' and the removal of the ovaries being said to produce an immediate improvement in driving skills. For many medical students, stereotyped ideas of this kind about women's inferiority may be an extension of beliefs which they (and most of their friends) have held to a greater or lesser extent all their lives. As a result, they can be easily absorbed to form the basis for their future professional practice.

Many women students keep silent, deciding to concentrate first on performing well:

I felt as a medical student you played by the rules of the game, otherwise you weren't going to keep moving.

Later, they plan to use their authority to challenge and perhaps change the distressing practices they saw as students. Unfortunately, medical training cuts so deeply into one's prior values that many women may well lose their desire to work for change. Others have no such desire.

Medical education is also extremely high pressure. Students have first to absorb enormous quantities of information. Junior doctor posts are gruelling, low paid, and often demand thirty-six-hour shifts and 100-hour weeks – conditions which are a danger to both doctor and patient and which effectively cut doctors off from everyday life. No wonder they emerge with little understanding of the emotional needs of their patients. This exhausting routine, originally set up for men who have women at home to take care of them, allows no flexibility for other commitments like family or sick relatives. Many women are unprepared for the deep isolation of the final years of training. They postpone having children or forgo motherhood entirely. Those who are mothers find it enormously stressful to combine childbearing and/or marriage with medical training. Part-time hospital jobs are few.

An equally challenging dilemma for many women is the effort to conform to male styles of emotional detachment. As Jean Baker Miller reports, most women carry with them the socialization to be highly sensitive to others.[42] However, the very qualities medical reformers claim they are seeking in students – sensitivity, empathy, honesty, humility – are instantly suspect if displayed by women, as signs of their possible clinical or intellectual incompetence. This tremendous resource that women bring to medical schools is being smothered by their training.

The emotional cost of medical training for most women is tremendous, more so than for most (white) men, because of discrimination, lack of support and intensity of outside demands. With these stresses added to the already dehumanizing training, many women emerge from the process expecting prestige and position just as men do. What's more, many are eager to prove that they can be as good as any male physician according to the male-centred criteria of the profession: clinical competence, emotional detachment and financial success. Since they have not chosen to question the underlying medical ideology, they are virtually indistinguishable from their male counterparts.

It is a mistake, therefore, to assume that women doctors are the answer to the inadequacies of the medical system. In fact, the public and the medical community have quickly elevated women doctors to the status of 'experts' on the feelings, experiences and health needs of all women. In health books, talk shows, conferences and magazines, female doctors are becoming the voices of women. Yet there are also women doctors who have survived the training, kept alive their warmth and compassion and remember what it's like to be a woman patient. They can make a great difference.

Some, like obstetrician gynaecologist Wendy Savage, suffer daily from the effort to put patients first. But for her own determination and the determination of women's groups who organized a campaign to defend her, Wendy Savage would certainly have been sacked by her health authority under pressure from her male colleagues who objected to her 'low-tech' approach to obstetrics (for her book about her fight, see Resources). The values of the 'old wives' can be brought into modern medicine but only if women in the community provide the support and protection which will allow these values to take root again.

SUPPORT ORGANIZATIONS FOR HEALTH-CARE WORKERS*

Organizations for Carers

Carers need practical help from domiciliary paramedical and nursing services in the community. Unfortunately, all these services are under strain from funding cuts. Nevertheless, we have a right to these services. Our social worker, health visitor and GP can all give us advice and assistance in getting the help we need.

We also need support for ourselves. Many organizations, such as the Carers' National Association, the Alzheimer's Disease Society, Age Concern and Mind, have established local groups to provide a place to go and renew our strength through sharing our worries with others; a lobbying group to put pressure on local health and social services; a self-help group to share tips on coping.

*See Resources for addresses.

CHALLENGING MEDICAL ATTITUDES

The students come to the session in the second week of obstetrics. This group of three, all men, arrive late. They are defensive, wary. When Penny asks them to imagine how it feels to be a mother, waiting in the ante-natal clinic, there is an embarrassed silence. Finally one student says, 'Most are just browned-off with waiting. They don't think at all about their pregnancy.'

Penny asks whether waiting time at the clinic could or should be reduced. Doctors often arrive late for it. The students deny this. One says defensively, 'We zip through the patients as fast as we can.' Penny asks whether that's a good thing. The students say that there's no choice; that women should discuss worries with their GPs and anyway a doctor's time is more important than a patient's.

He says that the monitor around his (narrow) stomach was uncomfortably tight, that he was confused by having so many people around the bed and passing through the room, and that people were pushing and shoving him so much that he became dizzy. The bed seemed too narrow and the pillow which should have supported him kept slipping down the rubber sheet.

The students agree that the room is bare, sterile, inhospitable and badly arranged so that those entering the room look directly at the baby being delivered. But, as the minutes pass, their empathy with the patient evaporates. The 'mother' ends up arguing that making the room more comfortable with carpets and cushions would be too unhygienic. There is criticism of patients, especially of those

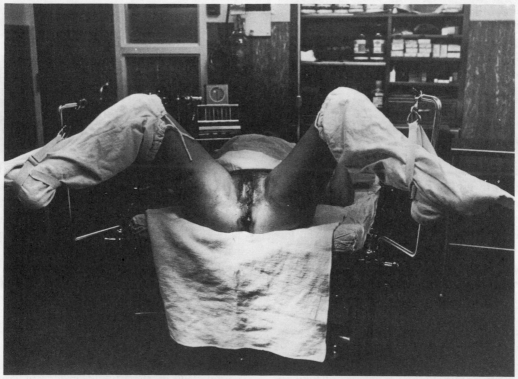

The obstetrician–gynaecologist's view of a woman

Penny announces that we are going to the labour ward for role-playing and there is a general groan. She is told that pretending to be a woman in labour is artificial and that students who have done it in the past have got nothing out of it. Ignoring this, Penny assigns one boy the role of mother, one becomes the father, one a midwife. The real midwife plays the part of doctor. As the 'mother' is hooked up to the monitor (a belt round 'her' stomach which measures the baby's heartbeats) the students begin to be caught up in their parts, despite themselves.

After twenty minutes the 'baby' has been delivered. The 'mother' is shaken by the experience.

who protest when unsupervised students are sent to sew them up after the birth. One student complains that the women who ask to give birth without drips and monitors can't explain why they want them off. Penny asks, 'Why do you want them on?' There is silence.

As the students leave, Penny asks them to make a contract with themselves – to do something, however small, to improve their patients' experience of giving birth. This group, unusually, has been resistant to new ideas, but Penny hopes that this at least is an appeal they will heed.

*An account of an obstetric training session with Penny Wallace of Hackney CHC Women's Health Group.

Organizations such as Age Concern are also setting up projects, using government funds, to provide respite care so that carers can get out regularly. As with many of these projects, they are set up more to massage the unemployment figures than to provide a real service. The personnel may be on the books only for a year, so their experience and usefulness will vary.

Organizations for Women Health Workers

Support and campaigning groups. Feminist nurses, midwives, health visitors and doctors have started to get together through setting up their own networks and conferences. *The Association of Radical Midwives* (ARM) was the first and has also had the highest profile. Its conferences attract midwives right across the spectrum and it has among its members many older midwives who see it as a welcome voice supporting the kind of professional, independent practice they remember from the early days of their careers. It is dedicated to fighting for an independent midwifery profession working alongside women to provide a sympathetic and supportive service before, during and after the birth.

Women in Medicine was established mainly as a forum for women medical students (though there were qualified women doctors involved). After much debate it has decided to open up to women alternative practitioners as well. WIM is concerned to campaign for changes in the organization of medical training and working patterns on the grounds that 'the present organization of the NHS does not meet the needs of women whether patients or professionals'.

Black Health Workers and Patients Group is made up of black people who have worked in the health service or have experienced its deficiencies as patients. Its primary concern is how racism adversely affects the working of the health service.

Trade Unions. There are a number of different unions organizing in the health service. They negotiate pay, help resolve disputes over working practices and provide a means by which the least powerful members of the service can combine together to protect their own interests and the interests of the people they care for. In recent years hospital cleaners, organizing through the *National Union of Public Employees* (NUPE), have begun raising issues about hospital hygiene and its relationship to their working conditions (Organizing for Change, p. 648). Nurses, increasingly, have seen the importance of belonging to a TUC-affiliated union rather than just the traditional professional bodies, and the *Confederation of Health Service Unions* (COHSE) has been involved in helping organize midwives against the increasing centralization of the maternity services and the fragmentation of their work. The *Medical Practitioners Union* (MPU), a branch of MSF, is the TUC-affiliated union for doctors.

The British Medical Association (BMA) is the best known of the organizations representing doctors. It seeks to represent the voice of medicine but it is mainly concerned with protecting the interests of its own members. Although it functions as a trade union, it is conservative in approach and has consistently backed private practice at the expense of the NHS. Since the government-induced cash crisis in the NHS, the BMA has shifted its ground. However, while it bewails the current attacks on the NHS it will inevitably collude with the privatization plans as long as they don't threaten their status and power.

Professional Bodies. Every branch of the medical profession has its own professional body, known as a *Royal College*, which organizes examinations to control the quality of practice. Nurses and midwives also have a Royal College, which seeks to act on behalf of their members rather like trade unions.

The Medical Women's Federation is regarded as the official voice of women doctors. However, it has represented a view of women as marginal to medicine and, in campaigning for special part-time posts (rather than attacking the absurd working hours of doctors in general), it in no way challenges the male monopoly of medicine.

SURVIVING THE SYSTEM: CHOOSING AND USING THE MEDICAL SYSTEM

To have some control over our lives and to be informed participants in our health and medical care, we need information about our bodies and about the care-giving system. Knowledge gives us the ability to make choices, and some of the control we desire.

Often when we visit doctors what we really come for is solid, factual information, not medical attention. When we have appropriate factual information and even a little skill or a few tools, or can get access to them quickly, we are in a much better position to cope with minor emergencies and to decide whether or not we really need to spend the time on a medical visit. Some illnesses can have serious complications, so we should be aware of the symptoms and get them treated early. Others are self-limiting and will get better without treatment. Many simple infections and even more complex ones like sexually transmitted diseases are to some extent preventable.

Today there is much more health and medical information available than there was ten years ago, some of it trustworthy, some of it not; this section offers guidance in selecting the most reliable sources. It is crucial for our health that we get information from sources which are both *reliable* and *independent* – that is, sources able to evaluate the material from technical, user *and* feminist perspectives.

LIVING WITH UNCERTAINTY

In giving up our unquestioning trust of the information we get from doctors and other medical personnel, we also give

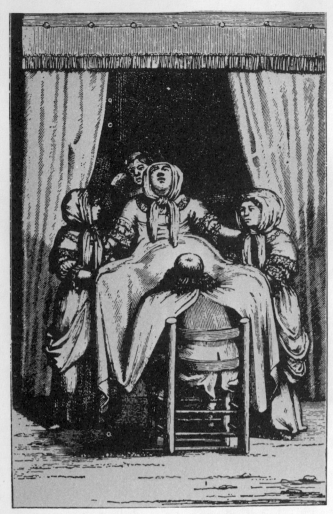

Doctor delivering under sheet, for modesty's sake

up the (often false) comfort that comes from their frequent reassurances that we are getting 'the best treatment possible'. Often we and our health practitioners have to make decisions without complete information, because no one, not even the 'experts', knows enough yet about certain problems to suggest that one approach is necessarily better than another. Yet physicians often believe that they have to act *sure* even when they are not. Especially when we are scared, it can be deeply reassuring to believe them. Learning about the controversies and alternatives rather than blindly trusting what our doctors tell us, therefore, may mean living without the particular kind of certainty or hope that they offer. Often what we need most is courage in the face of uncertainty.

WHERE TO FIND (AND NOT TO FIND) THE INFORMATION WE NEED

Ourselves

We know a lot about our bodies; we must listen to and trust what our bodies are telling us. Our awareness of change in ourselves or our children is the first and most important indicator of sickness. Most of what doctors learn about us we tell them. We learn much from the women in our lives: our mothers, sisters, aunts, grandmothers and friends.

Reading

Reading is important, but we must make sure that our sources are as accurate as possible. Magazines and newspapers, a common resource, have their problems (see opposite). Consumers can also look at *British National Formulary* or MIMS in local libraries to find out what the drug industry says about the drugs it manufactures. *Be sure to see consumer guides to drugs as well* (see Resources). Beware particularly of booklets and brochures that have

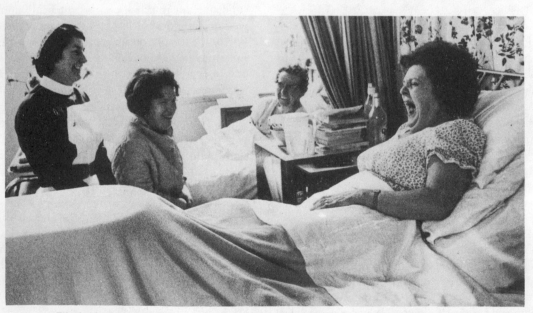

Elizabeth Garrett Anderson hospital, the only hospital in the UK run for and by women – saved from closure after a long campaign

been prepared by drug companies, and any publications that tend to downgrade non-medical or non-pharmacological approaches, and are slow to present innovative alternatives or prevention orientations.

The Media

These days the media carry more women's health and medical information than ever before. A few women's magazine articles and TV shows are excellent, well researched and responsible in their outlook. Most often, however, a 'medical expert' (usually a doctor) presents only the medical point of view, with no consumer representation. Reporters, awed by medical 'expertise', may spread inaccuracies by quoting as fact what are actually the doctor's opinions, or assuming the doctor is always up to date in her or his information. And the media cater to the human fascination with drama, highlighting the spectacular 'cures' and treatments, the most daring surgery, the most expensive and highly technical procedures. Media coverage usually perpetuates the mistaken assumption that medicine and spectacular medical technology create good health. Look for presentations that focus on what *you* can do. Remember that experts often disagree.

Self-help Groups

These are one of the most important sources of both courage and information. Different from medically-run support groups, these small informal groups of women meet to help each other learn about birth control, fertility awareness, menopause, breast cancer, cervical self-examination and many other topics.

Such groups are organized in ways which reflect values important to us. They are non-hierarchical; every member plays an equal part. Information is free. Implicit in these groups is the belief that we *can* understand medical information, that it 'belongs' rightfully to us. Group members' experiences are an important source of information about health, illness and treatment. By comparing notes and trading stories with other women, we learn best how to use the information we get from both medical and non-medical sources. Independent of medical-care institutions and professionals, these groups are not hampered in exploring non-medical therapies and practitioners, or in questioning, challenging and evaluating accepted ones.

When groups focus on one specific issue, they are often better able than many physicians to keep abreast of the most current research. Some groups already exist (see Resources in Chapter 28). We have to initiate others as the need arises. When you find one or two other women who want to get together, that is a good beginning.

Support Groups

These are growing up around many health issues and illnesses such as smoking, surviving MS, or discussing pregnancy and labour. Many of the groups which are initiated by doctors or health centres are very medically orientated and, though they may provide comfort and companionship, they are not usually designed to share

ideas about alternative treatments or to question medical opinions.

HEALTH INFORMATION RESOURCES*

The Women's Health and Reproductive Rights Information Centre (WHRRIC)

WHRRIC is the only national, independent, feminist health information centre. It sends out a regular newsletter and produces information leaflets on various aspects of health and reproductive rights. It also has a library of health material with a particular emphasis on non-medical treatments. The centre does not have the resources to deal with individual clinical advice or counselling, nor does it keep lists of clinics or practitioners. However, it does have a comprehensive listing of self-help groups. You can subscribe as an individual or as a group.

The College of Health

This is a consumer lobby in the health-care field. It produces regular bulletins and health information through publications and a tape-recorded 'Healthline'. It tries not to be too dominated by the medical model and focuses on helping the individual get the best from the system.

Health Education Departments

While many of these are medically- and establishment-orientated in the information they provide, some are very committed to providing a consumer-orientated service. It is worthwhile putting consumer pressure on all HEDs, as increasing lip-service is being paid to the importance of 'the community'. HEDs can be found in your telephone book under the name of your District Health Authority.**

Community Health Workers

They are employed in some urban areas, often by health education units, to work with the local community. They often initiate and facilitate self-help groups around specific health issues as well as general women's health groups. They are usually based in community centres and may have resources such as a 'health bus'. The information can be of very good quality, derived from individual experiences, with an emphasis on sharing information and advice. Groups set up by these health workers are usually encouraged to be questioning and challenge the assumptions of the medical system.

Community Health Councils

These are statutory bodies representing consumers (see p. 642). Some CHCs produce their own health education material. It varies in quality but there have been some

---

*See Resources for addresses.
**They should not be confused with the Health Education Authority (previously the Health Education Council) which is under the direct control of the Department of Health. The HEA provides HEDs with a certain amount of literature, which is of varying quality and understanding. In some areas the departments are called Health Promotion Departments.

excellent guides to local health resources and health issues such as *Having a Baby in Hackney* and *The Ricketts Report.* *

Health Visitors

Health visitors visit all new mothers from ten days after the birth and have a responsibility for children until they are five years old. They also have responsibility for elderly people. Although they are trained as nurses (with an extra year's specialist training) they rarely do any practical nursing. Their role is to support and advise and to put people in touch with other agencies where necessary. Health visitors who make real use of their access to women to listen and learn can provide a really valuable support service. The quality of the information they provide is extremely variable.

GETTING MEDICAL CARE IN THE NATIONAL HEALTH SERVICE**

Everyone who is resident in the United Kingdom for more than six months is entitled to free medical care. People from Common Market countries and countries with which the UK has a 'reciprocal agreement' are also entitled to free health care. However, visitors from countries not covered by agreements are now expected to pay as a private patient for any health-care services other than emergency treatment. Some hospitals have taken to demanding passports from any sick person who does not look 'English'. Black people have been particularly discriminated against and those whose immigration status is in any doubt will, of course, be deterred from seeking the health care they need.

General Practitioners

Everyone who is resident in the United Kingdom is entitled to be registered with a general practitioner (GP). Your GP (or family doctor) is usually the only health worker who has – in theory at least – an idea of you as a whole person. This then can be a very valuable relationship. A good GP should be able to help you make links between your mind, your environment and your body, treat minor illness, make the preliminary diagnosis for more serious problems, refer you for specialist help when necessary and help you to follow treatment. The non-specialist nature of this work is extremely valuable in a medical world in which bodies are increasingly fragmented into different 'specialities'. So establishing a relationship with a careful and caring GP can make the difference between good and indifferent medical care.

Probably the best way to find a good doctor is by word of mouth. Talk to neighbours and friends in the area. If that doesn't yield results, all GPs are listed in the Family Practitioner Committee (FPC) Medical List, which you can see at your local reference library or Community Health Council (see p. 642). Lists vary in the amount of information given but they will say if a doctor offers contraception or maternity services. If you want to find out more, you can select GPs living close to you and then look them up in the *Medical Directory*, which should be available at your reference library. This directory lists doctors in alphabetical order with information about their qualifications, research experience, and the year in which they qualified.

Questions to ask about GPs

- Is it a single or group practice? Single-handed GPs may provide a very personal service but they are more likely to use locum services to cover at nights and in holidays (you may be faced by a complete stranger when you most need a friend) and have fewer resources to call on in terms of midwives, community nurses, etcetera.
- Is it in a health centre? Both single-handed and group practices may work out of a health centre. This gives them access to a wide range of community resources such as ante-natal and child health clinics, dentists and community psychologists. You will find your health needs are more likely to be met under one roof here.
- Is there an appointment system? Some doctors still expect patients to turn up and wait in a queue; a system which further reinforces the inequality between the doctor (whose time is very precious) and you (whose time is limitless). The best practices combine an appointment system with an open system so that people can wait for a gap if they prefer to.

Questions to ask the receptionist/doctor

- If it's a group practice, can I choose a particular doctor?
- Are there any surgeries after working hours?
- Do doctors cover for each other? Is a locum service used?
- How far in advance do I have to make appointments?
- What arrangements are made for emergencies?
- Do they take private patients? (If so, you may hesitate to register with someone who provides a dual standard of care.)

Try to arrange to visit the doctor before you register (see below). It is better to get an idea of whether you will get on before you are already tied to one another. If you decide to register first, it is worth visiting when you are well, just so that you can discuss your medical history and establish contact. At this visit you might like to test out the doctor's attitude to such things as abortion or prescribing contraceptives to teenagers and try to find out whether s/he particularly likes/dislikes working with children or old people. Parents of young children often find doctors with children particularly helpful.

Registering. If you were born in the UK you will have been registered at birth with your family doctor. If you have lost your medical card you can write to your Family Practitioner Committee with your name, address, date of birth and the name and address of your last doctor, and they will issue a new one. If you have recently taken up residence in the UK you can approach the GP of your

---

*From Hackney and Haringey CHC respectively.

**For alternative and complementary medical care, see p. 83.

choice. If there is room on his/her list you should be given the necessary forms for registration.

If you move to a new area, ask your new doctor to fill in Part A of your medical card. This will then be returned to the Family Practitioner Committee which will then issue a new card. If you want to change to another doctor for any other reason, you are supposed to get your doctor to sign Part B of the card. However, you can just send the card back to the FPC saying you want to leave your doctor's list and they will send a new one. GPs have the right to refuse to accept you and don't have to say why. In some areas they are very reluctant to take on someone who has left her GP after a disagreement. This professional 'solidarity' may be used against women who are assertive about their own health care and it can be particularly difficult for women in areas where there are few doctors to choose from. However, the FPC is responsible for finding someone who will accept you, though it may not be the doctor you choose.

Questions to ask the doctor
- Go through the list of questions above if this is your first appointment.
- For subsequent appointments, make a list of *all* symptoms whether they appear to be related or not. Say what, if anything, you have done already. Don't allow yourself to be dismissed, or any conclusions to be drawn, until you've got through the list. Don't feel guilty about the others in the waiting-room. One thorough discussion at this stage may cut out future ones. It might help you to write down symptoms as they appear. It isn't always easy to remember when a pain or discharge, etc. actually started.
- If you are given a prescription, ask whether it will cure the condition or merely help symptoms, what it is, how to use it, and how long to take it for. Ask also whether to expect any side-effects. If you are unhappy about taking it, ask whether your condition can be managed any other way. Doctors can instruct the chemist to leave the label and instructions in the pack by ticking a box on the prescription form with the letters NP in it. They should be encouraged to do so.
- If you don't understand what your doctor is saying, never be ashamed to ask her/him to repeat it more slowly and simply.
- If you are worried or anxious you may forget what a doctor has said, take a notepad with you and write it down.
- If you don't feel confident, you might like to have someone with you to ask the questions you feel too confused to ask.

OTHER PRIMARY HEALTH-CARE WORKERS

Most primary health-care workers can be contacted directly if you need their services, though very often it will be your GP who arranges your first contact.

Midwives are trained to take full responsibility for women throughout a normal pregnancy, birth and for ten days thereafter. You are most likely to contact midwives through your GP, ante-natal clinic or at the hospital. However, if you want a home birth and either have difficulty finding a GP to 'cover' or would rather avoid it, you have the right to contact the Director of Midwifery and ask for a midwife to be assigned to you. It is likely that the Director of Midwifery would try to resist your request (see p. 354) but, if you insist, a midwife (or midwives) must be made available.

Practice nurses are employed by GPs to provide nursing services in the practice. Their jobs vary widely and so does their pay. Some are expected simply to do clerical work and take blood occasionally; others may run a well woman clinic, taking cervical smears, fitting IUDs and running support groups. There is no standard training; indeed some are known to be carrying out work far beyond the limits of their training. The nursing organizations are keen to see practice nurses employed direct by health authorities and given a standard training and standard terms of reference – a move which is opposed by doctors who prefer to control their work.

Nurse practitioners: this job could provide a whole new field of work for nurses who are keen to extend their role. According to a Marplan poll carried out for the Cumberledge Committee looking into nursing in primary care, the majority of people would like to have direct access to nurses to discuss minor medical matters and such things as pre-menstrual tension and depression. Some practices have already pioneered nurse-run clinics and have taken up the challenge of providing both adequate training and responsibility for nurses who wish to combine clinical and managerial work in the community. Once again, GPs are keen to retain control over these nurses and to pay them locally negotiated wages while claiming extra allowances for the work they do. The nursing organizations would prefer to see nurses employed by the health authority and working alongside doctors in a team.

Health visitors care for babies, young children and the elderly in the community. You can contact a health visitor direct through your local health centre (or your GP can give you the number). The health visitor's role is more social than medical but she can give advice on basic nursing matters and local facilities.

District nurses. They can also be contacted direct either at your health centre or via the nursing office of the health authority. The district nurse provides practical nursing services in your home. Most district nurses are over-stretched and visits may be limited to basic help such as turning a bed-bound invalid, helping with bathing, changing dressings, etc.

Chiropodists specialize in foot problems. If you are over sixty, under sixteen, handicapped or pregnant, you can go direct to a chiropodist. Otherwise you can be referred by a GP if necessary. Chiropodists usually work from health centres or special surgeries in hospitals. Find one in the Yellow Pages, via the health authority or your GP. If you are housebound you can be visited at home.

Community psychiatric nurses and psychologists are discussed in Chapter 8.

Clinics

Well woman clinics provide widely differing services. In some areas women have campaigned successfully for clinics which provide screening for a very wide range of problems including cervical smears, blood pressure and urine tests and breast self-examination. These clinics may provide counselling sessions and organize menopause or PMS support groups. Some of them provide health-care questionnaires to be filled in at the first visit to provide a baseline for discussion – a real whole person check-up. However, these comprehensive clinics are few and far between. In most cases a well woman clinic provides only cervical smear testing with possibly a blood pressure test thrown in. The clinics are allowed only to screen people; they cannot provide medication. You will almost always be referred back to your GP if a problem is discovered.

Well women centres are usually managed outside the NHS though often with some NHS funding. Usually established by local women's groups, they offer women-oriented information and support and are usually very encouraging to self-help groups.

Well baby clinics provide regular check-ups for all children up to the age of five. They will not treat sick children (they are referred back to their own doctors) but will provide routine inoculations and developmental tests provided by doctors and health visitors. You should be automatically referred to one when your baby's birth is registered.

Genito-urinary clinics (GU or VD clinics) are listed in the telephone book under VD. You do not have to be referred by a doctor (see p. 489).

Family Planning Clinics are also listed in the phone book (see p. 275).

Hospital Doctors

Consultants are doctors who have specialized in a particular branch of medicine and are in charge of a team of medical personnel. They have a great deal of power within the health service as they are answerable only to their employing authority. A consultant's team, or 'firm', usually includes *house officers*, who have just completed their training, *senior house officers*, who are non-specialist hospital doctors; *registrars*, who are specializing in this particular field; and *senior registrars*, who are often very experienced specialists waiting for a consultant position to become vacant. In a teaching hospital there will also be a group of students who will follow the consultant on his or her rounds. Often consultants treat their rounds simply as a part of their teaching and treat you, the patient, as though you were a rubber doll. If the consultant discusses your 'case' over your head without explaining what is going on, you can object. If you would rather not be used as teaching material, you can refuse altogether.

You cannot see a consultant unless you are referred by your GP. It is worth doing a bit of research first (talking to friends) and discussing various forms of possible treatment with your GP. (Unfortunately there is no feminist source of reference about doctors.) You can then ask for referral to a particular consultant. Changes in the organization of the health service could restrict this freedom. District Health Authorities will want the majority of people to attend hospitals with which the Authority has contracts rather than those chosen by the patients. Your GP can refuse but is not likely to.

Even if you have been referred you may not actually see the consultant of your choice. The NHS does not give you that right. You may end up being seen by a registrar but, as consultants usually choose their own registrars and run their departments according to their own medical philosophy, you will probably get the same kind of treatment. In fact, the registrar may be more approachable and easier to talk to, and a senior registrar may give you better medical care than the consultant.

Your GP is, officially, at the same level in the hierarchy as a consultant. This should mean that your own doctor can work as your advocate and interpreter if you don't understand what has been said or are unclear about the course of treatment. It is always useful to go back to your GP after a hospital appointment to 'de-brief' and make sure that you have fully understood what is going to happen. Unfortunately, many GPs are rather in awe of consultants and are loath to risk offending someone to whom they often refer patients. Once again the solidarity of the medical profession may prove stronger than the GP's sense of responsibility to his or her patient.

Other Hospital Services

These are provided by a whole range of specialists including *physiotherapists, speech therapists, dieticians,* and *occupational therapists.* If you think that one of these people can help you, ask your GP or consultant for a referral. In addition you can ask to see a hospital social worker, who is employed by social services but is based in the hospital.

Community Social Services

Social service departments have a duty to work with the health service and many of the community services which have a direct bearing on health.

Home helps work mainly with elderly people. They are extremely low paid but provide a valuable service, making it possible for many elderly and infirm people to live in their own homes. Their tasks cover cleaning, shopping and generally providing friendly support. A letter from your doctor or health visitor may be necessary in order to get a home help.

Day-centres for elderly and handicapped people provide companionship (not care) during the day. Transport can usually be arranged from your home.

Local authority day nurseries are primarily a service for parents and children living in particularly difficult circumstances. The provision is extremely varied throughout the country and nowhere is it sufficient. Your health visitor may be able to help you get a place.

Voluntary or Charitable Organizations

In some areas where the NHS has been particularly under-funded, voluntary and charitable institutions are still

ALLIED HEALTH WORKERS

Physical and *occupational therapists, nutritionists* and *other allied health workers* have such a low position in the medical care hierarchy in terms of pay and control that the public usually sees them as less skilled or valuable than doctors. Yet each is a profession separate from medicine, setting its own standards and training its own workers in distinct and vital skills. These workers can help us make the daily changes often necessary for a real cure or for preventing illness. Their techniques *can* speed healing, help us live with physical limitations and

ease the helplessness, loneliness and fear that often come with sickness. Yet they can rarely fully use their knowledge and skills. The system is set up so that patients do not have easy access to them, and often don't know their services exist unless their doctor tells them. We must learn more about what they do. Remember to ask to see some of these workers if you think they might be at all helpful to you.

making an important contribution. *Hospices* (see p. 587) provide high-quality care for people who are dying, they are mainly funded by public money and provide care for free; Marie Curie nurses are provided free by **Marie Curie Cancer Care Foundation** to care for people who are terminally ill with cancer at home. **Pregnancy Advisory Services** give help to women seeking abortion or artificial insemination.

With the growth of private practice and the desire of private companies to be seen as charitable, it is worth checking out the charitable status of organizations (particularly in the 'pregnancy advice' field) because some organizations that call themselves non-profit-making are simply private companies. All charities have an official number, given to them by the Charity Commissioners. It should be clearly visible on their literature.

OUR RIGHTS

We have few rights over our own bodies. We have the right to refuse treatment, to refuse to be used as teaching material and to be treated competently (as defined by doctors). We have the right to *ask* for a second opinion but our GP or consultant need not refer us if he or she deems it unnecessary. A Charter of Patients' Rights is currently under discussion in the EEC (see box p. 633) which could improve the position. However, it cannot become binding on member countries unless all member states agree to it. So far Britain has not.

INFORMED CONSENT AND THE LAW

The right to refuse treatment is meaningless if it does not also carry the right to information: if we do not fully understand the implications of treatment and we do not know whether we are in a trial, we have nothing on which to base a judgement about accepting or refusing. However, we have no absolute right to *informed* consent as it is defined in, for example, the USA and Canada. Legally a doctor is not supposed to touch us without consent

(otherwise there is the possibility that we could sue for assault). However, in most instances we are deemed to be giving *implied* consent to treatment just by walking into the doctor's surgery. The doctor has no absolute duty to inform us of the exact nature and risks of the treatment. Nor will he or she necessarily have to tell us if the treatment is part of a trial or not. Our consent will almost certainly be presumed unless we have expressly withheld it and, even then, doctors are well protected by the common assumption that they simply know better what is in our interests.

Only surgical treatment requires *express* consent by way of a signature on a *consent form.** The form usually ends with the words 'and follow', implying consent to any additional surgery deemed necessary for our welfare. In consenting to a form of treatment we do not necessarily have to know whether that is the standard treatment or a new one and we have the right to be informed *only of the risks which are reasonably probable, and serious in their consequences*. If a risk can be deemed 'improbable' by medical consensus, then the doctor who failed to inform us is legally protected, even if that problem actually occurs.

Things may be changing. The concept of *informed consent* does exist in common law, though it has only really been used in relation to property. For example, you have a right to know whether a house is scheduled for demolition before you buy it. Up until now common law has not been used to enforce the right to know whether you are dying in time to draw up a will. However, in a recent case which was taken to the House of Lords[43] the door was opened to the possibility of extending this definition of informed consent into the medical field. Future cases may well try this avenue and establish a right to informed consent in common law.

In the meantime, how do we protect ourselves? As Carolyn Faulder suggests, practice may start to change when doctors realize that we know what is going on:

---

*Consent may be waived in an emergency or if the patient is not considered capable of giving consent under the Mental Health Act, or in the case of certain specified, infectious diseases. In the case of someone under sixteen, the parent or guardian must give consent.

When you go into hospital don't be afraid to ask questions about your treatment, and whether you are being entered into a trial, and if so, exactly what the trial entails. If more people did this it would frighten doctors into thinking more positively about the whole issue of consent.[44]

In the meantime, never sign a consent form unless you are absolutely clear what you are consenting to; and if you are concerned about being included in a trial without your knowledge, insist on obtaining a straightforward answer on this question – preferably in writing – before signing the consent form. However, we have to face the fact that the information we need about new treatments and drugs depends largely on people consenting to Randomized Controlled Trials. This poses a dilemma between our personal desire for control and our belief that well-evaluated information is vital to the development of good medicine.

ACCESS TO RECORDS

The records which your doctor or midwife or other health worker writes are the property of the health authority. You have no right to see them (even as evidence in a case against your doctor), though many other people do: other doctors, social workers, health visitors, clerical workers – indeed, anyone whom your doctor feels has a legitimate interest in your health care. You need not be informed before this sharing of information takes place except in the case of reports written for insurance companies or employers. In these two cases only, you may see what your doctor has to say about you before the information is passed on, though doctors still have a limited right to withold information in some circumstances.

There are some radical practices which do allow people access to their notes, and pregnant women are sometimes asked to keep their notes. The evidence shows that they are less likely to get lost in our hands than in the hospital system, and the opportunity to read them at leisure increases the feeling of participation in treatment and the flow of information both ways.[45] Nevertheless, a BMA conference voted in 1986 to fight for an exemption for medical information from the Data Protection Act, which allows people access to computer records about themselves.

Doctors fear that if we can read their remarks it will either mean that they will no longer be free to speak their minds, or it will somehow damage vulnerable people. In fact, the information gathered by the Freedom of Information Campaign shows that, on the contrary, more people are more damaged by lack of access and inability to correct wrong information.

He [the specialist] seemed very angry when I asked whether and how any further treatment was indicated, and I can only suppose that his anger was based on the assumption that I was complaining, whereas the contrary was true. Since then I have moved twice within the area, but meet with nothing but hostility when I consult a doctor. I can only assume that something damning was written in the notes which have followed me from one health centre to another. The only clue I have as to what this may be came at my first encounter with one doctor who began by saying, 'I believe you don't like doctors' . . . The consequences . . . have been distressing to the point that, much as I hate to admit it, when I am ill I am terrified at the thought of consulting one.[46]

Elsewhere in the world, records have already been made accessible (including to people with mental health problems) with very good results:

We could identify no instance in which a patient was harmed by being offered his records. It seems likely that patients are better able to handle information than we usually assume.[47]

If doctors fear that people will be angry with them about the content of their medical notes then they should look to their consciences. If comments are justified then they should be open to challenge and, if necessary, alteration. If they are not justified then they shouldn't be there at all. Open notes may be a threat to the power of doctors; they are not a threat to the health of patients. The Freedom of Information Campaign wants all notes (not just computerized notes) to be open to patients (with some provisions for special cases). They feel that the tide among doctors is turning against secrecy.

ENFORCING OUR RIGHT TO COMPETENT TREATMENT

One way to safeguard your rights is to bring someone with you to medical encounters. It may be a friend, relative or women's health worker – anyone you trust enough to share confidential health information with and who will help you to be clear and assertive. Before your medical visit, discuss with this person what you expect – and what you *want* – to happen. Make sure you both understand what kinds of diagnostic tests, treatments or surgery are being proposed. Ask your friend to keep a record of events which occur while you are unable to be aware of them. Try to anticipate those situations which, in the past, made you feel powerless or inadequately informed. Make a list of the questions you want to ask. If there is more than one doctor involved in your case, your friend can help coordinate your care. If the medical staff raise questions about your emotional or psychiatric stability (and thereafter dismiss your concerns and complaints), your friend can speak up for you.

While some doctors do not mind the presence of a relative or friend during surgery visits or examinations, hospitals may be more restrictive. Be as firm as you can about wanting someone with you. If you have problems, contact your Community Health Council for support.

Patient advocates could be provided by Community Health Councils to act as 'friends' to those of us who need

RESOLUTION ON A EUROPEAN CHARTER ON THE RIGHTS OF PATIENTS

(a) the right to available treatment and care appropriate to the illness;

(b) the right to prompt treatment;

(c) the right to adequate social security cover to allow the rights set out in (a) to be exercised;

(d) the right to free choice of medical practitioner and health-care establishment;

(e) the right of access to hospital service within a reasonable travelling distance;

(f) the right to information concerning diagnosis, therapy and prognosis, the patient's right of access to his own medical data, and the patient's right to give his consent to or refuse the treatment proposed.

(g) the right to medical confidentiality, the only possible exceptions to which should be on a limited number of serious and well-defined grounds, having due regard for the integrity of the human person;

(h) the patient's right to lift the obligation of confidentiality completely or in part as regards his own medical records;

(i) the right to complaint based on 'damage to the interests of the patient';

(j) the right to an appeal procedure before the courts;

(k) the rights and duties of medical practitioners;

(l) the patient's right to be represented by independent associations and organizations;

(m) the definition of the legal status of the patient in a health-care establishment;

(n) the right to respect for private life and for religious and philosophical convictions;

(o) the right to a dignified death.

4. Considers that it may be necessary, in certain well-defined circumstances, to limit the rights of patients where they would involve a danger to public health.

5. Is of the opinion that the specific problems pertaining to the rights of the mentally ill and of children should not be dealt with in this context but in a special charter.

[Extract from RESOLUTION tabled by the European Parliament on 19 January 1984 and forwarded by the President to the Commission with the instruction to submit as soon as possible a European Charter on the Rights of Patients.]

support. In Hackney a patient advocacy service of this sort has been organized for non-English-speaking maternity patients. Similar schemes could be set up throughout the health service (see Chapter 28, p. 643).

COMPLAINTS PROCEDURES

If you are unhappy about the circumstances of your treatment – if, for example, you had to wait for seven hours for an ambulance, your GP refused to visit you at home (or send a locum) when requested, your midwife missed the birth of your baby or staff were unkind or careless in the treatment of a relative – you have a right to complain. However, if your complaint is about suspected negligence or a bad medical decision, this is considered to be a matter of 'clinical judgement'. This is dealt with on p. 634.

It is best to make your complaint in writing and to send a copy of the letter to your local Community Health Council. If you want help writing a letter, or information on where to send it, your CHC should be able to give both information and support. Not all CHCs are equally independent and some seem to see their role as NHS policemen keeping the public at bay. If you get this feeling from your local CHC secretary, you might do better to contact a Citizens Advice Bureau instead.

General Practitioner complaints should be sent to the Family Practitioner Committee* (to whom the GP is contracted) within six weeks of the incident. The GP will be contacted and given the opportunity to comment in writing. If the comments do not satisfy you and you wish to take the complaint further, the procedure may move to a hearing. If the FPC refuses a hearing, you have a right of appeal to the Secretary of State for Social Services. The GP may be warned, fined or have people removed from his/her practice list. Occasionally a reference may be made to an NHS tribunal, which has the right to dismiss him or her.

Midwives and nurses complaints. These should go to the district health authority or, if it is a matter of professional conduct, to the National Board for Nursing, Midwifery and Health Visiting (each region of the UK has its own board).

Hospital complaints. There is no single complaints system. You should ask, on admission, to see the leaflet setting out your hospital complaints procedure. If you have already left the hospital, it is usually best to write to the hospital administrator, unit general manager for the hospital or to the district general manager. A proper

*Primary Care Division of the Health Board in Scotland, and Central Services Committee in Northern Ireland.

investigation may be set up but you cannot count on this. Your complaint may seem to disappear without trace unless you or the CHC keep up the pressure.

Appeals against the investigation of any hospital, FPC or district health authority may be sent to the Health Service Commissioner, who can follow it up on your behalf.

Conduct, behaviour or ethical responsibility. If your doctor appears to be drunk, under the influence of drugs or has made sexual remarks or advances to you or another patient, complaints should be sent to the General Medical Council. The GMC also has the power to investigate a doctor itself, perhaps after a court case. The council wields the ultimate sanction: it can 'strike off' doctors from the medical register. However, it is more likely to use this power for sexual misconduct than for medical incompetence, and even then this is not something that is done readily. A warning or temporary ban is more likely. For the inside story on the GMC, see Jean Robinson's *A Patient View of the General Medical Council* (listed in Resources); you can use this book to pressure your MP for a change in the law so that the GMC might become more effective.

Clinical judgement cannot be dealt with through the standard hospital complaints system. The Health Service Commissioner is not able to intervene in such cases either. This is a major flaw in a very flawed complaints system and it means that doctors are virtually untouchable except through the law courts. Concern about this lack of accountability (from patient advocates) and the soaring cost of litigation and insurance against it (from doctors) has led to the development of an avenue for clinical complaints. It is rarely satisfactory and not often used. However, you can:

1. Write to the consultant asking for a meeting (or ask the ward sister to arrange it). Any other doctors involved should also attend. A written explanation should be sent to you.

2. If you are unsatisfied you may write to the Regional Medical Officer (RMO), who should discuss the matter and write back.

3. If you are still unsatisfied and can convince the RMO that you will not take legal action subsequently, two independent (so-called) consultants will be called in to review your case. You will not get any compensation but you *might* get the satisfaction of knowing that whatever happened to you won't happen again. However, in its first two years of operation, in spite of 13,373 recorded complaints, there were only 57 independent reviews.

USING THE LAW

Many people resort to legal action not so much for the money (which can be very useful if a medical accident has caused disability), but because it seems to be the only way to get satisfaction in the face of an unyielding system. However, the legal system is clumsy and costly. The effect of litigation, at least in America, has been a resort to greater medical intervention as doctors seek to protect themselves against possible future legal action. Doctors who seem to have taken every precaution in terms of tests and procedures are better protected in court than those who prefer to watch and wait, intervening only when clearly necessary.

This trend is certainly not in our interests and doctors have been quick to exploit the fear of litigation as an excuse for the increase in invasive procedures (see Caesareans, p. 394). Yet, in spite of endless discussion, no concrete plans for an alternative to legal action have yet been made. In New Zealand, for example, a system of 'no fault' compensation has been set up under which victims of medical accidents can claim compensation without needing to apportion blame. This system should release doctors from the fear of legal action and set up a climate of confidence in which they would feel able to discuss a case openly without insurance company lawyers breathing down their necks.

Until such a system is devised, and funded, the law may be the only avenue for dealing with clinical complaints. The Maternity Defence Fund (see Resources) (established by AIMS) is attempting to use the laws of assault to pressurize doctors into providing information rather than indulging in defensive intervention. They are collecting money to enable cases to be taken against doctors who fail to get *informed consent* before carrying out treatment, or who carry out treatment against the express wishes of women. If, for example, the administration of syntometrine during delivery (see p. 386), without consent, and in the absence of an emergency, can be proved to be a legal assault, the onus will be on doctors and midwives to explain fully all possible treatments and obtain consent for their use, prior to labour. While this could be reduced to a series of token 'consent forms', it could also open up the possibility of genuine partnership between women and their carers.

If you do decide to take legal action, it will be either over assault (described above) or negligence. To claim negligence there must be some obvious consequence of the negligence (the doctor operated on the wrong leg, for example) and the court will have to establish whether the doctor acted negligently. Other doctors will be called to give evidence of the action they would have taken in the circumstances. Only if the doctor clearly failed to act appropriately would negligence be proved. Only 30 to 40 per cent of cases are successful, partly because doctors tend to support one another and it is notoriously difficult to get a doctor to testify against a colleague. Most cases take four to five years to come to court. If you win, the level of damages will be decided by the judge. The doctor will not have to pay damages. All doctors are covered by medical insurance. Indeed, the doctor may simply return to do the same thing to someone else. Negligence is not considered by the General Medical Council to be grounds for action and the employing authority may not take action either.

Medical litigation is a complex field. You will need very good legal advice before you decide to proceed with a case and substantial funding to see it through. An inexperienced solicitor could well lose even a well-founded case. It is worth contacting the organizations listed below, who keep lists of solicitors specializing in this field. Action for the Victims of Medical Accidents also has a lawyers' support group so, if you prefer to use a solicitor you are familiar with, he or she can be helped to avoid the major pitfalls. You may be eligible for legal aid if you are on a low income. You should ask the solicitor or a Citizens Advice Bureau at the start.

There are two organizations offering advice to people contemplating legal action: **Action for the Victims of Medical Accidents** which offers free legal and medical advice and, crucially, has a panel of doctors who are willing to give independent medical opinions in court (in the past, accident victims have found it almost impossible to seek out doctors prepared to give evidence against their colleagues);

and the **National Association of Compensation Claimants,** which asks for a subscription and the return of money spent on your behalf if you are successful.

It may help also to make contact with your Community Health Council.

Within a socialized health system, recourse to the law should not be necessary in order to obtain either satisfaction or compensation. It is a measure of the power that doctors have been allowed that they can be approached only through complex and expensive legal procedures. They are as much a victim of the system as we are. In the next chapter we discuss ways in which accountability could be improved through the further democratization of our health service.

NOTES

1. A. Kinsey et al. *Sexual Behaviour in the Human Female*. New York: Simon and Schuster, 1953; W. H. Masters and V. E. Johnson. *Human Sexual Response*. Boston: Little, Brown, 1966.

2. N. Jeffcoate. *Principles of Gynaecology* (4th ed.). London: Butterworth, 1975, p. 568.

3. See Karen J. Armitage, Lawrence J. Schneiderman and Robert A. Bass. 'Response of Physicians to Medical Complaints in Men and Women', *Journal of the American Medical Association* (Brief Reports), vol. 241, no. 20, 18 May 1979, pp. 2186–7; Barbara Bernstein and Robert Kane. 'Physicians' Attitudes towards Female Patients', *Medical Care*, vol. 19, no. 6, June 1981, pp. 600–608.

4. Gena Corea. *The Hidden Malpractice: How American Medicine Mistreats Women* (new ed.). New York: Harper and Row, 1986, pp. 15–16; see also the discussion of the Pill in this book.

5. 'Legal Abortion, Family Planning Services; Largest Factors in Reducing Neonatal Mortality Rate', *Family Planning Perspectives*, vol. 13, no. 2, March/April, 1981.

6. Sir Douglas Black et al. *Inequalities in Health* (the Black Report). London: DHSS, 1980. Every attempt was made to suppress this report and only a few hundred copies were printed. However, a summary has now been published by Penguin; see Townsend and Davidson in Resources.

7. From GLC *report on Ethnic Minorities and the National Health Service in London*. London: GLC, 1985.

8. From Training in Health and Race, *Black Women and the Maternity Services* (available from National Extension College, 18 Brookland Avenue, Cambridge).

9. Male prisoners and volunteers are frequently used to test drugs. For nutrition research, see J. S. Garrow, *Energy Balance and Obesity in Man*. New York: Elsevier, and North Holland: Biomedical Press, 1978.

10. David H. Banta, Clyde J. Behney and Jane Sisk Wilkens. *Toward Rational Technology in Medicine*. New York: Springer, 1981.

11. Ann Oakley. *The Captured Womb*. Oxford: Basil Blackwell, 1985.

12. From Jill Rakusen and Nick Davidson. *Out of Our Hands*. London: Pan, 1982, p. 96.

13. 'Genetic Engineering Reprieve', *Journal of the American Medical Association*, vol. 220, no. 10, June 1972, p. 1355; quoted in 'Genetic Engineering. Evolution of a Technological Issue', US House of Representatives, 92 Congress, second session, 1972.

14. Rakusen and Davidson, op.cit., note 12.

15. For example, see Zola Irving. 'Medicine as an Institution of Social Control', in *Socio-Medical Inquiries - Recollections, Reflections, and Reconsiderations*. Philadelphia, PA: Temple University Press, 1983, p. 262ff.

16. People visiting their doctors for 'psychoemotional' problems form the third largest category of patients. See J. Fry. *Common Diseases* (3rd ed.). Cambridge MA: MIT Press, 1983, pp. 22–4, Table 1.4.

17. Bourne, Gordon. *Pregnancy*. London: Pan, 1975, p. 27.

18. See Janice Raymond. 'Medicine as a Patriarchal Religion', *Journal of Medicine and Philosophy*, vol. 7, 1982, pp. 197–216, for further explanation of this point.

19. Bourne, op. cit., note 17, p. 7.

20. For a thorough analysis of medicalization and iatrogenesis, see Ivan Illich. *Medical Nemesis: The Expropriation of Health*. London: Marion Boyars, 1975.

21. For more on this see Barbara Ehrenreich and Deirdre English. *For Her Own Good: 150 Years of the Experts' Advice to Women*. London: Pluto Press, 1979.

22. Mary Chamberlain. *Old Wives' Tales: Their History, Remedies and Spells*. London: Virago Press, 1981, p. 139.

23. Merlin Stone. *The Paradise Papers*. London: Virago Press/Quartet, 1976, p. 19.

24. Chamberlain, op. cit., note 22, p. 3.

25. Tom Richardson. *The Public and the Health Industry in the USA and Britain*. Oxfordshire CHC, 1980.

26. Federation of American Hospitals and Association of Investor-Owned Hospitals. *1983 Directory of Investor-owned Hospitals and Hospital Management Companies*. Little Rock, Ark. 1983.

27. Ben Griffith, Geoff Rayner and John Mohan. *Commercial Medicine in London*. GLC Industry and Employment Branch, 1985.

28. Letter to *Financial Times*, 25 February 1983, quoted in Griffith et al., op. cit., note 27.

29. For more about the drug industry and its international perspective, see Charles Medawar. *The Wrong Kind of Medicine*, London: Consumers' Association and Hodder and Stoughton, 1984; Charles Medawar. *Drugs and World Health*. London: Social Audit, 1984; and D. Melrose. *Bitter Pills: Medicine and the Third World*. Oxford: Oxfam, 1982.

30. Medawar, *The Wrong Kind of Medicine*, op. cit., note 29.

31. *Report of the Informal Working Group on Effective Prescribing* (the Greenfield Report). London: DHSS, 1982.

32. Quoted in F. Lesser. 'How We Keep Unsafe Drugs off the Market', *New Scientist*, 4 December 1980, pp. 634–5.

33. For more on this read Carolyn Faulder. *Whose Body is It Anyway? The Troubling Issues of Informed Consent*. London: Virago Press, 1985.

34. David Tuckett (ed.). *An Introduction to Medical Sociology*. London: Tavistock, 1979, p. 225.

35. Equal Opportunities Commission. *Who Cares for the Carers?* 1982, pp. 41–2.

36. Hilary Land. 'Who Cares for the Family?', *Journal of Social Policy*, vol. 7, no. 3, 1978.

37. Janet Finch and Dulcie Groves. 'Community Care and the Family: a

Case for Equal Opportunities?', *Journal of Social Policy*, vol. 9, no. 4, 1980.

38. Big Flame, Women's Struggle Notes, no. 6.

39. C. Hicks. 'Racism in Nursing', *Nursing Times*, 5 and 12 May 1982.

40. Quoted in Angela Phillips. 'Where Have all the Midwives Gone?', *Observer* Magazine, 8 July 1979.

41. Jean Robinson. *Journal of Medical Ethics*, no. 11, 1985, pp. 19–21.

42. Jean Baker Miller. *Toward a New Psychology of Women*. London: Penguin Books, 1978.

43. *Sidaway v. The Board of Governors of Bethlem Royal Hospital*, 1984.

44. Faulder, op. cit., note 33.

45. A. Lovell et al. *Why Not Give Mothers Their Own Notes? St Thomas's Maternity Case Note Study*. London: Cicely Northcote Trust, 1986.

46. M. Frankel and D. Wilson. 'I Want to Know What is in My File', Campaign for Freedom of Information, September 1985.

47. Goldetz et al. 'The Right to Know: Giving the Patient His Medical Record', *Archives of Physical Rehabilitation*, no. 57, 1976, pp. 78–81.

RESOURCES
PUBLICATIONS

Arditti, Rita et al. (eds). *Test Tube Women: What Future Motherhood?* London: Pandora Press, 1984. An international collection of feminist writings, mostly very critical of technological development.

Black Health Workers and Patients Group. *Black Health*. Bulletin of the BHWPG from 259a High Road, Tottenham, London N15.

Brent Community Health Council. *Black People and the Health Service*. Brent CHC, 1981.

Briggs, Anne and Judith **Oliver**. *Caring: Experiences of Looking After Disabled Relatives*. London: Routledge, 1985.

British National Formulary. London: BMA/The Pharmaceutical Press, 1988.

Cameron, Debbie et al. *Reproductive Wrongs – Male Power and the New Reproductive Technologies*. Leeds: FINRRAGE (Feminist International Network of Resistance to Reproductive and Genetic Engineering), 1984.

City and Hackney Community Health Council. *Multi Ethnic Women's Health Project, Health Advocacy for Non-English-speaking Women*. From City and Hackney CHC, 210 Kingsland Road, London E2 8EB.

College of Health. *Consumers Guide to Health Information*. London: College of Health, 1985.

College of Health. *Guide to Going into Hospital*. London: College of Health, 1985.

Consumers' Association/Patients' Association. *A Patient's Guide to the National Health Service*. London, 1983.

Corea, Gena. *The Mother Machine*. London: Women's Press, 1988. Takes a similar approach to reproductive technology as Arditti et al.

Cornwell, J. and P. **Gordon**. *An Experiment in Advocacy: the Hackney Multi-Ethnic Women's Health Project*. Published by City and Hackney CHC and the King's Fund Centre (126 Albert Street, London NW1 7NI), 1984.

Doyal, Lesley, with Imogen **Pennell**. *The Political Economy of Health*. London: Pluto Press, 1979.

Doyal, Lesley. *Unhealthy Lives, Being a Woman in London*. London: GLC Industry and Employment Branch, 1985. From Women's Studies Unit, The Polytechnic of North London.

Doyal, Lesley. 'Women, Health and the Sexual Division of Labour; a Case Study of the Women's Health Movement in Britain', *International Journal of Health Services*, vol. 13, no. 3, 1983.

Dreyfus, Claudia. *Seizing Our Bodies – the Politics of Women's Health*. New York: Vintage Books, 1977.

Ehrenreich, Barbara and Deirdre **English**. *For Her Own Good: 150 Years of the Experts' Advice to Women*. London: Pluto Press, 1979.

Elston, Mary Ann and Lesley **Doyal**. *Health and Medicine*. Milton Keynes: Open University course U221, Unit 14, 'The Changing Experience of Women'.

Faulder, Carolyn. *Whose Body Is It Anyway? The Troubled Issues of Informed Consent*. London: Virago Press, 1985.

Federation of Feminist Women's Health Centers. *How to Stay Out of the Gynecologist's Office*. USA: Peace Press, 1981.

Fightback and the Politics of Health Group. *Going Private, the Case Against Private Medicine*. London: Fightback and POHG. Available from 30 Camden Road, London NW1.

Frankel, M. and D. **Wilson**. *I Want to Know What is In My File*. London: Campaign for Freedom of Information, 1985.

Graham, Hilary. *Women, Health and the Family*. Brighton: Wheatsheaf Books, 1984. A sociological examination of the role of women as health carers in the family.

Greater London Council Health Panel. *Ethnic Minorities and the National Health Service in London*. London: GLC, 1985.

Griffith, Ben and Geoff **Rayner**. *Commercial Medicine in London*. London: GLC Industry and Employment Branch, 1985.

Health Rights. *Health Matters*. From c/o 344 South Lambeth Road, London SW8 1VQ. A regular journal on health issues available on subscription.

Hicks, Cherrill. *Who Cares?* London: Virago Press, 1988.

Holmes, Helen B. et al. (eds). *The Custom-made Child? – Women-centred Perspectives*. Clifton, NJ: Human Press, 1981. A thoughtful book, though somewhat out of date.

Illich, Ivan et al. *Disabling Professions*. London: Marion Boyars, 1985.

Johnson, M. *Race and Care: an Indexed Bibliography of Material on Multicultural Welfare Services*. Available from Centre for Research in Ethnic Relations, University of Warwick, Coventry CV4 7AL.

Kenner, Charmian. *No Time for Women: Exploring Women's Health in the 1930s and Today*. London: Pandora, 1984.

King's Fund Institute. *Medical Negligence: Compensation and Accountability*. London, 1988. Available from King's Fund Centre, 126 Albert Street, London NW1 7NF.

Landry, Charles et al. *What a Way to Run a Railroad: An Analysis of Radical Failure*. London: Comedia, 1987.

Leeson, Joyce and Judith **Gray**. *Women and Medicine*. London: Tavistock, 1978.

McKeith, Nancy. *The New Women's Health Handbook*. London: Virago Press, 1980.

Mares, Penny, Alex **Henley** and Carol **Baxter**. *Health Care in Multiracial Britain*. London: Health Education Council and National Extension College, 1985.

Medawar, C. *The Wrong Kind of Medicine?* London: Consumers' Association and Hodder and Stoughton, 1984.

Medawar, C. *Drugs and World Health*. IOCU 1985, available from Social Audit, PO Box 111, London NW1 8XG.

Mental Health Foundation. *Someone to Talk to Directory*. Mental Health Foundation, 1985. A directory of self-help and community support agencies in the UK and the Republic of Ireland.

Mitchell, Jeanette. *What Is To Be Done About Illness and Health? Crisis in the Eighties*. London: Penguin Books, 1984.

National Consumer Council. *Patients' Rights: a Guide for NHS Patients and Doctors*. London: HMSO, 1983.

Navarro, Vicente. *Class Struggle, the State and Medicine*. London: Martin Robertson, 1978.

O'Sullivan, Sue (ed.). *Women's Health – a Spare Rib Reader*. London: Pandora, 1987. Charts the development of feminist consciousness on health issues over the last fifteen years.

Overall, Christine. *Ethics and Human Reproduction, a Feminist Analysis*. London: Allen and Unwin, 1987.

Parish, P. *Medicine – A Guide for Everybody*, 6th rev. edn. London: Penguin Books, 1987. The best guide to drugs. Make sure you read the most up-to-date edition.

Patients' Association. *Rights of the Patient and Changing Your Doctor* and *Going Into Hospital: Using the NHS* and *Can I Insist?* Leaflets available from the Patients' Association (see Organizations).

Rakusen, Jill and Nick **Davidson**. *Out of Our Hands – What Technology Does to Pregnancy*. London: Pan, 1982.

Roberts, Helen (ed.). *Women, Health and Reproduction*. London: Routledge and Kegan Paul, 1981.

Roberts, Helen. *The Patient Patients: Women and their Doctors*. London: Pandora, 1984.

Robinson, Jean. *A Patient View of the General Medical Council*. London: Health Rights, 1988.

Salvage, Jane. *The Politics of Nursing*. London: Heinemann, 1985.

Sashidharan, S. *Race, Health and the Experts: a Critique of Two Views*. MRC Unit, Department of Psychiatry, University of Edinburgh.

Savage, Wendy. *A Savage Enquiry*. London: Virago Press, 1986.

Stanworth, Michelle (ed). *Reproductive Technologies – Gender, Motherhood and Medicine*. Oxford: Polity Press, 1988. A collection of feminist writings taking a different view from Arditti et al., though not necessarily less critical.

Stimson, Gerry and Carol Stimson. *Health Rights Handbook*. London: Penguin Books, 1980.

Torkington, Ntombenhle Protasia. *The Racial Politics of Health: a Liverpool Profile*. Merseyside Area Profile Group, Department of Sociology, University of Liverpool, 1983.

Townsend, P. and N. Davidson. *Inequalities In Health*. London: Penguin Books, 1982. An edited version of the government research paper known as the Black Report, which the incoming Conservative Government attempted to suppress.

Tyneside Women's Health Project. *Young Women and Health Issues* (available from Tyneside Women's Health Project, 313a High Street, Gateshead, Newcastle NE8 1EQ).

Victoria Health Authority, Paddington and North Kensington Health Authority. *Health Education Resources on Women's Health*. London: Victoria Health Authority, 1984.

Widgery, David. *Health in Danger – the Crisis in the National Health Service*. Basingstoke: Macmillan, 1979.

Winterson, Jeanette. *Fit for the Future: the Guide for Women Who Want to Live Well*. London: Pandora, 1986.

Wolfson, J. and R. Randall. *Taking Stock – A Whole Life Review*. Cambridge: National Extension College, 1983. Learning materials prepared along relatively holistic lines for the College of Health.

Women's Health and Reproductive Rights Information Centre. *The Newsletter*, no. 10, Winter edition, 1988. Special edition on well woman services. Available from WHRRIC (see Organizations).

Women's National Commission. *Report on Women and the Health Service*, 1984. (Available free from Government Offices, Great George Street, London SW1.)

PERIODICALS

Black Women's Newsletter (available from London Women's Centre – see Organizations).

British Medical Journal (see British Medical Association in Organizations).

Drugs and Therapeutics Bulletin, Consumers' Association, 14 Buckingham Street, London WC2 6AD.

Everywoman, 34A Islington Green, London N1 8DU. Monthly, 90p. Regular coverage of health and food issues.

In From the Cold, 49 Calorera Avenue, Virginia Water, Surrey GU2S 4HA. A liberation magazine for people with disabilities.

Jewish Feminist Newsletter, PO Box 39, c/o Sisterwrite (see overleaf): contact address for various Jewish groups.

The Lancet, 7 Adam Street, London WC2N 6AD.

London Black Women's Health Action Newsletter, London Black Women's Health Action Project (see Organizations).

New England Journal of Medicine, 13 Colina Road, London N15 3JA.

New Statesman and Society, 14–16 Farringdon Lane, London EC1R 3AV.

Nursing Times, Macmillan Journals, Farndon Road, Market Harborough, Leicestershire LE16 9NR.

Radical Community Medicine, 38 Weston Park, London N8..

Self Health, Journal of the College of Health (see Organizations).

Spare Rib, 27 Clerkenwell Close, London EC1R 0AP. Tel: 01-253 9792/251 1773. A women's liberation magazine, available on tape. Have lists of back copies on particular topics, including women's health.

WHRRIC Newsletter, Women's Health and Reproductive Rights Information Centre (see Organizations).

ORGANIZATIONS

Action for the Victims of Medical Accidents, 24 Southwark Street, London SE1 1TY. Tel: 01-403 4744.

Akina Mama Wa Africa, London Women's Centre, Wesley House, 4 Wild Court, London WC2B 5AU. Tel: 01–405 0678.

Asian Women's Network, London Women's Centre, Wesley House, 4 Wild Court, London WC2B 5AU.

Association of Community Health Councils for England and Wales, 30 Drayton Park, London N5. Tel: 01-609 8405.

Association of Northern Ireland District Committees, 25–27 Adelaide Street, Belfast BT2 8FH. Tel: 0232 224431.

Association of Radical Midwives (ARM) c/o Ishbel Kargar SRN, SCM, 62 Greetby Hill, Ormskirk, Lancashire L39 2DT. Tel: 0695–72776 (up to 9:30 p.m.)

Association of Scottish Local Health Councils, 21 Torphichen Street, Edinburgh EH3 8HX. Tel: 031-229 2344.

Black Community Against Women's Oppression, c/o London Women's Centre (as above).

Black Health Workers and Patients Group, 259a High Road, Tottenham, London N15. Tel: 01-809 0774.

British Medical Association, BMA House, Tavistock Square, London WC1N 9JP. Tel: 01-387 4499.

Camden Black Sisters, London Women's Centre (as above). Tel: 01-831 7897.

Campaign Against Health Fraud, Box CAHF. London WC1N 3XX. Tel: 01-673 4401. Started out as a campaign by orthodox practitioners against non-orthodox practitioners. With pressure, it could change.

Carers' National Association, 29 Chilworth Mews, London, W2 3R6. Tel: 01-724 7776.

Centre for Ethnic Minorities Health Studies, Field House Teaching Centre, Duckworth Lane, Bradford BD9 6RJ.

Child Poverty Action Group, 1 Macklin Street, London WC2B 5NH. Tel: 01-242 3224.

Children's Legal Centre, 20 Compton Terrace, Islington, London N1 2BR. Tel: 01-359 6251.

Citizen's Rights Office, 1 Bath Street, London EC1. Tel: 01-253 3406.

College of Health, 18 Victoria Park Square, London E2 9PF. Tel: 01-980 6263.

Commission for Racial Equality, Elliot House, 10–12 Allington Street, London SW1E 5EH. Tel: 01-828 7022. A statutory body working towards the elimination of race discrimination, towards equality of opportunity and good relations between people of different racial groups. Keeping under review the 1976 Race Relations Act.

Confederation of Health Service Employees (COHSE), Glen House, High Street, Banstead, Surrey SM7 2LH. Tel: 07373 53322.

Consumers' Association, 2 Marylebone Road, London NW1 4DX. Tel: 01-486 5544.

Equal Opportunities Commission, Overseas House, Quay Street, Manchester M3 3HN. Tel: 061-833 9244.

Family Practitioner Committees, in England and Wales; in Scotland, the **Primary Care Division of the Health Board**; in Northern Ireland, the **Central Services Committee**. Look in the telephone directory or ask directory inquiries for your local area office.

Family Rights Group, 62 Manor Gardens, Holloway Road, London N7 6LA. Tel: 01-263 4016/263 9724/272 7308. Produces research and lobbies for rights of families with children. Advice sessions Monday, Wednesday and Friday mornings.

Finrrage (*Feminist International Network of Resistance to Reproductive and Genetic Engineering*), Box 38, 59 Cookridge Street, Leeds 2 3AW. A campaigning rather than advisory organization, founded in 1984. Aims to monitor international developments in the area of reproductive technology, assess their impact on women's socio-economic position and well-being internationally, and bring together members of the network periodically. It is a non-funded, non-profit organization.

Freedom of Information Campaign, 3 Endsleigh Street, London WC1H 0DD. Tel: 01-278 9686.

General Medical Council, 44 Hallam Street, London W1N 6AE. Tel: 01-580 7642.

Health Education Authority, Hamilton House, Mabledon Place, London WC1H 9TX. Tel: 01-637 0930.

Healthline, PO Box 499, London E2 9PU. Tel: 01-980 4848 (recorded message service – 2 to 10 p.m., seven days a week). Recorded messages for a wide range of health problems and issues. Also lists UK self-help groups.

Health Service Commissioner (Ombudsman), Church House, Great Smith Street, London SW1P 3BW. Tel: 01-276 2035.

Health Service Commissioner for Scotland, 2nd Floor, 11 Melville Crescent, Edinburgh EH3 7LU. Tel: 031-225 7465.

Health Service Commissioner for Wales, 4th floor, Pearl Assurance House, Greyfriars Road, Cardiff CF1 3AG. Tel: 0222 394621.

Help for Health, The Grant Building, Southampton General Hospital, Southampton SO9 4XY. Tel: 0703 779091. One of the most comprehensive self-help databanks in the country.

Joint Council for the Welfare of Immigrants, 115 Old Street, London EC1V 9JR. Tel: 01-251 8706.

Law Centres Federation, National Office, 18–19 Warren Street, London W1P 5DB. Tel: 01-387 8570. Look in the telephone directory for your nearest office.

Law Society, for England and Wales: 113 Chancery Lane, London WC2A 1PL. Tel: 01-242 1222; for Northern Ireland: Law Society House, 90/106 Victoria Street, Belfast BT1 3JZ. Tel: 0232 231614; for Scotland: 26–7 Drumsheugh Gardens, Edinburgh EH3 7YR. Tel: 031-226 7411.

Local Government Health Rights Project, 344 South Lambeth Road, London SW8 1UQ. Tel: 01-720 9811/2.

London Black Women's Health Action Project, Wickham House, 10 Cleveland Way, London E1 4TZ. Tel: 01-790 2424 X343/432.

London Women's Centre, Wesley House, 4 Wild Court, London WC2B 5AU. Tel: 01-831 6946. This is a big resource for women in London, with meeting and conference rooms, video filming and editing facilities, and arts, sports and café facilities planned.

Low Pay Unit, 9 Upper Berkeley Street, London W1H 8BY. Tel: 01-262 7278.

Marie Curie Cancer Care, 28 Belgrave Square, London SW1X 8QG. Tel: 01-235 3325. Community nursing and residential care.

Maternity Defence Fund, 33 Castle Street, Hently-in-Arden, West Midlands.

Medical Practitioners' Union (MPU), c/o MSF, 79 Camden Road, London NW1 9ES.

Medical Women's Federation, Tavistock House North, Tavistock Square, London WC1 9HX. Tel: 01-387 7765.

National Association of Citizens' Advice Bureaux, 115–123 Pentonville Road, London N1 9LZ. Tel: 01-833 2181. They can tell you where your nearest bureau is.

National Association of Compensation Claimants, Durham House, 124 Old Christchurch Road, Bournemouth BH1 1NF. Tel: 0202 690937.

National Association for Patient Participation, Hazelbank, Peaslake, Guildford, Surrey GU5 9RJ.

National Association for the Welfare of Children in Hospital, (NAWCH), Argyle House, 29–31 Euston Road, London NW1 2SD. Tel: 01–833 2041.

National Council for Civil Liberties, 21 Tabard Street, London SE1 4LA. Tel: 01-403 3888.

National Council for Voluntary Organizations, 26 Bedford Square, London WC1B 3HU. Tel: 01-636 4066.

National Union of Public Employees (NUPE), 8 Aberdeen Terrace, London SE3. Tel: 01-852 2842.

Patients' Association, Room 33, 18 Charing Cross Road, London WC2H 0HR. Tel: 01-240 0671.

Public Health Alliance c/o Health Visitors' Association, 50 Southwark Street, London SE1 1UN. Aims to 'identify and publicize all risks to health, and to work for their reduction or complete removal'.

Radical Nurses Group, c/o 83 South View Road, Sheffield S7 1DB. Tel: 0742-580479.

Socialist Health Association, 195 Walworth Road, Southwark, London SE17 1RP. Tel: 01-703 6838.

Trades Union Congress, Congress House, Great Russell Street, London WC1B 3LS. Tel: 01-636 4030.

A Woman's Place, Hungerford House, Victoria Embankment, London WC2. Tel: 01-836 6081. Information, books, meeting place for women. Open Tuesday-Thursday 1-7 p.m.

Women in Medicine (WIM), 55 Mallard Point, Rain Hill Way, Bow, London E3.

Women's Health and Reproductive Rights Information Centre (WHRRIC), 52–54 Featherstone Street, London EC1 8RT. Tel: 01-251 6580/6332.

Women's International Resource Centre, 173 Archway Road, London N6.

BOOKSHOPS

If you have difficulty getting any of the books mentioned, these bookshops provide a mail order service:

Sisterwrite, 190 Upper Street, London N1. Tel: 01-226 9782. Produce a monthly booklist and back copies of this are also available. Send S.A.E.

West and Wilde Bookshop, 25A Dundas Street, Edinburgh EH1 3LE. Tel: 031-556 0079. Specialize in women's fiction, lesbian and gay books, and have a lot of American imports. Publish a lesbian booklist six times a year. Send S.A.E.

AUDIO LIBRARY

Feminist Audio Books, 52–54 Featherstone Street, London EC1Y 8RT. Tel: 01-251 2908/0713. A tape subscription library for blind, partially sighted and other women who have difficulty with the printed word.

AUDIO-VISUAL MATERIALS

Health Belongs to the People. War on Want, 467 Caledonian Road, London N7.

The following have a selection of videos and films on women's health:

BBC Enterprises Ltd, Education and Training Sales, Woodlands, 80 Wood Lane, London W12 0TT. Tel: 01-576-0237/0361.

Channel 4 Television, 60 Charlotte Street, London W1P 2AX. Tel: 01-631 4444.

PUBLISHERS

Arlen House, The Women's Press Publishers and Distributors, 69 Jones Road, Dublin 3. Tel: 0001-78 6913.

Onlywomen Press, 38 Mount Pleasant Street, London WC1X 0AP.

Pandora Press, 14 Leicester Square, London WC2H 7PH. Tel: 01-437 9011.

Sheba Feminist Publishers, 488 Kingsland Road, London E8 4AE. Tel: 01-254 1590.

Stramullion, 43 Candlemaker Row, Edinburgh EH1 2QB.

Virago Press, 20-23 Mandela Street, London NW1 0HQ. Tel: 01-383 5150.

Women's Press, 34 Great Sutton Street, London WC1V 0DX. Tel: 01-251 3007.

ORGANIZING FOR CHANGE

Prepared by
HELEN ROSENTHAL AND FIDELMA WINKLER

Getting the care, attention or treatment that we need is not always easy. Illness makes us vulnerable and saps both physical and emotional energy. Even when we are well, the cards are still frequently stacked against us by the medical system, as the last chapter showed. Those of us who are assertive may be able to improve things for ourselves, but it is only by acting collectively that we can make changes which will affect us all.

We need to find ways to translate our knowledge and individual experiences of struggling for what we need into clear demands and broad strategies for change in the NHS. We need to establish collective dialogues with the people who work in the NHS at all levels, as well as applying pressure, to ensure that our concerns are heard and responded to.

The examples in this chapter of women who have got together inside or outside the NHS to work for change show that change *is* possible. The examples also show that the process of negotiating for change, achieving and then monitoring and maintaining it are often very slow and arduous as much for health-service unions and community

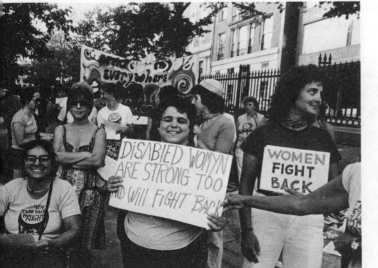

Sarah Putnam

health councils as for women in autonomous health groups and independent organizations.

THE WOMEN'S HEALTH MOVEMENT

There are thousands of women in the women's health movement both here in the UK and worldwide. Many of us began working on health issues with several other people. Some groups have remained small while others have expanded into much larger organizations. You will find excellent models on which to pattern your own group from the wide range of groups and organizations discussed here.

SELF-HELP GROUPS

People have always banded together to help one another deal with everyday problems. Feminist self-help means discussing feelings and experiences, supporting each other to learn together: finding out what we do know and what we do not know; deciding what we want to know, and exploring from there; demystifying the expertise of health professionals, and our own bodies; making choices based on our own experience and knowledge. Through sharing knowledge we develop certain skills which enable us to challenge the authority of doctors. Self-help also stresses that the way we learn – from one another in settings which make us feel equal, comfortable and respected – is as important as what we learn. Finally, self-help is political because it challenges the health-care providers and gives us more control over our own bodies.

The first feminist self-help groups were based on self-discovery. Each woman examined her vagina and cervix in a mirror, with a torch, seeing for the first time these formerly unmentionable parts of her body, and learning to monitor her own health. Some groups have been established around particular health concerns: the PID group (see p. 534) in London was established when two PID

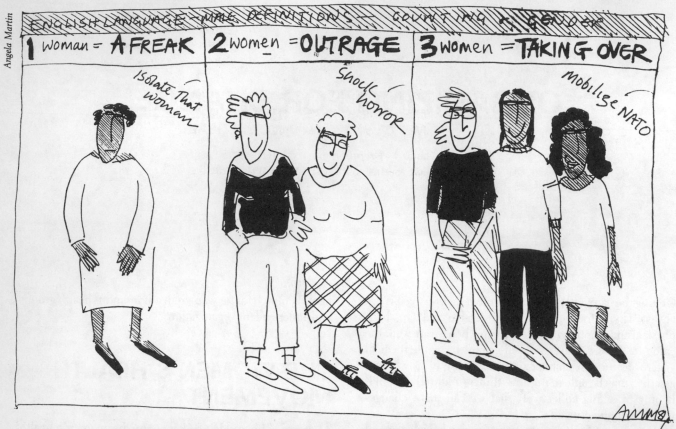

ENGLISH LANGUAGE — MALE DEFINITIONS — COUNTING X GENDER

1 woman = A FREAK   2 women = OUTRAGE   3 women = TAKING OVER

Isolate that woman

Shock horror

Mobilise NATO

Angela Martin

sufferers met at a party. Since then it has produced a newsletter and kept in touch with medical literature on the subject, providing both support and a reservoir of expertise for other women who join. Similar groups exist around endometriosis (see p. 534), herpes (see the Herpes Association, p. 534) and many others. Some groups have started around issues such as disability while others, such as the London Black Women's Action Group, focus on the needs of black women. Groups which have started as self-help

groups may grow into campaigns focusing on, for example, local abortion facilities. The principles of feminist self-help – lack of hierarchy, sharing of knowledge and concern for each other's needs – have found their way into the working practices of many more formally organized groups.

THE NATIONAL HEALTH SERVICE – HOW IT WORKS

While many of us will have developed an interest in health issues through our individual experiences, it soon becomes clear that the only way to achieve any real change in the provision of health care is to put pressure on the National Health Service. We may all feel tempted towards private solutions – perhaps as a step on the way to more radical change, as an example to the existing services or simply as a refuge from the sometimes apparently hopeless task of effecting change in so big a bureaucracy – but in the end our energies must be concentrated where we can make improvements for everyone and where the profit motive cannot distort the quality of care given.

The structure of the National Health Service is complex and difficult to understand. Even many members of staff don't know how the decision-making structure works. This is partly due to the constant reorganizations that have been taking place for almost two decades. The 1989 Health Service Review seems likely to be the most far-reaching change of all. Having spent a decade trying to cut NHS costs the Conservative Government decided, according to a senior civil servant, quoted in *The Independent*, to

MEDWAY WOMEN'S HEALTH CAMPAIGN*

We have been campaigning for a Well Women's Centre to be set up in the Medway Towns since 1982. The health authority has opposed it so we started to run our own information and discussion sessions on women's health. Eventually they did allow us to use a room in one of their clinics for this. Since then we have obtained more permanent accommodation in a building in the centre of Chatham. We are running a drop-in centre for women where they can get leaflets, information on health issues, plus a cup of tea and a chance to chat. We have also started to build up a reference library of women's health books and hold evening sessions devoted to particular health topics.

*From *Spare Rib*, no. 172, November 1986, p. 8.

ORGANIZING FOR CHANGE

1. *Find other people.* Talk to others at clinics, in schools, etcetera. Write a letter to your local paper or to the women's page of a national newspaper, or to a magazine such as *Spare Rib* or *Everywoman* (see p. 637) asking for others to contact you.

2. *Ensure diversity.* It is impossible to represent the interests of people whose needs are unknown to us. In establishing a group it is up to those of us who are initiators to ensure that we make contact with women from other groups. Our communities are divided and such contacts require effort and commitment if they are to rise above mere tokenism.

3. *Organize meetings.* Arrange meetings at times which are suitable for all and in locations which are accessible for people with disabilities. Make sure decisions happen at meetings and not in informal chats in the pub. People soon drop out if they do not feel fully involved.

4. *Inform yourselves.* Give everyone a task to do bringing information to the group: practical information, such as how and where to apply for grants; health-care information or information about local services. Contact your local health education unit, the Health Education Authority resources centre (see p. 637) if you live in London, Citizens Advice Bureaux, information units at your town hall, your Community Health Council; subscribe to the Women's Health and Reproductive Rights Information Centre (see p. 638) and take it in turns to read the newspapers and copy relevant articles. If you are working on a specific health issue it will help to read medical journals. You should find them in a good reference library (your district general hospital may allow access to its library). See Resources for names of journals. For information on using libraries and computer information services, read the *Consumers Guide to Health Information from the College of Health (see Resources, Chapter 27).*

5. *Inform others.* If you are campaigning for improved services you will need to contact people who can help your campaign and lobby the people with the power to make changes. Make a list of the organizations which share an interest in what you are doing: other women's groups, trade unions, voluntary organizations, etcetera. Many trade unions now have women's officers at their headquarters who can pass on information to the relevant people and tell you how the union could be useful to you.

6. *Use the press.* Local newspapers and local radio are usually thirsty for stories. Try to find the names of journalists who are likely to sympathize with your cause and then invite them to a private briefing. If the press show an interest in what you are doing, always give them *some* information. There is nothing that whets the journalistic appetite more than a secret. Groups that have tried to keep a low profile have sometimes found themselves being investigated and made to seem suspicious and cagey. At the same time, treat all journalists with caution until you are sure where they stand and then remember that they do not usually have control over the final shape of their story. Give only information which you want them to use. Try to present it in a lively way, if possible using quotes or case histories. Read the TUC guide to *How to Handle the Media* (from TUC, Congress House, Great Russell Street, London WC1).

7. *Write to your MP and to local councillors asking for their support.* Their replies make good news stories even if you do not get active involvement.

8. *Get to know the names of key people* in your health authority (see p. 644) and keep writing to them.

9. *Develop your personal skills.* Dealing with administrators, doctors and politicians requires confidence and clarity as well as information.

destabilize it and see what happened'. No one, least of all the Government, can really predict the outcome of this review.

Hospitals can 'opt out' and become self-governing, and financial control is to move from a planned model to one in which the market provides the major instrument of planning. District health authorities will have no control over which hospitals opt out, and limited control over the services they provide, be they abortion facilities or coronary care. If treatment is not available locally, we will have to travel in order to get it and bear the travelling costs ourselves. Some GPs may also 'opt out', take control of their own budgets and use their purchasing power to decide where their patients will be treated.

For most of us this new system would almost certainly limit choice. District health authorities and GPs can enter into contracts for treatment with various hospitals: their own, those that are opted out or even private ones. Since this review is essentially a cost-cutting exercise there will be little slack in budgets and GPs (whether opted out or not) will be under considerable financial pressure to use hospitals where special contracts mean that each item of care is cheaper, rather than opting for more expensive tailor-made referrals. There is likely to be little scope for shopping around for shorter waiting lists (or women gynaecologists) even for those of us who are able to travel.

If implemented the review would almost certainly create an even sharper divide between rich and poor. Beyond that we can, at this stage, only speculate. We do not know how the maternity services would be affected, we do not know how liaison between community and hospital would be organized. Clearly systems for monitoring health care will be vital within a fragmented service. We are not convinced that the plans for 'medical audit' (which in principle we welcome) will provide sufficient safeguards.

On the other hand the new system could also provide some opportunities for real innovation and improved care at a local level. This is a time when we need, more than ever before, to find our way into the organization of the service and use all the information we have at our disposal to ensure that women's interests are taken into consideration. If your aim is to get improvements to use the structure effectively as an individual or as a community group, then you have to learn the basics of the system. Of the eight bodies described below, three are particularly important: the community or local health council, the family practitioner committee, the district health authority. We have indicated how the structure will change if the 1989 Review comes into force.

THE COMMUNITY HEALTH COUNCIL

The community health council (CHC) has a statutory duty to represent the views of the community and user interests concerning the NHS.* There is one in each health district: 192 in England, 9 in Wales and 15 in Scotland. The councils are usually made up of between eighteen and twenty-four voluntary (unpaid) members, a paid secretary and small supporting staff. CHCs have rights to visit NHS premises, including NHS self-governing hospitals; to information about the NHS, and to be consulted on changes of use of NHS premises. They must publish a report of their work annually and meet the district health authority in public once a year.

For individuals and groups the first place to go for information about the NHS should be the CHC. They should be able to get the information for you or tell you where is the best place to get it. They also have access to an enormous amount of informal information that is essential for getting action.

What CHCs Can Do

They are *independent* of management and they do not have managerial responsibility; therefore, their role can be exclusively to represent the community and the users of the service. They should not have to weigh up various options and vested interests.

CHCs are limited by their resources. There are usually no more than two full-time paid staff, sometimes fewer, and much of the work is done by members on a voluntary basis. They should welcome involvement from groups, should act as your advocate, time and resources permitting, and should be able to put you in touch with other people and organizations inside and outside the NHS who share your concerns.

CHC Women's Groups

It is possible to establish a women's group under the auspices of a sympathetic CHC. The direct link with a statutory body will increase your ability to influence local services.

One group which has successfully achieved this is attached to City and Hackney CHC in London. The group has clear terms of reference to establish its identity and sense of direction.

The group is open to all women members of the CHC and to any interested woman in the district. Members are expected to show a commitment by coming to meetings regularly.

The main function of the group is to relate critically to the NHS locally, to engage with planners and providers and to campaign for improvements.

The group cannot be primarily a consciousness-raising or positive health group, though it will provide positive help in establishing other such groups.

The Women's Health Group is regularly asked to discuss proposals from the district health authority but it sets its own agendas and initiates as well as responds to ideas. For example, it initiated a successful campaign for a local day-care abortion service. The group regularly asks senior medical personnel to attend meetings at which the concerns of consumers are discussed. Meeting on CHC territory tends to tip the balance of power away from the professionals.

Through the CHC, more women have been channelled into the health service structures; for example, sitting on the Women's Health Planning Team and the Maternity Services Liaison Committee of the Health Authority. Women can be very isolated in these committees, but, as members of the women's group they are supported, they are accountable and they are independent of the system.

Small Successes
The Dean of St Bartholomew's Medical School has just agreed to review the practice of medical students going and repairing episiotomies. This is five years after the issue was raised by the local women's health group.

First the consultant obstetricians were asked to review the practice. They said it was unnecessary because, 'Medical students were always supervised properly.' We were told that it was necessary for medical students to learn this procedure so that they didn't have to learn it if they become house officers in obstetrics.

Over the years the women's group has continued to raise it in CHC reports and has held discussions with medical students. Medical students, we discovered, were on the whole very sympathetic. Examples of the awful consequences for women of 'bad repairs' were

*They are called local health councils in Scotland. In Northern Ireland the local district councils are the equivalent bodies.

collected and a particularly horrific example was raised at a meeting on medical education.

The Dean of the Medical School was in the Chair. He had not apparently, up until that moment, heard us on the subject and responded sympathetically to our request. The obstetricians present contributed with their tales of catastrophes brought about by medical students. The practice has not yet been stopped but, as with so much else, when powerful people have committed themselves to change, change is on the way, if they are 'pursued' by the women's group.

Limitations to Change

CHCs do not always work effectively on our behalf. Some CHCs even try to limit the involvement of community groups in the NHS. Some are as bureaucratic as the health authorities. Their policies reflect their membership and the prevailing political group in the community. If you find the CHC unhelpful you will have to identify and lobby

---

WOMEN-SENSITIVE SERVICES: ADVOCACY

The consultant sweeps into the examination room. The pregnant woman is on the couch. There is a male medical student and another woman in the room. The consultant announces that he wants to do an internal examination and indicates that he wants the woman made ready. He passes on to the next room. A typical scene in ante-natal clinics. This room is different. The other woman is a patient advocate. She asks the student if he considers the consultant's behaviour acceptable. The student looks shamefaced. When the consultant returns, the advocate asks him if he will please tell the woman why he wishes to examine her internally. The atmosphere changes. He looks at the woman's notes, then tells her that he doesn't think he needs to do an examination after all and proceeds with the consultation.

This minor example of the patient advocate reminding the staff to treat patients as human beings is part of the daily work of Hafize Ece and her colleagues on Hackney's Multi-ethnic Women's Health Project. On other occasions they may protect the woman in more significant ways by making sure that staff have fully explained all the available options to the woman or by requesting that the consultant discusses the course of treatment proposed before the woman makes a decision. If requests recur, for example for women doctors, then the issue will be taken to the medical staff and to the district health authority. They will keep lobbying until enough women doctors are appointed to the unit.

The workers on this project work specifically with non-English-speaking women. They are employed on a Community Health Council project which was set up as a direct result of women observing the poor service non-English-speaking women were getting. Their work is not a one-off campaign to get the service improved but a daily reminder to staff to deliver care according to the users' needs. They remain distinct from the staff, they are not part of

their hierarchy nor do they wear uniforms, but they work closely with them. They have as part of their brief advising the health authority of the policy changes necessary to make the service appropriate.

As many women's groups have noted, the service provided by these advocates would be just as useful to all women. We all suffer difficulties in communication with medical staff and have all felt patronized or put down at times. This project formalizes what has long been advocated by women's groups – take a friend with you – but the patient advocates have special advantages: they know how that particular unit works, they know the personnel, they can give women access to informal knowledge that is important but usually guarded by the professionals. They also have direct access via the CHC to those who make and can change policy.

Similar advocacy schemes are being set up elsewhere in various ways. The particular value of the Hackney scheme lies in the way it was established. It is run under the auspices of the CHC, which gives it access to health service premises. It is backed up by a steering group composed of health service professionals and members of the community in equal numbers. The group is responsible from day to day to the CHC secretary, and regular support sessions provide both training and a forum for discussing difficulties and ideas for change. It is the vital combination of access and independence which gives these women the power to do their job.

Given the lack of NHS resources, it is not likely that similar schemes will be made available, at least in the near future, to all NHS users. However, it is possible for women's groups and organizations to set up their own advocacy schemes, perhaps with CHC backing to provide access to the system. The National Childbirth Trust, for example, sends breastfeeding counsellors into hospitals in some areas. We could all lobby for hospitals to employ an advocacy officer whose job would be to liaise with local groups and to provide support, and training.

individual members who may be sympathetic. A good way to do this is to go to a CHC meeting: all are open to the public including all business and working group meetings from April 1989.) Then try to get your own members on to the CHC.

How to Become a Member of a CHC

Becoming a member means that you have access to information about the service and the ability to visit and ask questions about it. An informed, and assertive, member of a CHC can make sure that women's health issues are on agendas and can press for implementation of women-sensitive policies.

Half the members of a CHC are nominated by the local authorities (in practice by the dominant political party), one-sixth by the Regional Health Authority, from names received by it from organizations and individuals and the CHC secretary, and one-third are elected by voluntary organizations every two years. Make sure your group is on the list of organizations entitled to vote for CHC membership (consult the CHC secretary). CHCs can co-opt people on to their working groups, and on some CHCs a lot of the work is done by co-opted members. Tell the Secretary or Chair if you are interested in being involved in a working group.

THE FAMILY PRACTITIONER COMMITTEE

The FPC administers the contracts of general practitioners, dentists, chemists and opticians, and deals with complaints against GPs. It will also be responsible for quality and financial control of GPs. If you are campaigning for more women GPs, complaining about the location of GP premises, if you want a say in the choice of a new GP when one has retired, contact the administrator (soon to be General Manager), or Chair, and lobby FPC members. Write to members of the FPC asking for the issue to be put on the agenda for the next public meeting. Names and addresses of members should be available from the FPC and so too should times and dates of meetings. Usually these meetings have few members of the public present so a group attending would have some impact, as would the declared intention to issue a press release. (The local community health councils have observer status at these meetings. They can speak but not vote, so you should try to make sure that they will speak on the group's behalf.)

Limitations to Change

The powers of family practitioner committees are to be broadened, but essentially they reimburse small businessmen and women for the services they provide under contract to the FPC. What they do is further restricted by professional rights and associations. The local medical committee (which represents the doctors) has considerable influence on all FPCs, in part because of the fragmentation of the lay members and in part because of lay members' unwillingness to challenge doctors' opinions. FPCs, therefore, often give the impression of being primarily concerned about protecting the financial interests of contractees.

Little will change until users and community groups demand greater public accountability from FPC contractees and one good way of doing this is through FPC membership.

How to Become a Member of the FPC

The FPC chair is appointed directly by the Secretary of State. There are usually thirty members (which will be reduced to eleven). Half are nominated by the professions. The other half is made up of people from a variety of backgrounds.

If your group is particularly interested in services administered by the FPC you should ask for a nomination form for membership from the FPC administrator. The names go to the Secretary of State, but in future will go to the Regional Health Authority (RHA, see below), so it would also be worth writing to the RHA pointing out the need for representation from local women and getting other groups to put forward the same names as your group. There is no limit to the number of names you can put forward or for how many FPCs.

FPCs cover more than one health district and local authority. They are to be accountable to RHAs.

THE DISTRICT HEALTH AUTHORITY

The DHA is responsible for planning and managing the hospital service in the district and for the community health service – district nurses, health visitors, community midwives, health centres and the clinics in them, such as family planning clinics and child health clinics. They will also be responsible for administering the contracts of consultants. The officer responsible for the management of the services is the district general manager. Under him or her are unit general managers, who may be in charge of one hospital, several small ones, the community health services or psychiatric services.

The authority is made up of members who in theory are responsible for the management of the services and for setting the policy. Since the establishment of a new management system in 1984 much of that power and responsibility has passed to the district general managers. They are appointed on fixed-term contracts by the Regional Health Authority and their contract renewal depends on whether or not they fulfil the budgetary requirements laid down by ministers. In other words, a major reorganization took place in 1984, which left health authority members with less power, and the 1989 Review will reduce it further.

Limitations to Change

Districts must run their services within the money allocated for the year by the Regional Health Authority irrespective of need or local problems. They are penalized if they don't. DHA members, coming as they do from different backgrounds, don't often operate as a corporate body and the lay members are not always adequately briefed. The concentration of management power in the hands of general managers has called into question the role of the DHA which all too often acts simply as a rubber stamp on cost-cutting measures instigated centrally through the general manager.

A community group or women's group seeking to influence the care in hospitals, in community nursing or to get new services set up, would ideally need to develop contact with a significant number of DHA members to argue their case and lobby for them. The overwhelming majority of members are male. The community health council has an observer on the DHA who is allowed to speak but not to vote.

How to Become a Member of the DHA

The Chair of the district health authority is appointed by the Secretary of State and receives a salary. The members are appointed by the Regional Health Authority from nominations received from the professions and community organizations or individuals. Half the members appointed will be designated 'generalists', i.e. they do not represent the professions or local authority. Neither the nominating body nor the reason for appointments is made public. Until the 1989 review of the NHS, local authorities had been directly represented on DHAs. Now these places are to be abolished, which will block one of the most important points of access to the health service structure for health-care activists. It will be possible to join a DHA as a lay member only by getting nominations from existing DHA or RHA members or by getting support for your nomination from several organizations.

NHS HOSPITAL TRUSTS (SELF-GOVERNING HOSPITALS)

These are intended to come into effect as a result of the 1989 Government review. They will be managed by a board of directors, two of whom will be drawn from the local community and appointed by the RHA. Directors will have a managerial role, *not* a representative one, and trade union members are explicitly excluded. Only one meeting a year need be open to the public. The CHC role will be reduced to visiting only. Clearly, if a majority of hospitals opt for Trust status, democratic control and community involvement will be sharply reduced.

JOINT CONSULTATIVE COMMITTEES

Between hospital and the primary care service, between social service and health service, between statutory and private, between family/friends and professional care is community care.

Services delivered under the title of community care are increasingly crucial. Most women will be affected by the care or non-care provided under this service. Organizing for change relies on the same need to research the issue, galvanize the local forces. Only, in addition to learning

about the health service structure, you may well have to learn about the local authority's structures, particularly social services and housing.

The major committee responsible for joint planning between the various authorities and the voluntary sector is the Joint Consultative Committee. Elections are held among the community organizations for places on this committee. Again, your organization has to be on the list held at the Regional Health Authority to be eligible to vote. Check with your CHC or the Regional Health Authority who represents the voluntary sector and how to get on the list to stand for election.

In Northern Ireland there are four health and social services boards divided into units of management. In theory this should make community care easier to administer.

THE REGIONAL HEALTH AUTHORITY

Above the District Health Authority is the RHA, which is responsible for planning of services in the region. There are fourteen regions in England. Wales is the equivalent of one region, under the Welsh Office, similarly Scotland. The regions allocate finance to the districts according to a complex formula and plan, manage and fund capital developments, e.g., new hospitals. Members are appointed by the Secretary of State. Contact with a sympathetic member at the RHA is crucial if you are concerned about access to women doctors or getting members on your local DHA or CHC. CHCs should have a list of RHA members and be able to advise on who to contact.

SPECIAL HEALTH AUTHORITIES

There are fourteen of these authorities, mainly in London. They are seen as 'Centres of Excellence' and people come to them from all over the country. They get their funds directly from the government to provide specialist services, for example Queen Charlotte's Hospital is the responsibility of a special health authority, as is Great Ormond Street Hospital for Children. The Health Education Authority (previously the Health Education Council) was turned into a SHA to ensure more direct government control. Members are appointed by the Secretary of State, but they do have to meet in public.

THE DEPARTMENT OF HEALTH

The Department of Health is the government department responsible for the health service. It is headed by the Secretary of State, who is directly accountable to Parliament. Members of Parliament are therefore able to ask detailed questions in Parliament about the NHS. The NHS Management Board was set up in 1985 to provide a 'focus' for management of the NHS inside the department. It is chaired by the Minister of Health and seeks to make sure the Secretary of State's policies are implemented.

THE NHS IN ENGLAND 1989*

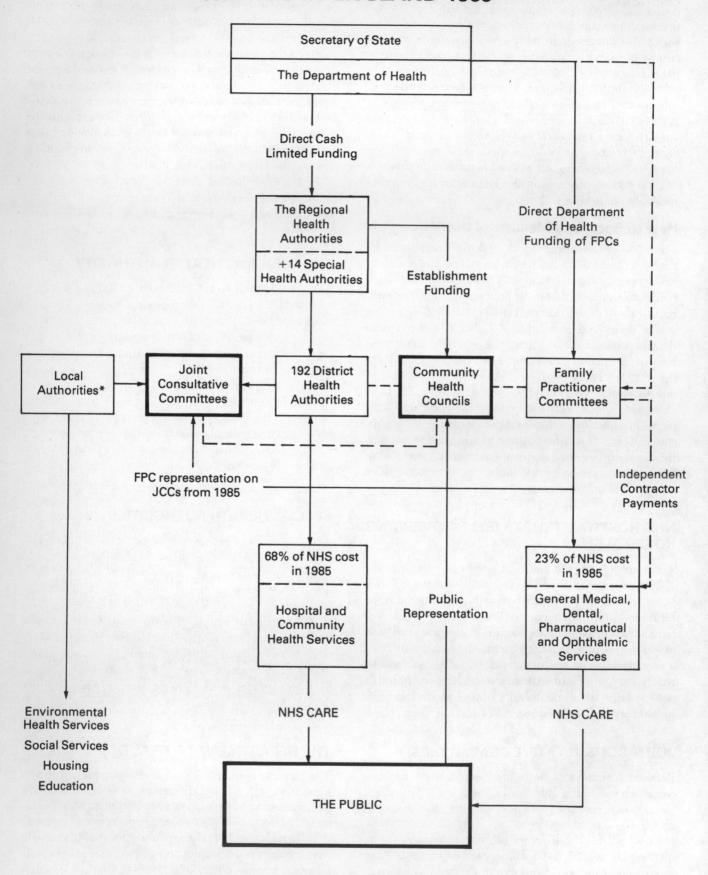

Source: From *Agenda for Health*. A Report of the Association of British Pharmaceutical Industry.

*For NHS Hospital Trusts, see page 645.

THE HEALTH SERVICE COMMISSIONER

The Health Service Commissioner is often referred to as the 'Ombudsman'. He (it has always been a he) is there to investigate individual complaints about the working of the NHS. He can deal only with individuals, who have the right to contact him direct (see p. 633 for more information).

INFLUENCING CARE SERVICES

Below district level – in the neighbourhood or patch – different professionals work side by side but are accountable to different authorities or employers. This can be confusing for groups seeking change.

If you want to influence a particular service, it will save you work if you begin by researching who is the appropriate person to introduce changes. With the most recent reorganization, management responsibility for community services in most areas has been gathered under a Community Unit General Manager. So, if you think, for example, there is a need for a community ante-natal clinic in your area or for a chiropody clinic, it might be appropriate to approach the Community Unit General Manager. However, if you think midwives are not competent or the health visitor's attitude unhelpful, a meeting with the Head of Midwifery or Health Visiting might be more useful. For a change in the GP service or dental service you will have to approach the FPC. Comments on receptionists or practice nurses should go to the GP who employs them, and problems with social workers should be addressed to the Director of Social Services.

GPs are independent contractors who have a contract to provide certain services; whether they agree to work with your group or respond to its request is entirely up to them. Some will have *patient participation groups* where patients can discuss practice arrangements or have talks about health-care problems. These have almost exclusively been set up because the GPs wanted them. If you think your GP should have one, ask him or her.

If it is the provision of local service you are concerned about, you will have to arrange (or get your CHC to arrange) a meeting bringing together the key people. If there is no response, it may help to get support from the patch councillors, the MP and the local press. You may then at least get an agreement to look at the issue. Then you'll have to keep nagging and pushing and monitoring until something happens. It is usually more difficult to achieve the reorganization of existing services than to get a new service set up. It helps to have supporters inside the system who will help.

INFLUENCING THE HOSPITAL

Women's health care is affected by access to clinics and hospital beds but also by the attitudes of the hospital managers and particularly the consultants. You may be intimidated by the thought of approaching consultants but since they rarely enter into face-to-face discussions with fully clothed women who are telling them what they want, it is worth remembering that even prestigious hospital consultants can feel threatened.

If you are concerned about clinical practice – a consultant who doesn't offer women choice, a consultant who you believe is doing excessive surgery on women – or you simply want to find out what the policy is in the obstetric unit or the infertility clinic, ask for a meeting with the consultants concerned or ask them to speak at one of your meetings. In the experience of City and Hackney CHC, a request for a meeting with a consultant, channelled through the CHC, has never been turned down.

But beware:

Consultants/doctors seem to have perfected the art of throwing red herrings on to the table, or responding to concerns with a personal anecdote to elicit sympathy, to show how difficult is their role. This usually means that the issue under discussion gets lost while everybody exchanges anecdotes. Women going to a meeting with doctors need to plan in advance how they will deal with this type of behaviour, how to stick to their agenda and not get side-tracked into discussing an individual experience unless it is agreed in advance.

Getting change in clinical practice will mean more than getting the consultants to change their practices. Women's groups seeking this sort of change will benefit if they can get the support of women working in the service. Do not expect that support to be automatic. Women workers are the least powerful members of the NHS hierarchy. A change in protocol handed down by a consultant may well be resented by someone who feels the burden of carrying out orders without sufficient involvement in decision-making. The very same 'bolshiness' that we value in midwives who have stood out against the indiscriminate use of technology can be turned against consumers who approach them in an insensitive and high-handed way.

As one midwife said:

The midwives feel caught between the consultants with their protocols and the women who want each delivery to be individual. They are expected to make constantly changing, sensitive and responsible decisions and yet they are given neither the recognition nor the pay they feel they deserve. Many of them have just stopped caring.

It may help to make your approach at two levels, through the management hierarchy and by asking to attend midwives' meetings, sisters' meetings or medical staff committees to discuss the issues that concern you. For most people these meetings are intimidating experiences and will require a lot of work and support for the women participating.

If sufficient women's groups did this in enough health

districts, women would know more about the health service, the health service would be more responsive and it would be easier to run national campaigns.

WORKERS ORGANIZING FOR BETTER SERVICES

Women working for change inside the system are often very isolated. We need to find ways of stretching across the professional divide if we are to succeed in improving services. There are different ways of approaching change.

UNIONS

Unions can provide the means of breaking down the isolation and tackling the power of the hierarchy. However, unions can also be a force against change. The difference lies in the attitude and involvement of ordinary rank-and-file members.

Jenny Koch decided to join the Confederation of Health Service Employees (COHSE) and persuaded her fellow midwives to join too when they discovered new attempts to streamline administration threatened the existence of community midwifery in High Wycombe, Buckinghamshire. The administration planned to bring all the community midwives into the GP unit where they would work rotating shifts; a plan which would destroy continuity of care as well as taking the heart out of their jobs. With the help of the union they successfully resisted restructuring. Jenny feels that union involvement was crucial:

Our union official knew we were completely green.

He managed to stall things for two years during which time we gained confidence and skill.

That battle was won but Jenny still finds the need to keep vigilant as the authority finds new ways of cost-cutting at the expense of women.

The experience of cleaners at the Barking Hospital in London was not so positive. They spent more than a year out on strike when the contractor who employed them cut costs by 40 per cent in an attempt to win a new contract. The changes drastically cut their wages and they were expected to work shifts which would have been totally incompatible with any child-care responsibility as well as being unsocial in every other sense. The strike raised the whole question of the role of cleaners. As one of them stated:

Domestics are part of a team, we care for patients too, the nurses rely on us.

During the strike, the work carried out by non-union labour was described in an independent report as:

So far deficient that routine cleaning will be insufficient to redress the situation.

Sadly, the strike was lost. In spite of initial enthusiasm, the union (the National Union of Public Employees) kept the control of the strike out of the hands of the strikers. Finally, the pickets were called off against their will. It would have been a hard battle to win in any case but the women were let down both by their own union and by their failure to appeal to NHS users whose health had been endangered by cost-cutting. The women did, however,

---

CHANGE COMES SLOWLY

To succeed in influencing the delivery of health care, a useful first step is for group members to attend as many committees as possible. Your ability to influence will depend:

1. on your knowledge and ability to put and sustain arguments against the professionals;

2. on your ability to develop an intelligence network – people who will keep you informed about what is happening (health service staff are often only too willing to provide members of health authorities or community groups with information although they may need reassurance about anonymity);

3. on your ability to make alliance with a variety of people who may have nothing in common with you but some vague concern for the NHS and fair play;

4. on the amount of time and energy you can put

into going to meetings and making informed contributions;

5. on the ability to make information public that the health authority would prefer to keep to itself (the ability to shame an authority or a powerful individual is a powerful weapon – as a minimum you should aim to produce a newsletter and have contacts with the local press);

6. on setting very limited goals to protect you from despair, because limited success will begin to give the group a sense of power – learning on the small issues will develop skill and expertise and contacts to take on the bigger issues;

7. on the other women's health groups and other women's groups being ready to help and to share their knowledge. (See also box on Organizing, p. 641.)

WOMEN-SENSITIVE SERVICES:
WELL WOMAN CLINICS

Campaigns for well woman clinics have been a major focus of women's health campaigns. The setting up of clinics has both shown that health services can be sensitized to women's needs and has challenged the rest of the system.

However, so far, even those clinics which are run by the health authorities remain on the edge of the health-care system, advising not treating, diagnosing but not continuing care. So women have to go to the GPs they didn't want to go to in the first place, for treatment or referral to consultants.

The answer to an insensitive service cannot lie simply in the setting up of a special facility. At worst, a well woman clinic may be merely a screening service and no more woman-sensitive than the rest of the system. At best it can demonstrate what a sensitive service can be, provide a short-term solution, help us develop our knowledge of the system and give us a sense of achievement. But we must not be conned into stopping there.

We must ask ourselves if, instead of campaigning for a well woman clinic, we would not do better to campaign for a place on the appointments panel for GPs; or to lobby group practices of GPs about the non-availability of women GPs or about their services for women. Perhaps we could challenge them to have a counsellor or social worker on their staff or a specially trained nurse. If there were sufficient numbers of sensitive GPs in our patch would we need well woman clinics?

If, having considered the options, a well woman clinic seems to be the best place to start, it is important to be absolutely clear about what we want. If we want health counselling and screening, with self-help groups attached, do we need a doctor in the clinic? Would a nurse practitioner/nurse counsellor be more appropriate? If we decide that we do need doctors in the clinic, do we not also want them to be able to treat us and to refer us to specialists? If so, should there be regular visits from appropriate specialists to the clinics, e.g. the consultant gynaecologist? This would give us opportunities to influence him or her as well as getting treatment. Should the clinic doctor be able to prescribe rather than sending women back to GPs they feel uncomfortable with?

In campaigns for services for women we must be wary of falling into a trap. We must make sure we are not left on the fringe.

---

write, with the help of the Labour Research Department, a 'Workers Plan' (see Resources) setting out just how a hospital should be cleaned to safeguard the health of patients.

MANAGEMENT

Getting into management is one way to influence decision-making. However, the struggle to reach a position high enough to acquire influence risks isolation from the needs of the people whose concerns we wish to affect, whereas change at a lower level may be temporary.

When feminists do get into positions from which they can make real changes, it is up to the rest of us to support and *pressurize* them so that they continue to feel accountable to users.

JOINT CAMPAIGNS

Joint campaigns can be far more powerful than any one group acting alone. Very often radical changes have been made through an alliance between a progressive consultant and an energetic local group. Broader campaigns have the potential for changing policy in more than one area which could outlive the enthusiasm of the person who initiated them.

The Association of Radical Midwives launched their document 'The Vision' with support from all the major maternity service user-groups. It suggests that midwives should be set up in community practices within the NHS as professional practitioners independent of doctors, seeing most women and referring to consultants only in response to a clear need. These radical plans are now being discussed throughout the health service by midwives, and the Royal College of Midwives has come up with a plan which is very similar. Together, midwives and mothers stand a better chance of influencing decision-makers. At the time of writing no moves had been made to link the RCM and ARM campaigns; however, a tripartite alliance between the ARM, maternity organizations and the unions would be a very strong force for radical change.

Useful alliances can also be made at a local level between different groups working outside the NHS. Working together can stimulate new thinking in each participant group, and creates powerful pressure for change. For example in Hackney, East London, the Town Hall Women's Unit and the City and Hackney CHC Women's Health Group joined forces to start a programme of health discussions at the town hall. Some Town Hall employees had become concerned about screening for cervical cancer, and had arranged for the district health authority's Mobile Screening Unit to visit the town hall. The CHC Women's Health Group had been looking at facilities for treatment of abnormal smears and cervical cancer, they were concerned

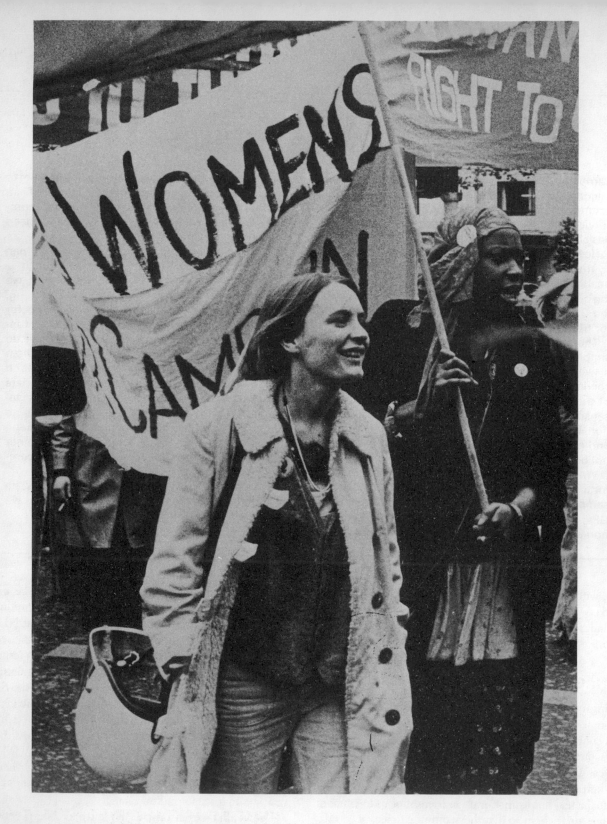

that publicity urging women to be screened should not only describe in detail what happens to you if you have an abnormal smear, but should also include what is known about causes of cervical cancer, and about its prevention.

The two groups got together and organized a mass meeting on these aspects of cervical cancer for all women employed by the local authority, and women in the community. They also prepared a detailed pamphlet on prevention, causes and how the local services work. The meeting was advertised through the pay packet of every local authority employee, in the local press and in the community. It was held over an extended lunchtime, and the unions negotiated time off where necessary for any employee wanting to attend. One speaker came from the Health District and the other was a feminist health researcher.

The success of the meeting lay in the fact that, far from a traditional health education exhortation telling women what to do, it provided detailed scientific information in a format which was understandable to women from all backgrounds.

Even when you get initial action, backsliding can start quickly. Women's groups need good sources of information and need to be frequently checking on apparent successes. Joint pressure from workers and consumers provides a measure of protection and monitoring, as the following experience in Hackney shows.

Women are always shocked when told that in many hospitals medical students are lined up in operating theatres to be taught how to examine women vaginally while they are unconscious. One nurse described seeing sixteen medical students lined up in this way. That this exercise is often carried out in an atmosphere of ribaldry further disgusts many nurses and medical students.

In Hackney the CHC asked for this procedure to be stopped unless women had given their permission in advance. Theatre staff and gynaecologists were asked to stop the practice of mass examinations. Two years later student nurses wrote to the Royal College of Nursing complaining about the practice. The General Manager, under threat of action from the RCN, told the Department of Obstetrics and Gynaecology the practice had to cease forthwith, and a policy document has since been issued banning the practice.

WORKING OUTSIDE THE HEALTH SERVICE

Some groups choose to work outside the health service, aiming to change policies and practices by publicity and by lobbying people in power. This approach can be effective with single issues, e.g. where a change in the law is needed. However, without support and representation at local level, such campaigns can easily become divorced from the real needs of the people they try to represent.

For example, in the early 1960s the Abortion Law Reform Association campaigned for liberalization of our restrictive abortion laws. Operating simply as a pressure group, without mass, grassroots support, they were forced to depend on sympathy for a minority of 'feckless women' to change the minds of MPs. As a result they had to agree to a law which gives doctors, rather than women, control over the decision to have an abortion.

In countries where abortion reform was the demand of a mass movement, with local and national involvement, much more radical legal changes were demanded, and won. Organizations arguing for a change in the delivery of existing services are even more dependent on local involvement, in order to keep in touch with the real needs of people using the services, and to provide channels for disseminating information, resources, expertise and support.

Where information exchange works well, the national dimension can provide a powerful focus for campaigning work. The expertise and public profile of the national office can effectively bring local concerns to a public forum with a speed and force which may be impossible for people running a small local campaign on a voluntary basis. Two organizations which operate nationally are the Maternity Alliance and the Association for Improvements in Maternity Services.

The Maternity Alliance

This is a national voluntary organization which campaigns for the improvements in rights and services of mothers, fathers and babies, and brings together a wide range of other organizations. The membership, which includes health professional organizations, voluntary organizations, unions and other pressure groups, reflects the view that changes in health and health-care depend on social, economic and political shifts.

The Maternity Alliance links housing and poverty with parental and child health. It campaigns on maternity and child benefits alongside the need for monitoring of caesarean births, on the needs of black and ethnic minority groups, on the effects of bad housing, on rights for working parents and their children, and on services for handicapped children and their families. An important tool, as in many pressure groups, is its bulletin and the reports, books and leaflets that it produces.

Until recently the Maternity Alliance worked mainly as a lobbying organization. It made contact with people through conferences and meetings attended largely by professionals. In campaigning, rather unsuccessfully, for improvements in maternity benefits and improved parental rights in employment, the Alliance recognized the need for more grassroots involvement. As a result it established a campaign (Maternity Emergency) with regional representation to fight for a major change in public consciousness on this issue.

The Association for Improvements in Maternity Services

AIMS is best known for its valuable and detailed independent critiques of research and technology in obstetrics. It has a regular newsletter produced by volunteers. In an attempt to fight for local implementation of the reforms they have been campaigning for nationally, regional AIMs groups have been established for women concerned to improve services locally. Women in local AIMs groups are encouraged to become active with their local community health councils. This way, the expertise and passionate concern of women willing to take on difficult areas of medical practice feeds into the user organization with its foot in the door of the local health services.

THE NHS IN CRISIS?

Since its inception the NHS has been short of money. Most of its staff have been underpaid, in some cases dramatically underpaid.

It has tried to provide twentieth-century medicine in under-capitalized Victorian hospitals. It has always raided the maintenance budgets to pay for day-to-day services. It has always provided comprehensive medical care on the cheap. Britain spends less on its health care than any other country in Europe except Greece. Its philosophy was always to provide a national service but, as in most things, the prosperous regions tended to have greater access to acute hospital care than other parts of the country. The general hospitals took the lion's share of the resources available, leaving mental illness, primary care, and services specifically for the elderly and mentally handicapped as the poor relations.

These problems have been aggravated in the 1980s by the inevitably increasing demands made on the services by

- an ageing population;
- medical technology that has made possible new and ever more expensive ways of diagnosing and treating our ailments, creating, in some cases, increased demand for more intervention;
- the private sector public-relations industry encouraging us to demand that the care be provided in better conditions;
- pressure from consumer organizations for a more responsive service;
- but most of all in recent years by the most serious underfunding ever, which is starving the NHS to death.

While the Government is looking for ways to control costs, it overlooks the fact that the NHS is the second cheapest system in Europe. Efficiency and better distribution of services cannot be achieved through the introduction of a market-orientated, cost-cutting system. In order to maintain a viable service, a significant amount of extra money is now needed.

A financial standstill, coupled with several major management reorganizations, has created the impression that the NHS is collapsing. This is further reinforced by Government promotion of insurance-based systems of health care; by its championing of private medicine in competition with the NHS; and by its insistence on privatization of services such as catering. There is a limit to the amount of major change any organization can take within a given period and the NHS has suffered continuous change for nearly two decades now. Little wonder that it has not had time, or money, to sort out the real management problems of health-care delivery at a local level.

However, the NHS has not collapsed. It still provides a superb service to many, in particular to the group that it has always served well – those suffering from acute conditions. The care that it gives to people who are elderly or mentally ill has always left much to be desired; so, too, do the conditions in which much good care is delivered.

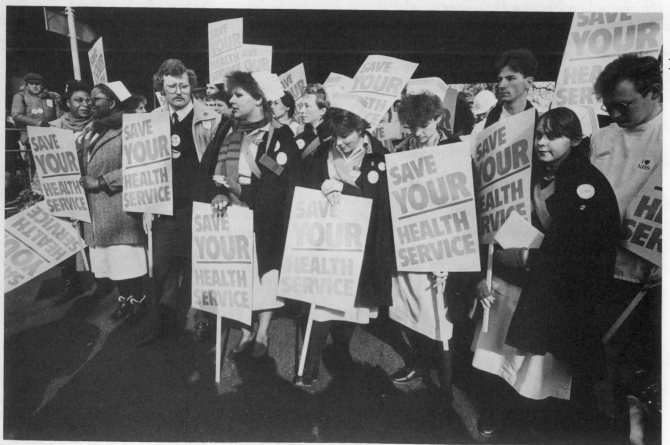

Times Newspapers Ltd

THE NHS WORKS: SAVE IT

ANGELA PHILLIPS

In the time it has taken to write this book there has been a radical change in thinking about the status of our National Health Service. As we started to work, the Conservatives were declaring that 'The NHS is safe in our hands.' As we finish, there is more and more talk of finding new sources of cash to prop up the system and a growing public assumption that health care is simply too expensive to provide through taxation. Edwina Currie, then junior Health Minister, told us that people will have to get used to paying for their own hip replacements instead of having a second holiday.

A system based on private cash would provide a first-class service to those of us who can afford second holidays. That does not include, for example, the one in every eight families who are headed by single parents (usually women). There is, in fact, no evidence that private sources of financing could improve the system as a whole. In fact, the reverse is true, as evidence from other countries clearly shows.

Indeed, Italy and Spain are moving away from insurance-based to tax-based health care simply because it is cheaper and more efficient to deliver. The Danish system is already tax-based.

The USA is always held up as the classic example of a country with an almost entirely private health-care system. Being private certainly hasn't made it efficient. The USA spends more money per head on health care than any other country. However, while the well-off and well-insured do pretty well out of the system, between 35 and 40 million people have no health insurance cover either public or private. They literally cannot afford to be ill. Many insurance policies do not cover maternity costs. A premature birth can be a total financial disaster. Parents of sick babies may be in debt for years paying back the cost of care.

Given these massive inequalities in health care, it is not surprising that the USA, the richest country in the world, has the fourth highest infant mortality rate (one of the most sensitive indicators of a nation's health) of the twenty-four OECD countries (Organization for Economic Cooperation and Development). Sweden and The Netherlands, both of which spend proportionately more public money on health care than we do, have the lowest rates. In Britain, as private health-care services have been growing, and public sector investment in healthcare has been shrinking, the infant mortality rate has started to rise for the first time in eighteen years.

The NHS has in the past been able to provide health care for everyone at a lower cost than many other countries. But, as a result of relentless under-funding by the Thatcher Government, the NHS now faces its biggest crisis ever. In spite of the much vaunted extra expenditure during the 1980s, the health-care services have suffered from a higher rate of inflation than other industries. Since government spending has not risen to cover this inflation, the actual amount left to spend has been declining at the rate of 1.5 per cent per year (see chart overleaf).

Over a period of several years this, together with the government's refusal to fund pay awards, has had a devastating effect: wards have closed, staff have been cut and morale destroyed. Far from being an inefficient service in need of wholesale reorganization and private investment, Peter Oppenheimer, an Oxford economist, contends that:

> One of the few visible sources of waste in Britain's hospital service today is the amount of health professionals' time taken up by futile corner-cutting in order to cope with real cuts imposed in the present decade.[1]

The situation is no different in the community-based services either. Since our public spending on health care is currently 10 per cent below the OECD average (1985), the remedy for the health service's ills lies very firmly in the hands of the government.

The NHS needs more money and we must fight for that. But that is not enough. As feminists we must find ways to feminize the health-care agenda. If choices are to be made, we must be there, applying pressure, participating in the decision-making. Do we want to spend more money on transplants or on care for the dying? On preventing sexually transmitted disease or paying for research into *in vitro* fertilization? As women we are close to the needs of carers and those they care for, and can make radical demands which others may not have thought of.

TOTAL HEALTH EXPENDITURE PER HEAD (1985)

USA	£992.17	Denmark	£421.78
Canada	£716.20	Italy	£378.77
Sweden	£654.74	**UK**	**£349.16**
France	£598.88	Spain	£254.74
Germany	£549.16	Greece	£140.78
Holland	£524.02		

OECD average   £473.74

HEALTH SPENDING AS % OF GDP (1985)

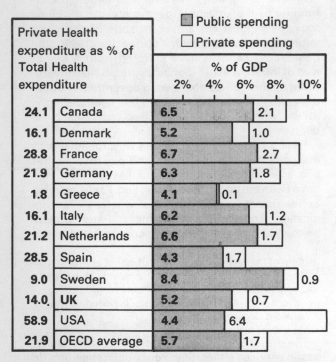

Private Health expenditure as % of Total Health expenditure		Public spending / Private spending — % of GDP
24.1	Canada	6.5 / 2.1
16.1	Denmark	5.2 / 1.0
28.8	France	6.7 / 2.7
21.9	Germany	6.3 / 1.8
1.8	Greece	4.1 / 0.1
16.1	Italy	6.2 / 1.2
21.2	Netherlands	6.6 / 1.7
28.5	Spain	4.3 / 1.7
9.0	Sweden	8.4 / 0.9
14.0	UK	5.2 / 0.7
58.9	USA	4.4 / 6.4
21.9	OECD average	5.7 / 1.7

Source: Nicholas Timmins, *The Independent*, 7 March 1988, p. 17.

When Wandsworth CHC read the GLC report on women as carers, we immediately picked up on one of the recommendations – that if people are going to care for others in the community they should be assisted to do so. One of the very basic things which might help families to care for their relatives might be the provision of 'hard white goods', like washing-machines and tumble-driers. Accordingly, our CHC wrote a proposal for funding from the Urban Programme for the purchase of washing-machines and similar aids and adaptations for people caring for their relatives in the community. We had tremendous arguments with the male administrator, who said 'surely everyone has one'. That was the first response, and then, 'My God! What on earth will that CHC come up with next.' But finally we got it through on the Urban Programme and the £50,000 has gone and we're hoping to get more.[2]

Women are involved in the NHS as users and low-paid workers, not as decision-makers. No matter how much money there is, feminists are going to have to work hard, analyse the service, raise the issues which concern us, and at the same time tackle sexism in medical cultures. We have made a start. There is a long way to go.

WELL, WOMAN?

When I am well, the joy of life wells up within
  me.
What is the source of spring?
Life springs from the earth; and from the earth's
  deep caverns
Water of life wells up, fresh, cold and clear.

I sit on the brim of the pool, looking at my
  reflection.
Is it my face I see, or the face of another?
Am I separated from myself?
It looks cool, strange, distant from me.
Moves as I move; turns as I turn.
But I do not feel it. Am I myself and yet another?

She regards me from deep waters, the woman of
  the well.

Is there not always another self, watching from the
  deep waters?
My being is here above the earth, acting my life.
But I know that in the deepest part of me I am
  distant,
Watching my life acted.
I am being above, and being below.
I reflect upon my life.

When I am full of joy and strength, I act as one
  being.
But when my strength ebbs, and my joys wane,
I am conscious of being watched and being the
  watcher.
The watcher is the woman of the well.
She is my well being.

If I am sad, the sadness is shared above and
  below.
A strong sadness makes my well being weep,
Even when my face is smiling.
When I have served someone ill, my well being is
  ashamed.
My face hides my shame, and laughs, or turns
  away.
But my well being is upset, and I cannot act as
  one.
I am divided until I face the truth.
My face looks on my reflection and acknowledges
  the wrong.

Then I am content and can act with sorrow,
To right the wrong.
When women are well they are whole,
  and not divided against themselves.

Sometimes when the moon is new,
And I am rested, and ready to begin new tasks,
I feel strength and hope well up in me.
My well being is rising up to act within me.
She is my will.

My will is strong, to act courageously.
Women will as woman needs, to take action;
To take part in every part of life.
To take a woman's part?

On reflection, we see ourselves,
And we see that we are not images on the surface
  of life;
Images for others to play with.
We are whole people.

And our part in life is to take part in all life;
To bring together all parts of life,
So that life is made whole.
It is the will of woman that the earth be made
  whole.

When we are divided against ourselves we are
  sick.
Health is wholeness.
To make whole is to heal.
To be whole is a holy thing.

© FREDA DAVIS

'will' and 'well' come from the germanic word 'wel'.
  'whole' is from the germanic word 'hailaz'
other words have grown from the same 'hailaz':
    'hale', 'heal' . . . written 'hailan'
    'hailitha' . . . that is 'health'
  also from health 'hailaz' comes 'hailagaz',
        which we say 'holy'.

NOTES

1. *The Independent*, 7 March 1988.
2. Caroline Langridge, CHC Secretary, Wandsworth CHC in Equal
Opportunity Policies.

DEVELOPING AN INTERNATIONAL AWARENESS

Rewritten by
KATH FRASER AND JILL RAKUSEN

As feminists, we feel a strong bond with all women. We believe that feminism as a political perspective must look across national boundaries to address all the issues which affect women's lives.

All of us have been systematically denied access to crucial information about our bodies, whether we live, for example, in Europe, Africa, Asia, Australia, Latin America or the USA. Denial of reproductive rights, domestic violence, rape, sexual harassment in the workplace or on the street, racism, sexism, repression of lesbians, occupational hazards, economic exploitation, poverty and the horrors of war – none of these respects national boundaries. From a rural women's health and education group in South India:

> When we read about women like us, rural, poor, from other parts of the world, we begin to feel women are similarly placed all over the world. The cultural contexts may differ, but the exploitation of women is the same everywhere.[1]

We have to take responsibility for the ways our countries' policies affect the lives of women elsewhere.

American and European feminists, by being uninformed about their sisters in other countries, contribute unwittingly to their exploitation.[2]

In 1956, in protest against the South African government's extension of its 'pass laws', 20,000 women marched on Pretoria singing:

Now you have tampered with the women
You have struck against rock
You have dislodged a boulder
You will be crushed.

On International Women's Day 1984, twenty-five women involved in Birmingham WONT (Women Oppose the Nuclear Threat) 'chained up' Hiatt's, a Birmingham factory which specializes in the manufacture of torture equipment. For 200 years the company has been exporting 'made-to-measure' gang-chains, leg-irons and handcuffs to South Africa, other African states and Middle East countries, for use in prisons to carry out torture and to perpetuate slavery.

They took this action on International Women's Day to express solidarity with and support for women all over the world who are tortured because they are involved in liberation struggles.

We leafleted neighbouring houses, passers-by and workers from other local factories, and got a fairly positive response to our protest. Although most Hiatt workers were told not to speak to us (most were women or young men who are non-unionized), some did come out in their lunch break and were not hostile to us.

We have publicly expressed our disgust at Hiatt's immoral trading practices, initially exposed in the *Daily Mirror* several weeks ago. This is part of our continuing campaign against militarism, and as part of our commitment to International Women's Liberation.[3]

For example, if we succeed in having dangerous contraceptives or other consumer products removed from the UK, manufacturers may dump them on Third World women, as was the case with high-oestrogen pills and hormonal 'pregnancy tests' (banned in Britain in 1975). Our activism must include organizing with women of other countries to prevent such abuses.

Opening our eyes to common issues and being aware and respectful of our different realities, women around the world can better understand and support one another.

Over 4,000 Finnish women of childbearing age are refusing to have children unless the government closes down the Finnish nuclear power stations (which produce 40 per cent of Finland's electricity) by 1990.

A protest document with the slogan 'Nuclear power shall not waste our children's lives' points out that 'Our security has up till now been decided by middle-aged men.'

COMMON ISSUES

Sexism, or discrimination on the basis of sex, is a universal problem. There are differences in the varying forms and degrees, but all patriarchal societies (dominated by men and organized around their activities and goals) circumscribe girls' and women's basic rights and opportunities.

Women around the world face the imperative to bear children. Western, Islamic and African cultures all value us as childbearers, homemakers and consumers above all. Yet we are not only childbearers: women's participation worldwide in the agricultural labour force is between 40 and 50 per cent.[4] Whatever work women do outside the home, it tends to carry a low status. For example, women run small businesses in Thailand – this is regarded as a lowly occupation.[5]

REPRODUCTIVE RIGHTS

Control of our bodies is a core feminist issue. Whether it is forced sterilization or its denial, illegal abortion or restricted availability of legal abortion, forced abortion, lack of maternity and infertility or contraceptive services, or wife-beating, sexual slavery, rape and harassment, 'crimes of passion', the meaning is the same: women are not free to control their own bodies. In the words of an Indian woman:

We are brought up to view our bodies with suspicion and contempt, and this gives us a poor self-image. We are taught to consider our very existence as women as a misfortune; we never understood the way our bodies functioned and always feared or were ashamed of natural happenings like menstruation, pregnancy, childbirth.

A healthy attitude towards our bodies would help us develop our self-respect, and such self-awareness is the first step towards playing an active role in our communities to change the unjust structures of which we are a part.[6]

When we say women must have reproductive freedom, we mean the possibility of controlling for ourselves, in a real and practical way – that is, free from economic, social or legal coercion – whether and under what conditions we will have children.[7]

Women all over the world increasingly see reproductive rights issues as central to self-determination.

The Women's Global Network on Reproductive Rights (formerly the International Contraceptive, Abortion and Sterilization Campaign – ICASC) grew out of women's struggles for the right to control our fertility. It is a network of local, national and regional women's campaigning groups, women's health centres and others working in their own countries for reproductive rights and joining together to fight the common battle internationally because the forces are international. Since the forces manipulating women's reproduction are many and powerful – governments, multinational corporations, organized religion, the pharmaceutical industry, population control agencies, the medical establishment and anti-abortion organizations – we need an international campaign to counteract them effectively.

Population control concretely violates our rights by determining our birth patterns through international and national policy. Many people see overpopulation as the world's priority issue, believing that it causes mass starvation, ecological destruction, social disruption, violence and poverty. On the contrary, we believe that it is not overpopulation but the inequitable distribution of the world's resources that has led to and perpetuated a cycle of poverty and misery for many of the world's peoples. Britain and other industrialized countries promote this inequity through our economic control over Third World economies, forcing them to produce for us instead of for themselves, not only goods but also interest payments on money we lend them (see also Development, p. 658). The USA alone consumes one-third of the world's resources to support only 6 per cent of the world's population.*

Those who advocate population control do not ask basic questions about the just distribution of resources. The Western ideology of 'population control' includes the use of family planning programmes, social and economic policies, foreign aid and educational materials to persuade people to reduce numbers of births. Often the programmes are aimed at particular groups within a country – usually the poor. This is very different from 'birth control', which we see as being every woman's right to control her fertility through birth control information and services. The population control establishment too often encourages

---

*See Resources for books by Mass, George, and Hartmann, and information from War on Want and Women's Global Network on Reproductive Rights. Organizations like Traidcraft buy *direct* from Third World producers, with a commitment to benefiting them.

drugs and techniques which may be dangerous, poorly researched or poorly monitored, rather than safer methods like the diaphragm, cap, condom or fertility observation. In many Third World countries money, food, clothing and other economic incentives are widely offered to women who accept IUDs, Depo Provera or sterilization, and are withheld when these are refused. Population control programmes to lower a country's birth-rate have little regard for local cultural, social and economic factors affecting the numbers of children born: for example, in the poorest rural areas up to half of all babies die in their first year.

Too often agencies do not consult users in the allocation of funds, and hire too few women to design, implement or evaluate their programmes. One of the better uses of money is in the training of traditional birth attendants who serve 90 per cent of women in developing countries. War on Want has given funds for additional training to midwives in Eritrea, Angola and Guatemala for example.

We must ask many questions about birth control programmes overseas: who controls the programme being offered? Who funds it, and what strings are attached? Are incentives or disincentives offered? Who distributes the contraceptives, and what kind? What kind of follow-up health care is provided? What kind of information and instructions are offered? Most important, what kinds of birth control do people really want?

Another form of population control is when economic and social policies dictate that an *increase* in the birth-rate is desirable. Policies aiming to increase as well as reduce births are both forms of social control, manipulating our choices to some political end. Pro-natalist policies may be punitive towards women who have no, or even a few, children. In Britain we are hearing the ugly idea raised again that certain types of women (i.e. those who are white and middle class) should do their duty by their country and breed more while the rest of us should breed less. This represents the thin end of a wedge that leads to pernicious policies like drastic abortion restrictions in Hungary, and those of Singapore, where higher-educated women were encouraged to have more children and others penalized for it by threats to their housing and benefits.

Although abortion restrictions often conflict with population control, abortion is subject to religious taboos. Largely because of the power of organized religion, it is illegal in parts of Europe and Asia, all Latin America, and in most of Africa. Even where it is legal, as in India, few women may be aware of this, rural women have no access to medical facilities, and those who do manage to obtain an abortion receive deplorable treatment. In Italy many doctors refuse to perform abortions on grounds of 'conscience', but manage to overcome their scruples if a woman pays them privately. In the USA poor women are denied access to Medicaid for legal abortions. Illegal abortions are second only to childbirth as the world's major cause of maternal death. We deplore the carnage that results from the unavailability of safe procedures.

EXPORTING MISGUIDED PRIORITIES

DEVELOPMENT

The word 'development' usually means modernization and industrialization. Development theory is based on the history of Western industrialization, and assumes that Third World countries could and would choose to follow the same path of economic growth. 'Development experts', mostly Western males, study poverty, low productivity and unemployment as 'problems of underdevelopment'. They conceptualize programmes to alleviate these 'problems' after, at most, limited consultation with men in the countries involved. They then try to get individual governments or international/multinational agencies like the United Nations or the World Bank (to which they often belong) to fund these programmes either with low-interest loans or free assistance. The end products of such aid are often extremely high levels of debt for 'developing' nations and dependency on foreign goods, expertise and money.* The result is *under*-development.

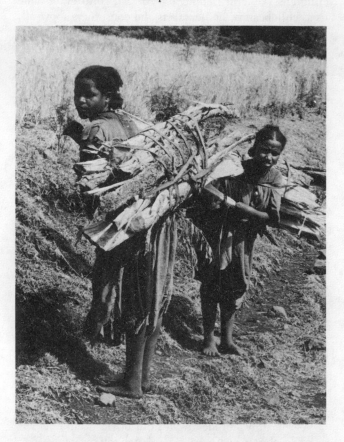

Women produce between half and two-thirds of the world's food, are integral to local distribution systems, food

*Even worse, the USA sometimes includes arms in foreign aid package deals.

processing and storage, and in many cultures have an important role as traders of foodstuffs. And yet this kind of development policy largely ignores such traditional roles. In newly irrigated, cleared areas, land titles are usually controlled by agribusiness – making local women and men into waged labourers. Where women work thus, it is usually on wages of less than half those of men, in the most manually intensive, back-breaking work, for example planting, weeding, fertilizing if this is done by hand, harvesting – e.g. of tea, sugar, coffee, fruits. Meanwhile many women are pushed off their traditional farming lands and forced to grow their subsistence food in less fertile, remote areas with reduced yields and increased workloads. The health of the whole community then suffers.

Planners find it hard to grasp that women need paid work. An Indian woman writes:

> There is a prevailing myth that women live like parasites off the earnings of their husbands, but we found the reverse to be true. The women who came to Saheli [a women's resource centre in Delhi] were women who had worked before and after their marriage – they earned their own living and had often built assets (i.e. dowry) for their new homes – yet when the marriage broke up, they usually lost all these assets.[8]

Development programmes generally offer extension programmes and training only to men, thereby denying women opportunities for learning new skills.

> Society's acceptance of male domination pervades development work. Though much lip service is paid to the equal participation of women in the male-dominated development circles, there is little thought of real effort towards genuine power sharing with women.[9]

Where women have been displaced from their traditional role in the countryside this leads to drifting towards towns, where shortage of paid work forces many women into prostitution to feed themselves and their children. With the spread of HIV (see p. 501), this economic dislocation can become a death sentence, particularly in parts of Africa. In spite of safer sex campaigns, condoms are not always readily available.

In Britain in 1985 a new National Women's Network, highly critical of racism and sexism in aid policies, recommended increased funding for aid programmes giving women rights and access to land, credit and technical training, and for women's groups organizing for women's rights. Prevalent theory in large-scale aid is the 'integration' of women into development – no real change needed, in other words. We need instead a theory which both acknowledges women's central role in production *and* challenges the economic and political systems which oppress women.

More women in every country must be involved in designing and implementing flexible programmes to meet women's needs and to reflect their productive roles both inside and outside the home.

MULTINATIONAL CORPORATIONS

The multinational corporations (MNCs) have played a major role in the process of 'development' or 'underdevelopment' of Third World countries. The MNCs we are discussing here are those which have branches in different countries but retain concentration of capital and authority in the industrialized West. Even though they are often women's only source of paid employment, they have a primarily negative effect on Third World women's lives.

The MNCs force women to compete with one another. For example, women in the US and Britain buy products produced by the toil of Third World women under sweatshop conditions. Whenever women (in South Korea, for example) begin to organize for better wages and working conditions, industries pick up and move to another community. There is no job security when high technology makes immediate relocation possible.

Free Trade Zones (FTZs) are areas which have been set up to process goods for export since the 1950s, especially in newly-industrializing countries. They are government-established industrial development areas within which the country's normal legislation and labour protection codes do not apply. They are often in remote areas of a country and guarded by security forces; typically the operating companies are Western or Japanese owned, and enjoy special tax concessions. At least half of the FTZs are in Asia, and up to 85 per cent of employees are young women.[10]

Textiles, electronics and agribusiness are three industries which locate in developing countries because of tax incentives and the promise of cheap and docile labour. Women perform 80 to 90 per cent of low-skilled assembly jobs. The MNCs pay low wages for long hours in unhealthy working conditions and then claim they are 'liberating' women by giving them work.

> In the Philippines . . . starting wages in US-owned electronics plants are between $36 and $46 a month, compared to a 'cost of living' of $37 a month; in Indonesia the starting wages are actually about $7 a month less than the 'cost of living'. 'Living' is interpreted minimally: a diet of rice, dried fish, and water, lodging in a room occupied by four or more people.[11]

Female workers worldwide earn 40 to 60 per cent less than their male counterparts. Single women enlist for these new jobs often at the insistence of their families, who desperately need their earnings. Their move to urban areas means an upheaval – they lose their kin and community networks and in return receive no wage protection, work benefits, priority or seniority. They are the most exploited section of the formal labour force.

Health hazards abound in MNC workplaces. Often MNCs move processes which have been classified as dangerous to a Third World country, or simply ignore the safety regulations enforced in the originating country. Most electronics factories are kept clean to protect the microelectronics components. And yet the health risks are such that most women workers are laid off at about twenty-five years of age. Potential damage to fetuses of pregnant women is great, and MNC managers in South-East Asia respond by sacking pregnant women.

Electronics workers often lose the twenty/twenty vision needed for the job of peering through a microscope at tiny wires for seven to nine hours at a time to meet quotas; their pay rate is less than £1 per day. One study of South Korean electronics assembly workers found that, after only one year of employment, 88 per cent had chronic conjunctivitis, 44 per cent had become near-sighted and 19 per cent had developed astigmatism. In one stage of the electronic assembly process, workers have to dip the circuits into open vats of acid. In Penang, Malaysia, women wear gloves and boots to do dipping, but when these leak, burns are common, and the workers sometimes lose fingers in painful accidents.[12]

In Malaysia, mass hysteria has become a form of resistance. One young woman sees a *Hantu* or *jin* (hideous varieties of ghosts) and, screaming, falls to the floor in convulsions, and within minutes the hysteria spreads up and down the assembly line. Sometimes the plant has to close for a week or more to exorcise the spirits. Malaysian academics point out that the attacks are likely to be preceded by a speed-up or a tightening of plant discipline.[13] The women's actions release tension as well as delay production.

Stress is probably the most invidious health hazard. Stomach-aches and nervous problems reflect internalized anxieties and pressures of meeting production quotas. The death-rate among sixteen to thirty-year-old workers for the Ricoh Philippines Watch Company is very high, the most common causes being stomach ulcers and heart attacks. Management actually encourages a high turnover rate in many industries; because wages rise with seniority, it is cheaper to train a new batch of teenagers than to pay for an experienced 'older' (i.e. twenty-three or twenty-four-year-old) woman.

Textile and garment industry conditions rival those of any nineteenth- or twentieth-century Western sweatshop. Workers are packed into poorly lit rooms where summer temperatures rise above a hundred degrees; textile dust, which can cause permanent lung damage, fills the air; rush orders require forced overtime of as much as forty-eight hours at a stretch, with the management supplying pep pills and amphetamine injections as needed. In her diary, published in a magazine now banned by the government, a thirty-year-old South Korean sewing-machine operator describes conditions in the garment factory where she works from 7 a.m. to 11.30 p.m.

When apprentices shake the waste threads from the clothes, the whole room fills with dust, and it is hard to breathe. Since we've been working in such dusty air, there have been increasing numbers of people getting tuberculosis, bronchitis, and eye diseases . . . It seems to me that no one knows our blood dissolves into the threads and seams, with sighs and sorrow.[14]

The MNCs say they are contributing to development, but they come into a country for one thing – cheap labour. The MNCs started leaving Western countries when good unionization pushed up the cost of labour. Wherever the labour stops being so cheap, they move on. What kind of development is it that depends on people staying poor? Saralee Hamilton, an organizer of a 1978 conference on 'Women and Global Corporations', says:

The multinational corporations have deliberately targeted women for exploitation. If feminism is going to mean anything to women all over the world, it's going to have to find new ways to resist corporate power internationally.[15]

BABY FOOD

After the post-war baby boom when birth-rates were declining in the West, baby food companies looked to the relatively untouched Third World markets. Convinced by aggressive and often unethical advertising practices that a bottlefed baby will be healthier and more likely to survive than a breastfed baby,* millions of Third World mothers stopped breastfeeding, but were unable to maintain the sanitary conditions for mixing and storing the baby food, and often couldn't afford to purchase it in sufficient quantities. The result has been 10 million cases of severe malnutrition each year and approximately 3 million infant deaths.[16]

The baby food industry promotes the idea that women's bodies cannot keep babies healthy and that they need an expert, often a male doctor, to tell them what to do.

People around the world have organized a major campaign to stop these unethical practices. The Infant Formula Action Coalition (INFACT) and International Baby Food Action Network (IBFAN) began a boycott against Nestlé, a Swiss company, which is the world's largest multinational food corporation and generates almost half of all baby food sales in the developing world.[17] The demands: an end to direct consumer advertising; an end to promotion through and to members of the health-care professions; an end to company 'milk nurses'; and an end to free samples.

---

*Baby food manufacturers use a large repertoire of promotion tactics, including hoardings and posters showing healthy children next to company products. They send sales personnel dressed in nurses' uniforms to offer mothers advice on infant feeding and give them free samples. Taking advantage of the medicalization of childbirth, they vigorously promote their products to and through health-care providers, especially in hospitals.

The boycott has had an economic impact. In 1978 the Norwegian Dairy Sales Association cancelled its exclusive contract with Nestlé for the distribution of Jarlsberg cheese. The greatest success has been in consumer education, which has brought the whole issue to the international governmental-agency level for serious debate and action. As a result, the World Health Organization (WHO) developed an 'International Infant Formula Code of Marketing Behaviour' for the industry. When the World Health Assembly voted on the code in May 1980, every country voted in favour of it except the US, whose representatives stated that it infringed upon the free enterprise system.

It's not enough to attack baby food manufacturers. Women need adequate diets in order to breastfeed fully. Diet depends on rights and access to land – MNC control of food production and emphasis on cash crops creates poverty. Breastfeeding is not always possible when women have to work full time outside the home, in Western or Third World countries. Women's fight is not only against a technological culture which says it's better to bottlefeed, but also for increased maternity leave with pay during the breastfeeding months or workplaces where breastfeeding is routine, and acceptance of the fact that women have a right to make choices in these matters. As a Senegalese woman puts it:

> It's not enough to talk about the natural superiority of breast milk and the advantages to both the mother and infant. We have to create the conditions to make it possible for women to do this. Yes to breastfeeding, but . . . how?[18]

The Baby Food Action Coalition is a British-based group active on these issues; see p. 668.

DRUGS – THE IMPACT OF THE INTERNATIONAL DRUG INDUSTRY ON THIRD WORLD WOMEN

Some of the most powerful and profitable multinational corporations operate in the pharmaceutical industry. In 1976 the US accounted for one-fifth of this trade, Western Europe controlling most of the rest. By 1980 the total value of UK drug exports reached about £600 million, 40 per cent going to Third World and OPEC countries (Nigeria and the Gulf states). In Bangladesh in 1982, 75 per cent of the market was controlled by only eight multinational companies, including Fisons, Glaxo and ICI. The companies sometimes spend more on promotion in a Third World country than that country spends on its whole health budget.

Third World women are increasingly the targets for psychoactive drugs in particular. For example, tranquillizers are being pushed to silence women's complaints, building dependency problems as in the West. Potentially dangerous drugs are advertised as completely safe (contrary to the International Federation of Pharmaceutical Manufacturers' Association's voluntary code of practice): a 1983 survey by the International Organization of Consumers Unions (OUCU) found nine anabolic steroid products in use in Indonesia, Bangladesh, Malaysia, Philippines, Thailand and India, listing *no* side-effects. These drugs were being produced specifically for children to stimulate growth: in fact, after an initial growth spurt, the ultimate effect is to stunt bone development. Food is the best treatment for malnutrition.

It becomes extremely difficult for 'developing countries' to provide essential medicines for most of their populations – local industry is suppressed by the competition of MNCs (who often control the raw materials for production of essential drugs), the drugs most sold are those most profitable to the MNCs rather than essential to health (so the governments cannot then *afford* drugs for diseases that have been eliminated in the West), and the created dependence on imported technology stultifies local research and development.

Regulations governing clinical testing are much looser than in industrialized countries, mainly because of cost. This means Third World peoples are more likely to be used as guinea pigs in trials. The birth control pill was first tested on women (mostly poor and illiterate) in Puerto Rico and later in El Salvador, sometimes without their knowledge and with severe consequences for their health.

In many instances, drugs that are available only on prescription here are sold over the counter in the Third World. For example, in Peru, Italian-produced chocolate flavoured 'sweeties for diarrhoea' are sold to children at the corner shop. These contain two antibiotics – chloramphenicol, which has toxic side-effects, and tetracycline, which is not given to children under twelve years in the UK.

In a BBC radio broadcast in 1979 George Teeling Smith, Director of the Office of Health Economics, stated the situation plainly:

> The reason multinational companies try to grab as much profit as possible out of the less developed countries is frankly because they are suspicious of the future stability of their operation there. I would just be talking rubbish if I were to say that the multinational companies were operating in the less developed countries for the welfare of those countries.

In 1982 the Bangladesh government instituted a Drug Control Ordnance which listed 250 essential drugs, banned 237 products deemed to be harmful, and ordered that 1,500 others – non-essential – be phased out. The Ordnance had to be modified in response to MNC and US government pressure. Even the World Health Organization's support for the Bangladesh initiative was muted – despite having drawn up its own essential drugs list in 1977 – perhaps because 25 per cent of its budget comes from the US. Nevertheless, the Bangladesh health minister in 1984 said production of essential drugs had increased, local companies now supplied three-quarters of them, and prices had fallen.

At the World Health Assembly in Geneva in 1984, the US was the only country to oppose the 'Rational Use of Drugs' resolution. This calls for unbiased drug information for developing countries, and a meeting between governments, pharmaceutical industries and patients' and consumers' organizations. More governments, for example in Thailand and the Philippines, seem to be trying to tighten up legislation to restrict the activities of the drug MNCs, although all efforts are limited by governments' dependence on foreign investments.

Women's and consumer groups have contributed to the change of climate. Health Action International (HAI) was established in Geneva in May 1981 to coordinate activities and share ideas and resources internationally among consumers and development and public interest groups, as well as to provide the framework for international campaigns. HAI has set up an international clearing-house for information on the drug industry's structure, ownership and marketing practices, and has established an international consumer product warning network, 'The Consumer Interpol'. They have the pharmaceutical industry worried. The companies, of course, say they prefer to monitor themselves internally. Most worrying for them is the possibility that HAI may influence the WHO to adopt a regulatory drug code similar to the one for baby food marketing. For more discussion about the role of the drug industry, see Chapter 27.

WESTERN MEDICINE VS. INDIGENOUS SYSTEMS

We export Western medicine all over the world, under the guise of sharing 'expertise' (the so-called 'transfer of technology'). A tragic result is the devaluation and breakdown of indigenous health systems. For example, health-care planning in newly independent India (in 1948) assumed a need for increased Western medical science and technology, in spite of the historical existence and availability of the traditional Indian system of Ayurveda and yoga. Ayurvedic medicine, through its holistic approach, provides effective prevention for a range of health problems untouched by Western medicine. Ayurveda, like many traditional systems, is decentralized, giving individuals more control over their own health, a crucial factor in a country like India where 85 per cent of the people live in rural areas.[19] Infectious diseases are still prevalent; public health measures like clean water, sanitation and a proper diet (i.e. control of own food production) could prevent much more ill health than new machines and Western-style hospitals ever will.

Women all over the world suffer when governments accept physicians' monopoly over the direction of health policy. Two centuries ago the medical establishment in the industrialized world began to ostracize and persecute women healers, the midwives and abortionists who had

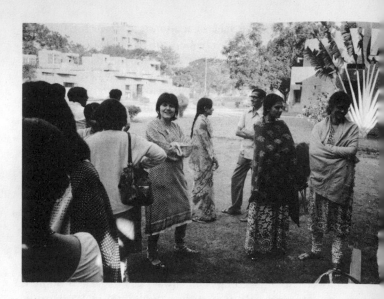

always served poor and rural women. 'Development' often means a similar shift in the Third World. Most countries need to keep health in the hands of community health providers, traditional healers and village health workers and to use doctors as auxiliaries or consultants, the role they should have in any case, based on their narrow, highly technical training.

FEMALE CIRCUMCISION

Female circumcision involves various types of genital mutilation. It is practised in many Arab and African communities. Between 20 and 74 million African females – mostly girls – undergo some form of genital removal every year. Traditional circumcision, or *sunna*, removes the hood of the clitoris. This is the mildest form. Excision, or *clitoridectomy*, involves cutting off part or all of the clitoris and the adjacent labia minora without actually closing the vulva. The most extreme and less common form is *infibulation* – Pharaonic circumcision – in which the clitoris and adjacent labia are completely removed and the two sides of the vulva stitched together, leaving a small opening for the flow of menstrual blood and urine. Traditionally, an infibulated woman is 'reopened' before her wedding night by a traditional midwife or in a clinic, or sometimes by her husband's repeated attempts at penetration. Women may be sewn up again after the birth of each child in some communities.

The health and medical consequences, particularly of clitoridectomy and infibulation, can be serious: haemorrhage, shock, tetanus from unsterilized tools, chronic vaginal and/or urinary infections, very painful periods, cysts as large as grapefruits, scar tissue, pain during intercourse, urinary incontinence or retention (often due to shock, fear and pain). There may be problems giving birth:

totally obstructed birth, which can result in the death of mother and/or baby (in the case of infibulation there is always a need to cut through the sewn tissues of the vulva); also the second stage of labour may be delayed. Circumcision done in a hospital may reduce some of the risks involved.

Although the practice of female circumcision is very old and culturally rooted, and it is practised by Muslims and Christians, among others, there is no basis for it in any religion. It is often regarded as a basic part of growing up. Many young women believe that uncircumcised girls will not find a husband, so they dare not risk that rejection. Men believe female circumcision gives more sexual pleasure to them and they may use their religion as a weapon of persuasion.

African opposition to the practice now includes growing numbers of public health workers. Many countries have passed laws against female circumcision. In Britain the Prohibition of Female Circumcision Act came into force in 1985. The London Black Women's Health Action Project (LBWHAP; see Resources) believes that legislation alone will not change people's attitudes to circumcision and that the practice will continue underground or girls be taken to countries where it is legal. Moreover, the Act contains racist implications in its clause 2:

> In determining . . . whether an operation is necessary for the mental health of a person, no account shall be taken of the effect on that person of any belief on the part of that or any other person that the operation is required as a matter of custom or ritual.

This slant confuses the issue when groups like the LBWHAP are trying to encourage debate about the dangers of female circumcision.

The LBWHAP is a grassroots organization which publishes a newsletter providing a platform for discussion, provides support and counselling for women and their families, and hopes to promote research into all aspects of female circumcision in Britain. They say:

> We take care not to impose Western practice as superior, but place female circumcision in the universal context of women's oppression and stress our opposition, to all forms of sexual violence.

Further, they ask the pertinent question:

> Can one isolate this physical act against women's sexuality and attempt to abolish it without changing the whole social fabric of the society?

TOURISM

Tourism is an increasingly important source of income in the Third World, in some cases the third or fourth largest source of foreign currency. A strong incentive for tourism is the availability of women in these countries either explicitly as prostitutes or disguised as hospitality girls, massage and bath attendants, performers in sex shows, hostesses and waitresses in clubs. Closely related to the sex-tourism industry is the 'rest and relaxation' (R-and-R) business which has grown up around many permanent US military bases in Asia. The sex-tourism and R-and-R industries exploit the vast majority of their employees both sexually and economically. Women enter this type of employment out of economic necessity and because there are often no alternatives for them.

> In Thailand the gap in incomes and opportunities between the city and countryside is enormous, setting the way for rural–urban migration. For women from poor rural backgrounds, migration provides an earning power which is simply astounding compared to normal rural budgets. Two or three years' working as a masseuse/prostitute enables a [woman's] family to build a house of size and quality few people in the countryside could hope to achieve with the earnings of a lifetime. Many families, indeed entire villages, have raised their standard of living through the bodies of their daughters.[20]

Most of the money generated by sex-tourism goes to tourist agencies, hotels, club owners, tour operators, pimps and other organizers of the business. Tourist agencies and airlines in industrialized countries reap huge profits. Because they see it as an important source of income, some governments condone or encourage sex-tourism outright: some officials even exhort their women to prostitution as a form of patriotism! The most blatant examples are in the Philippines, South Korea and Thailand. Some 200,000 to 300,000 women work in Bangkok's massage parlours, teahouses, nightclubs, brothels and disco-restaurants. From a Dutch travel agency's promotional material:

> Thailand is a world full of extremes and possibilities are unlimited. Anything goes in this exotic country, especially when it comes to girls . . . However, it may be a problem for visitors to Thailand to find the right places where they can indulge in unknown pleasures. It is frustrating to have to ask the hotel receptionist in broken English where you can pick up pretty girls. Rosie has done something about this. For the first time, you can book a trip to Thailand with erotic pleasures included in the price . . .[21]

Dutch men board charter flights from Amsterdam to

SISTERHOOD IS POWERFUL; INTERNATIONAL SISTERHOOD IS EVEN MORE POWERFUL

The decades of the 1970s and 1980s can be called the decades of women's organizing. Here are just a few examples of what women have been doing to link internationally over the past decade.

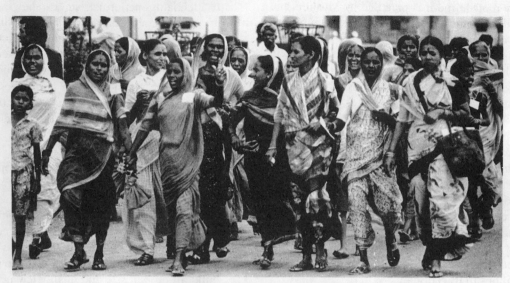

Striking domestic workers of Poona

1974 ISIS began as a resource and documentation centre in the international women's movement. It makes material from local women's groups available to women all over the world and publishes a quarterly *Bulletin*.

1975 Designated by the United Nations as International Women's Year. The official conference took place in Mexico; there was an unofficial parallel conference, called the Tribunal, to which non-governmental organizations and women's groups sent delegates.

1976 to 1985 UN International Women's Decade. Countries were instructed to look at their national priorities in development and to include women.

1976 International Tribunal of Crimes Against Women, Brussels. Out of this conference the International Feminist Network (IFN) was established. The IFN, coordinated by ISIS, is a communication channel through which women in one country can ask those in others for help – for instance, in the form of telegrams and letters expressing solidarity with an action they are taking.

1977 First International Women and Health Meeting, Rome.

1979 Feminist Conference, Bangkok. Third World women participants decided to embrace the term 'feminism', despite its distorted media image. They recognized an 'indigenous feminism' which was partly comprised of Third World women questioning the whole concept of 'development' and asking whether women *wanted* integration into this process, no matter how 'equally'. These women defined feminism in terms of two long-term goals: first, the achievement of women's equality, dignity and freedom of choice, through power to control our bodies and lives, inside and outside the home; secondly, the removal of all forms of inequity and oppression through the creation of a more just social and economic order, nationally and internationally.

1979 International Campaign for Abortion Rights set up in London. In 1980 the name was changed to ICASC (International Contraception, Abortion and Sterilization Campaign) to reflect a broadening of the issues involved. Following the Fourth International Women and Health Meeting (1984), the name was again changed to Women's Global Network on Reproductive Rights (WGNRR). There are autonomous groups in every continent, working on some or all aspects of women's right to decide if and when to have children and against population control policies.

1980 Mid-decade UN Conference on Women, Copenhagen. There was also a parallel

Continues opposite

	conference which 8,000 women attended. The theme was 'Development, Equality, and Peace'.	**1985**	rights and population control, organized by ICASC (see above). Attended by about 400 women from sixty-five countries.
1980	Second International Women and Health Meeting, Hanover, Germany.	**1985**	International Women's Conference, Nairobi, Kenya, to mark the end of International Women's Decade; 12–13,000 women attended the NGO Forum, including thousands from African countries. The decade primarily made us more deeply aware of the vast extent of women's *exclusion* from the political process in every continent. It will be up to us to monitor how real any 'progress' in women's lives has been.
1981	Third International Women and Health Meeting, Geneva.		
1981	First Latin American/Caribbean Feminist Meeting, Bogota, Colombia. Then held every other year, successive ones in Lima, Peru; São Paulo, Brazil.		
1983	WHO (European Region) Conference on Women and Health, in Peebles, Scotland. Attended by over eighty delegates from campaigning groups, women's health centres, academics and health professionals throughout Europe and North Africa.	**1986**	Second International Lesbian Conference in Geneva.
		1986	Meeting of women living under Muslim law, from many countries.
1984	Fourth International Women and Health Meeting in Amsterdam, on reproductive	**1987**	Fifth International Women and Health Meeting, San Jose, Costa Rica.

Bangkok, where they can buy a woman for twenty-five guilders (under £10) a night, a hundred guilders a week. The 'girls', on the other hand, earn about eighty guilders a month when they can find work. The AIDS crisis is likely to have more effect on this industry than any concern for women.

Japanese businessmen often fly on one-night *Kisaeng* (i.e. sex) tours to South Korea. The following appeared in a Japanese magazine:

> There are only two types of people who don't sleep with South Korean women; those with no money and those with something wrong with a certain part of their body.[22]

Prostitution in the Philippines has always flourished where there is a heavy concentration of foreigners, for example, in the row of 'clubs' adjacent to the US military bases in Angeles City and Olongapo. About 65,000 American military and civilian personnel come to Olongapo every day for R-and-R. Average monthly earnings for an Olangapo hostess are between 500 and 600 pesos (£50–£60). Some girls start work at age thirteen or fourteen through arrangement with club owners and managers, and women work until their late forties or fifties, or as long as the owners will allow it. Upon retirement, most have no savings or social security benefits, and end up as economically vulnerable as when they began. Analysts have predicted that as long as the US naval base remains, the profitable and powerful existing R-and-R trade will continue.

Women's and church groups in Asia have begun to protest against these activities, many seeking international solidarity. For example, the Third World Movement Against the Exploitation of Women has headquarters in the Philippines and groups in all South-East Asian countries.

South Korean women organized a demonstration at the airport where the *Kisaeng* airplanes land. They carried placards in Japanese saying: 'We will throw you beyond the sea, Japanese sex monsters!'[23]

Spurred on by this, women's groups in Japan have organized information campaigns and actions against the Japanese tourist agencies involved.

TO TALK FEMINISM IS NEVER TO TALK NONSENSE*

International women's organizations, along with hundreds of local groups on every continent, point to feminist efforts in organizing a strong women's international presence. We must nurture and expand these groups so that we may truly learn about the lives of our sisters by exchanging information, experiences and hopes. The numerous feminist magazines further these goals. *Broadsheet* (New Zealand),

*Donna Awatere, a Maori woman, New Zealand.

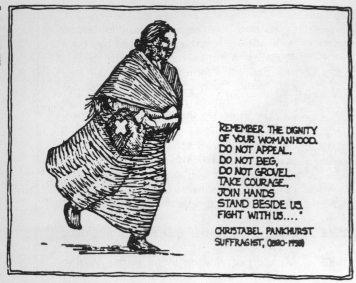

Karen Norberg

'REMEMBER THE DIGNITY OF YOUR WOMANHOOD. DO NOT APPEAL, DO NOT BEG, DO NOT GROVEL. TAKE COURAGE, JOIN HANDS STAND BESIDE US, FIGHT WITH US....'
CHRISTABEL PANKHURST
SUFFRAGIST, (1880-1958)

Manushi (India), *La Revuelta* (Mexico), *Off Our Backs* (USA) and *Spare Rib* (UK) are just a few of our important 'spokeswomen'. This kind of exchange can help diminish some of the barriers of region, race, class and fear that now divide us, and can strengthen the similarities we share.

As one woman in India said:

We will be able to derive strength for all our efforts if all women stand united, convinced of our worth, and angry at our oppression.[24]

NOTES

1. Sundari Ravindran. *Women's Camp*, 30 July to 3 August 1981, p. 35 (available from Rural Women's Social Education Centre and Rural Development Society, 15/1 Peria Melmaiyur, Chingleput, 603 002, Tamilnadu, South India).

2. *ISIS International Bulletin*, no. 3, April 1977, p. 3.

3. From a report by Birmingham WONT, *Spare Rib*, no. 142, May 1984.

4. Anita Anand. 'Rethinking Women and Development: the Case for Feminism', in *Women and Development Resource Guide*. ISIS (PO Box 50, 1211 Geneva, Switzerland), 1983, p. 7.

5. Jane Goldsmith, Women's Campaign World at the World University Service, quoted in the *Guardian*, 5 November 1984.

6. Ravindran, op. cit., note 1, p. 33.

7. *International Women and Health Resource Guide*, Boston, MA: BWHBC and ISIS, 1980, p. 51. Available from Boston Women's Health Book Collective.

8. *Saheli*, Indian Women's Resource Centre (10 Mazamudeen East, New Delhi 110013, India).

9. Anand, op. cit., note 4, p. 6.

10. War on Want, 'Women Working Worldwide', Conference Report, London 1983.

11. Barbara Ehrenreich and Annette Fuentes. 'Life on the Global Assembly Line', *MS Magazine*, January 1981, p. 55.

12. Ibid., p. 56.

13. Ibid., p. 55.

14. Ibid., p. 57.

15. Ibid., p. 60.

16. Sally Austen Tom. 'Hazards of Infant Formula', *Heresies*, vol. 4, no. 1 (issue 13), 1980, p. 74.

17. Fred Clarkson. 'Growing Nestlé Boycott Haunts Infant Formula Makers', *WIN Magazine*, 1 March 1981, p. 12; see also Andy Chetley. *The Baby Killer Scandal* (rev. ed.). London: War on Want, 1979.

18. Marie-Angelique Savane. 'Yes to Breastfeeding, But . . . How?' *Assignment Children*. UNICEF 49/50, Spring 1980, p. 82.

19. J. Bandyopadhya and V. Shiva. 'Alternatives for India, Western or Indigenous Science', *Science for the People*, vol. 13, no. 2, March/April 1981, pp. 22–8.

20. Pasuk Phongpaichit. 'Bangkok Masseuses: Holding Up the Family Sky', in 'Tourism: Selling Southeast Asia', *Southeast Asia Chronicle*, issue 78, April 1981, p. 23.

21. 'Tourism and Prostitution', *ISIS International Bulletin*, no. 13, November 1979, p. 9.

22. Ibid., p. 22.

23. Ibid., p. 8.

24. Ravindran, op. cit., note 1, p. 36.

RESOURCES
PUBLICATIONS

Here we can give only an indication of the range of books now available

Allison, Helen et al. *Hard Cash: Man-made Development and its Consequences. A Feminist Perspective on Aid*. London: Change, 1986.

Arditti, Rita et al. (eds). *Science and Liberation*. Boston, MA: South End Press, 1980.

Ashworth, Georgina. *An International Evaluation of the Decade for Women. Special Issue of Women's Studies International Forum*. London: Pergamon, 1985.

Atiya, Nayra. *Khul Khaal: Five Egyptian Women Tell Their Stories*. Syracuse, NY: Syracuse University Press, 1982.

Barry, Kathleen. *Female Sexual Slavery*. New York: Avon Books, 1981.

Beale, Jenny. *Women in Ireland, Voices of Change*. London: Macmillan Education, 1986. Chapters on contraception, abortion, sexuality.

Bernstein, Hilda. *Death is Part of the Process*. Chichester: Sinclair Browne, 1984. A group of black and white South Africans fight against apartheid.

Bhagat, Mukarram. *Aspects of the Drug Industry in India*. Bombay: Centre for Education and Documentation (3 Suleman Chambers, 4 Battery Street, Bombay 400 039, India), February, 1982.

Boston Women's Health Book Collective. *Our Bodies, Ourselves*. Over fourteen foreign-language editions. BWHBC, 47 Nichols Avenue, Watertown, MA 02172.

Bowles, Gloria and Renate **Duelli Klein** (eds). *Theories of Women's Studies*. London: Routledge and Kegan Paul, 1983. Feminists from different Western countries speak.

Bronstein, Audrey. *The Triple Struggle: Latin American Peasant Women*. WOW Campaigns Ltd, 1982. Available from Third World Publications, 151 Stratford Rd, Birmingham B11 1RD.

Burgos-Debray, Elisabeth. *I . . . Rigoberta Menchu: An Indian Woman in Guatemala*. London: Verso, 1984.

Chen, Martha Alter. *The Quiet Revolution: Women in Transition in Rural Bangladesh*. Lexington, MA: Schenkman Publishing Co., 1983.

Chetley, Andy. *The Baby Killer Scandal* (rev. ed.). London: War on

Want, 1979. Investigation into the promotion and sale of powdered baby milks in Third World.

Chetley, Andy. *The Crisis in Infant Feeding*. London: War on Want, 1981. Traces development of the 'baby foods campaign'.

Chetley, Andy. *Bangladesh: Finding the Right Prescription*. London: War on Want, 1983.

Chetley, Andy. *Information Pack on Pharmaceuticals*. London: War on Want, 1984.

Clarke, Gillian. *Letter from a Far Country*. Manchester: Carcanet Press, 1982. Poetry from a Welsh feminist.

Cock, Jacklyn. *Maids and Madams: the Conditions of Black Women Domestic Servants in South Africa*. New York: Raven Press, 1982.

Commission for Human Rights and War on Want. *Women in El Salvador*. London: Zed Press, 1985.

Cutrufelli, Maria Rosa. *Women of Africa: Roots of Oppression*. London: Zed Press, 1983.

Deighton, Jane et al. *Sweet Ramparts: Women in Revolutionary Nicaragua*. London: Change, 1983.

Desphande, Shashi. *Roots and Shadows*. Hyderabad: Sangam Books, 1983. On an Indian woman's conflict between pressures of traditional family life and strivings for independence.

Eisen, Arlene. *Women and Revolution in Vietnam*. London: Zed Press, 1984.

El-Saadawi, Nawal. *The Hidden Face of Eve: Women in the Arab World*. London: Zed Press, 1980.

El-Saadawi, Nawal. *Two Women in One*. London: Al Saqi Books, 1985. The story of a young Egyptian woman.

El-Saadawi, Nawal. *Women at Point Zero*. London: Zed Press, 1984. The story of one Arab woman.

Fairweather, Eileen, Roisin McDonough and Melanie McFadyean. *Only the Rivers Run Free – Northern Ireland: the Women's War*. London: Pluto Press, 1984.

First, Ruth. *117 Days* (new ed.). London: Penguin Books, 1982. About confinement and interrogation in South Africa.

George, Susan. *How the Other Half Dies, The Real Reason for World Hunger*. London: Penguin Books, 1976.

George, Susan. *A Fate Worse than Debt*. London: Penguin Books, 1988.

Glasgow Women's Studies Group. *Uncharted Lives*. Glasgow: Pressgang, 1983. Lives and history of Scottish women.

Hartman, Betsy. *Reproductive Rights and Wrongs*. New York: Harper & Row, 1987. About population control.

Hay, Margaret J. et al (eds). *African Women: South of the Sahara*. London: Longman, 1984. Essays covering economic, social and political roles of women in Africa.

Hayter, Teresa. *Aid as Imperialism*. London: Penguin Books, 1974. An early work exploring aid to developing countries by a World Bank analyst.

Heller, Tom. *Poor Health, Rich Profits: Multinational Drug Companies and the Third World*. Nottingham: Spokesman Books (Bertrand Russell Peace Foundation Ltd, Bertrand Russell House, Gamble Street, Nottingham), 1977.

Hosken, Fran P. *The Hosken Report: Genital and Sexual Mutilation of Females*. Lexington, MA: WIN News (187 Grant Street, Lexington, MA 02173), 1979.

Hosken, Fran P. *Universal Childbirth Picture Book*. WIN News (see address above).

Huston, Perdita. *Third World Women Speak Out*. New York: Praeger, 1979.

Huston, Perdita. *Explorations in Feminism Collective: an Introduction to Feminist Geography*. London: Hutchinson, 1986. Challenges current thinking about geographic research and teaching.

International Defence and Aid fund for S. Africa. *Women Under Apartheid*, 1981.

Irish Feminist Information Publications Ltd. *Missing Pieces – Women in Irish History. Vol I: Since the Famine*. Community Press.

ISIS. *Women in Development: A Resource Guide for Organization and Action*. Order from ISIS (see Organizations). A good feminist source with excellent, detailed resource sections.

Jayawardena, Kumari. *Feminism and Nationalism in the Third World*. London: Zed Press, 1986.

Jordan, Brigitte. *Birth in Four Cultures*. Montreal: Eden Press, 1978.

Keane, Molly. *Time after Time*. London: Abacus, 1984. Novel about three sisters living in southern Ireland.

Kishwar, Madhu and Ruth Vanita. *In Search of Answers: Indian Women's Voices from 'Manushi'*. London: Zed Press, 1984.

Latin American and Caribbean Women's Collective. *Slaves of Slaves: The Challenge of Latin American Women*. London: Zed Press, 1980.

Leghorn, Lisa, and Katherine Parker. *Women's Worth; Sexual Economics and The World of Women*. London: Routledge and Kegan Paul, 1981.

Leghorn, Lisa, and Mary Roodkowsky, *Who Really Starves? Women and World Hunger*. Friendship Press, 1977.

Lipman, Beata. *We Make Freedom: Women in South Africa*. London: Pandora, 1984.

Mamdani, Mahmood. *The Myth of Population Control: Family, Caste and Class in an Indian Village*. New York and London: Monthly Review Press, 1972.

Mamonova, Tatyana. *Women and Russia*. Oxford: Basil Blackwell, 1984.

Mass, Bonnie. *Population Target: The Political Economy of Population Control in Latin America*. Toronto: Women's Press, 1976.

Medawar, Charles. *Insult or Injury: An Inquiry into the Marketing and Advertising of British Food and Drug Products in the Third World*. London: Social Audit Ltd, 1979.

Medawar, Charles. *The Wrong Kind of Medicine?* London: Consumers' Association and Hodder and Stoughton, 1984.

Melrose, Diana. *Bitter Pills: Medicines and the Third World*. Oxford: Oxfam, 1982.

Morgan, Robin. *Sisterhood is Global*. London: Penguin Books, 1985. Anthology of the international women's movement.

Mukhopadhyay, Maitrayee. *Silver Shackles: Women and Development in India*. Oxford: Oxfam, 1984.

Murray, Maggie and Buchi Emecheta. *Our Own Freedom*. London: Sheba, 1981.

Nash, June and Helen Icken Safa (eds). *Sex and Class in Latin America*. South Hadley, MA: J. F. Bergin, 1980.

Newland, Kathleen. *Infant Mortality and the Health of Societies*, Worldwatch Paper no. 47. Washington, DC: Worldwatch Institute, 1981.

Newland, Kathleen. *The Sisterhood of Man*. New York and London: W.W. Norton, 1979.

Niethammer, Carolyn. *Daughters of the Earth: Lives and Legends of American Indian Women*. New York: Collier Books, 1977.

Nwapa, Flora. *One is Enough*. Nigeria: Tana Press. A novel in which a childless wife must decide whether to remarry for respectability, or continue away from her first husband in the face of criticism.

Nwapa, Flora. *Wives at War and Other Stories*. Nigeria: Tana Press

O'Kelly, Charlotte G. *Women and Men in Society*. New York, Toronto, London and Melbourne: Van Nostrand, 1980.

Omvedt, Gail. *We Will Smash This Prison: Indian Women in Struggle*. London: Zed Press, 1980.

Patterns for Change: Rural Women Organizing for Health. Washington, DC: National Women's Health Network, 1981.

Randall, Margaret. *Sandino's Daughters: Testimonies of Nicaraguan Women in Struggle*. Vancouver, BC: New Star Books, 1981.

Randall, Margaret. *Women in Cuba: Twenty Years Later*. New York: Smyrna Press, 1981.

Rao, Shanta Rameshwar. *Children of God*. Hyderabad: Sangam Books. Novel told in first person by woman of 'untouchable' caste about the suffering the caste system imposes.

Reiter, Rayna R. *Toward an Anthropology of Women*. New York and London: Monthly Review Press, 1975.

Rogers, Barbara. *The Domestication of Women: Discrimination in Developing Societies*. London and New York: Tavistock, 1980.

Rosaldo, Michelle Zimbalist and Louise Lamphere (eds). *Women, Culture, and Society*, Stanford CA: Stanford University Press, 1974.

Sakala, Carol. *Women of South Asia: A Guide to Resources*. Millwood, NY: Kraus International Publications, 1980.

Sawer, Marian and Marion Simms. *A Woman's Place: Women and Politics in Australia*. London: Allen and Unwin, 1984.

Seager, Joni and Ann Olson. *Women in the World: an International Atlas*. London: Pan, 1986.

Seedat, Aziza. *Crippling a Nation: Health in Apartheid South Africa*. International Defence and Aid Fund for South Africa, 1984.

Silverman, Milton et al. *Prescriptions for Death: Drugging in the Third World*. Berkeley, CA: University of California Press, 1982.

SNDT Women's University. *Women in India*. Bombay: SNDT (see Periodicals for address).

Tweedie, Jill. *Internal Affairs*. London: Penguin Books, 1987. Comic novel about a Western-funded birth control programme enacted upon poor women in a South-East Asian dictatorship.

Turshen, Meredith. *Women, Food and Health in Tanzania: The Political Economy of Disease*. London: Onyx Press, 1980.

War on Want. *Women Working Worldwide*. London: WOW, 1987.

War on Want. *We Carry a Heavy Load*. Zimbabwe Women's Bureau, 1981. Rural women on the status of women, land ownership, healthcare, education, work and community participation.

War on Want. *For a Few Dollars . . . More*. London: WOW, 1981.

Werner, David. *Donde No Hay Doctor* (Where there is no doctor). The Hesperian Foundation, Box 1692, Palo Alto, CA 94302. In Spanish, English, Portuguese, Swahili, Hindi.

PERIODICALS

Broadsheet, Box 5799, Wellesley Street, Auckland, New Zealand. An excellent in-depth coverage of women's health issues in New Zealand.

Healthsharing, Women Healthsharing, Box 230, Station M, Toronto, Ontario M6S 4T3, Canada. A quarterly newsletter covering a wide range of women's health concerns. On file at WHRRIC (see Organizations, Chapter 27).

Manushi, C/1202 Lajpat Nagar 1, New Delhi 110024, India. A feminist magazine (manushi means 'woman') which encourages women to write in and tell their stories as well as analyse their situations and move towards a shared understanding. Lively, interesting and sometimes very grim, as it reflects the Indian woman's often harsh reality. Available in UK from Sisterwrite bookshop (see Resources, Chapter 27).

Quest – A Feminist Quarterly, P.O. Box 8843, Washington, DC 20003, USA. Interesting articles on a wide range of topics relevant to women internationally.

SNDT Research Unit on Women's Studies at SNDT Women's University, Sir Vithaldas Vidyavihar, Juhu Road, Santacruz West, Bombay 400 049, India. An excellent newsletter on research being done at the university as well as feminist activities in and around Bombay. The studies cover education, health, employment, women's organizations, etc. Write to them if you are interested in an exchange of newsletters.

ORGANIZATIONS

ACHAN (Asian Community Health Action Network), Flat 2B, 144 Prince Edward Road, Kowloon, Hong Kong.

Akina Mama Wa Africa, London Women's Centre, Wesley House, 4 Wild Court, London WC2B 5AU. Tel: 01–405 0678.

Asian Women's Association, Post Restante, Shibuya Post Office, Tokyo, Japan. One of the major groups involved in campaigns against sex tourism. Their newspaper, *Asian Women's Liberation*, continually brings up the issue and reports on actions taking place.

Baby Milk Action Coalition, 34 Blinco Grove, Cambridge CB 1413. Tel: 0223 210094.

Campaign for the Demilitarization of the Indian Ocean, c/o Jaya, 30 Stonedene Close, Forest Row, East Sussex RH18 5DB. Tel: 034282-4603.

Change (International Reports: Women and Society), PO Box 824, London SE24 9JS. Tel: 01-274 4043. An educational charity that has produced a variety of reports since 1980 including ones on women in Bangladesh, Caribbean, Peru, Lesotho, Israel, Russia, Thailand and Uganda.

FORWAARD (Foundation for Women's Health Research and Development), 38 King Street, London WC2 8JT. Tel: 01-379 6889. For creating a network between European and African women.

Health Action International (HAI) c/o International Organization of Consumers' Unions, P.O. Box 1045, 10830 Penang, Malaysia; or Brederodestraat 5, 1054 MP, Amsterdam, Netherlands. An international 'antibody' set up in 1981 to resist ill treatment of consumers by multinational drug companies. It is a broad-based network of consumer and professional groups whose main concern is to look into contraceptive drugs and pharmaceutical companies' activities in this field. Produces *HAI News*, a bimonthly newsletter. HAI also has a women's group: WEMOS/HAI. International Group on Women and Pharmaceuticals, P.O. Box 4263, 1009 AG Amsterdam, Netherlands.

Interfaith Center on Corporate Responsibility (ICCR), 475 Riverside Drive, Room 566, New York, NY 10115, USA. A sponsored related movement of the US National Council of Churches, ICCR tries to make corporations responsible for their policies. They bring stockholder resolutions to try and change policies they don't agree with. They have produced an information/action packet on the whole issue of pharmaceutical marketing in the Third World. Write to them if you are interested in receiving this packet.

International Defence and Aid Fund for Southern Africa, Canon Collins House, 64 Essex Road, London N1 8LR. Tel: 01-359 9181.

ISIS International, Via San Saba 5, 00153 Rome, Italy. Tel: 010-39-6-5746479. Information and communication services with resource and documentation centres and networks of thousands of contacts throughout the world. Its publications are excellent and include the ISIS *International Women's Journal*, *Women in Action* (a supplement to the journal), and ISIS-WICCE's *Women's World*. It also provides technical assistance and training, and much else.

Jewish Feminist Newsletter, PO Box 39, c/o Sisterwrite, 190 Upper Street, London N1. This is a contact address for all the various Jewish groups including *Jewish Women Support the Palestinians*.

London Black Women's Health Action Project, Wickham House, 10 Cleveland Way, London E1 4TZ. Tel: 01-790 2424 or 01-980 3439. Active on health generally and particularly involved in female circumcision issue about which they have produced a lot of literature and operate a 24-hour counselling service.

Medico Friend Circle Bulletin, c/o National Institute of Nutrition, PO Jamai Osmania, Hyderabad 500007, India. A monthly newsjournal providing a radical critique of health services and policies in India. Has a membership organization of mostly doctors and health workers with some nurses, social workers and activists. The group meets annually to discuss a previously planned topic in depth. Has published an excellent book on health in India called *Health Care, Which Way to Go?*

National Women's Network ('for international solidarity'), Address c/o War on Want. Provides networking service for women in UK concerned with international issues.

Oxfam, 274 Banbury Road, Oxford OX2 7DZ. Tel: 0865-56777. A development organization with charitable status that produces many excellent publications.

Philippine Asia Resource Center, P.O. Box 40090 D, Berkeley, CA 94704, USA. Publishes *Philippine Monitor* and stocks back issues of *Philippine Report* and *Southeast Asia Chronicle*, an excellent bimonthly journal on developments in Vietnam, Laos, Kampuchea, Thailand, Malaysia, Indonesia and the Philippines.

Rural Women's Social Education Centre (RWSEC), Plot No. 19, Periya Melamaiyur, Vallam Post, Chengalputta 603 002, South India. A group of rural Indian women who meet regularly and plan literacy programmes and health education programmes for their respective villages. They give primary health care to village women and their children and also build awareness of how women can obtain basic health services from the government.

Saheli Women's Resource Centre, under Defence Colony Bridge (South Side), New Delhi 110024, India. Tel: 010-91-11 616485. It began as a group organizing against dowry burnings and tortures and now covers a broad range of women's issues. They run workshops and exhibits on health, consciousness raising and family violence and provide counselling to women on legal matters.

Traidcraft, Unit 123 Kingsway, TVTE, Gateshead, Newcastle-upon-Tyne. Tel: 091-491 0591.

US National Women's Health Network, 1325 G Street, NW (lower level), Washington, DC 20005, USA. 'Umbrella' of the US women's health movement. Group and individual members receive *Network News*, 'newsalerts' about issues that need immediate attention, and access to the Network's clearing house. The Network also publishes a series of health resource guides.

War on Want, 37–9 Great Guildford Street, London SE1. Tel: 01-620 1111. WOW is a Third-World oriented charity which produces many excellent publications. They also have a women's section, open to all women members and supporters, with groups in London and Manchester.

WISER LINKS (Women's International Self-Education and Resources Links), 173 Archway Road, London N6. A women's international information exchange project involving Third World and Western women.

Women's Global Network on Reproductive Rights (formerly ICASC), P.O. Box 4098 Minahassastraat, 1009 AB Amsterdam, Netherland. Tel: 010-30-20 92 39 00. Set up in 1978, aims to fight for women's reproductive rights all over the world. They organize international solidarity, including international days of action in support of the struggle for reproductive rights of women, and publish a quarterly newsletter.

Women's International League for Peace and Freedom, British section, 17 Victoria Park Square, London E2. Tel: 01-980 1030.

Women's International Resource Centre (WIRC) 173 Archway Road, London N6 5BL. Tel: 01-341 4403. A women's international information exchange project involving Third World and Western women. Development, education and resources. Library.

Women Working for a Nuclear Free and Independent Pacific, c/o Jane Graham, 58 High Lane, Chorlton, Manchester M21 1DZ.

ZATAR c/o 44 Sussex Road, Harrow, Middlesex HA1 4LX. Tel: 01-863 2294. A British-based organization concerned with Palestinian women, organizing financial and technical assistance.

DIRECTORIES

AUSTRALIA

ABORTION CLINICS
NEW SOUTH WALES

Most clinics offer pregnancy testing and counselling. Proof of age is needed for young women aged between 14 and 16 years. Parental consent is needed for girls under 14 years old. Contraception advice and contraceptives are available.

Bessie Smyth Foundation (Powell Street Clinic), cnr Powell Street and Wentworth Road, Homebush, NSW 2140. Tel: (02) 764 4886. Abortion with local anaesthetic up to 12 weeks' pregnancy. Small centre which offers personal, supportive counselling and is comparatively inexpensive.
Dr N. Marinko (private practice), 195 Macquarie Street, Sydney, NSW 2000. Tel: (02) 221 1933 (all hours). Abortion up to 20 weeks' pregnancy under local anaesthetic (awake or asleep), and painkillers as necessary.
Mediguide Family Planning (private), 237 Longueville Road, Lane Cove, NSW 2066. Tel: (02) 427 4275 (all hours). Abortions up to 12 weeks, local and general anaesthetic, counselling.
Preterm Foundation, 50 Cooper Street, Surry Hills, NSW 2010. Tel: (02) 699 9211.
Woollahra Clinic (private), 18 Ocean Street, Woollahra, NSW 2025. Tel: (02) 328 6911 (all hours). Abortion up to 18 weeks' pregnancy, local and general anaesthetic, accommodation at a reasonable rate arranged for country and interstate women.

VICTORIA

Services similar to those offered in NSW.

Fertility Control Clinic (private), 118 Wellington Parade, East Melbourne, Vic. 3002. Tel: (03) 419 2992/3449 (after hours). Abortions up to 20 weeks' pregnancy.
Melbourne Family Planning Clinic (private), 338 Dandenong Road, East St, Kilda, Vic. 3182. Tel: (03) 527 2992). Abortions up to 14 weeks' pregnancy.

Planned Parenthood Clinic (private, feminist), 341 High Street, Prahran, Vic. 3181. Tel: (03) 529 5899. Abortions up to 12 weeks' pregnancy, personal counselling and support.
Yarra Park Clinic, 395 Punt Road, Richmond, Vic. 3121. Tel: (03) 428 1273. Offers local anaesthetic up to 12 weeks' pregnancy.

SOUTH AUSTRALIA

Contact an abortion referral service first before visiting a hospital of your choice. Most hospitals except Queen Elizabeth use general anaesthetic.

Flinders Medical Centre, Flinders Drive, Bedford Park, SA 5042. Tel: (08) 275 9216.
Modbury Hospital, Smart Road, Modbury, SA 5092. Tel: (08) 264 6000. Requires an overnight stay.
Queen Elizabeth Hospital, Woodville Road, Woodville South, SA 5011. Tel: (08) 45 0222.
Queen Victoria Hospital, 160 Fullarton Road, Rose Park, SA 5067. Tel: (08) 332 4888.
Royal Adelaide Hospital, North Terrace, Adelaide, SA 5000. Tel: (08) 223 0230.

WESTERN AUSTRALIA

Most abortions performed in WA are presently carried out by two private clinics in Perth (see below).

King Edward Memorial Hospital for Women, Bafot Road, Subiaco, WA 6008. Tel: (09) 380 4444. Women are required to attend a gynaecologist at the out-patients' department and may see students or doctors who are opposed to abortion. Women may also be asked to see a psychiatrist.
Nanyarra Medical Group (private), 2 Cleaver Terrace, Riverdale, WA 6103. Tel: (09) 277 6070.
Zera Medical Centre (private), 8 Sayer Street, Midland, WA 6056. Tel: (09) 274 4166.

QUEENSLAND

Brisbane Fertility Control Clinic, 8 Ridge Street, Greenslopes, Brisbane, Qld 4120. Tel: (07) 397 1211 (all hours). For consultations and follow-up. Abortions up to 16 weeks' pregnancy, general anaesthetic only.
Planned Parenthood, 63–71 Wills Street, Townsville, Qld 4810. Tel: (077) 72 5533. Abortions up to 16 weeks' pregnancy, sterilization.
Tweed Heads Medical Centre, 127 Wharf Street, Tweed Heads, Qld 2485. Tel: (075) 36 1626.

TASMANIA

Phone **Women's Information Service** (feminist) first for advice and referral information. Tel: (002) 34 2166 (all hours).
Hobart Women's Health Centre, 9 Pierce Street, Moonah, Tas. 7009. Tel: (002) 28 0997.
Private Hospitals.
Very few perform abortions; contact **Women's Information Service** (above).
Royal Hobart Hospital and Launceston General Hospital will perform abortions for women shown to have severe psychological or medical problems.

ACT

Few abortions are performed in Canberra and most women go to either Sydney or Melbourne.

Royal Canberra Hospital, Acton, Canberra, ACT 2601. Tel: (062) 43 2111. General anaesthetic only.
Woden Valley Hospital, Yamba Drive, Garran, Canberra, ACT 2605. Tel: (062) 81 0433. General anaesthetic only.

NORTHERN TERRITORY

Abortions can be carried out only by specialist obstetricians or gynaecologists, so most are performed in public hospitals.

Alice Springs Hospital, Gap Road, Alice Springs, NT 5750. Tel: (089) 50 2211.
Royal Darwin Hospital, Rocklands Road, Casuarina, Darwin, NT 5792. Tel: (089) 20 7211.
Both hospitals offer general anaesthetic only. Hospital policy is to try to obtain husband's approval, although this is not required by law.

ABORTION COUNSELLING REFERRAL
NEW SOUTH WALES

Birth Control and Related Medical Services, 23 Newland Street, Bondi Junction, NSW 2002. Tel: (02) 389 7733. Contact social workers of general or women's hospitals for information.

Every Woman's Health Centre, 164 Flood Street, Leichhardt, NSW 2040. Tel: (02) 569 9522.
Family Planning Association, 161 Broadway, Broadway, NSW 2007. Tel: (02) 211 0244. Contact Broadway centre for information on your nearest FPA clinic.
Women's Health Centres (feminist). See Health Department of NSW for centres in your district.

VICTORIA

Action Centre, 268 Flinders Lane, Melbourne, Vic. 3000. Tel: (03) 654 4766. Particularly for women under 20 years old, confidential counselling and support, financial help with contraception.
Family Planning Association, 270 Church Street, Richmond, Vic. 3121. Tel: (03) 429 1177. Contact Richmond centre for information on your nearest FPA clinic.
Women's Liberation Switchboard and **Women's Abortion Action Campaign**, c/o Women's Liberation House, 295 Victoria Street, West Melbourne, Vic. 3003. Tel: (03) 329 8515/2374.
Contact social workers at women's or general hospitals for information.

SOUTH AUSTRALIA

See **Women's Health Centres** (feminist).
Family Planning Association, 17 Phillips Street, Kensington, SA 5068. Tel: (08) 31 5177. Contact the Kensington Centre for information about your nearest FPA clinic.
Pregnancy Support, 597 South Road, Everard Park, SA 5035. Tel: (08) 297 4422.

WESTERN AUSTRALIA

Abortion Information Service (feminist), PO Box 397, Subiaco, WA 6008. Tel: (09) 401 9661. Free telephone and personal counselling, advice on which doctors will perform abortions in private/general hospitals.
Family Planning Association, 104 Colin Street, West Perth, WA 6005. Tel: (09) 321 2701. Referral only.
Pregnancy Help, 459 Hay Street, Perth, WA 6000. Tel: (09) 325 5592.
Women's Health Care House (feminist), 92 Thomas Street, West Perth, WA 6005. Tel: (09) 321 2383.

QUEENSLAND

Children by Choice, 237 Lutwyche Road, Windsor, Qld 4030. Tel: (07) 357 5377. Provides counselling service for women with unplanned/unwanted pregnancies.
Family Planning Association, 100 Alfred Street, Fortitude Valley, Brisbane, Qld 4006. Tel: (07) 52 5151.
Planned Parenthood (private), 63–71 Will Street, Townsville, Qld 4810. Tel: (077) 72 5533. Abortion counselling and clinic.
Women's House Shelter Information (feminist), Victoria Street, West End, Qld 4101. Tel: (07) 844 4008 (after hours recorded message with alternative phone number).

TASMANIA

Women between 18 and 35 years of age cannot easily obtain abortions in Tasmania. Very few abortions are done in private hospitals, while the Royal Hobart and Launceston General Hospitals will do abortions only in cases of extreme medical or psychological distress, supported by a psychiatric report. Most women go to Melbourne.

Family Planning Association, 73 Federal Street, North Hobart, Tas. 7000. Tel: (002) 34 7790. Counselling available and referral if required.
Women's Information Service (feminist). Address changeable. Tel: (002) 34 2166 (all hours). Pregnancy counselling and referral; most women are referred to Melbourne.

ACT

Abortion Counselling Service (feminist), 3 Lobelia Street, O'Connor, Canberra, ACT 2601. Tel: (062) 47 8070. (Recorded message gives home phone numbers of counsellors for immediate contact.) Free service, pregnancy testing and information about referrals for abortion, sympathetic doctors. Pre- and post-abortion counselling, face-to-face or by telephone.
Family Planning Association Health Promotion Centre, Childers Street, Canberra, ACT 2601. Tel: (062) 47 3077. Social workers at community health centres will be able to give advice.

NORTHERN TERRITORY

Family Planning Association, PO Box 1107, Alice Springs, NT 5750. Tel: (089) 52 5571.
Family Planning Association, 133 Mitchell Street, Larrakeyal, NT 5790; PO Box 3158, Darwin, NT 5794. Tel: (089) 81 5335.
Also contact general hospitals and community health centres for information.

ACCOMMODATION

Contact Women's Houses and Centres for assistance with accommodation, and look up 'Hostels' in the phone book. The YWCA (Young Women's Christian Association) also offers accommodation ranging from cheap to fairly expensive, and the YMCA may be able to provide rooms when the YWCA is full. The Country Women's Association may also be able to advise on or provide accommodation. (See also **Refuges**.)

NEW SOUTH WALES

Guthrie House, 9 Liberty Street, Enmore, Sydney, NSW 2042. Tel: (02) 516 5588 (all hours). Referral from court or jail, self-referral, drug and alcohol problems, half-way house for women only.

People's Palace, 400 Pitt Street, Sydney, NSW 2000. Tel: (02) 211 5777; 61 Pittwater Road, Manly, NSW 2095. Tel: (02) 977 6177/6211. Mixed, single or families, short- or long-term.
Ruby Rich, 25 Bland Street, Ashfield, Sydney, NSW 2131. Tel: (02) 660 7695. Ask for welfare officer. Prisoner half-way house for women on parole, probation or bail.
Samaritan House, 6 O'Laughlin Street, Surry Hills, NSW 2010. Tel: (02) 211 5794 (all hours). Single women, temporary accommodation, small charge for meals, free if necessary.
Satyananda Ashram, RMB 4820, Mangrove Mountain, Gosford, NSW 2240. Tel: (043) 77 1171 (seven days). Mixed, relaxed – for retreat or nervous tension and stress, vegetarian, cheap.
Young Cross Country Traveller Association, 25 Hughes Street, Kings Cross, NSW 2011. Tel: (02) 358 1143. Mixed, cheap accommodation, shared rooms.
YWCA, 5 Wentworth Avenue, Darlinghurst, NSW 2012. Tel: (02) 264 2451. Single women or families up to two months. Referral is required for a longer period.
Women and Girls Emergency Centre, Rooms 16 and 17, 401A Pitt Street, Sydney, NSW 2000. Tel: (02) 264 7114. Provides referral for accommodation and other needs.
Women's Housing Co-operative, 34 Liverpool Street, Sydney, NSW 2000. Tel: (02) 264 7439. Waiting list, single women on low income, very cheap.

VICTORIA

Mary Anderson Lodge (Salvation Army), 4 Burnley Street, Richmond, Vic. 3121. Tel: (03) 428 7728 (all hours). For women and children, small charge if it can be afforded.
Women's Refuge Referral Service, PO Box 70, Elsternwick, Vic. 3185. Tel: (03) 329 8433. Accommodation and refuge information.
YWCA, 353 Church Street, Richmond, Vic. 3121. Tel: (03) 428 6349. Long-term accommodation for single women, cheap rates.

SOUTH AUSTRALIA

Elouera YWCA Emergency Accommodation, PO Box 360, Whyalla, SA 5600. Tel: (086) 49 1957.
Emergency Housing Office, 38 Waymouth Street, Adelaide, SA 5000. Tel: (08) 51 6801.
Helping Hand Centre Inc., Mary Seymour Houses, 93 Tynte Street, North Adelaide, SA 5006. Tel: (08) 267 3927. Run by Uniting Church for young women 15–25 years old.
ITRA (Independent Therapeutic Residence for Adolescents), 18–20 Penola Street, Kilkenny, Adelaide, SA 5009. Tel: (08) 268 8371 (all hours). Two houses offering long-term placement for girls and boys 12–18 years old; referral from social worker or crisis care needed.
St Joseph's Centre, 82 Wattle Street, Fullerton, Adelaide, SA 5063. Tel: (08) 272 6811. For single, pregnant women.
YMCA, 76 Flinders Street, Adelaide, SA 5000. Tel: (08) 223 1611. Mixed accommodation.

WESTERN AUSTRALIA

Aboriginal Accommodation Service. Tel: (09) 328 3722. Referral for single women or families.

Country Women's Association, Hay Street, West Perth, WA 6005. Tel: (09) 321 6081.

Mothercraft Home and Training Centre, 1 Jarrah Road, South Perth, WA 6151. Tel: (09) 367 7855. For mothers and small children or pregnant single women, cost dependent on finances.

'Willong' Aboriginal Women's Shelter, 119 Aberdeen Street, Northbridge, Perth, WA 6000. Tel: (09) 328 1115 (all hours).

YMCA, Goderich St, Perth, WA 6000. Tel: (09) 325 1085. Mixed accommodation, reasonable rates.

QUEENSLAND

Anglican Women's Hostel, Moray Street, New Farm, Qld 4005. Tel: (07) 229 3831. For single women only, no children.

Black Community Housing Group, Paris Street, West End, Qld 4101. Tel: (07) 844 4006.

Jane Arnold Hostel, 155 Moray Street, New Farm, Qld 4005. Tel: (07) 358 2694. For single women or women with children.

Opal, 2331 Pacific Highway, Eight Mile Plains, Qld 4123. Tel: (07) 341 5510. Cost depends on circumstances.

Queensland Country Women's Association Female Hostel, 5 Brisbane Street, Ipswich, Qld 4305. Tel: (07) 281 3701 (all hours). For girls 16–25 years old.

Yumba Hostel, 55 Gray Street, Hill End, Qld 4101. Tel: (07) 844 3721. Will take young single Aboriginal women who have money or jobs.

TASMANIA

Centacare Family Welfare, 44 Sandy Bay Road, Hobart, Tas. 7000. Tel: (002) 27 8878 (all hours). Cheap, shared, mixed accommodation.

City Mission, 50 Barrack Street, Hobart, Tas. 7000. Tel: (002) 310966. Flat available, free, limited time period.

Elim Centre (Salvation Army), 17 Lansdowne Crescent, West Hobart, Tas. 7000. Tel: (002) 34 1898 (all hours). Emergency shelter for women and children, fortnight limit, bed and board only, small charge.

Gateway Youth Hostel, 4 Bilton Street, Claremont, Tas. 7011. Tel: (002) 49 5486. For 16–25-year-olds, mixed, up to six weeks only, will help find alternative accommodation; small charge.

Salvation Army, 24 View Road, Burnie, Tas. 7320. Tel: (004) 31 5791 (all hours). For families or individuals.

Salvation Army Emergency Shelter, William Street, Devonport, Tas. 7310. Tel: (004) 24 2513 (all hours). For homeless families and individuals, charges dependent on finances.

ACT

Ainslie Village, Quick Street, Ainslie, Canberra, ACT 2602. Tel: (062) 48 6931. Cheap accommodation.

Housing Assistance Programs. Government-owned rental housing is made available to families and single persons in need. Enquiries to Allara House, London Circuit, Canberra, ACT 2601. Tel: (062) 75 8111.

YWCA, Bougainville Street, Manuka, ACT 2603. Tel: (062) 95 6775.

NORTHERN TERRITORY

YWCA, 119 Mitchell Street, Darwin, NT 5790. Tel: (089) 81 8644 (seven days). Reasonable rates, referral for cheap accommodation.

CHILD ABUSE
NEW SOUTH WALES

Contact your local office of the NSW Department of Youth and Community Services (YACS) or write to the Sydney office for information on country offices.

Blacktown Family Crisis Service. Tel: (02) 622 0522. (Parramatta and Western Suburbs.)

Child Abuse Prevention Service, Room 17, 33 Bundock Street, Randwick, NSW 2031. Tel: (02) 344 5111/7646 (all hours). For parents who fear they may physically or emotionally abuse their children (including sexual abuse), anonymity given if requested.

Hunter Region Child Protection Unit, 266 Lawson Street, Hamilton South, Newcastle, NSW 2303. Tel: (049) 69 4699.

Illawong Child Protection and Family Crisis Unit, 107 Murphy Avenue, Keiraville, NSW 2500. Tel: (042) 28 4000 (all hours).

Montrose Child Protection Unit. Tel: (02) 745 2233 (all hours). All suburbs except Parramatta and Western Suburbs family crisis service, residential assessment unit, day program, training and education service.

YACS, Child Protection and Family Crisis Centre. Tel: (02) 818 5555 (24 hours); (008) 42 5288 (toll free).

YACS, Child Protection Unit. Tel: (02) 745 2233.

VICTORIA

Child Protection Unit. For information about the nearest regional CPU, contact **Community Services of Victoria**. Tel: (03) 654 4222.

Community Policing Squad, 380 William Street, Melbourne, Vic. 3000. Tel: (03) 667 1911/1663/1664 (24 hours). Part of the Victoria police force with fourteen squads throughout Victoria to answer calls concerning child abuse and other family problems. Ring head office, (03) 320 3333, for information about country squads.

Parents Anonymous. Tel: (03) 654 4654 (all hours). Confidential support and counselling for parents who feel their children are at risk.

SOUTH AUSTRALIA

If you suspect a case of child maltreatment, contact your local district of the Department of Community Welfare by looking in the telephone directory.

Child Protection Panel: These panels review action taken by the Department of Community Welfare, play a role in the education of the community and provide information.
Central Eastern Region, 4–8 Angas Street, Kent Town, S A 5067. Tel: (08) 332 9966.
Central Northern Region, 87 John Street, Salisbury, S A 5108. Tel: (08) 258 9988.
Central Southern Region, 1 Malwa Street, Glandore, S A 5037. Tel: (08) 297 5799.
Central Western Region, PO Box 154, Port Adelaide, S A 5015. Tel: (08) 47 8777.
Mt Gambier District Office, PO Box 1160, Mt Gambier, S A 5290. Tel: (087) 25 6200.
Murray Bridge Regional Office, PO Box 721, Murray Bridge, S A 5253. Tel: (085) 32 3055.
Port Augusta Regional Office, PO Box 1137, Port Augusta West, S A 5700. Tel: (086) 42 2211.

WESTERN AUSTRALIA

Child Protection Society, 286 Beaufort Street, Perth, W A 6000. Tel: (09) 328 7047.
Children's Protection Service, Department of Community Welfare, 91 Hensman Street, Subiaco, Perth, W A 6008. Tel: (09) 382 1266.
Incest Parent Support Group. Tel: (09) 361 5903 (all hours). Feminist, experienced counsellors give support and help to deal with the problem.
Parent Help Centre, 15 Glendower Street, Perth, W A 6000. Tel: (09) 328 3266 (all hours). Service for parents worried about their feelings and behaviour towards their young children.

QUEENSLAND

Contact your local office of the Department of Children's Services with any queries or reports, and ask for the Child Protection Unit. Otherwise contact the Brisbane Child Protection Unit for information about your local office.

Child Protection Unit, PO Box 153, North Quay, Brisbane, Qld 6061. Tel: (07) 227 7111.
Family Life Centre (incest only), St Andrew's Church, 1 Wickham Terrace, Brisbane, Qld 6000. Tel: (07) 229 4090. Support group for incest victims and parents.

TASMANIA

Child Protection Assessment Board, Knopwood House, Montpelier Retreat, Battery Point, Hobart, Tas. 7000. Tel: (002) 30 2921/3660 (after hours for recorded alternative numbers). For protection of children from physical abuse.
Social Welfare Department, 12 Murray Street, Hobart, Tas. 7000. Tel: (002) 30 8011. Reports of child abuse, incest and maltreatment are made by this department after contact with a social welfare worker who reports to the Child Protection Unit.

ACT

Family Crisis Unit, ACT Administration Centre, cnr London Circuit and Constitution Avenue, Civic 2601. Tel: (062) 75 8214/8417/95 0053 (24 hours).

NORTHERN TERRITORY

Department of Health and Community Services, Welfare Service Branch. Tel: (089) 20 3268/41 1644 (24 hours).
Welfare Offices:
Alice Springs, Tio Building, Todd Street. Tel: (089) 50 3260/52 3146 (after hours).
Alyangula, Groote Eylandt Welfare Office. Tel: (089) 87 1013.
Casuarina, Ethos House, Trower Road. Tel: (089) 27 5022.
Darwin, 60 Cavenagh Street. Tel: (089) 81 4733.
Katherine, First Street. Tel: (089) 72 2555.
Nhulunbuy. Tel: (089) 87 2366.
Palmerston, Shop 8, Baywood Plaza. Tel: (089) 32 1055.
Remote Areas Team, Casuarina Plaza. Tel: (089) 20 3302.
Tennant Creek, cnr Haddock and Peko Roads. Tel: (089) 62 2442.

CHILDBIRTH
NEW SOUTH WALES

Childbirth Education Association, 127 Forest Road, Hurstville, N S W 2220. Tel: (02) 57 4927. Pre-natal classes, referrals, newsletter, literature, post-natal advice and education, discussion groups for new parents, films, practical assistance, miscarriage counselling.
Homebirth Access, PO Box 66, Broadway, N S W 2007. Tel: (02) 630 3017. Newsletter, free home help, meetings, midwife contact, literature, education.
Homebirth Australia, PO Box 107, Lawson, N S W 2783. Tel: (047) 82 2008.
Nursing Mothers' Association of Australia, 2 Queens Road, Asquith, N S W 2078. Tel: (02) 477 5934 (all hours with recorded message of phone numbers of rostered counsellors). Information on breast-feeding, literature, referral, community education, country centres.

Parents' Centres Australia, PO Box 398, Parramatta, NSW 2150. Tel: (02) 633 5899. Pre-natal classes, newsletter. Counselling for miscarriage, still birth, neo-natal death and grieving. Library. Contact Sydney office for interstate and country centres.

VICTORIA

Homebirth Register, c/o 1 Terana Crescent, Bayswater, Vic. 3153. Tel: (03) 729 0026.

Nursing Mothers' Association of Australia, 5 Glendale Street, Nunawading, Vic. 3131. Tel: (03) 878 3304.

SOUTH AUSTRALIA

Childbirth Education Association Adelaide (Inc.), 1140a South Road, Clovelly Park, SA 5042. Tel: (08) 276 9810.

Homebirth Network of South Australia, PO Box 703, Unley, SA 5061. Tel: (08) 272 7351.

Nursing Mothers' Association of Australia (SA), 11 Oliver Street, Crafers, SA 5152. Tel: (08) 339 6783/332 4094. Breast-feeding information, mothercraft instruction, literature, support groups, counselling.

Single Pregnancy and After Resource Centre, 64b Pennington Terrace, North Adelaide, SA 5006. Tel: (08) 267 4511. Support services for single-parent families, counselling, information, referrals, support group.

WESTERN AUSTRALIA

Australian Early Childhood Association, PO Box 15, West Perth, WA 6005. Tel: (09) 321 7930.

Birthplace Support Group, PO Box 1070, Fremantle, WA 6160. Tel: (09) 382 1940. Newsletter, home-birth information, midwife referral.

Home Birth, 3 Cedus Place, Menora, WA 6050. Tel: (09) 272 2531.

Nursing Mothers' Association of Australia, 41 Lichfield Street, Victoria Park, WA 6100. Tel: (09) 361 5716, or refer to telephone directory for your local centre.

QUEENSLAND

Airlea Beach Homebirth Association. Tel: (079) 46 1121.

Cairns Homebirth Association. Tel: (070) 55 9056.

Gold Coast Homebirth Association. Tel: (075) 33 9217.

Home Midwifery Association, PO Box 29, Red Cliff, Qld 4020. Tel: (07) 283 1810/285 5453.

Nursing Mothers' Association, Ross Street, Northgate, Qld 4013. Tel: (07) 266 3119. Refer to telephone directory for your local centre or phone Northgate number.

TASMANIA

Childbirth Education Association, 212 Roslyn Avenue, Blackman's Bay, Tas. 7152. Tel: (002) 29 5211.

Homebirth Tasmania, 27 Wentworth Street, South Hobart, Tas. 7000. Tel: (002) 23 5348.

Nursing Mothers' Association of Australia. Tel: (002) 48 6738 (for counselling)/29 5461 (enquiries).

ACT

Canberra Homebirth Association, PO Box 88, O'Connor, ACT 2601. Tel: (062) 41 2692.

Childbirth Education Association, PO Box 54, Woden, ACT 2606. Tel: (062) 82 3614.

Nursing Mothers' Association. Tel: (062) 58 8928 (all hours).

NORTHERN TERRITORY

Childbirth Education Association, PO Box 542, Alice Springs, NT 5750. Tel: (089) 52 7290.

Childbirth Education Association, PO Box 42162, Casuarina, NT 5792. Tel: (089) 27 2575/1731 (after hours).

Darwin Homebirth Group, PO Box 41252, Casuarina, NT 5792. Tel: (089) 88 1580.

CHILD CARE

Check first with your local council or else contact:

Community Child Care, 405–411 Sussex Street, Sydney, NSW 2000. Tel: (02) 212 4600/4144 for Australia-wide referral, including Sydney.

NEW SOUTH WALES

Aboriginal Children's Services, 31 Cope Street, Redfern, NSW 2016. Tel: (02) 699 9835.

Development Unit (ethnic), 142 Addison Road, Marrickville, NSW 2204. Tel: (02) 569 1855/1288. For training of child care workers.

Dial-a-Mum Association of Australia (parent support), PO Box 241, Wahroonga, NSW 2076. Tel: (02) 477 6777 (all hours).

Lady Gowrie Child Centre, Elliott Avenue, Erskineville, NSW 2043. Tel: (02) 517 2755.

Playgroup Association, 145 Wellington Street, Sefton, NSW 2162. Tel: (02) 645 1910.

VICTORIA

Community Child Care, 191 Brunswick Street, Fitzroy, Vic. 3065. Tel: (03) 419 1148.

Lady Gowrie Child Centre, 36 Newry Street, North Carlton, Vic. 3054. Tel: (03) 347 6388.

Playgroup Association, 94 Howard Street, North Melbourne, Vic. 3051. Tel: (03) 329 6277.

SOUTH AUSTRALIA

Early Childhood Resource and Advisory Unit, 72 Edmond Avenue, Unley, SA 5061. Tel: (08) 271 9705.

Lady Gowrie Child Centre, 39a Dew Street, Thebarton, SA 5031. Tel: (08) 352 5520.

Playgroup Association, 95 Palmer Street, North Adelaide, SA 5006. Tel: (08) 267 3695.

Remote and Isolated Children's Exercise (RICE), PO Box 1729, Port Augusta, SA 5700. Tel: (086) 42 4827.

WESTERN AUSTRALIA

Aboriginal Child Care Agency, 66 Brewer Street, East Perth, WA 6000. Tel: (09) 328 3888.

Children's Activity Time Society, 76 Boulton Street, Dianella, WA 6060. Tel: (09) 275 5171.

Lady Gowrie Child Centre, 3 Yarall Place, Karawara, WA 6152. Tel: (09) 450 5411.

Out of School Child Care Association, PO Box 437, Claremont, WA 6010. Tel: (09) 384 6233.

Playgroup Association, GPO Box 616, West Perth, WA 6005. Tel: (09) 321 3028.

QUEENSLAND

Crèche and Kindergarten Association, 14 Edmondstone Street, Newmarket, Qld 4051. Tel: (07) 356 7444.

Family Day Care, PO Box 709, Mount Isa, Qld 4825. Tel: (077) 43 3009.

Keeping in Touch Children's Centre, PO Box 1337, Cairns, Qld 4870. Tel: (070) 54 1424.

Lady Gowrie Child Centre, 228 St Paul's Terrace, Fortitude Valley, Qld 4006. Tel: (07) 52 2667.

Migrant Resource Centre, 149 Melbourne Street, Brisbane, Qld 4101. Tel: (07) 844 8144. Drama and circus groups for 10–13-year-olds.

Playgroup Association, 396 Milton Road, Auchenflower, Qld 4066. Tel: (07) 371 8253.

TASMANIA

Child Health Association, PO Box 27, Lindisfarne, Tas. 7015. Tel: (002) 44 1355. Branches in most towns, with trained sisters from the Health Department; free.

Community Services Division, Child Care
Bell. Tel: (002) 30 3204.
Burnie. Tel: (004) 30 2246.
Devonport. Tel: (004) 24 5644.
Glenorchy. Tel: (002) 30 6624.
Hobart. Tel: (002) 30 2000.
Launceston. Tel: (003) 32 2376.

Lady Gowrie Child Centre, 17 Runnymede Street, Battery Point, Tas. 7000. Tel: (002) 34 9833.

Playgroup Association, PO Box 799, Launceston, Tas. 7250. Tel: (003) 31 6599.

ACT

ACT Resource Centre, PO Box 23, Barker Centre, ACT 2603.

Australian Early Childhood Association, Knox Street, Watson, ACT 2602. Tel: (062) 41 6900.

Child Health Clinic in each suburb – contact Child Health Clinic (central office), cnr Alinga and Moore Streets, Canberra, ACT 2601. Tel: (062) 45 4111.

Occasional Care Centres in Civic, Manuka, Charnwood, Weston, Woden and Melba, c/o Marcus Clarke Street, Canberra, ACT 2600. Tel: (062) 48 5697.

NORTHERN TERRITORY

Family Day Care, PO Box 2260, Darwin, NT 5794. Tel: (089) 81 4611.

Playgroup Association, PO Box 41405, Casuarina, NT 5792. Tel: (089) 27 2144.

Welfare Office, PO Box 40596, Casuarina, NT 5792. Tel: (089) 81 4733.

COMMUNITY HEALTH CENTRES

Generally these are free and provide various services, information and referral. See the front of white pages of telephone directory under your State Government section:

New South Wales Health Department
Victoria Health Commission
South Australia Health Commission
Western Australia Public Health Department
Queensland Health Department
Tasmania Health Services Department
Northern Territory Health Department.

DRUG AND ALCOHOL SERVICES
NEW SOUTH WALES

AA Central Coast Intergroup Office, Suite 11, 412 The Entrance Roads, Lons Jetty, NSW 2261. Tel: (043) 331 1866.

AA Central Office (Lower Hunter and Newcastle), Room 7, St Peters Hall, Dixon Street, Hamilton, NSW 2303. Tel: (049) 69 2196.

AA Wollongong and Shoalhaven District, 14 Station Street, Wollongong, NSW 2500. Tel: (042) 29 5241/8177.

Al-Ateen and Al-Anon (for adolescents and families of alcoholics), 262 Pitt Street, Sydney, NSW 2000. Tel: (02) 264 9255. Self-help group meetings, emotional support.

Alcoholics Anonymous, 127 Edwin Street North, Croydon, NSW 2132. Tel: (02) 799 1199.

Langton Clinic, Centre for Education and Information on Drugs and Alcohol, cnr Nobbs and South Dowling Streets, Surry Hills, NSW 2010. Tel: (02) 331 2196.

Leichhardt Women's Health Centre, 54 Thorley Street, Leichhardt, NSW 2040. Tel: (02) 560 3011. Minor tranquillizer withdrawal clinic, counselling, referral, literature.

McKinnon Unit, Rozelle Hospital, PO Box 1, Rozelle, NSW 2039. Tel: (02) 810 9461 (all hours). Treatment centre, information, referral, education and training, drug-free withdrawal, Alcoholics Anonymous and Narcotics Anonymous.

NSW Drug and Alcohol Authority, PO Box K700, Haymarket, NSW 2000. Tel: (02) 217 6666. Funding of drug and alcohol services, education and training, information and research, policy advice.

Women's Place, PO Box 1196, Potts Point, NSW 2011. Tel: (02) 357 3186 (seven days). Refuge for drug/alcohol-dependent women, counselling, information, referral.

VICTORIA

Al-Ateen and Al-Anon Family Groups, Area Office, 238 Flinders Lane, Melbourne, Vic. Tel: (03) 650 3368. (After hours answering service).
Northern Districts: PO Box 81, Mooroopna, Vic. 3629. Tel: (058) 25 1160.

Alcohol and Drug Centre, Montclair Private Hospital, 18 Montclair Ave. Brighton North, Vic. 3186. Tel: (03) 596 6357.

Alcohol and Drug Dependence Recovery Centre, 36 Pine Cres., Boronia, Vic. 3155. Tel: (03) 762 4200 for counselling service.

Alcohol and Drug 'Direct' Line. Tel: (03) 614 1999 (24-hour service).

Alcohol, Drug and Forensic Branch, 555 Collins Street, Melbourne, Vic. 3000. Tel: (03) 616 7777. Information, education and training, co-ordination of treatment, rehabilitation, library, referral.

Alcohol and Drug Foundation, 153 Park Street, South Melbourne, Vic. 3205. Tel: (03) 690 6000. Information, referral, education and training, occupational drug and alcohol program, counselling, library.

Alcoholics Anonymous, Central Service Office, Floor 1, 658 Bridge Road, Richmond, Vic. 3121; PO Box 136, East Melbourne, Vic. 3002. Tel: (03) 429 1833.

Ballarat Regional Alcohol and Drug Dependence Association, 1001 Main Street, Ballarat, Vic. 3350. Tel: (053) 31 5333. Counselling, referral and other services.

Overeaters Anonymous, GPO Box 1102J, Melbourne, Vic. 3001. Tel: (03) 898 7852 (all hours hotline – recorded information and alternative phone numbers). Self-help group for compulsive overeaters.

Palm Lodge Rehabilitation Centre, 25 David Street, Horsham, Vic. 3400. Tel: (053) 82 3113. In- and out-patient, counselling and other services.

Women's Addiction Council on Homelessness and Addiction, PO Box 291, Brunswick, Vic. 3056. Tel: (03) 329 8515.

SOUTH AUSTRALIA

Al-Anon Family Groups, Floor 1, 31 Gilbert Place, Adelaide, SA 5001. Tel: (08) 51 2959 (after hours answering service).

Alcoholics Anonymous, AA House, 11 Rundle Road, Kent Town, SA 5067. Tel: (08) 42 2977. One group for women only.

Aboriginal Health Organization of South Australia, 62 Beulah Road, Norwood, SA 5067. Tel: (08) 218 3529. Outpatient treatment centre, information, referral, education and training, client representation in court, rehabilitation, education, counselling, library, home visiting, hospital liaison.

Aboriginal Sobriety, 128 Wakefield Street, Adelaide, SA 5000. Tel: (08) 223 4204; after hours (08) 43 8524.

Drug and Alcohol Service Council (DASC), 3/161 Greenhill Road, Parkside, SA 5063. Tel: (08) 274 3333. Administration headquarters, education, driver assessment clinic, training, library, research and information.

Narcotics Anonymous, PO Box 479, Norwood, SA 5067. Tel: (08) 223 7228.

WESTERN AUSTRALIA

Al-Anon Family Groups, 2nd Floor, 251 Hay Street East, Perth, WA 6000. Tel: (09) 325 7528 (after-hours answering service).

Alcohol and Drug Information Service, 79 Collins Street, West Perth, WA 6005. Tel: (09) 481 1088.

Alcoholics Anonymous, 2nd floor, 251 Hay Street East, Perth, WA 6000. Tel: (09) 325 3566 (all hours).

Narcotics Anonymous, PO Box 668, Subiaco, WA 6008. Tel: (09) 328 1619.

Overeaters Anonymous, PO Box 203, Double View, WA 6018. Tel: (09) 341 2708; 128 Walderton Avenue, Balga, WA 6061. Tel: (09) 349 2407.

QUEENSLAND

Al-Anon Family Groups, 308 Edward Street, Brisbane, Qld 4000. Tel: (07) 229 2501 (24 hours).

Alcohol and Drug Dependence Service, 270 Roma Street, Brisbane, Qld 4000. Tel: (07) 229 67566 (24 hours). In- and out-patient centre, information, referral, education and training, court program, counselling, library, special teenage and Aboriginal groups.

Alcohol and Drug Foundation, 119 Leichhardt Street, Spring Hill, Qld 4004. Tel: (09) 832 3798.

Alcoholics Anonymous, Central Service, 453 Ann Street, Brisbane, Qld 4000. Tel: (07) 221 7920.

Industry Co-Ord Program, PO Box 320, North Brisbane, Qld 4000. Tel: (07) 221 3045. Industrial program, education and training, consultant to employer/employee, information, referral, library, resource material, speakers.

Overeaters Anonymous, Gympie High School, Cootharabar Road, Gympie, Qld 4570. Meetings on Mondays 8 pm.

Women and Addiction Centre, 767 Stanley Street, Wooloongabba, Qld 4102; PO Box 248, Wooloongabba, Qld 4102. Tel: (07) 393 1175 (Tues. evening), (07) 369 3743 (most other times). Self-help and support centre.

TASMANIA

Al-Anon Family Groups, PO Box 293, Sandy Bay, Tas. 7005. Tel: (002) 23 4244.

Alcohol and Drug Dependence Board, Box 1403P, Hobart, Tas. 7000. Tel: (002) 30 8022.

Alcoholics Anonymous, Box 317D, GPO Hobart, Tas. 7000. Tel: (002) 34 8711.

Alcoholics and Drug Dependency Services, John Edis Hospital, Creek Road, New Town, Tas. 7008. Tel: (002) 28 8220 (all hours). Detoxification unit.

Caroline House, 19 Carr Street, New Town, Tas. 7008. Tel: (002) 28 7118 (all hours). Live-in, cost negotiable, homeless women with children for short terms, half-way house.

Division of Health, 34 Davey Street, Hobart, Tas. 7000. Tel: (002) 30 3652. Drug education program, prison program, training, library.

ACT

Al-Ateen and **Al-Anon Family Groups**, Health Promotion Centre, Childers Street, Canberra City, ACT 2600. Tel: (062) 48 8651. (After hours recorded message).

Alcohol and Drug Dependence Foundation, Health Promotion Centre, Childers Street, Canberra City, ACT 2600. Tel: (062) 47 4747. Information, referral, education and training, emphasis on prevention and early intervention counselling.

Alcoholics Anonymous, Health Promotion Centre, Childers Street, Canberra City, ACT 2600. Tel: (062) 49 1340.

Occupational Assistance Service, PO Box 214, Civic Square, Canberra, ACT 2601. Tel: (062) 48 6066. Counselling, referral, for employers to send employees.

We Help Ourselves Fellowship, 19 Keira Street, Narrabundah, ACT 2604. Tel: (062) 95 6865.

NORTHERN TERRITORY

Al-Anon and **Al-Ateen Family Groups**, Alice Springs Hospital. Tel: (089) 50 2211 (phone for meetings only).

Alcoholics Anonymous, 2 Water Street, Northcliffe, NT 5790. Tel: (089) 85 4479 (24-hour emergency service).

Darwin and Districts Alcohol and Drug Dependence Foundation Inc., 155 Stuart Highway, Parap, NT 5790. Tel: (089) 81 8030.

NT Drug and Alcohol Bureau, 79 Smith Street, Darwin, NT 5790. Tel: (089) 80 2911.

Overeaters Anonymous, Casuarina Library, Darwin, NT 5790. Meetings on Wednesdays 7 pm.

FAMILY PLANNING ASSOCIATIONS

Hundreds of clinics throughout Australia offering various services: contraception, gynaecological treatment, sexuality, counselling, male sterilization, education, literature, library, resources and referral.

NEW SOUTH WALES

Family Planning Association of NSW, 161 Broadway, Broadway, NSW 2007. Tel: (02) 211 0244 (administration), (02) 698 9499 (enquiries for counselling).

VICTORIA

Family Planning Association of Victoria, 259 Church Street, Richmond, Vic. 3121. Tel: (03) 429 1868/6871. (Training and Education Unit.)

SOUTH AUSTRALIA

Family Planning Association of South Australia Inc., 17 Phillips Street, Kensington, SA 5068. Tel: (08) 31 5177.

WESTERN AUSTRALIA

Family Planning Association of Western Australia, 104 Collins Street, West Perth, WA 6005. Tel: (09) 321 6607.

QUEENSLAND

Family Planning Association of Queensland, 100 Alfred Street, Fortitude Valley, Qld 4006. Tel: (07) 52 5151.

TASMANIA

Family Planning Association of Tasmania, 73 Federal Street, North Hobart, Tas. 7002. Tel: (002) 34 7200.

ACT

Family Planning Association of ACT, Health Promotion Centre, Childers Street, Canberra City, ACT 2605. Tel: (062) 47 3077.

NORTHERN TERRITORY

Family Planning Association of NT, 133 Mitchell Street, Lawwakeyah, NT 5790. Tel: (089) 81 5335.

LESBIAN GROUPS

Check what each centre can provide: social events, library, counselling information, resources, political action.

NEW SOUTH WALES

Clover Business Woman's Club, PO Box 28, St Leonards, NSW 2065. Tel: (02) 810 1558 (after 6 pm). Non-political, non-sectarian, businesswomen's club.

Gay Counselling Service, 51 Holt Street, Surry Hills, NSW 2010. Tel: (02) 211 1177. (Sydney *Gay Guide* available from this address.)

Homosexual Acceptance Centre, 57 Hold Street, Surry Hills, NSW 2010. Tel: (02) 212 5247.

Lesbian Line (feminist), PO Box 247, Rozelle, NSW 2039. Tel: (02) 810 5630.

VICTORIA

Gay Advisory Service, McLachlan Street, Northcote, Vic. 3070. Tel: (03) 489 2059.

Gayline Support Service, Box 1801, GPO, Melbourne, Vic. 3001. Tel: (03) 329 5555.

Lesbian Line (feminist), 295 Victoria Street, West Melbourne, Vic. 3003. Tel: (03) 329 8515. Information and referral service. Social events, discussion, counselling.

SOUTH AUSTRALIA

Gayline, PO Box 459, North Adelaide, SA 5006. Tel: (08) 268 5577.

Women's Liberation (feminist), 234a Rundle Street, Adelaide, SA 5000. Tel: (08) 223 1005. Groups, discussion.

WESTERN AUSTRALIA

Camp WA, GPO Box 1031, Perth, WA 6001. Tel: (09) 328 9044/386 255.

Gay Counselling Service, GPO Box G406, Perth, WA 6000. Tel: (09) 328 9044.

QUEENSLAND

Homosexual Counselling and Welfare Service, Brunswick Street, Fortitude Valley, Qld 4006. Tel: (07) 852 1414.

Lesbian Feminist Network, c/o University of Queensland, PO Box 279, Ashgrove, Qld 4060. Tel: (07) 371 1611 ext 233.

TASMANIA

Lesbian Line. Tel: (002) 34 5839.

ACT

Contact Women's Health Centres for counselling, information, resources, contacts, etc., or:

ACT Gay Contact, PO Box 214, Woden, ACT 2606. Tel: (062) 47 2726.

Lesbian Line, c/o Women's Centre, 3 Lobelia Street, O'Connor, ACT 2601. Tel: (062) 47 8882.

MIGRANT SERVICES

In the white pages of the telephone directory, various migrant services are listed alphabetically under 'M' for migrant. Major hospitals have an ethnic services co-ordinator. State Departments of Health have all services: advisers, interpreters, translations, health education personnel, health promotion, training.

NEW SOUTH WALES

Ethnic Affairs Commission, Floor 1, 164 Liverpool Road, Ashfield, NSW 2131. Tel: (02) 797 8244. Liaising, research, increasing accessibility of services, information for migrant women.

Interpreter Services:
Leichhardt Women's Centre. Tel: (02) 560 3011.
Liverpool Women's Centre. Tel: (02) 601 3555.
Telephone Interpreter Service. Tel: (02) 221 1111.

VICTORIA

Migrant Resource Centre, 575 Elizabeth Street, Melbourne, Vic. 3000. Tel: (03) 328 2421.

Migrant Women's Officer (Welfare Department), Ethnic Affairs Unit, Department of Immigration, Local Government and Ethnic Affairs, cnr Spring and Latrobe Streets, Melbourne, Vic. 3000. Tel: (03) 669 2978. To link migrant women to the services available to them in the Commonwealth Government.

SOUTH AUSTRALIA

Migrant Women's Officer, Department of Immigration and Ethnic Affairs, Floor 6, 150 North Terrace, Adelaide, SA 5001. Tel: (08) 216 7111. To link migrant women in the community to the services available to them.

Telephone Interpreter Service. Tel: (08) 213 1999 (all hours, seven days). Free, information, referral, interpreting service, over fifty languages. Contact with interpreters can be arranged in special circumstances. Whyalla callers: 45 3033. For the price of a local call, you will be transferred to the Adelaide Interpreter Service.

Women's Information Switchboard, 122 Kintore Avenue, Adelaide, SA 5000. Tel: (08) 223 1244 (7 days); (008) 188 158 toll-free for country callers. Speak various languages, counselling information. See Women's Health Centres for more information.

WESTERN AUSTRALIA

Migrant Resource Centre, 186 High Street, Fremantle, WA 6160. Tel: (09) 335 9588.

Migrant Women's Officer, Department of Immigration and Ethnic Affairs, 12–14 St Georges Terrace, Perth, WA 6000. Tel: (09) 325 0521. To link migrant women in the community to the services available to them.

Telephone Interpreter Service. Tel: (09) 325 9144 (all hours – can reverse-charge calls).

QUEENSLAND

Migrant Telephone Interpreter Service. Tel: (07) 225 2233 (after hours switched through to Sydney). Local phone call charged only – can reverse-charge call from country areas.

Migrant Women's Officer (Welfare Department), Department of Immigration and Ethnic Affairs, 100 Edward Street, Brisbane, Qld 4000. Tel: (07) 233 6033. To link migrant women in the community to services available to them.

TASMANIA

Migrant Resource Centre, 75 Cameron Street,

Launceston, Tas. 7250. Tel: (003) 31 2470; 222 Elizabeth Street, Hobart, Tas. 7000. Tel: (002) 34 9411.
Migrant Telephone Interpreter Service. Tel: (002) 34 3599 (all hours).

ACT

Migrant Women's Officer (Welfare Department), Department of Immigration and Ethnic Affairs, Chan Street, Belconnen, ACT 2617. Tel: (062) 64 1111. To link migrant women in the community to the services available to them.
Telephone Interpreter Service. Tel: (062) 49 8555 (all hours). If calling from Albury/Wodonga, phone 24 5122 for cost of local call.

NORTHERN TERRITORY

Migrant Women's Officer (Welfare Department), Department of Immigration and Ethnic Affairs, PO Box 864, Darwin, NT 5794. Tel: (089) 81 4566. To link migrant women in the community to the services available to them.

OCCUPATIONAL HEALTH CENTRES

Independent non-profit research and information centres concerned with widespread but largely neglected problem of occupational illness and injury. Workers' Health Centres and other Centres involved in occupational health povide information on health and safety to unions, workers and the community.

NEW SOUTH WALES

Workers' Health Centre, 27 John Street, Lidcombe, NSW 2141. Tel: (02) 646 3233/643 1851. Library, information, referral, treatment, groups, support re injury or health, education, research, speakers.

VICTORIA

Western Region Community Health Centre, 72–78 Paisley Street, Footscray, Vic. 3011. Tel: (03) 689 4888.
Western Region Working Women's Centre, 93 Cowper Street, Footscray, Vic. 3011. Tel: (03) 689 3273/8758.
Workcare, Occupational Health and Safety, 80 Collins Street, Melbourne, Vic. 3000. Tel: (03) 651 0011.

SOUTH AUSTRALIA

Adelaide Women's Health Centre, 64 Pennington Terrace, North Adelaide, SA 5006. Tel: (08) 267 5366.

QUEENSLAND

Brisbane Worker's Health Centre, 16 Peal St, South Brisbane, Qld 4101. Tel: (07) 846 2719.

UNION CENTRES
NEW SOUTH WALES

NSW Labor Council, Occupational Health Unit, 377–383 Sussex Street, Sydney, NSW 2000. Tel: (02) 264 1691.
Occupational Health and Safety Officer, AMWU, 136 Chalmers Street, Surry Hills, NSW 2010. Tel: (02) 698 9988.
Trade Union Medical Centre, 2nd Floor, 515 Kent Street, Sydney, NSW 2000. Tel: (02) 267 8120.

VICTORIA

ACTU/VYHV Occupational Health Unit, Trades Hall, 54 Victoria Street, Melbourne, Vic. 3000. Tel: (03) 662 3511.
Occupational Health and Safety Officer, AMWU, 174 Victoria Parade, East Melbourne, Vic. 3053. Tel: (03) 662 1333.

RAPE CRISIS ASSISTANCE
NEW SOUTH WALES

Rape Crisis Centre (feminist). Tel: (02) 819 6565 (24 hours, reverse-charge calls to centre). Counselling/talk/support, will accompany a woman to hospital, police and court if she chooses; basic information on medical, legal, restraining orders; self-defence classes; refuge contact; speakers go to schools or women's groups.
Rape/Sexual Assault Clinics can be found at the following hospitals:
    Blacktown Hospital, Blacktown, NSW 2148. Tel: (02) 622 1111; (02) 622 6111 (after hours).
    King George V Hospital, Missenden Road, Camperdown, NSW 2050. Tel: (02) 516 6111.
    Prince of Wales Children's Hospital, High Street, Randwick, NSW 2031. Tel: (02) 399 0111.
    Royal North Shore Hospital, Pacific Highway, St Leonards, NSW 2065. Tel: (02) 438 7111.
    St George's Hospital, Belgrave Street, Kogarah, NSW 2217. Tel: (02) 588 1111 (all hours).
    Westmead Hospital, Westmead, NSW 2145. Tel: (02) 633 6333 (all hours).

If wanting to report rape to police, the least traumatic way is to ring Rape Crisis Centre or a hospital (listed above), where you will see a social worker, forensic evidence will be taken, and medical treatment will be given as necessary; you are given time to think and then the police are contacted.

VICTORIA

Sexual Assault Clinic, Queen Victoria Medical Centre, 172 Lonsdale Street, Melbourne, Vic. 3000. Tel: (03) 665 5111 (24 hours).

SOUTH AUSTRALIA

Rape Crisis Centre (feminist), PO Box 230 Woodville, SA

5011. Tel: (08) 363 0233 (crisis). Emergency and on-going support, information about VD, tests, abortion; will accompany woman to hospital, police or courts; referrals to doctors, lawyers or others; teaches self-defence and assertiveness; general information about women and rape; provides speakers for community groups.

Sexual Assault Referral Centre, Queen Elizabeth Hospital, Woodville Road, Woodville, SA 5011. Tel: (08) 45 0222 (all hours).

Rape Enquiry Unit, Police Department. Tel: (08) 218 1212.

WESTERN AUSTRALIA

Princess Margaret Hospital, Roberts Road, Subiaco, WA 6008. Tel: (09) 382 8222. For children under 12 years old.

Rape Crisis Assistance, Sexual Assault Referral Centre, Sir Charles Gardner Hospital, Nedlands, WA 6009. Tel: (09) 389 3333 (all hours). Woman doctors on call and sympathetic counsellors.

Sexual Assault Referral Centre, 411 Barker Road, Subiaco, WA 6009. Tel: (09) 382 3323.

QUEENSLAND

Mater Hospital, Raymond Terrace, Brisbane, Qld 4000. Tel: (07) 240 8111. Will admit children on suspicion of rape or incest and do child analysis.

Rape Crisis Centre. Tel: (07) 844 4008 (24 hours).

Royal Brisbane Hospital, Herston Road, Herston, Qld 4006. Tel: (07) 253 8111. Will admit children on suspicion of rape or incest and do child analysis.

TASMANIA

Hospitals:

Calvary Hospital, 49 Augusta Road, Lenah Valley, Tas. 7008. Tel: (002) 28 0331.

Royal Hobart Hospital, 48 Liverpool Street, Hobart, Tas. 7000. Tel: (002) 38 8308.

Rape Crisis Information Centre. Tel: (002) 34 7200.

Women Against Rape (feminist), c/o Women's Phone Information Service, Department of the Prime Minister, 169 Liverpool Street, Hobart, Tas. 7000. Tel: (002) 34 2166.

ACT

Rape Crisis Line. Tel: (062) 47 2525.
Public Hospitals.

NORTHERN TERRITORY

Hospitals.

REFUGES
NEW SOUTH WALES

Amelie House, Como, NSW 2266. Tel: (02) 528 9426.

Blacktown Community Cottage, Blacktown, NSW 2148. Tel: (02) 621 8253.

Bonnie Women's Refuge, PO Box 57, Canley Heights, NSW 2166. Tel: (02) 609 3939.

Bringa Women's Resource Centre, PO Box 556, Dee Why, NSW 2099. Tel: (02) 981 1971.

Butler Lodge Women's Refuge, Glebe, NSW 2037. Tel: (02) 660 1274/692 0857.

Cawarra Women's Refuge, PO Box 20, Mt Druitt, NSW 2770. Tel: (047) 21 8922.

Delvena Women's Shelter, PO Box 495, Lane Cove, NSW 2066.

Elsie Women's Refuge, Glebe, NSW 2037. Tel: (02) 660 1371.

Essie Women's Refuge, PO Box 62, Rooty Hill, NSW 2766. Tel: (02) 625 7503/622 0522.

Homeless Persons Information Centre, 5th floor, 449 Pitt Street, Sydney, NSW 2000. Tel: (02) 211 4653/4415.

Marian Villa, Arncliffe, NSW 2205. Tel: (02) 599 7776 (all hours). Women and children.

Penrith Refuge, PO Box 55, Penrith, NSW 2750. Tel: (047) 32 2318.

Women's Emergency Refuge (Salvation Army), La Perouse, NSW 2036. Tel: (02) 398 9057 (all hours).

VICTORIA

Women's Refuge Referral Service (feminist), PO Box 382, North Melbourne, Vic. 3066. Tel: (03) 329 8433 (should contact this number first, not the refuge).

Aboriginal Refuge, c/o Aboriginal Advancement League, 219 Westgarth Street, Northcote, Vic. 3070.

Brenda, PO Box 65, East Doncaster, Vic. 3109.

Emma, PO Box 547, Warrnambool, Vic. 3280.

Latrobe Refuge (feminist), PO Box 108, Churchill, Vic. 3842.

Maroondah, PO Box 12, Ringwood, Vic. 3134.

Matilda, PO Box 4054, Melbourne, Vic. 3001.

Mordialloc Refuge, PO Box 219, Mentone, Vic. 3194. Tel: (03) 584 7539.

Mountain Refuge, PO Box 260, Belgrave, Vic. 3160.

Peninsula, PO Box 512, Frankston, Vic. 3199.

Robinson Refuge, PO Box 66, Blackburn, Vic. 3130.

Sheila, PO Box 53, Footscray, Vic. 3011.

Western Region, PO Box 45, Mooney Ponds, Vic. 3039.

Yarra Valley, PO Box 188, West Heidelberg, Vic. 3081.

SOUTH AUSTRALIA

Bramwell House Emergency Units (Salvation Army). Tel: (08) 79 7614.

Christies Beach Women's Shelter, PO Box 111, Christies Beach, SA 5165. Tel: (08) 382 0004/0066. Women and children.

Hope Haven Women and Children Emergency Shelter. Tel: (08) 344 6011. Women and children.

Irene Women's Shelter. Tel: (08) 293 4488; (08) 297 9698 (after hours). Women and children.

Para Districts Women's Shelter, PO Box 326, Elizabeth, SA 5112. Tel: (08) 255 3469. Women and children, run by religious institution.

Western Area Women's Shelter, PO Box 252, Woodville, SA 5011. Tel: (08) 268 7897.

Women's Emergency Shelter (feminist). Tel: (08) 267 5982; (08) 267 4982 (after hours). Women and children, counselling, health care.

QUEENSLAND

Brisbane Youth Service, 97 Wickham Street, Fortitude Valley, Qld 4006. Tel: (07) 229 6661. Employs street workers, Christian.

Kalparrin Women's Refuge, PO Box 780, Fortitude Valley, Qld 4006.

Koolkuna, PO Box 373, Redcliffe, Qld 4020.

Legion of Mary Hostel, Indooroopilly, Qld 4068.

Mary and Martha's, 12 Hawthorne Street, Woolloongabba, Qld 4102; PO Box 48, Holland Park, Qld 4121.

Redcliffe Women's Refuge, PO Box 144, Margate, Qld 4109.

Ringsfield Women's Refuge (Lifeline), PO Box 108, Fortitude Valley, Qld 4006.

Youth Emergency Shelter, 25 Thorne Street, Windsor, Qld 4030.

TASMANIA

Annie Kenny Young Women's Refuge (feminist), PO Box 115, North Hobart, Tas. 7002. Tel: (002) 34 6359. For homeless women.

ELIM (Salvation Army), 17 Lansdowne Crescent, West Hobart, Tas. 7000. Tel: (002) 34 1898.

Gireh House Women's Shelter (Uniting Church), Kingston, Tas. 7150. Tel: (002) 29 3750.

Hobart Women's Shelter (feminist), PO Box 367, Sandy Bay, Tas. 7005. Tel: (002) 34 6323 (all hours). Half-way house for women.

ACT

Canberra Women's Refuge, PO Box 203, Kingston, ACT 2604. Tel: (062) 95 9618.

Caroline Chisholm (Catholic), 23 Aurora Close, Mawson, ACT 2607. Tel: (062) 86 2173. Women and children.

Queanbeyan Women's Refuge, PO Box 810, Queanbeyan, ACT 2620. Tel: (062) 97 6070.

Single Women's Shelter, PO Box 75, Watson, ACT 2602. Tel: (062) 47 2438. Women without children.

Youth Refuge, Downer, ACT 2602. Tel: (062) 47 0330. Mixed.

NORTHERN TERRITORY

Women's Refuge, PO Box 41744, Casuarina, NT 5792. Tel: (089) 27 4581.

WOMEN'S CENTRES
NEW SOUTH WALES

See telephone directory.

Aquarius Youth Service, 196 Palmer Street, Darlinghurst, NSW. Tel: (02) 357 6270.

South Sydney Women's Centre (feminist), 231 Abercrombie Street, Chippendale, NSW 2008. Tel: (02) 699 7494.

Washhouse (feminist), 30 Myrtus Crescent, Bidwill, NSW 2770. Tel: (02) 628 3008.

Women and Girls' Advisory Centre, 401a Pitt Street, Sydney, NSW 2000. Tel: (02) 264 7114. Drop-in, resource and reference, welfare assistance.

Women's Action Alliance (Australia), c/o PO Box 1165, North Sydney, NSW 2060. To strive to advance and benefit women within the community.

Women's Liberation House (feminist), 62 Regency Street, Chippendale, NSW 2008. Tel: (02) 699 5281.

VICTORIA

Women with Disabilities Feminist Collective, 38 Larnook Street, Prahran, Vic. 3181. Tel: (03) 534 7231.

Women's Action Alliance (Australia), Suite 6, 493 Riversdale Road, Camberwell, Vic. 3124. Tel: (03) 82 8809.

Women's Advisory Service, Office of Women's Affairs, Department of Premier and Cabinet, 1 Treasury Place, Melbourne, Vic. 3002. Tel: (03) 651 1703. To provide an information and referral service for women by telephone.

Women's Centre (feminist), 295 Victoria Street, West Melbourne, Vic. 3003. Tel: (03) 329 8515.

SOUTH AUSTRALIA

St Peter's Women's Community Centre, 64 Nelson Street, Stepney, SA 5065. Tel: (08) 42 6571. Free service, information, resources, library, child care, craft, discussion and groups.

Women's Action Alliance (Australia), PO Box 301, Unley, SA 5061.

Women's Information Switchboard, 122 Kintore Avenue, Adelaide, SA 5000. Tel: (08) 223 1244 (reverse-call charge for country women). Free, provides information and counselling; accompanies women when they deal with government departments; government managed; multi-lingual; drop-in centre.

Women's Liberation Centre (feminist), 234a Rundle Street, Adelaide, SA 5000. Tel: (08) 223 1005. Information, various groups, political, counselling referral; pregnancy testing.

WESTERN AUSTRALIA

Campus Women's Groups, c/o Student Guild, Murdoch University. Tel: (09) 323 2158.

Campus Women's Groups, c/o Student Guild, Western

Australian Institute of Technology. Tel: (09) 451 8611. Ask for women's room or women's officer.

Women's Action Alliance (Australia), 9 Durant Way, Brentwood, WA 6153. Tel: (09) 364 4286.

QUEENSLAND

Women's Action Alliance, 243 Brunswick Street, Fortitude Valley, Qld 4006. Tel: (07) 52 7078.

Women's House, 54 Browning Street, West End, Qld 4101. Tel: (07) 44 4008 (after hours recorded message with alternative number).

TASMANIA

Community Resource Centre and Women's Room, 290 Murray Street, Hobart, Tas. 7000. Tel: (002) 34 6397. Ask for women's room.

Women's Action Alliance, PO Box 53, Glenorchy, Tas. 7010. Tel: (002) 44 4679.

Women's Information Service. Tel: (002) 23 6547.

ACT

Women's Action Alliance, 10 Scarlett Street, Melba, ACT 2615.

Women's Centre (feminist), 3 Lobelia Street, O'Connor, ACT 2601. Tel: (062) 47 8070.

Women's Shopfront Information Service, Ground Floor, CML Building, Darwin Place, Canberra, ACT 2600. Tel: (062) 46 7266.

NORTHERN TERRITORY

Women's House/Crisis Centre, PO Box 3219, Alice Springs, NT 5750. Tel: (089) 52 6075. Information groups, health issues, abortion referral, counselling.

WOMEN'S HEALTH CENTRES

These centres generally provide information on any issue of women's health, contraceptives, gynaecological treatment, counselling/support, talking, referral; resource centre, literature, library groups of many kinds, migrant workers, drug/alcohol workers. The list goes on and on. Ring about anything you want help on, and they'll probably be able to help.

NEW SOUTH WALES

Bankstown Women's Health Centre (feminist), 74 Restwell Street, Bankstown, NSW 2200. Tel: (02) 70 1378.

Darling Street Women's Health Centre (feminist), 323 Darling Street, Balmain, NSW 2041. Tel: (02) 818 2364/ 2994. Abortion, contraceptives, gynaecological treatment.

Leichhardt Women's Community Health Centre (feminist), 164 Flood Street, Leichhardt, NSW 2040. Tel: (02) 560 3011. Free service.

Liverpool Women's Community Health Centre (feminist), 273 George Street, Liverpool, NSW 2170. Tel: (02) 601 3555. Free service.

Women's Healing Centre (feminist), 119 Trafalgar Street, Annandale, NSW 2038. Tel: (02) 660 4316. Alternative health services, e.g. massage, naturopathy, etc.

VICTORIA

Women's Health Group, c/o Collingwood Community Health Centre, 145 Sackville Street, Collingwood, Vic. Tel: (03) 419 6155.

Women's Health Information Centre, Royal Women's Hospital, 132 Grattan Street, Carlton, Vic. 3053. Tel: (03) 344 2650. Drop-in, information, resource.

Women's Health Line, Emergency Department, Royal Women's Hospital. Tel: (03) 344 2650. (Referral only, all hours.)

Women's Health Resource Collective (feminist), 199–201 Sydney Road, Brunswick, Vic. 3056. Tel: (03) 380 9974.

SOUTH AUSTRALIA

Adelaide Women's Community Health Centre (feminist), 64 Pennington Terrace, North Adelaide, SA 5006. Tel: (08) 267 5366. Free services, counselling, gynaecological health, information and literature, groups, speakers, occupational health concerns.

Elizabeth Women's Community Health Centre (feminist), cnr Woodford Road and Elizabeth Way, Elizabeth, SA 5112. Tel: (08) 252 3711. Free services, groups, health care, information and referral, pregnancy tests, counselling, literature.

WESTERN AUSTRALIA

Aboriginal Medical Service, 154 Edward Street, East Perth, WA 6000. Tel: (09) 328 3888 (all hours, emergency).

East–West Acupuncture Centre. Tel: (09) 381 9518.

Women's Health Care House, 92 Thomas Street, West Perth, WA 6005. Tel: (09) 321 2383.

QUEENSLAND

Aboriginal and Islander Community Health Service, 10 Hubert Street, Woolloongabba, Qld 4102. Tel: (07) 393 0055; 10 Poinciana Street, Inala, Qld 4077. Tel: (07) 372 1235. Free dental, medical, maternal and child welfare service, information.

TASMANIA

Hobart Women's Health Collective (feminist), GPO Box 1053, Hobart, Tas. 7000. Group only, working on funding.

ACT

Women's Health Service (feminist), 3 Lobelia Street, O'Connor, ACT 2601. Tel: (062) 47 8070. Referral, information.

Women's Health and Family Planning, Department of Health, PO Box 100, Woden, ACT 2606. Adviser to provide advice on family planning and other health matters of special significance to women.

MENTAL HEALTH
NEW SOUTH WALES

Aftercare Association of NSW, 3/3 Wharf Road, Leichhardt, NSW 2040. Tel: (02) 810 7878. Accommodation and rehabilitation training for people suffering from psychiatric or intellectual disabilities.

Louisa Lawson House, 112 West Botany Street, Arncliffe, NSW 2205. Tel: (02) 59 4251. Groups, resources, therapy, information, referral, counselling, support, talking.

National Grow, 209A Edgeware Road, Marrickville, NSW 2204. Tel: (02) 516 3733.

PALA, 119 Birrell Street, PO Box 153, Waverly, NSW 2024. Tel: (02) 389 5806.

VICTORIA

GROW, 29 Erasmus Street, Surrey Hills, Vic. 3127. Tel: (03) 890 9846. Community mental health movement.

SOUTH AUSTRALIA

GROW, 354 Marion Road, Plympton, SA 5037. Tel: (08) 297 6933.

WESTERN AUSTRALIA

Association of Relatives and Friends of the Mentally Ill, 311 Hay Street, Subiaco, WA 6008. Tel: (09) 381 4747.

GROW, 146 Beaufort Street, Perth, WA 6000. Tel: (09) 328 3344.

QUEENSLAND

GROW, PO Box 178, Holland Park, Qld 4121. Tel: (07) 394 4344.

TASMANIA

GROW, Hampden House, 82 Hampden Road, Battery Point, Tas. 7004. Tel: (002) 23 6284.

ACT

GROW, Grow House, Canberra, ACT 2600. Tel: (062) 95 7791.

WOMEN'S HOSPITALS
NEW SOUTH WALES

King George V Hospital, Missenden Road, Camperdown, NSW 2050. Tel: (02) 516 6111.

Royal Hospital for Women, 188 Oxford Street, Paddington, NSW 2021. Tel: (02) 339 4111.

VICTORIA

Mercy Maternity Hospital, Clarendon Street, East Melbourne, Vic. 3002. Tel: (03) 411 0261.

Monash Medical Centre, 246 Clayton Road, Clayton, Vic. 3168. Tel: (03) 550 1111. Birthing centre.

The Royal Women's Hospital, 132 Grattan Street, Carlton, Vic. 3053. Tel: (03) 344 2000. Birthing centre.

SOUTH AUSTRALIA

Mother's and Baby's Health Association, Mothercraft Hospital, 293 South Terrace, Adelaide, SA 5000. Tel: (08) 223 2477.

Queen Victoria Hospital for Women, 160 Fullarton Road, Rose Park, SA 5067. Tel: (08) 332 4888. No birthing centres in SA.

WESTERN AUSTRALIA

King Edward Memorial Hospital for Women, Bagot Rd, Subiaco, WA 6008. Tel: (09) 380 4444. Has 'natural birth room' used at discretion of woman and her doctor.

QUEENSLAND

Royal Women's Hospital, Bowen Bridge Road, Brisbane, Qld 4029. Tel: (07) 253 8111. There are no home-birth centres within hospitals in Queensland.

TASMANIA

Queen Alexandra Hospital for Women, 31 Argyle Street, Hobart, Tas. 7000. Tel: (002) 38 8308.

ACT

No women's hospitals so contact general hospitals:
Calvary Hospital. Tel: (062) 52 9111.
John James Memorial Hospital. Tel: (062) 81 8100.
Queanbeyan District Hospital. Tel: (062) 97 2266.
Royal Canberra Hospital. Tel: (062) 43 2111.
Woden Valley Hospital. Tel: (062) 81 0433.
No home-birth centres in ACT.

NORTHERN TERRITORY

No separate women's hospitals in the Northern Territory. No home-birth centres within the general hospitals though they have delivery facilities.

VD CLINICS
NEW SOUTH WALES

Prince of Wales Hospital, High Street, Randwick, NSW 2031. Tel: (02) 399 2455. Phone for appointment.
Sexual Health Clinic, The Parramatta Hospital, 158 Marsden Street, Parramatta, NSW 2150. Tel: (02) 635 0333. Phone for appointment.
Sexually Transmitted Diseases Clinic, 93 Macquarie Street, Sydney, NSW 2000. Tel: (02) 217 5990 (male); (02) 217 5993 (female). Phone for appointment.
STD Clinic, Royal North Shore Hospital, Pacific Highway, St Leonards, NSW 2223. Tel: (02) 438 0411. Phone for appointment.

VICTORIA

Communicable Diseases Centre, 364 Little Lonsdale Street, Melbourne, Vic. 3000. Tel: (03) 602 4900.
Sexually Transmitted Diseases Clinic, Queen Victoria Medical Centre, Lonsdale Street, Melbourne, Vic. 3000. Tel: (03) 665 5111.
STD Clinic, Western General Hospital, Gordon Street, Footscray, Vic. 3011. Tel: (03) 317 0211 ext. 473.

SOUTH AUSTRALIA

Port Adelaide Community Health Services, Special Clinic for Venereal Diseases, 32 Nile Street, Port Adelaide, SA 5015. Tel: (08) 47 1715/7811/7634.
STD Clinic, Flinders Medical Centre, Microbiology Department, Level 5, Bedford Park, SA 5042. Tel: (08) 275 9911. (Contact for hours.)
Venereal Diseases Control Centre, 275 North Terrace, Adelaide, SA 5000. Tel: (08) 218 3557.

WESTERN AUSTRALIA

King Edward Memorial Hospital for Women Consultation Clinic, Bagot Road, Subiaco, WA 6008. Tel: (09) 380 4444.
Queen Elizabeth II Medical Centre, Room 12, Link B, Diagnostic Unit, Nedlands, WA 6009. Tel: (09) 380 1122 ext. 3327.
STD Clinic, 69 Moore Street, Perth, WA 6000. Tel: (09) 325 6466.

QUEENSLAND

STD Special Clinic, 484 Adelaide Street, Brisbane, Qld 4000. Tel: (07) 224 5634 (male); (07) 229 8264 (female).

TASMANIA

Special Clinic, Royal Hobart Hospital, Liverpool Street, Hobart, Tas. 7000. Tel: (002) 38 8441/8442.

ACT

STD Clinic, Woden Valley Hospital, Garran, ACT 2605. Tel: (062) 81 0433.

NORTHERN TERRITORY

Any Community Health Centre in the Northern Territory is equipped to deal with STD patients, but only the Alice Springs Centre is designated as an STD Clinic.

Casualty Department, Casuarina Hospital, Casuarina, NT 5792. Tel: (089) 20 7211.

AIDS (Acquired Immune Deficiency Syndrome)
NEW SOUTH WALES

Albion Street Centre, 150 Albion Street, Surry Hills, NSW 2010. Tel: (02) 332 4000.

VICTORIA

AIDS Clinic, Communicable Diseases Centre, 364 Little Lonsdale Street, Melbourne, Vic. 3000. Tel: (03) 602 4900.
AIDS Hotline. Tel: (03) 347 3000 (counselling, advice and information).
AIDS Support Group, The Peter Knight Centre, 117 Johnston Street, Collingwood, Vic. 3066. Tel: (03) 417 1759.

SOUTH AUSTRALIA

Sexually Transmitted Disease Services, 275 North Terrace, Adelaide, SA 5000. Tel: (08) 218 3668.

WESTERN AUSTRALIA

AIDS Information Line. Tel: (09) 11 642 (for advice, counselling and information).

QUEENSLAND

Venereal Disease Clinic, 484 Adelaide Street, Brisbane, Qld 4000. Tel: (07) 227 7095 (female); (07) 227 7091 (male).

TASMANIA

AIDS Hotline. Tel: (008) 005 188 (toll free) – information and counselling.

ACT

AIDS Reference Centre, Woden Valley Hospital, Yamba Drive, Garran, ACT 2605. Tel: (062) 842184/842231.

NORTHERN TERRITORY

NT Aids Clinical Advisory Group, Royal Darwin Hospital, Rocklands Drive, Tiwi, NT 5792. Tel: (089) 20 7211.

NEW ZEALAND

This New Zealand directory does not claim to be a thoroughly comprehensive list in all categories, but every effort has been made to provide the latest information. Citizens Advice Bureaux (listed in local telephone directories) are a good source of information throughout New Zealand.

WOMEN'S GROUPS: GENERAL

If you are seeking further information on specific health issues and groups not covered in the individual listings, the following women's organizations will be able to refer you to the appropriate sources and address.

Broadsheet (feminist magazine), PO Box 5799, Auckland.
Citizens Advice Bureaux. See local phone directory.
Maori Women's Counselling & Support, 27A Garland Rd, One Tree Hill, Auckland. Tel: 595–431.
Maori Women's Health Centre, PO Box 8696, Symonds St, Auckland. Tel: 397–790.
Maori Women's Support, Hamilton. Tel: (071) 557–282.
Maori Women's Support, Wellington. Tel: (04) 848–116.
Ministry of Women's Affairs, Private Bag, Wellington.
New Zealand Working Women's Council, PO Box 27–215, Wellington.
NOW, PO Box 2946, Auckland.
Social Works Department at Public Hospitals throughout New Zealand.
Society for Research on Women, PO Box 13–078, Johnsonville, Wellington. Tel: 766–468.
West Auckland Women's Centre, 11 McLeod Rd, Henderson. Tel: 836–6381.
Womanline, 63 Ponsonby Road, Auckland. Tel: 765–173. Telephone listening, information and referral service.
Women Against Pornography, 10 Kensington St, Wellington. Tel: 846–340.
Women's Studies Association, PO Box 5067, Auckland.
Women's Support Centre, PO Box 909, Papakura.

ABORTION COUNSELLING AND SERVICES

ACWAR (Action Council for Women's Abortion Rights), PO Box 1236, Auckland.
ALRANZ (Abortion Rights):
  PO Box 33–135, Takapuna, Auckland.
  PO Box 13–129, Armagh Street, Christchurch.
  PO Box 1289, Dunedin.
  PO Box 19–052, Wellington. Tel: 758–450.
Auckland Medical Aid Centre:
  283–289 Dominion Rd, Mt Eden, Auckland. Tel: 686–041.
  Epsom Day Hospital, 5 Warborough Avenue, Epsom, Auckland. Tel: 501–191.
  Parkview Clinic, Coromandel Street, Newtown, Wellington. Tel: 894–136.
Sisters Overseas Service (SOS)
  PO Box 47–090, Auckland.
  PO Box 884, Christchurch. Tel: 796–970.
  PO Box, Dunedin.
  PO Box 28–099, Wellington.
WONAAC (Abortion Rights), 154 Colombo Street, Christchurch.

CHILD CARE AND MOTHER SUPPORT

Auckland Birth Mother Support Group. Tel: 303–2441.
Anglican Trust for Women & Children, Auckland. Tel: 276–3729.
Barnardos General. Tel: 275–4481.
Council for the Single Mother and Her Child, PO Box 47090, Auckland. Tel: 760–476.
Family Care, 66 Mayfield Avenue, St Albans, Christchurch.
Federation of New Zealand Parents Centres (Inc.), PO Box 11310, Wellington. Tel: 766–950.
La Leche League NZ (Inc.), PO Box 2307, Christchurch.
New Mother Support Groups (Inc.), PO Box 9600, Courtenay Place, Wellington. Tel: 847–103.
Parent Help. Tel: 276–331.

Parents Association of the Mentally Handicapped. Tel: 889–721.

Pregnancy Help (Inc.), cnr Dixon and Taranaki Sts, PO Box 13–012, Johnsonville, Wellington. Tel: 847–979.

CHILD AND WOMAN ABUSE

Battered Women's Support Line, PO Box 1560, Hamilton.

Battered Women's Support Group, PO Box 2720, Christchurch.

Coalition Against Violence on Women, PO Box 884, Christchurch.

HELP, PO Box 16129, Wellington. Tel: 892–472.

HELP (Counselling for Victims of Sexual Assault), PO Box 68–152, Newtown, Auckland. Tel: 399–185 (all hours).

Salvation Army. See local directories.

Supportline for Abused Women, PO Box 6192, Auckland. Tel: 694–949.

Women Against the Sexual Abuse of Children, PO Box 3260, Wellington.

Women Against Violence Against Women, PO Box 475, Wellington.

FAMILY PLANNING CLINICS

Family Planning Association, National Office, PO Box 11–515, Wellington. Tel: 844–349.

The New Zealand Family Planning Association runs thirty-five clinics in twelve cities. The address of your closest clinic is listed under 'Family Planning' in your local telephone directory.

MAIN CENTRE CLINICS

Alice Bush Clinic, 214 Karangahape Road, Newton, Auckland. Tel: 775–049.

Christchurch Arts Centre, 301 Montreal Street, PO Box 2137, Christchurch. Tel: 790–514.

Family Planning Association, National Office, PO Box 11–515, Wellington. Tel: 844–349.

First Floor, NML Building, The Octagon, PO Box 5298, Dunedin. Tel: 775–850.

45 Tory St, PO Box 9574, Wellington. Tel: 849–743.

New Zealand Association of Natural Family Planning (Inc.), Mater Hospital, Auckland. Tel: 605–451 (for enquiries about other centres).

HEALTH CENTRES

Auckland Women's Health Centre, 63 Ponsonby Road, PO Box 47090, Auckland. Tel: 764–506.

Collective for Women, PO Box 8044, Dunedin. Tel: 771–229.

Devonport Women's Centre, 18 Kerr St, Devonport. Tel: 453–068.

Glenfield Health Collective, PO Box 40112, Glenfield. Tel: 444–4618.

Glenn Innes Women's Centre, 99 Leybourne Circle, Glenn Innes. Tel: 521–1404.

Hamilton Women's Centre, PO Box 7205, Hamilton.

Hecate Women's Health Centre, PO Box 19–117, Wellington. Tel: 842–732.

Mangere Women's Centre, 7 Hair St, Mangere East. Tel: 276–4574.

Maori and Pacific Islanders Women's Health Collective, 63 Ponsonby Rd, Auckland. Tel: 766–838.

Nelson Women's Centre, 94 Collingwood St, Nelson. Tel: 89–874.

New Zealand Women's Health Network (Inc.), PO Box 2312, Tauranga.

Palmerston North Women's Centre, 51 Waldegrove St, Palmerston North.

THAW (Health Alternative for Women), PO Box 884, Christchurch. Tel: 796–970.

LESBIAN GROUPS

Gayline, Gay and Lesbian Support Group and Information, Auckland. Tel: 303–3584.

LMDG (Lesbian Mothers' Defence), PO Box 11–009, Dunedin.

Wellington Lesbians, PO Box 427, Wellington.

MENTAL HEALTH

Anorexia and Bulimia Group, PO Box 21–489, Henderson, Auckland.

Community Addiction Services, 77 Carrington Rd, Auckland. Tel: 860–868.

Mental Health Foundation, PO Box 37–438, Auckland. Tel: 303–1517.

Women's Mental Health Project, PO Box 2312, Tauranga.

RAPE CRISIS ASSISTANCE

Auckland Rape Crisis. Tel: 764–404. See also **Help** (Counselling for Victims of Sexual Assault) under **Child and Woman Abuse**.

Christchurch Rape Crisis and Incest Group. Tel: 796–202 (all hours telephone counselling).

Dunedin Rape Crisis Centre, PO Box 5424, Dunedin. Tel: 741–592.

Gisborne Rape Crisis Centre, PO Box 1398, Gisborne. Tel: 79–967.

Hamilton Rape Crisis Centre, PO Box 1560, Hamilton. Tel: 394–433.

Rape Education Groups Inc., Auckland. Tel: 860–504.

Wellington Rape Crisis Centre, PO Box 9563, Wellington. Tel: 859–880.

Whangarei Rape Crisis Group, PO Box 913, Whangarei. Tel: 486–962.

REFUGES

See also **Child and Woman Abuse.**

Dunedin Women's Refuge, PO Box 282, Dunedin. Tel: 771–229.

Gisborne Women's Refuge, PO Box 1398, Gisborne.

Hastings Women's Emergency Centre, PO Box 328, Hastings.

Lower Hutt Family Refuge, PO Box 31–073, Lower Hutt. Tel: 691–040.

Manukau Women's Refuge, PO Box 593, Papakura. Tel: 298–0996.

Marlborough Emergency Refuge, PO Box 607, Blenheim. Tel: 84–099/82–144.

Napier Women's Emergency Centre, PO Box 4142, Marewa, Napier. Tel: 436–515.

Nelson Women's Emergency Centre, PO Box 832, Nelson. Tel: 87–566.

Palmerston North Women's Refuge, PO Box 573, Palmerston North.

Rotorua Women's Refuge, PO Box 1652, Rotorua. Tel: 476–210.

South Auckland Family Refuge, PO Box 22–039, Otahuhu. Tel: 279–8868.

Tauranga/Bay of Plenty Women's Refuge, c/o PO Box 753, Tauranga. Tel: 84–012.

Upper Hutt Family Refuge Centre, PO Box 40–051, Upper Hutt.

Wellington Women's Refuge Group, Courtenay Place, PO Box 16–079, Wellington. Tel: 736–280.

West Auckland Women's Refuge, PO Box 45–063, Auckland. Tel: 834–4119.

Whangarei Women's Refuge, PO Box 826, Whangarei.

Women's Refuge Centre, PO Box 7299, Christchurch.

SEXUALLY TRANSMITTED DISEASES CLINICS

AIDS, Burnett Clinic, Auckland. Tel: 33124.

AIDS Hotline. Tel: 395–560 (toll-free).

STD Clinic, Auckland Hospital. Tel: 797–440.

Herpes Support Network, Auckland. Tel: 771–050 (24 hours).

SPECIALIST WOMEN'S BOOKSHOPS

Kate Sheppard Women's Bookshop, 202 High Street, PO Box 22–659, Christchurch. Tel: 790–984.

The Women's Bookshop, 288 Dominion Rd, Auckland. Tel: 607–162.

WOMEN'S HOSPITALS

See local directories.

INDEX